D1489524

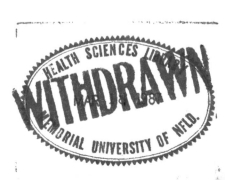

Current Guidelines for the Management of Cancer

Current Guidelines
for the Management
of Cancer

EDITED BY

Rene A. Khafif, M.D., F.A.C.S.
Attending in Charge, Division of Head and Neck
  Surgery and Surgical Oncology
Maimonides Medical Center
Brooklyn, New York
and Associate Clinical Professor
State University of New York
Downstate Medical Center
Brooklyn, New York
and Visiting Staff Attending, Division of Head and
  Neck Surgery
Long Island Jewish Hillside Medical Center
New Hyde Park, New York
and Consultant, Division of Head and Neck
  Surgery
Wyckoff Heights Medical Center
Brooklyn, New York
and Chairman, Management Guidelines
  Committee
Brooklyn Community Hospital Oncology Program
Brooklyn, New York

Sameer Rafla, M.D., Ph.D.
Chief, Department of Radiation Therapy
The Methodist Hospital
Brooklyn, New York
and Lutheran Medical Center
Brooklyn, New York
and Maimonides Medical Center
Brooklyn, New York
and Clinical Professor, Radiation Oncology
State University of New York
Downstate Medical Center
Brooklyn, New York
and Principal Investigator, Cancer and Leukemia
  Group B-SUNY
and Principal Investigator, Brooklyn Community
  Hospital Oncology Program

Samuel Kopel, M.D.
Assistant Director, Division of
  Hematology/Oncology
Maimonides Medical Center
Brooklyn, New York

1986

ACADEMIC PRESS, INC.
Harcourt Brace Jovanovich, Publishers

Orlando   San Diego   New York   Austin
Boston   London   Sydney   Tokyo   Toronto

ACADEMIC PRESS, INC.
Orlando, Florida 32887

United Kingdom Edition published by
ACADEMIC PRESS INC. (LONDON) LTD.
24–28 Oval Road, London NW1 7DX

Library of Congress Cataloging in Publication Data

Current guidelines for the management of cancer.

Includes index.
 1. Cancer—Treatment—Collected works. I. Khafif,
Rene A. II. Rafla, Sameer. III. Kopel, Samuel.
[DNLM: 1. Neoplasms—therapy. QZ 266 C976]
RC270.8.C87 1985   616.99'406   84-24161
ISBN 0—12—406020—X (alk. paper)

PRINTED IN THE UNITED STATES OF AMERICA

86 87 88 89   9 8 7 6 5 4 3 2 1

This book is dedicated to our wives,
Amy Khafif, Marie Jacqueline Rafla, and Sharon Kopel,
for their support, understanding, tolerance,
and endurance through this project.

Contents

Contributors   xi
Foreword   xvii
Preface   xix

Section 1   Tumors of the Head and Neck

   I. Early Detection and Screening   5
  II. Pretreatment Evaluation and Work-Up   7
 III. Preoperative Preparation   10
 IV. Therapeutic Management: General Considerations   23
  V. Therapeutic Guidelines: Site Specific   29
 VI. Adjuvant Use of Chemotherapy in Head and Neck
     Cancer   44
 VII. Treatment of the Advanced Head and Neck Cancer
     Patient   45
VIII. Postoperative Care, Evaluation, and Rehabilitation of
     the Head and Neck Cancer Patient   47
 IX. Management Algorithms for Head and Neck Cancer   53
     Suggested Readings   53

Section 2   Carcinomas of the Breast

   I. Early Detection and Screening   67
  II. Preoperative Evaluation and Preparation   71
 III. Therapeutic Management   76
 IV. Carcinoma of the Breast in Pregnancy   80
  V. The Role of Radiotherapy in the Treatment of Breast
     Cancer   82
 VI. Adjuvant Chemotherapy for Breast Cancer   83
 VII. Guidelines for the Treatment of Advanced Breast
     Cancer   85
VIII. Postoperative Care, Evaluation, and Rehabilitation   90
 IX. Management Algorithm for Cancer of the Breast   93
     Suggested Readings   93

Section 3   Carcinomas of the Skin

   I. Early Detection and Screening   99
  II. Pretreatment Evaluation and Work-Up   100
 III. Therapeutic Management of Nonmelanoma Skin Cancer 102
 IV. Malignant Melanomas of the Skin   113
  V. Other Select Skin Tumors   118
 VI. Postoperative Care, Evaluation, and Rehabilitation of
     the Patient with Skin Cancer   122
 VII. Management Algorithm for Skin Melanoma   123
     Suggested Readings   123

Section 4   Tumors of the Endocrine Glands

Part A Tumors of the Adrenal Gland

   I. Primary Hyperaldosteronism   133
  II. Cushing's Syndrome   136
 III. Pheochromocytoma   142
 IV. Neuroblastoma   148
     Suggested Readings   153

Part B Pancreatic Tumors

   I. Insulinoma   157
  II. Gastrinoma (Zollinger-Ellison Syndrome)   160
 III. Glucagonoma (Hyperglycemia Syndrome)   163
 IV. Vipoma (Pancreatic Cholera, the WDHA Syndrome, or
     Verner-Morrison Syndrome)   166
     Suggested Readings   169

Part C Parathyroid Tumors

   I. Early Detection and Screening   173
  II. Pretreatment Evaluation and Work-Up   174
 III. Preoperative Preparation   175
 IV. Therapeutic Management   176
  V. Postoperative Care, Evaluation, and Follow-Up   178
 VI. Management Algorithm for Parathyroid Tumors   178
     Suggested Readings   180

Part D Paraneoplastic Endocrine Syndromes (Ectopic Hormone Producing Tumors)

   I. Evaluation of the Patient 184
  II. Preoperative Preparation 185
 III. Therapeutic Management 186
     Suggested Readings 188

Part E Multiple Endocrine Neoplasia

   I. Multiple Endocrine Neoplasia, Type I (MEN-I or Werner's Syndrome) 191
  II. Multiple Endocrine Neoplasia, Type II (Sipple's Syndrome) 193
 III. Prognosis 194
     Suggested Readings 194

Part F Apudomas

   I. APUD Cell Characteristics 197
  II. Classification 197
     Suggested Readings 199

Part G Carcinoid Tumors

   I. Clinical Considerations 203
  II. Pathological Considerations 204
 III. Early Detection and Screening 204
 IV. Pretreatment Evaluation and Work-Up 205
  V. Therapeutic Management 207
 VI. Postoperative Care, Evaluation, and Follow-Up 210
 VII. Management Algorithm for Carcinoid Tumors 211

Section 5   Tumors of the Skeletal System

   I. Introduction 217
  II. Early Detection and Screening 226
 III. Pretreatment Evaluation and Work-Up 227
 IV. Therapeutic Management 234
  V. Postoperative Care, Evaluation, and Rehabilitation 243
 VI. Management Algorithm for Bone Tumors 248
     Suggested Readings 248

Section 6   Soft-Tissue Sarcomas

   I. Early Detection and Screening 255
  II. Pretreatment Evaluation and Work-Up 256
 III. Preoperative Preparation 258
 IV. General Management Guidelines 258
  V. Therapeutic Guidelines: Type-Specific 266
 VI. Postoperative Care, Evaluation, and Rehabilitation 269

 VII. Management Algorithm for Soft-Tissue Sarcoma 271
     Suggested Readings 271

Section 7   Tumors of the Central Nervous System

   I. Early Detection and Screening 277
  II. Pretreatment Evaluation and Work-Up 278
 III. Pretreatment Preparation 283
 IV. Therapeutic Management 283
  V. Specific Neurologic Tumors 291
 VI. Postoperative Care, Evaluation, and Rehabilitation 304
 VII. Management Algorithm for Brain Tumors 307
     Suggested Readings 307

Section 8   Pediatric Tumors

Part A Solid Tumors

   I. Early Detection and Screening 315
  II. Pretreatment Evaluation and Work-Up 316
 III. Preoperative Preparation 319
 IV. Therapeutic Management 319
  V. Postoperative Care, Evaluation, and Rehabilitation 320
 VI. Solid Pediatric Tumors: Type-Specific 322
     Suggested Readings 338

Part B Leukemias and Lymphomas

   I. Leukemias of Childhood 341
  II. Lymphomas in Childhood 346
     Suggested Readings 349

Section 9   Neoplastic Disorders of the Blood, Bone Marrow, and Lymphatic System

Part A Hodgkin's Disease and Non-Hodgkin's Lymphomas and Related Disorders

   I. Early Detection and Screening 355
  II. Pretreatment Evaluation and Work-Up 356
 III. Therapeutic Management of Hodgkin's Disease 362
 IV. Therapeutic Management of Non-Hodgkin's Lymphoma 369
  V. Other Specific Types of Lymphoma and Related Disorders 376
 VI. Follow-Up Evaluation and Rehabilitation of the Patient with Lymphoma 378

VII. Management Algorithm for Lymphomas   379
     Suggested Readings   379

Part B Leukemias

   I. Acute Leukemias   385
  II. Chronic Myelocytic Leukemia   391
 III. Chronic Lymphocytic Leukemia   394
  IV. Hairy Cell Leukemia   398
     Suggested Readings   399

Part C Multiple Myeloma

   I. Definition and Clinical Considerations   403
  II. Pretreatment Evaluation and Work-Up   403
 III. Therapeutic Management   404

Part D Other Neoplastic Disorders of the Blood

   I. Polycythemia Vera   411
  II. Myelofibrosis and Myeloid Metaplasia 413
 III. Acute Myelofibrosis   415
  IV. Essential Thrombocythemia   415

Section 10 **Chest Tumors**

Part A Cancer of the Lung

   I. Early Detection and Screening   421
  II. Pretreatment Evaluation and Work-Up   422
 III. Preoperative Preparation   431
  IV. Therapeutic Management   431
   V. Postoperative Care, Evaluation, and Rehabilitation   437
  VI. Management Algorithm for Chest Tumors 439

Part B Tumors of the Mediastinum

   I. General Considerations   443
  II. Early Detection and Screening   445
 III. Pretreatment Evaluation and Work-Up   446
  IV. Therapeutic Management   447

Part C Pleural Tumors (Mesotheliomas)

   I. General Considerations   455
  II. Pretreatment Evaluation and Work-Up   455
 III. Therapeutic Management   456

Part D Cancer of the Esophagus

   I. Epidemiology   461
  II. Pathological Considerations   461
 III. Pretreatment Evaluation and Work-Up   462
  IV. Preoperative Preparation   462
   V. Therapeutic Management   463
  VI. Postoperative Care and Evaluation   467
 VII. Management Algorithm for Cancer of the Esophagus   468

Section 11 **Carcinomas of the Alimentary Tract**

Part A Carcinoma of the Stomach

   I. Early Detection and Screening   475
  II. Pretreatment Evaluation, Work-Up, and Preparation   476
 III. Therapeutic Management   478
  IV. Postoperative Care, Evaluation, and Rehabilitation   483
   V. Management Algorithm for Cancer of the Stomach   484
     Suggested Readings   484

Part B Colorectal Cancer and Tumors of the Anus and Small Intestine

   I. Early Detection and Screening of Colorectal Cancer   489
  II. Preoperative Evaluation and Preparation of Patients with Colorectal Cancer   490
 III. Pathological Considerations of Colorectal Carcinoma   492
  IV. Therapeutic Management of Colorectal Carcinoma   496
   V. Postoperative Care, Psychosocial Support, Rehabilitation, and Evaluation of Patients with Colorectal Carcinoma   499
  VI. Carcinoma of the Anus   501
 VII. Neoplasms of the Small Intestine   504
     Suggested Readings   504

Part C Carcinoma of the Pancreas (Eccrine Gland) and the Biliary Tree

   I. Early Detection and Screening for Pancreatic Carcinoma   509
  II. Pretreatment Evaluation and Work-Up for Patients with Pancreatic Carcinoma   510
 III. Preoperative Preparation of Patients with Pancreatic Carcinoma   513
  IV. Therapeutic Management of Carcinoma of the Pancreas and Periampullary Region   514
   V. Postoperative Care and Evaluation of Patients with Pancreatic Carcinoma   520
  VI. Management Algorithm for Pancreatic Carcinoma   520
 VII. Therapeutic Management of Carcinoma of the Gallbladder and Extrahepatic Biliary Tree   522
     Suggested Readings   525

Part D Malignant Tumors of the Liver

   I. Early Detection and Screening   529
  II. Pretreatment Evaluation and Work-Up   529
 III. Pretreatment Preparation   532
  IV. Therapeutic Management   532

Section 12 **Gynecologic Malignancies**

   I. Early Detection and Screening   541
  II. Pretreatment Evaluation and Work-Up   543

III. Pretreatment Preparation 545
IV. Therapeutic Management: Carcinoma of the Vulva 546
V. Therapeutic Management: Carcinoma of the Vagina 555
VI. Therapeutic Management: Carcinoma of the Cervix 556
VII. Therapeutic Management: Carcinoma of the Uterus 560
VIII. Therapeutic Management: Carcinoma of the Ovary 562
IX. Postoperative Care, Evaluation, and Rehabilitation 566
X. Management Algorithms 566
Suggested Readings 567

Section 13 Tumors of the Genitourinary System

Part A Tumors of the Kidney

I. Early Detection and Screening 575
II. Pretreatment Evaluation and Work-Up 576
III. Preoperative Preparation 578
IV. Therapeutic Management 581
V. Postoperative Care and Evaluation 583
VI. Management Algorithm for Renal Tumors 585

Part B Tumors of the Bladder

I. Early Detection and Screening 589
II. Pretreatment Evaluation and Work-Up 590
III. Pretreatment Preparation 591
IV. Therapeutic Management 592
V. Postoperative Care, Evaluation, and Rehabilitation 597
VI. Management Algorithm for Bladder Tumors 597

Part C Tumors of the Prostate

I. Early Detection and Screening 601
II. Pretreatment Evaluation and Work-Up 601
III. Preoperative Preparation 604
IV. Therapeutic Management 607
V. Treatment of Advanced Prostate Cancer 610
VI. Postoperative Care, Evaluation, and Rehabilitation 611
VII. Management Algorithm for Prostate Cancer 613

Part D Testicular Tumors

I. Introduction 617
II. Early Detection and Screening 618
III. Pretreatment Evaluation and Work-Up 619
IV. Preoperative Preparation 620
V. Therapeutic Management 620
VI. Chemotherapy for Advanced Testicular Cancer 624
VII. Postoperative Care, Evaluation, and Rehabilitation 625
VIII. Management Algorithm for Testicular Tumors 625

Part E Penile Tumors

I. Early Detection and Screening 629
II. Pretreatment Evaluation and Preparation 629
III. Therapeutic Management 630
IV. Postoperative Care 631
V. Management Algorithm for Penile Tumors 632
Suggested Readings 632

Index 635

Contributors

Numbers in parentheses indicate the pages on which the authors' contributions begin.

ASSOCIATE EDITORS

LASZLO BIRO, M.D., F.A.C.P. (95), Chief of Dermatology, Department of Medicine, Lutheran Medical Center, Brooklyn, New York 11220, and Clinical Professor, Division of Dermatology, State University of New York, Downstate Medical Center, Brooklyn, New York 11203, and Chief of Dermatology, The Brooklyn Hospital, Brooklyn, New York 11209, and Consultant, Department of Dermatology, Veterans Administration Hospital, Brooklyn, New York, and Chairman, Skin Subcommittee, Management Guidelines Committee, Brooklyn Community Hospital Oncology Program (B-CHOP)

MICHAEL GOLDING, M.D., F.A.C.S. (417), Director of Surgery, Lutheran Medical Center, Brooklyn, New York 11220, and Clinical Professor of Surgery, and Attending Surgeon, State University of New York, Downstate Medical Center, Brooklyn, New York 11203, and Attending Surgeon, Kings County Medical Center, Brooklyn, New York 11203, and Consultant in Surgery, The Methodist Hospital, Brooklyn, New York 11215, and Chairman, Pulmonary Subcommittee, Management Guidelines Committee, Brooklyn Community Hospital Oncology Program (B-CHOP)

NICHOLAS LEONE, M.D., F.A.C.A.[1] (351), Chief of Oncology Department and Attending in Medicine and Hematology, Cancer Activities Committee, The Methodist Hospital, Brooklyn, New York 11215, and Attending in Department of Medicine and Clinical Assistant Professor, State University of New York, Downstate Medical Center, Brooklyn, New York 11203, and Associate Attending in Medicine and Hematology/Oncology, Lutheran Medical Center, Brooklyn, New York 11220, and Victory Memorial Hospital, Brooklyn, New York 11228, and Chairman, Lymphoma/Leukemia Subcommittee, Management Guidelines Committee, Brooklyn Community Hospital Oncology Program (B-CHOP)

[1]Deceased. Requests for offprints should go to Rene A. Khafif, 2219 Ocean Avenue, Brooklyn, New York 11229.

ROBERT LERNER, M.D., F.A.C.S. (127, 251), Director of Department of Surgery, Interfaith Medical Center (Brooklyn Jewish Site), Brooklyn, New York, and Clinical Professor of Surgery, State University of New York, Downstate Medical Center, Brooklyn, New York 11203, and Chairman, Endocrine Subcommittee and Subcommittee on Soft Tissue-Tumors of the Management Guidelines Committee, Brooklyn Community Hospital Oncology Program (B-CHOP)

AARON MILLER, M.D. (273), Director of Division of Neurology, Maimonides Medical Center, Brooklyn, New York 11219, and Associate Clinical Professor of Neurology, State University of New York, Downstate Medical Center, Brooklyn, New York 11203, and Visiting Assistant Professor of Neurology, Albert Einstein College of Medicine, Bronx, New York 10461, and Chairman, Neurological Subcommittee, Brooklyn Community Hospital Oncology Program (B-CHOP)

HUBERT S. PEARLMAN, M.D., F.A.C.S. (213), Attending in Charge, Division of Orthopedic Surgery and Chief of Orthopedic Surgical Training Program, Maimonides Medical Center, Brooklyn, New York 11219, and Chief of Orthopedic Surgery, Lutheran Medical Center, Brooklyn, New York 11220, and Consultant, Orthopedic Surgery, Methodist Hospital, Brooklyn, New York 11215, and St. John's Episcopal Hospital, Brooklyn, New York, and Brooklyn Hospital, Caledonian Hospital, Brooklyn, New York, and Adjunct Professor of Health Sciences, Long Island University, Brooklyn, New York 11201, and Associate Clinical Professor, Division of Orthopedic Surgery, State University of New York, Downstate Medical Center, Brooklyn, New York 11203, and Chairman, Bone Subcommittee, Management Guidelines Committee, Brooklyn Community Hospital Oncology Program (B-CHOP)

GILBERT WISE, M.D., F.A.C.S. (571), Director, Division of Urology, Maimonides Medical Center, Brooklyn, New York 11219, and Director, Department of Urology, Coney Island Hospital, Brooklyn, New York 11235, and New York Clinical Professor, Department of Urology, State University of New York, Downstate Medical Center, Brooklyn, New York 11203, and Consultant in Urology, Brooklyn Hospital, Caledonian Hospital, Brooklyn, New York 11226, and the Methodist Hospital of Brooklyn, Brooklyn, New York 11215, and Attending in Urology, Metropolitan-Jewish Geriatric Center, Brooklyn, New York 11215, and Chairman, Urology Subcommittee, Management Guidelines Committee, Brooklyn Community Hospital Oncology Program (B-CHOP)

CONTRIBUTORS

JOHN ADDRIZZO, M.D. (417), Attending, Pulmonary Disease, the Methodist Hospital of Brooklyn, New York 11215, and State University of New York, Downstate Medical Center, Brooklyn, New York 11203, and Lutheran Medical Center, Brooklyn, New York 11220, and Victory Memorial Hospital, Brooklyn, New York 11228, and Director of Environmental Medicine/Pulmonary St. Vincent's Medical Center, Staten Island, New York 10310, and Director of Medicine, Doctor's Hospital, Staten Island, New York, and Consultant, Baley-Seton, Staten Island, New York

MARGARET AMATO, R.N., M.S. (213, 351), Clinical Specialist, Oncology, The Methodist Hospital of Brooklyn, New York

MARIO ANSELMO, M.D., F.C.A.P. (1, 213), Assistant Attending, Department of Pathology, Maimonides Medical Center, Brooklyn, New York 11219

ISSAM ARNUK, M.D., F.A.C.S. (63), Attending, Surgery, The Methodist Hospital of Brooklyn, Brooklyn, New York 11215, and Attending and Associate Chief, General Surgery, Lutheran Medical Center, Brooklyn, New York 11220, and Clinical Assistant Professor, Surgery, State University of New York, Downstate Medical Center, Brooklyn, New York 11203, and Clinical Assistant Professor, Surgery, New York Medical College, New York, New York 10029

MICHAEL BASHEVKIN, M.D. (1, 273), Assistant Attending, Hematology/Oncology, Maimonides Medical Center, Brooklyn, New York 11219

ALFREDO BRAND, M.D. (95), Clinical Assistant Professor, Dermatology, State University of New York, Downstate Medical Center, Brooklyn, New York 11203, and Assistant Attending, Dermatology, The Brooklyn Hospital, Brooklyn, New York 11201, and Lutheran Medical Center, Brooklyn, New York 11220, and The Methodist Hospital of Brooklyn, Brooklyn, New York 11215

AURELIA CACATIAN (571), Chief, Medical Oncology, Lutheran Medical Center, Brooklyn, New York 11220

RICHARD CALAME, M.D. (537), Director, Gynecological Oncology, Brooklyn Cumberland Medical Center, Brooklyn, New York 11205, and Consultant, Gynecological Oncology, The Methodist Hospital, Brooklyn, New York 11215, and Lutheran Medical Center, Brooklyn, New York, and Clinical Professor, Obstetrics and Gynecology, State University of New York, Downstate Medical Center, Brooklyn, New York 11203

FREDERICO CAPOZZI, M.D.[2] (1, 63), Chief, Head and Neck Surgery, The Methodist Hospital of Brooklyn, Brooklyn, New York 11215, and Assistant Attending, Surgery, Lutheran Medical Center, Brooklyn, New York 11220

ANDREW CATANIA, M.D. (1), Chief, Dentistry, Coney Island Hospital, Brooklyn, New York 11235, and Associate-in-Charge, Dentistry, Maimonides Medical Center, Brooklyn, New York 11219, and Consultant, Dentistry, Interfaith Medical Center, Brooklyn, New York 11238, and Associate Attending, Dentistry, Jewish Chronic Disease Hospital, New York

RAFAEL CINELLI, M.D. (95), Attending Plastic Surgeon, Surgery, Maimonides Hospital, Brooklyn, New York 11219, and Medical Arts Hospital, New York, New York 10019, and Assistant Attending Plastic Surgeon, Surgery, Coney Island Hospital, Brooklyn, New York 11235

DENNIS CIRILLO, M.D. (63), Assistant Attending and Chief of Plastic Reconstructive Surgery, Lutheran Medical Center, Brooklyn, New York 11220, and Courtesy Staff, New York Eye & Ear Hospital, New York, New York 10003, and Clinical Instructor, New York State University Hospital, Kings County Hospital Center, Brooklyn, New York 11203

BERTRAM D. COHN, M.D. (309), Director, Pediatric Surgery, Maimonides Medical Center, Brooklyn, New York 11219, and Clinical Associate Professor of Surgery, State University of New York, Downstate Medical Center, Brooklyn, New York, and Attending-in-Charge, Pediatric Surgery, Staten Island Hospital, Staten Island, New York 10305, and Attending Pediatric Surgeon, University Hospital, Brooklyn, New York 11203

ALAN M. CRYSTAL, M.D., F.A.C.S. (213), Assistant Attending, Orthopedic Surgery, Maimonides Medical Center, Brooklyn, New York 11219, and Attending, Orthopedic Surgery, Community Hospital, Brooklyn, New York 11229, and Visiting Attending Surgeon, Kings County Hospital, Brooklyn, New York 11203, and Clinical Instructor, Orthopedic Surgery, State University of New York, Downstate Medical Center, Brooklyn, New York 11203

[2]Deceased. Requests for offprints should go to Rene A. Khafif, 2219 Ocean Avenue, Brooklyn, New York 11229.

CAROLYN DICKSON, R.N., M.S. (571), Nurse Oncologist, Lutheran Medical Center, Brooklyn, New York 11220

MARILYN DRAXTON, R.N., M.A. (471), Assistant Administrator/Director of Nursing, The Methodist Hospital, Brooklyn, New York 11215

ADOLFO ELIZALDE, M.D. (351), Chief, Hematology/Oncology Division, The Methodist Hospital of Brooklyn, Brooklyn, New York 11205, and Assistant Clinical Professor, State University of New York, Downstate Medical Center, Brooklyn, New York 11203

IRVING ENQUIST, M.D. (471), Director, Surgery, The Methodist Hospital of Brooklyn, Brooklyn, New York 11215, and Visiting Surgeon, Kings County Hospital, Brooklyn, New York 11203, and University Hospital, Brooklyn, New York, and Consultant Surgeon, Veterans Administration Hospital of Brooklyn, Brooklyn, New York 11209

ARI FEIBEL, M.D. (213, 251, 273), Chief, Rehabilitation Medicine, Coney Island Hospital, Brooklyn, New York 11235, and Associate Clinical Professor of Rehabilitation Medicine, Albert Einstein College of Medicine, Bronx, New York 10461, and Former Director Rehabilitation Medicine, Maimonides Medical Center, Brooklyn, New York 11219

FELIX FELDMAN, M.D., F.A.A.P. (309), Director of Pediatric Services and Director of the Division of Pediatric Hematology-Oncology, Maimonides Medical Center, Brooklyn, New York 11219, and Professor Clinical Pediatrics, State University of New York, Downstate Medical Center, Brooklyn, New York 11203, and Attending Pediatrician, Pediatrics, Coney Island Hospital, Brooklyn, New York 11235, and Kings County Hospital, Brooklyn, New York 11235, and Consultant, Pediatric Hematology-Oncology, The Methodist Hospital of Brooklyn, Brooklyn, New York

LAWRENCE FEUERMAN, M.D. (63), Attending, Surgery, Maimonides Medical Center, Brooklyn, New York 11219, and Attending, Surgery, Kings Highway Hospital, Brooklyn, New York 11234

JOSEPH GIOVANIELLO, M.D. (471), Attending Radiologist, Director Radiology, The Methodist Hospital of Brooklyn, Brooklyn, New York 11215

SUSAN GOLDFINE, M.D. (309), Director of Pediatric Radiology, Maimonides Medical Center, Brooklyn, New York 11219

BERNARD GUSSOF, M.D., F.A.C.P. (417, 527), Attending Physician, Hematology/Oncology, Lutheran Medical Center, Brooklyn, New York 11220, and Clinical Associate Professor of Medicine, State University of New York, Downstate Medical Center, Brooklyn, New York 11203, and Kings Highway Hospital, Brooklyn, New York 11234

AIZID HASHMAT, M.D., F.R.C.S., F.A.C.S. (127), Chief, Urology, Interfaith Medical Center, Brooklyn, New York 11238, and Assistant Professor Urology, State University of New York, Downstate Medical Center, Brooklyn, New York 11203

HOSSEIN HEDAYATI, M.D. (1), Chief, Head and Neck Surgery, Attending Surgeon, The Methodist Hospital of Brooklyn, Brooklyn, New York 11215, and Victory Memorial Hospital, Brooklyn, New York 11220

EDWARD HEILMAN, M.D., F.A.A.D. (95), Assistant Professor Dermatology/Pathology, State University of New York, Downstate Medical Center, Brooklyn, New York 11203, and Attending Dermatologist, Kings County Hospital, Brooklyn, New York 11203

BURTON HERZ, M.D. (127), Chief, Surgical Services, Coney Island Hospital, Brooklyn, New York 11235, and Associate Director of Surgery, Maimonides Medical Center, Brooklyn, New York 11219, and Attending Surgeon, Manhattan Veterans Administration Hospital, New York, New York 10010, and Assistant Attending Surgeon, Bellevue Medical Hospital, New York, New York 10016

ROBERT HOLTZMAN, M.D. (273), Assistant Clinical Professor, Neurosurgery, State University of New York, Downstate Medical Center, Brooklyn, New York 11203, and Assistant Attending, Neurosurgery, Beth Israel Medical Center, New York, New York 10003

VENKIT S. IYER, M.D. (251), Chief Gastroenterology, Interfaith Medical Center, Brooklyn, New York 11238

KARL JINDRAK, M.D. (63, 451, 417, 471), Attending, Pathology, The Methodist Hospital of Brooklyn, Brooklyn, New York 11203, and Clinical Assistant Professor, Pathology, State University of New York, Downstate Medical Center, Brooklyn, New York 11203

MARSHALL KEILSON, M.D. (273), Associate Director Division of Neurology, and Director EEG Laboratory, Maimonides Medical Center, Brooklyn, New York 11219, and Assistant Clinical Professor, Department of Neurology, State University of New York, Downstate Medical Center, Brooklyn, New York

RENE A. KHAFIF, M.D., F.A.C.S. (1, 63, 95, 127, 213, 251, 471), Attending-in-Charge, Head and Neck Surgery, Surgical Oncology, Maimonides Medical Center, Brooklyn, New York 11219, and Associate Clinical Professor, State University of New York, Downstate Medical Center, Brooklyn, New York 11203, and Visiting Staff Attending, Head and Neck Surgery, Long Island Jewish Hillside Medical Center, New Hyde Park, New York 11040, and Consultant, Head and Neck Surgery, Wyckoff Heights Medical Center, Brooklyn, New York and Chairman, Management Guidelines Committee, Brooklyn Community Hospital Oncology Program (B-CHOP)

FARIDA KHAN, M.D. (127), Chief, Endocrinology and Metabolism, Interfaith Medical Center, Brooklyn, New York 11238, and Assistant Professor of Medicine, State University of New York, Downstate Medical Center, Brooklyn, New York 11203, and Visiting-Staff-Attending, Medicine, Kings County Hospital, Brooklyn, New York 11203, and State University Hospital, Brooklyn, New York 11203

BAROUKH KODSI, M.D., F.A.C.P. (471), Attending-in-Charge, Gastroenterology, and Associate Professor of Clinical Medicine, Maimonides Medical Center, Brooklyn, New York 11219

SAMUEL KOPEL, M.D. (63, 95, 213, 251, 417, 471, 537, 571), Assistant Director, Division of Hematology/Oncology, Maimonides Medical Center, Brooklyn, New York 11219

KRISHNARAJ G. LINDSAY, M.D., F.A.C.S. (571), Chief, Urology, Coney Island Hospital, Brooklyn, New York 11235, and Attending, Urology, Maimonides Medical Center, Brooklyn, New York 11219, and Associate Clinical Professor, State University of New York, Downstate Medical Center, Brooklyn, New York 11203

RICHARD LOPCHINSKY, M.D., F.A.C.S. (1), Assistant Attending, Head and Neck Surgery and General Surgery, Maimonides Medical Center, Brooklyn, New York 11219, and Brookdale Hospital, Brooklyn, New York 11212, and The Methodist Hospital of Brooklyn, Brooklyn, New York 11215, and Clinical Instructor, State University of New York, Downstate Medical Center, Brooklyn, New York 11203, and Booth Memorial Medical Center, Flushing, New York 11355, and Flushing Hospital Medical Center, Flushing, New York 11355

HELEN MCCARTHY, R.N., B.S. (251), Director of Cancer Communications, Oncology Nurse Coordinator, The Brooklyn Hospital–Caledonian Hospital, Brooklyn, New York 11226

CHANCHAL MALHOTRA, M.D. (309), Assistant Attending, Department of Pathology, Maimonides Medical Center, Brooklyn, New York 11219

MICHAEL MARTUSCELLO, M.D. (95), Attending, General, Thoracic, and Vascular Surgery, Lutheran Medical Center, Brooklyn, New York 11220, and Victory Memorial Hospital, Brooklyn, New York 11228, and Jamaica Hospital, Brooklyn, New York 11418

IRVIN MODLIN, M.D. (127), Assistant Professor, Surgery, State University of New York, Downstate Medical Center, Brooklyn, New York 11203, and Director of Surgery, Woodhull Hospital, Brooklyn, New York 11206, and Associate Professor and Vice Chairman, Department of Surgery, Yale University School of Medical, New Haven, Connecticut 06510

RANDI MOSKOWITZ, R.N., M.S. (1, 63, 95, 251, 273, 351, 537), B-CHOP Project Administrator, The Methodist Hospital, Brooklyn, New York 11215

ISMAT NAWABI, M.D. (351), Director, Hematology/Oncology, Maimonides Medical Center, Brooklyn, New York 11219, and Assistant Professor, State University of New York, Downstate Medical Center, Brooklyn, New York 11203

ANN NELSON, R.N., A.A.S. (63, 95), Head Nurse, Radiotherapy Department, Lutheran Medical Center, Brooklyn, New York 11220

KAPILA PARIKH, M.D. (95, 537), Assistant Attending, Radiation Therapy, The Methodist Hospital, Brooklyn, New York 11215, and Lutheran Medical Center, Brooklyn, New York 11220, and Maimonides Medical Center, Brooklyn, New York 11219, and Beekman Downtown Infirmary Hospital, New York, New York, and Clinical Instructor, State University of New York, Downstate Medical Center, Brooklyn, New York 11203

MUKUND R. PATEL, M.D. (213), Assistant Clinical Professor, Surgery/Orthopedics, State University of New York, Downstate Medical Center, Brooklyn, New York 11203, and Attending, Orthopedic Surgery and Hand Surgery, Maimonides Medical Center, Brooklyn, New York 11219, and Brooklyn Hospital, Brooklyn, New York 11201, and The Methodist Hospital of Brooklyn, Brooklyn, New York 11215, and Lutheran Medical Center, Brooklyn, New York 11220, Clinical Professor of Health Sciences, Long Island University, Brooklyn, New York 11201, and Long Island University, Brooklyn, New York 11201

ELY PRICE, M.D., F.A.C.P. (95), Attending-in-Charge, Dermatology, Maimonides Medical Center, Brooklyn, New York 11219, and Clinical Associate Professor, Dermatology, State University of New York, Downstate Medical Center, Brooklyn, New York 11203, and Consultant, Dermatology, Lutheran Medical Center, Brooklyn, New York 11220

MARILYN QUISBERT, R.N., M.A. (1), Oncology Nurse Coordinator, Hematology/Oncology, Maimonides Medical Center, Brooklyn, New York 11219

SAMEER RAFLA, M.D., PH.D. (1, 213, 251, 351, 417), Chief, Department of Radiation Therapy, The Methodist Hospital, Brooklyn, New York 11215, and Lutheran Medical Center, Brooklyn, New York 11220, and Maimonides Medical Center, Brooklyn, New York 11219, and Clinical Professor, Radiation Oncology, State University of New York, College of Medicine, Brooklyn, New York, and Principal Investigator, Cancer and Leukemia Group B-SUNY, and Principal Investigator, Brooklyn Community Hospital Oncology Program (B-CHOP)

ANTHONY RAIA, M.D., F.A.C.S., F.I.C.S. (1), Chief, Otolaryngology, Facial Plastic and Head and Neck Surgery, Victory Memorial Hospital, Brooklyn, New York 11228, and Clinical Assistant Professor of Otolaryngology, State University of New York, Downstate Medical Center, Brooklyn, New York 11203, and Visiting Attending Otolaryngologist, Kings County Hospital, Brooklyn, New York 11203, and Assistant Attending Surgeon, Otolaryngology, Manhattan Eye, Ear and Throat Hospital, New York, New York 10021, and Otolaryngology, Long Island College Hospital, Brooklyn, New York 11203, and Cabrini Medical Center, New York, New York 10021

HOWARD RASI, M.D., D.D.S.[3] (1), Chief, Plastic Surgery, The Methodist Hospital of Brooklyn, Brooklyn, New York 11215, and Assistant Clinical Professor, State University of New York, Downstate Medical Center, Brooklyn, New York 11203

RAMIRO REQUENA, M.D., F.A.C.S. (127), Associate Director Surgery, Interfaith Medical Center, Brooklyn, New York, and Assistant Clinical Professor of Surgery, State University of New York, Downstate Medical Center, Brooklyn, New York 11203

THOMAS REYNOLDS, M.D. (471), Medical Oncologist, Interfaith Medical Center, Brooklyn, New York 11238

LINDA ROGANDO, R.N. (417), Nursing Care Coordinator, Lutheran Medical Center, Brooklyn, New York

HOSNY SELIM, M.D. (63, 471, 537), Attending, Radiation Therapy, The Methodist Hospital, Brooklyn, New York 11215, and Attending, Radiation Therapy, Lutheran Medical Center, Brooklyn, New York 11220, and Clinical Assistant Professor, Radiation Oncology, State University of New York, Downstate Medical Center, Brooklyn, New York 11203

FELIX A. SIEGMAN, M.D., F.A.C.S. (471), Attending in Charge of Vascular Surgery, Maimonides Hospital, Brooklyn, New York 11219, and Assistant Attending, Surgery, Coney Island Hospital, Brooklyn, New York 11235, and Clinical Assistant Professor, State University of New York, Downstate Medical Center, Brooklyn, New York 11203

ARNOLD SILVERBERG, M.S. (127), Attending in Charge, Endocrinology, Maimonides Medical Center, Brooklyn, New York 11219, and Clinical Associate Professor of Medicine, State University of New York, Downstate Medical Center, Brooklyn, New York 11203, and Attending Physician in Medicine and Endocrinology, Kings Highway Hospital, Brooklyn, New York 11203, and Consultant, Medicine and Endocrinology, Victory Memorial Hospital, Brooklyn, New York

CARMENCITA SORIANO, M.D. (251), Associate Pathologist, Interfaith Medical Center (Site B), Brooklyn, New York 11238

IRENE SWEENEY, M.D. (351), Assistant Attending, Radiology, The Methodist Hospital of Brooklyn, Brooklyn, New York 11215

JEROME TEPPERBERG, M.D. (273), Physician in Charge, Child Neurology, Maimonides Medical Center, Brooklyn, New York 11219, and Clinical Associate Professor, Neurology, State University of New York, Downstate Medical Center, Brooklyn, New York 11203, and Consultant Child Neurologist, Staten Island Hospital, Staten Island, New York, and Coney Island Hospital, Brooklyn, New York 11235

EZZAT YOUSSEF, M.D. (273, 417, 571), Associate Attending, Radiation Therapy, The Methodist Hospital, Brooklyn, New York 11215, and Lutheran Medical Center, Brooklyn, New York 11220, and Maimonides Medical Center, Brooklyn, New York 11219, and Clinical Instructor of Radiation Oncology, State University of New York, Downstate Medical Center, Brooklyn, New York 11203

[3]Deceased. Requests for offprints should go to Rene A. Khafif, 2219 Ocean Avenue, Brooklyn, New York 11229.

Foreword

The editors, associate editors, and contributors to this encyclopedic work are due great praise and credit. They have rendered a tremendous service to all who treat patients with malignant disorders. They have assembled and organized in a most understandable manner the outstanding points pertaining to the prevention, early detection, diagnosis, treatment, and rehabilitation of patients with cancer.

This is a book obviously written by individuals with considerable clinical experience and good practical judgment. While there are indeed controversial points made, especially concerning such subjects as the value of thin-needle biopsies, the treatment of *in situ* cancers of the breast, and the place of elective regional lymph node dissections for malignant melanoma, these subjects are the kind on which no unanimity of opinion can be found among oncologists today. The forthright statements made in this work simply serve to indicate the up-to-date nature of this endeavor and its honesty. The points made are very well taken.

The Preface states that this endeavor is "not intended to teach the surgeon surgical techniques or the medical oncologist how to administer chemotherapy." This is a great understatement of the methods and approaches set forth. Indeed there is much information here which will be of great value to knowledgeable teachers as well as to students who are just learning the subject of oncology. The content of this work ranges from statistical data and the prevention of those tumors for which such knowledge is available to early diagnosis where possible.

Sensible and very good judgment is displayed in the step-by-step approach to therapy and all the many and varied disciplines that can contribute to the best possible end result for the patient. Flow charts are included which simplify the understanding of the methods to be employed.

The authors are to be commended for continually stressing the choice of the least complicated way of treatment which will give the most acceptable quality of survival for the patient. Nor do the authors overlook the importance of nutritional requirements, relief of pain, physical rehabilitation, and psychological support. These subjects are very frequently neglected.

This is indeed a work of distinction and one which should be of great help to all who treat patients with malignant disorders.

STEPHEN L. GUMPORT
—President
American Cancer Society
New York City Division
—Professor of Surgery
New York University School of Medicine
—Consultant
Division of Oncology
and
Director
Cancer Rehabilitation Service
New York University Medical Center

Preface

"Current Guidelines for the Management of Cancer" is presented as a comprehensive, practical guide to the physician at large, regardless of his or her level of expertise in the field of oncology. This publication is not intended to teach the surgeon surgical techniques or the medical oncologist how to administer chemotherapy, nor is it "geared" to the superspecialist. It is primarily aimed at the general physician, the family practitioner, the physician-in-training (residents, fellows, etc.), the internist, the general surgeon, and any other physician who, at one point or another, is presented with a cancer patient and may not have readily available all the information necessary for optimum management of that patient at a particular phase of his or her illness. This publication will also provide the physician with the ability to properly explain the disease to the patient, as well as the family, and to make the proper sequence of referrals.

The text makes use of what we feel is probably the most important element today in achieving the best result, i.e., the multidisciplinary approach to the patient and his or her illness, coupled with balanced judgment. No one individual physician can offer the patient the expertise available in the varied disciplines that are recognized today as being instrumental to the ultimate well-being of the patient. The epidemiologist, pathologist, surgeon, plastic surgeon, nurse oncologist, psychiatrist, social worker, physical therapist, and many more physicians and support professionals have extremely valuable contributions to make to patient care, and all these talents must be utilized to achieve the optimum results in terms of cure, survival, and, most of all, quality of life. Every section of this text was prepared with the input of all the disciplines believed instrumental in the treatment of each specific cancer site. Furthermore, recognizing the controversial nature of a number of the various therapeutic approaches, the lack of definitive answers to several problems in cancer care, and the multitude of effective methods of treatment in many cases, several specialists, often with divergent opinions, were asked to participate in establishing the guidelines for each site. The recommendations in the pages that follow are the end result of lengthy discussion and debate among the various contributors, and sometimes we let stand varying approaches recommended as acceptable options.

In compiling this publication, we attempted to keep the format of presentation the same throughout the text for easier identification of specific points. All facets of management of the cancer patient are covered, including early detection and screening; pretreatment evaluation (including confirmation of diagnosis, staging of the primary tumor, and a global assessment of the patient); therapeutic management (including the goals of treatment, complications and pitfalls, available therapeutic modalities, sequence, and use of adjuvant therapy); postoperative care and rehabilitation; and long-term evaluation and follow-up care of the treated patient. In addition, each section includes a "site-specific data form" with mapping for that particular tumor and staging instructions, as well as a therapy algorithm. At this juncture, at least, we plan to produce an updated volume at appropriate intervals to keep pace with the rapidly changing concepts in cancer management as well as the flow of investigational data that is continuously ebbing.

It will be obvious to the reader that no bibliography is referred to in the text and that few specific references are made to identify the source of any material. This is deliberate, since every contributor was specifically asked to present the concepts and methods that govern his or her approach to the specific tumor rather than report on publications already available to the reader. Most contributors did conduct an extensive literature review prior to putting their own thoughts on paper, and many of them have chosen to list some landmark publications as "suggested readings" rather than refer to them in the text of their contributions.

This publication is a product of the efforts of the Management Guidelines Committee of the Brooklyn Community Hospital Oncology Program (B-CHOP).[4] This organization is a federally sponsored program, promoted and funded by the National Cancer Institute in an attempt to decentralize the efforts at improving the care of the cancer patient and to place them in the hands of the local communities. The B-CHOP spans a total of seven major hospitals and medical centers in the southeastern section of Brooklyn, New York. Five of these hospitals are voluntary university-affiliated medical centers, one is a large city hospital, and the last is a smaller community hospital. The total bed capacity of these institutions is in excess of 3000 acute-care beds, servicing a population of more than 2,000,000 inhabitants. As a major function of the B-CHOP, and in addition to a large number of varied programs intended to evaluate and improve a broad spectrum of cancer care components (including screening and detection, cancer nursing, rehabilitation, physician education, hospice and terminal care, community relations, public education, etc.), the Management Guidelines Committee was established to create a set of guidelines for the management of various cancers, to promote the utilization of these guidelines, and to evaluate the results of the program.

The editors, associate editors, and contributors to this publication were all selected because of their active experience in the clinical management of patients with cancer. Most of them are involved in one or more major clinical investigative projects related to cancer, and most have participated in one or more of the nationwide clinical trial groups.

The editors, associate editors, and contributors gratefully acknowledge Mrs. Diane Savattieri and Mrs. Gertrude Gilligan, our executive secretaries, without whose efforts this project could not have been completed. We also wish to thank Mrs. Randi Moskowitz, R.N., the B-CHOP Project Administrator, for her sustained support.

[4]Supported in part by NCI contract no. 1-CN-25589.

Section 1

Tumors of the Head and Neck

RENE A. KHAFIF

With Contributions by

Sameer Rafla	Radiotherapy
Hossein Hedayati	Head and Neck Surgery
Richard Lopchinsky	Head and Neck Surgery
Frederico Capozzi	Head and Neck Surgery
Michael Bashevkin	Medical Oncology
Anthony Raia	Otolaryngology
Howard Rasi	Plastic Surgery
Andrew Catania	Oral Surgery
Mario Anselmo	Pathology
Marilyn Quisbert	Oncology Nursing
Randi Moskowitz	Oncology Nursing

1

Section 1. Tumors of the Head and Neck

I. Early Detection and Screening   5
  A. Patient Education
  B. Predisposing Factors and Cancer Prevention
  C. Regular Dental and Medical Checkups
  D. Early Signs of Head and Neck Cancer
    1. Mouth
    2. Larynx and Hypopharynx
    3. Nasal Cavities, Sinuses, and Nasopharynx
    4. Skin
    5. Neck
  E. Mass Screening
II. Pretreatment Evaluation and Work-Up   7
  A. History
    1. History of Present Illness
    2. Social History
    3. Family History of Carcinoma
    4. Past Medical History
  B. Clinical Examination
  C. Office Endoscopy
  D. Diagnostic Radiology
  E. Other Selected Evaluations
  F. Cytology
  G. General Medical Evaluation
  H. Operative Endoscopy
  I. Tissue Diagnosis
  J. Multidisciplinary Consultation
  K. Site-Specific Data Sheets
    1. Oral Cavity and Oropharynx
    2. Larynx and Hypopharynx
    3. Nasal Cavity, Paranasal Sinuses, and
       Nasopharynx
    4. Salivary Gland Tumors
    5. Thyroid Cancer
III. Preoperative Preparation   10
  A. Nutritional Support
    1. Nutritional Depletion
    2. Assessment of Nutritional Status
    3. Methods of Nutritional Support
      a. Enteral Hyperalimentation
      b. Parenteral Hyperalimentation
  B. Hematologic Considerations
  C. Respiratory Considerations
  D. Antibiotics
  E. Psychiatric Considerations
  F. Preparation of the Oral Cavity
    1. Dental Maintenance
    2. Functional Restoration of Teeth
    3. Preradiation Dental Extraction
    4. Mouth Cleansing
  G. Preparation of Prosthetic Devices and/or Skin Flaps

IV. Therapeutic Management: General Considerations   23
  A. Introduction and Statistical Data
  B. Management Goals
  C. Common Pitfalls
    1. Unwarranted Delay in Treatment
    2. Inadequate Biopsy
    3. Inadequate Surgery
    4. Inadequate Radiotherapy
    5. Failure to Recognize Certain Biological Facts
  D. Complications of Treatment
  E. Selection of the Modality of Treatment
    1. Histological Nature of the Tumor
    2. Location of the Tumor
    3. Size and Stage of the Tumor
      a. Small Lesions
      b. Intermediate Lesions
      c. Massive Lesions
    4. Other Factors
      a. Age
      b. Medical Status
      c. Social Factors
      d. Occupation
      e. Coexisting Tumors
      f. Psychological Factors
  F. Special Treatment Modalities
    1. Laser Surgery
    2. Fulguration
    3. Cryosurgery (or Freezing in Situ)
    4. Mohs's Technique
    5. Immunotherapy
  G. Treatment of the Neck Nodes
    1. Biopsy
    2. Guidelines for Treatment
      a. Clinically Positive Node with a Known
         Primary
      b. Metastatic Neck Node with an Unknown
         Primary
      c. Nonpalpable Lymph Node
    3. Radical Neck Dissection
      a. Standard Operation
      b. Partial Neck Dissection
      c. Conservation Operations
V. Therapeutic Guidelines: Site-Specific   29
  A. Lesions of the Oral Cavity and Oropharynx
    1. Leukoplakia and Erythroplasia
    2. Lip
    3. Buccal Mucosa
    4. Alveolar Ridge
    5. Floor of the Mouth
    6. Anterior Two-Thirds of the Tongue

7. Base of Tongue
8. Hard Palate
9. Soft Palate
10. Tonsillar Pillar and Tonsillar Fossa
11. Oropharyngeal Tumors
B. Lesions of the Larynx, Hypopharynx, Cervical
Esophagus, and Cervical Trachea
1. Larynx
  a. Supraglottic Larynx
  b. Vocal Cords (Glottic Larynx)
  c. Subglottic Larynx
2. Hypopharynx
  a. Early Lesions
  b. Larger Lesions
3. Cervical Esophagus
4. Cervical Trachea
C. Tumors of the Nasal Fossa, Paranasal Sinuses and
Nasopharynx
1. Nasal Fossa
2. Paranasal Sinuses
  a. Clinicopthological Considerations
  b. Biopsy
  c. Therapeutic Considerations
  d. Surgical Considerations
3. Nasopharynx
  a. Surgery
  b. Radiotherapy
D. Tumors of the Salivary Glands
1. General Principles
2. Histopathological Considerations
  a. Mucoepidermoid Carcinoma
  b. Adenocarcinoma
  c. Adenoid Cystic Carcinoma (Cylindroma)
  d. Malignant Mixed Tumors
  e. Epidermoid Carcinoma
  f. Acinic Cell Carcinoma
3. Modality of Treatment according to Site
  a. Parotid Tumors
  b. Submaxillary Gland Tumors
  c. Minor Salivary Gland Carcinomas
4. Chemotherapy for Advanced Disease
E. Carcinoma of the Thyroid
1. General Considerations
  a. Epidemiology
  b. Histological Types
  c. Mode of Spread
  d. Etiologic Factors
2. Diagnosis of Thyroid Carcinoma
  a. Thyroid Radioisotope Scanning
  b. Sonography
  c. Needle Biopsy
  d. X-ray
  e. Other
3. Treatment
  a. Surgical Treatment
  b. Non-Surgical Treatment

F. Other Head and Neck Cancers
VI. Adjuvant Use of Chemotherapy in Head and Neck
Cancer 44
VII. Treatment of the Advanced Head and Neck Cancer
Patient 45
A. Chemotherapy
B. Radiotherapy
C. Surgery
D. Supportive Measures
1. Nutritional Support
2. Relief of Pain
3. Psychological Support
4. Support Care Team
VIII. Postoperative Care, Evaluation, and Rehabilitation of the
Head and Neck Cancer Patient 47
A. Evaluation and Care of the Postoperative Patient
1. Vital Signs
2. Tracheostomy Care
3. Analgesics, Tranquilizers, and Narcotics
4. Antibiotics
5. Oral Hygiene
6. Wound Care and Vacuum Tube Drains under
  Skin Flaps
7. Tube Feedings
8. Laryngectomy Care
9. Postmaxillectomy Care
10. Post-thyroidectomy and/or Parathyroidectomy
   Care
B. Pre- and Post-therapy Care of the Irradiated Patient
C. Reconstructive Measures
1. Local Flaps
2. Distant Flaps
3. Muscle and Musculocutaneous Flaps
4. Gastric Transposition and Pull-Up Operations
5. Free Flaps
D. Prosthetic Rehabilitation
E. Psychiatric Support
F. Follow-Up Evaluation
G. Rehabilitation
1. Mouth and Teeth
2. Deglutition
3. Speech
4. Airway
5. Physical Therapy
6. Cosmetic Rehabilitation
IX. Management Algorithms 53
A. Oral Cavity and Oropharynx
B. Larynx and Hypopharynx
C. Maxillary Sinus and Paranasal Sinuses
D. Nasopharynx
E. Salivary Glands
F. Thyroid Gland

Suggested Readings 53

While head and neck cancer is rather rare as a whole (< 30 per 1000,000 population and $< 10\%$ of all cancers) (Table I), it is of great importance because of its impact on the special sense organs (eyes, ears, nasal cavity), its proximity to, and potential invasion of vital organs (brain and spinal cord), and the devastating cosmetic effects both of the disease and of ill-conceived therapy.

I. EARLY DETECTION AND SCREENING

A. Patient Education

The most basic aspect of early cancer detection is patient education. Such education in the case of head and neck cancers should be carried out by the physician, the nurse oncologist, the dentist, or the dental hygienist. The American Cancer Society through its publications and/or media advertising, and the hospital through one of its multiple agencies involved in community education, can offer much support in the educational process. Patient education must be in the form of a three-pronged attack: cancer prevention, regular dental and medical checkups, and identification of early signs and symptoms of head and neck cancer.

B. Predisposing Factors and Cancer Prevention

The use of tobacco in any of its forms is undoubtedly the most important predisposing factor in the development of cancers of the upper aerodigestive tract. The intense epidemiologic studies carried out in an attempt to uncover a cause of cancer have yet to come up with evidence that links any agent to cancer in as incontrovertible a way as that linking tobacco to mouth, larynx, and lung cancer. Any program of patient education geared to cancer prevention, especially head and neck cancer, cannot overemphasize the importance of discontinuing any kind of smoking and tobacco chewing.

Heavy intake of alcohol has also been identified as an important factor in head and neck cancer, particularly for mouth, pharynx, and larynx cancers. Furthermore, there seems to be a synergistic effect between smoking and heavy drinking in elevating the cancer risk.

Other factors that seem to affect the incidence of head and neck cancer include exposure to asbestos, nickel, and wood dust.

C. Regular Dental and Medical Checkups

Early detection of mouth cancer can be promoted most readily by encouraging patients to have thorough regular annual mouth examinations by a competent, alert dentist. Most tumors of the mouth are readily visible and palpable and can be detected very early during such examinations. Furthermore, a large number of mouth cancers are linked to certain oral lesions such as leukoplakia and erythroplasia; early detection of these will prevent the occurrence of carcinoma. Examination of the oral cavity should include not only dental examination but systematic inspection and palpation of the gums, floor of mouth, buccal mucosa, palate, tongue, and pharynx. Adequate lighting is paramount, and an oral mirror is extremely useful in identifying blind spots. Dental hygiene, correction of caries, periodontal scraping, filing of jagged teeth, denture adjustments, etc. should all be done during these dental checkups. Any persistent anomalous finding (persistent granulations, loose teeth, asymmetry, poorly fitting dentures, and leukoplakia, etc.) should be promptly investigated, and early consultation and biopsy should be considered. During those dental checkups, patients should be instructed in self-inspection of the mouth at the same time as they are instructed on brushing and flossing their teeth.

Early detection of head and neck cancers other than those of the oral cavity remains the responsibility of the primary care physician; a complete examination of the head and neck should be a part of every physical examination whether done during a routine check up or during consultation for unrelated complaints; it should be thoroughly and systematically carried out.

Table I

Annual Incidence of Head and Neck Cancer in the United States[a]

	Rate per 100,000 population	Percentage of head and neck[b] cancers	Percentage of all cancers	Number of cases in United States (1978)
Oral cavity				
Tongue	2.1	13	0.7	4,600
Lip	1.9	12	0.6	4,200
Floor of mouth	1.0	7	0.3	2,200
Rest of oral cavity	1.8	13	0.5	3,900
Oropharynx	1.6	10	0.5	3,500
	8.4	55	2.6	18,400
Nasopharynx	0.6	4	0.2	1,300
Nose and paranasal sinuses	0.7	4	0.2	1,500
	1.3	8	0.4	2,800
Larynx	4.2	25	1.4	9,200
Hypopharynx	0.8	5	0.3	1,800
Cervical esophagus	0.35	3	0.4	800
Cervical trachea	0.05	—	—	100
	5.4	33	2.1	11,900
Thyroid	3.6		1.2	7,900
Salivary glands	1.1	7	0.4	2,400
Melanoma of skin of head and neck	1.3		0.4	2,900
Lymphomas of head and neck	2.9		1.0	6,400
Unknown primary	0.35	2	.2	800
Other	1.1		0.4	3,400
(Ear, eye, endocrine, soft tissues, bone, brain)	4.7		1.6	10,300

[a]Figures taken from "Management Guidelines for Head and Neck Cancer." U.S. Department of Health, Education and Welfare, Public Health Service, NIH, Washington, D.C., 1979.

[b]Exclusive of thyroid, brain, skin, soft tissues, and lymphomas.

The mouth, pharynx, hypopharynx, and nasopharynx must be examined by inspection and palpation. The skin, nose, ears, and neck must likewise be carefully examined. Any asymmetry, distortion, discoloration, or tumefaction should be noted. Indirect laryngoscopy should also be part of a comprehensive examination, particularly in the elderly.

The use of toluidine blue dye to identify early cancers of the oral cavity and oropharynx has been reported on several occasions and is based on the fact that early mucosal cancer will stain, whereas normal mucosa or areas of benign dysplasia will not. This method has been emphasized recently for use as a tool to identify the nature of surface changes in the mouth and pharynx that are otherwise not impressive. It may also be used as a rapid mass-screening technique for high-risk patients such as heavy smokers or drinkers. The patient rinses his mouth with mild acetic acid followed by water and then rinses with the toluidine blue dye. This is followed by a repeat acetic acid

and water rinse. Areas that stain dark blue must be suspected of harboring malignant changes.

D. Early Signs of Head and Neck Cancer

Any persistent complaint in or about the mouth or throat and any lump in the neck should arouse suspicion and the patient should be referred for consultation. The most common symptoms that might indicate the presence of a tumor in the head and neck are as follows:

1. Mouth

- Persistent sore in the mouth, tongue, or lips.
- Any nodule, mass, or fungating exophytic lesion in the mouth.

- Any bleeding from the mouth and throat, or blood-streaked sputum.
- Persistent sore throat, especially when localized to one area.
- Any discoloration of the mucosa, whether white (leukoplakia), red (erythroplasia), or black (melanosis).
- Limitation of tongue movement.
- Ill-fitting dentures, loose teeth, or periodontal granulations.

2. Larynx and Hypopharynx

- Hoarseness. By and large, the most important early sign of cancer of the larynx in an elderly individual.
- Chronic irritative cough.
- Soreness or a feeling of "lump in the throat."
- Blood-streaked sputum.
- Dysphagia, dyspnea, or stridor.

3. Nasal Cavities, Sinuses, and Nasopharynx

- Stuffed nose.
- Swelling of face and loss of facial skin folds.
- Ocular signs: oculomotor palsy, exophthalmos, double vision, etc.
- Nosebleeds.
- Pain.
- Earache or persistent headache.
- Trismus.
- Persistent serous otitis or hearing loss.

4. Skin

- Sores or persistent crusting of skin.
- Bleeding.
- Discoloration.
- Lumps.
- Changes occurring within a pigmented lesion.

5. Neck

- Mass or nodes.
- Asymmetry.
- Evidence of cranial nerve involvement.
- Facial paralysis.
- Oculomotor paralysis.
- Dropped shoulder.
- Referred pain.
- Thyroid mass.
- Parotid mass.

These symptoms need to be publicized to the population at large and reinforced to the patients and the general physicians, to increase their awareness as to the significance of these early warning signs.

E. Mass Screening

In addition to regular dental and medical checkups, which effectively screen a significant percentage of the population, mass screening should be encouraged through widely publicized annual Mouth Cancer Days, Smoker's Days, and Head and Neck Cancer Days. These could be established at various hospitals, clinics, union centers, industrial complexes, and the like. Examinations of the mouth and oropharynx can then be done on a large segment of the population that presents itself. Such programs can be publicized effectively by several methods:

- Posters, judiciously placed.
- Notices distributed to clinic patients.
- Mailings of flyers to community members.
- Radio announcements.
- Local speaker announcements.
- Word of mouth.

The screening should be done by dentists, otolaryngolosists, and/or head and neck surgeons, all of whom are attuned to cancer detection. Any positive findings should be immediately reported to the patient and his regular physician so that appropriate action can be undertaken.

The same screening process is available through the various organizations that offer comprehensive, general physical examinations to patients who present themselves voluntarily for such an examination, or through organizations specifically designated for cancer detection (e.g., the Strang Clinic in New York).

More intensive screening of selected groups of patients should be encouraged in certain circumstances:

- Patients having received radiotherapy to the head and neck.
- Patients who were treated successfully for a prior head and neck cancer, since multiple synchronous or metachronous cancers of the upper aerodigestive tract are quite common.
- Heavy smokers and/or drinkers who continue to abuse their habits.
- Patients in certain high-risk occupations or who are in contact with carcinogenic agents (e.g., cabinetmakers for maxillary sinus carcinoma).
- Certain racial predilection (e.g., Southeast Asians for nasopharyngeal carcinoma.)

II. PRETREATMENT EVALUATION AND WORK-UP

The pretreatment evaluation of the patient with head and neck cancer should include the following comprehensive work-up before any definitive decision is made.

A. History

1. History of Present Illness

- Duration of symptoms.
- Pain, bleeding, odor.
- Dysphagia, dyspnea, dysarthria, hoarseness.
- Loose teeth, poorly fitting dentures.
- Skin changes, sores, pigmentation.
- Masses in the face or neck.
- Other.

2. Social History

- Race.
- Occupation.
- Smoking history.
- Drinking history.

3. Family History of Carcinoma

4. Past Medical History

- History of cancer.
- Previous therapy.

B. Clinical Examination

A complete examination of the head and neck must always be done to evaluate properly the primary tumor and areas of potential spread and to identify any second primary and/or other pathology. The examination should include the following:

1. Complete Examination of the Mouth and Pharynx

Examination includes inspection and palpation.

2. Identification of the Characteristics of the Lesion

- Location of the lesion, sites involved.
- Size.
- Type: ulcerating or submucosal, superficial, exophytic or fungating, infiltrating.
- Mobility: fixed to skin or fixed to deep tissues.
- Tongue mobility.
- Bone involvement (describe extent).

- Condition of teeth.
- Periodontal granulations, caries, etc.

It is important to investigate thoroughly vague and seemingly innocuous complaints:

- Edema and/or prolonged inflammation, etc.
- Asymmetry.
- Salivary pooling (pyriform sinus tumors).
- Slurred speech.
- Identification of skin changes.
- Tracheal deviations, etc.

3. Examination of the Neck, Identification of Node Metastases

- Number.
- Size.
- Mobility.
- Attachment to skin, base of skull, or deep structures.

4. Examination of Other Organs

- Thyroid.
- Parotid.
- Ears.
- Nose, etc.

5. Evidence of Cranial Nerve Involvement

- Facial paralysis.
- Dropped shoulder.
- Hoarseness of voice.
- Deviation of tongue or palate.
- Others: loss of hearing, diplopia, ocular deviations, loss of sense of smell, facial skin paresthesia, etc.

C. Office Endoscopy

- Nasopharyngoscopy.
- Indirect laryngoscopy: evaluation of the valleculae and base of tongue, epiglottis, pyriform sinsuses, pharynx, larynx, and postcricoid area; identification of any masses, ulcers, polyps, or fixation of the cords.
- Direct laryngoscopy (fiberoptic flexible or telescopic).

D. Diagnostic Radiology

- Soft-tissue x-rays. Good anteroposterior (AP) and lateral views of the head and neck region utilizing an appropriate x-ray unit can give valuable information. A study of the air column and a search for calcifications are important.

- Dental x-rays and panorex views. These are particularly important in evaluating patients with mouth cancer; they offer a definition of detail in the mandible and maxilla that is not available with routine radiological study.
- Special views for sinuses and a submentovertical view for the nasopharynx.
- Skull and facial bones. Erosions of the base of the skull, alteration of the various foramina, bone saucerization or destruction, etc.
- Tomograms. Plain linear tomography (AP and lateral) will offer a great deal of detail particularly relevant to the larynx, sinuses, and orbit.
- Laryngogram (air or contrast studies). This is rarely done today and has been supplanted by the computerized axial tomography.
- Cinefluoroscopy. This modality is of use only in evaluating the swallowing mechanism or the mobility of the larynx and vocal cords. Distendibility of the valleculae and pyriform sinuses can also be assessed.
- Computerized axial tomography (CAT) scan. The advent of the CAT scan has revolutionized the evaluation of the patient with head and neck tumors. It is of particular value in the assessment of patients with tumors of the paranasal sinuses, pterygoid region, larynx, and orbit. In all these sites, the CAT scan will identify the exact extent of the tumor and its stage, the extent of bone involvement and the status of the orbit and ethmoid cells, extensions toward the pterygoid or temporal fossae, and any intracranial extension. In the larynx, the details of tumor extension may be clearly demonstrated; subglottic, commissure, subarytenoid, or preepiglottic extension may be identified. Cartilage involvement and extralaryngeal extensions may also be seen, and better therapy planning can thus be made, especially if one contemplates conservation procedures. The CAT scan in head and neck tumors is also useful in identifying soft-tissue masses, displacement of structures, and even on occasion enlarged lymph nodes (over 1 cm in size). The study, however, needs to be thorough, with slices every 2–5 mm in both coronal and sagital planes, using high-resolution units.
- Pharyngograms, esophagrams, or tracheobronchograms.

E. Other Selected Evaluations

These evaluations are of a more specific nature relevant to tumors of certain special head and neck organs:

- Thyroid function tests, ^{131}I studies, technetium scan, sonography (thyroid tumors).
- Sialography in the evaluation of selected salivary gland tumors (rarely of benefit).

- Noninvasive vascular evaluation of the carotid artery, including ocular plethysmography (to assess the status of the collateral circulation in cases where one artery may have to be ligated) and digital radiographic subtraction procedures.
- Selective angiography and venous catheterization.
- Parathormone determinations (hyperparathyroidism).
- Calcitonin determinations (medullary carcinoma, thyroid).
- Barr-Epstein antibodies (nasopharyngeal tumors).

F. Cytology

- Aspiration (aspiration of cysts, needle aspiration of tumors).
- Smears (ulcerated tumors).
- Needle biopsy (deep-seated masses).
- Punch biopsy (ulcerated tumors).

G. General Medical Evaluation

- Medical consult, if indicated, or complete physical examination.
- Complete blood cell count (CBC).
- Multichannel biochemical profile (SMA-12), serum chemistries.
- Other pertinent studies, as indicated (e.g., thyroid function tests).
- EKG, in any patient over a certain age (suggested over 40).
- Chest x-ray.
- Search for metastases. In most cases, the above work-up is sufficient for screening of metastatic disease. If metastases are strongly suspected (in advanced cases or where specific findings are suspicious of possible metastases), additional selective work-up could be indicated (e.g., bone scan, brain scan, etc.).

H. Operative Endoscopy

Operative endoscopy should be done whenever pertinent and must include

- Direct laryngoscopy.
- Nasopharyngoscopy.
- Bronchoscopy.
- Esophagoscopy.

This is particularly true when a search for an unidentified primary is being carried out, and it should be done prior to the biopsy of cervical nodes. Endoscopic biopsy must also be done whenever indicated. It has even been suggested that a panendoscopy, as listed above, be carried out prior to the treatment of any cancer of the upper aerodigestive tract in order to detect a possible second primary.

I. Tissue Diagnosis

In almost all cases, a tissue diagnosis must be obtained prior to instituting treatment. Repeat biopsies and pathology consultation may even sometimes be desirable. The following guidelines for biopsies in head and neck tumors are recommended:

- Open biopsies should be done only after complete evaluation of the patient and just prior to instituting therapy.
- The simplest and least disturbing method of obtaining a tissue diagnosis should be attempted first (smears, aspirations, needle biopsies, and punch biopsies).
- If an open biopsy is necessary, it is strongly recommended that this be carried out after consultation with the physician responsible for the definitive treatment and preferrably by the consultant himself whenever possible.
- *Neck incisions must be planned carefully so as not to interfere with the definitive therapy.*
- Small lesions that are easily excised should be totally excised for biopsy (e.g., small tongue lesions, small basal cell cancers of the skin, etc.).
- Biopsy of a metastatic mass should be avoided unless the primary cannot be found; it is always preferable to biopsy the primary tumor.
- Biopsies of specific sites.
  Antral lesion: Caldwell-Luc operation.
  Laryngeal lesions: during direct endoscopy.
  Melanomas: preferably excisional biopsy.
  Parotid tumors: no biopsy necessary prior to definitive surgery.
  Thyroid tumors: no biopsy necessary prior to definitive surgery (except in rare cases).

J. Multidisciplinary Consultation

The need for a multidisciplinary approach for consultation, evaluation, and treatment of the patient with cancer is paramount.

Such an approach is essential in head and neck cancer and must include several specialties whose importance must be emphasized. Besides the three traditional specialists involved in the care of the patient—head and neck surgeon, radiation oncologist, and medical oncologist—other specialists offer the patient with cancer of the head and neck an expertise that is not always available within the three primary groups. To wit: otolaryngologist, pathologist, oral surgeon, and other specialists within dentistry (preventive dental care, dental hygiene, and prostodontics): plastic surgeon; nurse oncologist; rehabilitation physician and physiatrist (with particular emphasis on speech and deglutition rehabilitation); and finally, occupational therapist, speech therapist, and psychiatrist. All

these specialists are essential at one stage or another in the care of the cancer patient.

The primary care physician must coordinate the total care of the patient and insure that every specialist will be available at the proper time. His or her knowledge of, and relationship with, the patient places him or her in a unique and invaluable position to serve the best interest of the patient. Although it is conceivable that one highly specialized individual caring for the head and neck patient may be able to utilize the above mentioned specialists appropriately at the time they are needed, evaluation and advice prior to treatment by representatives of several of those disciplines would be of great value.

K. Site-Specific Data Sheets
(see pp. 11–19)

It is desirable, prior to instituting therapy, to document all findings using a site-specific data sheet for each patient with head and neck cancer. The sheet should include all pertinent data on the patient and his tumor, his preoperative work-up, mapping of the lesion, and staging. Recommended site-specific data sheets for the more common head and neck cancer sites are presented.

III. PREOPERATIVE PREPARATION

A. Nutritional Support

1. Nutritional Depletion

There are many reasons to emphasize the importance of nutritional support of the head and neck cancer patient. Many of these patients have poor nutrition and have been in a negative balance for long periods of time. Dietary indiscretions are common in the typical head and neck patient, especially in the smoker and drinker. In addition, the tumor may further decrease the intake of food, either directly by causing dysphagia and/or obstruction of the food passageways, or indirectly by systemically weakening the patient and causing anorexia. Malnutrition is often worsened by the therapy that the patient must undergo. Surgery often decreases the food intake mechanically; radiation and chemotherapy may cause temporary mucositis and stomatitis in addition to some decrease in the quantity and quality of saliva. In order to enable these poorly nourished patients to tolerate the further stresses of therapy, they must be brought to a positive balance.

Experimentally, it has been shown that chronic protein deprivation will decrease the T-cell immunity. Head and neck cancer patients tend to have an anergic response to antigenic stim-

SITE-SPECIFIC DATA FORM—ORAL CAVITY AND OROPHARYNX

HISTORY

Age: _____

Symtoms

_____ Pain

_____ Mass

_____ Bleeding

_____ Infection

_____ Dyspnea

_____ Loose tooth

_____ Poor-fitting dentures

_____ Ulceration

_____ Odor

_____ Weight loss ____ lb.

Other _____

Symptom duration: _____

Social history

Occupation: _____

Race: ____White ____Black ____Oriental ____Other

Smoker: ____Yes ____No   How much? _____

Drinker: ____Yes ____No   How often? _____

Family history of carcinoma

Relation: _____ Site: _____

Previous history of carcinoma

____ No ____Yes Site: _____

Rx: _____

Previous treatment (Describe):
(Surgery, radiation, chemotherapy, tracheostomy, etc.)

_____

_____

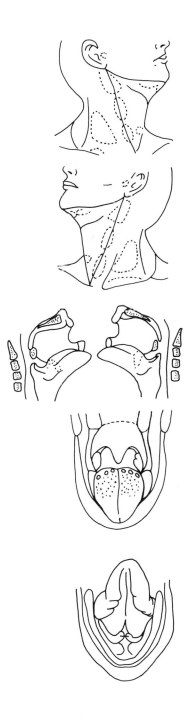

PHYSICAL EXAMINATION

Site of tumor and extension: ____Left ____Right

	Site of origin	Extension to		Site of origin	Extension to
Oral cavity			Oropharynx	_____	_____
Lips: upper	_____	_____	Tonsillar pillar	_____	_____
lower	_____	_____	Tonsil	_____	_____
Buccal mucosa	_____	_____	Soft palate	_____	_____
Floor of mouth	_____	_____	Lat. pharyngeal	_____	_____
Oral tongue	_____	_____	Post. pharyngeal	_____	_____
Hard palate	_____	_____	Base of tongue	_____	_____
Gingiva: upper	_____	_____	Also invades		
lower	_____	_____	Nasopharynx		_____
Retromolar trigone	_____	_____	Pterygoid muscles		_____
			Nasal cavity		_____
			Maxillary antrum		_____
			Soft tissues of neck		_____
			Bone		_____

Size: ____<2 cm ____2-4 cm ____>4 cm ____Massive

Characteristics: _____ Superficial   _____ Skin involvement

_____ Exophytic   _____ Extension to bone

_____ Moderate infiltration   _____ Erosion of bone

_____ Deep infiltration   _____ Bone invasion

Regional lymph nodes: _____ Palpable _____Nonpalpable

		Side		Size (cm)			Number of nodes
		R	L	3	3-6	>6	
_____ Soft	Jugulo-omohyoid	_____	_____	_____	_____	_____	_____
_____ Rubbery	Upper deep cervical	_____	_____	_____	_____	_____	_____
_____ Hard	Lower deep cervical	_____	_____	_____	_____	_____	_____
_____ Fluctuant	Submaxillary	_____	_____	_____	_____	_____	_____
_____ Ulcerated	Submental	_____	_____	_____	_____	_____	_____
	Parotid	_____	_____	_____	_____	_____	_____

Distant metastases: ____No ____Yes ____Lung ____Liver ____Bone ____Other

Histologic diagnosis: _____

PREOPERATIVE WORK-UP (Check, if done)

Views of mandible: ____Routine: Involvement ____Yes ____No

____Panorex

Endoscopy: ____Yes ____No

	Neg.	Pos.	Suspicious		Neg.	Pos.	Suspicious
Barium swallow	_____	_____	_____	Bone scan	_____	_____	_____
Chest x-ray	_____	_____	_____	Bone survey	_____	_____	_____
Tomogram (chest)	_____	_____	_____	Biopsies	_____		
Liver chemistries	_____	_____	_____	CAT scan	_____		
Liver scan	_____	_____	_____	Other	_____		

Classification: ____T ____N ____M

Stage: _____

Signature: _____

Countersignature: _____

Date: _____

Classification of Cancer of the Oral Cavity and Oropharynx

Tumor Classification

TX   Tumor cannot be assessed
T1S Carcinoma *in situ*
T1   Tumor 2 cm or less in greatest diameter
T2   Tumor >2 cm but <4 cm
T3   Tumor >4 cm in greatest diameter
T4   Massive tumor >4 cm in diameter with deep invasion to involve antrum, pterygoid muscles, root of tongue, skin of neck, or bone

Nodal Classification

NX   Cannot be assessed
N0   No clinically positive nodes
N1   Single clinically positive homolateral node <3 cm
N2a Single clinically positive homolateral node >3 cm and <6 cm
N2b Multiple clinically positive homolateral nodes, none >6 cm
N3a Clinically positive homolateral node(s), one >6 cm
N3b Bilateral clinically positive nodes: *stage each neck separately*
N3c Contralateral clinically positive node(s) only

Metastatic Classification

MX   Cannot be assessed
M0   No metastatic disease
M1   Metastasis present

Summary of Stage Groupings

Stage I   T1, N0, M0
Stage II   T2, N0, M0
Stage III   T3, N0, M0;
            T1, T2, or T3, N1, M0
Stage IV   T4, N0, M0
            Any T, N2, M0
            Any T, any N, M1

Additional Classification (for All Carcinomas)

Residual tumor
R0   No residual tumor
R1   Microscopic residual disease
R2   Gross residual tumor

Tumor grading
G1   Well differentiated
G2   Moderately differentiated
G3   Poorly differentiated
G4   Undifferentiated

Host Performance Status

		Zubrod scale	Karnofsky scale (%)
H0	Normal activity	0	90–100
H1	Symptomatic, care for self	1	70–80
H2	Ambulatory more than 50% of time—needs some assistance	2	50–60
H3	Partially ambulatory, needs nursing care	3	30–40
H4	Bedridden	4	10–20

SITE-SPECIFIC DATA FORM—LARYNX AND HYPOPHARYNX

HISTORY

Age: _____

Symtoms

_____ Hoarseness   _____ Infection
_____ Pain   _____ Dyspnea
_____ Mass   _____ Dysphagia
_____ Bleeding   _____ Odor
_____ Sore throat   _____ Weight loss ____ lb.

Other _____

Symptom duration: _____

Social history

Occupation: _____

Race: ___ White ___ Black ___ Oriental ___ Other

Smoker: ___ Yes ___ No   How much? _____

Drinker: ___ Yes ___ No   How often? _____

Family history of carcinoma
   Relation: _____ Site: _____
Previous history of carcinoma
   ___ No ___ Yes   Site: _____
Rx: _____
Previous treatment (Describe):
(Surgery, radiation, chemotherapy,
tracheostomy, etc.)

_____
_____

PHYSICAL EXAMINATION

Site of tumor and extension: ___ Left ___ Right

Larynx	Site of origin	Extension to
Supraglottis		
ventricular band	_____	_____
arytenoid	_____	_____
suprahyoid epiglottis	_____	_____
infrahyoid epiglottis	_____	_____
aryepiglottic fold	_____	_____
Glottis: vocal cords	_____	_____
Subglottis	_____	_____

Hypopharynx	Site of origin	Extension to
Pyriform sinus-med. wall	_____	_____
Pyriform sinus-lat. wall	_____	_____
Vallecula	_____	_____
Postcricoid area	_____	_____
Posterior pharyng. wall	_____	_____
Also invades		
Base of tongue	_____	_____
Pre-epiglottic space	_____	_____
Trachea	_____	_____
Soft tissue or skin	_____	_____

Size: ___ <2 cm ___ >2 to <4 cm ___ >4 cm ___ Massive

Characteristics: _____ Superficial   _____ Impaired cord mobility
           _____ Exophytic   _____ Cord fixation
           _____ Infiltrating   _____ Cartilage or bone involvement
           _____ Skin involvement   _____ Tracheal invasion

Cervical nodes: _____ Palpable ___ Nonpalpable

	Side		Size (cm)			Number of nodes
	R	L	3	3-6	>6	
_____ Soft Jugulo-omohyoid	_____	_____	_____	_____	_____	_____
_____ Rubbery Upper deep cervical	_____	_____	_____	_____	_____	_____
_____ Hard Lower deep cervical	_____	_____	_____	_____	_____	_____
_____ Fluctuant Submaxillary	_____	_____	_____	_____	_____	_____
_____ Ulcerated Submental	_____	_____	_____	_____	_____	_____
Parotid	_____	_____	_____	_____	_____	_____

Distant metastases: ___ Yes ___ No ___ Lung ___ Liver ___ Bone ___ Other

Histologic diagnosis: _____

PREOPERATIVE WORK-UP (Check, if done)

	Neg.	Pos.	Suspicious
Soft-tissue x-rays	_____	_____	_____
Tomograms	_____	_____	_____
CAT scan	_____	_____	_____
Laryngogram	_____	_____	_____
Esophagogram	_____	_____	_____
Laryngoscopy	_____	_____	_____
Esophagoscopy	_____	_____	_____
Bronchoscopy	_____	_____	_____
Biopsy	_____	_____	_____

	Neg.	Pos.	Suspicious
Metastatic survey			
Chest x-ray	_____	_____	_____
Tomogram (chest)	_____	_____	_____
Liver chemistries	_____	_____	_____
Liver scan	_____	_____	_____
Bone scan	_____	_____	_____
Bone survey	_____	_____	_____
Other	_____	_____	_____

Classification: ___ T ___ N ___ M

Stage: _____

Signature: _____

Countersignature: _____

Date: _____

Right | Left

Hypopharynx

T1S	Carcinoma *in situ*
T1	Tumor confined to site of origin
T2	Extension of tumor to adjacent site or region, without fixation of hemilarynx
T3	Extension of tumor to adjacent site or region, with fixation of hemilarynx
T4	Massive tumor invading bone or soft tissue of neck

Supraglottis

T1S	Carcinoma *in situ*
T1	Tumor confined to site of origin, with normal mobility
T2	Tumor involves adjacent supraglottic site(s) or glottis, without fixation
T3	Tumor limited to larynx, with fixation and/or extension to involve postcricoid area, medial wall of pyriform sinus, or pre-epiglottic space
T4	Massive tumor extending beyond larynx to involve oropharynx or soft tissues of neck or destruction of thyroid cartilage

Glottis

T1S	Carcinoma *in situ*
T1	Tumor confined to vocal cord(s), with normal mobility (includes involvement of anterior or posterior commissures)
T2	Supraglottic and/or subglottic extension of tumor, with normal or impaired cord fixation
T3	Tumor confined to larynx, with cord fixation
T4	Massive tumor, with thyroid cartilage destruction and/or extension beyond confines of larynx

Subglottis

T1S	Carcinoma *in situ*
T1	Tumor confined to the subglottic region
T2	Tumor extension to vocal cords, with normal or impaired cord mobility
T3	Tumor confined to larynx, with cord fixation
T4	Massive tumor, with cartilage destruction or extension beyond confines of larynx

Nodal Classification

N0	No clinically positive node
N1	Single clinically positive homolateral node <3 cm
N2a	Single clinically positive homolateral node >3 cm and <6 cm
N2b	Multiple clinically positive homolateral nodes, none >6 cm
N3a	Clinically positive homolateral node(s), one >6 cm
N3b	Bilateral clinically positive node(s); *stage each neck separately*
N3c	Contralateral clinically positive node(s) only

Metastatic Classification

M0	No metastatic disease
M1	Metastasis present

Summary of Stage Groupings

Stage I	T1, N0, M0
Stage II	T2, N0, M0
Stage III	T3, N0, M0
	T1 or T2 or T3, N1, M0
Stage IV	T4, N0, M0
	Any T, N2, M0
	Any T, any N, M1

SITE-SPECIFIC DATA FORM—NASAL CAVITY, PARANASAL SINUSES, AND NASOPHARYNX

HISTORY

Age: _____

Symptoms

_____ Mass: cheek

_____ Mass: nose

_____ Mass: mouth

_____ Mass: pharynx

_____ Mass: neck

_____ Odor

_____ Pain

_____ Visual disturbances

_____ Headache

_____ Bleeding

_____ Exophthalmus

_____ Cranial nerve deficit

    Which nerve? _____

_____ Facial anesthesia

_____ Trysmus

_____ Weight loss

Nasal symptoms

_____ Bleeding

_____ Discharge

_____ Obstruction

Ear symptoms

_____ Pain

_____ Serous otitis

_____ Drainage

_____ Hearing loss

Other _____

Symptom duration: _____

Social history

Occupation: _____

Race: ____ White ____ Black ____ Oriental ____ Other

Smoker: ____ Yes ____ No   How much? _____

Drinker: ____ Yes ____ No   How often? _____

Family history of carcinoma

Relation: _____ Site: _____

Previous history of carcinoma

_____ No _____ Yes Site: _____

Rx: _____

Previous treatment (Describe):
(Surgery, radiation, chemotherapy, tracheostomy, etc.)

_____

PHYSICAL EXAMINATION

Site of tumor and extension: _____ Left _____ Right

	Site of origin	Extension to
Antrum		
Infrastructure		_____
Suprastructure	_____	_____
Both	_____	_____
Nasal cavity		
Septum	_____	_____
Roof	_____	_____
Lateral wall	_____	_____
Floor	_____	_____
Ethmoid		
Anterior	_____	_____
Posterior	_____	_____
Nasopharynx		
Posterosuperior	_____	_____
Lateral wall	_____	_____

Also invades

Skin _____

Palate _____

Cribriform plate _____

Orbit _____

Base of skull _____

Pterygoid muscles _____

Pterygoid bone _____

Sphenoid sinus _____

Frontal sinus _____

Cranial nerves _____

Size: _____ <2 cm _____ 2-4 cm _____ >4 cm _____ Massive

Characteristics: _____ Superficial _____ Skin involvement

_____ Exophytic _____ Extension to bone

_____ Moderate infiltration _____ Erosion of bone

_____ Deep infiltration _____ Bone invasion

Cervical nodes: _____ Palpable _____ Nonpalpable

		Side		Size (cm)			Number of
		R	L	3	3-6	>6	nodes
_____ Soft	Jugulo-omohyoid	_____	_____	_____	_____	_____	_____
_____ Rubbery	Upper deep cervical	_____	_____	_____	_____	_____	_____
_____ Hard	Lower deep cervical	_____	_____	_____	_____	_____	_____
_____ Fluctuant	Submaxillary	_____	_____	_____	_____	_____	_____
_____ Ulcerated	Submental	_____	_____	_____	_____	_____	_____
	Parotid	_____	_____	_____	_____	_____	_____

Distant metastases: _____ Yes _____ No _____ Lung _____ Liver _____ Bone _____ Other

Histologic diagnosis: _____

PREOPERATIVE WORK-UP (Check, if done)

	Neg.	Pos.	Suspicious
X-rays/facial bones/sinuses	_____	_____	_____
Tomograms	_____	_____	_____
CAT scan	_____	_____	_____
Nasopharyngogram	_____	_____	_____
Endoscopy	_____	_____	_____
Caldwell-Luc	_____	_____	_____
Other biopsies	_____	_____	_____

	Neg.	Pos.	Suspicious
Metastatic survey			
Chest x-ray	_____	_____	_____
Tomogram (chest)	_____	_____	_____
Liver chemistries	_____	_____	_____
Liver scan	_____	_____	_____
Bone scan	_____	_____	_____
Bone survey	_____	_____	_____
Other	_____	_____	_____

Classification: _____ T _____ N _____ M

Stage: _____

Signature: _____

Countersignature: _____

Date: _____

Tumor Classification: Nasopharynx

TX	Tumor cannot be assessed
T1S	Carcinoma *in situ*
T1	Tumor not visible or confined to one site of nasopharynx
T2	Tumor involving two sites (both posterosuperior and lateral walls)
T3	Extension of tumor into nasal cavity or oropharynx
T4	Tumor invasion of skull and/or cranial nerve involvement

Tumor Classification: Maxillary Sinus

TX	Tumor cannot be assessed
T1	Tumor confined to the antral mucosa of the infrastructure, with no bone erosion or destruction
T2	Tumor confined to the suprastructure mucosa, without bone destruction, or to the infrastructure, with destruction of medial or inferior bony walls only
T3	More extensive tumor invading skin of cheek, orbit, anterior ethmoid sinuses, or pterygoid muscle
T4	Massive tumor with invasion of cribiform plate, posterior ethmoids, sphenoid, nasopharynx, pterygoid plates, or base of skull

Note: Ohngren's line, a theoretical plane joining the medial canthus of the eye with the angle of mandible, may be used to divide the maxillary antrum into the anterior inferior portion (the infrastructure) and the super posterior portion (suprastructure).
No tumor classification for nasal cavity, sphenoid, and sinuses.

Nodal Classification

NX	Nodes cannot be assessed
N0	No clinically positive node
N1	Single clinically positive homolateral node <3 cm
N2a	Single clinically positive homolateral node >3 cm and <6 cm
N2b	Multiple clinically positive homolateral nodes, none >6 cm
N3a	Clinically positive homolateral node(s), one >6 cm
N3b	Bilateral clinically positive nodes: *stage each neck separately*
N3c	Contralateral clinically positive node(s) only

Metastatic Classification

MX	Cannot be assessed
M0	No metastatic disease
M1	Metastasis present

Summary of Stage Groupings

Stage I	T1, N0, M0
Stage II	T2, N0, M0
Stage III	T3, N0, M0
	T1 or T2 or T3, N1, M0
Stage IV	T4, N0, M0
	Any T, N2, M0
	Any T, any N, M1

SITE-SPECIFIC DATA FORM—SALIVARY GLAND TUMORS
HISTORY

Age: _____

Symptoms
_____Mass
_____Pain
_____Ulceration
_____Bleeding
_____Facial paralysis
Other _____

Symptom duration: _____
Rate of growth _____

Social history
Occupation: _____
Race: ____ White ____ Black ____ Oriental ____ Other
Smoker: ____ Yes ____ No   How much? _____
Drinker: ____ Yes ____ No   How often? _____

Family history of carcinoma
  Relation: _____ Site: _____
Previous history of carcinoma
  ____ No ____ Yes Site: _____
Rx: _____
Previous treatment (Describe):
(Surgery, radiation, chemotherapy,
tracheostomy, etc.)

_____
_____

PHYSICAL EXAMINATION

Site of tumor and extension: ____ Left ____ Right

Gland:		Extension to:	
Parotid	_____	Skin	_____
Submaxillary	_____	Bone	_____
Sublingual	_____	Parapharyngeal space	_____
		Hypoglossal nerve	_____
Palate	_____	Lingual nerve	_____
Maxillary sinus	_____	Facial nerve	_____
Larynx	_____		

Size: ____ <2 cm ____ >2-<4 cm ____ >4-<6 cm ____ Massive

Characteristics:
_____ Mobile   _____ Hard
_____ Limited mobility   _____ Soft
_____ Fixed   _____ Cystic
_____ Attached to bone   _____ Smooth
_____ Ulcerated   _____ Irregular
_____ Skin involvement

Nerve involvement:
_____ Facial
_____ Hypoglossal
_____ Lingual
_____ Vagus
Other _____

Cervical nodes: (Check) ____ Palpable ____ Nonpalpable

		Side		Size (cm)			Number of multiples
		R	L	3	3–6	>6	
_____ Soft	Jugulo-omohyoid	_____	_____	_____	_____	_____	_____
_____ Rubbery	Upper deep cervical	_____	_____	_____	_____	_____	_____
_____ Hard	Lower deep cervical	_____	_____	_____	_____	_____	_____
_____ Fluctuant	Submaxillary	_____	_____	_____	_____	_____	_____
_____ Ulcerated	Submental	_____	_____	_____	_____	_____	_____
	Parotid	_____	_____	_____	_____	_____	_____

Distant metastases: ____ Yes ____ No ____ Lung ____ Liver ____ Bone ____ Other

Histologic diagnosis: _____

Grade: ____ 1 ____ 2 ____ 3 ____ 4

PREOPERATIVE WORK-UP (Check, if done)

	Neg.	Pos.	Suspicious		Neg.	Pos.	Suspicious
Soft-tissue x-rays	____	____	____	Metastatic survey			
Tomograms	____	____	____	Chest x-ray	____	____	____
CAT scan	____	____	____	Tomogram (chest)	____	____	____
Sialogram	____	____	____	Liver chemistries	____	____	____
Biopsy	____	____	____	Liver scan	____	____	____
				Bone scan	____	____	____
				Bone survey	____	____	____
				Other	____	____	____

Classification: ____ T ____ N ____ M

Stage: _____

Signature: _____
Countersignature: _____
Date: _____

Parotid gland – – –
Sublingual gland – –
Submaxillary gland – – –

17

Classification of Salivary Gland Tumors
(Applies Only to Parotid Gland)

TNM Classification

Primary tumor (T)

TX   Tumor cannot be assessed
T1   Tumor 0–2 cm in diameter; solitary; freely mobile, facial nerve intact
T2   Tumor 2–4 cm in diameter; solitary; freely mobile, reduced mobility, or skin fixation; and facial nerve intact
T3   Tumor 4–6 cm in diameter, or multiple nodules, skin ulceration, deep fixation, or facial nerve dysfunction
T4   Tumor >6 cm in diameter and/or involving mandible and adjacent bones

Nodal involvement (N)

NX   Nodes cannot be assessed
N1   No clinically positive nodes
N2   Single clinically positive homolateral node, <3 cm in diameter or multiple clinically positive homolateral nodes, none >6 cm in diameter
N2a   Single clinically positive homolateral node, 3–6 cm in diameter
N2b   Multiple clinically positive homolateral nodes, none <6 cm in diameter
N3   Massive homolateral node(s), bilateral nodes, or contralateral node(s)
N3a   Clinically positive homolateral node(s), >6 cm in diameter
N3b   Bilateral clinically positive nodes (in this situation, each side of the neck should be staged separately; that is, N3b; right; N2a: left, N1)
N3c   Contralateral positive node(s) only

Distant metastasis (M)

MX   Not assessed
M0   No (known) distant metastasis
M1   Distant metastasis present (specify)

Specify sites according to the following notations:

Pulmonary	PUL	Lymph nodes	LYM	Skin	SKI
Osseous	OSS	Bone marrow	MAR	Eye	EYE
Hepatic	HEP	Pleura	PLE	Other	OTH
Brain	BRA				

Stage Grouping

No stage grouping is recommended at present

Histological Classification

Histologic type and grade of tumor must be included in any classification of salivary gland tumors.

G1   Well differentiated
G2   Moderately well differentiated
G3   Poorly differentiated
G4   Undifferentiated

Residual tumor status and host performance is the same as all other tumors.

SITE-SPECIFIC DATA SHEET—THYROID CANCER

HISTORY

Age: _____
Symptoms
_____ Mass
_____ Pain
_____ Hoarseness
_____ Dysphagia
_____ Dyspnea
_____ Hypothyroidism
_____ Hyperthyroidism
Other _____
Symptom duration: _____
Social history
Occupation: _____
Race: ____ White ____ Black ____ Oriental ____ Other
Previous radiation therapy to head and neck: ____ No ____ Yes. If yes, indicate type:
_____

Family history of carcinoma
  Relation: _____ Site: _____
Previous history of carcinoma
  ____ No ____ Yes Site: _____
  Rx: _____
Previous treatment (Describe):
(Surgery, radiation, chemotherapy,
tracheostomy, etc.)
_____
_____

PHYSICAL EXAMINATION

Site of tumor and extension: _____ Right lobe _____ Left lobe _____ Isthmus
Extension to:

Substernal extension	_____	Vocal cord paralysis	_____
Tracheal deviation	_____	Strap muscle involvement	_____
Tracheal invasion	_____	Fixation	_____
Esophageal involvement	_____	Skin involvement	_____

Size: _____ <3 cm _____ >3 cm _____ Massive
      _____ Single nodule _____ Multicentric
Regional lymph nodes: _____ Palpable _____ Nonpalpable

		Side		Size (cm)			Number of
		R	L	3	0–5	>5	nodes
_____ Soft	Jugulo-omohyoid	_____	_____	_____	_____	_____	_____
_____ Rubbery	Upper deep cervical	_____	_____	_____	_____	_____	_____
_____ Hard	Lower deep cervical	_____	_____	_____	_____	_____	_____
_____ Fluctuant	Submaxillary	_____	_____	_____	_____	_____	_____
_____ Ulcerated	Submental	_____	_____	_____	_____	_____	_____
	Parotid	_____	_____	_____	_____	_____	_____

Distant metastases: ____ Yes ____ No ____ Lung ____ Liver ____ Bone ____ Other

PREOPERATIVE EVALUATION (Check, if done)

X-rays of neck:	_____ Negative	_____ Positive	_____ Suspicious
Thyroid scan:	_____ Cold nodule	_____ Warm	_____ Hot
Sonogram:	_____ Cystic	_____ Solid	_____ Mixed
Thyroid functions:	_____ Hyperthyroid	_____ Hypothyroid	_____ Euthyroid
Calcitonin:	_____ Negative	_____ Positive	_____ Suspicious
Antithyroid antibodies:	_____ Negative	_____ Positive	_____ Suspicious

METASTATIC SURVEY

	Negative	Positive	Suspicious
Chest x-ray	_____	_____	_____
Liver chemistries	_____	_____	_____
Bone scan	_____	_____	_____
Other			

Classification
Histological typing: _____ Papillary _____ Follicular _____ Medullary
                     _____ Undifferentiated _____ Giant cell _____ Spindle cell
                     Grade: _____ 1 _____ 2 _____ 3 _____ 4
_____ T _____ N _____ M   Signature: _____
Stage: _____   Countersignature: _____
                               Date: _____

19

Tumor Classification

TX   Tumor cannot be assessed
T0   No evidence of primary tumor
T1   Tumor 3 cm or less in greatest diameter
T2   Tumor >3 cm in greatest diameter
T3   Multiple intraglandular foci of tumor
T4   Invasion through the thyroid capsule or fixation of the tumor

Nodal Involvement

NX   Nodes cannot be assessed
N0   No clinically (or histologically in case of postsurgical classification) involved nodes
N1   Nodes involved

Distant Metastases

MX   Not assessed
M0   No known metastases
M1   Distant metastases present
      Site: _____

   Because of the great prognostic importance of the patient's age and the histologic nature of the tumor in the behavior of the disease, these factors must be taken into account in any staging of thyroid cancer.

Histologic Types

Papillary carcinomas (with or without follicular foci)
Follicular carcinomas
Medullary carcinomas
Undifferentiated carcinomas

Stage Grouping

   The grouping of thyroid cancer is most complex and takes into account the patient's age and the histology of the tumor, as well as the TNM classifications.

Stage I
   Under age 45   Any papillary or follicular tumor with N0, M0
   Over age 45   Papillary carcinoma with any T with N0, M0; or T1, N1, M0
                    Follicular carcinoma with T1, N0, M0

Stage II
   Under age 45   Any papillary or follicular carcinoma with N1
                    Any medullary carcinoma with M0
   45 years and over Papillary carcinoma with T2—T4, N1, M0
                    Follicular carcinoma with T2—T4, N0, M0

Stage III
   45 years and over Any follicular carcinoma with N1, M0
                    Any medullary carcinoma with M0

Stage IV
   Any age   Any undifferentiated carcinoma
                    Any medullary carcinoma with M1
   45 years and over Any papillary or follicular carcinoma with M1

ulation, indicating a certain degree of immune deficiency. Restoring the nutritional status of these patients is necessary to improve their physical well-being, as well as their metabolic and immunologic status.

2. Assessment of the Nutritional Status

It is important a priori, to establish which patients require nutritional support and how well they respond to the therapy. The most obvious sign of poor nutritional status is *weight loss;* weight loss of more than 15 pounds is indicative of a severe catabolic state. Various physical measurements have been shown to correlate with a severe catabolic status, but these are cumbersome and unfamiliar. They include

- The triceps skin fold thickness (TSFT) (< 12.5 mm ♂ or 16.5 mm ♀).
- The mid-upper arm circumference (> 29 cm ♂ or 28.5 cm ♀).
- The mid-upper arm muscle circumference: = arm circ. − ($0.314 \times$ TSFT mm) (> 25 ♂ or 23 ♀).

Poor nutrition will also manifest itself in abnormal laboratory tests:

- Hemoglobin (< 14 ♂ or 12 ♀).
- Serum albumin (< 3.5 gm %).
- Serum transferrin (< 200 mg %).
- Serum cholesterol (< 150 mg %).

It is also desirable to test these patients for their cell-mediated immunity with skin tests (including Varidase, candida, mumps, PPD, and dermatophytin). The total lymphocyte count as well as the T-cell component may also be used as an indicator of the immunologic status of the patient.

3. Methods of Nutritional Support

For those patients who are nutritionally depleted or who will require stressful therapy, nutritional support should be instituted as soon as feasible, Normal nutritional maintenance requires about 35 kcal per kg per day. To create an anabolic state, 45 kcal per kg per day is required. Nitrogen should be supplied in a ratio of approximately 1 g per 150 nonprotein calories.

a. Enteral Hyperalimentation

The ideal means of providing nutrition is through the gastrointestinal tract. When the oral intake is limited because of dysphagiga (related directly or indirectly to the tumor), a feeding tube is placed below the tumor into the distal esophagus or directly in the stomach. Avoidance of a tube passing through the gastro–esophageal junction will prevent reflux and esophagitis; furthermore, an undisturbed gastro–esophageal

junction is of value in preventing aspiration of gastric contents. Sitting the patient up for the feedings and keeping him thus for 30 min after the feedings will also help prevent aspiration. The feedings can be either of a blenderized diet or of any of the nutritional supplements or elemental diets commercially available. The elemental diets must be started cautiously and at one-quarter strength, as they may cause an osmotic diarrhea. Most patients will tolerate ordinary dietary supplements more readily, although milk-based products may also cause diarrhea. The best tolerated feedings include that of a blenderized hospital or house-prepared diet with calculated protein and caloric intake. Generally, these are easily prepared and inexpensive.

Patients should be instructed as to the function and necessity of a feeding tube, if it will be used postoperatively. This knowledge will facilitate the patient's acceptance and reduce the tendency to pull it out, an accident that may prove nutritionally disastrous, especially in the presence of a pharyngeal suture line.

For those patients who require additional nutritional support beyond that administered through tube feedings, peripheral parenteral nutrition may be given using a fat emulsion together with amino acids and dextrose as a supplement to oral intake.

b. Parenteral Hyperalimentation

Intravenous hyperalimentation (IVH) is recommended when oral intake or tube feeding is not feasible. This must be given through a centrally placed venous catheter because of the high osmolarity of the solution. Combinations of amino acids and glucose are given thus at about 1 cal per cubic centimeter until maximum tolerance is achieved; as much as 4000 cc per day may be administered. Various mineral and vitamin solutions including trace elements must be either added in the solution or given separately. Complications of this therapy are frequent, and patients must be closely monitored; electrolyte abnormalities, water overload, glucose intolerance, and catheter-related problems are the most frequent complications. The first three are especially noted when IVH is utilized too rapidly in patients who are extremely malnourished. Catheter insertion complications include pneumothorax or hydrothorax, catheter sepsis, and dislodgement of the catheter. For these reasons, central IVH should be reserved for those patients who cannot be managed with a combination of enteric and peripheral alimentation.

B. Hematologic Considerations

Most patients with carcinomas of the oral cavity are somewhat volume depleted and may require several units of packed cells once they have been hydrated. As these large volume changes take place, the patients should be closely observed for electrolyte imbalance and fluid overload. Since many head and neck cancer patients are alcoholics, a check of their coagulation profile should be carried out, and any deficiency should be corrected. Preoperative patients should not be permitted aspirin since this may cause qualitative platelet defects that are not ordinarily detected on routine coagulation screening; as a result, this could cause bleeding tendencies that might prove disastrous with the large flaps employed in the head and neck region.

C. Respiratory Considerations

All patients undergoing major head and neck surgery, especially those with heavy smoking histories, should receive preoperative instructions regarding proper pulmonary toilet and the necessity for clearing secretions. If feasible, patients should be instructed on self-suctioning so that they can actively participate in their postoperative care.

Patients being prepared for total laryngectomy should, if possible, see a speech therapist preoperatively so that a personal rapport can be established between them. This will help to alleviate the enormous fear experienced by patients prior to operation and permit them to familiarize themselves with the postoperative rehabilitation program.

D. Antibiotics

All patients having aerodigestive tract surgery should have prophylactic perioperative antibiotics suitable for treating the oral flora as well as the nosocomial hospital flora. Patients undergoing major head and neck surgery following radiotherapy should also be considered as candidates for such perioperative antibiotic therapy in preparation for surgery. Massive bone resections and procedures that require entrance into the cranial fossa (e.g., maxillectomies) should be covered by broad-spectrum antibiotics. Likewise, patients who require reoperation in the same field should receive perioperative antibiotics.

E. Psychiatric Considerations

All patients who are about to have extensive, potentially multilating or disabling procedures should have such procedures thoroughly explained to them. Often, a visit by a previously treated patient with the same type of tumor or disability can go a long way toward reassuring apprehensive patients. These patients may benefit from preoperative contact with a social worker or psychiatric nurse or, if necessary, a psychiatrist. One must be careful not to underestimate the psychological impact that the disease and its treatment can have on pa-

tients and preoperative assessment and preparation is far more valuable than any postoperative therapy.

F. Preparation of the Oral Cavity

The oral cavity and teeth ought to be brought to an optimum level of hygiene and cleanliness prior to the institution of therapy.

1. Dental Maintenance

A thorough evaluation by a dentist, including cleaning of the teeth and gums, should be mandatory. Instructions regarding oral hygiene, plaque control, and daily topical fluoride application should be carried out. Teeth fluoridation is a particularly useful precaution prior to and during radiotherapy.

2. Functional Restoration of Teeth

As many teeth as possible should be retained during and after therapy. They are essential for retention of prostheses and dentures. Salvageable teeth should be brought to an optimum condition prior to treatment. Cavities should be filled; periodontal scraping and cleaning must be done; and any periodontal or pulp pathology that can be expeditiously corrected should be corrected preoperatively.

3. Preradiation Dental Extraction

If extraction of some of the teeth that are within the field of radiation therapy is necessary because of dental problems, this must be carried out prior to treatment. It must be remembered that extraction of teeth following heavy radiation has the potential complication of osteonecrosis. The extraction should be done under proper antibiotic coverage, and the teeth should be removed with the least possible trauma.

The lapse of time between extraction and radiotherapy and the need for selective or total teeth extraction prior to therapy are both subject to controversy and should be decided jointly by the oral surgeon and the therapist. It is, however, not advocated to remove mandibular impacted molars or maxillary teeth, except when absolutely necessary. The large bony defects created by these extractions require prolonged healing and delays, which may be ill advised. Excision of symptomatic operculum over partially erupted third molars is a safer approach.

4. Mouth Cleansing

Mouth cleansing with antiseptic and/or deodorizing solutions and other methods of local cleansing of the mouth and tumor should be encouraged and actively carried out in the immediate period prior to therapy.

G. Preparation of Prosthetic Devices and/or Skin Flaps

Preparation of dental molds, fixation devices, retaining molds, maxillary obturators, or even facial prostheses must be planned and preferably done prior to therapy so that they can be available to use during or immediately following surgery. The patient must be seen by the prosthodontist before surgery in order to take the necessary impressions and prepare the desired prosthesis. On rare occasions, pedicle skin flaps must be raised, delayed, lined, or otherwise prepared prior to definitive therapy.

IV. THERAPEUTIC MANAGEMENT: GENERAL CONSIDERATIONS

A. Introduction and Statistical Data

It is quite probable that nowhere else in the body do malignant lesions require as much rational judgment and careful evaluation prior to selecting the therapeutic modality best suited for the patient, than in specific lesions of the head and neck.

Lesions that appear identical clinically will require a totally different therapeutic approach if they have different histological types. Likewise, the same lesion located but 1 cm away will behave in a totally different manner and requires a totally different treatment. Also, the therapy will vary considerably in the same tumor depending on its size and stage. It is, therefore, essential to have a thorough understanding of the different biologic behaviors of various tumors in order to rationally apply a therapeutic plan.

A multidisciplinary approach is of the greatest importance in head and neck surgery. Although the final therapeutic responsibility will invariably rest in the hands of the head and neck surgeon or the radiotherapist, optimum care requires that they avail themselves of the knowledge and expertise of other specialities.

Males are more prone to develop cancers in the head and neck region; the overall male/female ratio is about 3 : 1, with rates as high as 9 : 1 in the larynx and 11 : 1 in lip cancer. The age incidence increases markedly beyond age 50.

Overall results in the treatment of head and neck cancer vary considerably according to the size, histology, area, and stage. They are, however, encouraging in most areas when a multidisciplinary, well-organized plan of treatment is instituted early. An average cure rate of 50–60% can be expected. An

Table II

Five-Year Relative Survival[a,b]

	Localized	Regional	Distant	All stages
Tongue	52	22	7	33
Lip	89	57	—	86
Floor of mouth	65	31	18	45
Other oral cavity	61	29	18	44
Oropharynx	44	23	11	28
Larynx	73	30	11	57
Hypopharynx	20	14	12	15
Cervical esophagus	25	21	6	—
Nasopharynx	44	25	10	26
Nasal fossa and paranasal sinuses	59	20	10	40
Salivary glands	87	51	23	69
Thyroid	96	84	24	83

[a]Data taken from "Management Guidelines for Head and Neck Cancer." U.S. Department of Health, Education, and Welfare, Public Health Service, NIH, Washington, D.C., 1979.

[b]Percentage of observed survival rate compared to expected survival rate of individuals in the general population with same age, sex, race, and calendar year studied.

annual death rate of 13,000 patients per year results from head and neck cancer. Table II gives a few examples of five-year relative survivals.

B. Management Goals

Biopsy of the lesion, using the least disruptive modality but allowing adequate identification of the tumor and its grade, is mandatory before a definitive multidisciplinary decision requiring therapy can be made. The goal of effective therapy encompasses the following factors:

- Effective control of the lesion with the least disabling consequences.
- Concern over the quality of life, at least as much as concern over the prolongation of life.
- Early application of rehabilitative measures in order to return the patient to a normal social existence within a reasonable period of time.
- Acceptance of the fact that some tumors are beyond the hope of cure and offering palliation for such patients rather than heroic measures that are doomed to failure.

C. Common Pitfalls

The following are some of the departures from sound clinical management that are most frequently encountered and that one must avoid:

1. Unwarranted Delay in Treatment

- Prolonged treatment of lesions of the mouth with local applications, antibiotics, or dental adjustments, in the face of obvious failure.
- Prolonged watch-and-wait attitude in the face of asymptomatic masses.
- Hoarseness that is ignored for a prolonged period of time.

2. Inadequate Biopsy

- Incisional biopsy of a leukoplakia or erythroplasia of the mouth, which is not representative of the whole lesion.
- Acceptance of a single biopsy with a benign report, to override a clinical diagnosis of carcinoma.
- Failure to review slides of tissues from previous operations that could bear a relationship to the present illness or treatment decision.
- Incomplete evaluation of the patient prior to biopsy and failure to obtain necessary x-rays, endoscopy, or other studies.
- Open biopsy of a neck mass prior to an attempt at identifying a primary tumor.

It is always desirable for the physician who will ultimately be responsible for treating the patient to do the biopsy or, at the very least, to evaluate the patient prior to the biopsy.

3. Inadequate Surgery

- Tailoring the extent of surgery to the ability of the surgeon, rather than to the disease.
- Compromising the ablative phase of the procedure in order to accommodate reconstruction.
- Compromising the margins of resection grossly, with the hope of subsequent salvage by adjunctive radiotherapy or chemotherapy. Although radiation may affect cure in some such cases, the necessary use of high doses following surgery may result in excessive morbidity.
- Carrying out partial resection of a tumor that is obviously not totally removable.
- The utilization of unproven conservation operations rather than time-honored more radical procedures.
- Performing radical procedures where conservation operations have been demonstrated to be equally effective.

4. Inadequate Radiotherapy

The most important and common reasons for radiation failure due to inadequate treatment are

- Poor case selection. Certain biologic factors preclude the use of radiotherapy as a single curative modality; these in-

clude bone or cartilage involvement by cancer and massive epidermoid lesions; fixed lesions also respond relatively poorly.
- Poor timing. Preoperative or postoperative radiotherapy must be designed jointly with the operating surgeons if optimum results are to be obtained.
- Inadequate volume treated. This causes geographic failures and reseeding.
- Insufficient dosages.
- Poor treatment planning. Low biologic dose (e.g., a modest dose given over long time periods), lack of attention to treatment plan and verifying films (causing either hot spots or cold spots), and an unduly long delay between surgery and radiotherapy are among the more important factors. For optimum results, no more than 3 weeks should elapse between surgery and subsequent radiation, or 4–6 weeks between radiation and surgery in patients selected for preoperative radiotherapy.
- Inadequate observation. Failure to watch the patient carefully during the course of treatment may result in excessively early or late reactions that could be otherwise avoided.

5. Failure to Recognize Certain Biological Facts

- ''Condemned mucosa'' in the mouth, frequently associated with specific carcinogens (smoking) or genetic in nature. This is not an uncommon condition in which multiple areas of the oral mucosa display evidence of malignant and premalignant changes synchronously or metachronously.
- Multiplicity of primaries of the aerodigestive tract, synchronous or metachronous.
- The biologic behavior of the various specific histological entities (e.g., papillary versus anaplastic thyroid cancer; adenoid cystic carcinomas of the salivary gland with their intense ability to spread and metastasize, yet compatible with long survivals; limited radiosensitivity of certain cancer cell types such as the verrucous squamous cell carcinoma of the mouth, etc.).

D. Complications of Treatment

It must be kept in mind that both surgery and radiation have long-term complications. For surgery, these can be cosmetic or functional and are related to the organ or part that is resected, its location, its size, and the ability to reconstruct and rehabilitate. For radiotherapy, the long-term complications are related to dryness of the mouth, mucous membrane and gum atrophy, loss of taste, dental caries, and osteonecrosis. Though rare, the potential of a second malignancy related to the radiotherapy must be kept in mind.

E. Selection of the Modality of Treatment

There are two curative modalities in head and neck cancer—surgical or radiotherapeutic—and both are based on the elimination of the tumor and its potential sites of spread. Recently, the safe combination of both modalities has been found to yield better results in the more advanced lesions and seems to be advisable in select cases. The inclusion of chemotherapy either prior to or after local treatments has been under study and shows promise.

The selection of radiotherapy or surgery for any specific tumor must take several factors into consideration.

1. Histological Nature of the Tumor

The histology of the lesion will often dictate the optimum type of treatment. Generally, undifferentiated carcinomas (poorly differentiated epidermoid carcinoma, anaplastic thyroid carcinoma, undifferentiated parotid cancer) are more radiosensitive than the well-differentiated lesions. For example, verrucous carcinoma of the oral cavity (a well-differentiated epidermoid carcinoma) and papillary or follicular thyroid cancers are considered relatively radioresistant. On the other hand, the well-differentiated lesions are usually more localized, slower growing, and more amenable to surgical extirpation.

Salivary gland tumors and other glandular malignancies, though reported to be less radiosensitive than epidermoid cancers, are amenable to control by radiotherapy but will require high doses of radiation. Radiotherapy combined with surgery, particularly for larger lesions, seems to produce better results.

Sarcomas of the bones and soft tissues are also not very sensitive to radiotherapy. Several of these lesions (e.g., embryonal cell rhabdomyosarcoma), have been found to be extremely sensitive to chemotherapeutic agents; others (e.g., osteogenic sarcomas) seem to do better if resected following high doses of chemotherapy. Most sarcomas will require combined therapy.

Skin cancers, with the exception of malignant melanomas, are highly radiocurable.

Lymphomas, not infrequently seen in the head and neck, are treated according to the lymphoma guideline.

2. Location of the Tumor

The location of the tumor and the inaccessibility of the lesion to the surgeon or radiotherapist often dictates the choice of treatment and the preferred modality. The following guidelines indicate the preferred treatment modality according to the location of the lesion.

a. Oral Cavity and Oropharynx

Lesions of the mouth in close proximity to or involving bone are preferably treated by surgery whenever possible, often utilizing radiotherapy as an adjunctive postoperative modality in the more sizable lesions.

Lesions in the posterior third of the mouth, oropharynx, and nasopharynx are preferably treated by radiotherapy whenever possible. Tumors in these sites, particularly when rich in lymphocytic components (for example in lymphoepithelial carcinomas), are extremely radiosensitive. Primary surgery in these locations (e.g., base of tongue, tonsillar fossa, soft palate, and oropharynx) is rather formidable and should be reserved for those cases in which radiotherapy did not elimate the disease completely. The surgery could then be carried out either as a planned postradiotherapy resection or as a more limited resection of the residual disease.

b. Paranasal Sinuses

Lesions within the paranasal sinuses are preferably treated with a combination of radiotherapy and surgery. Usually radiotherapy is given as a full preoperative course.

c. Larynx

Lesions within the larynx, in areas that cannot be easily visualized, are usually not the best candidates for radiotherapy since it is difficult to evaluate the patient during and after radiation because of the reaction (edema and discoloration) that results from the therapy; failures could be missed for long periods of time. Early lesions of the vocal cords, without fixation of same, are, however, candidates for primary radiotherapy.

3. Size and Stage of the Tumor

The size and stage of the disease also governs the choice of treatment. For example, all other factors being equal, the following general guidelines apply.

a. Small Lesions: T1 and Early T2 Tumors

These tumors, less than 3 cm in size, can be cured effectively by surgery or radiotherapy. Lesions easily accessible to the surgeon, (e.g., tongue or floor of mouth) are those readily treated by resection, whereas small lesions in difficult anatomic locations (e.g., larynx, pharynx, etc.) often respond well and with less disability, to radiotherapy.

b. Intermediate Lesions: Larger T2 and Early T3 Tumors

These tumors, between 3 and 5 cm in size, can be equally well treated by either modality in most cases. The choice of treatment will then be dependent on the histopathology and the exact location of the lesion; the morbidity of surgery for these larger tumors often exceeds that of radiotherapy, and a joint decision is absolutely essential in order to offer the patient the optimum treatment. Radiotherapy is usually not recommended as a primary modality, however, when the tumor has extended into the bone or cartilage.

c. Massive Lesions: T3 and T4 Tumors

Local control rate for these tumors is poor with either modality alone. Combination treatment is almost always necessary to achieve acceptable results. Preoperative radiotherapy is preferably used in cases of questionable operability, whereas postoperative radiotherapy is selected for those lesions that are easily resectable, or whenever surgical complications after preoperative radiotherapy are increased (e.g., hypopharynx tumors or cases where a bone-conservation operation is contemplated). Postoperative radiotherapy is also preferred in lesions that have limited radioresponsiveness and in those cases where the unrecognized extent of the lesion resulted in inadequate surgical margins. More recently, preoperative or anterior chemotherapy has been effectively used in advanced head and neck cancer as an adjuvant, with radiotherapy given postoperatively.

Whenever radiotherapy is selected, either as the sole modality or as a preoperative approach, the patient must be closely observed; if the lesion is judged to be of poor radioresponsiveness, a change in the course of therapy to early surgery must be considered. The addition of chemotherapy in such cases may also be helpful.

4. Other Factors

Several other factors must be considered in the selection of treatment of a specific cancer of the head and neck.

a. Age

The age of the patient is usually not a contraindication to surgery in itself. A single surgical procedure, regardless of its magnitude, may be better tolerated by an elderly patient than a protracted course of treatment with radiotherapy or chemotherapy.

b. Medical Status

On the other hand, severe medical illnesses may preclude radical surgery, leaving radiotherapy (alone or with salvage surgery) as the only alternative. Poor respiratory function may limit the surgical options; for example, partial laryngectomies are contraindicated in such patients, even if the local lesion invites it.

c. Social Factors

Smoking is an undesirable habit, more so if the patient is unable to stop. It may jeopardize the patient's chances by increasing the complications of treatment with either radiotherapy or surgery. Likewise, an unreliable, noncompliant patient is not a suitable candidate for radiotherapy and may not complete the course of treatment. The patient's nutritional state is also of paramount importance for either surgery or radiotherapy.

d. Occupation

In certain circumstances, special occupations would almost prohibit surgery as a therapeutic modality because of the disability that would result from the surgery. It must be kept in mind at all times that the objective of treatment is to return patients to a normal social existence and not just to rid them of their disease.

e. Coexisting Tumors

If a patient has two or more carcinomas, either in the mouth or in other areas of the body, the decision whether to treat with radiotherapy or surgery must take into account the therapy of both lesions.

f. Psychological Factors

The psychological trauma of the disease and the potential disability that might be caused by the treatment must be carefully considered throughout.

F. Special Treatment Modalities

In addition to surgery, radiotherapy, and chemotherapy, which constitute the mainstream of cancer therapy, a number of more recently developed procedures, or procedures under study and development, may at times be advantageous.

1. Laser Surgery

This surgery may be useful in eye and laryngeal tumors.

2. Fulguration

Mentioned just to be condemned, cauterization or fulguration of tumors should be done only for palliation and possibly reduction of bulky tumors in patients who cannot tolerate (or who refuse) any other mode of treatment.

3. Cryosurgery (or Freezing in Situ)

This method, which produces local destruction of tissue without excision, can, at times, achieve satisfactory results in well-selected cases. It might be considered as a reasonable alternative in

• Nonmelanoma skin cancers.
• Very high surgical risk patients with limited surface disease.

- Desire to conserve bone in certain selected cases of mouth cancer.
- Small oropharyngeal lesions, especially if inaccessible to surgical resection and reconstruction.
- For palliation of residual local disease, following the more conventional methods of treatment.

4. Mohs's Technique

This is a very effective method of resecting difficult tumors of the skin (e.g., rodent ulcers) while preserving the maximum amount of normal tissue. The procedure involves fixing tissues *in situ* and then resecting the tumor minimally with careful mapping and pathological study of the margins. The procedure is repeated as often as necessary until the entire tumor is removed. Wounds are usually allowed to heal by secondary intention but sometimes require skin grafts or plastic reconstruction at a later stage. The procedure requires an experienced dermatologist and pathologist and should only be carried out in specialized centers. More recently, the laser has been used in combination with Mohs's technique, and a fresh tissue technique without *in situ* fixation has been gaining popularity (see § 3, p. 109).

5. Immunotherapy

Enhancement of host immune responses (specific or nonspecific) and efforts to correct various defects in immune systems in cancer patients are actively being investigated but remain confined to the research area. On the other hand, assessment of the patient's immune competence is an important prognostic tool. The tests usually employed are delayed cutaneous hypersensitivity tests and lymphocyte counts (total and T-cell) and blastogenic responses.

G. Treatment of the Neck Nodes

1. Biopsy

Patients who have known carcinomas of the head and neck and who present with enlarged cervical lymph nodes must be assumed to have metastatic disease to the neck; preliminary biopsy of those nodes is rarely indicated and should be avoided in order not to violate a virgin field and open up planes that might permit undesirable spread of tumor prior to definitive surgery. On rare occasions, a needle biopsy may be done if the diagnosis is very doubtful in a patient where surgery appears risky.

2. Guidelines for Treatment

a. Clinically Positive Cervical Lymph Node with a Known Primary

It has been generally agreed that significantly enlarged metastatic lymph nodes in the neck are not radiocurable, though recent studies showed that they might, at times, be radiosensitive. It is advisable, therefore, when enlarged cervical lymph nodes coexist with an identifiable primary malignant tumor in the head and neck, that the nodes be treated by radical neck dissection. There are circumstances, however, where radiotherapy is the preferred primary modality for the treatment of cervical node metastases; those include cases in which the primary tumor is preferably treated by radiotherapy. In these cases, the neck nodes are usually included in the field, and surgery is reserved for those patients in whom nodes persist after completion of treatment (e.g., carcinoma of the tonsillar fossa or soft palate with positive lymph nodes). The neck dissection may then be performed in conjunction with resection of any residual tumor at the primary site; or alone, if the primary tumor is totally controlled.

b. Metastatic Neck Node with an Unknown Primary

In about 10–15% of patients with metastatic epidermoid carcinoma in a neck node, extensive evaluation will fail to reveal the primary source of the tumor. Several areas in the oropharynx are "blind spots" where a small primary cancer might be hidden for long periods of time. These sites include the base of the tongue and valleculae, the pyriform sinuses, the ventral surfaces of the epiglottis, the subglottic larynx, and the nasopharynx. A thorough search for the primary must be carried out before starting therapy or doing an open biopsy of the node. Investigations should include a complete x-ray evaluation with CAT scans and direct panendoscopy (laryngoscopy, nasopharyngoscopy, bronchoscopy, and esophagoscopy).

The location of the metastatic node might serve as a guide to the primary:

- The highest spinal accessary node in the mastoid vicinity may be indicative of nasopharyngeal cancer.
- Submandibular nodes usually occur with carcinomas of the anterior tongue, gums, and floor of mouth.
- Upper jugular and jugulodigastric nodes frequently signify the presence of a tumor of the base of the tongue or hypopharynx.
- Jugular nodes are often enlarged with thyroid cancer.
- Supraclavicular nodes are most often an indication of a primary tumor below the clavicle (e.g., lung, breast, gastrointestinal tract, ovary, etc.)

Despite exhaustive investigation, however, a significant number of patients will not have the primary identified. Treatment should be instituted as soon as the evaluation is completed, even though the search for the primary will continue and be repeated regularly.

Metastatic epidermoid carcinoma of the neck with no identifiable primary is generally treated with radiotherapy to the neck, preferably including those areas where a possible primary site is suspected based on the location of the node. It is necessary to perform repeated examinations of the head and neck over a period of 3 months (during the radiotherapy and during the waiting period) in an attempt to identify the occult primary tumor. In this category of patients, surgery should be carried out in the following circumstances:

• For nodes that fail to respond adequately to radiotherapy and/or appear to be getting larger during treatment.
• In cases where the primary is found and is better treated surgically.
• Whenever neck disease persists (or recurs) after completion of radiotherapy.

Many surgeons have recommended carrying out radical neck dissections as the primary treatment in these patients and using radiotherapy postoperatively, claiming the end results to be essentially like those of the reverse approach just described.

c. Nonpalpable Lymph Node

Depending on the histological type of the tumor and the site of the primary, carcinomas of the head and neck have a more or less significant propensity for spread to the cervical lymph nodes. The incidence of metastatic nodes, both clinically obvious or occult, increases with the size and stage of the primary lesion; furthermore, certain locations have a higher incidence of spread to the lymph nodes because of their rich lymphatic drainage (e.g., base of tongue and tonsillar fossa as opposed to hard palate or maxilla; similarly, supraglottic laryngeal tumors as opposed to vocal cord tumors).

The following is a brief guideline for the recommended treatment of clinically nonpalpable nodes in the various head and neck cancers:

• Oral cavity and oropharynx. In T1 and early T2 lesions (lesions less than 4 cm in size), the incidence of lymph node metastases in a clinically negative neck is less than 15%, and no treatment of the cervical nodes is required, either by radiotherapy or by surgery. For patients with larger, deeply infiltrating or poorly differentiated lesions, one must consider treating the occult neck at the same time along with the primary. This may be done by an elective radical neck dissection, preferably modified to preserve function and cosmetic appearance, or by prophylactic radiotherapy to the ipsilateral neck.
• Larynx and hypopharynx. The high incidence of node metastases in supraglottic carcinomas (valleculae, pyriform sinus, epiglottis) makes a radical neck dissection an integral

part of the treatment of these tumors. Vocal cord lesions, on the other hand, rarely spread to nodes, and no elective neck dissection is indicated unless the tumor has broken through the thyroid cartilage and extended into the soft tissues of the neck.
• Maxilla. Maxillary tumors rarely spread to nodes, and elective radical neck dissection is not indicated. When nodes are clinically involved, the prognosis is usually quite dismal; yet node treatment is indicated.
• Nasopharynx. Nasopharyngeal carcinoma has a very high incidence of neck node metastases, and these nodes should always be included in the irradiated field whether they are palpable or not.
• Salivary glands. Parotid carcinomas, although often involving the parotid group of nodes, do not usually metastasize to the lower nodes except in the poorly differentiated, or anaplastic, tumors. Elective radical neck dissection is, therefore, not indicated as a rule. Submaxillary gland carcinomas, on the other hand, are often associated with metastatic nodes, and a radical neck dissection (partial or total) should always be performed.
• Skin. The incidence of clinically undetected metastatic nodes in skin cancer is significant only in melanomas and then only in level III lesions or deeper. Elective neck dissection has been routinely recommended in these lesions, though it appears to have more of a prognostic than a therapeutic value. Some surgeons even recommend doing only partial node dissections for melanomas of the head and neck, rather than a complete radical neck dissection, based on the conviction that there is no sacrifice in therapeutic efficacy.
• Thyroid. Only papillary thyroid carcinomas have a high incidence of occult neck nodes (as high as 70–80% with lesions over 1 cm in size). Elective radical neck dissections have therefore been recommended by some for papillary thyroid cancer. Because of the very low grade biologic behavior of this tumor, however, node dissection is only justifiable if it can be carried out with minimal cosmetic and functional morbidity, and even then, only a modified radical neck dissection should be done. Elective neck dissections should be deferred in thyroid cancer if the tumor is in the midline or is bilateral, or if it is small or sclerosing in nature. A midline node dissection (pretracheal, paratracheal, and superior mediastinal) must be carried out together with the thyroidectomy in all cases of thyroid cancer regardless of size or histology.

Although elective radical neck dissection has been the traditional method of treatment for occult lymph node metastases in the neck, recently, the use of elective radiotherapy to the neck has yielded excellent prophylactic results and may be considered as an effective alternative. It is particularly indicated in the following circumstances:

- The contralateral neck when a primary tumor is extensive enough to spread to both sides of the neck.
- Midline primaries when both sides of the neck need to be treated.
- Tumors that are particularly radiosensitive.

3. Radical Neck Dissection

a. Standard Operation

A radical neck dissection is, by definition, a total cervical lymphadenectomy with removal of all the neck nodes within the first and third layers of the deep cervical fascia, together with the jugular vein, sternomastoid muscle, spinal accessary nerve, cervical plexus, and submaxillary gland. Although the standard neck dissection as defined above is still the basic operation, particularly when large metastatic nodes are present, its morbidity, both cosmetic and functional, has prompted a large number of modifications that are today widely employed, particularly when the operation is done for subclinical disease.

b. Partial Neck Dissection

Partial neck dissections are not desirable for the treatment of metastatic neck nodes. Tumors of the head and neck have often been reported to skip adjacent nodes and involve groups that are at some distance from the primary. Partial dissections, however, are recommended in certain specific circumstances:

- For evaluation of the first echelon of nodes where metastases may occur but are not common.
- To obtain a better margin during excision of a bulky primary tumor (e.g., carcinoma of salivary glands excised along with a suprahyoid node dissection).
- When the compartment in point has to be opened for exposure of the primary (e.g., carcinoma of the floor of the mouth and suprahyoid node dissection).
- To establish a prognostic outlook (e.g., in melanomas).

c. Conservation Operations

These procedures are becoming gradually more popular and have, in many circumstances, been shown to be as effective as the standard radical neck dissection in achieving local and regional control of the disease, especially when combined with radiotherapy. The modifications described are endless; most, however, tend to preserve one or more of the following structures:

- The spinal accessory nerve, to avoid the dropped shoulder and pain that occurs after its sacrifice.
- The sternomastoid muscle, to maintain the contour of the neck.
- The submaxillary gland, to avoid the submental indentation.

- The jugular vein, to avoid facial and intracranial edema (especially in bilateral neck dissections).
- Part or all of the cervical plexus, to obviate the numbness and paresthesias that follow a standard radical neck dissection.

It must be clearly understood that the above recommendations for management of the various cancers of the head and neck, as well as the site-specific guidelines that follow, are strictly general guidelines. Treatment must always be individualized to suit the specific patient; all factors must be kept in mind, and a multidisciplinary approach designed to fulfill all of the patient's needs should always be used.
Furthermore, variations in treatment according to the expertise of the treating physician and the available facilities must be accepted. Finally, it is clear, that with the rapid developments in the various modalities of treatment, these guidelines cannot be a permanent document and will require updating as the field of head and neck surgery, radiotherapy, and chemotherapy evolves.

V. THERAPEUTIC GUIDELINES: SITE SPECIFIC

The general considerations discussed in the previous section apply to and complement the following brief presentation of the site-specific management of head and neck cancer. The reader is, therefore, referred back to that section before reading any of the site-specific treatments in this section.

A. Lesions of the Oral Cavity and Oropharynx

1. Leukoplakia and Erythroplasia

These lesions are the premalignant counterparts of mouth cancer and will present histologically with varying degrees of aggressiveness, which often conform to their clinical appearance. On inspection, leukoplakia will range from the totally innocous glistening, poorly defined, smooth, whitish plaque of little importance to the thick, corrugated, irregular, infiltrating white lesion that is often eroded and frequently harbors a carcinoma *in situ*. Erythroplasia, which presents as areas of deep reddening and atrophy of the mucosa often associated with thick leukoplakia, is even more threatening and aggressive than leukoplakia and must be considered a carcinoma *in situ* until proven otherwise.
Histologically these lesions display various degrees of hyperkeratosis with or without dysplasia. Progression of the changes

may lead to a carcinoma *in situ* or even an invasive cancer; these changes may be present in a limited segment of the entire lesion so that a partial biopsy of a leukoplakia is of little value since it could easily miss the area of malignant change. A decision to excise the lesion must be made on clinical grounds, and a total excision should then be carried out, with adequate but minimal margins whenever possible. The clinically innocuous leukoplakia may be left alone and observed; it is important to identify any potential cause of irritation and eliminate it (e.g., chronic biting, jagged teeth, preference for scalding foods, etc.); smoking or tobacco chewing must be stopped, and the patient should be warned about the serious implications of this type of lesion if smoking is continued.

Several specific white lesions of the mouth mucosa may be seen that are indicative of specific diseases unrelated to dysplasia or cancer. Lichen planus is undoubtedly the most common of these and must be clinically recognized since its treatment is nonsurgical and it almost never develops into cancer. Candida, particularly in its chronic indolent form, and pemphigus are other white lesions of the mouth that must be distinguished from the hyperkerotic leukoplakia.

2. Lip

Small lip cancers are often easily excised by a V-wedge excision with primary closure or by a small lip-shave operation. Radiotherapy is also extremely effective and is especially useful in the poor-risk patients.

Larger lesions require a more extensive resection with immediate reconstruction by one of several local flap methods. Cosmetic results following adequate surgery are highly satisfactory and may even be less disfiguring than those following ill-planned high-dose radiotherapy. Radiotherapy, though, is equally effective in eliminating the tumor and is indicated in selected cases.

Carcinoma of the lip is readily curable by local treatment in over 85% of the patients. It must be pointed out, however, that some lesions are extremely aggressive with a high rate of local recurrence, rapid progression, and high incidence of node metastases. These patients must be treated aggressively by combined methods including wide radical excision with reconstruction, radical neck dissection when indicated, and radiotherapy.

3. Buccal Mucosa

Buccal mucosa carcinomas, unless extremely small or occurring in areas of leukoplakia, are better treated by radiotherapy as the primary modality. Surgery should be reserved for the following types of lesions:

- The small, easily resectable tumor that requires no reconstruction.

- Radiotherapy failures.
- Verrucous carcinomas.
- Those cancers arising in areas of leukoplakia.
- Massive through-and-through tumors and those involving bone that may require combined-modality therapy with flap reconstruction.

4. Alveolar Ridge

Carcinomas of the alveolar ridge and adjacent mucosa are ordinarily treated by surgery.

- T1 or early T2 lesions (lesions less than 2 or 3 cm in size), can be treated with limited local resection, marginal mandibulectomy, and primary closure. If much mucosa must be removed from the adjacent floor of mouth or lip, a skin graft or small flap may be used to reconstruct the gutter, or a secondary sulcus augmentation procedure may be planned for a later date.
- Larger lesions of the lower alveolus will often require a composite resection of one type or another to include excision of the primary tumor in the mouth as well as that adjacent segment of mandible and a radical neck dissection in continuity. Radiotherapy is often indicated as a postoperative adjunctive modality in these more extensive tumors; it is not usually recommended as primary treatment in alveolar ridge lesions because of the proximity and frequent involvement of the underlying bone.
- Extensive lesions of the upper alveolar ridge often present as maxillary carcinomas and require partial maxillectomy, which may be combined with radiotherapy when indicated.

5. Floor of the Mouth

Carcinomas of the floor of mouth are managed either by surgery or radiotherapy. Radiotherapy can be administered as interstitial implants, external radiotherapy, or through an intraoral cone and is particularly indicated when no bone involvement is identified.

It should be kept in mind that preservation of the arch of the mandible is most important in rehabilitation of the mouth cancer patient; every attempt should be made to preserve some rim of mandible at the arch, if this can be done without compromising the total removal of the tumor. A special problem occurs when tumors of the lower alveolar ridge or floor of the mouth are extensive and midline, requiring total resection of the arch of the mandible; this type of procedure (the so-called Andy Gump operation), results in an extremely difficult cosmetic and functional rehabilitative problem. Recent developments in reconstructive surgery, particularly the advent of composite flaps and the use of free transfer of tissue with microvascular anastomoses, have made these lesions more amenable to surgery.

6. Anterior Two-Thirds of the Tongue

These tumors are treated equally effectively by surgery or radiotherapy, and the choice of treatment is often dictated by other factors such as size, location, infiltration, involvement of adjacent structures, etc. (see §1.IV.E).

If surgery is carried out, function and cosmesis must be kept foremost in mind. Conservation surgery must be contemplated whenever possible:

- Wide-wedge resection or partial or hemiglossectomy are often sufficient in early tumors.
- Pull-through procedures, with or without marginal mandibulectomy may also be done whenever the tumor has not involved the bone itself.
- Even in composite resections, as much conservation as possible is always in order, provided one can accomplish total tumor removal. Preservation of the tip of the tongue greatly facilitates rehabilitation of speech and eating. Preservation of as much of the mandible as possible is also desirable, and at times, mandibular section with rewiring can be done.
- Where resection of metastatic nodes is indicated, a modified neck dissection should be employed whenever possible.
- Transverse skin incisions should be favored over any vertical or trifurcate incision.

If radiotherapy is selected as the definitive therapeutic modality, the use of external irradiation followed by interstitial implant or small-volume electron therapy is usually the most profitable approach. Careful treatment planning and attention to detail is necessary for success and to keep treatment complications to a minimum. Wedge filter plans may be used with beam-directing devices to afford a small-volume, high-dose approach necessary to control the lesions.

When radiotherapy and surgery are combined, the treatment should be planned in advance in order to achieve the best chance of cure with the least possible morbidity or functional damage.

7. Base of Tongue

Resection of lesions of the base of the tongue frequently requires an extended composite operation, and often a laryngectomy as well. Flap reconstruction is frequently necessary, complicated, associated with an increased morbidity, and not always of the best cosmetic quality. Furthermore, surgical cure rates in these areas are rather low. It is therefore preferable, in general, to opt for radiotherapy as the primary mode of treatment.

External irradiation using a supervoltage beam (linear accelerator or well-collimated ^{60}CO) is the primary modality of treatment. The treatment volume must include the primary draining nodes. The secondary nodes are also included, especially in lymphoepithelial or large lesions (T3 and T4). The dose given must be cancericidal (6500 rads in 7 weeks) regardless of early tumor response or even complete disappearance. Dental care prior to and during radiotherapy, good mouth hygiene, and elimination of focuses of infection are important ancillary measures.

Extensive lesions of the base of the tongue often require combined therapy in order to achieve acceptable cure rates. In these cases, radiotherapy is often selected as a preoperative mode, with surgery carried out for residual disease.

8. Hard Palate

Malignant tumors of the hard palate are, in a large proportion of cases, of minor salivary gland origin. For the small minor salivary gland carcinomas, as well as the early epidermoid carcinomas, a wide local excision, including periosteum and sometimes underlying bone, is often sufficient. Closure is unnecessary, and healing occurs rapidly by secondary intention. More deeply infiltrating tumors, both glandular and epidermoid, behave as an antral carcinoma and are treated as such. Most often, treatment consists of a full course of radiotherapy first, followed by surgical extirpation. The poorly differentiated (or high-grade) lesions are notoriously aggressive, and combined modality therapy is strongly recommended.

9. Soft Palate

Carcinomas of the soft palate behave and respond in a way akin to those of the tonsillar fossa. It is important, however, to be sure that such lesions are not extensions of a primary nasopharyngeal carcinoma. Radiotherapy is the treatment of choice, with surgery reserved for radiation failures. One must bear in mind the function of the soft palate as a mobile diaphragm that separates the nasal cavities from the oral cavities during deglutition and phonation; sacrifice of the soft palate usually results in nasal regurgitation and a nasal and sometimes incomprehensible voice.

10. Tonsillar Pillar and Tonsillar Fossa

Tumors of the tonsillar fossa are reputed to be extremely radiosensitive, and primary treatment of any lesion in that area should be a full course of radiotherapy. Surgical management consists of extended composite resections and should be reserved for patients who fail radiotherapy.

T3 and T4 lesions (lesions over 4 cm in size) will most often require combined therapy, and some surgeons have opted to carry out a composite resection first and use radiotherapy postoperatively to avoid the complications of postirradiation surgery.

11. Oropharyngeal Tumors

Carcinomas of the oropharynx, other than those of areas previously discussed (base of tongue, tonsillar area, soft palate), are extremely rare. Tumors of the oropharyngeal wall, when limited in nature (e.g., to the posterior pharyngeal wall), can be treated either with radiotherapy or with a local surgical excision and a split-thickness skin graft. Exposure can be obtained through the open-mouth approach or by a median labioglossotomy approach or a mandibular swing operation. Larger lesions of the pharyngeal mucosa are better treated by radiotherapy; in these patients, surgery is a formidable procedure with poor results and should be reserved for radiation failures.

B. Lesions of the Larynx, Hypopharynx, and Cervical Esophagus, and Cervical Trachea

Carcinomas of the larynx and adjacent sites are grouped together because the tumor as well as the therapy will frequently encompass several sites simultaneously.

1. Larynx

Because of the very specific nature of the behavior and mode of spread of the various different tumors of the larynx, the treatment of carcinoma of the larynx depends on the exact site and stage of the lesion. Fur purposes of rational understanding of the biologic behavior of cancers in the larynx, the organ is conventionally divided into three distinct zones.

a. Supraglottic Larynx

By definition, the supraglottic larynx includes the ventricles, ventricular bands, aryepiglottic folds, and epiglottis. Lesions of the valleculae and pyriform sinuses, although properly identified as tumors of the hypopharynx, are often included in the supraglottic larynx for the sake of discussion.

Lesions of the supraglottis are usually silent for long periods of time and frequently manifest themselves by neck metastases or symptoms of advanced local extension. It is the rare lesion that is identified early, usually in a patient undergoing routine repeated examinations of the head and neck for previous carcinomas.

Early supraglottic lesions, particularly those limited to the epiglottis, can usually be managed by a local resection, which ordinarily entails a supraglottic laryngectomy. This conservation operation, which strives at preservation of the vocal cords and maintainance of speech, is a most desirable operation but carries a high degree of morbidity resulting from the loss of the normal ability to close the airway during deglutition. Varying periods of aspiration invariably occur after supraglottic laryngectomy, and these, at times, defy any attempt at rehabilitation. The selection of patients for supraglottic laryngectomy should, therefore, be discriminating, and—although some have extended its indications to a large variety of lesions including those with involvement of the pyriform sinus, valleculae, and even part of the vocal cords, with apparently good results—we favor a more cautious approach. The indications for the procedure must be dictated by several factors:

- Extension of the lesion; proximity or involvement of the anterior commissure or a vocal cord must contraindicate the procedure.
- Significant involvement of the valleculae and/or base of the tongue, which requires substantial resection of the base of the tongue and thus makes rehabilitation of deglutition much more complex, is also a relative contraindication.
- The patient's age; older patients (over 55 years of age) suffer a distinct disadvantage, since almost all will aspirate for varying periods of time after supraglottic laryngectomies. Older patients do not tolerate aspiration as well as younger patients and should therefore not be selected for supraglottic laryngectomies.

When conservation surgery is not feasible in early supraglottic laryngeal cancer, radiotherapy should be considered as the primary modality of treatment. Total laryngectomy should be reserved for radiation failures.

In the more advanced supraglottic lesions (T3 or T4) involving fixation of the larynx or extension to the postcricoid area, pyriform sinus, oropharynx, or soft tissues of the neck, total laryngectomy must be carried out and is usually combined with postoperative radiotherapy. The incidence of neck node metastases is high in these cases and often bilateral; treatment must, therefore, include therapy for the neck nodes, either by surgery if the nodes are enlarged or on the side where the primary tumor predominates, or by radiotherapy when the nodes are clinically negative (or for the contralateral neck).

b. Vocal Cords (Glottic Larynx)

Lesions of the glottic larynx usually present early because of the almost immediate onset of hoarseness that is associated with any nodule, ulceration, or impaired mobility of the vocal cord. Treatment of carcinoma of the vocal cord varies greatly with the stage of the lesion:

i. Carcinoma in Situ. A large number of unanswered questions have plagued the surgeon who is responsible for treating carcinoma *in situ* of the vocal cord:

- Is carcinoma *in situ* just one further stage of keratosis and marked dysplasia, or are these two totally distinct entities?

- Is carcinoma *in situ* an early malignant lesion, or is it just an indication of a "condemned mucosa" that will give rise to invasive cancer, if exposure to carcinogens continues?
- Will carcinoma *in situ* invariably progress to invasive cancer, or is it a process than can be reversed?

It has been suggested by some that a more generic term be used inclusively for all the various stages of vocal cord dysplasias that are not clearly invasive cancers; they have been grouped together under the name "intraepithelial neoplasia." Histologically, in order to call one of these lesions "carcinoma *in situ*," it is necessary to identify cellular atypia of the epithelium; these changes will, when untreated, progress to true invasive cancer in the large majority of cases, though they have been reported to regress if the causative agent (smoking) is removed. Treatment is by local excision through a laryngofissure or preferably, endoscopically using the operating microscope, with or without laser. The biopsy itself is often sufficient to eliminate the disease, but a thorough evaluation of the cord is necessary to identify other lesions; toluidine blue dyes can help pinpoint areas that should be biopsied. Radiotherapy should be reserved for patients with a T1 lesion or those with widespread disease.

ii. T1 Tumors. T1 tumors are those confined to one cord with normal mobility. Radiotherapy is the ideal treatment of early carcinoma of the vocal cord with unimpaired mobility of the cord. Surgery (cordectomy performed endoscopically by microsurgical techniques, laser excision, or surgical resection with laryngofissure) should be reserved for *in-situ* carcinomas or for patients who are very difficult to evaluate and where postradiation recurrences would be difficult to detect. Patients with verrucous carcinomas might also be considered candidates for surgery.

iii. T2 and T3 Tumors. These are tumors confined to the larynx but with extension to the supraglottic or subglottic larynx and/or instances where there is cord fixation. Though surgery is the primary approach in the treatment of T2 and T3 vocal cord carcinomas, these patients do respond favorably to radiation therapy. Partial laryngectomies (vertical hemilaryngectomy or a combination of vertical and supraglottic laryngectomy) must be contemplated whenever possible. While total wide-field laryngectomy is curative in most cases, the subsequent loss of normal voice and function makes its application less than ideal. The primary use of radiotherapy is advisable, with surgery reserved for failures. Over half of the patients may thus escape with normal voices.

iv. T4 Tumors. T4 tumors are those that have extended beyond the larynx proper or have resulted in thyroid cartilage destruction. Patients with these lesions usually require combined therapy, with radiotherapy preferably used postoperatively to avoid increased postoperative complications that may occor in the preoperatively irradiated patient. A total wide-field laryngectomy with ipsilateral radical neck dissection is performed and followed by radiotherapy.

With the exception of patients with T4 lesions, neck node metastases are rare in vocal cord carcinomas, and elective radical neck dissection need not be considered.

c. Subglottic Larynx

The pure subglottic carcinoma that is not an extension from a vocal cord lesion is rare compared with glottic or supraglottic cancer. In contradistinction to higher laryngeal lesions, where the histology is almost always squamous cell carcinoma, subglottic cancers are not infrequently of minor salivary gland origin.

Subglottic cancers are usually not detected until the vocal cords have been involved (T2 or T3), and the disease is usually extensive at the time of diagnosis. Furthermore, these lesions are generally thought to be relatively radioresistant compared with glottic lesions. Therapy, therefore, is mainly surgical. Likewise, it is recognized that lymphatic spread of subglottic lesions, or lesions with a significant subglottic component, is common and frequently bilateral. Surgery must include a larygnectomy with a thyroid lobectomy and a pre- and paratracheal node dissection on the side of the tumor; a radical neck dissection (modified, if possible) should be considered on one or both sides, depending on the site and extent of the tumor and nodes. The neck may also be treated by radiotherapy, if there are no clinically involved nodes.

Postoperative radiotherapy must always be considered in the following cases:

- Inadequate margins of resection.
- Extensive node involvement, especially when the capsule is breached.
- Extension to the tracheoesophageal area.
- Patients who had a tracheostomy performed prior to the laryngectomy.

Tracheostomy for carcinoma of the larynx should be avoided whenever possible, a markedly increased incidence of tracheal stoma recurrence has been demonstrated when tracheostomy precedes the definitive surgery. If a diagnosis can be confirmed by endoscopy and frozen section, emergency laryngectomy must be considered. If the patient can be intubated atraumatically, this should be done and the tube kept in place (about 24 hours) until a definitive diagnosis can be established and the patient prepared for surgery. In the more urgent situation or when intubation is not possible, a tracheostomy under local anesthesia may be performed and followed immediately, or as soon as possible, by laryngectomy. In any case, if tracheostomy is done, definitive surgery must be done as soon as possible and must include resection of the tracheostomy tract. Postoperative radiotherapy should always be administered to these patients.

2. Hypopharynx

a. Early Lesions: T1 Tumors Limited to One Site without Involvement of the Larynx

Lesions of the hypopharynx remain silent for long periods of time. They produce dysphagia and odynophagia, frequently with pain radiating to the ear (a sign of poor prognosis), only after the tumor has grown quite sizable and has invaded the pharyngeal musculature. The serendipitous finding of an early pharyngeal wall lesion located in the posterior or lateral pharyngeal wall is rare; the lesion can be treated either by limited surgery or radiation therapy. If the lesion was discovered during a routine follow-up examination in a patient with a past history of head and neck cancer, surgery is the preferred modality, since the patient may be developing field cancerization and other primaries might develop in the future that might require radiotherapy. Radiotherapy may selectively be used if it had not been used the first time; treatment by radiotherapy frequently results in an unacceptable degree of tissue damage, is often unsuccessful, and should be avoided.

Surgically, the lesions can be approached through

- A transhyoid or suprahyoid approach.
- A lateral or posterior pharyngotomy approach.
- A median or paralingual labiomandibuloglossotomy approach.

There is a very high propensity for node metastases in hypopharyngeal cancer, and consideration must be given to elective treatment of the neck nodes even in these early lesions.

b. Larger Lesions: T3 or T4 Tumors or Tumors of the Pyriform Sinus or Postcricoid Area

These tumors will always require a laryngopharyngectomy with total laryngectomy and plastic reconstruction for closure of the pharynx. These patients will be candidates for postoperative radiotherapy much as in laryngeal carcinomas. Clinically involved ipsilateral cervical nodes demand a radical neck dissection at the time of laryngopharyngectomy, but even in the clinically negative neck, elective treatment of the nodes by surgery or radiotherapy is indicated and should be directed at both sides since the larger lesions frequently metastasize bilaterally. In patients with bilateral neck node metastases, the more extensively affected side should be treated by node dissection at the time of the resection of the primary. Surgery to the other side should be deferred 2–3 weeks; or treatment may be primarily by radiotherapy for 5 weeks, followed by surgery if nodes do not resolve completely. Simultaneous bilateral neck dissection should be avoided to obviate the serious sequelae of this operation (increased intracranial pressure and facial edema).

3. Cervical Esophagus

The natural history of carcinoma of the cervical esophagus is similar to that of the remainder of the hypopharynx in its silent presentation, its propensity for node metastases and wide submucosal extension. Early lesions are controllable by radiotherapy, but extensive tumors are best treated by combined therapy. The surgery is rather extensive, and a realistic assessment of the probability of cure must be carried out beforehand. The procedure usually requires a circumferential resection of the esophagus, with or without pharyngolaryngectomy depending on the level of the tumor and its extent. Preservation of the larynx is rarely possible but should be considered in lower esophageal lesions. The extent of the resection should include at least two centimeters of normal mucosa beyond the clinically identifiable tumor. The margins of resection must be monitored by frozen section examination prior to starting the reconstruction. Radical neck dissection, or postoperative irradiation to the neck and upper mediastinum, must be considered, even in the absence of clinically palpable lymph nodes.

Reconstruction of the gullet is almost always necessary following resections of the hypopharynx and cervical esophagus and can be accomplished by one of several methods:

- Mucosal shifts with primary closure (for small noncircumferential resections, especially in the hypopharynx).
- Tubed deltopectoral skin flaps, if the lower anastomosis is in the neck.
- Tubed myocutaneous pectoralis major flap (likewise in the neck).
- Skin graft over wire mesh.
- Gastric pull-up operations or colonic transposition (with or without thoracotomy), if the tumor extends down below the thoracic inlet. The gastric pull-up operation is rapidly becoming the preferred procedure with the lowest rate of failure and complications.
- Free jejunal interposition with microvascular anastomosis.

One-stage repairs should preferably be selected since they shorten the postoperative recovery period and facilitate early institution of postoperative radiotherapy.

If a combined approach by radiation and surgery is deemed necessary, it must be planned carefully. Generally, radiotherapy is best used postoperatively because of the complexity of the surgical procedures and the risk of increased postoperative morbidity following radiotherapy. However, a sandwich approach where surgery is carried out after a short preoperative course of radiotherapy followed by further postoperative radiation is claimed by some to be highly effective.

Further discussion of the treatment of carcinoma of the esophagus may be found in §10.

4. Cervical Trachea

This disease is extremely rare, and cases must be investigated carefully to rule out the presence of intrathoracic primaries. The treatment of choice in most cases is surgical resection. Sizable resections can be done with primary end-to-end anastomosis by using a variety of maneuvers: supralaryngeal release, flexion of the neck, mediastinal freeing, section of the fascia between several tracheal rings, etc. Permanent tracheostomy may, however, be necessary and often requires resection of a portion of the manubrium or sternum to allow exteriorization of the stoma; it is even necessary, at times, to construct a skin tube to reach a low tracheal transsection.

C. Tumors of the Nasal Fossa, Paranasal Sinuses, and Nasopharynx

1. Nasal Fossa

Tumors of the nasal cavity are rather rare and most often benign. Histologically they may be divided into:

- Nasal polyps.
- Squamous papillomas (inverted or Schneiderian).
- Nasopharyngeal angiofibroma.
- Squamous carcinoma (infiltrating or verrucous).
- Adenocarcinoma.
- Minor salivary gland or mucous cell carcinoma (with all their subtypes).
- Small-cell carcinoma.

It is important to recognize the various benign tumors of the nasal cavity; the simple hyperplastic or allergic nasal polyp is of little significance and is easily managed by local resection with a snare or cautery. One must, however, rule out the nasopharyngeal angiofibroma, lest castastrophic hemorrhage occur during biopsy or an attempt at resection. These latter tumors, usually arising from the nasopharynx, are extremely vascular, difficult to excise, and require special preparation and exposure. Carotid angiography will confirm the diagnosis and, at times, identify a major feeding vessel. Preoperative estrogens have been shown to cause significant decrease in the size of nasopharyngeal angiofibroma, and radiotherapy has been attempted by some, though it should only be considered as a last resort. Wide surgical exposure is necessary to control potential bleeding: a transpalatal approach; a transnasal approach with lateral rhinotomy, a retromaxillary approach; or

any combination of these approaches may be used for resection of these nasopharyngeal angiofibromas. Squamous papillomas (or inverted Schneiderian papillomas) are rare and unusual papillary lesions that have a high potential for local recurrence and malignant degeneration. They may arise from the paranasal sinuses and must be treated aggressively.

Malignant tumors of the nasal fossa proper are most often squamous cell carcinoma and are usually similar to the other squamous cell cancers of the mucous membranes. They can be treated either by local excision (sometimes requiring lateral rhinotomy for exposure and skin grafting for reconstruction) or radiotherapy. Radiotherapy is particularly effective in tumors of the nasal vestibule; when applied carefully and successfully, the cosmetic results are very satisfying. Most often, malignancies of the nasal fossa are actually paranasal sinus carcinomas that have broken into the nasal fossa; a thorough investigation of the sinuses must be carried out prior to treatment of what appears to be a carcinoma of the nasal fossa.

Adenocarcinomas or salivary gland tumors of the nasal fossa are less common but must be treated aggressively by surgery and postoperative radiotherapy.

Small-cell cancers include a large variety of tumors that may be difficult to identify: lymphoma, melanoma, olfactory neuroblastoma, and undifferentiated carcinoma. An attempt at clearly identifying the lesion must be made both radiologically and histologically by all available means (including electron microscopy) before undertaking therapy.

2. Paranasal Sinuses

a. Clinicopathological Considerations

Carcinoma of the paranasal sinuses most often involves primarily the maxillary sinus, more rarely the ethmoids, and only affects the other sinuses (sphenoid or frontal) by contiguous extension. It is a relatively rare disease that requires a careful and methodical multidisciplinary approach, intensive preoperative planning and preparation, combined therapy, and a comprehensive program of postoperative rehabilitation.

Carcinomas of the maxillary sinus are most often epidermoid in nature (80–90%), although salivary gland carcinomas (e.g., adenocarcinomas, mucoepidermoid carcinomas, and cylindromas) are seen in a significant number of cases (4–8%). More rarely, lymphomas, or tumors arising from the bony framework, can be identified.

Early symptoms are rare and often nonspecific (see §1.D), and the disease is usually identified after significant local spread has occurred. This must be carefully assessed and evaluated preoperatively to design the best possible therapeutic course. A good CAT scan and polytomogram in various planes can give a most accurate picture of the exact extent of local spread to the contiguous areas: orbit, pterygoid or temporal spaces, sphenoid or intracranial extension. Lymph node metastases are not common but when present usually denote a dismal prognosis. Routine or elective node dissections are not recommended; therapeutic neck dissections should be deferred until after the primary tumor has been resected (performance of maxillectomy following radical neck dissection with ligation of the internal jugular vein can result in massive bleeding from the pterygoid plexus due to the increased venous pressure).

b. Biopsy

Biopsy of lesions of the maxilla must be done prior to planning a therapeutic approach. In lesions that present through the skin, in the nasal cavity or through the palate, a punch or small incisional biopsy is usually adequate. Whenever the lesion presents entirely within the sinus, a Caldwell-Luc operation with complete mucosal stripping and drainage of the sinus is necessary.

c. Therapeutic Considerations

The last 15 years have seen a strong trend toward combining both radiotherapy and surgery for the treatment of carcinomas of the paranasal sinuses in order to achieve optimum local control. There is still some controversy as to whether radiotherapy should be given preoperatively or postoperatively. Preoperative radiotherapy has the advantage of being given in a virgin field with less fibrosis and better oxygen saturation; it decreases the size of the tumor, making surgery easier and more complete, and it reduces the viability of the peripheral areas of the tumor and thus diminishes the chances of seeding and tumor implantation. Furthermore, preoperative radiotherapy permits more time for a thorough evaluation and preparation of the patient, the teeth, and the prosthesis, without delaying the institution of therapy. Postoperative radiotherapy, on the other hand, is of particular value for the treatment of residual disease at the margins of resection. The following guidelines seem appropriate and reasonable in most cases:

i. Early Lesions. For T1 infrastructure tumors with no bone involvement, surgery alone is often adequate, with radiotherapy utilized only if surgical margins are inadequate.

ii. Moderately Advanced Lesions. For T2 and T3, all-suprastructure tumors and lesions involving bone, skin, or pterygoid muscles, preoperative radiotherapy is strongly recommended and should only be deferred for patients with poor tolerance to radiotherapy.

iii. Advanced T4 Lesions. These tumors involving the posterior ethmoids, the cribriform plate, the base of the skull, the sphenoid sinus, or the pterygoid plates must be carefully evaluated before undertaking any treatment. Criteria for inoperability are

- Bilateral tumors, especially those affecting the suprastructures.
- Destruction of the base of the skull at the middle fossa, or brain involvement.
- Substantial infiltration of the nasopharynx.
- Inoperable cervical nodes.
- Distant metastases, although in a patient who is relatively well (particularly in salivary gland carcinomas) a palliative resection might be indicated.
- Massive pterygoid fossa involvement is also a relative contraindication.
- Skin edema and lymphangitic involvement of a diffuse nature.

Cribriform plate and orbital involvement are not contraindications for surgery, only poor prognostic signs. In patients deemed inoperable, radiotherapy in combination with chemotherapy may offer effective palliation for short periods of time. Methotrexate and 5-fluorouracil (5-FU) infusions have been reported to be quite effective in conjunction with radiotherapy.

An important radiotherapeutic consideration is the necessity for very accurate planning, and the use of supervoltage sharp beams to avoid damage to surrounding sensitive structures (eye, brain, etc). Such care will also keep radiation reaction within the limits of tolerance and allow timely subsequent surgery with acceptable morbidity.

d. Surgical Considerations

Maxillectomy, which by definition implies resection of the facial bones, is the term loosely applied to resections of carcinomas of the paranasal sinuses. Its extent can range from a limited resection of a segment of the hard palate and/or maxillary tuberosity, to the massive craniofacial resections required for lesions affecting the cribriform plate, ethmoids, and orbit. The surgical procedure must be tailored to the extent of the disease. The cosmetic and functional importance of all structures in this area make it mandatory to be as conservative as possible, while being as radical as the tumor demands. Plastic and prosthetic rehabilitation must always be an integral part of the total treatment plan.

The basic operations used for various lesions of the maxilla are

- Local resections for small lesions of the hard palate or upper gum.
- Partial transoral maxillectomy for more infiltrative lesions.
- Subtotal maxillectomy, preserving the floor of the orbit whenever possible. This is the procedure most frequently performed. Preceded by an external carotid artery ligation to diminish operative blood loss, it is completed by a reconstruction employing a skin graft in the operative cavity and a previously prepared dental plate and obturator as a prosthesis.

- Total maxillectomy. This implies sacrifice of the floor of the orbit. The eye can still be preserved if uninvolved and the orbital floor reconstructed with a muscle, fascial, or cartilage sling prior to the skin grafting.
- Total maxillectomy with orbital exenteration. This procedure is indicated whenever the orbit is extensively involved by tumor.
- Craniofacial resections. This operation is reserved for those cases where the tumor has extended into the cribriform plates and/or the dura. Primary ethmoid carcinomas often require this type of procedure, although at times, curetting of the ethmoid during maxillectomy might suffice. It is usually desirable to start these procedures intracranially (a neurosurgeon is essential during this phase) to determine operability prior to carrying out the maxillofacial resection.

3. Nasopharynx

By virtue of its anatomic relationships, the nasopharynx is a rather inaccessible area to the surgeon. The frequently silent nature of the primary makes it unlikely that the tumor will be identified before one of the many complications of nasopharyngeal carcinomas has occurred:

- Bone erosion at the base of the skull.
- Cranial nerve involvement by extension of the tumor through the foramen lacerum (third, fourth, fifth, and sixth cranial nerves) or by direct infiltration through the lateral pharyngeal wall and roof of the nasopharynx (ninth, tenth, eleventh, and twelfth cranial nerves).
- Invasion of the cavernous sinus.
- Involvement of the nasal fossa or orbital cavity.
- Extensive nodal disease.

Finally, the marked radiosensitivity of nasopharyngeal carcinomas in most cases and the lack of accessibility to surgical excision, makes radiotherapy almost always the treatment of choice.

More than 80% of nasopharyngeal carcinomas are epithelial in nature: squamous cell carcinomas (of different degrees of differentiation) or lymphoepithelial carcinomas (where lymphoid proliferation is an important element). Lymph node metastases are present in over 80% of cases and are often the presenting symptom. Any therapeutic modality must, therefore, include the neck nodes bilaterally. Lymphomas comprise about 10% of all cases.

a. Surgery

The role of surgery is limited, in the majority of cases, to the establishment of the diagnosis and the assessment of the exact extent of the tumor. Several surgical approaches have been designed for selected cases and are utilized primarily for the resection of the very small early tumor or for those cases where a residual tumor after radiotherapy is still resectable; these approaches include

- Palatal fenestration or palate-splitting procedures.
- Lateral or, preferably, posterior pharyngotomy procedures.
- Trans- or suprahyoid approaches.

The range of resections carried out is:

- Fulguration or cryosurgery (mostly for palliation).
- Local resection with or without skin grafting for the very small lesions.
- Radical composite resections with primary closure or with some type of reconstructive substitution (forehead flap, deltopectoral flap, myocutaneous flap, gastric transposition, etc.).

Surgery for residual neck nodes, on the other hand, is necessary when radiotherapy has apparently controlled the local disease but not the neck nodes. Bilateral radical neck dissection may be required, in which case, it should be staged, with, if at all possible, preservation of one internal jugular vein.

b. Radiotherapy

Radiotherapy is the mainstay of treatment of nasopharyngeal carcinoma. The treatment volume usually encompasses the nasopharynx as well as the draining lymph nodes on both sides, since node involvement occurs frequently very early and often extensively. Carcinoma of the nasopharynx is generally radiosensitive, which makes the delivery of tumoricidal doses (about 6500 rads in 7 weeks) to this large volume possible and curative in about one-third of patients. Radiotherapy technique is rather important when treating these sites to avoid damage to the spinal cord and surrounding sensitive organs. The use of meticulous treatment planning and sharp, well-collumated supervoltage beams is necessary.

D. Tumors of the Salivary Glands

1. General Principles

The salivary glands, comprising the parotid glands, the submandibulary glands, the sublingual glands, and the minor salivary glands, are widely distributed in the upper aerodigestive tract. The therapeutic management of malignant tumors of the salivary glands must take into account the fact that histological confirmation of the diagnosis or type of malignancy is, in the majority of cases, not available prior to surgery. Some surgeons have recommended the use of fine-needle biopsy of salivary gland tumors prior to surgery. Although the technique may be useful in establishing the diagnosis, it is usually unnecessary since the surgery is ordinarily no different for benign or malig-

38 **1. TUMORS OF THE HEAD AND NECK**

nant tumors and the risk of tumor seeding and implantation (even in benign mixed tumors) is possibly significant.

The following guidelines should, therefore, govern the approach to all tumors of the salivary glands:

- All salivary gland tumors should be totally excised for biopsy.
- Excision should always include an adequate margin of normal salivary gland tissue around the tumor. It is not necessary or possible to carry out an operation based on arbitrary anatomic boundaries (i.e., superficial lobectomy, total parotidetomy, etc.). In the case of minor salivary gland tumors, an adequate margin of mucosa and soft tissues around the tumor must be excised. Where the lesion is in the parotid gland, the facial nerve must always be identified (in part or in whole) to permit a safe and adequate excision of the tumor.
- Dissection of the facial nerve is recommended from its trunk forward in large tumors or in those presenting posterior to the vertical ramus of the mandible, whereas small peripheral tumors or tumors of the tail of the parotid can be approached by dissecting one or more of the peripheral branches just enough to clear the tumor. Only in cases of Warthin's tumors or parotid nodes of small size is it sometimes safe to enucleate the tumor without exposing the facial nerve.
- In the absence of clinical facial nerve paralysis, sacrifice of part or all of the facial nerve should only be carried out if, during dissection of the nerve, it is found to be involved by the tumor. In this case, an open biopsy of the tumor with frozen section should be carried out to confirm the diagnosis of malignancy before sacrificing the nerve, and only those branches of the nerve that are actually involved should be sacrificed. The need to sacrifice an uninvolved facial nerve because of the malignant nature of the tumor or its tendency to perineural spread is moot, since the rate of local recurrence after such a step does not seem to be diminished; furthermore, the use of adjuvant postoperative radiotherapy has significantly improved local control of the disease and thus makes conservation of the uninvolved nerve perfectly acceptable.
- Primary repair of a sacrified branch or trunk of the facial nerve should always be attempted. This may be carried out by direct end-to-end suturing if a small segment was excised, or may require interposition or crossover nerve grafts. The use of magnifying loops or an operating microscope is extremely useful for such nerve anastomoses.
- Submaxillary gland tumors should always be approached by doing an excisional biopsy of the entire gland, with a suprahyoid node dissection. This permits a safer dissection of the various important anatomic structures in the submaxillary triangle that must be preserved, allows for adequate margins around the tumor, and permits excision of the first echelon of nodes (most submaxillary tumors are malignant and readily spread to nodes).
- Large tumors of the minor salivary glands must be biopsied prior to carrying out the radical procedures that are often required for their excision.

2. Histopathological Considerations

There is a large histopathological variety of malignant salivary gland tumors, and the nature of the tumor has important implications for the behavior of the disease. It is necessary, therefore, prior to discussion of the management of salivary gland tumors, to mention the histological types of these tumors, their mode of behavior, and their malignant potential.

a. Mucoepidermoid Carcinoma

This type of carcinoma constitutes 30% of all salivary gland tumors. It is more prevalent in women and is also one of the most common cancers of the parotid gland.

Mucoepidermoid carcinomas have been divided into three categories depending on their degree of differentiation and the extent of epidermoid metaplasia identified in the tumor:

- Low-grade mucoepidermoid carcinomas. These are well-differentiated lesions that are predominantly mucinous and have little evidence of invasion. They are not aggressive lesions, and some pathologists are reluctant to call them "cancers." The treatment is local excision, and the results are excellent.
- Medium-grade mucoepidermoid carcinomas.
- High-grade mucoepidermoid carcinomas. These lesions are extremely aggressive and difficult to control. They are predominantly epidermoid and metastasize readily to local lymph nodes and distant organs, often recurring locally and involving the facial nerve. Consequently, treatment needs to be aggressive, with as radical a local resection as is necessary, together with a node dissection, and followed by radiotherapy.

b. Adenocarcinoma

Pure adenocarcinomas of salivary glands constitute 18% of all malignant tumors of these organs. This figure, however, may include other types of cancers (adenoid cystic, acinic cell) that are not recognized by the pathologist as such. These tumors may also be of low- or high-grade potential but do not spread to node as readily. Treatment will generally be along the lines previously discussed. Since these tumors have a relatively long natural history, careful observation for the development of distant metastases must be carried out for long periods of time.

c. Adenoid Cystic Carcinoma (Cylindroma)

These tumors are histologically characteristic and occur with some prevalancy in minor salivary glands (oral cavity, palate, sinuses, larynx, trachea, etc.). In spite of a slow growth rate, cylindromas have a marked propensity for invasion and spread through perineural pathways. This increases the risk of local recurrence as well as metastatic spread (mainly to the lungs). Even when pulmonary metastases do occur, however, long-term survivals are not uncommon.

Local treatment of cylindromas is thus of great importance and must be carried out even if only for palliation. Because of the propensity for perineural spread, sacrifice of the facial nerve has been recommended by some surgeons in all cases of cylindromas of the parotid gland; as previously mentioned, this is not always necessary, and the use of postoperative radiotherapy in the treatment of cylindromas has significantly decreased the incidence of local recurrences even when conservation procedures are carried out.

d. Malignant Mixed Tumors (Pleomorphic Adenocarcinoma)

This entity has been reported with a greater or lesser incidence by various groups and seems to depend largely on meticulous examination of the specimen and on the interpretation of the reviewing pathologist. Poorly differentiated mucoepidermoid carcinomas, adenoid cystic carcinomas, and adenocarcinomas can at times be confused with malignant mixed tumors or vice versa!

There undoutedly is, however, a category of truly malignant mixed tumors with both local malignant characteristics and an ability to spread to lymph nodes or distant organs. Patients usually present with a tumor of long-standing duration (20–40 years) with recent acceleration of growth, or with a long history of multiple inadequate surgical resections for a locally recurring, apparently benign "mixed tumor." For this reason, it is most important to scrutinize a "mixed parotid" tumor very carefully before pronouncing it to be a benign pleomorphic adenoma.

Malignant mixed tumors are extremely aggressive lesions; treatment should be much the same as that of adenoid cystic carcinomas: radical local surgery followed by radiotherapy. Node dissections are only indicated in submaxillary gland carcinomas or when metastatic nodes are clinically identified.

Prevention of this entity must, however, be an important consideration and may be achieved by adequate early resection of all benign mixed tumors to prevent their malignant transformation.

e. Epidermoid Carcinoma

This type of malignancy, in its pure form, is quite uncommon in salivary glands. It is, however, an extremely aggressive lesion locally and will often metastasize to regional nodes. Wide local excision with neck dissection is usually indicated, and it should be followed by radiotherapy.

f. Acinic Cell Carcinoma

An uncommon tumor of salivary glands, this tumor is very specific and well defined and is characterized by the presence of zymogen granules in its cytoplasm. Acinic cell carcinomas may metastasize locally or distantly but are often low grade and localized. Treatment is usually confined to a wide local excision of the tumor and observation. Postoperative radiotherapy should be considered in large lesions.

3. Modality of Treatment according to Site

Surgery is generally accepted as the preferred primary method of treatment of nearly all malignant salivary gland tumors. The choice of operation, the need for a neck dissection, the necessity to sacrifice the facial nerve, the use of adjunctive therapy, etc., remain, however, controversial.

a. Parotid Tumors

i. Local Resection. The small malignant tumor of about 2 cm (T1) can be treated successfully with subtotal parotidectomy with exposure and preservation of the facial nerve.

Larger tumors (T2 tumors, 2–4 cm in size, mobile, with no nerve paralysis) require a conventional subtotal parotidectomy. Identification and preservation of the facial nerve branches is still possible if the nerve branches are not actually involved by the tumor. Frozen section can sometimes help one make a decision if the nerve appears to be involved. In low-grade carcinomas, a tedious dissection to preserve all branches of the facial nerve should be attempted. In high-grade malignancies, a more radical excision is required, and sacrifice of some or all segments of the facial nerve may at times be indicated.

In massive tumors (T3 or T4 tumors, over 4 cm in size, where there is facial nerve dysfunction, fixation, and bone or adjacent skin involvement), radical surgery, including resection of the overlying skin, masseter muscle, mandible, and part or all of the facial nerve may be necessary and must be carried out whenever these structures are involved. These patients should always receive postoperative radiotherapy.

ii. Radical Neck Dissection. A therapeutic radical neck dissection is indicated for patients with palpable cervical lymph nodes that are suspicious of metastases. Elective radical neck dissection is indicated only when the tumor is very bulky and extends into the neck and in cases of large, high-grade mucoepidermoid or epidermoid carcinoma. In all other cases, node metastases are rare, and elective radical neck dissection should be deferred.

iii. Postoperative Radiotherapy. Postoperative radiotherapy has, in recent years, proved to be a most valuable adjunct in the treatment of malignant salivary gland tumors. The rate of local and regional control of the disease following the use of postoperative radiotherapy has been reported as being 91% over 3 years and 41% over 5 years, as compared with historical controls of 58% and 25% respectively when no radiotherapy was used. The indications for radiotherapy are

- High-grade histological types: adenoid cystic carcinoma (cylindroma), epidermoid carcinoma, adenocarcinoma, and high-grade mucoepidermoid carcinoma.
- All T4 tumors with involvement of nerve, skin, muscle, bone, or cartilage.
- Deep-lobe tumors and cases where the tumor has to be peeled off the nerve.
- Cases in which residual disease is suspected: unresectable gross tumor, microscopically positive margins, close resections, nerve conservation operations.
- Cases with positive lymph node metastases or lymphatic invasion.

Radiotherapy must be carefully planned and utilize beam-directing devices and particle beams such as electron beam therapy.

b. Submaxillary Gland Tumors

i. Local Resection. Extension into and involvement of the mandible, floor of mouth, lingual nerve, and hypoglossal nerve, though very rare, should be evaluated preoperatively; the exact extent of the surgical resection, however, can only be determined at the time of surgery. Any neighboring structures, such as skin, periosteum, mandible, lingual nerve, hypoglossal nerve, and/or underlying musculature should be included within the scope of the resection if they appear to be involved by the tumor. Even if the tumor appears to be benign, a total resection of the entire gland with a suprahyoid node dissection constitutes the minimum extent of resection; further surgery will depend on the result of frozen section or the final pathology report.

ii. Radical Neck Dissection. Radical neck dissection is always done for carcinomas of the submaxillary gland with clinically palpable metastatic neck nodes. Elective radical neck dissection along the lines described earlier should also be considered in most carcinomas of the submaxillary gland.

iii. Postoperative Radiotherapy. Recommended for patients in whom

- The resection margin is not free of tumor.
- The nerve is involved by tumor.
- The carcinoma is high grade.
- The neck nodes are clinically positive.

c. Minor Salivary Gland Carcinomas

Over 60% of all minor salivary gland tumors are malignant. Adenoid cystic carcinomas (cylindromas) are the most common and most aggressive type of minor salivary gland tumors. The most common site is the palate; however, they can be seen in the lip, retromolar trigone, buccal mucosa, tongue, larynx, paranasal sinuses, and/or nasal mucosa.

Early lesions of minor salivary glands are treated with a wide local excision as the primary procedure. This serves as a biopsy, removes the disease, and is often sufficient therapy in small lesions. The defect can be left to heal by secondary intention or, if possible, may be sutured primarily.

Larger, bulky, and infiltrating tumors require radical local resections (including at times maxillectomies or mandibulectomies) that must be combined with radiotherapy, either preoperatively or postoperatively. Radical neck dissections are not indicated in carcinomas of the minor salivary glands unless metastatic nodes can be clinically identified.

4. Chemotherapy for Advanced Disease

Experience in the chemotherapy of metastatic salivary gland carcinoma is still rather limited. Active agents and combinations are, however, available and should be used in appropriate clinical settings (see §1.VII.A on treatment of the advanced head and neck cancer patient). The following regimens have been used with some degree of success:

- CMF (cyclophosphamide, methotrexate, 5-fluorouracil)
- CAF (cyclophosphamide, adriamycin, 5-fluorouracil)
- CAV (cyclophosphamide, adriamycin, vincristine)
- CAP (cyclophosphamide, adriamycin, *cis*-platinum)

E. Carcinoma of the Thyroid

1. General Considerations

a. Epidemiology

Thyroid carcinoma is a malignant tumor characterized by slow growth and generally low morbidity and mortality. It does, however, cause death in a sufficient number of patients when treatment is delayed or inadequate. Good therapy is based on early diagnosis. The disease most often presents as a "thyroid nodule," which is a lump easily found either by the patient or by the examining physician. It is estimated that 15–30% of all solitary nodules are malignant; 5–10% of multinodular goiters are malignant; and less than 1% of all thyrotoxic glands are malignant.

The disease presents most often in younger people, which is of great importance since a failure of therapy, even in this slow-growing cancer which may take 10–30 years to kill, will result in death at a relatively young age. While most cancers in young adults and children have a poorer prognosis than their counterpart in adults, cancer of the thyroid gland behaves in the opposite manner, offering a much better prognosis at younger ages. The prognosis worsens at the age of 40 for males and 50 for females, with failure rates of about 30% instead of the 5–10% failures reported in younger patients. It has been often postulated that the poor prognosis of thyroid cancer in the elderly patient results from a tumor that may have been present for 20–30 years.

Sex also plays some role in prognosis. In younger patients, the prognosis is slightly worse in males. In older patients, the prognosis is slightly worse in females.

b. Histological Types

i. Follicular Carcinoma.   This is the typical most differentiated malignant tumor of the thyroid, where the histology so resembles the normal thyroid follicles that it is often difficult, even histologically, to make the diagnosis with certainty. Only when one can identify capsular or angioinvasion is the diagnosis certain. Pure follicular carcinoma is rare (5–10% of cases) and most often presents with areas of papillary changes; in its pure form it does not tend to spread to lymph nodes but does, in its aggressive angioinvasive form, result in distant metastases.

ii. Papillary Carcinoma.   Pure, this tumor carries the best prognosis of all thyroid cancers. It has the longest natural history, slow growth, but frequent occurrence of lymph node metastases (reported in as high as 80% of cases).

iii. Mixed Papillary and Follicular Carcinoma.   This carcinoma behaves much like the pure papillary carcinoma with a favorable prognosis but high risk for lymph node metastases.

iv. Medullary Carcinoma (Isolated or Familial).   This type of carcinoma is a special tumor that originates from the interstitial C cell of the thyroid gland (which derives from the neural crest). These cells produce calcitonin, and although this function is rudimentary in humans under normal circumstances, in medullary carcinomas an elevated calcitonin level is often identified.

Medullary carcinoma of the thyroid may be sporadic or familial. The latter type is the less frequent but has been the subject of intensive study. The disease is inherited as a Mendelian autosomal dominant trait, and when investigative studies of the pedigrees of patients with medullary carcinoma is done, large numbers of occult cases can be detected. Furthermore, in patients with elevated calcitonin levels in whom no tumor is found in the thyroid, it is not unusual to identify hyperplasia of the C cells. The familial type of medullary carcinoma of the thyroid is most often associated with other endocrine tumors and is grouped in multiple endocrine adenopathy (MEA), Type IIa (hyperparathyroidism, medullary carcinoma of the thyroid, and pheochromocytoma) or Type IIb (without hyperparathyroidism but with a marfanoid habitus; neuromas of the tongue, lips, and eyelids; and intestinal ganglioneuromatosis in addition to the pheochromocytoma and medullary thyroid carcinoma).

Medullary thyroid carcinoma is an aggressive tumor (especially within the context of the MEA, Type IIb) that infiltrates rapidly and spreads to nodes in all directions.

The evaluation of serum calcitonin levels by immunoreactive measurement is of great value in the diagnosis and follow-up of patients with medullary carcinoma of the thyroid; although baseline levels may be elevated in a variety of conditions besides medullary carcinoma (lung cancer, renal failure, Zollinger-Ellison syndrome, acute pancreatitis, and hypercalcemia from a variety of causes other than hyperparathyroidism), the marked increase in levels seen following provocative tests with calcium and pentagastrine or glucagon is usually diagnostic of medullary carcinoma.

v. Anaplastic Carcinoma.   This is the most aggressive type of cancer of the thyroid. It represents only 5% of thyroid carcinoma and is seen only in older patients. The patients often present with a long-standing history of a tumor in the thyroid, sometimes even following resection of a well-differentiated thyroid cancer in the past. Most anaplastic thyroid cancers appear to arise from, or are associated with, a neglected or poorly treated well-differentiated thyroid carcinoma that has been permitted to progress over many years or even decades. The outcome of anaplastic thyroid cancer is quite dismal, with most patients dying within 6 months to 1 year, and only about 10% surviving longer.

Several histological types of anaplastic thyroid cancer are described: small-cell, spindle cell, giant-cell, or undifferentiated; the former seems to have a slightly more favorable prognosis and appears to respond well to radiotherapy.

c. Mode of Spread

Thyroid carcinoma spreads in a variety of ways.

- Intraglandular pathways
  By direct extension through the capsule of the tumor into the surrounding normal thyroid tissue.
  Via the thyroid lymphatics to produce multifocal carcinomas throughout the thyroid gland.
- Extraglandular pathways.
  Direct invasion of the surrounding structures (strap muscles, jugular vein, pharynx, larynx, esophagus, trachea, recurrent laryngeal nerve, and vagus nerve).

Lymphatic spread to the pretracheal nodes, cricothyroid (Delphian) node, paratracheal nodes, internal jugular nodes, superior mediastinal nodes, or retropharyngeal nodes (at base of skull). The disease can then spread to more distant nodes via regular lymphatic channels.

Hematogenous spread. The most common sites are the lung and bone.

d. Etiologic Factors

- A biologic predisposition seems to be present in patients with Blood Type A, while Type O individuals show a decreased tendency to develop thyroid carcinomas.
- Experimentally, cancer of the thyroid has been produced in the laboratory by prolonged TSH stimulus (e.g., severe iodine restriction, or subtotal resection of the thyroid). It is clinically well recognized that most thyroid cancers are TSH dependent.
- Radiation effect. Exposure to radiation (atomic explosion or external irradiation) of the head and neck area is now recognized to be of great importance as a cause of thyroid cancer. Young children treated by external irradiation to the neck for tonsillar disease or acne display a considerable increase in the rate of thyroid carcinoma, which is noted from 5 to 30 years after irradiation. It appears that the risk is only increased in patients who receive small doses of irradiation to the head and neck.

2. Diagnosis of Thyroid Carcinoma

The diagnosis of thyroid cancer is often only established at the time of surgery. It is, however, most important to try and identify those nodules that are potentially malignant long before obvious signs of malignancy present. A striking statistical difference in survival has repeatedly been reported in thyroid cancers over 5 cm in diameter, and it is therefore desirable to identify thyroid nodules with a high risk of malignancy before they reach a large size. The following are some guidelines for early surgery in patients with thyroid nodules:

- Solitary noncystic nodules.
- Nonfunctioning nodules (cold on scan).
- Solitary nodules in males or children.
- Any thyroid nodule or nodules that exhibit a sudden change in size.
- History of exposure to radiation several years previously.
- Hoarseness that persists, especially if laryngoscopy confirms a vocal cord paralysis in the presence of a thyroid mass.
- Any local finding suggestive of malignancy in a nodule: hard, irregular, fixed, attached to the overlying muscles or skin, tracheal involvement.
- Palpable cervical nodes. Occasionally cancer of the thyroid

presents as one or more enlarged cervical nodes without a palpable mass in the thyroid.

- Transillumination is not very useful since cancer has been found in colloid cysts and since papillary carcinomas are at times partially cystic.

The following tests are sometimes used to assist in establishing a diagnosis:

a. Thyroid Radioisotope Scanning (^{131}I or Tc Pertechnetate)

This is undoubtedly the most useful test in trying to identify thyroid carcinomas. Of solitary cold nodules, 20–30% are malignant, while a hot nodule or a warm autonomous nodule is hardly ever malignant.

b. Sonography

This is of little value, except when it identifies a totally cystic lesion; if this lesion can be aspirated and totally evacuated without refilling, then carcinoma may be ruled out with reasonable assurance; if however, the lesion cannot be totally evacuated or refills, or if the contents of the cyst are hemorrhagic, carcinoma should be considered.

c. Needle Biopsy

The use of needle biopsy of the thyroid, either by aspiration or by core tissue biopsy, is still very controversial. Supporters of its use cite as its advantages the simplicity of the technique and the early histological confirmation so easily obtained. Opponents suggest that the tissue obtained is scarce, requiring a skilled pathologist for interpretation, and that the findings can be misleading if negative because the amount of tissue may not be representative of the whole tumor and may be so well differentiated that one might not be able to read cancer within it. The technique is most useful, however, to rule out carcinoma in patients with suspected Hashimoto's thyroiditis or to establish a diagnosis prior to surgery in the clinically obvious carcinoma of the thyroid.

d. X-ray

Plain films of the neck may reveal tracheal stenosis, displacement, or invasion by the tumor. They are also important in the detection of calcification in the thyroid region (psammoma bodies are common in papillary and follicular carcinoma, and calcifications in the thyroid region are also found in medullary carcinoma).

The value of CAT scans in the identification of thyroid cancer has not been clearly identified as yet.

e. Other

- Thyroid function tests are useless in the detection of thyroid cancer.

- Serum calcitonin is useful to identify medullary carcinoma in patients with a family history of medullary carcinoma or a multiple endocrine syndrome.

3. Treatment

Treatment of thyroid carcinoma continues to be controversial and includes a variety of surgical and nonsurgical modalities selected according to the patient's age, histological type, stage of the tumor, and the surgeon's preference.

- Surgical treatment of the primary includes the following: Lobectomy, with or without isthmusectomy.
  Near-total thyroidectomy.
  Total radical thyroidectomy with pre- and paratracheal node dissection.
- Surgical treatment of neck nodes may include
  Elective neck dissection (standard or modified).
  Therapeutic neck dissection.
- Nonsurgical treatment
  TSH suppression with thyroid hormones.
  Systemic ^{131}I.
  External irradiation.
  Chemotherapy.

a. Surgical Treatment

i. Local Surgery. When a solitary nodule of the thyroid is operated upon, a lobectomy and isthmusectomy is usually carried out as the preliminary procedure; frozen section is obtained and, if the report indicates a papillary, mixed papillary, or follicular carcinoma, definitive surgery can then be carried out. Some surgeons elect to quit at this point and place the patient on postoperative thyroid suppression. Other surgeons carry out a near-total thyroidectomy, removing the opposite lobe but leaving a small portion of the posterior capsule with the parathyroid glands behind. Others yet will carry out a radical total thyroidectomy with pre- and paratracheal node dissection.

Because of the extremely high rate of multicentric focuses of cancer throughout the thyroid gland (reported in as much as 60–80% of cases) and the frequent involvement of paratracheal nodes, we believe that the latter approach is warranted for all cases of differentiated thyroid cancer (papillary or follicular). A bilateral total thyroidectomy with pre- and paratracheal node dissection is therefore the preferred operation, provided it can be carried out with reasonable assurance that the parathyroid glands can be preserved together with their blood supply in order to obviate the serious complication of permanent postoperative hypoparathyroidism.

When a medullary tumor is found, a total thyroidectomy as just described should also be carried out. Node dissection is usually indicated in medullary cancer of the thyroid and must include the superior mediastinal nodes, where this disease often seems to spread.

If anaplastic carcinoma is found, a concerted effort should be made to try and resect all gross tumor; in many cases, this may not be possible, and a debulking procedure is all that can be carried out. If tumor is left in the area around the trachea, a tracheostomy is mandatory. Surgery must in all cases be followed by radiotherapy.

An attempt should always be made to remove all gross disease in the advanced thyroid cancer, regardless of its histological nature; this might require sacrificing portions of the esophagus, trachea (or tracheal cartilage), larynx, muscles, recurrent laryngeal nerve, and/or parathyroid glands. Furthermore, in the case of the well-differentiated thyroid cancer, it is recommended that all functioning thyroid tissue be removed in order to make it possible to use therapeutic doses of radioactive iodine in the patient whose distant metastases are found to pick up ^{131}I.

At times, the pathologist cannot determine on frozen section if a well-differentiated thyroid tumor (follicular or papillary) contains malignancy. In these cases, the wound is closed after the lobectomy and isthmusectomy, and the decision for definitive treatment will have to be made upon study of the parafin sections of the specimen.

Reoperation, if it is to be carried out, should be done as soon as possible (within 48 hours and no later than 5 days) after the original operation to avoid the technical operative difficulties that result from postoperative edema, fibrosis, discoloration, and adhesions.

ii. Treatment of Neck Nodes. Therapeutic neck dissection, in the presence of enlargement of cervical lymph nodes and/or extensive local spread, must be carried out. The radical neck dissection in the case of thyroid carcinoma should preferably be a modified neck dissection which attempts to preserve the sternocleidomastoid muscle, the spinal accessory nerve, the internal jugular vein (especially if bilateral neck dissection is necessary), and the suprahyoid neck contents. The procedure has an excellent cosmetic and functional result and should always be attempted in patients under age 40. The standard neck dissection, however, must be done when extensive clinical nodes are present.

The subject of elective neck dissection is an extremely controversial one. Statistically, several reports seem to indicate that 65–80% of patients with papillary or mixed papillary and follicular carcinomas greater than 1 cm in size will have metastatic nodes in the ipsilateral neck identifiable histologically, even if not clinically palpable. Furthermore, some studies indicate a lower survival if the surgery is deferred until clinically positive nodes develop. It would thus seem reasonable to consider doing an elective node dissection in all patients with papillary thyroid cancers over 1 cm in size. Most surgeons, however, elect not to do neck dissection routinely for thyroid cancer but prefer to wait for clinical evidence of metastases. We recommend doing an elective neck dissection for large papillary or mixed thyroid cancers, but only if it can be done with no cosmetic or functional morbidity; with a modified radical neck dissection carried out meticulously, this can be accomplished and is therefore desirable. Elective neck dissection is not indicated in "pure" follicular thyroid cancer since these rarely spread to nodes.

b. Nonsurgical Treatment

i. Radioactive Iodine Therapy. It has been stated by some that it is almost impossible to perform a total thyroidectomy and that technically some tissue is always left behind, as demonstrated by postoperative scans. To obliterate that residual thyroid tissue and increase the iodine pickup in distant metastases, ablation of that residual thyroid tissue after thyroidectomy can be carried out with one dose of 30–60 millicuries (mCi) of ^{131}I depending upon the amount of residual thyroid tissue. This is necessary if there are metastases and if functioning tissue can be demonstrated in the neck, since it is only in the absence of normal thyroid tissue that distant metastases become avid for iodine and susceptible to treatment with ^{131}I. Following the administration of the ablative dose of ^{131}I, and after the patient has been off any thyroid hormones for at least 4 weeks, a dose of 1–5 mCi of ^{131}I is given, and a total body scan is obtained after TSH stimulation to identify any functioning metastatic thyroid tissue. If uptake is identified in any distant site, radioactive iodine therapy can then be started. The dose varies from 100 to 200 mCi and is repeated at 3-month intervals until total ablation of the metastasis is achieved. Usually, the maximum total dose is 500 mCi. In the absence of distant metastases, it is unnecessary to ablate with ^{131}I the residual thyroid function that may be identified postoperatively within the thyroid bed; this is invariably due to tiny fragments of thyroid tissue left behind by the surgeon and is not an indication of metastases or residual cancer.

ii. TSH Suppression Therapy. Since most thyroid cancers are TSH dependent, thyroid suppression therapy is given to all patients after completion of the primary therapy. It is achieved by administration of exogenous thyroid hormones in large doses to induce total TSH suppression. This is started with small amounts and progressively increased to tolerance. Older patients usually do not respond to suppressive therapy as well as the younger ones. It is important to note, however, that metastatic carcinoma often regresses when treated with exogenous thyroid.

iii. External Irradiation. For the well-differentiated thyroid carcinoma, there is no room for the primary use of radiotherapy. Its use is limited to postoperative adjunctive treatment of residual disease or palliative treatment of inoperable disease. Treatment of metastatic disease by radiotherapy follows the same lines designed for other metastases. .

For anaplastic carcinomas, however, especially in the small-cell type, radiotherapy used postoperatively is of utmost importance and must be carefully planned and administered. High doses (5000–6000 rads) must be delivered if a beneficial effect is to be accrued.

iv. Chemotherapy. Of all drugs continuously tried, adriamycin appears to be the only one with any promise in the control of thyroid cancer. It can be administered at a dose of 60 mg per square meter of surface area.

F. Other Head and Neck Cancers

Other tumors of the head and neck are discussed in various appropriate sections of these volumes:

- Parathyroid tumors: see §4, Part C.
- Soft-tissue tumors: see §6.
- Lymphomas: see §9.
- Melanomas: see §3.

VI. ADJUVANT USE OF CHEMOTHERAPY IN HEAD AND NECK CANCER

Patients with locally advanced carcinomas of the head and neck (late Stages III and IV) currently have a poor prognosis. After surgery and/or radiotherapy, 50–80% of patients have a recurrence at 2 years, and less than one-third survive 5 years. This is due to the failure of standard local treatments (surgery and/or radiation therapy) at both the regional and the distant metastatic sites. Recurrent or residual disease is the usual cause of failure, which subsequently results in distant metastases.

Combination chemotherapy may offer a potential to improve treatment results. These combinations have been more effective when used as an initial treatment in locally advanced cases (anterior or induction chemotherapy) than when used in the treatment of recurrent or metastatic disease. For instance, the combination *cis*-platinum, bleomycin, and methotrexate only achieved 8% complete response and 38% partial response in the treatment of recurrent or metastatic disease, as compared with an 18% complete response and a 55% partial response in patients with locally advanced disease treated primarily with chemotherapy. These improved therapeutic results may be attributed to better tumor vascularity, better host nutrition, and favorable immune status in the untreated patients. It must be understood, however, that responses to chemotherapy are usually temporary; accordingly, it seems logical to incorporate preoperative or preirradiation chemotherapy into the management of locally advanced disease in order to maximize the efficacy of treatment.

Induction chemotherapy, to be effective, must be used in compliance with certain basic requirements:

- A combination of drugs must be used, and *cis*-platinum appears to be essential in the regimen.
- All drugs must have been demonstrated to be active.
- Ideally, the combination should yield an 80% response rate (complete and partial), with at least 20% complete responses.
- The patient must receive two or three preoperative courses at 3-week intervals, and surgery or radiation may be performed as early as 2 weeks after the last course, provided the white blood count and platelets are satisfactory.
- Treatment should be limited to the advanced disease (Stages III and IV) only.

Potential benefits of induction chemotherapy include reduction in the size of the local tumor, which, in some cases, renders patients initially believed to be inoperable, eligible for definitive surgery. In addition, such therapy may decrease the incidence of distant failures.

Price and Hall tested this hypothesis by administering chemotherapy, prior to surgery and radiotherapy, to 76 newly diagnosed patients. (Chemotherapy consisted of vincristine, bleomycin, methotrexate, hydrocortisone, and 5-fu). Some remission occurred in 75% of the patients. Although this report, as well as several other uncontrolled studies, suggests potential benefit from primary chemotherapy, its ultimate worth in terms of relapse-free survival, as determined by prospectively randomized studies, remains uncertain; the indications for its use, therefore, remain at the discretion of the treating physician. Nevertheless, based on the results of studies like those cited above, it now seems reasonable to integrate primary (i.e., preoperative and preirradiation) chemotherapy into the treatment of locally advanced head and neck carcinoma.

Regimens such as high-dose methotrexate; *cis*-platinum and bleomycin, with or without vincristine; 5-FU infusion or bolus with various combinations, etc., are currently undergoing clinical trials and are being used as adjunctive modalities in selected patients with T3 and T4 disease.

The long-term impact of induction chemotherapy used before surgery or radiation is still not entirely clear. There seems to be little doubt that local responses can be achieved in a high percentage of patients thus treated; whether this will reflect itself in improved survival is still controversial. Two major medical centers (Roswell Park in Buffalo, New York, and the Dana-Farber Cancer Institute in Boston) are now reporting

significant improved survival rates. Others, however, have not succeeded in supporting this finding.

All the recommended drugs are cytotoxic, and treatment complications, including mucositis, bone marrow depression, and vomiting, may tax these patients, especially those whose general condition is marginal. Obviously, performance and nutritional status play an important role in the selection of patients for this multimodality type of treatment. Hyperalimentation may also be necessary prior to, during, or following chemotherapy in order to reverse the nutritional deficits cause by the disease and its treatment.

VII. TREATMENT OF THE ADVANCED HEAD AND NECK CANCER PATIENT

Patients with advanced head and neck cancer fall into two different categories: those with uncontrolled local disease, whether primary or nodal spread, and those with distant metastases. Although most patients who die of head and neck cancer will have visceral metastases, mainly to lung or bones, the majority will in fact die from the result of the inability to control local disease.

Treatment of the incurable patient with head and neck cancer is strictly of a palliative nature, and one must keep in mind the quality of life and not only its prolongation. Surgery, chemotherapy, and radiation therapy all have definite roles in managing the problems of the patient with incurable head and neck cancer. In addition, assistance from a large number of paramedical professionals is most important in providing the patient with a host of services: nutritional, psychological, clerical, rehabilitative, occupational, etc. The inclusion of a well-organized supportive care team in the approach to the terminal patient is of the greatest importance.

A. Chemotherapy

Active chemotherapeutic agents include *cis*-platinum, bleomycin, 5-FU, methotrexate, vincristine, and vinblastine. Treatment with these agents, either singly or in combination, results in response rates of 25–50% with less than 7% of patients achieving complete regression. Furthermore, responses are short lived, usually lasting an average of 3 months before relapse occurs. Chemotherapy should be considered, however, particularly when failure is due to distant metastases, and treatment should be instituted in selected patients in an attempt to achieve temporary disease regression and prolongation of life. Treatment decisions should be based on the nutritional and functional status of the patient; chemotherapy is usually of no benefit in bedridden or severely malnourished patients and should, in these cases, be avoided.

Certain specific chemotherapeutic modalities used for palliation (or at times as adjunctive procedures) must be mentioned:

- Agents that enhance the effects of radiotherapy
  Hydroxyurea: increases cells in G2 phase that are most radiosensitive.
  Actinomycin D and adriamycin: inhibit protein synthesis and reduce the Sutton-Elkind curve of radiation.
  Bleomycin: is syngergistic to radiotherapy.
- Administration of chemotherapy by infusion or isolation perfusion. A vogue of the early 1960s and 1970s, these procedures used to be extremely complex, requiring prolonged hospitalizations and resulting in a significant morbidity and mortality. Furthermore, they were found, in fact, to be no more effective than some of the newer combination drugs currently administered systemically. Today, however, with the newer, portable, totally implantable infusion pumps (e.g., Infusaid), interest in regional chemotherapy is being rekindled.

B. Radiotherapy

Treatment of the unresectable primary tumor, or one that recurs and is not resectable, is primarily carried out by radiotherapy. The treatment offers excellent palliation at the primary site, as well as in areas of troublesome metastatic deposits that produce pain, obstruction, or bleeding. Pain, especially when related to bone metastases, responds to radiation within 10 days of treatment initiation and reaches its zenith about 4–6 weeks later. Pain due to other etiologies, such as neurological or muscular invasion, does not usually respond as well. Bleeding, when related to an oozing malignant lesion, usually responds within a few days and, if a sufficient dosage (about 4,000 rads) is given, may be kept in abeyance for long periods.

C. Surgery

Palliative surgical extirpation can also be of great usefulness but should be reserved for patients who have failed radiotherapy and chemotherapy. Such resections should always conform to two basic principles:

- Total excision of all visible tumor; one should never undertake to carry out a surgical resection for palliation unless one is reasonably sure that a total excision of the disease is possible. Otherwise, quick recurrence within a matter of weeks is liable to occur, creating an even worse dilemma.
- Possible rehabilitation of the patient within a reasonable period of time after the surgery.

Often, formidable resections are justified in order to eliminate massive tumor sites and rid the patient of associated pain

and odor. One must, however, ascertain that surgical reconstruction within a reasonably short period of time is feasible, and it must be possible to return the patient to his family and a relatively normal social existence; otherwise, palliation, in the real sense, has not been achieved. If it appears that total removal of the tumor-bearing tissue is not technically feasible, it is preferable to avoid surgery.

D. Supportive Measures

Within the scope of supportive management of the advanced head and neck cancer patient, nutritional support, pain relief, and psychological support are essential goals.

1. Nutritional Support

Nutritional support can be carried out in several ways. If the patient is hospitalized, total intravenous hyperalimentation, nasogastric tube feedings, esophagostomy, or gastrostomy are all acceptable options. The latter two procedures should be used only when direct oral tube feeding is impossible. The intravenous route should be reserved for patients with gastrointestinal problems prohibiting enteric alimentation, or when such feedings are impractical. For ambulatory patients, the preferred method of hyperalimentation is either oral or via a nasogastric tube, which the patient can learn to manage himself and insert intermittently for his meals.

2. Relief of Pain

Radiotherapy is an effective method of palliating pain due to bone metastases. However, relief of pain from other reasons (e.g., nerve involvement) can be extremely difficult because of the inability to block or transect easily accessible sensory nerves. Various analgesics, both oral and parenteral, are available and must be administered in whatever dose and frequency is required to alleviate pain. Oral methadone has proven especially useful because of its prolonged half-life and consequent sustained blood level and analgesic activities. Various cocktails mixing multiple drugs with different target organs are often more effective than simple analgesics (e.g., methadone, prednisone, tricyclic antidepressant, sedatives, caffein, etc.). It must be stressed that it is totally unconscionable for a patient with terminal disease to be denied relief of pain, regardless of the drug that might be required, the amounts necessary, and its rate of administration.

3. Psychological Support

This aspect of patient care is of utmost importance at this stage of the disease and is often neglected. Although the responsible attending physician or the patient's primary physician may be of great help in offering comfort, solace, and at times, some degree of hope to the patient, more professional assistance is often needed and can often be better administered by specialized personnel who have more time and more experience in dealing with such problems.

4. Supportive Care Team

The participation of a supportive care team especially dedicated to assist the terminally ill cancer patient is the ideal way of offering the patient and his family the multidisciplinary services that may be necessary at this stage of the illness. The team should include

- A nurse oncologist who may help the patient with whatever nursing care and counseling is necessary.
- A nutritionist to ensure adequate nutritional support.
- A psychiatric liaison nurse or psychiatrist.
- An oncologist.
- An anesthesiologist to assist in the problems of relief of pain.
- A physiotherapist and an occupational therapist.
- A social worker to advise the patient and his family what agencies or social services are available and what type of financial support can be obtained from various organizations. The social worker can also help in placing the patient in special terminal care facilities when the time comes.
- A clergy member.

Time, compassion, and patience are essential in relating to the terminally ill patient and his family. This period of time in his illness is, by and large, the most trying one for the patient, his family, and the physician as well.

VIII. POSTOPERATIVE CARE, EVALUATION, AND REHABILITATION OF THE HEAD AND NECK CANCER PATIENT

A. Evaluation and Care of the Postoperative Patient

1. Vital Signs

These should be monitored carefully. Head and shoulders should be kept elevated 60–90° as soon as the blood pressure is stabilized to prevent excessive postoperative edema and improve respiration. Monitoring of cardiac and respiratory status is a must. Blood gas determinations, tidal volumes, blood electrolytes and blood chemistries, CBCs and hematocrits, etc.

should be obtained as often as possible when indicated. Corrective measures for electrolyte disturbances or blood volume deficits should be taken as soon as possible.

2. Tracheostomy Care

Tracheostomy tubes should be sutured in place for the first few days after surgery. A tracheostomy ribbon should be tied loosely around the neck to prevent pressure on the skin flaps, which could lead to necrosis of the flap and edema of the head and neck. Tracheostomy cuffs should only be inflated when positive pressure breathing is required and during feedings; at other times, it is important not to inflate the cuff because it may lead to serious injury to the trachea, stenosis, and even necrosis. The inner tube of the tracheostomy tube should be removed and cleaned at least every 4 hours. The entire tube can be removed and replaced only after a tract has been formed, which takes approximately 5–6 days. Oxygen and humidity can be given through a mist collar. Suctioning of the tracheobronchial tree should be done as frequently as necessary. Tracheostomies should be terminated as soon as the patient's condition permits, and tubes should be removed as soon as possible.

3. Analagesics, Tranquilizers, and Narcotics

These medications are often prescribed but must be used with discretion. Patients should not be so heavily sedated as to impair their ability to breathe and cough effectively and must be encouraged to be as active as possible.

4. Antibiotics

Antibiotics should be given to the patient in the following circumstances:

- Surgery that communicates with the aerodigestive tract (mouth, antrum, esophagus, etc.).
- Extensive surgery, which involves bones.
- Surgery following irradiation.
- Reoperation.
- Whenever the cranial fossa is entered.

5. Oral Hygiene

Oral hygiene is very important following surgery involving the oral cavity and oropharynx. A mixture of hydrogen peroxide and saline can be best used for irrigation and is better administered by a power atomizer. During the oral irrigation, it is best for the patient to be in a sitting position to prevent aspiration and so that the irrigating solution may be satisfactorily suctioned.

6. Wound Care and Vacuum Tube Drains under Skin Flaps

Suction drains, if used, should be kept on suction and patent at all times to result in adherence of the skin flaps to the underlying structures. Suture lines of the skin may be covered only by a thin layer of antibiotic ointment, although a fluffy pressure dressing is preferred by some. The neck wound should be carefully examined for any evidence of fluid accumulation, hemorrhage under the flaps, or infection; prompt evacuation of any accumulation is mandatory. If the drainage contains mucous, it suggests an oropharyngeal fistual arising from a mucosal suture-line disruption; in such a case and in cases of abscess formation, the incision must be laid open, irrigated, and packed.

When the carotid artery is exposed, vigorous and meticulous wound care should be given; if a segment of the vessel seems pale and avascular and becomes dark and dried up, it indicates impending rupture. Ligation of the carotid artery should be performed if it is irretrievably necrotic or as soon as any bleeding occurs.

7. Tube Feedings

Whenever oral intake of food is going to be delayed for any reason, feedings may be administered by means of a nasoesophageal or nasogastric tube. Nasoesophageal intubation is preferable because it prevents gastroesophageal reflux.

High-caloric liquid feedings can be given through the feeding tube starting the first day following surgery. The amount of feeding can be increased gradually to the point of tolerance. Feedings can be given every 3–4 hours, up to 300–400 cc each time, or one may utilize the continuous-drip method. (It is advisable to omit the 3–4 A.M. feeding.) The feeding tube should be irrigated after each feeding of formula and/or medication in order to prevent blockage of the tube by inspissated material.

In a fresh postoperative patient, do not attempt to reinsert a feeding tube that was inadvertently removed, since the reinserted tube may lead to disruption of the suture line.

8. Laryngectomy Care

The stoma needs almost the same care as that described for a tracheostomy. The laryngectomy tube should be removed, cleaned, and replaced at least twice a day. The suture lines should be cleaned, and antibiotic ointment should be applied to the suture line. When an adequate stoma can be constructed, it is often preferrable not to put a tube in at all, or to remove it within 12–24 hours. Crusting must be thoroughly cleaned as often as necessary.

9. Postmaxillectomy Care

Prosthetic devices that have been prepared preoperatively should be put in and secured at the time of the operation; this permits early oral feedings and obviates the need for tracheostomies.

Maxillary-cavity packing (soaked with tincture of benzoin or Betadine solution) should be kept in place over the skin graft for 5–7 days. Upon removal of the packing, the prosthesis should be augmented with an obturator to fill in the cavity, retain the skin graft, and prevent contractures. Frequent local cleansing of the cavity should be done; removal of crusts, irrigation, and debridement must be meticulously carried out until total healing of the graft occurs. The maxillary prosthesis must be adjusted as often as necessary until permanent rehabilitation is possible.

10. Post-thyroidectomy and/or Parathyroidectomy Care

Close monitoring of the serum calcium level must be done, but calcium should be administered only if the patient becomes symptomatic; allowing the serum calcium to be low is the only stimulus available to increase the function of the remaining normal parathyroids. These patients should also be watched very closely for respiratory distress, which might result from various local complications (laryngeal edema, bleeding, vocal cord paralysis, etc.); these need to be immediately corrected by the administration of corticosteroids, reintubation if necessary, and evacuation of hematoma under pressure when indicated.

B. Pre- and Post-therapy Care of the Irradiated Patient

The preradiotherapy care of teeth, gums, and oral hygiene has been mentioned earlier and is mentioned again for emphasis.

Care of the mucous membranes is most important in the irradiated patient. The use of various mild anesthetic solutions (Gly-Oxide, Xylocaine viscus, and others) to control the mucositis and relieve the discomfort is recommended by some. However, these measures are often ineffective, and mouth hygiene in addition to analgesics (aspirin in solution or something similar) is often enough. Rarely, stronger pain killers (e.g., Percodan) are needed. Adequate fluid intake to correct the thickening of the saliva and dryness of the mouth is also important.

Skin care and treatment of erythema and desquamation is easily accomplished by the use of measures that leave the skin clean and dry (e.g., dusting powder or cornstarch). Desquamation on a substantial scale almost never occurs after properly planned and executed radiotherapy. Small patches of moist desquamation are easily controlled by dressing with a mixture of Desitin and antibiotic ointment, and Corticosteroid ointments have been used by some. This reaction must be watched carefully until it heals. Rarely, patients may display unusual sensitivity to irradiation resulting in marked early reactions; daily dose reduction in these cases may be necessary, but the biologic basis of radiation effect and the importance of delivering a cancericidal dose must be respected at all times. Such increased reaction is sometimes noted in patients who have received earlier chemotherapy (e.g., adriamycin).

The long-term care after a course of irradiation is very important if late sequelae such as excessive fibrosis or tissue necrosis are to be avoided.

Smoking must be totally avoided since it is liable to cause mucositis and increased dryness; this, in addition to its carcinogenic effect, makes complete abstinence from smoking essential. Liquor and spicy foods should also be avoided.

Dryness of the mouth often lasts for many months if a high dose of radiation is delivered to a large volume. The use of artificial saliva and frequent fluid intake (such as water) is a simple and effective solution.

Skin areas irradiated should be protected from sunlight (especially, for example, the summer sun on a beach, which may be combined with a troublesome wind effect). Keeping the skin covered with simple petroleum jelly or any ointment with an effective sunscreen will often prevent excessive skin drying and epithelial denudation.

Heavy irradiation of the mandible may result in late bone necrosis and sequestration that can be painful and terribly troublesome. This is especially noticeable after heavy irradiation combined with poor mouth hygiene. The trauma of impacted teeth removal may trigger the process. It is important for the dentist to consult closely with the radiation therapist before embarking on any procedure after radiation of the mouth. Generally, conservative procedures are well tolerated under an antibiotic cover, but unnecessary extensive procedures are frowned upon. If bone necrosis is noted, it is strongly advised that no sequestrectomy be done until there is complete separation of the sequestrum, which is then removed atraumatically. Appropriate use of antibiotics and careful mouth and teeth hygiene will reduce the incidence of such sequelae to a negligible rate.

C. Reconstructive Measures

One of the most important criteria for treatment of patients with head and neck cancer is that no therapy is acceptable unless it can permit the patient to return to a near normal social and functional existence. The assistance of the plastic surgeon and the great strides recently made in reconstructive surgery have permitted heretofore unacceptable operations to be carried out with a reasonable assurance that the patient can be rehabilitated surgically.

Many operations are available to us today to help reconstruct a patient after various formidable resections. These can be divided into five categories, as follows:

1. Local Flaps

Useful local flaps are

- Abbé and Estlander lip-switch flaps, often used following resections of over one-third of the lip.
- Fan flaps and cheek-advancement flaps, most useful following resections of skin lesions; can be fashioned in such ways as to minimize the scarring.
- Nasolabial flaps, which have been of great help in reconstructing the alveolar areas, as well as the floor of the mouth, following marginal resections for limited tumors. They are also extremely useful for coverage of skin defects, particularly in the nose.
- Vermillion flaps and tongue flaps, which are particularly helpful following resections of limited areas in the buccal mucosa, palate, and pharynx.

2. Distant Flaps

Useful distant flaps are

- Forehead flap, which for many years was the workhorse of the head and neck surgeon. Its main disadvantage was the unsightly cosmetic appearance of the grafted forehead and the need for a two-stage operation.
- Deltopectoral flap, which had, until recently, largely replaced the forehead flap. Its versatility and reach are excellent, and it has been used for anything from replacement of neck skin to reconstruction of the mouth, pharynx, esophagus, etc. It is only hampered by the need for a second stage to sever the pedicle and by the vulnerability of the flap, with its significant rate of failure when used without delay. It has been largely replaced by the musculocutaneous flaps.
- Cervical flap, shoulder flap, posterior occipital flap, acromial flap, acromiothoracic flap, bipedicle flap from the abdomen carried to the area on a forearm attachment, etc., all of which are less reliable and less commonly used; they suffer from the need for delays and staging but can still come in handy on occasion.

3. Muscle and Musculocutaneous Flaps

The demonstration of the vascular cutaneous territories of muscles carried on their vascular pedicles has led to the development of single-stage reconstruction to replace the multistage reconstructive procedures of the past. The pectoralis major, sternocleidomastoid, trapezius, temporalis, and latissimus dorsi muscles may be used to carry sizable surfaces of skin at great distances, permitting relatively simple one-stage procedures that have revolutionized reconstruction of the head and neck cancer patient.

4. Gastric Transposition and Pull-Up Operations

These procedures, as well as colon interposition operations, are particularly useful in the reconstruction of the gullet after extensive pharyngoesophagectomy.

5. Free Flaps

Advances in microsurgical techniques have lead to the development of several procedures for the rehabilitation of the head and neck patient using free-tissue transfer. Groin flaps, dorsalis pedis flaps, and latissimus dorsi flaps can be used for soft-tissue reconstruction. Compound flaps (e.g., rib flaps, iliac crest flaps) for reconstruction of soft tissue and bone in a one-stage procedure have also been attempted. Finally, free jejunal interpositions have been successfully used for esophageal reconstruction. Free flaps are not as safe as muscular and musculocutaneous flaps and require an expertise in microsurgical techniques that is not always available.

More complex, but still feasible, is the bony reconstruction, which is sometimes necessary following extensive mandibular resections. The use of various methods for mandibular replacement (Kirschner pin, various acrylic molds, steel mesh, titanium molds with or without bone graft, rib grafting, etc.) goes back several decades. Although none of these procedures has proven uniformly successful, and complication and failure rates are high, their use has permitted sizable mandibular resections, including resection of the mandibular arch, to be carried out with a reasonable assurance that cosmetic and functional rehabilitation is possible.

D. Prosthetic Rehabilitation

Rehabilitation of the head and neck patient can often be carried out with great ease, rapidity, and considerable effectiveness by the use of prosthetic devices. These are often much easier than cumbersome multistage plastic surgery procedures and frequently fill needs that defy the ability of the surgeon. The following prosthetic devices are available for use in the rehabilitation of the patient following head and neck surgery:

- Maxillary prostheses following maxillectomy.
- Dental prostheses for the rehabilitation of various types of

mandibulectomy (e.g., sliding-plane dentures or other maintenance devices to correct the mandibular shift that follows segmental mandibulectomy, mandibular implants procedures for denture retention, etc.).
- Prosthetic troughs to guide and direct food and salivary secretions in a desired direction (to avoid chronic aspirations).
- Palate obturators to prevent nasal regurgitation in patients after resection of palatal tumors.
- Facial prostheses, when sizable segments of skin are resected with maxillectomy.
- Artificial eyes.
- Voice rehabilitation prostheses (e.g., Blom-Singer tube, Panje button, and other types of artificial larynx)

E. Psychiatric Support

This part of the patient's care cannot be overemphasized. Although frequently it is effectively carried out by the treating physician (surgeon or oncologist) in concert with the patient's primary care physician, in many cases, sociopsychiatric help may be necessary. This is particularly so in

- Severely mutilating or disabling operative procedures.
- Operations that require a change of lifestyle or occupation.
- Disadvantaged patients with a poor social background, an unfavorable family environment, poor nutritional status, and/or difficult financial situation, etc.

Support from a social worker, nurse oncologist, psychiatric nurse, and even a psychiatrist himself can be of great value in the post-therapy care of the cancer patient.

F. Follow-Up Evaluation

It is essential in the aftercare of the head and neck cancer patient to establish a routine of regular scheduled examinations. The high incidence of local recurrences and the potential for multiple primaries in carcinomas of the aerodigestive tract make frequent follow-ups essential. This is particularly important considering that recurrences of head and neck cancer, if detected early enough, are often still curable.

Tables III and IV supply a schedule that seems reasonable in the follow-up of these patients.

G. Rehabilitation

Rehabilitation of the head and neck cancer patient after completion of therapy is of utmost importance and should be carried out as soon as possible.

Table III

Follow-Up Evaluation of the Head and Neck Cancer Patient:
Cancer of the Oral Cavity and Oropharynx; Maxillary Tumors; and Nasopharynx, Larynx, Hypopharynx, and Cervical Esophagus Carcinoma

Management	First 3 months: monthly	First year–third year				Fourth year and thereafter	
		3 Months	6 Months	9 Months	12 Months	Every 6 months	Annually
History							
Complete[a]	X	X	X	X	X		X
Tobacco	X	X	X	X	X	X	
Snuff	X	X	X	X	X	X	
Alcohol	X	X	X	X	X	X	
Pain	X	X	X	X	X	X	
Bleeding	X	X	X	X	X	X	
Anorexia	X	X	X	X	X	X	
Weight loss	X	X	X	X	X	X	
Eating ability	X	X	X	X	X	X	
Cough	X	X	X	X	X	X	
Palpable masses	X	X	X	X	X	X	
Physical							
Complete[a]			X		X		X
Oral cavity	X	X	X	X	X	X	
Oropharynx	X	X	X	X	X	X	
Indirect laryngoscopy	X	X	X	X	X	X	
Cervical nodes	X	X	X	X	X	X	
Skin	X	X	X	X	X	X	
Abdomen/liver	X	X	X	X	X	X	
Investigation							
CBC			X		X	X	
SMA-12			X		X		X
X-ray, chest			X		X		X
Bone scan			As indicated				
CAT scan			As indicated				
Liver scan			As indicated				
Dental prophylaxis[b]	X	X	X	X	X	X	

[a]For detection of other tumors.
[b]In mouth cancer patients and those who received radiotherapy.

1. Mouth and Teeth

Rehabilitation of the mouth and teeth is essential for cosmetic purposes and good nutritional status.

2. Deglutition

Rehabilitation of deglutition can be most difficult but must be taken into account. An intensive attempt at reeducating the patient to swallow without aspirating must be done whenever the problem occurs (following extensive oropharyngeal resection or extended radical neck dissection where several cranial nerves had to be sacrificed). In some cases (e.g., partial laryngectomy or pharyngectomy), drastic measures may become necessary to rehabilitate swallowing if aspiration persists: surgical intervention, laryngectomy, or permanent tube alimentation may be necessary.

3. Speech

Speech rehabilitation following laryngectomy may be carried out by one of several methods:

Table IV

Follow-Up Evaluation of the Head and Neck Cancer Patient:
Long-Term Follow-Up Schedule for Parotid and Thyroid Tumors

Management	First 3 months: monthly	First and second year				Third–fifth year		Thereafter: every 12 months
		3 Months	6 Months	9 Months	12 Months	Every 6 months	Annually	
History								
Complete[a]	X	X	X	X	X		X	X
Pain	X	X	X	X	X	X		X
Bleeding	X	X	X	X	X	X		X
Anorexia	X	X	X	X	X	X		X
Weight loss	X	X	X	X	X	X		X
Eating ability	X	X	X	X	X	X		X
Cough	X	X	X	X	X	X		X
Palpable masses	X	X	X	X	X	X		X
Drainage	X							
Physical								
Complete[a]			X		X		X	X
Local site	X	X	X	X	X	X		X
Cervical nodes	X	X	X	X	X	X		X
Skin	X	X	X	X	X	X		X
Abdomen/liver	X	X	X	X	X	X		X
Search for hypothyroidism (in thyroid cases)	X	X	X	X	X		X	X
Investigation								
CBC			X		X	X		X
SMA-12			X		X		X	X
X-ray, chest					X		X	X
Bone scan		As indicated						
Thyroid function tests and [131]I		As indicated						
Serum calcium and phosphates		As indicated						
Provocative calcitonin		As indicated						

[a]For detection of other tumors.

- Electronic devices.
- Esophageal speech training.
- The use of a voice prosthesis (Blom-Singer tube or Panje button).
- Surgical neoglottic methods may even be attempted in selected cases.

Voice and speech training in cases of loss of free oral and tongue mobility, or in cases of laryngeal nerve sacrifice or vocal cord resections, is most important. Rehabilitation of speech in these cases may even require endoscopic Teflon injections into the vocal cord or surgical reinnervation of a paralyzed cord by a nerve–muscle pedicle graft (Tucker's operation).

4. Airway

Arytenopexy or arytenoidectomy may be indicated in patients where respiratory embarrassment results from vocal cord paralysis.

5. Physical Therapy

Physical therapy for shoulder and neck disabilities following surgery is also useful.

6. Cosmetic Rehabilitation

Cosmetic and prosthetic rehabilitation should be seriously considered whenever it would help return the patient to a normal social existence or whenever it would appear to be psychologically indicated.

Rehabilitation of a facial nerve palsy is at times important and might require nerve grafting or crossover, tarsorrhaphy, canthoplasty, or facial sling operations, etc.

The head and neck oncologist must, at all times, have, as the foremost priority, the need to return the patient to as normal a social existence as soon as is possible and must, therefore, utilize any available medical, surgical, prosthetic, reconstructive, rehabilitative, psychiatric, and social modality that is available to help him achieve this goal.

IX. MANAGEMENT ALGORITHMS FOR HEAD AND NECK CANCER

(see pp. 56–61)

SUGGESTED READINGS

(see list following for full reference)

Early detection and screening: (27, 33, 41, 45, 53, 54, 84, 86)
Pretreatment Evaluation
    Radiology: 52, 60, 67
    Staging: 6
Multidisciplinary approach—combined therapy: 35, 51, 83
Preoperative preparation
    Nutritional: 9, 19, 20
    Medical: 26
    Emotional: 42
Therapeutic management
    Problems related to surgery: 43, 48, 61
    Problems related to Radiotherapy: 7, 8, 11, 32, 49
Selection of modality based on
    Histology
        Salivary: 36, 58, 74, 78, 79, 80
        Thyroid: 13, 21, 37, 50
    Site (squamous cell)
        Lip: 62
        Oral cavity: 15, 68
        Tongue: 76
        Supraglottic larynx: 17, 34
        Larynx: 40, 85
        Hypopharynx: 69, 71
        Paranasal sinuses: 47, 65, 70
        Nasopharynx: 22, 46, 73
        Ear: 55
    Special treatment modalities
        Laser: 81
        Cryosurgery: 10, 24, 30
        Mohs's chemotherapy: 56
Reconstruction: 1, 4, 18, 25, 44
Chemotherapy: 14, 16, 22, 28, 29, 31, 38, 57, 63, 74, 75
Rehabilitation: 34, 59, 66, 72, 82

Readings List

1. Ariyan, S. The pectoralis major myocutaneous flap. *Plast. Reconstr. Surg.* **63,** 73–81 (1979).
2. Attie, J. N., and Khafif, R. A. Presentation of parathyroid glands during total thyroidectomy. *Am. J. Surg.* **130,** 399–403 (1975).
3. Attie, J. N., Khafif, R. A., and Steckler, R. M. Elective neck dissection for papillary carincoma of the thyroid. *Am. J. Surg.* **122,** 464–471 (1971).
4. Back, S., Bitler, H. F., Krespi, Y. P., and Lawson, W. The pectoralis major myocutaneous flap for reconstruction of the head and neck. *Head Neck Surg.* **1,** 293–300 (1979).
5. Batsakis, J. G. "Tumors of the Head and Neck: Clinical and Pathological Consideration," 2nd ed. Williams & Wilkins, Baltimore, Maryland, 1979.
6. Beahrs, O. H., and Myers, M. "Manual for Staging of Cancer," 2nd. ed. American Joint Committee for Cancer, Staging and Result Reporting. Lippincott, Philadelphia, Pennsylvania (1983).
7. Beumer, J., III, Curtis, T., and Harrison, R. E. Radiation therapy of the oral cavity: Sequelae and management. *Head Neck Surg.* **1,** 301–312 (1977).
8. Bird, R. J., and Bryce, D. P. Long term effects of heavy irradiation to the neck. *J. Otolaryngol* **9,** 18–22 (1980).
9. Brennan, M. F. Total parenteral nutrition in the cancer patient. *N. Engl. J. Med.* **305,** 375–382 (1981).
10. Carpenter, R. J., and Synder, G. G., III. Cryosurgery: Theory and application to head and neck neoplasia. *Head Neck Surg.* **2,** 129–142 (1979).
11. Case Records of the Massachusetts General Hospital. *N. Engl. J. Med.* **296,** 94–100 (1976).
12. Case Records of the Massachusetts General Hospital. *N. Engl. J. Med.* **297,** 652–660 (1977).
13. Case Records of the Massachusetts General Hospital. *N. Engl. J. Med.* **301,** 559–605 (1979) (anaplastic cancer).
14. Chiuten, D., Vogh, S. E., Kaplan, B. H., and Greenwald, E. Effective outpatient combination chemotherapy for advanced cancer of the head and neck. *Surg., Gynecol. Obstet.* **151,** 659–662 (1980).
15. Chu, W., Litwin, S., and Stravitz, J. G. Resection and radiation in the control of cancer within the mouth. *Surg., Gynecol. Obstet.* **146,** 38–42 (1978).
16. Clifford, P. The role of cytotoxic drugs in the surgical management of head and neck malignancies. *J. Laryngol. Otol.* **93,** 1151–1180 (1979).
17. Coates, H. L., DeSanto, L. W., Devine, K. D., and Elveback, L. R. Carcinoma of the supraglottic larynx: A review of 221 cases. *Arch. Otolaryngol.* **102,** 686–689 (1976).
18. Conley, J., and Baker, D. C. The surgical treatment of extratemporal facial paralysis: An overview. *Head Neck Surg.* **1,** 12–23 (1978).
19. Copeland, E. M., III, Daly, J. M., Ota, D. M., and Dudrick, S. J. Nutrition, cancer and intravenous hyperalimentation. *Cancer* **43,** 2108–2116 (1979).
20. Copeland, E. M., III, Daly, J. M., and Dudrick, S. J. Nutritional concepts in the treatment of head and neck malignancies. *Head Neck Surg.* **1,** 350–364 (1979).
21. Cortes, E. P., Amin, V. C., Khafif, R. A., Wolk, D., Attie, J., Aral, I., and Eisenbud, L. Bleomycin infusion with cyclophosphamide, methotrexate and 5-fluorouracil in head and neck carcinoma. *Proc. Am. Assoc. Cancer Res.* **19,** 558 (1978).
22. Cortes, E. P., Amin, V. C., Attie, J., Eisenbud, L., Khafif, R. A., Wolk, D., Aral, I., Sciubba, J., and Akbiyik, N. Combination low dose bleomycin (bleo) followed by cyclophosphamide (C), methotrexate (M) and 5-fluorouracil (F) for advanced head and neck cancer. *Proc. Am. Assoc. Cancer Res.* **20,** 259 (1979).
23. Crile, G., Jr. Diagnosis and management of thyroid cancer. *Hosp. Med.* July, pp. 48–63 (1977).
24. DeSanto, L. W. Application of cryosurgery and otolaryngology. *Minn. Med.* **53,** 29–32 (1970).
25. DeSanto, L. W., and Carpenter, R. J. Reconstruction of the pharynx and upper esophagus after resection for cancer. *Head Neck Surg.* **2,** 369 (1980).
26. Diener, C. F. Evaluation of disability and assessment of operative risk. *Med. Clin. North Am.* **57,** 763–770 (1973).
27. Editorial. Snuff dipper's cancer. *N. Engl. J. Med.* **304,** 778–779 (1981).
28. Einhorn, L. H., and Williams, S. D. The Role of cis-platinum in solid tumor therapy. *N. Engl. J. Med.* **300,** 289–291 (1979).
29. Elias, E. G. Chemotherapy prior to local therapy in advanced squamous cell carcinoma of the head and neck. *Cancer* **43,** 1025 (1979).
30. Elton, R. F. Cryo corner: Wisdom of subsequent biopsies. *J. Dermatol. Surg. Oncol.* **3,** 386 (1977).

31. Ervin, T. J., Werchselbau, R. R., Posner, M. R., Fabian, R. L., and Miller, D. Multimodality treatment of advanced squamous cell carcinoma of the head and neck. Presented at the American Society for Head and Neck Surgery, March (1983).
32. Farris, M. J., Schneider, A. B., *et al.* Thyroid carcinoma owing as a late consequence of head and neck irradiation. *N. Engl. J. Med.* **294,** 1019.
33. Fitzpatrick, M. B. The biologic effects of solar radiation on skin. *J. Dermatol. Surg. Oncol.* **3,** 199 (1979).
34. Fletcher, G. H., Jesse, R. H., Linberg, R. D., and Koons, C. R. The place of radiotherapy in the management of squamous cell carcinoma of the supraglottic larynx. *Am. J. Roentgenology* **198,** 19–26 (1970).
35. Fu, K. K., Eisenberg, L., Deds, H. H., and Philips, T. L. Results of integrated management of supraglottic cancer. *Cancer* **40,** 2874–2881 (1977).
36. Fu, K. K., Leibel, S. A., Levine, M. L., Friedlander, L. M., Boleo, R., and Philips, T. Z. Carcinoma of the major and minor salivary glands. *Cancer* **40,** 2882–2890 (1977).
37. Graze, K., Spile, I. *et al.* Natural history of familial medullary thyroid carcinoma. *N. Engl. J. Med.* **299,** 980–985 (1978).
38. Green, M. R. Chemotherapy of head and neck cancer. *Head Neck Surg.* **1,** 75–86 (1978).
39. Harrison, R. E. Prosthetic management of maxillectomy. *Head Neck Surg.* **1,** 366–370 (1979).
40. Harwood, A. R., Deboer, G., and Kaxim, F. Prognostic factors in T3 glottis cancer. *Cancer* **47,** 367–372 (1981).
41. Henderson, B. E., Louie, E., Jing, J. S., Buell, P., and Gardner, M. B. Risk factors associated with nasopharyngeal carcinoma. *N. Engl. J. Med.* **295,** 1101–1106 (1976).
42. Herzon, F. S., and Boshier, M. Head and neck cancer—emotional management. *Head Neck Surg.* **2,** 112–119 (1979).
43. Hill, J. H., and Olson, N. R. The surgical anatomy of the spinal accessory nerve and the internal branch of the superior laryngeal nerve. *Laryngoscope* **89,** 1935–1942 (1979).
44. Jabaley, M. E. Reconstruction of patients with oral and pharyngeal cancer. *Curr. Prob. Surg.* **14** (1977).
45. Kaufman, J. A., and Shapshay, S. M. Detection of oral cancer. Letters to the Editor. *N. Engl. J. Med.* **297,** 841 (1977).
46. Khafif, R. A. Resection of carcinoma of the oropharynx and nasopharynx—a new approach. *Am. J. Surg.* **134,** 479–488 (1977).
47. Khafif, R. A. Surgery for tumors of the maxila and related structures. *In* "Head and Neck Surgery," 2nd ed. Appleton, New York, 1979.
48. Looser, K. G., Shah, J. P., and Strong, E. W. The significance of "positive" margins on surgically resected epidermod carcinoma. *Head Neck Surg.* **1,** 107–111 (1978).
49. MacComb, W. S. Necrosis in the treatment of intraenteral cancer by radiation therapy. *Am. J. Roentgenol., Radium Ther. Nurel. Med.* **87,** 431–440 (1962).
50. Makeshwari, Y. K., Hill, C. S., Jr., Hayne, T. P., III, Hickey, R. C., and Samaan, N. A. I^{131} therapy in differentiated thyroid carcinoma. *Cancer* **47,** 664–671 (1981).
51. Malaken, K., Robson, F., and Schipper, H. Combined modalities in the management of advanced head and neck cancers. *J. Otolaryngol.* **9,** 24–30 (1980).
52. Mancuso, A. A., and Hanafee, W. N. A comparative evaluation of computed tomography and laryngography. *Radiology* **133,** 131–138 (1979).
53. Mashberg, A. Erthyroplasia versus leukoplakia in the diagnosis of early asymptomatic oral squamous carcinoma. Editorial. *N. Engl. J. Med.* **297,** 104–110 (1977).
54. Mashberg, A. Re-evaluation of toluidine blue application as a diagnostic adjunct in the detection of asymptomatic oral squamous carcinoma. *Cancer* **46,** 758–763 (1980).
55. Mladnick, R. A. The core resection: Composite regional ear resection. *Clin. Plast. Surg.* **3,** 397–402 (1976).
56. Mohs, F. E. Chemosurgery: Microscopically controlled surgery for skin cancer, -past, present and future. *J. Dermatol. Surg. Oncol.* **4,** 41–54 (1978).
57. Murphy, R. *et al.* Cisdischolordiamine-platinum, methotrexate, and bleomcyin chemotherapy for patients with advanced squamous cell carcinoma of the head and neck. *Proc. Am. Assoc. Cancer Res.* **21,** 166 (1980).
58. Nigro, M. F., and Spiro, R. H. Deep lobe parotid tumors. *Am. J. Surg.* **134,** 523–527 (1977).
59. Olson, M. L., and Shedd, D. P. Disability and rehabilitation in head and neck cancer patients after treatment. *Head Neck Surg.* **1,** 52–59 (1978).
60. Parsons, A., Chapman, P., Corinter, R. T., and Grundy, A. The role of computed tomography in tumors of the larynx. *Clin. Radio.* **31,** 529–533 (1980).
61. Pascl, R. R., Hobby, L. W., Lattes, R., and Crikelair, G. F. Prognosis of "incompletely excised" versus "completely excised," basal cell carcinoma. *Plast. Reconstr. Surg.* **41,** 328–332 (1968).
62. Petrovich, Z., Knishe, H., Tobochnik, N., Hittle, R. E., Barton, R., and Jose, L. Carcinoma of the lips. *Arch. Otolaryngol.* **105,** 187–191 (1979).
63. Price, L. A. *et al.* Kinetically based combination chemotherapy for head and neck cancer: Implication for improved survival. *Proc. Am. Soc. Clin. Oncol.* **21,** 472 (1980).
64. Rafla, S., and Rotman, M. "Introduction to Radiotherapy; A Textbook" and Mosby, St. Louis, Missouri, 1974.
65. Ritter, F. "The Paranasal Sinuses: Anatomy and Surgical Techniques." Mosby, St. Louis, Missouri, 1978.
66. Salmon, S., and Goldstein, L. P. "Artificial Larynx Handbook." Grune & Stratton, New York, 1978.
67. Scheible, F. W., and Leopold, G. R. Diagnostic imaging in head and neck disease: Current applications of ultrasound. *Head Neck Surg.* **1,** 1–12 (1978).
68. Shah, J. P., Cendon, R. A., Farr, H. W., and Strong, E. W. Carcinoma of the oral cavity: Factors affecting treatment failure at the primary site of neck. *Am. J. Surg.* **132,** 504–507 (1976).
69. Shah, J. P., Shaha, A. R., Spiro, R. H., and Strong, E. W. Carcinoma of the hypopharynx. *Am. J. Surg.* **132,** 439–443 (1976).
70. Shah, J. P., and Galicich, J. H. Caraniofacial resection for malignant tumors of the ethmoid and anterior skull base. *Arch. Otolaryngol.* **103,** 514–517 (1977).
71. Silver, C. E. Surgical management of neoplasms of the larynx, hypopharynx and cervical esophagus. *Curr. Probl.* **14**(9) (1977).
72. Singer, M. I., and Glom, E. D. An endoscopic technique for restoration of voice after laryngectomy. *Ann. Otol., Rhinol., Laryngol.* **89,** 529–533 (1980).
73. Sinka, P. P., and Aziz, H. I. Juvenile nasopharyngeal angiofibroma. *Radiology* **127,** 501–505 (1978).
74. Spanos, G. Preoperative chemotherapy for giant cell carcinoma of the thyroid. *Cancer* **50,** 2252–2256 (1982).
75. Spaulding, M. B., Vasques, J., Khan, A., and Lore, J. M. A non-toxic adjuvant protocol for advanced head and neck cancer. Presented at the American Society of Head and Neck Surgery, March (1983).
76. Spiro, R. H., and Strong, E. W. Surgical treatment of cancer of the tongue. *Surg. Clin. North Am.* **54,** 759–765 (1974).
77. Spiro, R. H., Alfonso, A. E., Farr, H. W., and Strong, E. W. Cervical node metastasis from epidermoid carcinoma of the oral cavity and oropharynx. *Am. J. Surg.* **128,** 562–567 (1974).
78. Spiro, R. H., Hayden, S. I., and Strong, E. W. Tumors of the submaxillary gland. *Am. J. Surg.* **132,** 463–468 (1976).
79. Spiro, R. H., Huvos, A. G., and Strong, E. W. Acinic cell carcinoma of salivary origin. *Cancer* **41,** 924–935 (1978).
80. Spiro, R. H., Lewis, J. S., Hayden, S. I., and Strong, E. W. Mucous gland tumors of the larynx and laryngopharynx. *Ann. Otol., Rhinol., Laryngol.* **85,** 498–503 (1976).

81. Strong, M. S. *et al.* Transoral management of localized carcinoma of the oral cavity using the CO_{60} laser laryngoscope. *Laryngoscope* **89,** 897–900 (1979).

82. Tucker, H. M. Reinnervation of a paralyzed larynx: A review. *Head Neck Surg.* **1,** 235–243 (1979).

82a. U.S. Department of Health, Education, and Welfare. "Management Guidelines for Head and Neck Cancer." Public Health Service, National Institutes of Health, Washington, D.C. (1979).

83. Vikram, B. Importance of the time interval between surgery and postoperative radiation therapy in the combined management of head and neck cancer. *Int. J. Radiat. Oncol., Biol. Phys.* **5,** 1837–1840 (1979).

84. Vrabec, D. P. Multiple primary malignancies of the upper aerodigestive system. *Ann. Otol., Rhinol. Laryngol.* **88,** 846–854 (1979).

85. Wang, C. C. Treatment of squamous cell carcinoma of the larynx by radiation. *Radiol. Clin. North Am.* **16,** 209–218 (1978).

ALGORITHM FOR CANCER OF THE ORAL CAVITY AND OROPHARYNX

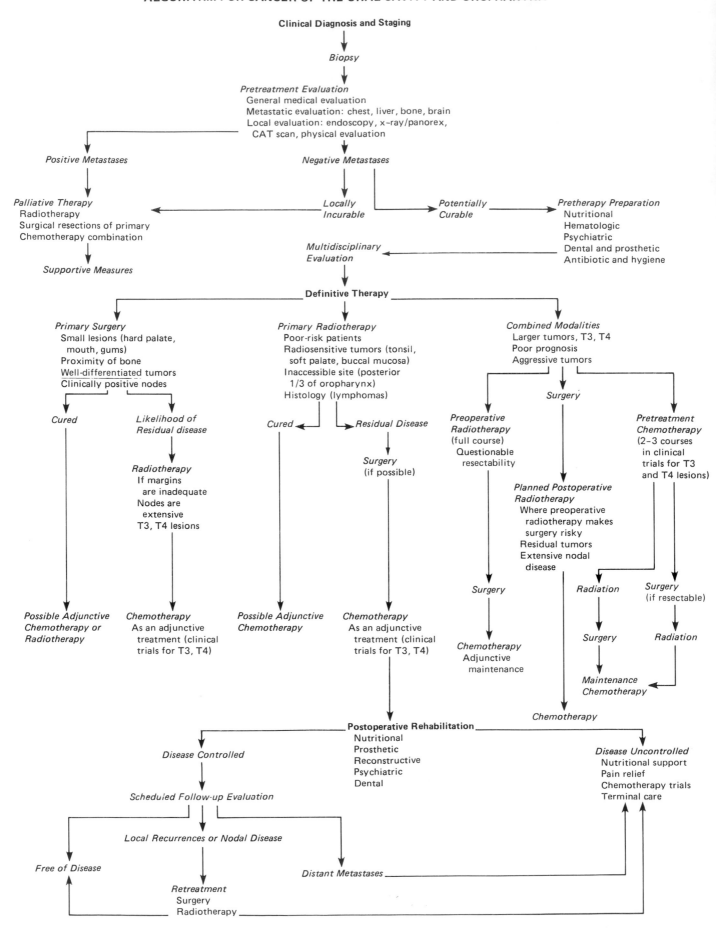

ALGORITHM FOR CANCER OF THE LARYNX AND HYPOPHARYNX

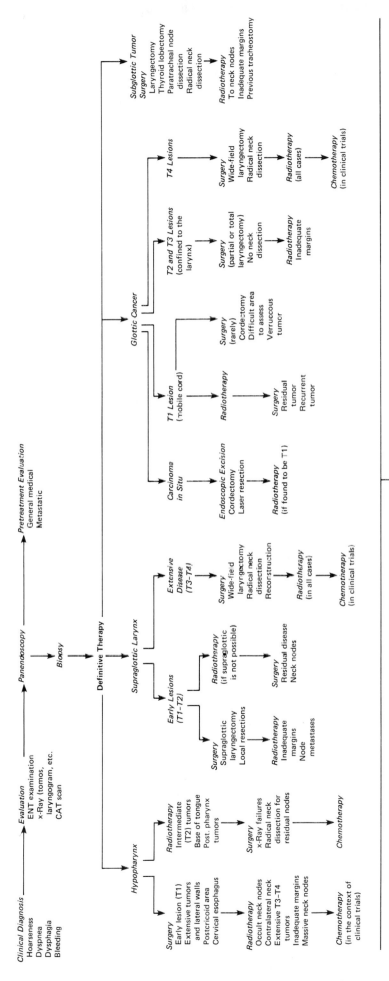
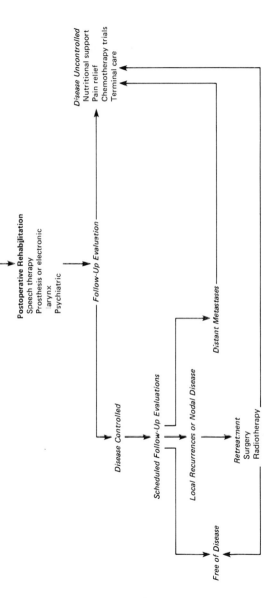

ALGORITHM FOR CANCER OF THE PARANASAL SINUSES

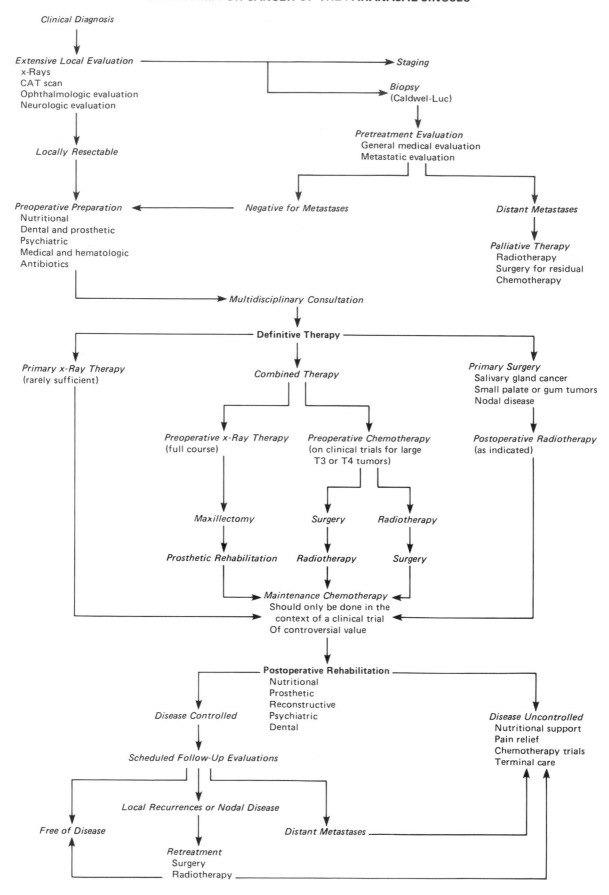

Clinical Diagnosis

Extensive Local Evaluation ⟶ *Staging*
  x-Rays
  CAT scan
  Ophthalmologic evaluation
  Neurologic evaluation

Biopsy
(Caldwel-Luc)

Pretreatment Evaluation
  General medical evaluation
  Metastatic evaluation

Locally Resectable

Negative for Metastases   *Distant Metastases*

Preoperative Preparation   *Palliative Therapy*
  Nutritional   Radiotherapy
  Dental and prosthetic   Surgery for residual
  Psychiatric   Chemotherapy
  Medical and hematologic
  Antibiotics

Multidisciplinary Consultation

Definitive Therapy

Primary x-Ray Therapy   *Combined Therapy*   *Primary Surgery*
(rarely sufficient)   Salivary gland cancer
                                                     Small palate or gum tumors
                                                     Nodal disease

Preoperative x-Ray Therapy   *Preoperative Chemotherapy*   *Postoperative Radiotherapy*
(full course)   (on clinical trials for large   (as indicated)
                                   T3 or T4 tumors)

Maxillectomy   *Surgery*   *Radiotherapy*

Prosthetic Rehabilitation   *Radiotherapy*   *Surgery*

Maintenance Chemotherapy
  Should only be done in the
  context of a clinical trial
  Of controversial value

Postoperative Rehabilitation
  Nutritional
  Prosthetic
  Reconstructive
  Psychiatric
  Dental

Disease Controlled   *Disease Uncontrolled*
                           Nutritional support
                           Pain relief
                           Chemotherapy trials
                           Terminal care

Scheduled Follow-Up Evaluations

Local Recurrences or Nodal Disease

Free of Disease   *Distant Metastases*

Retreatment
  Surgery
  Radiotherapy

ALGORITHM FOR CANCER OF THE NASOPHARYNX

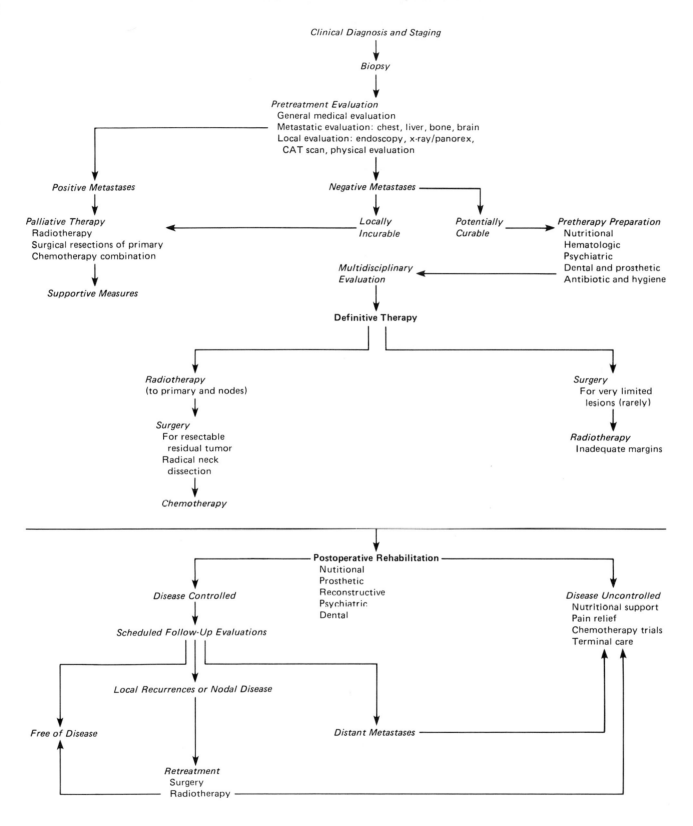

Clinical Diagnosis and Staging

Biopsy

Pretreatment Evaluation
General medical evaluation
Metastatic evaluation: chest, liver, bone, brain
Local evaluation: endoscopy, x-ray/panorex,
CAT scan, physical evaluation

Positive Metastases

Negative Metastases

Palliative Therapy
Radiotherapy
Surgical resections of primary
Chemotherapy combination

Locally Incurable

Potentially Curable

Pretherapy Preparation
Nutritional
Hematologic
Psychiatric
Dental and prosthetic
Antibiotic and hygiene

Supportive Measures

Multidisciplinary Evaluation

Definitive Therapy

Radiotherapy
(to primary and nodes)

Surgery
For very limited
lesions (rarely)

Surgery
For resectable
residual tumor
Radical neck
dissection

Radiotherapy
Inadequate margins

Chemotherapy

Postoperative Rehabilitation
Nutitional
Prosthetic
Reconstructive
Psychiatric
Dental

Disease Controlled

Disease Uncontrolled
Nutritional support
Pain relief
Chemotherapy trials
Terminal care

Scheduled Follow-Up Evaluations

Local Recurrences or Nodal Disease

Free of Disease

Distant Metastases

Retreatment
Surgery
Radiotherapy

ALGORITHM FOR CANCER OF THE SALIVARY GLANDS

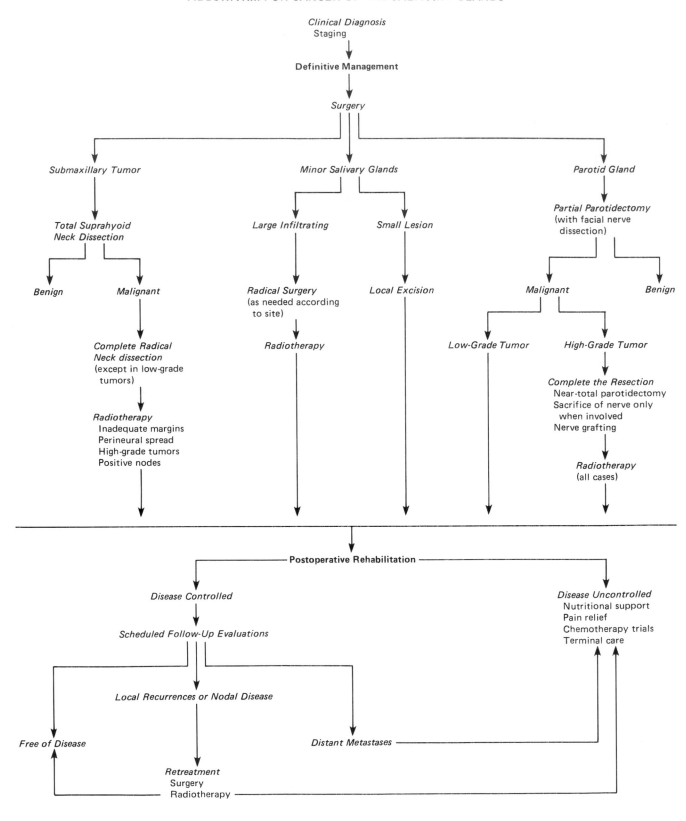

ALGORITHM FOR CANCER OF THE THYROID

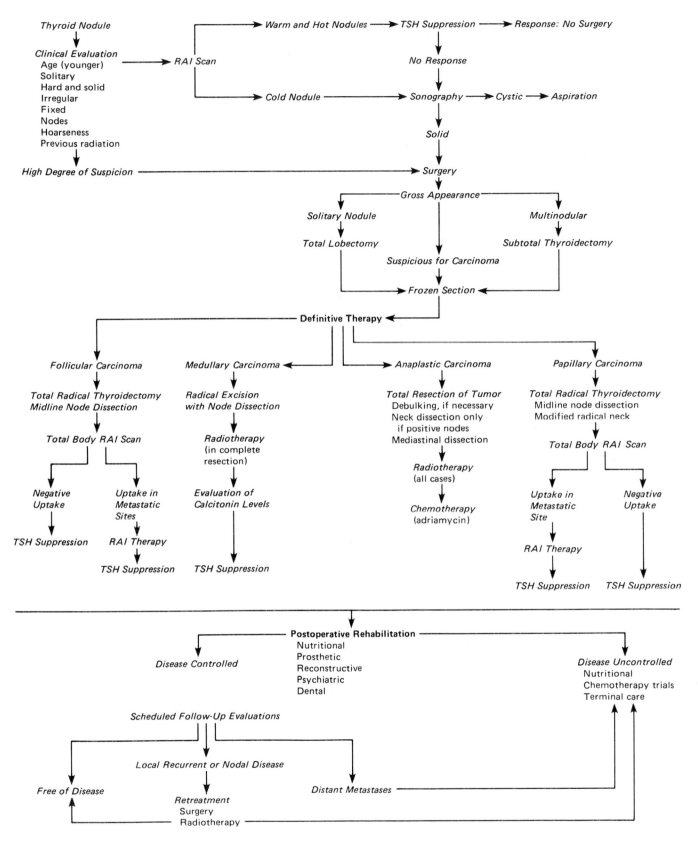

Section 2

Carcinomas of the Breast

RENE A. KHAFIF

With Contributions by

Frederico Capozzi	Surgical Oncology
Lawrence Feuerman	Surgery
Issam Arnuk	Surgery
Hosny Selim	Radiation Oncology
Samuel Kopel	Medical Oncology
Karl Jindrak	Pathology
Dennis Cirillo	Plastic Surgery
Ann Nelson	Nursing Oncology
Randi Moskowitz	Nursing Oncology

CURRENT GUIDELINES
FOR THE MANAGEMENT OF CANCER

Copyright © 1986 by Academic Press, Inc.
All rights of reproduction in any form reserved.

Section 2. Carcinomas of the Breast

I. Early Detection and Screening   67
  A. Predisposing Factors
  B. Early Detection
  C. Patient Education
  D. Breast Self-Examination
    1. Technique of Breast Self-Examination
    2. What to Look for during BSE
  E. Early Signs of Breast Cancer
  F. Signs of More Advanced Disease
  G. Screening of Breast Cancer
    1. Breast Self-Examination
    2. Routine Clinical Checkup
    3. Mammography
      a. Indications for Mammography
      b. Diagnostic Features of Mammography
      c. Value of Mammography in Predicting Risk
         Factors
    4. Thermography
    5. Diaphynography
    6. Sonography
II. Preoperative Evaluation and Preparation   71
  A. Physical Evaluation
    1. Breast "Lump" of Undetermined Nature
    2. Breast Mass of Suspicious Nature
  B. Biopsy
    1. Needle Biopsy
    2. Open Excisional Biopsy with Frozen Section
    3. Two-Step Procedure
  C. Assessment of Possible Metastatic Disease
    1. Stage I
    2. Stage II
    3. Stage III
  D. Preoperative Preparation
  E. Site-Specific Data Form for Cancer of the Breast
  F. Multidisciplinary Consultation and Evaluation
III. Therapeutic Management   76
  A. Definition of the Various Surgical Procedures
    1. Lumpectomy
    2. Segmental Mastectomy or Quarterectomy
    3. Simple Mastectomy
    4. Modified Radical Mastectomy
    5. Radical Mastectomy
    6. Supraradical Mastectomy
  B. Treatment according to the Stage of Disease
    1. Carcinoma *in Situ*
    2. Stage I
    3. Stage II
      a. Supraradical Mastectomy with Dissection of
         the Internal Mammary Nodes

      b. Standard Radical Mastectomy
      c. Modified Radical Mastectomy
      d. Simple Mastectomy
      e. Lumpectomy or Segmental Mastectomy
    4. Stage III
    5. Stage IV
  C. Histological Nature of the Disease and Its Therapeutic
     Implications
    1. Pathological Varieties of Breast Cancer
    2. Types of Mammary Carcinomas (Ackerman)
    3. Grading of Mammary Carcinoma
    4. Pathological Description of the Specimen
  D. Cosmetic Considerations
IV. Carcinoma of the Breast in Pregnancy   80
  A. Management of the Breast Tumor
  B. Management of the Pregnancy
  C. Endocrine Ablation
V. The Role of Radiotherapy in the Treatment
   of Breast Cancer   82
  A. Radiotherapy as Adjuvant Modality
  B. Radiotherapy as a Primary Modality
    1. Stage I
    2. Stage III
    3. Recurrent Breast Cancer
  C. Palliative Therapy
VI. Adjuvant Chemotherapy for Breast Cancer   83
  A. Concepts and Rationale
    1. Breast Cancer: An Early Systemic Disease
    2. Tumor Cell Kinetics
    3. Adjuvant Trials in Humans
  B. Guidelines for Adjuvant Chemotherapy
    1. Stage I
    2. Stage II
      a. Premenopausal Patients
      b. Postmenopausal
    3. Stage III
VII. Guidelines for the Treatment of Advanced
   Breast Cancer   85
  A. Evaluation of the Extent of Disease
  B. Prognostic Factors
  C. Assessment of Treatment Response
  D. Chemotherapy
  E. Hormonal Manipulation
  F. Management of Selected Complications and Specific
     Types of Metastases
    1. Bone Metastases
    2. Brain Metastases
    3. Pleural Effusions
    4. Hypercalcemia

5. Cutaneous and/or Regional Recurrence
6. Systemic Recurrence in the Estrogen-Receptor-Positive Patient
7. Systemic Recurrence in the Estrogen-Receptor-Negative Patient
8. Systemic Recurrence in the Estrogen-Receptor-Unknown Patient
9. Systemic Recurrence following Previous Adjuvant Chemotherapy
VIII. Postoperative Care, Evaluation, and Rehabilitation   90
   A. Immediate Postoperative Care
   B. Psychological Support
   C. Coordination of Postoperative Therapy

D. Follow-Up Evaluation
E. Rehabilitation
   1. Immediate Postoperative Rehabilitation
   2. Management of Lymphedema
   3. External Prosthetic Appliances
   4. Reconstructive Surgical Procedures
   5. Treatment of the Other Breast and High-Risk Prophylactic Surgery
F. Nursing Role in Rehabilitation
IX. Management Algorithm for Cancer of the Breast   93

Suggested Readings   93

I. EARLY DETECTION AND SCREENING

A. Predisposing Factors

Breast cancer has the highest incidence rate of all cancers in women (85.6% for 100,000 population) and is the leading cause of cancer death among women. It is estimated that 1 out of 11 women will develop breast cancer in her lifetime. It is also estimated that there will be 114,900 new cases diagnosed and 37,500 deaths from breast cancer this year. The median age of the patients with breast cancer is 55, with about one-third of cases appearing before age 50 and the majority of cases presenting between the ages of 45 and 54. Recently, however, there appears to be an increasing number of cases among young women in their 20s and 30s.

Although a great deal of statistical analysis and many investigative studies have been carried out to try and determine specific predisposing factors and to identify premalignant states in breast cancer, little of substance has evolved. The following risk factors have been identified:

- Family history of breast cancer, particularly when the family member is the mother or a sibling, and when the occurrence was premenopausal.
- Childbirth history. Nulliparity or first childbirth at a late age are probably the most significant factors associated with an increased incidence of breast cancer.
- Menstrual history. Early age of menarche and late menopause seem to be significant risk factors in relation to the incidence of breast cancer.
- High-dose radiation exposure.
- History of benign breast disease. Although several reports seem to suggest that chronic cystic mastitis predisposes to breast cancer, the issue is quite controversial, and it would seem that only those patients with atypical duct hyperplasia or papillomatosis have a clearly higher risk of breast cancer.
- Socioeconomic factors. It has been suggested that single women, obese patients, Jewish females, and women in a higher socioeconomic level are at greater risk for breast cancer.
- Diet and alcohol consumption. A diet high in animal fats and low in fiber, along with increased alcohol consumption, seem to be associated with a higher incidence of breast cancer.
- Use of oral contraceptive hormones or estrogen replacement therapy. This has probably been the issue most emotionally discussed but yet not clearly resolved. There seems to be mounting evidence that the use of oral contraceptives neither increases nor decreases the incidence of breast cancer. Increased incidence has been demonstrated, however, in selected subgroups:
  - Use of birth control pills for 6 years or more in patients with benign breast disease (twofold increase reported).
  - Use of birth control pills in the nulliparous woman.
  - Use of birth control pills for over one year in women with a family history of breast cancer (threefold increase reported).

  Likewise, several studies failed to identify a significant correlation between postmenopausal estrogen replacement usage and the development of breast cancer. There appears to be an increased risk in this group, however, when the analysis is made after 10 years of usage and in certain subgroups of patients, namely those with benign breast disease.
- Other risk factors suggested include use of hair dyes, use of some antihypertensive drugs, and abortion in the first trimester. These factors seem to be of dubious importance.

Extensive studies conducted by the Department of Epidemiology and Statistics of the American Cancer Society in New York seem to indicate that the risk increases with the presence of more risk factors, with an annual incidence of the disease ranging from 134.8 per 100,000 population between 30 and 54 years of age with one risk factor, to 264.1 per 100,000 population in women over age 54 with four or more risk factors. It must be pointed out, however, that the clinical importance of these risk factors is extremely limited, and most are factors over which neither the physician nor the patient has much control. Furthermore, over three-quarters of all breast cancers cannot be attributed to any of the known specific factors, and potential control of the disease by control of these factors is not likely. Greater emphasis needs to be put, therefore, on early detection and screening for breast cancer, rather than on prevention.

B. Early Detection

Few cancers have undergone such revolutionary changes in concepts and therapy in recent years as has breast cancer. This is primarily a result of the earlier detection of the disease in a larger proportion of patients, with improvement in prognosis in spite of the more conservative therapy often applied today. Earlier detection of breast cancer has resulted from a multitude of factors:

- Patient education.
- Breast self-examination.
- Recognition of early signs of breast cancer.
- Screening by various modalities.

C. Patient Education

The mass media—newspapers, magazines (especially those directed at women), radio, and television—have, in the past few years, effectively undertaken to educate the public at large on a variety of subject matters related to breast cancer. This has naturally heightened the awareness of the public as to the importance of early detection. Such a vital subject, however, should not be totally delegated to lay reporters, who often distort the facts in search of sensationalism, but rather should be undertaken by those who are best able to serve the patient.

Education should be carried out, or at least directed, by physicians or nurse oncologists and should be directed primarily at early detection, identification of the early signs and symptoms, importance and place of screening procedures, and breast self-examination. A plethora of educational material and pamphlets is available from the American Cancer Society, the National Cancer Institute, and the American Medical Association; these could be effectively used for reference or for distribution. In addition, volunteers from the American Cancer Society or from one of their informed lay groups (e.g., Reach-to-Recovery) could be extremely helpful in the education of the public.

In addition to heightening the public awareness of the disease and encouraging early detection, it is also necessary to dispel the myth that every breast lump is a death warrant, to inform the public at large that most breast lumps are benign and that, when malignant, most are totally curable if detected and treated early. This education would thus encourage the public to seek professional help promptly.

D. Breast Self-Examination

The importance of the anatomy of the breast and the technique of breast self-examination (BSE) should be stressed to all women. Breast anatomy is best taught in conjunction with menstraul teaching around the age of puberty. Self-examination can be taught at the time of the first pelvic examination by the age of 20, or sooner in the increased-risk population. This education can be carried out in one of several ways:

- On a one-to-one basis by the physician with the patient.
- In small groups by a physician or nurse oncologist. Such groups can be arranged by hospitals, clinics, community groups, churches, large industry, etc. Teaching aids from the American College of Surgeons or the Reach-to-Recovery program, in the form of pamphlets, films, or Betsi-models or Spenco are available for use in such programs.
- On a larger scale by the news media or through distribution of pamphlets by mail.

1. Technique of Breast Self-Examination

Breast self-examination should be done monthly. In premenopausal women, it should be planned 7–10 days after the onset of the menses when the breasts are least engorged and tender and when cystic changes are at a minimum. The examination should be done during a shower or bath when the skin is wet, enabling the fingers to glide easily over the breasts.

The woman should begin the examination by using the flat part of her fingers. Using the right hand to examine the left breast and placing the left hand on the head with the elbow at about a 45° angle, she should glide her fingers gently but firmly in a circumferential motion, starting from the periphery, working her way to the center, making sure to cover the entire breast. The left hand should then be used to examine the right breast, placing the right hand on the head with the elbow at a 45° degree angle.

After drying, the woman is to stand in front of a well-lighted mirror with arms at the sides and then raise them high over the head while observing herself in the mirror. She should take note of any asymmetry or visible abnormality, especially if not identified on a previous BSE. The breast must then be inspected during various strain maneuvers.

Resting the palms on the hips, she should then press down firmly to flex the chest muscles. This can also be achieved by grabbing the fingers of both hands and pulling so that the chest muscles contract.

To palpate the breast more effectively, the woman should then lie either on a bed or on the floor. Using a small pillow or folded towel placed under the right shoulder, she should place the right hand under the head so that the breasts are flattened. Pressing down gently on the right breast with the fingers of the left hand, she should work them around the outermost circle of the breast in small circular motions. Now working inward, she repeats the examination three times until the entire breast has been examined. The same maneuver is then carried out for the left breast.

Squeezing the nipple between the thumb and index finger while still lying on a flat surface, the woman should look for any signs of discharge or bleeding.

2. What to Look for during BSE

During BSE, one should check for any discoloration, swelling, or asymmetry (breasts may not match exactly, few women's do!). Retraction of the skin in one area must arouse suspicion. Likewise, thickening of the skin and dimpling (often called "pig skin" or "peau d'orange") should be noted. One must look for retraction of the nipple, although some women may normally have a retracted nipple. A change from one examination to the next is a significant sign. Crusting of the nipple or erosion should also arouse suspicion. Any enlargement of veins should also be noted.

On palpation, one tries to identify any newly occurring lumps, either in the breast or in the armpit. The woman must learn the usual consistency of her own breasts; there are many irregularities and thickenings that are normal; she is to keep track of them and note any changes.

If squeezing the nipple produces a discharge, one should note the color of the discharge. The clear, watery, milky, or greenish discharge is often of little importance, particularly when it is multicentric and when no masses are felt. The serosanguinous or bloody discharge is a red flag suggesting the possibility of neoplasia. In the young woman, especially in the absence of a mass, it usually identifies a benign intraductal papilloma; over the age of 50, or when there is a palpable mass, carcinoma must be considered given that 80% of these cases are malignant.

The most important advice to give the patient is DO NOT HESITATE TO CONSULT YOUR PHYSICIAN AND BRING TO HIS OR HER ATTENTION ANY DISTURBING FINDINGS AS EARLY AS THEY ARE SUSPECTED.

E. Early Signs of Breast Cancer

- Lump in the breast, most often painless.
- Nipple discharge.
- Nipple retraction.
- Nipple crusting or erosion.
- Retraction of the skin or change of contour or shape of the breast.
- "Peau d'orange," dimpling, or thickening of the skin.

F. Signs of More Advanced Disease

- Edema or erythema of the breast
- Ulceration of the skin.

- Lump in the axillae.
- Arm swelling.

G. Screening of Breast Cancer

1. Breast Self-Examination

Most breast masses are identified by the patient herself, and it is, therefore, obvious that the most useful, least harmful, and least expensive screening method is the BSE. This should be encouraged early on in life and carried out on a monthly basis.

2. Routine Clinical Checkup

Beyond BSE, women should be encouraged to have their breasts examined at regular intervals by their primary physician or gynecologist; this should be done every 3 years in women between 20 and 40 years of age and on a yearly basis in all women over the age of 40. Patients in a moderate- or high-risk category should be checked every 6 months, or even every 3 months if possible.

3. Mammography

a. Indications for Mammography

The value of mammography as a screening procedure is still a volatile subject. The clinical indications for diagnostic mammography, however, are better defined. Diagnostic mammography is indicated in the following cases:

- Fullness or questionable mass in the breast, especially in opulent breasts that are difficult to evaluate.
- Lumpy, highly cystic or dense breasts and breasts scarred from previous surgery.
- Nipple discharge, nipple retraction, or crusting in the absence of a mass.
- Palpable axillary nodes without breast masses.
- Presence of a suspicious mass, especially for evaluation of the contralateral breast.

Physicians must be aware of the limitations of mammography, bearing in mind that the x-ray is a complimentary and valuable modality in evaluating the breast but must not, even when negative, preclude a biopsy when one is indicated by the physical findings.

Mammography for screening should be more selective and must be considered according to the risk of breast cancer.

i. High-Risk Patients. Patients at a significantly greater risk of developing breast cancer include patients with

- Previous carcinoma in one breast.

- Strong family history of carcinoma of the breast, especially if the carcinoma occurred in the mother and/or sisters and particularly if it was found prior to menopause.
- Patients with premalignant disease (e.g., papillomatosis). These patients should be advised to have, in addition to their quarterly physical examination, a yearly mammogram regardless of their age.

A screening mammography should be recommended for these patients at greater risk as part of their yearly physical examination every year, or at times even more often.

ii. Intermediate-Risk Patients. These include the following:

- Patients with extensive cystic mastitis, especially where previous surgery identified significant hyperplasia or atypia.
- Family history in distant relatives.

A baseline mammogram should be obtained in these patients at the time of their first examination. This can then be repeated every 3 years until age 40 or 45. After that age, mammography may be obtained yearly.

iii. Low-Risk Patients. Although patients in the following categories are actually at low risk, they might have a slight increase in incidence of breast cancer compared with the rest of the population at large. The indication for screening mammography in these cases must be individualized.

- Age. Predilection seems to be for women over 45, with the incidence increasing with advancing age.
- Menses. Women who have started to menstruate early and have a late menopause seem to be at higher risk.
- Childbearing. Risk is higher for those women who have never been pregnant or those who had their first pregnancy after age 30.
- Obesity or, possibly, dietary fat content.
- Drugs. No definite evidence exists to incriminate birth control pills, but the use of estrogens at menopause seem to lead to a higher incidence of breast cancer 15–20 years later.
- X-ray exposure of the breasts, particularly if exposure occurred between ages 10 and 19.

iv. Mass Screening. The use of a mammography for screening of broad segments of the population has been recommended on and off by some authorities who have conducted large-scale studies (the Health Insurance Plan of Greater New York and the Brooklyn Breast Cancer Demonstration Network, or BBCDN). The BBCDN study of 280,000 women detected 3557 cases of breast cancer, 41.6% of these were discovered by mammography only, and an additional 47.3% had palpable masses that could be demonstrated by mammography as well. Most important is the fact that 32.4% of the

cancers detected were either noninvasive or less than 1 cm in size. With the emergence of better x-ray equipment, delivering smaller doses of radiation (between 0.04 and 1 rad per study), it is felt by these groups that the risk is small and the yield worthwhile, and the most recent publications have recommended mammography on a yearly basis in all women over the age of 40. We believe that a bseline mammography, with additional studies done periodically according to the risk factor or specific indications is sufficient in women between 30 and 45. It seems more reasonable to limit the use of yearly screening mammography to patients over age 45.

b. Diagnostic Features of Mammography

Findings identified on mammography that are suggestive of carcinoma fall within a broad range of changes, some clearly diagnostic, others only suspicious. The following are some of the features suggestive of breast cancer:

- A mass with irregular borders and extensions into the adjacent parenchyma.
- Skin thickening and loss of definition of the subcutaneous fat layer.
- Skin retraction and/or dimpling.
- Stippled punctate calcifications within a mass or even in the absence of a mass.
- Venous engorgement.

Since mammography screening may detect a substantial number of tumors in the absence of a clinically identifiable mass, biopsy might have to be carried out on the basis of the radiological findings. The following recommendations should be followed in those circumstances:

- Repeat the mammography.
- Advise the patient of the blind nature of the procedure.
- Utilize some method of localizing the tumor prior to surgery in order to avoid large excisions. Several methods are available, including multiple projections with a grid or marker, needle localization during fluoroscopy, introduction of a hooked wire in the vicinity of the lesion under x-ray control, preoperative injection of the tumor site with a mixture of toluidine blue and Lipiodol with x-ray control.
- X-ray the specimen to insure that the removed tissues include the radiologically suspicious area.
- Defer definitive surgery until adequate study of the specimen is completed, unless a grossly identifiable carcinoma is found in the excised specimen and confirmed by frozen section.

c. Value of Mammography in Predicting Risk Factors

Identification of women at high risk for breast cancer on the basis of parenchymal patterns identified on mammography is a highly controversial issue. Although Wolfe's classification basing the risk on radiographic images indicating mammary dysplasia and prominent ducts is supported by a correlation of the histological studies and radiographic appearance of the breast parenchyma, there is not enough evidence to support sufficiently the "high-risk" contention in this group of patients in order to utilize mammographic patterns as indicators of a high-risk group that would require closer screening.

Wolfe's classification is as follows:

- N1. Predominantly fatty breast, no duct response. Extremely low-risk pattern.
- P1. Epithelial elements compose 25% of the breast and are predominantly subareolar. Low-risk pattern.
- P2. Entire breast contains epithelial components, both ductal or lobular, with prominent duct patterns. Great risk of incident cancers.
- DY. Extremely dense parenchyma, homogeneous with difficult-to-define duct patterns. Predominant in young glandular breasts and difficult to assess in terms of risk.

The P2 category can be further separated into three subsets: P2a with linear fibrotic shadows, P2b with nodular densities associated with severe lobular hyperplasia and atypia, and P2c, which includes both. The latter two types are considered to harbor the highest risk of incident breast cancer. The utilization of this type of "pattern" classification in clinical practice may be useful in selecting a subgroup of women (those with a P2 or DY pattern), particularly in the younger age group, that might benefit from closer follow-up. However, a significant number of N1 and P1 patterns present with carcinoma of the breast, making screening based on mammographic patterns an unrealistic concept.

4. Thermography

Although commonly done, especially in mass screening, its accuracy and interpretation leaves a great deal to be desired.

5. Diaphynography

The use of transillumination with photo recording of the image is a newer modality of identification of breast lesions. Its simplicity and safety make it desirable, but not enough experience has been accumulated to identify its value, either as a diagnostic tool, or for screening use.

6. Sonography

This has been also recommended by some, but its accuracy and yield have also been unpredictable and it appears to be of little usefulness.

II. PREOPERATIVE EVALUATION AND PREPARATION

A. Physical Evaluation

A distinction needs to be made between the patient with a "lump in the breast" of undetermined nature and the one with a suspicious or documented carcinoma of the breast.

1. Breast "Lump" of Undetermined Nature

In these cases, a good history with physical evaluation of the breast, axilla, and neck, aided by mammography, is the primary step. The risk factors should be assessed by obtaining a complete history, menstrual and gestational history, history of previous irradiation or hormonal intake, as well as history related to the breast itself:

- Pain, premenstrual tension, or swelling.
- Cyclic occurrence and changes related to the menstrual cycle.
- Past history of breast trauma, mastitis, or surgery.
- Nipple discharge, its character and site.
- Duration of the mass.

The physical examination must clearly define the characteristics of the mass as well as the texture of the rest of the breast:

- Description of the breasts.
- Location of the mass and its size.
- Consistency, shape, and borders.
- Mobility.
- Involvement of surrounding tissues (skin or muscle).
- Skin retraction, dimpling, or peau d'orange.
- Nipple retraction, erosion, or ulceration.
- Nipple discharge and its characteristics.

The axilla and neck must also be examined for nodes.

Reexamination at a different phase of the menstrual cycle, or needle aspiration of a suspected cystic lesion, can aid in the differential diagnosis and avoid an unnecessary operation. Mammography will also be of help in ruling out a carcinoma, but only when there is no clear-cut indication for a biopsy on clinical grounds. Biopsy of a "lump in the breast" of an undetermined nature will be dictated by:

- The presence of a discreet, definite mass on palpation, even if it is believed that this is benign.
- A suspicious mammographic finding.
- Any finding suggestive of carcinoma (e.g., retraction, peau d'orange, nipple erosion, bloody discharge, etc.).
- Even a poorly defined area in high-risk patients.

2. Breast Mass of a "Suspicious" Nature

In the patient with a suspicious or confirmed carcinoma of the breast, the preoperative evaluation of the patient can be divided into four phases:

- Physical evaluation of the tumor. Thorough evaluation of the breast, the axilla, the neck, and the tumor itself in order to define accurately the tumor, its stage, and its local extent is, of course, mandatory (see §2.II.E).
- Mammography is extremely important in order to define the lesion, evaluate the contralateral breast, and identify multicentricity or bilaterality of tumors.
- A complete physical examination is also mandatory to assess the patient's general condition, her ability to tolerate the projected therapy, and the presence of metastases.
- Biopsy.

B. Biopsy

Regardless of the clinical certainty of the diagnosis, no definitive therapy for breast cancer should ever be contemplated without positive tissue diagnosis. The biopsy may be one of three types.

1. Needle Biopsy

Needle biopsy, preferably done shortly before the projected definitive treatment, and using a large-bore tissue needle rather than a "needle aspiration" technique, is the preferred method of biopsy. This offers several advantages:

- It provides a firm diagnosis prior to hospitalization, thus facilitating planning.
- It enables the patient to know her diagnosis prior to being anesthetized and offers the surgeon the opportunity to discuss more specifically the diagnosis, prognosis, and various therapeutic options available, thus allowing the patient to participate in the decision as to the type of treatment or extent of surgery that she might have.
- It does not open up tissue planes, permits better planning of the incision and the surgery, and allows less skin sacrifice than if the mastectomy is done following an open biopsy.
- It may yield sufficient tissue for estrogen receptor and progesterone receptor studies by using qualitative immunofluorescent techniques for identification of the receptors.

2. Open Biopsy with Frozen Section

An open biopsy, preferably excisional, with frozen section is the age-old procedure that is still the most commonly employed type of biopsy. This technique, however, suffers primarily from the disadvantage of having to tell all patients about the possibility of a mastectomy. It also calls for a significant prolongation of anesthesia time and might complicate the mastectomy to a certain extent. An adequate open biopsy is, however, mandatory in the inoperable patient in order to establish the exact diagnosis and obtain enough tissue for proper receptor-site studies.

3. Two-Step Procedure

A two-step procedure, with a biopsy followed within a few days by the definitive therapy, is becoming more and more acceptable and offers most of the advantages of the needle biopsy except that it requires two anesthesias and a larger excision at the time of mastectomy. Furthermore, the delay between the biopsy and the definitive surgery could be detrimental in terms of tumor spread, especially if it exceeds 30 days. In addition, the psychological trauma of having to be told postoperatively that the tumor was malignant and that the patient must return to the operating room for definitive surgery, may even exceed the stress of having to sign a preoperative consent for "possible mastectomy."

It must be stressed that a most important part of the assessment of the tumor besides the establishment of a histological diagnosis, is the measurement of the estrogen and progesterone receptor proteins of the tumor. This must always be done on the biopsy, or on the mastectomy specimen in cases where only a needle biopsy has been done for diagnosis. More than any other factor besides the stage of the disease, the presence or absence of estrogen and progesterone receptors in the tumor determines the prognosis of the disease and guides the physician as to the type of adjunctive or palliative measures that might be helpful to the patient. Patients with negative receptors or low values generally have a poorer prognosis and are not likely to benefit from any endocrine ablation or hormonal manipulation, regardless of their menstrual status.

C. Assessment of Possible Metastatic Disease

The evaluation of a patient for possible metastases depends on the tumor and its natural history, the stage of the disease, and the yield of various tests as compared with their cost effectiveness. Bones, lungs and liver are, in this order, the most commonly affected organs in metastatic breast cancer. In aggressive breast cancer, metastatic spread occurs in a high percentage of patients and it is, therefore, incumbent upon the surgeon to try to identify such spread prior to definitive therapy.

II. PREOPERATIVE EVALUATION AND PREPARATION

1. Stage I

All patients with breast cancer, including those with Stage I disease (T1, N0: tumors less than 2 cm with negative axilla) must have a complete blood count (CBC) and urinalysis, chest x-ray, and a multichannel biochemical profile (SMA-12) with special attention paid to serum phosphatase and liver enzymes. If these determinations are all within normal limits, it is unlikely that further evaluation will result in a significant yield. At this stage of the disease, the incidence of distant metastases is rather low, and no further testing is necessary unless suggested by a symptom or physical finding.

2. Stage II

With an incidence of bone metastases as high as 80% being reported in some retrospective studies, it is wise in all patients with Stage II disease (T2, N0 or T1 or T2 each with N1: tumors between 2 and 5 cm with or without movable axillary lymph nodes) to obtain a bone scan. If a suspicious lesion is identified on a scan, it should be confirmed by other methods (e.g., bone x-rays). The yield and accuracy of liver scanning is disappointing, and it should be obtained only in patients whose liver enzymes are consistently elevated or whose livers are enlarged on palpation, suggesting possible liver metastases.

Other specific tests need to be ordered whenever symptoms suggest the possibility of other types of metastases (e.g., bone pains, neurological complaints, hypercalcemia, chronic cough, etc.) A computerized axial tomography (CAT) scan or conventional tomograms of the chest, although extremely accurate, are not cost effective on a routine basis; they must be obtained, however, if routine x-rays of the chest show the slightest abnormality or in patients whose clinical symptoms suggest pulmonary metastases.

3. Stage III

The cure rate in this category of patients is such that, most often, treatment is only palliative. One must, therefore, go to all lengths to identify metastases in order to avoid unnecessary mutilating procedures. SMA-12, chest x-ray, tomograms or CAT scan of the lung, bone scan and bone survey of any suspicious area, liver scan and any other test that might be indicated by unexplained signs or symptoms, CAT scan of the brain, bone marrow biopsy, etc. must all be done prior to undertaking any definitive procedure in patients with Stage III disease (any T3 lesion with N0 or N1, and any T with N2: tumors over 5 cm or those tumors with skin or chest-wall fixation or those with attached axillary nodes). These tests can be deferred when a clean-up ("toilet") mastectomy is contemplated as a preliminary therapeutic step; they can then be obtained while the patient is recovering from her surgery.

D. Preoperative Preparation

Most operable patients with breast cancer are in a satisfactory general condition and only rarely require any preoperative support such as nutrition, electrolyte repletion, or blood transfusion. On the other hand, psychological support is most important in these patients; not only are they frightened by the prospect of "cancer" or the unknown of "surgery," but they also need to face the possibility of "mastectomy" with its defeminizing and cosmetic implications. This type of support often can be adequately given by the surgeon and the primary care physician but requires several patient, unhurried, honest, and warm encounters. A nurse oncologist can, on admission, be most helpful in offering the patient explanations, answers, and much needed support prior to the surgery. Some patients might even benefit from more formal evaluation and support by a psychiatric nurse or a psychiatrist, and when a mastectomy is definitely going to be done, a preoperative visit by a volunteer from the "Reach-to-Recovery" program could go a long way in aiding and reassuring the patient. It is often necessary to continue these contacts postoperatively to the extent indicated by the patient's needs.

Patients with advanced Stage IV disease, especially when bone or brain metastases are clinically apparent, may require correction of certain specific physiological aberrations prior to instituting therapy:

- Serum calcium may have to be controlled in a patient with acute hypercalcemia from bone metastases; hydration with diuretics, corticosteroids, mithramycin, dialysis, etc. may be necessary to reduce the serum calcium.
- Corticosteroids may also be necessary to reduce cerebral edema in cases of brain metastases.
- Nutritional and blood volume support might be required.
- Fixation of impending fractures may be desirable in selected cases.

It goes without saying that patients who require preparation as a result of a preexisting medical condition should have such preparation prior to surgery. For example, diabetes control, restoration of coagulation defects, effective compensation of cardiac status, inhalation therapy, physiotherapy, etc. should all be carried out prior to undertaking the definitive treatment of the cancer.

E. Site-Specific Data Form for Cancer of the Breast (see p. 74)

SITE-SPECIFIC DATA FORM—BREAST CANCER

HISTORY

Age: _____

Lump detected by: _____ patient _____ on routine exam
_____ other health professional _____ mammogram

Duration of history: _____

Previous history of:
_____ Breast trauma
_____ Mastitis
_____ Breast surgery
_____ Nipple discharge
_____ Benign tumor

Previous history of carcinoma
Site: _____
Rx: _____

Obstetrical history
_____ Para
_____ Breast fed
_____ Last menstrual period

Menstrual history
Onset: Age: _____
Duration: _____
Periodicity: Every _____ days
Menopause: Date: _____
Type: _____ natural
_____ surgical

Medication history (duration)
_____ Estrogen _____
_____ Progesterone _____
_____ Androgen _____
_____ Contraceptives _____
_____ Other _____

Family history (complete only if applicable):
Carcinoma of breast: _____ Mother _____ Sister _____ Daughter _____ Aunt _____ Grandmother
When: _____ Premenopausal _____ Postmenopausal
Carcinoma of other site (specify site):
Previous biopsy: _____ No _____ Yes _____ Type _____ Report

PHYSICAL EXAMINATION

Size
_____ Carcinoma *in situ*
_____ Paget's disease without tumor mass
_____ >0.0 and <2.0 cm diameter
_____ >2.0 and <5.0 cm diameter
_____ >5.0 cm diameter

Extent
_____ Fixation to underlying fascia or muscle
_____ Fixation to chest wall
_____ Skin changes: edema, ulcer, satellite nodules
_____ Inflammatory carcinoma (microscopic dermal lymphatic permeation)
_____ Edema of arm

Consistency of afflicted breast
Breast mass is _____ Mobile _____ Fixed _____ Erythema _____ Dimpling _____ Satellite nodules
Nipple has _____ Discharge _____ Retraction _____ Neither

RIGHT

A
B C
F
D E

LATERAL

NP

LEFT

G
J H
M
L K

LYMPH NODES

_____ Palpable _____ Nonpalpable

	Side		Size (cm)				
	R	L	0–2	2–4	>4	Fixation	Number
Low axillary	_____	_____	_____	_____	_____	_____	_____
Middle axillary	_____	_____	_____	_____	_____	_____	_____
Axillary apex	_____	_____	_____	_____	_____	_____	_____
Interpectoral	_____	_____	_____	_____	_____	_____	_____
Infraclavicular	_____	_____	_____	_____	_____	_____	_____
Ipsilateral supraclavicular	_____	_____	_____	_____	_____	_____	_____

Distant metastases: _____ No _____ Yes _____ Lung _____ Liver _____ Bone _____ Other
Histologic diagnosis: _____

PREOPERATIVE WORK-UP (Check, if done)

	Neg.	Pos.	Suspicious		Neg.	Pos.	Suspicious
Calcium	_____	_____	_____	Bone survey	_____	_____	_____
Alkaline phosphatase	_____	_____	_____	Liver chemistry	_____	_____	_____
Chest x-ray	_____	_____	_____	Liver scan	_____	_____	_____
Chest tomogram or CAT	_____	_____	_____	Bone marrow			
Mammogram				Aspiration	_____	_____	_____
(ipsilateral)	_____	_____	_____	Biopsy	_____	_____	_____
(contralateral)	_____	_____	_____	Other	_____	_____	_____
Bone scan	_____	_____	_____				

Classification:
_____ T (local tumor)
_____ N (regional lymph node)
_____ M (distant metastases)
Stage: _____

Signature: _____
Countersignature: _____
Date: _____

Primary Tumor

TX   Tumor cannot be assessed

T1S   Preinvasive carcinoma (carcinoma *in situ*), noninfiltrating intraductal carcinoma or Paget's disease of the nipple with no demonstrable tumor

T0   No demonstrable tumor in the breast

T1   Tumor 2 cm or less in greatest dimension

T1A   With no fixation to underlying pectoral fascia and/or muscle

T1B   With fixation to underlying pectoral fascia and/or muscle

T2   Tumor more than 2 cm but not more than 5 cm in its greatest dimension

T2A   With no fixation to underlying pectoral fascia and/or muscle

T2B   With fixation to underlying pectoral fascia and/or muscle

T3   Tumor more than 5 cm in greatest dimension

T3A   With no fixation to underlying pectoral fascia and/or muscle

T3B   With fixation to underlying pectoral fascia and/or muscle

T4   Tumor of any size with direct extension to the chest wall or skin. Note: Chest wall includes ribs, intercostal muscles, and serratus anterior muscle, but not pectoral muscle

T4A   With fixation to chest wall

T4B   With edema (included peau d'orange), ulceration of the skin of the breast, or satellite skin nodules confined to the same breast

T4C   Both of above

Dimpling of the skin, nipple retraction, or any other skin changes except those in T4B may occur in T1, T2, or T3 without affecting the classification.

Regional Lymph Node

NX   Regional lymph nodes cannot be assessed clinically

N0   No palpable homolateral axillary nodes

N1   Movable homolateral axillary nodes

N1A   Nodes not considered to contain growth

N1B   Nodes considered to contain growth

N2   Homolateral axillary nodes considered to contain growth and fixed to one another or to other structures

N3   Homolateral supraclavicular or infraclavicular nodes considered to contain growth or edema of the arm
      Note: Edema of the arm may be caused by lymphatic obstruction, lymph nodes may not then be palpable.

Distant Metastases

MX   Not assessed

M0   No evidence of distant metastases

M1   Distant metastases present, including skin involvement beyond the breast area

Stage Groupings

T1S—Carcinoma *in situ*
Invasive carcinoma

Stage I	T1, N0, M0
Stage II	T1, N1, M0
	T2, N0 or N1
	M0
Stage III	Any T3 with any N
	Any T4 with any N
	Any T with any N2 } M0
	Any T with N3
Stage IV	Any T, any N with M1

F. Multidisciplinary Consultation and Evaluation

The need for a multidisciplinary approach to consultation and evaluation, and even to treatment, of the patient with breast cancer is obvious and paramount. The use of such a multidisciplinary approach should be encouraged; it can only be carried out, however, after implementation of a program where a multidisciplinary consultation and evaluation of an advisory nature is available and established.

A multidisciplinary approach in breast cancer is essential and includes a number of specialties, the importance of which must be emphasized. The primary care physician must be included as part of the team; his or her knowledge of and intimacy with the patient, as well as the patient's trust and personal relationship with him or her is extremely important. This physician's help will be required in all phases of treatment and must be utilized. Beside the traditional treating specialties of breast surgery, radiotherapy, and medical oncology, other specialties also offer the patient with breast cancer an expertise that is not always available within the three primary treating disciplines. Among these specialties are pathology, nursing oncology, psychosocial services, rehabilitation medicine, prosthetic rehabilitation, and plastic and reconstructive surgery. All these specialties are essential at one or another stage in the care of the cancer patient. It is conceivable that one highly specialized individual caring for the breast cancer patient may be able to utilize these specialties at the proper time and with discrimination, particularly when dealing with the simpler types of tumors; for most situations, however, evaluation and advice prior to treatment by representatives of several of these disciplines would be of great value.

III. THERAPEUTIC MANAGEMENT

The surgical treatment of the local tumor-bearing area in the patient with operable breast cancer is undoubtedly one of the most controversial issues in surgical oncology today. Furthermore, few areas in surgical oncology are undergoing such rapid changes, both in concepts and methodology—changes often resulting from large, multi-institutional, randomized prospective clinical trials. Challenges have been raised to the most elementary, basic principles of cancer surgery, such as

- The danger of spread during the period between biopsy and definitive surgery.
- The importance of monobloc resection of the primary tumor and its first area of spread.
- The need to remove the first echelon of lymphatics, in a tumor in which lymphatic invasion is an important mode of spread.

- The importance of wide total removal of the tumor-bearing organ, particularly with a tumor that has a tendency to be multicentric.

Often these challenges have been supported by large-scale clinical trials. Some leading figures in the field of breast cancer have even made statements that indicate that the treatment of the primary tumor in breast cancer patients makes little or no difference to the outcome.

Notwithstanding such extreme positions, however, and taking into account all of the above changes in concepts and the current controversies, it is nevertheless important to examine the subject rationally and establish guidelines for the treatment of the patient with breast cancer. It is also of value to try to identify indications for the various surgical procedures currently employed.

A. Definition of the Various Surgical Procedures

1. Lumpectomy

Removal of the actual tumor with a small margin of normal tissues around it, as is done during an excisional biopsy.

2. Segmental Mastectomy or Quarterectomy

Removal of a large segment of the breast ranging from 25–40% of the breast gland. This might include excision of an ellipse of overlying skin and usually extends in depth to and beyond the pectoralis fascia.

3. Simple Mastectomy

This procedure involves a total removal of the breast gland and could be done in one of three ways depending on the indication:

- Subcutaneous mastectomy with preservation or reimplantation of the nipples. This is the procedure of choice in the rare case where one is performing a prophylactic mastectomy (contralateral mastectomy) or a mastectomy performed for extensive recurrent fibrocystic disease; it has also been suggested by some in carcinoma *in situ* or diffuse papillomatosis.
- Amputation of the breast. This may be carried out for palliation in an elderly poor-risk patient under local anesthesia or in Stage III or IV disease, when it is sufficient for clean-up mastectomy.
- Simple mastectomy for cure. This procedure includes removal of the subcutaneous lymphatics by raising the usual flaps and excision of the pectoralis fascia. It is often combined with sampling, or at times, excision of some or all of

the axillary nodes for prognosis and planning of adjuvant therapy.

4. Modified Radical Mastectomy

A modified radical mastectomy involves performing a simple mastectomy as described above in continuity with a total axillary dissection but with preservation of the pectoralis major (and at times the pectoralis minor) muscle.

5. Radical Mastectomy

The standard Halsted radical mastectomy is a monobloc procedure where the breast, the axillary lymphatics and all intervening tissues (namely the pectoral muscles and interpectoral nodes) are removed.

6. Supraradical Mastectomy

Various procedures have been described where the standard radical mastectomy is extended to resect additional lymphatic reservoirs that have been identified to be the site of spread in selected cases of breast cancer. Thus, in addition to radical mastectomy, the following procedures are added: supraclavicular dissection and dissection of internal mammary nodes.

Three main factors seem to influence the decision as to which procedure is best suited for a specific patient:

- The stage of the disease.
- The histological nature of the tumor, which often helps predict its behavior.
- The cosmetic disability resulting from therapy, which influences the patient and physician to select one modality over another.

B. Treatment according to the Stage of Disease

Most important in selecting the type of surgical procedure best suited to the patient is an accurate classification of the tumor and its stage.

1. Carcinoma *in Situ*

Two main controversies exist in reference to the treatment of carcinoma *in situ* (whether these be lobular carcinomas *in situ* or noninvasive intraductal carcinomas):

- The need for total mastectomy. This seems to be dictated by the multifocal nature and multicentricity of the disease. Although the use of local excision and radiotherapy has been advocated by some, most feel that a wide total subcutaneous mastectomy (with or without preservation of the nipple) should be done and can easily be followed by reconstruction.
- The bilaterality of the disease. This has raised some questions as to the treatment of the opposite breast. Bilateral mastectomy or elective contralateral mastectomy appears hard to justify in the presence of premalignant disease but has been hotly debated in the invasive and infiltrating lobular and intraductal carcinoma, where the same multicentricity and bilaterality has been demonstrated.

2. Stage I

Stage I breast cancer includes T0 and T1 tumors with N0, that is tumors less than 2 cm in size without evidence of any clinically involved axillary nodes. As a result of early detection and mass screening, more patients are being seen with early breast cancer today than ever before. Those are the patients best suited for conservation surgery. A mounting number of series are being reported suggesting that lumpectomy or quarterectomy, with axillary sampling or node dissection, followed by radiotherapy if the nodes are negative and/or chemotherapy if the nodes are positive, is as effective as mastectomy (approximately 85% long-term cure rates were reported by Veronesi in over 700 cases). This option may, therefore, be offered to patients with T1, N0 disease; more time however, needs to elapse before any dogmatic statement can be made as to the exact value and place of lumpectomy in the treatment of breast cancer and before it can be recommended on a routine basis. Until then, the treatment of choice for patients with Stage I breast cancer remains similar to that for Stage II.

3. Stage II

This stage includes patients with any T2, N0 or with any T0, T1, or T2 with N1, that is, tumors up to 5 cm with or without evidence of clinically involved movable nodes in the axilla.) These are the patients about whom the greatest controversy exists, with procedures being recommended ranging from supraradical mastectomy to lumpectomy.

In addition to the surgical treatments described in the following sections, the need for adjuvant chemotherapy in Stage II disease is today well recognized and must be encouraged. There is still some controversy as to whether radiotherapy and/or chemotherapy is the best choice of adjuvant treatment, especially in the T2, N0 patients or patients with medial or subareolar lesions where a high incidence of internal mammary nodes, demonstrated to be usually radiosensitive, might be anticipated. Several reports, however, seem to demonstrate that chemotherapy is equally effective in controlling local recurrence and has the advantage of also being systemic therapy. This will be discussed in a later section of these guidelines.

a. Supraradical Mastectomy with Dissection of the Internal Mammary Nodes

This operation was devised to overcome the failures resulting from the high incidence of internal mammary node metastases (30–60%) in patients with medial and subareolar tumors. The morbidity and mortality associated with this procedure, coupled with the ability to control node metastases of small size by radiotherapy, have caused this procedure to be almost totally abandoned.

b. Standard Radical Mastectomy

For several decades, this has been the standard procedure for the treatment of breast cancer, and it complies with all the basic requirements of a "good" cancer operation. Recently, however, it has been challenged because of the cosmetic disability that ensues. Besides the loss of the breast, the additional loss of the pectoral muscles causes a subclavicular indentation that is difficult to cover with the usual prosthetic devices or wearing apparel. Over the past decade, modified radical mastectomy has largely replaced the standard radical mastectomy, and although many specific instances of local failure may well be attributable to the modified radical mastectomy, large-scale statistical studies indicate no difference in long-term results. Radical mastectomy, however, could still be carried out in the following circumstances:

- Patients with large nodes, particularly high in the axilla or deep to the muscle.
- Medial lesions, especially if large or deep in the breast and, particularly, in small breasts.
- Attachment of the tumor to the muscles or the fascia makes a radical mastectomy almost mandatory.

c. Modified Radical Mastectomy

This procedure is today the most widely used operation for Stage II breast cancer. The preservation of the pectoralis major muscle offers a better cosmetic result and, more importantly, permits an easier and more effective surgical reconstruction of the breast if this is desired by the patient at a later date.

d. Simple Mastectomy

This approach offers little or no cosmetic or functional advantage over the modified radical mastectomy. Although it could be effective if associated with an axillary node dissection (called "extended simple" by some, "modified radical" by others) and/or adjunctive radiotherapy or chemotherapy, the sacrifice of the breast makes it of little value as a conservation operation, and it therefore has little place in the treatment of Stage II breast cancer.

e. Lumpectomy or Segmental Mastectomy

More recently, attempts at preserving the breast have encouraged numerous clinical trials in which less than a total mastectomy has been carried out along with axillary node sampling followed by radiotherapy and chemotherapy if the nodes are positive. This approach is still in an investigative stage, particularly for patients with clinically involved nodes; it can, however, be used if the patient so wishes after being informed of the risk.

4. Stage III

This stage includes patients with T3, T4, or any T with N2 or N3—that is, patients with tumors over 5 cm in size or tumors fixed to the skin or chest wall and patients with matted or fixed nodes but no demonstrable distant metastases. It is well recognized that the survival and cure of such patients is not usually much influenced by the local treatment. Therapy therefore, must include measures designed for systemic disease in addition to the treatment planned for control of the primary. Attempts at avoiding breast amputations by the use of radiotherapy for control of the primary disease are reasonable.

Surgery should be limited to patients in whom radiotherapy and chemotherapy have failed to control the local disease; segmental, simple, or even radical mastectomy for residual tumors in the breast or axilla are selectively indicated. Clean-up mastectomy is also indicated in cases where it would facilitate the total care of the patient and/or the administration of radiotherapy.

5. Stage IV

Stage IV disease, where distant metastases can be identified, is obviously incurable, and any consideration of surgical intervention must be based on its palliative nature. Open biopsy to establish the histological nature and status of hormone receptors of the tumor must always be done.

Clean-up mastectomy is sometimes indicated after chemotherapy and/or radiotherapy, to eliminate residual disease that threatens to cause serious local problems. The end stage of local disease, with an ulcerating, exophytic, foul-smelling lesion or with wide-spreading *en cuirasse* disease is undoubtedly one of the most distressing situations for the patient; it should be prevented, whenever possible. It is sometimes preferable to carry out a clean-up mastectomy prior to chemotherapy whenever the breast or the tumor is so large as to preclude effective use of radiotherapy; in addition, the reduction of the bulk of the tumor might enchance the chemotherapy effect on distant disease.

Local resection of skin recurrence is often indicated in conjunction with chemotherapy. Extensive local resections of various types, requiring at times formidable reconstructive procedures, are even occasionally indicated to eliminate deeply infiltrating and destructive local disease (particularly after radiotherapy) in a patient who is otherwise well controlled with systemic therapy.

With the exception of oophorectomy, which is still often the primary therapeutic step in the management of a premenopausal patient with metastases and elevated estrogen/progesterone receptors, endocrine ablative procedures (adrenalectomy, hypophysectomy) are today rarely necessary and have been widely replaced by hormonal manipulation and hormonal antagonists (i.e., Tamoxifen or aminoglutethimide).

C. Histological Nature of the Disease and Its Therapeutic Implications

1. Pathological Varieties of Breast Cancer

Although most breast cancers fall into the broad category of the infiltrating duct cell adenocarcinoma or scirrhous carcinoma, there are several other different histological types that display slightly different behaviors that might justify some alteration in the therapeutic approach.

The following less common tumors, seem to have a slightly less aggressive course and a lower incidence of metastatic nodes:

- Medullary carcinomas.
- Colloid, or pure mucinous, carcinomas.
- Papillary carcinomas.
- Tubular carcinomas.

In addition, the following tumors have specific characteristics that will impact on their treatment:

- Paget's disease of the nipple, with or without a palpable tumor, behaves exactly like the infiltrating duct cell tumors and should be treated in the same manner.
- Lobular carcinoma must be recognized as a slightly lower grade tumor but with a high propensity for bilaterality. A reported incidence of simultaneous bilateral lobular carcinoma of 11–13% (in the absence of contralateral clinical findings) has encouraged some surgeons to carry out contralateral random or mirror-image biopsies in all patients with lobular carcinoma of the breast. This approach has not been widely accepted. It is mandatory, however, to carry out very close follow-up evaluations of these patients and to consider an early wide biopsy of the contralateral breast at the slightest suggestion of a mass or irregularity identified on clinical or mammographic examinations.
- Invasive intraductal carcinoma is also fraught with a very high incidence of multicentricity and bilaterality and must

be approached in a similar fashion as the invasive lobular carcinoma.
- Cystosarcoma Phyllodes is an entirely different tumor than the duct cell carcinoma. It seems to represent a variant of a giant fibroadenoma and can histologically be benign or malignant. These tumors rarely spread to lymph nodes, are almost never multicentric, and when malignant, will spread mainly through the bloodstream. The recommended treatment is, therefore, a wide local excision in the smaller and/or benign lesions, a total mastectomy for the more common large tumors and/or the malignant ones.

In addition to the histological nature of the tumor, its type and grading are extremely important in evaluating the prognosis and determining how aggressive the treatment needs to be. Tumors should be typed according to Ackerman's typing and graded according to their degree of differentiation, and the identification of vascular, perineural, or lymphatic involvement should be noted. The use of adjuvant therapy is often determined by these characteristics as well as by the stage of the disease. Some have even recommended adjuvant chemotherapy in Stage I patients if their tumors are identified as very aggressive.

2. Types of Mammary Carcinoma (Ackerman)

- TYPE I: all *in-Situ* Carcinomas
  - Intraductal carcinoma with or without Paget's disease.
  - Intraductal papillary carcinoma.
  - Lobular carcinoma *in situ*.

(Numerous blocks should be obtained in all Type I tumors to rule out invasion.)

- TYPE II: low-grade carcinoma
  - Pure mucinous carcinoma.
  - Well-differentiated tubular carcinoma.
  - Invasive papillary carcinoma.
  - Medullary carcinoma.
- TYPE III: Ordinary invasive carcinoma
  - Invasive duct cell carcinoma.
  - Intraductal carcinoma with invasion.
  - Invasive lobular carcinoma.
  - All carcinomas not classified as Types I, II, and IV.
- TYPE IV: undifferentiated carcinomas, signet-ring carcinoma, all tumors with blood vessel invasion.

3. Grading of Mammary Carcinoma

The grading by the World Health Organization is based on

- Tubule formation (1–3 points).
- Hyperchromatism and mitoses (1–3 points).
- Irregularity of size, shape, and staining of nuclei (1–3 points).

The following summarizes the relation between tumor grade and survivals.

	Survival %	
Grade	5 Years	10 Years
I (3–5 points)	75	45
II (6–7 points)	53	27
III (8–9 points)	31	18

4. Pathological Description of the Specimen

Each description of surgical specimens of mammary carcinoma should contain the following information:

- Gross

    Size of tumor in centimeters (less than 1 cm, favorable; over 2 cm, unfavorable).

    Location of tumor within the breast (middle quadrants, unfavorable).

    Size of the breast.

    Relationship of tumor to the skin (unfavorable if the skin is involved).

    Relationship of tumor to the fascia and muscle (unfavorable if involved).

- Microscopic

    Description of cell type.

    Type of tumor (Type I, favorable), Types II, III, and IV, increasingly unfavorable).

    Grade of tumor (progressively unfavorable with higher grade).

    Evidence of lymphatic and blood vessel invasion (unfavorable).

    Lymphoplasmocytic infiltrates around the tumor (favorable).

    Margins of tumor (pushing, favorable; rootlike, unfavorable).

    Number of lymph nodes identified and examined.

    Number of lymph nodes involved by carcinoma.

    Extranodal extension of lymph node metastases (unfavorable).

    Presence of sinus histiocytosis within the lymph nodes (favorable).

    Involvement of the nipple (unfavorable).

    Secondary focuses of carcinoma in the same breast specimen (unfavorable).

Such data has been found by various authors to have a prognostic significance in large groups of patients studied. Favorable ratings in any individual patient should not cajole the treating physician into omitting essential steps in breast cancer therapy. Unfavorable ratings, on the other hand, should urge the physician to apply, without unnecessary delay, vigorous means of therapy.

D. Cosmetic Considerations

The impact of the loss of a breast on a woman—the cosmetic and potentially defeminizing effect that it can have and its associated psychological effect—has forced both patients and physicians to reassess their approach to breast cancer. From this have evolved

- The more commonly utilized conservation procedures (modified mastectomy, lumpectomy).
- The heightened awareness of the public at large, promoted by wide media exposure, of the various options available.
- The attempt at allowing patients to participate in the final decision making and the recognition of the fact that the patient has the right to opt for a compromise approach after being told the possible consequences.
- Promotion of early reconstructive procedures.

Although it may appear at times that this has hampered the choice of treatment of certain patients, in an overall setting with an intelligent patient and a patient surgeon and the assistance of the primary care physician, it does work toward a better total end result, not only in terms of cure, but also in terms of the cosmetic and psychological rehabilitation of the patient.

IV. CARCINOMA OF THE BREAST IN PREGNANCY

Management of the patient with breast cancer during pregnancy demands immediate concerted action on the part of all concerned. Carcinoma of the breast is recognized as being hormonal dependent to a great extent, and the extremely high levels of estrogens present during gestation have been known to result in wild progression of the disease in patients with untreated breast tumors, as well as in patients with subclinical metastatic disease many years following what appeared to be successful control of the cancer by mastectomy or other local regional therapy.

A. Management of the Breast Tumor

The presence of any discrete mass in the breast in a patient that is pregnant requires immediate evaluation and identification; engorgement of the breasts, cystic changes, nodularity, and breast abscesses that are all so common during gestation must be identified and appropriately ruled out by aspiration, antibiotics, supportive measures, incision and drainage, etc. Any persistent mass, regardless of its apparent benign nature (e.g., fibroadenoma), must be biopsied or, preferably, excised without delay. This can be done under local anesthesia as an office procedure and need not threaten the pregnancy in any way. If a diagnosis of carcinoma is clinically suspected or identified at the time of biopsy or excision of an apparently benign tumor, appropriate management of the breast cancer must immediately be instituted, regardless of the stage of the pregnancy. Treatment will be along the same lines as that previously described for breast cancer in general.

B. Management of the Pregnancy

Handling of the pregnancy is more difficult, although it would seem reasonable to interrupt the pregnancy simultaneously with or immediately before the treatment of the breast cancer. Such an approach is not always practical and depends to a great extent on the patient's wishes and needs, as well as on various emotional, social, and religious circumstances. It is often necessary for the treating physician to understand the needs of the patient and sometimes to compromise in what he or she believes is the ideal method of treatment. Nevertheless, certain recommendations seem appropriate:

- In all patients where gestation has gone far enough to result in a viable baby, delivery should be carried out immediately either by induction of labor or by cesarean section, and treatment of the cancer should be initiated shortly thereafter.
- In the first 12 weeks of gestation, especially in a young woman who can still bear a child 2 or 3 years later, it is prudent to carry out an abortion, preferably by suction curettage, and to proceed with the treatment of the cancer without delay.
- In other patients where religious convictions do not stand as an obstacle and where the ability to bear children a few years hence exists, or where the need and desire to have an additional child are not overwhelming, termination of the pregnancy is advised regardless of the stage of gestation and by whatever method is deemed advisable by the obstetrician at that stage of gestation.
- In those women in their second trimester where the desire to continue the gestation to a viable fetus is keen or where religious convictions prohibit abortion under ordinary circumstances, the physician must evaluate several parameters before attempting to convince the patient or obtain religious dispensation for an interruption of the pregnancy:

  The patient's religious beliefs and the intensity of her convictions.

The patient's age and parity. A patient in her late 30s or 40s, without other children might be permitted to take a calculated risk.

Socioeconomic conditions and marital harmony must be taken into account, and the husband's feelings and wishes kept in mind.

The stage and type of disease is of some importance; for example, a patient with a noninvasive intraductal or lobular carcinoma *in situ*, might well be allowed to complete her pregnancy after her mastectomy, whereas a patient with a T3 carcinoma with vascular invasion identified microscopically would not.

The need for adjuvant therapy, whether radiotherapy or chemotherapy (large, bulky tumors, or Stage II disease) would militate against the wisdom of permitting continuation of gestation.

The reliability of the patient and the ability to keep a very close observation is most important if one permits continuation of the pregnancy.

The status of estrogen and progesterone receptors is also extremely important.

- In patients who are irrevocably opposed to interruption of pregnancy for any one of a number of reasons, it is incumbent on the treating physician to respect the patient's and her family's decision. Surgical treatment of the cancer must be carried out and is safe at almost any phase of the pregnancy. Adjuvant therapy may, however, have to be deferred to avoid injury to the fetus, and the patient must be very closely observed. Resumption of treatment, use of adjuvant therapy, interruption of the pregnancy, and even oophorectomy must all be considered if the disease recurs or metastases appear.

C. Endocrine Ablation

The indication for oophorectomy for carcinoma of the breast during pregnancy has also been a subject of great controversy. In the case of Stage III disease or greater where interruption of the pregnancy is being carried out, or in a patient who may already have several children or is in a perimenopausal age, an oophorectomy during the cesarean section would appear indicated and desirable and should be carried out if the patient consents. In all other cases, the oophorectomy will have the same moral and psychological implications as the abortion, and again all the factors discussed above must be taken into account.

The advisability of allowing further pregnancies in a patient who is apparently cured of breast cancer is also not clear-cut. The decision must weigh the stage of the disease and the likelihood of recurrence or metastases, as against the age and parity of the patient and her need for additional children. In any case, it is ordinarily recommended that the patient wait a minimum of 2–3 years after treatment before considering becoming pregnant again.

It must be made perfectly clear that, because of the nature of the controversies that govern the management of breast cancer, the guidelines outlined above for the treatment of breast cancer must by necessity be extremely broad. Diametrically opposed approaches are being promoted by surgeons of expertise with claims of equally effective results. Furthermore, because of the large number of clinical trials being carried out nationwide and the various recommendations resulting from these studies, the treatment of breast cancer is changing everyday, and any guideline manual will have to be updated at frequent intervals to be of any value.

V. THE ROLE OF RADIOTHERAPY
IN THE TREATMENT
OF BREAST CANCER

A. Radiotherapy as an Adjuvant Modality

A certain group of patients with operable breast cancer have a higher incidence of local and/or regional recurrences. These include

- Patients with lesions larger than 5 cm in diameter or those with deep involvement of the muscle or involvement of the skin.
- Tumors that show widespread lymphatic permeation.
- Tumors in the medial half of the breast or those centrally located tumors where internal mammary nodes are often involved.
- Patients with large metastatic axillary nodes, in whom the tumor extends beyond the capsule of the lymph nodes and invades the surrounding tissues.
- Patients with positive lymph nodes at the apex of the axilla.

Postoperative radiotherapy in these cases will reduce the incidence of postoperative local and/or regional recurrences. The extent of the treatment to be given will depend on the reason for giving the postoperative therapy (e.g., patients with medial or central lesions should receive treatment primarily to the internal mammary chain). Moderate doses of radiotherapy in the order of 5000 rads in 5 weeks are adequate to control microscopic disease in the high-risk areas irradiated postoperatively and should be delivered as soon as possible after surgery, unless the patient is receiving adjuvant chemotherapy.

B. Radiotherapy as a Primary Modality

1. Stage I

A large number of series reported recently from several major centers have shown that radiotherapy following lumpectomy with axillary sampling in T1 and early T2 disease (those tumors that are less than 2 cm or between 2 and 5 cm without nodal involvement) offers results as good as those obtained by the standard radical mastectomy and yet has the advantage of preservation of the breast. This option, therefore, may be offered to patients with clinical T1, N0 and T2, N0 disease. Radiotherapy is given to the breast and all draining lymph node areas to a dose of 5000 rads in 5 weeks, followed by a booster dose to the site of the primary tumor in the breast, giving an additional 1000–1500 rads in 1–1.5 weeks. Careful treatment planning is important in order to be able to get a good cosmetic result, which is the most important factor in planning this type of treatment.

2. Stage III

Patients with Stage III disease (where the tumor is either over 5 cm or attached to the chest wall, or when axillary nodes are matted and attached) have a much higher incidence of local recurrence if local disease is managed by surgery alone. Therefore, these patients should either be treated primarily by radiotherapy, or by surgery (where surgery results in the removal of the bulk of the disease in the breast) followed by postoperative radiotherapy. If radiotherapy is used as the primary modality of treatment, high doses are required to control areas of gross disease (doses in the order of 6000–7000 rads in 6–7 weeks). Systemic therapy should be instituted as soon as possible in these patients, as they are at high risk for disseminated disease.

3. Recurrent Breast Cancer

Patients with recurrent disease, either locally on the chest wall or involving the regional lymph nodes in the axilla, supraclavicular fossa, or internal mammary region, should be treated primarily by radiotherapy. The interaction of the different chemotherapy drugs with radiotherapy and the possibly greater intensity of local reactions following chemotherapy should be kept in mind when administering radiotherapy to these patients. Once a patient shows local recurrence, she should receive radiotherapy to the entire chest wall and all draining lymph node areas, irrespective of the site of recurrence; the latter site will however have to receive an additional boost to control the gross recurrent disease. The surgical removal of the local recurrence to confirm the diagnosis and to check the estrogen receptor status should, when technically possible, be carried out.

Systemic chemotherapy and/or hormonal therapy is essential in these patients.

C. Therapy as a Palliative Modality

Radiotherapy plays a major role in the palliation of the various symptoms of metastatic breast cancer. Pain from metastatic bone disease responds to radiotherapy much faster than to chemotherapeutic agents and/or hormones. The occurrence of pathological fractures, especially in weight-bearing bones, can be averted by local radiotherapy along with proper orthopedic procedures; this also helps in the process of recalcification of the bone. Radiotherapy to the spine is also imperative when metastases are identified in the vertebrae, to obviate the serious complication of cord compression.

Radiotherapy is also of definitive palliative value in cases of metastatic disease to the skin and soft tissues and the central nervous system.

For management of metastatic disease to the viscera (e.g., liver or lung) one should rely more on systemic therapy (chemotherapy and/or hormonal therapy) rather than on radiotherapy. Radiotherapy, however, could be given to isolated large lesions that are causing or threatening to cause symptoms (e.g., mediastinal masses and superior vena caval obstruction).

VI. ADJUVANT CHEMOTHERAPY FOR BREAST CANCER

A. Concepts and Rationale

Despite 75 years of experience with various methods developed for the control of local and regional disease in breast cancer, noteworthy gains relative to long-term survival have not occurred in the past three decades. There is increasing awareness that most patients have disseminated disease at the time of diagnosis and that any further improvement in survival (i.e., "cures" of micrometastases) is likely to result only from the employment of effective systemic therapy in conjunction with the classic modalities used for local control. This awareness is based on a number of clinical and biologic observations.

1. Breast Cancer: An Early Systemic Disease

This contention is supported by analysis of the sites and incidence of treatment failures at 10 years following standard mastectomy. Even patients who have no metastases in the axillary nodes are at a 20–25% risk of failure in 10 years, indicating that this apparently localized tumor was already disseminated at the time of diagnosis, although the metastases were beyond detection at presentation. The incidence of relapse at 10 years is strongly related to the number of axillary nodes found to be positive at presentation, a finding especially significant when the number of positive nodes is four or more. Thus axillary node involvement is a reliable indication that systemic spread of the disease has probably already occurred.

A tumor that has gone through 40 doublings has generally reached its end stage and is usually lethal; a 1-cm tumor in the breast, a size below which it is usually not detectable, has already undergone 30 doublings and has had adequate opportunity to metastasize during that interval. In addition, it has been shown that excision of the primary implanted tumor in mice does not result in cure unless effective systemic therapy is given at the same time. Numerous animal studies are available to support this hypothesis.

2. Tumor Cell Kinetics

A number of concepts in cell kinetics are important and are summarized as follows:

a. Doubling Time

Considering that growth fractions and doubling times of primary tumors may differ from those in clinically undetectable micrometastases, it is thought likely that the latter are more sensitive to chemotherapy because of the fact that a higher proportion of their cells are in the growth fraction than is the case in the clinically detectable stages.

b. Micrometastases

Micrometastases probably have better relative vascular supply, allowing for tumoricidal drug levels to accumulate in the tumor bed, whereas larger tumors often have necrotic centers in which cancer cells may find sanctuary. Thus, micrometastases should be more amenable to total, or near-total, eradication by systemic therapy than would be gross disease, since the number of viable tumor cells in the former are far fewer in number and more excessible to the drugs.

c. Animal Models

Experimental animal model systems suggest that better results are obtained by a combination of surgery followed by chemotherapy. It has also been established that the chemotherapy must be given shortly after the surgery, that is, before a significant regrowth of tumor has occurred, in order to be effective.

Cell kinetics models suggest various techniques of using chemotherapy: either a long period of chemotherapy with consideration given to "late intensification" (with dose escalation) or, if the micrometastases are very sensitive to the agents employed, a shorter course of chemotherapy might be just as effective.

3. Adjuvant Trials in Humans

Influenced by the low cure rates for patients with positive axillary nodes and by the development, in the past two decades, of effective combination chemotherapy programs for metastatic breast carcinoma, a number of investigators have set out to apply the principles of adjuvant chemotherapy interacting with high-risk breast cancer.

Trials with short-term immediate postoperative therapy using thiotepa (in the United States) and cyclophosphamide (in Scandinavia) were carried out in the 1960s. The initial results seemed inconclusive, but long-term follow-up has shown significant gains in the treated groups.

In 1969 Cooper reported a low recurrence rate in a series of women with breast cancer who had four or more positive axillary nodes treated adjunctively with a five-drug combination chemotherapy program. His series, however, was uncontrolled. The National Surgical Adjuvant Breast Project (NSABP) thereafter inaugurated a program employing phenylalanine-mustard (L-PAM) versus placebo in a prospectively randomized trial of women with Stage II breast cancer who had just undergone radical mastectomy. At the same time, the National Cancer Institute of Italy in Milan started a similar trial, using a three-drug combination of Cytoxan, methotrexate, and 5-fluorouracil (CMF) versus a no treatment control arm for Stage II breast cancer.

Subsequent reports of these studies carried in the United States and Italy (published in 1976) provided important confirmation that there was a potential efficacy in the employment of postoperative chemotherapy. Thus it was shown that the results of adjuvant therapy using L-PAM or CMF were impressive in premenopausal patients but not demonstrably superior in postmenopausal patients. In a retrospective analysis, however, it seemed that postmenopausal patients who received more than 85% of the scheduled dose of drug had apparently benefited to the same extent as the premenopausal patients. It must be kept in mind, however, that the latter conclusion is based on a rather small sample of patients and is a retrospective observation.

A number of other groups have demonstrated the efficacy of postoperative chemotherapy in both pre- and postmenopausal patients. These include series from the M. D. Anderson Hospital, the University of Arizona, the Cancer and Leukemia Group B, the Southwest Oncology Group, and several trials in Europe.

Furthermore, studies conducted by the NSABP in the United States showed that there appeared to be a significant advantage accruing to postmenopausal patients whose tumors are estrogen and progesterone receptor positive when tamoxifen (an antiestrogen agent) is added to the chemotherapy. It must be remembered that a majority of postmenopausal patients are estrogen receptor positive, whereas premenopausal patients are usually estrogen receptor negative.

It appears, therefore, that adjuvant chemotherapy continues to show consistent improvements over the results achievable with local-regional treatments alone. The following questions are still, however, not fully answered and await further clarification and studies:

- The optimum chemotherapy regimen.
- The use of one or more combinations in sequence, including combinations of chemotherapy and hormonal agents.
- The proper length of treatment by chemotherapeutic agents postoperatively.
- The possible extension of chemo or chemohormonal therapies to patients with early breast cancer where the disease shows unfavorable patterns, (e.g., negative estrogen receptors, poor histology, vascular or lymphatic invasion, high-grade or anaplastic tumor, etc.).
- The possible use of hormonal agents (tamoxifen) alone for estrogen-receptor-positive elderly postmenopausal patients versus chemotherapy or chemohormonal treatment.

In addition, it will be necessary to maintain all patients treated with adjuvant chemotherapy under close observation in the future in order to detect potential late sequelae of chemotherapy. By definition, "adjuvant" chemotherapy is given to patients at a time immediately after "definitive" surgery and/or radiotherapy, when the patient is apparently disease free but at high risk for relapse. This implies that a certain percentage of patients will be treated unnecessarily, as they have already been cured by surgery. If the risk of recurrence is high and the risk of treatment-related toxicity is low, the risk/benefit ratio favors treatment. If, however, the expected gain of adjuvant chemotherapy proves modest and a substantial fraction of patients is likely to have been already cured by surgery, late sequelae, should they develop, may outweigh short-term advantages of early chemotherapy. Well-conceived and controlled clinical studies are necessary to answer these highly important questions.

B. Guidelines for Adjuvant Chemotherapy

Adjunctive treatment refers to an ancillary therapy applied immediately or shortly after "definitive" local measures, to patients at high risk of relapse. As currently practiced, adjunctive therapies most commonly consist of postoperative radiotherapy, chemotherapy, hormonal therapy, or any combination thereof.

Because a large number of unanswered questions still remain, it is difficult to make precise recommendations. Furthermore, adjuvant therapies, especially chemotherapy, are, as of this writing, actively undergoing clinical trials in many centers. Therefore, it is strongly urged that whenever a patient's case fits the eligibility criteria for inclusion into such trials, physicians should consider participation.

Nevertheless, adequate information is already available to make a number of recommendations:

1. Stage I

Adjuvant chemotherapy should be considered only in the context of a clinical trial for patients deemed at high risk of recurrence. This includes patients with

- T2 lesions (ordinarily classified as Stage II but believed by some to really fit better with the Stage I patients).
- Vascular, lymphatic, or perineural invasion.
- Anaplastic histology.
- Estrogen-receptor-negative tumors.

With these exceptions, patients with Stage I breast cancer (tumors less than 2 cm with clinically uninvolved nodes) are curable in a high percentage (85%) of cases by local and regional treatment, and no adjuvant chemotherapy is warranted.

2. Stage II

a. Premenopausal Patients

Chemotherapy is advised for premenopausal patients with positive axillary nodes. The agents used, the combinations, the sequence and dosages, and the duration of treatment are all subject to great debate and are in a state of active investigation. The choice, then, depends on the preference of the treating chemotherapist or the design of an available clinical trial.

b. Postmenopausal Patients

In this category of Stage II patients (those with tumors between 2 and 5 cm in size or movable axillary nodes), no firm recommendation can be made at this time, although adjuvant chemotherapy or chemohormonal therapy seems to offer an edge. Once again, clinicians are urged to consider clinical trials for eligible patients. In the absence of such trials, the decision of whether to use or not to use adjuvant chemotherapy and/or hormonal therapy will depend on the extent of the local disease, the number of nodes involved, the patient's age and general condition, the status of the tumor's receptor proteins, the inclination of the treating physician, and the patient's disposition.

Postoperative radiotherapy in Stage II breast cancer has been the historical traditional practice, but its indications and value have been challenged recently. It is still a widely used modality and may be indicated, either by itself or following two and possibly three courses of chemotherapy, for patients at high risk for local recurrence and/or for those who are suspected of having metastases to the internal mammary nodes (very large lesion, proximity or involvement of the overlying skin, medial or central tumors, and microscopic evidence of lymphatic involvement). This is particularly true in those patients in whom adjuvant chemotherapy is not used for one reason or another.

3. Stage III

Most patients at this stage (with tumors larger than 5 cm or fixed to the skin or chest wall, or with nodes that are matted or attached) will not be cured by local treatments alone. If it proves possible to remove the local disease completely, follow-up treatment with chemotherapy and/or hormonal therapy with or without radiotherapy is recommended.

If the local lesion cannot be excised, radiotherapy with or without chemotherapy is suggested for local control. If the tumor becomes operable after radiotherapy and chemotherapy, clean-up mastectomy may then be considered. Systemic chemotherapy and/or hormonal manipulation should follow completion of local therapies since these patients must be considered to have systemic disease, even though it may not be readily demonstrable. The type of systemic therapy to be used depends on many factors (see the next heading).

If the radiotherapy is employed as the primary therapy, it is obviously excluded from use as adjunctive treatment as defined in these guidelines.

VII. GUIDELINES FOR THE TREATMENT OF ADVANCED BREAST CANCER

The current state of the art of the treatment of far-advanced breast cancer is such that significant, worthwhile palliation is commonly achievable, but cure hardly ever. The vast majority of patients whose disease recurs, or is primarily inoperable, will die of their disease. This should not be taken to mean that the situation is always hopeless, for significant long-term remissions can be induced with prolongation and improvement of the quality of life. Combination chemotherapy, formerly considered to be a last-resort treatment reserved for those patients who had failed surgery, radiotherapy, and hormonal manipulations, has been developed as a powerful tool.

The proper integration of the various modalities available for the treatment of advanced breast cancer presupposes thorough familiarity with the natural history of the disease, the modalities of treatment available, and the complications of such treatments and an appreciation of the treatment of the patient as a whole. It also requires an accurate evaluation of the extent of the disease, the criteria for assessing response to treatment, and the essential role of prognostic factors.

A. Evaluation of the Extent of Disease

A careful history, thorough physical examination, and selected laboratory studies, as in the following list, are mandatory in order to select appropriate therapy. Any complaints, particularly those relating to pain in various areas, especially osseous, demands prompt investigation.

- Routine x-rays (chest, bone, etc., as indicated).
- Blood counts and serum chemistries.
- If routine x-rays of painful areas are negative, tomograms may detect additional lesions. Whole-lung tomograms or CAT scan are indicated in selected cases, especially if the patient has respiratory complaints.
- Bone scans are indicated, both as baseline studies and for the detection of asymptomatic areas of possible involvement. It must be remembered that bone scans, while more sensitive, are not as specific as radiographic studies. Any suspicious site discovered on a bone scan should receive radiological follow-up.
- Liver scan is suggested if the liver is enlarged or if abnormal liver chemistries are present.
- Careful attention should be directed at the opposite breast, as well as the supraclavicular and axillary areas. Manual palpation of the skin of the chest and back is important in detecting subcutaneous nodules. Suspicious nodules should be approached by excisional biopsy for diagnosis and hormonal receptor studies.
- Thorough neurological examination is very important. Complaints of weakness in the legs should never be ascribed to the simple effects of progressive carcinomatosis or to the use of narcotic analgesics unless a careful examination is performed. In addition to the usual radiographic examination of the spine, it may be necessary to perform myelography in order to rule out spinal cord compression. Symptoms such as changes in affect and behavior should not simply be ascribed to the natural depression that often accompanies advanced malignant disease, but brain scan must be ordered to rule out metastases.
- Brain scan and CAT scans should be done as indicated.
- Metastases to the retina or to the retro-orbital fossa are not uncommon in breast cancer, and an orbital CAT scan, as well as a special ophthalmologist examination, may be necessary.

B. Prognostic Factors

The extent and location of the recurrent or metastatic disease at the time of its discovery are important in determining the prognosis. Familiarity with different prognoses related to different presentations is important in determining the type of treatment to be instituted. For instance, hormonal manipulations have a long lag period (4–8 weeks) before response is seen; they are, therefore, not appropriate for patients whose disease presentation is such that their life is imminently in danger. Other presentations with prognostic significance are as follows:

- Patients with massive involvement of the liver and brain have a very poor prognosis. This is also true for the patient with lymphangitic metastases to the lung.
- The prognosis is better in patients whose recurrence is in the local soft tissues and/or bone.
- The interval between the time of the initial mastectomy and the time of recurrence is also of significant prognostic value: The longer the disease-free interval, the better the prognosis.
- Patients who are perimenopausal are said to respond less frequently to chemotherapy than those who are definitely pre- or postmenopausal.
- The performance status of the patient is likewise important. Patients who spend a good part of their day in bed as a result of progressive disease are less likely than those patients who remain ambulatory to respond to any treatment.
- Finally, the estrogen receptor content of the tumor is of utmost importance, not only in the prognosis (estrogen-receptor-positive tumors have a better prognosis), but also in determining the choice of treatment to employ in any particular case. Patients with estrogen and progesterone negative tumors should not be subjected to hormonal manipulations, since they are unlikely to respond. Likewise, patients with a high level of estrogen and progesterone receptors in their tumors and whose disease presentation is not immediately life threatening are ideal candidates for hormonal manipulations. Evidence has accrued suggesting that the presence or absence of estrogen receptor protein correlates with the prognosis as an independent variable. It should be kept in mind that estrogen receptor content is not simply a positive–negative test. The absolute amount of estrogen receptor protein and the presence or absence of progesterone receptors are also very likely to have prognostic importance.

C. Assessment of Treatment Response

It is important for the members of the multidisciplinary team who care for patients with breast cancer to employ a common language so that the assessment of treatment responses remains consistent and agreed upon. Accepted terminology is as follows:

- A *complete response* should indicate complete disappearance of all known disease as well as relief of all disease-related symptoms. In the case of lytic bone metastases, these must be shown to have recalcified.
- A *partial response* is greater than a 50% decrease in the bidimensional measurement of any individual lesion with no contemporaneous increase in the size of any lesion.
- A *minor response* is a decrease in the size of between 25 and 50%.
- *No change* should indicate a less-than-25% change in the size of the lesion.
- *Progression* indicates new lesions appearing, or a greater-than-25% increase in the measurement of any particular lesion.
- *Evaluable but nonmeasurable disease* includes osteoblastic metastases, lung infiltrates, lymphedema, and pleural effusions. For evaluation of these, serial evidence of appreciable change must be documented by objective means such as x-rays or photographs.

D. Chemotherapy

It has been shown by a number of studies that combination chemotherapy is superior to single-agent treatment. Table I lists the most commonly used single agents and their relative response rates (partial and complete).

It must be stressed that the use of these agents is associated with serious potential complications and that familiarity with their indications, means of administration, side effects, toxic effects, metabolism, and mechanism of action is of the utmost importance. It is suggested that their use be supervised by personnel trained in the field of chemotherapy.

Currently, there is no agreement as to the best overall reg-

Table I

Useful Single Agents in the Treatment of Breast Cancer[a]

Drug	Dosage and schedule	Response rate (%)
Adriamycin	60–75 mg/m^2 IV every 3 weeks	37
Cyclophosphamide	100 mg/m^2 p.o. daily 500 mg/m^2 IV weekly	34
L-PAM	6.0 mg/m^2 p.o. × 5 days every 4–6 weeks	23
5-Fluorouracil	600 mg/m^2 IV weekly	26
Methotrexate	20 mg/m^2 IV or i.m. twice weekly	34
Vincristine	1.0 mg/m^2 IV weekly	21
Mitomycin C	20 mg/m^2 IV every 4–6 weeks	38

[a]By permission from Carbone and Davis (3).

Table II

Useful Drug Combination in the Treatment of Breast Cancer[a]

Regimen		Drug dosage and schedule	Response rate[b]
CMFVP	Cyclophosphamide	80 mg/m^2 p.o. daily	62
	Methotrexate	20 mg/m^2 IV weekly	
	Fluorouracil	500 mg/m^2 IV weekly	
	Vincristine	1.0 mg/m^2 IV weekly	
	Prednisone	30 mg/m^2 p.o. daily × 15 (then taper)	
CMF	Cyclophosphamide	100 mg/m^2 p.o. days 1–14	53
	Methotrexate	60 mg/m^2 IV days 1 and 8	
	5-Fluorouracil (Repeat cycles every 4 wk)	600 mg/m^2 IV days 1 and 8	
CMF (P)	Cyclophosphamide	100 mg/m^2 p.o. days 1–14	63
	Methotrexate	60 mg/m^2 IV days 1 and 8	
	5-Fluorouracil	600 mg/m^2 IV days 1 and 8	
	Prednisone (Repeat cycles every 4 wk)	40 mg/m^2 p.o. days 1–14	
AV	Adriamycin	75 mg/m^2 IV day 1	52
	Vincristine (Repeat cycles every 3 wk)	1.4 mg/m^2 IV days 1 and 8	
CA	cyclophosphamide	200 mg/m^2 p.o. days 3–6	74
	Adriamycin (Repeat cycles every 3–4 wk)	40 mg/m^2 IV day 1	
CAF	Cyclophosphamide	100 mg/m^2 p.o. days 1–14	82
	Adriamycin	30 mg/m^2 IV day 1	
	Fluorouracil (Repeat cycles every 4 wk)	500 mg/m^2 IV days 1 and 8	
DAV	Dibromodulcitol	150 mg/m^2 p.o. days 1–10	71
	Adriamycin	45 mg/m^2 IV day 1	
	Vincristine	1.2 mg/m^2 IV day 1	

[a]By permission from Carbone and Davis (3).
[b]Includes complete and partial response rate.

imen. However, it is reasonable to combine several agents with convergent effects on the tumor but divergent toxicities on the host. The issue of continuous versus intermittent treatment has also not been satisfactorily answered, but most current investigations employ intermittent schedules that allow for patients to rest between treatments; it is also felt that intermittent chemotherapy may be less immunosuppressive.

Table II lists several of the more commonly utilized combinations of drugs and their relative response rates. It must be stressed that the doses indicated are only suggestions and that different patients will require modification of doses based on the extent of the disease, amount of bone marrow involvement, amount of previous radiation and chemotherapy administered, size, weight of the patient, amount of body fat, etc.

That a large number of unsettled questions still exist should not come as a surprise in a disease as heterogeneous as breast cancer, one in which responses vary according to many factors (menstrual status, level of estrogen receptors, etc.). Well-designed, properly controlled clinical studies are attempting to answer several of these questions. These studies should be widely publicized and deserve encouragement and support with patient referrals on the part of all physicians treating breast cancer.

E. Hormonal Manipulation

- Therapeutic oophorectomy has been employed in the management of advanced breast cancer for premenopausal patients for many years and is still recommended in the premenopausal patients with estrogen-receptor-positive tumors.
- Hypophysectomy is indicated in selected patients.
- Additive hormonal therapy with estrogens, androgen, or progesterone is useful, especially in postmenopausal patients. Androgens are said to be particularly useful for osseous metastases.
- Antiestrogens. More recently, the antiestrogen tamoxifen has found an important place in our armamentarium. Currently approved for use in postmenopausal patients, it has also been shown to be effective in some premenopausal patients. In fact, it has been claimed that response to tamoxifen, or lack of same, is as important as the presence or absence of estrogen receptors in predicting response to any further hormonal therapies.
- Adrenalectomy has been largely supplanted by the use of medical therapy, such as the adrenal steroid inhibitor aminoglutethimide.

The most important development in the hormonal therapy of breast cancer has been the demonstration that the presence of estrogen receptor protein in a tumor specimen is very highly predictive of the likelihood of response to hormonal manipulation of any kind. Consequently, attempts should be made, whenever possible, to obtain tissue for evaluation of estrogen receptor content. This is particularly important if such information is not available from the tumor removed at the time of the original mastectomy. A biopsy of a recurrent or metastatic nodule for hormonal evaluation may have merit; some reports have shown that the estrogen receptor content of the metastasis is not necessarily consistent with the result obtained at the

original mastectomy (divergence is noted in up to 15% of cases).

F. Management of Selected Complications and Specific Types of Metastases

1. Bone Metastases

In addition to being very painful, metastatic lesions that involve osseous structures, especially those that bear weight, are highly susceptible to fracture. Radiation therapy is indicated in these cases and results in effective pain relief in the majority of patients. Prevention of ultimate fracture may also be achieved with the use of radiation. If fracture occurs or appears imminent, internal fixation or even total joint replacement may prove indicated. This has the important benefit of allowing the patient to remain ambulatory and reducing the risk of infections, hypercalcemia, pneumonia, and venous thrombosis. The presence of multiple areas of metastatic involvement is *not* a contraindication to such surgery.

Compression of the spinal cord due to pathological fracture or epidural involvement of the spinal canal is quite frequent. A careful neurological examination is mandatory in all cases; myelography, if indicated, and neurological consultations should not be delayed. Laminectomy and radiation therapy are the treatments of choice. During early cord compression, the use of high-dose corticosteroids is indicated.

2. Brain Metastases

Most chemotherapy and hormonal agents do not achieve effective concentrations of antitumor drug in the central nervous system. Consequently, radiation therapy remains the treatment of choice for any patient with proven brain metastases. Intrathecal administration of drugs such as methotrexate or cytosine arabinoside (ARA-c) may prove of benefit to patients with meningeal carcinomatosis. It must be remembered that visual disturbances may occur as a consequence of metastases in any one of a number of sites: retina, retro-orbital space, cerebrum, or meninges.

3. Pleural Effusions

Following a diagnostic tap, appropriate systemic therapy should be undertaken. If this fails to control the effusion, intrapleural instillation of sclerosing agents such as tetracycline or, if that fails, nitrogen mustard, following closed-tube thoracostomy should be undertaken. Sometimes the use of a radioactive material (e.g., colloidal gold, ^{198}AU, or ^{32}P) may achieve some control of pleural metastases.

4. Hypercalcemia

It is necessary always to be alert to the possibility of hypercalcemia. The treatment of this complication involves general medical measures of fluid replacement, diuretics, corticosteroids, and encouraging the patient to ambulate. Oral phosphates and calcitonin can also be tried, and in more severe or refractory cases, the use of mithramycin is indicated. Maintenance of the ambulatory state, as well as attention to adequate hydration, is most important.

5. Cutaneous or Regional Recurrence

About 5–15% of patients develop single or multiple lesions located within the mastectomy site as the initial manifestation of recurrence, especially when no regional radiation was used; this without any demonstrable evidence of widely disseminated disease after thorough evaluation. These patients have a very high likelihood of having microscopic metastatic disease in other sites, however, and less than 10% are likely to survive 10 years. At present, there is no standard approach to the management of this situation. Most authors agree that surgical removal of the recurrence is indicated, both for diagnostic purposes and for evaluation (or reevaluation) of the estrogen receptor content. Radiotherapy should be used a priori if it has not been previously used. In premenopausal patients with an estrogen-receptor-positive tumor, oophorectomy followed by chemotherapy for at least 2–3 years is also recommended. For the older patients, local treatment alone with surgery and/or radiation therapy (depending on the merits of the case) might be sufficient. The use of hormonal manipulations (for estrogen-receptor-positive patients) or chemotherapy might well be reserved until such time as systemic metastases are manifest.

6. Systemic Recurrence in the Estrogen-Receptor-Positive Patient

In premenopausal patients whose estrogen and progesterone receptor assay is strongly positive, a surgical (or radiation-induced) ovarian ablation should be done. There is no unanimity of opinion regarding the use of chemotherapy or tamoxifen immediately after the oophorectomy. Many authors suggest that for certain subgroups of premenopausal patients (by definition, young), the use of intensive chemotherapy following oophorectomy may well be beneficial and may result in prolonged remission.

For postmenopausal patients with estrogen- and progesterone-receptor-positive tumors and a favorable disease presentation, the use of hormonal manipulation is appropriate. Estrogen, androgens, or tamoxifen appear to be interchangeable as far as the likelihood of inducing a response is concerned. Other considerations are:

- Estrogen (diethylstilbestrol) at 15 mg per day has the advantage of being a drug with which many are familiar and which is inexpensive but which is associated with an appreciable incidence of fluid retention, cardiovascular or thromboembolic complications, and hypercalcemia.
- Androgens suffer from the side effects of virilization and possible hepatic toxicity.
- Tamoxifen is quite well tolerated but at present is quite expensive.
- Some studies suggest increased efficacy for combinations of hormonal agents, e.g., diethylstilbestrol or tamoxifen with androgens.
- Aminoglutethimide (plus hydrocortisone replacement) is still considered investigational as of this writing.

In the patient whose clinical presentation is dire or life threatening, the use of combination chemotherapy instead of hormonal manipulations is suggested. Once a response is established, the addition of hormonal agents to the chemotherapy regimen may be considered. At present, the concurrent administration of hormones and chemotherapy remains investigational.

In the hormone-receptor-positive patient more than 65 or 70 years of age, hormonal therapy continues to be the favorite modality of treatment. Upon failure of one hormonal manipulation following a response, another hormonal manipulation may well prove to be of further benefit. The decision regarding the specific choice of the second hormonal therapy must be based on the experience of the physician and the medical condition of the patient.

Surgical ablative procedures are probably not indicated in any patient who has failed to manifest a response to additive hormonal therapy. For such patients, the use of chemotherapy is indicated.

7. Systemic Recurrence in the Estrogen-Receptor-Negative Patient

In such patients, whether pre- or postmenopausal, the use of hormonal manipulations is unlikely to result in clinical benefit. Chemotherapy remains the treatment of choice in both of these subgroups. Those patients who fail to respond to the initial chemotherapy regimen, or who relapse following the achievement of an objective response, should be treated with alternate drug combinations. In some fragile and elderly patients, it may still be appropriate to use a single agent as initial therapy.

8. Systemic Recurrence in the Estrogen-Receptor-Unknown Patient

In the event that the estrogen receptor content of the original tumor is unavailable and there is no tissue readily available at the time of detection of metastatic disease for determination of hormone receptor content, the choice of treatment to employ must take into account the patient's condition, the sites and extent of disease recurrence, the length of the disease-free interval, and the menopausal status of the patient. Thus, additive hormonal manipulations are indicated for elderly patients with generally slow-growing disease, and combination chemotherapy programs are indicated for younger patients with more aggressive disease. Obviously, breast cancer presents a wide spectrum of diseases, and various combinations of treatments will be appropriate in different subsets of patients.

9. Systemic Recurrence following Previous Adjuvant Chemotherapy

In the past 5 years, more and more women have been treated with chemotherapy immediately after mastectomy in the hopes of preventing recurrence. For those women who do recur, the selection of therapy should once again be based on several factors, including estrogen receptor status, menstrual status, extent of disease, the chemotherapy combinations already used, etc.

Oophorectomy is indicated if the patient is still menstruating and if her tumor was hormone (estrogen/progestrone) receptor positive or unknown. If the interval between the completion of the adjuvant chemotherapy program and the finding of dissemination is in excess of 1 year, reinstitution of the same chemotherapy might prove beneficial. If the interval, however, has been short, a different combination of drugs should be employed. In any patient whose tumor is hormone receptor positive and whose clinical condition permits, hormal manipulation is obviously indicated. Thus, a postmenopausal patient with an estrogen/progesterone-receptor-positive tumor that recurred following adjuvant chemotherapy should be treated with hormonal manipulation. The combination CMF has been shown to be effective after failure with melphalan; and adriamycin-containing combinations have been shown to be effective following failure with CMF. These regimens, therefore, might be appropriate therapeutic options for either pre- or postmenopausal patients whose estrogen receptor content was negative.

In conclusion, it is necessary to recognize that metastatic breast cancer presents the treating physician with a heterogeneous group of problems. The choice of the appropriate therapy at any particular time is necessarily a complex decision and must be based on an appreciation of several factors. Many studies will need to be done and analyzed before one may hazzard firm recommendations. Treatment will have to be individualized for different subgroups of patients at different stages of the disease. The only hope for increasing the reliability of guideline suggestions stems from analysis of current and future clinical studies. It should be remembered that the very

patients these guidelines are intended to serve, themselves serve as subjects for such studies. The participation of physicians and patients in well-designed and properly controlled studies is, therefore, an obligation for all.

VIII. POSTOPERATIVE CARE, EVALUATION, AND REHABILITATION

A. Immediate Postoperative Care

After stabilization of the patient in the immediate postanesthesia period, the vital signs should be monitored frequently. Other measures include

- The patient should be in the semi-Fowler position, with IV in place until the patient tolerates oral diet without difficulty.
- Suction drains used for drainage as well as adherence of skin flaps should be maintained at least 4–5 days, or as otherwise determined by the amount of drainage. This should be charted at the bedside every shift.
- CBC should be performed ad lib depending upon the operative circumstances.
- Bulky pressure dressing may be avoided as it might embarrass the vascularity of skin flaps. A light dressing of Xeroform and 4- by 4-inch gauze with minimal paper tape extended to regions outside the undermined area will provide adequate coverage. The wound is sealed in 24 hours. Hematomas, if present, should be evacuated under sterile conditions.
- Prophylactic antibiotics should be avoided.
- Elevation of the arm on the affected side should be maintained on two pillows, and this arm should not be used for IV cannulation. Exercises should not begin before the fourth or fifth postoperative day.
- Deep breathing and coughing should be encouraged as often as necessary.
- Analgesics and tranquilizers may be utilized, avoiding, however, having the patient become too heavily sedated.

B. Psychological Support

Recognizing that all patients will be affected to some degree by the trauma of the disease and treatment, a formally structured program should be presented to the patient at the onset. If the patient is aware that professionals are available for these "usual" sequelae, the magnitude of the difficulties may be reduced. The continuous educational program, which should be invoked immediately, serves as an excellent vehicle for monitoring patients responses. Psychiatric social workers should be included in the educational program to prevent the usual sequelae and, at the same time, to evaluate the patient's need for further professional help. All this can be performed under the physician's supervision and without violating the very important physician–patient relationship. Reach-to-Recovery can be of great help to the patient by offering solace, advice, and equipment. Contact between their member and the patient should be encouraged as early as possible.

The patient's consort (husband) must offer the greatest amount of support, indicating his love and affection. Sexual activity should be started as early as possible to dispel the patient's impression that she has lost her appeal. Family members and/or close friends should be incorporated in the support program, both for immediate and for long-range benefit to the patient. Ongoing general lecture series and/or open forums for affected patients should include all interested persons and should continue long after recovery.

C. Coordination of Postoperative Therapy

Patients may enter the program for any of the treatment modalities: surgery, chemotherapy, or radiation therapy. The initial treatment modality should, however, include consideration of further therapy in the other areas. The timing and order will be dependent upon the individual circumstances. Individual patient's reaction to a treatment mode, especially chemotherapy, may require reassessment of the original plan. Consultations and suggestions from each of these areas should be available to all people involved in the care of the patient. This should be channeled through the treating physician to maintain continuity of care.

D. Follow-Up Evaluation

Long-term follow-up evaluation of the patient following breast cancer therapy must be carried out periodically and diligently. The schedule given in Table III is recommended.

E. Rehabilitation

1. Immediate Postoperative Rehabilitation

Arm exercises and physical therapy should be started as soon as possible under the direction of the physical therapy department. This will, of course, be guided by the type of procedure performed, but at least 4 days are required for operations

Table III

Long-Term Follow-Up Schedule for Breast Cancer

Management	First-through third year (in months) 3	6	9	12	Fourth-through fifth year Semi-annually	Annually	Thereafter, annually for life
History							
Complete				X		X	X
Soft tissue masses	X	X	X	X	X	X	X
Bone pain	X	X	X	X	X	X	X
Cough, dyspnea, chest pain	X	X	X	X	X	X	X
Weight loss, anorexia, weakness	X	X	X	X	X	X	X
Self-examination: breast	X	X	X	X	X	X	X
Headache, falls, seizure	X	X	X	X	X	X	X
Performance status	X	X	X	X	X	X	X
Other symptoms	X	X	X	X	X	X	X
Physical							
Complete				X		X	X
Mastectomy area	X	X	X	X	X	X	X
Remaining breast	X	X	X	X	X	X	X
Lymph nodes	X	X	X	X	X	X	X
Abdomen–liver, masses	X	X	X	X	X	X	X
Chest, bones	X	X	X	X	X	X	X
Skin	X	X	X	X	X	X	X
Investigations							
CBC, urine		X				X	X
SGOT, LDH		X				X	X
Alkaline phosphatase and calcium phosphate		X				X	X
X-ray, chest		X				X	X
Mammogram		X				X	X
Scans and other examinations	As indicated from history and physical exam						

where the pectoralis muscles are removed. If skin grafting is necessary, a longer period of immobilization may be required.

Education as to postoperative skin care, whether or not there is radiation and/or chemotherapy, is especially important for the comfort of the patient.

2. Management of Lymphedema

Lymphedema is a common complication of mastectomy, particularly when a thorough axillary dissection was performed and if postoperative radiotherapy is administered; the degree of lymphedema varies considerably from slight increase in circumference measurement to the disabling elephantiasis type of lymphedema.

Preventative hygienic measures are most important and include

- Elevation.
- Exercises.
- Avoiding dependent weight carrying.
- Meticulous hygienic care and avoidance of infections.
- Early use of antibiotics in even minor infections in the hand or arm.

Treatment of the acute stage of lymphedema, which is most often related to infection, should include the most active management of the septic process. Diuretics may also be used on a short-term basis.

The more chronic and progressive lymphedema will require the use of elastic pressure sleeves or even intermittent (2–3 times a week) or continuous (24–48 hours) use of aerodynamically produced pressure using a Jobst or Lymphapress type of pump.

Various surgical procedures have been described over the years to treat the most severe types of lymphedema. They are usually complex and frought with a high morbidity. More recently, a promising approach using lymphovenous anastomoses in the arm under microscopic control has been tried with encouraging preliminary results.

3. External Prosthetic Appliances

In the immediate postoperative period, should chemotherapy and/or radiation therapy not be contemplated, prosthetic devices of the external variety can help immeasurably in the emotional support of the patient. With minimal care and with special consideration for the underlying skin to avoid the possibility of irritation and vascular compromise, they can be used safely. There are many types of prosthetic devices, and this should be incorporated in the educational program. In certain cases, this may be the only reconstructive consideration necessary, as most patients will be quite satisfied with the use of an external prosthesis and will not request any surgical reconstructive procedure. If radiotherapy is instituted, the use and timing of such prosthesis should be planned carefully to avoid undue problems to the skin.

4. Reconstructive Surgical Procedures

Education as to the availability or feasibility of reconstructive surgery should be started preoperatively. The knowledge that reconstruction is available has increased participation in screening programs and early detection. Patients should be made aware that a normal-appearing reconstruction is available, especially when a lesser procedure is performed in situa-

tions of early diagnosis. The type of procedure will be dependent upon the cancer operation performed; all defects, from the extended radical mastectomy to the simple mastectomy, can be greatly improved with today's available procedures and prostheses.

Surgical reconstruction using internal prosthesis can be done with one of several types of devices:

- Inflatable silicone shells, where normal saline is used to inflate the prosthesis.
- Liquid silicone shell combinations of silicone prosthetics with inflatable compartments.
- Custom prosthetics made with varying consistencies of silicone gel to simulate muscle in the subclavicular defects.

There have been no incidents of cancer after implantation of these materials, and they do not obscure the follow-up with any of the current modalities of testing. More recently, external custom-made prosthetic molds have been prepared and used in selected cases; they simulate the normal skin and breast and attach to the patient's body with a special surgical glue. These molds are not always available but offer new prospects in terms of external prostheses.

Surgical flaps are now often carried out at the time of insertion of the prosthesis. Myocutaneous flaps are performed to correct the subclavicular defects of the total mastectomy, while allowing formation of a breast mound and permitting a more natural "sagging" of the breast. If a skin graft was necessary in the extirpative procedure, this can be effectively reconstructed as well. The rehabilitation also includes one of several methods of reconstructing the nipple and areola complex and frequently necessitates an augmentation or reduction mammoplasty of the contralateral side to achieve symmetry.

More recently, transposition of free muscle skin flaps with microvascular anastomoses has been successfully carried out using the gluteal muscle, and cosmetic results seem to be extremely promising. Likewise, a rectus abdominus myocutaneous flap reconstruction without the use of a prosthesis is rapidly becoming a favorite method of breast reconstruction, yielding a very satisfactory cosmetic result.

The timing of reconstruction will depend on the extent of the cancer surgery. Postoperative chemotherapy and/or radiation therapy also weigh heavily upon the timing of the reconstructive procedures. It is usually recommended, however, that the patient wait 6 months for adequate tissue recovery and psychological stabilization, before surgical reconstruction is carried out. Primary reconstruction at the time of mastectomy has been recommended by some and is desirable in selected cases.

5. Treatment of the Other Breast and High-Risk Prophylactic Surgery

Since breast cancer patients are at high risk for developing carcinoma in the contralateral breast, especially if the histological diagnosis and family history provide additional risks, prophylactic removal of the opposite breast may conceivably be considered in carefully selected patients, provided it is thoroughly explained to the patient and psychologically well received. Here, a subcutaneous mastectomy with immediate reconstruction is possible with excellent cosmetic results.

This type of prophylactic procedure may also be recommended for high-risk patients who have undergone multiple biopsies for fibrocystic disease. The ability to follow these patients effectively is decreased in many instances, and the incidence of obscure carcinoma is increased. Subcutaneous mastectomy for those high-risk patients would decrease the incidence of clinical carcinoma.

F. Nursing Role in the Rehabilitation of the Breast Cancer Patient

Rehabilitation actually begins at the time the diagnosis is made. The nurse needs to know the modalities of treatment that the patient will receive, as well as the effect of the treatment upon the rehabilitation process.

The nurse needs to establish the rehabilitation contacts and to learn what is available and when to use these resources according to the attending physician's recommendations. A large number of rehabilitation resources are available, including the following:

- American Cancer Society. Reach-to-Recovery program, educational publications, financial aid, counseling, and supplies and dressings.
- Cancer Information Service. Access to cancer information, provision of support, local resources, provision of fact sheets, and free mailed pamphlets upon request.
- Cancer Care Incorporated. Counseling and guidance, financial assistance, and supportive services: prosthetics, equipment, supplies, information, and referral.
- Visiting Nurse Association. Home care nursing, family education, and supportive services.
- Social Service Department. Advice in reference to the availability and use of the above-mentioned agencies; assistance with referrals to various outside agencies, along with health facility (extended care facility) placement; and assistance in obtaining home health services.

There is a need for the physician, nurse, social worker, psychological and vocational counselors, and physical and occupational therapists to work together to provide continuity of care for the patient from the time of diagnosis, up to and through the process of rehabilitation.

IX. MANAGEMENT ALGORITHM FOR CANCER OF THE BREAST (see p. 94)

SUGGESTED READINGS

1. Bland, K. I. A clinicopathologic correlation of mammographic parenchymal patterns and associated risk factors for human mammary carcinoma. *Annu. Surg.* **195** (5), 584–594 (1982).
2. Bonadonna, G., Valagussa, P., Rossi, A., Zucali, R., Tancini, G., Bajetta, E., Brambilla, C., DeLena, M., DiFronzo, G., Banfi, A., Rilke, F., and Veronesi, U. Are surgical adjuvant trails altering the course of breast cancer? *Semin. Oncol.* **5** (4), 450 (1978).
3. Carbone, P. P., and Davis, T. E. Medical treatment for advanced breast cancer. *Semin. Oncol.* **5** (4), 417 (1978).
3a. Cooper, R. G. Combination chemotherapy in hormone resistant breast cancer. *Proc. Am. Assoc. Cancer Res.* **10**, 15 (1969).
3b. Cooper, R. G., Holland, J. F., and Glidwell, O. Adjuvant chemotherapy of breast cancer. *Cancer* **44**, 793–795 (1979).
4. Crile, G., Jr. Management of breast cancer: Limited Mastectomy. *JAMA, J. Am. Med. Assoc.* **230**, 95 (1974).
5. Cronin, T. D. Reconstruction of the breast after mastectomy. *Plast. Reconstr. Surg.* **59**, 1 (1977).
6. Degenshein, G. A. Estrogen and progesterone receptor site studies as guides to the management of advanced breast cancer. *Breast* **3**, 29 (1977).
7. Egan, R. L. Mammography, an aid to early diagnosis of breast carcinoma. *JAMA, J. Am. Med. Assoc.* **182**, 839–843 (1962).
8. Fechner, R. E. Breast cancer—role of oral contraceptives and estrogen replacement therapy. Review of endocrine related cancer. *Cancer* **7**, 5–12 (1980).
9. Fisher, B. The surgical dilemma in the primary therapy in invasive breast cancer—a critical appraisal. *Curr. Probl. Surg.* **2**, 1–53 (1970).
10. Fisher, B., and Gebhardt, M. C. The evolution of breast cancer surgery: Past, present and future. *Semin. Oncol.* **5** (4), 385 (1978).
11. Gershon-Cohen, J., and Berger, S. M. Detection of breast cancer by periodic x-ray examinations: A five year survival. *JAMA, J. Am. Med. Assoc.* **176**, 1114. (1961).
12. Haagensen, C. D. "Disease of the Breast." Saunders, Philadelphia, Pennsylvania, 1971.
13. Handley, R. S., and Thackery, A. C. Conservative radical mastectomy (Patey's operation). *Ann. Surg.* **157**, 162–164 (1963).
14. McGuire, W. L. Hormone receptors: Their role in predicting prognosis and response to endocrine therapy. *Semin. Oncol.* **5** (4), 428 (1978).
15. McWhirter, R. Treatment of cancer of the breast by simple mastectomy and radiotherapy. *Arch. Surg. (Chicago)* **59**, 830 (1979).
16. Rush, B. F., Jr. Axillary dissection in breast cancer: A staging procedure. *Surgery (St. Louis)* **77**, 478 (1975).
17. Salmon, S. E., and Jones, S. E., eds. "Adjuvant Therapy of Cancer," III, pp. 305–492. Grune & Stratton, New York, 1981.
18. Seidman, M. B. A. A different perspective on breast cancer risk factors—some implications of the non-attributable risk. *Cancer* **32**, 301–312 (1982).
19. Urban, J. A. Bilaterality of Cancer of the Breast: Biopsy of the opposite breast. *Cancer* **20**, 1867–1870 (1967).
20. Veronesi, U. Adjuvant combination chemotherapy with CMF in primary mammary carcinoma. *World J. Surg.* **1**, 337 (1977).
21. Veronesi, U., Saccozzi, R. *et al.* Comparing radical mastectomy with quadrantectomy, axillary dissection, and radiotherapy in patients with small cancers of the breast. *N. Engl. J. Med.* **305**, 6–11 (1981).
22. Wise, L., Masdn, A. Y., and Ackerman, L. V. Local excision and irradiation: An alternative method for the treatment of early mammary cancer. *Ann. Surg.* **174**, 382–401 (1971).
23. Wolfe, J. N. Risk for breast cancer development determined by mammographic parenchymal patterns. *Cancer* **37**, 2486–2492 (1976).

ALGORITHM FOR CANCER OF THE BREAST

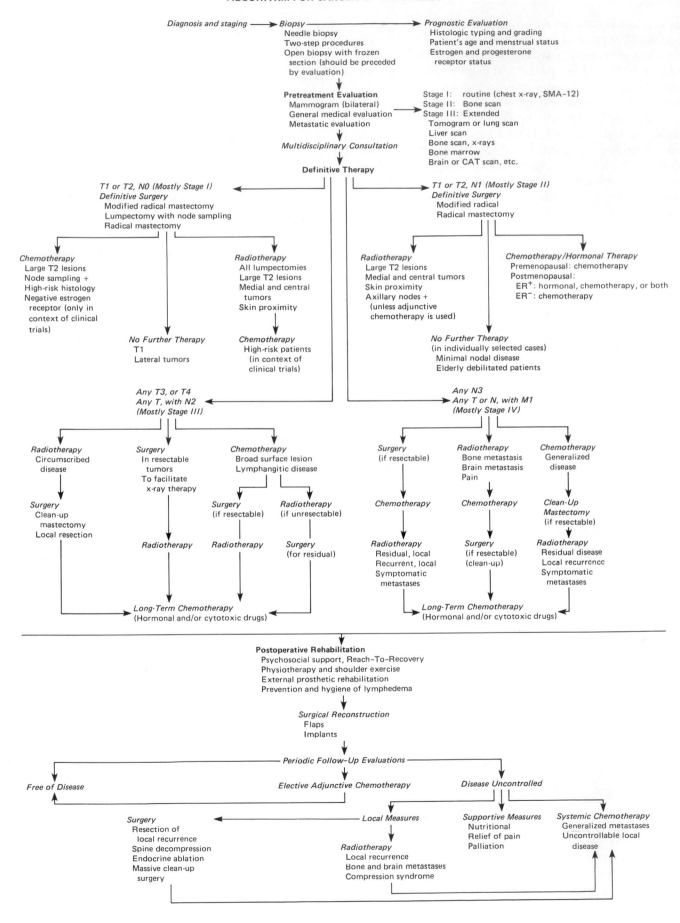

Diagnosis and staging ⟶ *Biopsy*
Needle biopsy
Two-step procedures
Open biopsy with frozen
  section (should be preceded
  by evaluation)

⟶ *Prognostic Evaluation*
Histologic typing and grading
Patient's age and menstrual status
Estrogen and progesterone
  receptor status

Pretreatment Evaluation
Mammogram (bilateral)
General medical evaluation
Metastatic evaluation

Stage I: routine (chest x-ray, SMA–12)
Stage II: Bone scan
Stage III: Extended
  Tomogram or lung scan
  Liver scan
  Bone scan, x-rays
  Bone marrow
  Brain or CAT scan, etc.

Multidisciplinary Consultation

Definitive Therapy

T1 or T2, N0 (Mostly Stage I)
Definitive Surgery
  Modified radical mastectomy
  Lumpectomy with node sampling
  Radical mastectomy

T1 or T2, N1 (Mostly Stage II)
Definitive Surgery
  Modified radical
  Radical mastectomy

Chemotherapy
Large T2 lesions
Node sampling +
High-risk histology
Negative estrogen
  receptor (only in
  context of clinical
  trials)

Radiotherapy
All lumpectomies
Large T2 lesions
Medial and central
  tumors
Skin proximity

Radiotherapy
Large T2 lesions
Medial and central tumors
Skin proximity
Axillary nodes +
  (unless adjunctive
  chemotherapy is used)

Chemotherapy/Hormonal Therapy
Premenopausal: chemotherapy
Postmenopausal:
  ER+: hormonal, chemotherapy, or both
  ER−: chemotherapy

No Further Therapy
T1
Lateral tumors

Chemotherapy
High-risk patients
  (in context of
  clinical trials)

No Further Therapy
(in individually selected cases)
Minimal nodal disease
Elderly debilitated patients

Any T3, or T4
Any T, with N2
(Mostly Stage III)

Any N3
Any T or N, with M1
(Mostly Stage IV)

Radiotherapy
Circumscribed
disease

Surgery
In resectable
tumors
To facilitate
x-ray therapy

Chemotherapy
Broad surface lesion
Lymphangitic disease

Surgery
(if resectable)

Radiotherapy
Bone metastasis
Brain metastasis
Pain

Chemotherapy
Generalized
disease

Surgery
Clean-up
mastectomy
Local resection

Surgery
(if resectable)

Radiotherapy
(if unresectable)

Chemotherapy

Chemotherapy

Clean-Up
Mastectomy
(if resectable)

Radiotherapy

Radiotherapy

Surgery
(for residual)

Radiotherapy
Residual, local
Recurrent, local
Symptomatic
metastases

Surgery
(if resectable)
(clean-up)

Radiotherapy
Residual disease
Local recurrence
Symptomatic
metastases

Long-Term Chemotherapy
(Hormonal and/or cytotoxic drugs)

Long-Term Chemotherapy
(Hormonal and/or cytotoxic drugs)

Postoperative Rehabilitation
Psychosocial support, Reach–To–Recovery
Physiotherapy and shoulder exercise
External prosthetic rehabilitation
Prevention and hygiene of lymphedema

Surgical Reconstruction
Flaps
Implants

Periodic Follow-Up Evaluations

Free of Disease

Elective Adjunctive Chemotherapy

Disease Uncontrolled

Surgery
Resection of
  local recurrence
Spine decompression
Endocrine ablation
Massive clean-up
  surgery

Local Measures

Radiotherapy
Local recurrence
Bone and brain metastases
Compression syndrome

Supportive Measures
Nutritional
Relief of pain
Palliation

Systemic Chemotherapy
Generalized metastases
Uncontrollable local
  disease

Section 3

Carcinomas of the Skin

LASZLO BIRO

With Contributions by

Edward Heilman	Dermatology and Pathology
Rene A. Khafif	Surgical Oncology
Alfredo Brand	Dermatology
Ely Price	Dermatology
Kapila Parikh	Radiotherapy
Samuel Kopel	Medical Oncology
Rafael Cinelli	Plastic Surgery
Michael Martuscello	Surgery
Ann Nelson	Nursing Oncology
Randi Moskowitz	Nursing Oncology

CURRENT GUIDELINES
FOR THE MANAGEMENT OF CANCER

Copyright © 1986 by Academic Press, Inc.
All rights of reproduction in any form reserved.

Section 3 Carcinomas of the Skin

I. Early Detection and Screening 99
  A. Cancer Precursors
  B. Predisposing Factors
  C. Patient Education
  D. Screening
II. Pretreatment Evaluation and Work-Up 100
  A. History and Physical Examination
    1. History
      a. Present Illness
      b. Social History
      c. Family History of Skin Cancer
      d. Past History
    2. Physical Examination
      a. Inspection and Palpation of the Skin Lesions
      b. Palpation of Regional Lymph Nodes
  B. Biopsy
    1. Basal Cell Carcinoma
    2. Squamous Cell Carcinoma
    3. Keratoacanthoma
    4. Melanoma
  C. Metastatic Evaluation
  D. Pretreatment Preparation
  E. Multidisciplinary Evaluation
  F. Site-Specific Data Form for Skin Cancer
III. Therapeutic Management of Nonmelanoma
Skin Cancer 102
  A. Management Goals
    1. Tissue Diagnosis
    2. Selection of Type and Extent of Therapy
  B. Common Pitfalls
    1. Unwarranted Delay in Treatment
    2. Lack of Biopsy or Inadequate Biopsy
    3. Selection of Inappropriate Surgical Technique
    4. Failure to Recognize Biological Facts
  C. Complications of Treatment
  D. Selection of Treatment
    1. Histological Nature of the Tumor
    2. Location of the Tumor
    3. Size of the Tumor
    4. Multiple Tumors
    5. Age of the Patient
    6. Psychological Factors
  E. Specific Therapeutic Modalities
    1. Desiccation and Curettage (Electrosurgery)
    2. Cryosurgery
    3. Excision Surgery
    4. Radiation Therapy
      a. Volume
      b. Modalities
      c. Dose
    5. Mohs's Surgery

    6. Laser Surgery
    7. Topical Chemotherapy (5-Fluorouracil)
  F. Guidelines for Treatment according to Histology
    1. Superficial Basal Cell Carcinoma
    2. Nodular, Noduloulcerative, Cystic, and
      Pigmented Basal Cell Carcinoma
    3. Morphea-Type Basal Cell Carcinoma
    4. Keratoacanthoma
    5. Bowen's Disease
    6. Squamous Cell Carcinoma
  G. Therapeutic Management: Site Specific
  (Nonmelanoma)
    1. Head and Neck
      a. Eyelids
      b. Nose
      c. Lips
      d. Ears
      e. Scalp
      f. Neck
      g. High-Risk Factors and Metastases
    2. Trunk and Extremities
IV. Malignant Melanomas of the Skin 113
  A. Prevention, Screening, and Early Detection:
  The Benign Nevus
    1. Benign Nevus and Its Precancerous Potential
    2. Recommendations for Elective Resection of
      Benign Nevi and Pigmented Lesions
      a. Giant Congenital Hairy Nevi
      b. Lentigo Maligna
      c. Pigmented Lesions from Patients with
        Xeroderma Pigmentosa
      d. Benign Juvenile Melanomas
      e. Atypical Melanocytic Lesions
      f. Nevi in Specific Sites
      g. Nevi Subjected to Chronic Trauma
    3. Early Signs of Malignant Transformation
  B. Evaluation of the Patient
    1. Biopsy
    2. Staging
    3. Metastatic Evaluation
  C. Therapeutic Management
    1. Excision of the Primary Site
      a. Width of Excision
      b. Depth of Excision
      c. Skin Graft
    2. Treatment of Lymphatic Drainage Sites
      a. Therapeutic Lymphadenectomy
      b. Elective Lymphadenectomy
    3. Adjuvant Therapy
      a. Radiotherapy
      b. Immunotherapy

        c. Systemic Chemotherapy
        d. Regional Chemotherapy
    D. Chemotherapy of Malignant Melanoma
        1. Systemic Chemotherapy
        2. Immunotherapy
        3. Regional Perfusion
V. Other Select Skin Tumors   118
    A. Malignant Tumors of the Skin Appendages
        1. Classification
            a. Benign Appendage Tumors with Associated
               Cutaneous Malignancy
            b. Malignant Skin Appendage Tumors
        2. Therapeutic Management
            a. Surgery
            b. Radiotherapy
    B. Mycosis Fungoides and Sézary Syndrome
        1. Pathogenesis, Incidence, and Prognosis
        2. Clinical Manifestations
            a. The Premycotic Phase
            b. Patch-Plaque Lesions

        c. Tumors and Nodules
        d. Erythroderma
        3. Staging
        4. Therapeutic Management
            a. Topical Nitrogen Mustard or BCNU
            b. Electron Beam Therapy
            c. PUVA
            d. Systemic Chemotherapy
    C. Kaposi's Sarcoma (Multiple Idiopathic
       Hemorrhagic Sarcoma)
VI. Postoperative Care, Evaluation, and Rehabilitation
    of the Patient with Skin Cancer   122
    A. Postoperative Care
    B. Evaluation
    C. Rehabilitation
        1. Functional rehabilitation
        2. Cosmetic rehabilitation
        3. Psychiatric rehabilitation
VII. Management Algorithm for Skin Melanoma   123

Suggested Readings   123

I. EARLY DETECTION AND SCREENING

A. Cancer Precursors

Skin cancers are among the few malignant tumors where precancerous lesions and specific predisposing factors are well recognized. Skin cancers usually arise on skin surfaces exposed to sunlight and to a much lesser degree on the protected truncal regions of the body and extremities. Thus, most skin cancers are found about the face, ears, hands and scalp.

Precancerous lesions include

- Actinic keratoses.
- Arsenical keratoses.
- Radiation dermatitis that results from chronic, often inadvertent exposure such as was the case in early workers with radioactive materials.
- Large congenital nevi.
- Chronic dermatitis following exposure to any low-grade, long-term trauma.

Should any of these lesions present with any deviation from its natural history, or should it undergo changes such as rapid growth or slow progressive changes, ulceration, color changes, bleeding, or nodule formation, biopsy is strongly indicated.

B. Predisposing Factors

Predisposing factors contributing to the causation of skin cancer include

- Ethnic factors (especially Celtics and other fair-skinned individuals).
- Exposure to sun.
- Exposure to certain chemicals (arsenic, hydrocarbons).
- Radiotherapy.
- Chronic repeated trauma.
- Chronic indolent ulceration and infection.

Caucasians, particularly of Celtic and northern European origin, with light complexion and blue eyes, are known to have the highest incidence of melanoma and nonmelanoma skin cancer.

Ultraviolet (UV) exposure from natural or industrial sources can induce skin cancer. Certain chemicals, mainly products of distillation of petroleum, are carcinogenic in their own right but can also potentiate the effects of UV radiation on the skin. Individuals with outdoor occupations, such as gardeners, construction workers, fishermen, farmers, and pipeline and railroad workers, are exposed to excessive natural UV radiation in the form of sunlight. Welders, maintenance workers, and plasma torch operators, on the other hand, are exposed to welding-arc industrial sources; pharmaceutical industry workers are exposed to germicidal lamps; and workers involved in curing and drying wood are also exposed to industrial UV sources. All these individuals are at a higher risk of developing skin cancer. Workers in outdoor occupations are advised to wear protective clothing and use sunscreens such as those containing para-aminobenzoic acid to block out the harmful effects of ultraviolet radiation.

Industrial exposure to coal tars and pitch as well as distillation products of aromatic hydrocarbons can, after prolonged exposure, have a carcinogenic effect on the skin. Certain industrial oils formerly used in cotton mills have been banned in this country because of their carcinogenicity. Regulations that require showering and changing of clothing on entering and leaving industrial plants have eliminated many of the problems associated with petroleum products and oils.

Occupational exposure to inorganic arsenic, especially if ingested, can produce squamous cell carcinoma, superficial basal cell carcinoma, and Bowen's disease. Orchard workers and workers in trades involved with copper and lead smelting are exposed to arsenic.

Chronic radiodermatitis, which often results in a variety of skin cancers, can be the result of professional or inadvertent long-term exposure. Dentists, fluoroscopists, dermatologists and orthopedists were once among those in the medical profession most likely to develop skin cancer because of their indiscriminate use of x-ray machines. This is rarely seen today because of the strict regulations, increased awareness, and protective measures used.

Marjolin's ulcer, arising in chronic scars, sinus tracts, burns, chronically infected skin, stasis ulcers, osteomyelitis, etc., are known to predispose to skin cancer. These tumors are extremely aggressive and difficult to treat.

C. Patient Education

Patient education is of utmost importance in the prevention and early detection of skin cancer. Such education can be carried out through a variety of methods:

- Educational materials in the form of pamphlets, magazines, newspaper articles, books, etc.
- Mass media information.
- Lectures directed at special segments of the population, especially in the various industrial settings where the risk is increased.

Educational efforts should be directed primarily at highlighting preventive measures. The recognition of various predisposing factors and occupational hazards and the means of combating them (use of sunscreens, shields, industrial hygiene, and protective measures, etc.) need to be emphasized. Self-examination should be encouraged, and premalignant lesions identified. Early signs of skin cancers should be taught: lumps, sores, crusting, bleeding, changes in pigmented moles. Finally, patients should be encouraged to seek professional advice early.

D. Screening

Screening is easier for skin neoplasia than for any other organ since the surface of the body may be examined rapidly by inspection, by either the patient or the physician, as part of a multiphasic screening, or as a specific skin cancer screening that may be set up and organized in one of many ways. It can be promoted by various groups such as a Lions Club or a church group, which carries out the first or preparatory phase. This consists of placing posters in hospitals and in the community or sending mass mailings. The posters indicate the time and place of the screening and the characteristics of people at risk for whom the screening is intended. It has been found that by limiting skin cancer screenings to populations at increased risk, such as those over 60 years of age, individuals with fair skin, persons who have a suspected lesion in the skin, or groups of individuals exposed to any of the earlier indicated hazards, the yield will be considerably greater than screening the general public.

The second phase of the screening program requires four or five small treatment rooms with good lighting, an administrative staff from the sponsoring group to conduct traffic, and dermatologists assisted by other physicians, possibly residents in training, to conduct and supervise the examinations. Patients are requested to disrobe completely (if only screened areas are available, they disrobe partially and remove final clothing at the time of examination) and are thoroughly examined. To avoid missing melanomas, it is essential that all parts of the body be examined, including hairy areas (scalp, axilla, pubis, etc.), nails, interdigital areas, and hidden areas (ears, nose, etc.).

The third phase of the screening entails referrals for biopsy, treatment, and follow-up. If a positive finding is identified, consent is obtained from the patient examined to send a full report to his family physician. The screening physician must be in contact with the family physician to follow up on the particular finding.

A screening of this type has been conducted in Brooklyn, New York, on 855 patients (sun exposed areas only were examined). The yield for the 855 patients was 90 basal cell carcinomas, 6 squamous cell carcinomas, 1 melanoma, and 172 precancerous lesions that included actinic keratoses, leukoplakias, and melanotic freckles.

It is estimated that there are over 500,000 nonmelanoma skin cancers treated per year in the United States. Melanoma cases amounted to 14,500 in 1980.

Mortality attributed to skin cancer is primarily related to malignant melanoma and some nonmelanoma skin cancers such as squamous cell carcinomas and some aggressive or poorly managed basal cell carcinomas. These may be responsible for a total of 6900 deaths per year (1980 estimate).

II. PRETREATMENT EVALUATION AND WORK-UP

The pretreatment evaluation of a patient with skin cancer should include the following work-up prior to making any therapeutic decisions.

A. History and Physical Examination

1. History

a. Present Illness

- Duration of present lesion.
- Pain.
- Bleeding.
- Itching.
- Tenderness.
- Changes in size.
- Changes in pigmentation.
- Recurrent infection.

- Ulceration.
- Other.

b. Social History

- Race.
- Occupation.
- Smoker.
- Drinker.
- Outdoor recreational activities.
- Skin pigmentation, freckles, etc.

c. Family History of Skin Cancer

d. Past History

- History of previous skin cancer.
- Previous therapy for skin cancer including radiation therapy, cryotherapy, surgical procedures, topical therapy, or Mohs's chemosurgery.
- Excessive exposure to UV light, e.g., phototherapy or psoralen with UV light (PUVA) for psoriasis.
- Prior irradiation for internal malignancies, e.g., thyroid or neck lesions.
- Previous scars, fistulas, or chronic ulcers.
- History of ingestion of certain medications, e.g., those containing arsenic.
- History of possible exposure to industrial carcinogens.
- History of heart disease, pulmonary insufficiency, renal disease, diabetes, etc.
- Allergies.

2. Physical Examination

A complete examination of the skin should be done with particular attention to those areas exposed to the sun.

a. Inspection and Palpation of the Skin Lesions

- Location of lesion.
- Size and shape, consistency, smooth or rough, regular or irregular borders.
- Flat, depressed, raised, nodular, verrucous.
- Color, solidly pigmented or mottled.
- Scaly or crusted, eroded, ulcerated.
- Hairy or nonhairy, associated telangiectasia.
- Mobility or infiltration.
- Encroachment of mucocutaneous borders or adjacent structures.
- Encroachment on the ear canal, conjunctiva, or lacrimal ducts.

b. Palpation of Regional Lymph Nodes

The physical examination includes palpatation of the regional lymph nodes.

c. Peripheral Vascular and Neurological Exam

This examination should be carried out, if indicated.

B. Biopsy

All skin lesions that are to be treated by any type of excision or curetting must have tissue sent for histology. If the lesion is suspected of being neoplastic, biopsy must be carried out before an adequate therapeutic regimen can be outlined. An adequate and representative biopsy should be obtained. A negative biopsy from a clinically suspicious lesion is an indication for rebiopsy. It is always advisable for the biopsy to be performed by the physician who performs the ultimate definitive surgery. The simplest biopsy technique should be considered, providing it yields adequate tissue and orientation.

Small lesions that can be easily excised should be totally excised for biopsy. For larger lesions, the biopsy technique may be any of the following:

- Punch biopsy.
- Shave biopsy.
- Curette biopsy. This method should be discouraged since it does not allow proper orientation of the specimen or full evaluation of the depth of the lesion.
- Incisional biopsy.
- Excisional biopsy.

The following characteristics, when identified by the pathologist, are of great help to the clinician:

1. Basal Cell Carcinoma

Variants of this tumor must be identified since they have varying prognoses and require specific therapeutic considerations:

- A morphea-type component within the basal cell carcinoma.
- A superficial basal cell carcinoma.
- Deep infiltration.
- A markedly atypical squamous cell component within a basal cell carcinoma.

2. Squamous Cell Carcinoma

The following features should be noted:

- Grade of differentiation.
- Depth of invasion.
- Presence or absence of solar elastosis.
- Presence or absence of spindle cell components.
- Perineural invasion.

Squamous cell carcinoma *in situ* must also be identified. The presence of solar elastosis implies a good prognosis. It can, however, be associated with exposure to carcinogens such as arsenic and may be associated with internal malignancies; this type of tumor usually presents in surfaces not normally exposed to sun.

3. Keratoacanthoma

This rapidly growing benign lesion is seen mostly in the elderly on sun-exposed areas of the skin. It presents clinically as a nodular lesion with overhanging edges around a central crater containing keratinizing material. A proper biopsy and sampling of a full-thickness slice from the center will differentiate it from squamous cell carcinoma. Clinical and pathological features must be correlated for an accurate diagnosis.

4. Melanoma

Pathologists are urged to section the specimen in thin contiguous layers whenever presented with a complete excisional biopsy. This will provide the necessary information for accurate pathological classification of the tumor and will also provide a prognostic index.

Melanomas are classified as follows:

- Superficial, spreading malignant melanoma.
- Nodular melanoma.
- Lentigo maligna (Hutchinson's, or melanotic, freckle).
- Acral lentiginous melanoma.

In addition, it is essential to identify the following features before selecting the appropriate therapy:

- Clark's level of invasion.
- Depth of invasion, using Breslow's micromeasurements.
- Presence or absence of ulceration.
- Presence or absence of satellitosis within the biopsy specimen.
- Presence or absence of lymphatic spread.
- Presence or absence of mononuclear cell infiltrate below the lesion.

C. Metastatic Evaluation

Nonmelanoma skin lesions almost never develop distant metastases, and generally no metastatic work-up is indicated. A good history and physical examination is sufficient for most cases. In patients with extensive, infiltrative, or recurrent tumors, particularly squamous cell carcinomas, and in cases where node metastases are identified, a chest x-ray and a multichannel biochemical profile (SMA-12) are advisable as a baseline work-up prior to therapy.

Malignant melanoma, on the other hand, spreads widely often and early, necessitating a full metastatic evaluation before deciding on a plan of management.

D. Pretreatment Preparation

Patients with nonmelanoma skin cancers are not usually effected by their tumor and rarely need any systemic preparation. Older patients, however, or patients with other intercurrent illnesses, should have a good medical evaluation and correction of any medical problems identified.

E. Multidisciplinary Evaluation

Nonmelanoma skin cancer is mostly diagnosed, biopsied, and treated in an office setting. Often the anatomic location of the tumor will prompt the patient to seek help of a particular specialist (such as an opthalmologist, a head and neck surgeon, a plastic surgeon, an otolaryngologist, or a dermatologist). Selection of therapy should be based on two sets of criteria: patient factors (such as patient's age, complexion, sex, medical status, distance from the nearest medical facility, etc.) and tumor factors (such as size of the tumor, its histological type, its location, etc).

In order to assure the optimal therapeutic approach for melanomas and the difficult and extensive nonmelanoma skin cancer, a multidisciplinary forum consisting of surgical and nonsurgical specialists should evaluate the individual problem based on all the criteria already mentioned. This forum should represent dermatology, plastic surgery, general surgery, pathology, radiotherapy, chemotherapy, nursing, and social service, particularly in the case of melanomas. Decisions are better made jointly, and full therapeutic planning should be established including rehabilitation of the patient. The apparent simplicity of most skin lesions, e.g., basal cell and squamous cell carcinomas, should not deter such an approach.

F. Site-Specific Data Form for Skin Cancer

(see p. 103)

III. THERAPEUTIC MANAGEMENT OF NONMELANOMA SKIN CANCER

The most common primary skin cancers, exclusive of malignant melanoma, include

- Basal cell carcinoma.
- Squamous cell carcinoma.

SITE-SPECIFIC DATA FORM—SKIN

HISTORY

Age: _____

Symptoms

_____ Pain _____ Itching
_____ Ulceration _____ Infection
_____ Crusting _____ Change in pigment
_____ Bleeding _____ Change in size
_____ Nodule

Other _____

Social history

Occupation: _____

Race: _____ White _____ Black _____ Oriental _____ Other

Exposure to sun _____

Allergies: _____ Arsenic ingestion _____

Family history of carcinoma
　Relation: _____ Site: _____
Pevious history of carcinoma
　_____ No _____ Yes Site: _____
　Rx: _____
Previous treatment (describe):
(Surgery, radiotherapy, chemotherapy,
PUVA, phototherapy, etc.)

PHYSICAL EXAMINATION

Site of tumor and extenson: _____ Left _____ Right

SITE OF ORIGIN (Check)

Trunk		Nose		Genitalia	
Chest	_____	Dorsum	_____	Scrotum	_____
Abdomen	_____	Alae	_____	Penis	_____
Back	_____	Collumella	_____	Vulva	_____
Buttock	_____			Extends to	
		Ear		Salivary glands	_____
		Pinna	_____	Eyes	_____
Upper extremity		Meatus	_____	Bone	_____
Arm	_____			Sinuses	_____
Forearm	_____	Eyelid		Cranial nerves	
Hand	_____	Upper	_____	VII	_____
Finger	_____	Lower	_____	IX	
				X	_____
		Perioral	_____	XI	_____
Lower extremity		Forehead	_____	XII	_____
Thigh	_____	Cheek	_____	Tendon	
Leg	_____	Chin	_____	Bone	_____
Foot	_____	Scalp	_____	Nerves	_____
Toes	_____	Neck	_____		

Size: (in centimeters) _____

Characteristics:

_____ Exophytic	_____ Hard	_____ Depressed
_____ Superficial	_____ Soft	_____ Flat
_____ Infiltrating	_____ Cystic	_____ Nodular
_____ Ulcerated	_____ Mobile	_____ Scaly or crusty
_____ Verruccous	_____ Fixed	_____ Hairy

Pigmented: _____ Lentigo _____ Superficial spreading _____ Nodular _____ Unclassified
(Melanomas only) Satellite lesions: _____ No _____ Yes _____ Number
_____ Within 2 cm of primary _____ More than 2 cm

REGIONAL LYMPH NODES

_____ Palpable _____ Nonpalpable

		Side		Size (cm)		Number of multiples
		R	L	0-5	>5	
_____ Soft	Juguloomohyoid	_____	_____	_____	_____	_____
_____ Rubbery	Upper deep cervical	_____	_____	_____	_____	_____
_____ Hard	Lower deep cervical	_____	_____	_____	_____	_____
_____ Fluctuant	Submaxillary	_____	_____	_____	_____	_____
_____ Moveable	Submental	_____	_____	_____	_____	_____
_____ Fixed	Parotid	_____	_____	_____	_____	_____
	Axilla	_____	_____	_____	_____	_____
	Groin	_____	_____	_____	_____	_____

Histologic diagnosis: _____

PREOPERATIVE EVALUATION (For melanomas only)

Biopsy: _____ Excisional _____ Incisional
Depth of invasion (mm): _____ 0-0.75 _____ 0.76-1.5 _____ 1.151-4.0 _____ >4.0
Levels: _____ I _____ II _____ III _____ IV _____ V

METASTATIC SURVEY

	Neg.	Pos.	Suspicious		Neg.	Pos.	Suspicious
Chest x-ray	_____	_____	_____	Liver scan	_____	_____	_____
Tomogram (chest)	_____	_____	_____	Bone scan	_____	_____	_____
Liver chemistries	_____	_____	_____	Brain scan	_____	_____	_____
Bone survey	_____	_____	_____	Other	_____	_____	_____

Distant metastases: _____ No _____ Yes _____ Lung _____ Liver _____ Bone _____ Other

Classification: _____ T _____ N _____ M

Signature: _____
Countersignature: _____

Stage: _____

Date: _____

I. Melanomas

Clarke levels of invasion

Level I   *In situ* melanoma, no invasion of the epidermal–dermal interface
Level II   Papillary dermis invasion, superficial
Level III   Invasion of full thickness of the papillary dermis down to, but not involving, the reticular dermis
Level IV   Invasion of reticular dermis
Level V   Invasion through the dermis into the subcutaneous fat

Levels of invasion have been correlated with measured thickness of infiltration by occular micrometry, the measurement extending from the level of what would be the normal basement membrane to the deepest level of the tumor seen microscopically (Breslow's measurements).

TNM classification

This can only be done accurately after excisional biopsy of the tumor and the measurement of depth of invasion and levels.

TX   Tumor cannot be assessed
T0   Melanoma *in situ* (level I)
T1   0–0.75 mm in depth (level II) papillary dermis invasion
T2   0.76–1.5 mm in depth (level III) invasion down to the papillary reticular dermal interface
T3   1.51–4.0 mm in depth (level IV) invasion of reticular dermis
T4   >4.0 mm in depth (level V) invasion of subcutaneous tissues, or satellite nodules within 2 cm of the primary

Nodal classification

NX   Nodes cannot be assessed
T0   No regional nodes
N1   Involvement of one regional lymph node station, moveable nodes (<5 cm in size) or negative nodes
         but fewer than five intransit skin metastases
N2   Any of the following: more than one regional lymph node station; nodes >5 cm in size or fixed;
         or five or more intransit metastases

Distant metastases

MX   Cannot be assessed
M0   No known metastases
M1   Involvement of skin or subcutaneous tissues beyond the primary lymphatic station
M2   Visceral metastases

Stage groupings

Stage I   T1 or T2, N0, M0
Stage IIa   T3 with N0, M0
Stage IIb   T4 with N0, M0
Stage III   Any T with N1, M0
Stage IV   Any T with N2 or M1 and 2

Histopathologic classification

Grade 1   Well differentiated
Grade 2   Moderately well differentiated
Grade 3   Poorly differentiated
Grade 4   Undifferentiated

Types

Lentigo malignant
Superficial spreading melanoma
Nodular melanoma

II. Nonmelanoma: Skin Cancer

TNM classification

T1   Tumor 2 cm or less in its largest dimension, strictly superficial or exophytic
T2   Tumor more than 2 cm but not more than 5 cm in its largest dimension, or with minimal infiltration
         of the dermis, irrespective of size
T3   Tumor more than 5 cm in its largest dimension, or with deep infiltration of the dermis, irrespective of size
T4   Tumor involving other structures such as cartilage, muscle, or bone

No node classification or stage grouping is recommended for skin cancers other than melanomas.

- Adnexal neoplasms (eccrine gland carcinoma and sebaceous gland carcinoma).

Basal cell and squamous cell carcinomas have the highest incidence among the malignant neoplasms of the skin. In most cases they are invasive only locally. An array of therapeutic modalities may be used to extinguish or destroy these tumors, and the overall cure rate is between 90 and 95% when treatment is performed by an experienced physician in a timely fashion. Unlike other neoplasms, most skin cancers are treated in the physician's office; it is, therefore, often the operator's personal expertise and available office equipment that determines the patient's therapy. Under optimal conditions, a multidisciplinary consultation should be obtained for the difficult tumors prior to starting therapy.

A. Management Goals

1. Tissue Diagnosis

It is important to biopsy all lesions where the slightest suspicion of skin cancer exists. Furthermore, any tissues removed from a patient, by any modality whatsoever, must be sent for histological evaluation, regardless of its apparent clinical insignificance, in order to determine its histological nature and exact content. With both the clinical diagnosis and its histological confirmation, one has a more complete view of the tumor and is better able to select the appropriate therapeutic modality.

2. Selection of Type and Extent of Therapy

An attempt should be made to control the lesion by the therapeutic modality that will cause the least morbidity while at the same time achieving the highest possible cure rate. Because many skin cancers are located in important visible areas (i.e., face and neck), the cosmetic end result is an important determining factor. A given lesion can be treated by various therapeutic modalities with varying cosmetic results; when selecting among the various techniques, we should favor those that will give the patient the most desirable cosmetic result as well as one that best fits his or her psychological needs.

Patients with the highest incidence of skin cancers—the elderly—are often undertreated because of their low expected longevity. Their skin cancers are often neglected for many years, resulting in increased size, deeper infiltration, and marked difficulties in the projected therapeutic approach. Since we really cannot predict longevity of a patient, these tumors should be effectively treated while they are small.

B. Common Pitfalls

The following are some of the departures from sound clinical management that are most frequently encountered:

1. Unwarranted Delay in Treatment

- Prolonged watch-and-wait attitude.
- Prolonged topical medications (over the counter and prescription).
- Prolonged delay due to expectation of short-term patient survival.

2. Lack of Biopsy or Inadequate Biopsy

This may lead to acceptance of a biopsy report that is not in keeping with the clinical picture.

3. Selection of Inappropriate Surgical Technique

- Failure to recognize the cosmetic implications of the various modalities.
- Tailoring the extent of surgical procedure to the ability of the surgeon.
- Inadequate margins of resection.

4. Failure to Recognize Biological Facts

- The relatively limited invasiveness and slow progression of skin cancers. On the other hand, certain types will display a very aggressive behavior (e.g., squamous cell carcinomas and some adnexal malignant neoplasms).
- The aggressiveness of local recurrences, which result in an increased morbidity and mortality.
- The potential spread of some tumors to nodes (e.g., lower lip lesions, squamous cell carcinomas).

C. Complications of Treatment

Since many of these skin tumors can be treated by a variety of therapeutic modalities, one must recognize the advantages and disadvantages of each in order to make the proper selection. The postsurgical complications of treatment can be divided into early and late complications.

- Early complications.
  Infection.
  Postcryosurgical edema.
  Vascular complications, bleeding, hematoma formation.
  Wound dehiscence.
  Graft necrosis.

- Late complications.
  Scarring and keloid formation.
  Loss of pigment.
  Marjolin's ulcer.
  Complications due to the special function of certain specific surgically treated sites (e.g., ectropion and tearing secondary to eyelid treatments).
- Complications of topical chemotherapeutic agents.
  Discomfort, pain, pruritus.
  Erythema.
  Local hyperthermia.
  Oozing.
  Skin necrosis.
  Treatment failure. These agents may conceal a deep recurrence.
- Complications of radiotherapy.
  Early excessive erythema and moist desquamation, especially if a high dose was used.
  Skin pigmentation and photosensitivity, skin thinning and atrophy, telangiectasia, fibrosis, contracture, chronic ulceration and necrosis, and Marjolin's ulcer are complications of very unusual circumstances (e.g., heavy or repeated irradiation, unusual sensitivity of skin following arsenic ingestion, chronic irritation, and infection).

Recurrences can occur after treating these tumors by any modality.

D. Selection of Treatment

A number of therapeutic choices are available for the treatment of nonmelanoma skin cancers. The selection of one technique over another will depend on the following:

- Patient factors: age, occupation, ethnic factors, sex, complexion, predisposing factors, etc.
- Tumor factors: size, location, histology, and histological behavior.
- Physician factors: physician's speciality and expertise.

1. Histological Nature of the Tumor

Nonmelanoma skin cancer refers basically to two tumors: basal cell carcinoma and squamous cell carcinoma. Both of these tumors tend to have a slow rate of growth with a very low incidence of metastases which, when they do occur, are primarily limited to draining nodes.
Basal cell carcinomas can be of various types:

- Superficial.
- Nodular.
- Cystic.
- Pigmented.
- Nodular ulcerative.
- Morphea type.

Most of these basal cell cancers can be treated by any of the therapeutic modalities available, the exception being the morphea type, for which excision is strongly recommended.

Squamous cell carcinomas may be more agressive and can, at times, metastasize, primarily to lymph nodes. Margins of therapy need to be slightly wider, and regional nodes must be carefully evaluated. Bowen's disease (which is a squamous cell carcinoma *in situ*) and squamous cell carcinomas located on sun-damaged skin tend to have a very low potential for metastases but a high degree of multicentricity. When located on non-sun-exposed areas or mucous membranes, these lesions may be neglected and thus acquire a higher potential for metastases; excisional surgery is recommended for these lesions.

2. Location of the Tumor

The anatomic location of the tumor is very important when selecting the appropriate therapeutic modality. We must, for example, be very discriminating in the selection of the appropriate modality when treating lesions of the face, in order to offer the best cosmetic result and maintain a high cure rate. The individual sites and the proper choice of treatment will be dealt with in §3.III.G.

3. Size of the Tumor

In general, lesions smaller than 2 cm can be treated by any of the therapeutic modalities:

- Desiccation and curettage.
- Excision surgery.
- Cryosurgery.
- Radiation therapy.

For lesions greater than 2 cm, excision surgery should be the first consideration unless there are medical contraindications or the patient refuses. Radical radiotherapy is also highly curative, but treatment should be planned carefully to achieve good cosmesis.

Recurrent lesions should be treated by Mohs's surgery, or if such is not available, they should be reexcised with adequate margins; this will sometime require grafts or skin flaps for closure. Radiation therapy is an acceptable alternative choice. Certain neglected or recurrent lesions may reach extensive dimensions and become life threatening by virtue of invading a neighboring vital organ. Such a lesion needs all the ingenuity and expertise of both a surgeon and a radiotherapist to devise and execute a combined approach in order to eliminate the tumor successfully.

4. Multiple Tumors

Patients may present with multiple tumors over their entire body surface as a result of extensive actinic damage to the skin. Excision surgery for all these tumors is impractical. Electrosurgery or cryosurgery is probably the better alternatives in such cases. Such lesions may necessitate the use of several modalities depending on the characteristics and location of each lesion.

5. Age of the Patient

Subconsciously, one tends to be more concerned with the cosmetic impact of therapy on a young patient. Physicians also tend to be more conservative when treating tumors in the older age group. Thus a higher recurrence rate is often noted in both these age groups.

For the elderly patient (more than 65 years old), radiation therapy is often a good modality. Some patients in this age group, however, are not ambulatory enough to receive radiotherapy, in which case, cryosurgery is an excellent alternative. In the debilitated, handicapped, or medically ill patient, one must select the simplest and fastest modality of treatment (i.e., electrosurgery or cryosurgery).

6. Psychological Factors

The psychological trauma of the disease and potential scarring caused by treatment must be carefully considered. The patient will occasionally insist on a newer, more fashionable technique; the consulting physician should use an unbiased opinion in advising for or against such requests.

E. Specific Therapeutic Modalities

Table I summarizes the various treatment modalities for nonmelanoma skin cancer.

Table I

Treatment Modalities for Nonmelanoma Skin Cancer

	Indications	Contraindications	Disadvantages
Desiccation and curettage (electrosurgery)	Multiple lesions Superficial lesions Keratoses and premalignant lesions	Pacemaker patients Compromised blood supply Morphea-type basal cell Sensitivity to local anesthetics History of keloid formation	Depigmented scar
Cryosurgery	Eyelids, ear, nose Pacemaker patients To local anesthesia sensitivity Bedridden patients	Aggressive lesions Cryoglobulinemias Tumors of fingers, scalp Patients with impaired vascularity	Oozing and edema Delayed healing (4–6 weeks) Depigmented scar
Excisional surgery	Morphea-type basal cells Infiltrating lesions and recurrent tumors Unavailable Mohs's surgery High cosmetic expectations	Sensitivity to local anesthetic agents Poor surgical risk	
Radiotherapy	Older patients Lesions of face, eyelids, canthi, nose Extensive lesions in poor-risk patients	Extremity lesions Proximity to bone Trunk lesions	Acute and chronic radiodermatitis
Mohs's surgery	Recurrent lesions or very extensive lesions Previous irradiation Morphea-type basal cell Areas where conservation is important: fingertips, eyelids, etc.		Highly specialized technique, requires special skills and facilities
Laser surgery	Small lesions In conjunction with Mohs's surgery to avoid bleeding		Expense and bulk of equipment
Topical chemotherapy	Multicentric lesions Sun-damaged skin, keratoses Superficial basal cell carcinoma	Deep infiltrating lesions	Oozing, erythema, pain

1. Desiccation and Curettage (Electrosurgery)

This technique can be used to treat most types of superficial skin cancers. Its drawback lies in the fact that it does not permit histological confirmation of the effectiveness of the therapy. The literature has shown, however, that this technique, used by experienced physicians, can yield a 95% cure rate. Malignant neoplasms have a different consistency than normal surrounding skin; by skillful curettage, one can remove malignant tissues only, since normal skin resists the cutting edge of the curette. Curettage and electrodesiccation must be repeated three times in one single visit in order to obtain this high cure rate.

Desiccation and curettage is contraindicated in patients with pacemakers, areas with a compromised blood supply, morphea-type basal cell carcinoma, and hypersensitivity to local anesthetics. The advantages of this technique are that multiple lesions can be treated in one visit; there is no need for hospitalization; and normal skin is not sacrificed when removing the malignant neoplasm. The main disadvantage of the technique is that it may leave a depressed, depigmented scar at the treated site.

2. Cryosurgery

Cryosurgery is another form of surgery where the results are based on clinical observation rather than histological confirmation. The procedure has immediate sequelae, which are edema and oozing, but these resolve within a week or two, and healing occurs by secondary intention within 4–6 weeks.

There are selected sites where cryosurgery offers distinct advantages: the eyelids, the ears, and the nose. Liquid nitrogen spares the lacrimal system and the normal cartilage, making unnecessary extensive surgical procedures that would require excision and deformity of the external ear or nose. This technique has other advantages: it can be used for patients with pacemakers; no local anesthetics are necessary in patients who are sensitive to these agents; and due to the ease of transportation of the equipment, it can be used for bedridden patients or patients in nursing homes. The technique has a cure rate of 95%, but cosmetic results are similar to those of electrosurgery, and a hypopigmented scar remains at the treated site. Cryosurgery should not be used in the digits or lower legs or wherever the microvasculature is compromised (diabetes, peripheral vascular disease, etc.).

3. Excision Surgery

When excisional surgery is selected as the treatment of a malignant skin neoplasm, histological confirmation of the nature and the extent of the tumor is obtained, and the adequacy of the resection can be checked histologically. This technique can be used in any of the skin tumors, but it is especially indicated in morphea-type basal cell cancer and recurrent skin tumors when Mohs's surgery is not available. It is especially suited for patients who insist on a superior cosmetic result. The procedure may be contraindicated in patients allergic to local anesthetics.

4. Radiation Therapy

This therapeutic modality is an excellent alternative, especially for the older age group and for large lesions in exposed areas. Radiation therapy is a field therapy; there is no histological confirmation of the destruction of the malignant neoplasm, but the treated area is usually well beyond the clinical extent of the tumor. This technique is especially suited for areas that are difficult to excise (eyelids, canthi, pinna, nose, and periauricular region) or those that would require extensive surgical grafting in a medically compromised patient with an extensive and deeply infiltrating lesion situated in a cosmetically critical area, e.g., the face. Radiotherapy is less desirable in the trunk and should preferably not be used on the extremities (hands and feet) because of the underlying osseous structures. Bone and cartilage absorb much more radiation than the skin if a low-voltage beam is utilized (< 200 kV unfiltered), which limits the use of radiation therapy when these structures are too close to the tumor. Radiotherapy is also suited for patients who are unwilling to have their tumors surgically removed. Radiation therapy should be used judiciously in areas where there is concern about slow healing or postradiation changes. When properly used, however, radiotherapy will control more than 90% of skin cancers with minimal ill effects. The vast majority of skin cancers treated by radiotherapy receive treatment through a single-incident beam, but many factors govern the choice of the radiation technique.

In order to treat skin cancer successfully by radiotherapy, a thorough knowledge of different technique alternatives and the availability of a wide array of treating units is necessary. Attention to detail in the design and execution of a course of radiotherapy is mandatory if one is to achieve a high cure rate with good cosmetic result. The following discussion of treatment technique is not intended to be comprehensive but, rather, illuminatory.

a. Volume

The estimation of the extent of a given lesion is by artful inspection using a lens and palpation in three dimensions. This determines the portal size, the normal tissue margin to be included in the field, and the energy of radiation to be used. Generally, the volume is kept limited to the lesion with a small safety margin. This volume and safety margin is usually increased in case of squamous cell carcinomas or recurrent rodent ulcers.

b. Modalities

These include external-beam radiation with photons (x-ray) and γ beam (^{60}Co). Other electrons (betatron- or accelerator-originated beams) and special interstitial implants may be used and are indicated in special circumstances. The most commonly used modalities nowadays are either electrons or external photon beam radiation with appropriate energies (60–200 kV) depending on the thickness of the lesion (0.5–1.0 cm). Deeply infiltrating and larger lesions require larger fields and more penetrating beams.

In advanced lesions that have infiltrated bone and cartilage, a better quality radiation (^{60}Co beam or high-voltage photons), as well as a combination of radiotherapy and surgery, may be necessary. Electrons can also be used for large lesions of the nose, pinna, and external ear. Furthermore, certain sites such as inner canthus or eyelids require special care and protection of the eye; this can be adequately achieved by the use of lead eye shields.

c. Dose

The daily dose depends upon the site and size of the lesions. Small lesions are treated with small fields and limited fractionation. Large lesions require large ports, higher energy, higher total doses, and greater fractionation. For example, for a 2-cm port (not overlying cartilage or eyelids) 4000 rads in 10 days is quite satisfactory. For lesions treated with large ports or lesions on the lids, canthi, or overlying cartilage, a dose of 5000 rads in 4 weeks gives excellent control and cosmetic results. Occasionally, aggressive lesions may need doses as high as 6500 rads for effective local control.

5. Mohs's Surgery

This is another highly specialized technique performed only by specially trained practioners with adequately equipped facilities and support services (pathology and plastic surgery). It is a very valuable technique, although tedious and costly. The procedure consists of microscopically controlled surgery with serial excisions of tumor tissues fixed *in vivo*. The lesion is mapped; horizontal sections of the neoplasm are cut; and frozen sections are immediately examined to determine the extent of the tumor. Those mapped horizontal sections where neoplasm is identified in the cut margins indicate sites in the patient where there would be residual tumor. These sites are immediately retreated by surgical removal of a subsequent level. The procedure is repeated until there is histological confirmation of the absence of tumor in all margins.

Over the last 10 years the fresh-tissue technique has gained popularity over the *in-situ* fixation method. This newer technique is essentially the same, but no *in-situ* fixation is necessary. The majority of the obvious tumor is destroyed with a curette or scalpel, and a tissue section of the remaining base is then excised somewhat like a saucerization. This saucer-shaped fragment is mapped, color coded, and examined "*en face*," using a cryostat–frozen section technique. If any tumor is left, the map is consulted for its exact location, and a second stage or even a third stage may be carried out to ensure a clear margin. This is repeated until a tumor-free margin is achieved.

Mohs's chemosurgery or Mohs's surgery (the fresh-tissue technique) is indicated in the following circumstances:

- Recurrent carcinomas of the skin.
- Anatomic sites where preservation of normal tissue is paramount (i.e., fingertip, eyelid, penis).
- Areas where the incidence of recurrences are highest, namely, around the inner canthus, ala nasi, and the pinna.
- It is also indicated for the aggressive morphea-like basal cell carcinomas.

Mohs's chemosurgery is an outpatient procedure and requires no general anesthesia. When expertly carried out, it provides the most effective removal of the tumor while sacrificing the least amount of normal tissues. The defects caused by Mohs's surgery are best allowed to heal by secondary intention. Occasionally, reconstructive plastic surgery is necessary. In certain situations, the defect may be covered by a local or regional flap or a suitable graft technique; this, however, carries the risk of an occult recurrence developing under the graft site and going undetected for a long time.

6. Laser Surgery

A new promising method not yet available in most institutions is laser surgery. The unique properties of lasers make them extremely useful in a variety of therapeutic applications. The carbon dioxide (CO_2) laser can be used for endophotoincisions and endophotocautery and is applicable for the treatment of skin cancer. The CO_2 laser utilizes a high-intensity infrared light source as energy. Since body soft tissue is 80–90% water, when the laser beam is focused on the tissue, intracellular water instantly vaporizes to steam. Tissue can thus be cut, evaporated, vaporized, or destroyed. The effects are localized and instantaneous, and the thermal changes induced by this light-source energy make it possible simultaneously to cauterize vessels and reduce blood loss, as well as cause thermal alterations of the proteins in the cells.

The CO_2 excision laser focuses the infrared beam through lenses and can be used to pinpoint small lesions. In the treatment of basal cell carcinoma for example, it may be used for cutting and has the advantage of simultaneously producing hemostasis and sealing lymphatics. In larger lesions, it can be used in conjunction with Mohs's fresh-tissue technique to avoid troublesome bleeding. Healing takes place by granulation.

The main disadvantage of the laser technique is that the unit is expensive and the handpiece bulky. The results of its applications (cure and cosmesis) are still not widely confirmed.

7. Topical Chemotherapy (5-Fluorouacil)

This technique is particularly useful when there is extensive sun-damaged skin associated with a number of premalignant lesions (e.g., actinic keratoses). It is also effective in the treatment of superficial spreading basal cell carcinoma. The procedure involves the topical application of 5-fluorouacil (5-FU) twice daily for 3–6 weeks. This causes moderate-to-severe discomfort manifested by oozing, erythema, local hyperthermia, and pain in the treated area. Ultimately, a scab forms, which falls off when healing is complete. The patient must be advised of these side effects prior to treatment to insure patient compliance. This treatment is also a field therapy where no histological confirmation of the total destruction of the tumor is assured, and close follow-up evaluation is necessary to identify residual or recurrent disease. The major shortcoming and risk of this technique is its superficial nature, which may lead to an apparent cure on the surface of the skin while a deep nodular recurrence remains concealed, only to recur months or years later.

F. Guidelines for Treatment according to Histology

1. Superficial Basal Cell Carcinoma

These lesions are often 1–2 cm in diameter, and they spread horizontally in a slow growth. The treatment alternatives are

- Electrosurgery.
- Cryosurgery.
- Excision.
- Topical 5-FU.
- Radiotherapy.

2. Nodular, Noduloulcerative, Cystic, and Pigmented Basal Cell Carcinoma

Two techniques are equally effective in dealing with these types of tumors:

- Electrosurgery and cryosurgery (for lesions under 2 cm).
- Excision surgery.

Individual preferences and other factors will be the determining factors. Radiation therapy and Mohs's surgery are reserved for the more extensive lesions or special cases.

3. Morphea-Type Basal Cell Carcinoma

The treatments of choice are:

- Excision with or without plastic reconstruction.
- Mohs's surgery with or without plastic reconstruction.
- Radiation therapy.

4. Keratoacanthoma

This is a pseudomalignancy. The treatments of choice are

- Electrosurgery.
- Local excision.
- Cryosurgery.
- Radiation (for recurrences in the head and neck area).

5. Bowen's Disease

Bowen's disease is an intraepithelial squamous cell carcinoma, often multicentric. The treatment modalities of choice, in order of preference, are

- Excision surgery.
- Cryosurgery.
- Curettage and electrodessication.
- Radiation therapy (rarely indicated).

6. Squamous Cell Carcinoma

The treatments of choice of squamous cell carcinoma of the skin are

- Excision surgery.
- Radiation therapy (particularly in the older age group).
- Cryosurgery.
- Mohs's surgery for the extensive or recurrent lesion, or in areas where conservation is essential.
- Electrosurgery for multiple small tumors in sun-damaged skin.

G. Therapeutic Management: Site-Specific (Nonmelanoma)

1. Head and Neck

Various areas of the head and neck require special individual attention because of the cosmetic importance of any interference with the normal features of the face and because of the unique structures present in this location.

a. Eyelids

The most common therapeutic choices for treating skin cancers of the eyelids are cryosurgery, excision surgery, and radiation therapy.

i. Cryosurgery. Cryosurgery is an excellent therapeutic modality for treating tumors of the eyelids; it does not destroy lacrimal system structures; it does not cause notching; cosmetic results are excellent; and recurrence rates are very low (between 3 and 5%). It does, however, cause loss of eyelashes when the treated area involves the eyelid margins. Lesions that are amenable to cryosurgery should be well defined, not infiltrating underlying structures, and should not invade the anterior conjunctival sac.

ii. Excision Surgery. The primary aim of treatment should be complete extirpation of the neoplasm with the least possible structural deformity and functional impairment of the eyelids. Surgical excision offers several advantages:

- A sectional examination of the surgical specimen provides microscopic evidence of the completeness of the surgical excision and provides a sound basis for accurate prognosis. Ideally, a frozen section should be done at the time of surgery to determine the existence of tumor-free margins.
- Previously irradiated lesions that develop recurrences can be treated by surgical excision.
- Excisional surgery is the treatment of choice for recurrent or new lesions in previously irradiated sites.
- When cosmetic effect and functional results are good, excisional surgery has minimal side effects.

iii. Radiation Therapy. Radiation therapy gives excellent results in periorbital cancers. The eye is shielded by placing a lead shield beneath the eyelids; this prevents any cataract development. When the lesion is on the inner canthus or involves the tear duct, stenosis of the duct can be prevented by inserting a Silastic tube prior to radiation therapy. Permanent loss of the eyelashes will occur after radiotherapy and is a cosmetic deformity to be considered, especially if the lid margin is involved with disease.

iv. Chemosurgery. Primary lesions of the inner canthus and recurrent lesions can be effectively treated by chemosurgery if this modality is available.

b. Nose

Malignant tumors of the nose can be treated by a number of therapeutic modalities. The most common choices are electrosurgery, cryosurgery, excision surgery, and radiation therapy. Both cryosurgery and electrosurgery, when performed on the free edge of the ala nasi, can cause notching. For tumors over 2 cm in diameter, where some infiltration in depth may be anticipated, the best treatment is by surgical removal, though this may require rotation of flaps for reconstruction.

Recurrent basal cell carcinomas of the nose are much more difficult to treat. They often receive inadequate treatment because the surgeon fails to appreciate the true extent of the invasion into adjacent skin. Furthermore, for the sake of preserving the cosmetic appearance, the surgeon often fails to resect sufficient tissues. In the treatment of recurrent lesions of the nose, Mohs's surgery has an impressive cure rate and, if available, seems to be the treatment of choice, preserving, as it does, the maximum amount of tissue.

Radiation therapy is an excellent therapeutic alternative but, because of the close proximity of the underlying nasal cartilage, needs special care in the choice of the treatment beam to avoid cartilage necrosis. Electron beam therapy—γ beams (^{60}Co) of short source–skin distance—may be particularly beneficial in this site, and shielding of the nares is useful to prevent crusting and contractures.

c. Lips

Local excision of tumors of the lip is the best choice of treatment. The excision is carried out with the intent of removing a margin of apparently normal tissue of between 0.5 and 1.0 cm. In the case of small tumors, the defect in the lip can be closed primarily in a straight line, or as a triangular-wedge resection, using a small step at the vermillion margin to prevent a scar contracture. For larger lesions, more extensive resections are necessary, and these will require more complex closures, sometimes using local mucosal or skin flaps (e.g., lip shave with mucosal advancement flap, Estlander flaps, Abbé flaps).

Radiation therapy is also effective in the management of some lip lesions, especially the large superficial ones that are curable by radiotherapy without the need for extensive surgical repair. When irradiation is used, the gums and teeth must be protected, using special shields.

d. Ears

Tumors of the ears can be treated by cryosurgery, excisional surgery, radiation therapy, or occasionally, electrosurgery.

i. Cryosurgery. Cryosurgery is of particular value in the treatment of tumors of the ear because liquid nitrogen does not destroy cartilage unless it has been invaded by tumor. Therefore, most tumors that are not fixed or that do not invade the underlying cartilage can be adequately treated with cryosurgery. When using the cryosurgical spray technique on the external ear, one should adequately shield the external auditory canal so as to avoid spraying liquid nitrogen into this area.

ii. Excisional Surgery. For small lesions of the auricle, excision can be done safely in the shape of a wedge resection followed by primary closure of the auricular defect. When carcinoma of the ear involves the external auditory canal, special problems arise. Carcinomas confined to the external auditory canal can usually be resected as a sleeve of tissue (with the adequacy of resection checked by frozen section) and the defect repaired by an inlay-free graft; stenosis of the canal is not a problem in this type of case. When, however, the carcinoma involves the bone, more massive resections, which could include the mastoid or temporal bone, may be required. A skin flap repair is usually indicated in these cases, and stenosis becomes a serious problem if an attempt is made to preserve the external auditory canal. Impairment of hearing on one side, even when it causes little concern to the patient, is a real threat. Because of the extent and complexity of this type of surgery, Mohs's surgery, when available, should be attempted initially. Extensive lesions of this type, however, will often necessitate a combination of surgery and radiotherapy in order to achieve cure with minimum tissue loss.

iii. Radiation Therapy. In skin cancer of the ear, radiation therapy has been blamed for chondronecrosis. This may occur when superficial therapy is used to treat infiltrating lesions extending to the cartilage. Electron beam, on the other hand, has several advantages and can be used for larger lesions as well as for carcinomas involving the external auditory canal. When good-quality radiation with careful fractions is used, chondritis becomes a rare complication.

iv. Electrosurgery. Electrosurgery may be effectively used for small tumors under 0.5 cm in diameter, not infiltrating cartilage.

e. Scalp

Excisional surgery is the preferred alternative for lesions in this location. The subaponeurotic space usually provides sufficient depth for excision of superficial cancers since this space is a very good barrier to deeper growth. When the excised specimen is larger than 2 cm in diameter, repair by direct approximation of the skin edges is virtually impossible on the scalp. Regional flaps or transposition of free grafts must be used.

Electrosurgery, in experienced hands, may be an alternative to excisional surgery. Cryosurgery, on the other hand, is not advised in this site due to the fact that higher recurrence rates have been observed when treating tumors in this location with cryosurgery. Radiation therapy is not recommended in the scalp since it is usually accompanied by irreversible alopecia in addition to slow healing at the treated site.

f. Neck

Malignant tumors of the neck can be accurately treated by a number of therapeutic modalities. The most common therapeutic choices are electrosurgery or surgical excision.

g. High-Risk Factors and Metastases

Certain high-risk factors affecting head and neck skin cancer in general are recognized. They include

- Critical locations: eyelids, canthus, pinna, nasolabial fold, and nasal alae.
- Size: greater than 2 cm in diameter.
- Histopathological types: morphea-type basal cell carcinoma and noduloulcerative basal cell carcinoma (rodent ulcer).
- Recurrent lesions; these are lesions possibly best treated by Mohs's surgery, if available.

These factors could justify a slightly more aggressive approach than that usually taken for other skin cancers.

The incidence of metastases to regional lymph nodes is small in nonmelanoma tumors of the head and neck. Only therapeutic lymph node dissection is indicated; prophylactic node dissection has no place in nonmelanoma skin cancer. Lymph nodes that are increasing in size or that are persistently enlarged in a patient with a definitely proven primary carcinoma of the skin are indications for a cervical lymphadenectomy.

2. Trunk and Extremities

Therapy of basal cell carcinoma is dictated by its two most important features: slow growth and absence of metastases. However, the lesion may extend on rare occasion to osseous or nerve tissue. Excision and grafts are rarely necessary in the trunk or extremities; the removal of the affected area without lymph node dissection is usually enough. As in other areas, simple elliptical excision with adequate margins is sufficient. Electrosurgery is a suitable alternative and is especially indicated when dealing with multiple tumors smaller than 2 cm in diameter. Cryosurgery can also be used to treat these tumors but is especially utilized in the presternal area where keloid formation is common after excision surgery or electrosurgery.

Squamous cell carcinomas of the skin tend to be slightly more aggressive. Squamous cell carcinoma on sun-damaged skin tends to cause fewer metastases than a similar lesion arising on a protected area. This factor has to be taken into account when considering a lymph node dissection; this, however, should only be performed in continuity with the primary tumor when nodal disease is clinically present, since few patients will actually have nodal metastases. The preferred therapeutic modality for most primary squamous cell carcinomas of the trunk is simple elliptical excision. Electrosurgery, cryosurgery, and radiation therapy are utilized less frequently but are selectively indicated in certain cases.

More aggressive treatment may, on rare occasions, be indicated when the tumor has infiltrated in depth, sometimes even affecting bone, neurovascular structures, etc. Amputations of digits or extremities might be necessary, and large locoregional flaps may be required to cover the defect of the excision in the site.

In treating lesions of the extremities, one must take into consideration the status of the patient's microvasculature, especially so in the elderly. The microvasculature is particularly important when selecting a therapeutic modality where the mode of healing is by second intention or when grafts are to be utilized. Patients with compromised microvasculature (i.e., diabetics and those with peripheral vascular disease) should preferably have their lesions removed by surgical excision.

IV. MALIGNANT MELANOMAS OF THE SKIN

Malignant melanomas constitute a disease entity that is distinctly different from all other skin cancers. Although they constitute a very small proportion of skin cancer (3–5% of skin cancers and less than 1% of all malignant tumors), they are of importance because of their potential seriousness. Unlike other skin cancers, malignant melanomas have a marked predilection for lymphatic as well as vascular spread, with possible distant metastases to any organ in the body.

A. Prevention, Screening, and Early Detection: The Benign Nevus

The presence of a preexisting pigmented lesion in a large number of patients with melanoma and the presence of discrete signs of early changes indicative of malignant transformation of these pigmented lesions, offer unique opportunities for prevention and early detection of malignant melanoma; this constitutes a significant aspect of the management of this tumor. It has been estimated that over 23% of melanomas unequivocally arise from preexisting benign nevi. Most individuals have several nevi (18–20 per person on the average), and the incidence of melanoma is only 1–2 per 100,000 population. Thus, it appears that only one nevus in a million will become malignant, and one must, therefore, try to narrow the selection to those nevi with some specific premalignant potential.

1. Benign Nevus and Its Precancerous Potential

Nevi are pigmented lesions of the skin caused by a proliferation of melanocytes within the lower epidermis, the dermis, or both. They are truly hamartomas but are considered by some to be neoplastic. The overwhelming majority of nevi are acquired and begin to appear sometime between the ages of 2 and 5, or during puberty; only a small proportion of melanocytic nevi

are truly congenital. When acquired nevi first appear, they go through a process of maturation, changing histologically and dermatologically from the "junctional nevus" of childhood (a small, regular, flat lesion that occupies the epidermo–dermal junction) through the "compound nevus" of adolescence (this has both junctional and dermal components) to the intradermal nevus, which is a mature lesion totally situated in the dermis. Acquired nevi are usually less than 1 cm in diameter, are homogeneously pigmented, and have uniform surface characteristics. Mature nevi can be flat, slightly elevated, verrucoid, polypoid, dome shaped, sessile, or papillomatous. Some may even have a prominent hairy component, and these are always benign lesions with no malignant potentials whatsoever. Likewise, the "blue nevus," which is made up of neuritic dermal melanocytes, is located in the deep dermis and is a benign lesion.

Some more specific nevi that do not fall precisely into the categories described above carry a greater potential for malignant transformation and must be considered precancerous:

- Congenital nevi. These are pigmented melanocytic nevi that are present at or very close to birth. They can be divided according to their size. The giant congenital nevus (giant hairy nevus, bathing-trunk nevus, etc.) is over 20 cm in its greatest diameter and has a well-recognized malignant potential. The medium-sized and small congenital nevi are less than 20 cm, and their malignant potential is controversial.
- Benign juvenile melanomas (spindle and/or epithelioid cell nevus, Spitz's nevus). This lesion, ordinarily found prior to puberty, tends to be a small, solitary eruptive papule that is biologically benign although histologically strongly suggestive of a malignant melanoma.
- Melanotic freckle (Hutchinson's freckle, or lentigo maligna). This is an easily recognizable, flat, pigmented lesion that usually appears in an older age group and is seen on sun-exposed skin areas (hands and face). It is a malignant melanoma *in situ* with a very long noninvasive growth phase. Resection of these lesions is strongly recommended in order to avoid later malignant complications.
- Nevi in patients with xeroderma pigmentosa.
- The dysplastic nevus syndrome (DNS) was originally described in the setting of familial melanoma where family members of patients with this disease were noted to have morphologically and histologically atypical nevi in large numbers throughout the body. The presence of these nevi identifies a subset of patients that are several hundred times more susceptibe to melanoma than the normal population. Subsequently, the same dysplastic lesion was noted to be present in one-third of patients previously treated for malignant melanoma and was identified as being the usual precursor of second melanomas in these patients. Clinically, the lesion presents as an irregular lesion over 5 mm in size with

varigated pigmentation and a macular component; histologically, it displays marked atypia in its epithelial component.

2. Recommendations for Elective Resection of Benign Nevi and Pigmented Lesions

The following nevi should be considered as having enough premalignant potential to warrant elective excision:

a. Giant Congenital Hairy Nevi

These might require multiple-stage excisions. The malignant potential of smaller congenital nevi is not clear; it is advisable however, that when the lesion can be removed with minimal cosmetic or functional deficit, it should be removed.

b. Lentigo Maligna

These lesions should be completely but conservatively excised. The margins are more easily defined with the aid of a Wood's light.

c. Pigmented Lesions from Patients with Xeroderma Pigmentosa

Although, these are sometimes so extensive and numerous that they defy any attempt at rational treatment, they should, whenever possible, be excised and must otherwise be closely observed and removed at the slightest indication of changes.

d. Benign Juvenile Melanomas

These should be conservatively but completely excised to allow for complete histopathological examination. These lesions can be difficult to interpret microscopically, but confusion will be avoided if the lesion is submitted *in toto;* furthermore, it is believed by some that if left *in situ* after puberty, they will often become aggressive malignant melanomas.

e. Atypical Melanocytic Lesions

In particular, those lesions presenting in patients with numerous pigmented lesions or in patients with a family history or past history of malignant melanoma (DNS) should be considered for elective excision. The indication for excision of dysplastic nevi is quite complex because of the very large number of these lesions in any one individual. They should be closely watched for any change by both the patient and the physician. Early excisions should be reserved for those lesions that show any change (particularly the appearance of black pigmentation) and for lesions in the scalp that are difficult to observe.

f. Nevi in Specific Sites

It is debatable whether unremarkable pigmented lesions of the palms and soles, interdigital creases, subungual areas, gen-

italia, and mucous membranes have any increased malignant potential. If the lesion is atypical in any way, it should be completely excised for biopsy. It is most important to note that any pigmented lesion that presents with any physical change whatsoever should be biopsied.

g. Nevi Subjected to Chronic Trauma

Nevi that are subjected to chronic trauma: bra line, belt line, hairline or scalp, shoe pressure points, etc., should be considered for excision. Excision of these nevi should be carried out surgically and completely but with minimal margins of normal skin and subcutaneous fat only. They must be submitted for histological study.

3. Early Signs of Malignant Transformation

Any pigmented lesion that presents with any of the following signs must be considered as already undergoing malignant transformation and is an absolute indication for a total excisional biopsy as described above for the benign nevi:

- Increase in size.
- Changes in color (deepening or blanching, mottling, appearance of a halo).
- Changes from a macular lesion to a papular or nodular one.
- Pain or pruritus.
- Inflammatory reaction.
- Bleeding.
- Ulceration or crusting.

B. Evaluation of the Patient with Malignant Melanomas

1. Biopsy

Before any extensive procedure is undertaken, a biopsy confirming the diagnosis of malignant melanoma must be done. This can be carried out by

- Smear or punch biopsy in ulcerated tumors.
- Incisional biopsy (preferably with frozen section) in large, spreading lesions.
- Total excisional biopsy with a minimal margin of normal tissue, whenever this is possible.

The latter method is the only one that permits accurate staging of the tumor according to the level and depth of invasion and is, by and large, the preferred method.

2. Staging

Identification of the depth of infiltration of the local lesion is the most important local factor in predicting the prognosis and in planning the appropriate therapy. Two methods are frequently used to measure the depth of the tumor: Clark levels, based on the penetration of the tumor to various levels of the skin, and Breslow's micromeasurements, based on the thickness of the tumor. These are described at length in §3.II.F. Staging is further dependent upon the presence or absence of regional nodes, and these must be clinically assessed with great care.

3. Metastatic Evaluation

Malignant melanomas constitute a group of lesions with a behavior that is most unpredictable. Patients with Level II disease (T1) have been known to present with generalized metastases after 18 years of disease-free follow-up subsequent to a local excision of the lesion, whereas patients with T4 (Level V) lesions have at times be known to remain free of disease for 10 years or more. Host immunity, seems to be of great importance in the outcome of the disease. Measurements of specific tumor immunity have been found to be positive in over 80% of the early melanomas but in less than 40% of the advanced cases.

Several studies seem to indicate little value to any intensive preoperative evaluation for metastases in clinically early malignant melanoma. A reasonable metastatic evaluation of the patient should be carried out prior to surgery, especially if radical procedures are being contemplated for cure. It is usually sufficient to start such an evaluation with the following:

• Routine urinalysis and blood count.
• A good-quality chest x-ray followed, if indicated, by a tomogram or CAT scan. This should be done routinely in advanced lesions or whenever the routine chest x-ray identifies any suspicious area.
• Serum chemistries and liver profile. In cases where liver chemistries are abnormal, a liver scan should be done.

Additional work-up may be warranted as dictated by specific symptoms.

C. Therapeutic Management

The treatment of malignant melanoma depends largely on the depth of penetration of the tumor and on the clinical stage of the disease, the location of the primary, its proximity to a predictable lymphatic drainage site, and the presence of palpable nodes.

Curative treatment is primarily surgical and must take into account the primary lesion, the lymphatic reservoir, and any available adjuvant treatment modalities. The following general criteria are suggested.

1. Excision of the Primary Site

a. Width of Excision

A wide excision of the confirmed melanoma, with a large margin of normal skin (to include in the specimen any microscopic satellite or intralymphatic tumor) is essential. It has historically been recommended to resect approximately 4–5 cm beyond the visible tumor; in some areas, such as in the head and neck (e.g., tumors in the cheek, eyelids, ear, etc.), this is often impractical, and one may have to settle for a 1- to 2-cm margin only. In addition, the width of excision must be guided by the depth of the melanoma; for Level I and superficial Level II melanomas, a conservative excision with a 0.5- to 2.0-cm margin will usually suffice. Furthermore, the need to perform wide resections with a 4–5 cm margin has been questioned recently. There is no convincing evidence that a 2- or 3-cm margin, for instance, results in a higher incidence of local recurrence or a lower total cure rate than the traditional wide margin. An intergroup study has been proposed to investigate this question in a prospectively randomized, controlled clinical trial.

b. Depth of Excision

A deep three-dimensional excision down to and including the underlying fascia, aponeurosis, or even periosteum must be carried out to include the subfascial lymphatics that may have been affected by lymphatic permeation (a mode of spread almost unique to melanomas).

c. Skin Graft

Skin grafting of the defect (or locoregional flap) is almost always necessary to close the defect after wide three-dimensional excisions. In some areas (e.g., in the abdomen or back), however, wide mobilization of the skin around the defect could permit primary closure. The extent of resection should, however, never be compromised in order to permit primary closure, at least until convincing evidence is available to suggest that smaller excisions are adequate.

2. Treatment of the Lymphatic Drainage Sites

One of the main avenues of spread of malignant melanoma is through lymphatic embolization to the first major echelon of lymph nodes. The indication to carry out a radical regional lymphadenectomy, however, must be based on a number of factors.

a. Therapeutic Lymphadenectomy

Therapeutic lymphadenectomy must always be considered an integral part of the treatment of malignant melanoma whenever regional lymph nodes are enlarged and suspected of harboring metastases. Whenever possible, this should be done in continuity with the resection of the primary in order to avoid leaving behind residual in transit disease that may have resulted from lymphatic permeation. If, however, there is a big distance between the primary and the nodal reservoir, a discontinuous procedure might have to be carried out.

b. Elective Lymphadenectomy

Elective lymphadenectomy in the absence of clinically involved nodes (Stages I and II of the disease) is a highly controversial issue. The decision to perform an elective node dissection must, therefore, be an individual decision by the treating surgeon; several factors are useful in trying to identify those patients who are at higher risk of having occult node metastases, and these must be assessed prior to making the final decision.

A major factor is the microscopic level of the tumor and thickness of infiltration. The incidence of occult node metastasis is in direct relation to the thickness and depth of invasion of the primary lesion. It has been suggested that elective radical lymphadenectomy (i.e., in the absence of clinically palpable nodes) is desirable in patients with lesions penetrating beyond the papillary dermis (Levels III and over) or lesions that are over 1.0 mm in thickness (Breslow's micromeasurements), i.e., in Stage II. On the other hand, Level I and II lesions (less than 1 mm in thickness), i.e., Stage I lesions, rarely spread to nodes and need no elective treatment to the nodes. There seems to be little discussion about the futility of elective node dissection in Levels I and II disease, nor about its need in Level V disease. Two recent reports emanating from a large multinational study conducted by the World Health Organization Melanoma Group (Veronesi and Cascinelli) appear to show no real advantage to elective node dissection in Stage II disease (Levels III and IV) of the extremities as compared with when the node dissection is deferred until the appearance of clinical node metastases. Several previous reports, however, had supported the use of elective node dissection on the basis of their own series (Davis and McCleod, Balch *et al.,* Breslow, Das Gupta, etc.). Furthermore, wide criticism of Veronesi's report on several grounds has been aired: the multinational nature of the group of patients treated, the lack of accurate histological documentation of the levels in 60% of the cases, and the small number of cases when they are divided into subsets by depth of invasion. The issue is obviously far from being resolved as yet, and the decision must remain in the hands of the treating surgeon. To help resolve these controversies, an intergroup study is currently being organized in the United States and Canada. Patients will be randomly allocated to have, or not to have, elective node dissections. At least 4–5 years follow up will be necessary before trustworthy conclusions are available.

Several factors other than the depth of invasion are of some value in aiding the surgeon to make a decision relevant to performing an elective lymphadenectomy in specific cases. One is location of the primary. Lymphadenectomy must be deferred if the lymphatic drainage cannot be predicted or in cases where several areas might be at risk (e.g., with lesions in the umbilical area; lesions in the waistline; midline lesions such as interscapular, midpubic, or presternal, etc.). Furthermore, one may be less inclined to do an elective lymphadenectomy when the lesion is very distant from the lymphatic reservoir (e.g., melanoma of the foot, subungueal melanoma, etc.). Local in-transit recurrences in the intercurrent area between the primary and the nodes are extremely difficult to manage and often occur when a discontinuous resection is done.

The yield in terms of positive nodes found, the end result of the elective lymphadenectomy, and the morbidity encountered in each specific site will also influence the decision.

i. Neck Dissection.
Elective neck dissection in patients where no nodes are clinically identifiable remains a rather controversial issue. Large randomized studies indicate very little difference in survival between patients who were found to have microscopically positive nodes during an elective neck dissection and those where therapeutic neck dissection was done after the clinical appearance of nodes. It seems that the identification of the positive nodes is more of a prognostic indicator than of a therapeutic value; some surgeons will now perform limited partial neck dissections for staging, rather than complete neck dissections for cure and reserve the total radical neck dissection for cases with clinically positive nodes.

The location of the lesion within the head and neck area is also of importance. Scalp lesions have a very high incidence of node metastases and require a parotidectomy and total neck dissection. Posterior scalp lesions also require an occipital node dissection as well. Lesions in the neck should have a concomitant neck dissection in continuity since the neck will be widely exposed during resection of the primary tumor and the use of flaps or grafts might make a secondary node dissection extremely difficult.

ii. Axillary Node Dissection.
In melanomas of the upper extremity, breast, and chest wall there appears to be a clear advantage in carrying out an axillary node dissection for lesions of Level III and deeper. The morbidity of axillary dissection is minimal, and the yield seems to justify recommending it, even in the absence of clinically involved nodes.

iii. Ilioinguinal Node Dissection.
This procedure is indicated primarily for deeply invasive malignant melanomas of the lower extremity, groin and perineum. It carries a rather high morbidity due to the frequent occurrence of skin sloughs, lymphorrhea, and especially lymphedema of the lower ex-

tremity. One must, therefore, advise it judiciously only in the deeply infiltrating lesions and should defer it in the elderly patients, in obese patients, and in those with any preexisting lower extremity disability (venous insufficiency, edema, vascular or trophic skin changes, or severe arthritis).

A compromise, which is often advisable in lesions that would otherwise warrant a radical groin dissection, is to carry out a superficial inguinal dissection and only complete the iliofemoral portion of the operation if the superficial nodes show metastases. There is some reported evidence, however, that a superficial groin dissection is not as effective therapeutically as a total groin dissection.

3. Adjuvant Therapy

Because of the notoriously poor results of local treatment in malignant melanomas of Stage IIb (T4, N0), Stage III (any T with N1), or Stage IV (any T with N2 or M1), a large number of clinical trials with various adjuvant modalities have been conducted.

a. Radiotherapy

Although radiotherapy is effective at times for palliation of large ulcerated tumors or brain metastases, it has not been promising as an adjuvant modality in this country. Reports from large European centers, however, seem to indicate some value and would justify some clinical investigation, especially for treatment of subclinical lymphatic disease sites.

b. Immunotherapy

Immunotherapy (nonspecific with BCG or specific with tumor antigens) is under extensive study but has not to date been widely accepted as an adjuvant modality.

c. Systemic Chemotherapy

A variety of agents, used singly or in combination, have been widely tried in advanced disease; positive results have been scanty and not predictable enough to warrant their use as adjunctive therapy. Dimethyl triazeno imidazole carboxamide (DTIC) is today the most effective agent available but is still under investigation in the adjuvant setting.

d. Regional Chemotherapy

Regional chemotherapy has been used by various investigators both by infusion and by isolation perfusion. The results have not been readily reproducible, and the morbidity is high. These techniques, therefore, are only used in special centers and are mostly investigational in nature. Recent reports from two centers that have been long involved with studying adjunctive isolation perfusion chemotherapy in malignant melanoma seem to show definite improvement in the end results of patients so treated.

Stehlin, in a report on 412 cases, showed a 10-year disease-free survival around 85% in Stage I patients, 60% in patients with local recurrences and in-transit disease, and 40% in patients with clinically positive nodes or Stage III disease. He even suggests that leaving the primary disease *in situ* for several months after the isolation perfusion might result in a stimulation of the host immunity by the destroyed melanoma cells, thus aiding in the control of systemic disease.

Bennett reported an 80% 10-year disease-free survival in 105 patients with lower extremity melanoma treated by 1-hour isolation perfusion of the femoral vessels with phenylalanine mustard, followed by a superficial groin dissection and removal of the primary. He recommends this approach for all patients with Level III lesions over 1 mm in thickness, Level IV patients, and all patients with satellite nodules or node metastases. The use of these techniques seems to be most desirable in patients with multiple local recurrences or in-transit metastases that are confined to one extremity.

D. Chemotherapy of Malignant Melanoma

1. Systemic Chemotherapy

Chemotherapy of malignant melanoma, whether as an adjuvant in the subclinical disease setting, or as a palliative modality for metastatic disease, remains entirely unsatisfactory. This is due to the paucity of active agents capable of affecting regression of tumor in more than 20% of patients. Of the available agents, only DTIC has been shown to yield an overall response rate (complete and partial remission) of 20–25% in over 1300 accumulated cases reported in the literature. Patients whose disease is localized to soft tissues or lymph nodes respond best (as high as 40%); patients with pulmonary metastases respond better than those with involvement of other visceral sites. Although only a small fraction of patients respond to treatment, the responding patients may derive substantial benefit as remissions may last as long as 6–12 months.

Innumerable other agents and combinations have been tried with response rates of 10–15%. Nitrosoureas have yielded an overall response rate of about 15%. Although DTIC and nitrosoureas are drugs with totally different mechanisms of action and different toxicities, such that it would seem reasonable to combine them, there is no real evidence for additive or synergistic interaction; the results of combining these two agents has not substantially increased the response rate. Although a number of uncontrolled single-institution studies have claimed response rates as high as 40% when DTIC and nitrosourea, plus or minus a vinca alkaloid or hydroxyurea, were combined, larger studies have failed to confirm such high response rates.

A miscellaneous group of agents with marginal activity includes the vinca alkaloids, procarbazine, hydroxyurea, cis-platinum, bleomycin, dactinomycin, and cyclophosphamide. All of these agents have response rates of 10% or less. A recent report claiming a response rate in excess of 50% with a combination of cis-platinum, vinblastine, and bleomycin still requires confirmation.

This absence of really active agents accounts for the poor results obtained to date when chemotherapy has been used as an adjuvant to surgery in Stage I or Stage II disease. Several reports in the literature seem to suggest apparently effective adjuvant regimens when the results obtained are compared with historical controls; only a prospectively randomized trial, however, can truly answer the question as to whether chemotherapy or possibly chemoimmunotherapy is beneficial as an adjuvant to potentially curative surgery. The World Health Organization trial for adjuvant chemotherapy in malignant melanomas has recently been reported: no advantage accrued to patients receiving either DTIC or BCG immunotherapy, or both, as compared with control patients receiving only surgery. Thus, it seems clear that adjuvant therapy cannot, at present, be recommended outside the context of a clinical trial.

2. Immunotherapy

Many features of the natural history and clinical behavior of melanoma suggest that immunologic factors play a significant role. For instance, long latent intervals in the growth of the disease have been well documented, and lymphocytic infiltration is not infrequently seen underneath the primary lesion and is thought to confer a better prognosis. Spontaneous regressions of melanoma have also been well documented, and it is possible to demonstrate the presence of antibodies that react with melanoma cells in the patient's serum, as well as in the serum of close relatives.

As early as 1970, reports became available suggesting that local injections of BCG organisms into recurrent skin nodules led to resolution of such nodules in a fair proportion of patients. As many as two-thirds of all injected nodules in the dermis are likely to respond and, in 20% of cases, even uninjected nodules near or at a distance from the area of injection will also undergo regression. It has been observed that only immunocompetent patients respond and that the response is seen generally in dermal lesions but not in subcutaneous lesions. Other immunostimulants such as dinitrochlorobenzene (DNCB), *Corynebacterium parvum,* methynol extractable residue of BCG (Bacillus Calmett Guerin) (MER), etc., have also been tried with similar results; the latter have the advantage of not using live organisms.

The response of metastatic lesions to direct injection of BCG has led to the institution of several studies that employ BCG as an active, nonspecific immunotherapeutic agent. In general,

immunization with BCG instead of direct tumor inoculation has been practiced as an adjuvant measure after completion of local treatment by whichever surgical procedure is indicated.

Again, while there is some evidence of efficacy, controlled series have to date not been able to confirm significant responses. Likewise, combining immuno- and chemotherapy still needs full evaluation.

3. Regional Perfusion

In view of the fact that a frequent problem with melanoma of the extremities is local recurrence and in-transit metastases, various attempts at regional perfusion of extremities with active chemotherapeutic agents have been attempted during the last 25 years. Such chemotherapy can be given by direct intra-arterial infusion of the active agent with occlusion of the draining veins to maintain the drug in the extremity for as long as possible, or else it can be administered by a method of isolation perfusion using a pump oxygenator. A variety of agents have been perfused including nitrogen mustard, dactinomycin, adriamycin, and others. The results are difficult to interpret in view of the fact that every patient has necessarily been preselected. Nevertheless, some dramatic responses have been observed, such that carefully selected patients with locally recurrent or in-transit disease may still be referred to centers where this technique is available.

The technique of regional perfusion has also been used as an adjuvant to surgery, both preoperatively and postoperatively. While it is very difficult to evaluate the results obtained, the overall impression is that the serious side effects and potential complications of the procedure override the possible benefits that might ensue. Nevertheless, several single institutions, as mentioned previously, have reported improved cure rates.

An approach that potentially offers some hope is the use of hyperthermia, either locally, through a perfusion mechanism, or systemically. This has been used in conjunction with chemotherapy and/or radiation therapy, and although still experimental, it seems to show some early promising results.

V. OTHER SELECT SKIN TUMORS

There are a large number of malignancies affecting the skin. Some are extremely rare but worthy of mention for the sake of completeness.

A. Malignant Tumors of the Skin
Appendages

These are exceedingly rare tumors, often presenting as skin nodules that are clinically difficult to identify. Some of them (syringocystadenoma, nevus sebaceus) are actually benign tumors that may be associated with basal cell carcinomas. Others are malignant tumors of varying aggressive tendencies.

1. Classification

a. Benign Appendage Tumors with Associated Cutaneous Malignancy

i. Syringocystadenoma Papilliferum. Clinically, this benign tumor is most commonly seen on the scalp as an isolated lesion. It is usually present at birth or appears shortly thereafter and presents as a plaque that becomes verrucous during adolescence. In approximately 10% of these tumors, an associated basal cell carcinoma is observed. The suggested therapeutic approach is surgical excision.

ii. Nevus Sebaceus. Nevus sebaceus is a benign tumor present at birth and most commonly found on the scalp. It presents as a yellow orange plaque that develops into a verrucous growth during adolescence. Basal cell carcinomas are also associated with this tumor in approximately 10% of the cases, and therefore, surgical excision is advisable.

b. Malignant Skin Appendage Tumors

i. Carcinoma of Eccrine Glands (Sweat Gland Carcinoma). Carcinomas of the sweat glands are quite rare. Metastases from these tumors are so infrequent that the tumors are often indifferently labeled "sweat gland adenoma." Clinically, they do not have a typical appearance and are only diagnosed on biopsy. A wide local excision is the usually accepted treatment.

ii. Carcinoma of the Apocrine Glands. Carcinomas of the apocrine glands are also seen infrequently. They most commonly occur in the axilla, nipples, vulva, and eyelids. These tumors are more aggressive and frequently metastasize. They do not have a characteristic clinical appearance and are usually diagnosed after excisional biopsy.

iii. Carcinoma of Sebeacous Glands. The most common presentation for this tumor is an ulcerated nodule, and the most common site is in the eyelids. Extensive metastases are common when the primary tumor is on the eyelids, and it is considered to be the most aggressive malignant skin appendage tumor.

Malignant tumors of the skin appendages are histologically akin to mucous gland tumors; cylindromas and mucoepidermoid tumors may occur in addition to clear adenocarcinomas.

2. Therapeutic Management

a. Surgery

The treatment of these tumors is primarily surgical and usually precedes the histological confirmation. If the diagnosis is suspected and the tumor is comfortably resectable, a wide local excision with primary closure is the treatment of choice. An adequate margin of normal subcutaneous tissue is important and must be confirmed histologically. For the larger or more infiltrative lesions, a preliminary biopsy is recommended, and definitive therapy must be planned; total wide excision is necessary, sometimes requiring resection of adjacent tissues (muscle, periosteum, bone, etc.). Plastic surgery reconstruction in the form of skin grafts, rotational or pedicled flaps, myocutaneous flaps, or even sometimes composite flaps, may be necessary. In those cases where the extent of resection appears inadequate, postoperative radiotherapy is indicated. When surgery is not desirable because of the location of the tumor or the general condition of the patient, other forms of therapy, such as chemosurgery, cryosurgery, primary radiotherapy, or the other modalities previously described in the treatment of the aggressive basal or squamous cell cancers of the skin could also be used as alternative modalities in treating skin appendage tumors.

b. Radiotherapy

Malignant tumors of skin appendages have many similarities to mucous gland tumors situated in the upper air and food passages; histologically their natural behavior and their response to radiotherapy is much the same.

Some share with the mucous gland type of tumor an ability to evade detection as malignant tumors by appearing to be relatively low grade in cytological appearance. They are all malignant, however, with varying abilities to spread to lymph nodes and other organs. It is because of this danger that they should be treated aggressively. After complete surgical excision (the recommended first step), postoperative radiotherapy to the primary site and occasionally to draining lymph node regions is recommended when the tumor is incompletely excised or in the case of poorly differentiated or anaplastic lesions. Very rarely, a situation might arise when surgery is not feasible because of the patient's general condition or because of the tumor (e.g., recurrent large tumor in the face). A high-dosage course of radiotherapy can then be given and will often result in substantial reduction of tumor size or even, in some instances, tumor disappearance.

Radiation modality used must be capable of treating the skin lesion with beam penetration to appropriate depths. The doses aimed at are usually high (about 6000 rads in 6 weeks for postoperative courses), but these are well tolerated if the volumes are kept reasonably limited.

B. Mycosis Fungoides and Sézary Syndrome

Mycosis fungoides is a malignant T-cell lymphoma with primary manifestations in the skin. It is an uncommon, progressive, and fatal disease, albeit interrupted by periods of remission.

1. Pathogenesis, Incidence, and Prognosis

The pathogenesis of this disorder is quite controversial. There is evidence to suggest that persistent exposure to industrial chemicals causing a chronic contact dermatitis is an important factor in the etiology of the disease.

Mycosis fungoides is seen approximately in a 1 : 1 ratio between men and women, and it occurs between the ages of 30 and 70, but most often between the fifth and seventh decade.

When it presents in its early stages, the prognosis is good, and survival rates are high. If there are tumors, ulcers, or lymph node involvement, the patients will usually not survive more than 2 years.

2. Clinical Manifestations

Patients may present with any one of the following stages of the disease.

a. Premycotic Phase

This stage consists of a long-standing erythematous, eczematous, or psoriasiform eruption usually on the trunk or proximal extremities. Parapsoriasis en plaque is a lesion that fits into this category, and many patients with parapsoriasis en plaque eventually develop mycosis fungoides. Skin biopsies will often show only a nonspecific inflammatory process, making it necessary to observe the patient closely and periodically rebiopsy the lesion. Clinicians may have difficulty in deciding whether to treat or observe patients that are suspected of having mycosis fungoides who present with this type of manifestation.

b. Patch-Plaque Lesions

These are widely distributed infiltrating patches and plaques of long-standing duration. Sometimes, the involved areas are atrophic with slight scaling and telangiectatic vessels (poikiloderma). The skin biopsy here will reveal the diagnostic features of mycosis fungoides, namely, nests of atypical lymphocytes in the epidermis (Pautrier's microabcesses).

c. Tumors and Nodules

This is characterized by ulcerating and nonulcerating fungating tumors that can present on the head, neck, and/or trunk. This is a very late stage of the disease.

d. Erythroderma

At this stage of the disease, the patient presents with 100% of the skin involved with severe erythema and generalized exfoliation.

In addition to these local manifestations, mycosis fungoides may present with systemic lymph node or visceral involvement in the later stages of the disease. A biopsy from an involved node will show a malignant lymphoma with a population of convoluted T lymphocytes. Other organs commonly involved at this stage include the spleen, lungs, and liver. The bone marrow is rarely involved.

3. Staging

- Stage I: Macules, papules, and/or plaques. No tumors or lymphadenopathy. This stage is subdivided as A or B, depending on whether less or more than 10% of the body surface is involved: (A) <10%, and (B) >10%.
- Stage II: (A) Nontumorous skin lesions plus lymphadenopathy, and (B) cutaneous tumors with or without adenopathy.
- Stage III: Erythroderma.
- Stage IV: Histologically documented extracutaneous mycosis fungoides. (A) Lymph node involvement, and (B) visceral involvement.

4. Therapeutic Management

a. Topical Nitrogen Mustard or BCNU

Parapsoriasis en plaque and the nontumorous form of mycosis fungoides can be adequately treated with a topical solution of mechlorethamine hydrochloride dissolved in water and applied to the whole body daily. Long-standing remissions can be induced with this modality. A number of patients will develop a contact dermatitis to this substance, but treatment can be continued by using more dilute solutions of the medication. If unsuccessful, topical BCNU (carmustine) can be used in a similar manner.

b. Electron Beam Therapy

The use of an electron beam of appropriate penetration to the whole body is effective in inducing remissions in most stages of mycosis fungoides. These high-energy electrons will clear the skin of the atypical lymphocytes and only penetrate to the prescribed depth (about 7 mm for 2 Mev). Total dosage can go as high as 3600 rads. Its use is limited to certain selected centers because of the relatively small number of these machines available. Side effects include nausea, severe pruritis, and alopecia (often temporary).

c. PUVA

Orally administered, psoralen in combination with whole-body UV light irradiation not only will induce a photosensitivity reaction in the skin but will induce remissions of mycosis fungoides. This treatment, however, needs to be given every other day and may be required for years; in addition, complications of PUVA include cataracts, itching and dryness of the skin, and the increased incidence of cutaneous squamous cell carcinomas reported with prolonged use. Furthermore, the response of deeper lesions is questionable.

d. Systemic Chemotherapy

Nitrogen mustard, cyclophosphamide, chlorambucil, and methotrexate among others have been used singly or in combination in the treatment of advanced mycosis fungoides. Such systemic therapy can induce a remission of the disease, but these remissions are usually incomplete and short lived. It is quite controversial whether they add significantly to the survival time of the patient. When the disease becomes a systemic lymphoma/leukemia type disease, it should be treated as such.

C. Kaposi's Sarcoma (Multiple Idiopathic Hemorrhagic Sarcoma)

Kaposi's sarcoma is a multifocal vascular neoplasm primarily affecting the skin, although involvement of other organ systems such as the gastrointestinal tract does occur. There is a higher incidence of this disease in southern and eastern Europe, and an endemic area has also been described in tropical Africa; the disease is strikingly frequent in Kenya, Tanzania, and Zaire. Some studies have shown the disease to be more common in Jews and people of Mediterranean origin. In the European variety, the most common age of onset is between 50 and 70. In Africa, the lesions may have their onset during childhood.

The cause of Kaposi's sarcoma is presently unknown. The skin manifestations are in the form of plaques, nodules, and tumors with a violaceous hue, and the lesions are most commonly seen on the lower extremities. Internal organs may be involved; the GI tract may be the site of similar tumors, and hemorrhages may occur from the nose and GI tract. The course of the disease is rather indolent and can last anywhere from 1 to 20 years, with an average of 6–8 years.

Localized tumors can be treated either by surgical excision, cryosurgery, or radiation therapy. Radiation is the preferred modality, however, since the lesions are highly radiosensitive. The use of radiotherapy in the treatment of localized Kaposi's sarcoma is highly effective, and if beams of enough penetration are used to deliver adequate doses (about 3000 rads in 3 weeks), results are very satisfactory both in terms of complete local control and low incidence of recurrence in the sites irradiated. Recurrences in unirradiated sites and/or systemic widespread disease do, however, continue to occur.

When the disease is widespread and can no longer be controlled by radiotherapy, chemotherapeutic agents may be employed; these patients typically have fungating recurrent lesions on the extremities and/or systemic involvement. Favorable results have been obtained with vinca alkaloids, particularly vinblastine, when used on a low-dose weekly or biweekly schedule (many of the patients are elderly with diminished tolerance); this type of chemotherapy will yield a significant response in terms of clearing of local lesions as well as objective regressions. Patients with systemic disease respond less favorable. Other agents reported to have some efficacy include dactinomycin, bleomycin, and nitrogen mustard. Studies in Uganda have shown optimal results with the use of actinomycin D and DTIC, but tumor relapses with this type of treatment are quire frequent. Experimental work on the use of other chemotherapeutic agents and immunotherapy is at present being done.

Since 1981 small clusters of cases of a particularly aggressive type of Kaposi's sarcoma seen in male homosexuals have been reported to the Center for Disease Control. Most of the reports have been from either New York or California, with a large number of homosexual men reported with this type of disease. The clinical course in these individuals mimics that of the aggressive varieties seen in Africa and is similar to Kaposi's sarcoma that has been described in immunosupressed renal transplant patients. More recently, hemophiliacs and drug addicts have also been reported to be prone to Kaposi's sarcoma, and Haitians seem to be particularly vulnerable.

Much circumstantial evidence points to an acquired immunodeficient syndrome (AIDS) or possibly a viral infectious disease as the etiologic agent in Kaposi's sarcoma. In this group of individuals, skin lesions are the most frequent complaint; they have erythematous macules and papules ranging from a few millimeters to 1.0 cm in size; some patients have violaceous or erythematous plaques up to 2.5 centimeters in diameter; some have lymph node involvement; and many have systemic involvement. Response to combination therapy is very poor, and most patients die within 18 months of diagnosis. Most of these patients have used a wide range of recreational drugs such as amyl or butyl nitrite, cocaine, and marijuana and most have had a multitude of sexually transmitted diseases such as gonorrhea, hepatitis B, syphilis, amebiasis, condyloma accuminatum, and herpes simplex progenitalis. Immunologic studies have shown a decreased cell-mediated immune response, and immunogenetic studies have shown a significant increase in the frequency of human lymphocyte antigen (HLA) DR-5. Frequent secondary infections by opportunistic agents have been observed in this group of patients, including pneumonia caused by *Pneumocystis carinii*. The cause of the alteration in immune response that predisposes to opportunistic infections in homosexual men is subject to intensive investigation. Much excitement has been generated recently by the announcements, from the National Cancer Institute and a group of French investigators, of the isolation and identification of a new virus as the probable etiologic agent of AIDS. This retrovirus is related to the previously described human T cell virus (HTLV I), an agent implicated in the pathogenesis of a rare form of human leukemia/lymphoma. The putative AIDS-inducing virus has been called HTLV III by American investigators and is probably the same virus identified by the French group. The virus has been grown from tissues of AIDS patients, and antibodies to HTLV III are found in a significant fraction of such patients. Much effort is being expended to develop screening tests for the presence of viral antigens in blood products. Even greater efforts are underway to develop a vaccine to be used for high-risk populations. As of the beginning of 1985, a screening test for blood products has just appeared and is actively being tested for efficacy. A vaccine has not yet been produced.

Kaposi's sarcoma has been reported in patients receiving renal transplants who are maintained on immunosuppressive therapy. Discontinuation of the immunosuppressive measures results in regression of the disease in these patients.

VI. POSTOPERATIVE CARE, EVALUATION, AND REHABILITATION OF THE PATIENT WITH SKIN CANCER

A. Postoperative Care

The care of a patient following treatment for skin cancer will vary depending on the site of the lesion, its nature, the method of treatment, and/or the extent of therapy. If the patient is treated by electrodesiccation, cryosurgery, topical chemotherapy, or chemosurgery, it is imperative that the patient be informed of the post therapy sequelae (burning, pain, oozing, edema, redness, or delayed healing depending on the type of treatment) that can be anticipated as well as the time it will take for complete healing. Proper wound care must be explained to the patient, and the patient should be checked often enough to ensure that this is carried out.

Lesions treated by primary surgical excision require practically no postoperative care. Sutures are removed 3–10 days later (depending on the site of excision), and no further care is needed.

Skin grafts and flaps require the usual care: stenting, bolus dressings, observation for and drainage of seromas or hematomas, immobilization, suction drainage, etc. The care of radical lymphadenectomies is also standard, requiring suction drainage for 5–7 days.

Certain specific sites require additional care:

- Rib, pleura, or chest wall resection. Reconstruction is often recommended primarily. Pleural-space drainage must be uti-

lized, and follow-up x-rays are essential to insure proper inflation of the lungs and drainage of the pleural space.
- Anal region lesions. Wounds there are often left open for drainage, and the patient will require sitz baths and emollients regularly until healing is complete.

Radiation therapy for skin cancer requires practically no care with the exception of local hygienic measures.

B. Evaluation

Follow-up care of the patient with skin cancer is of utmost importance, especially when dealing with melanomas and with the more aggressive basal or squamous cell carcinomas.

The ordinary basal cell carcinoma or early superficial squamous cell carcinoma require little follow-up evaluation. Patients should be seen monthly the first 3 months, every 3 months for the first year, and every 6–12 months thereafter. The examiner needs only to check the site of the original lesion, the adjacent skin, and the regional lymphatics; examination of the integuments and especially the sun-exposed areas should be carried out, and biopsies should be performed whenever indicated. No other physical or laboratory evaluation is necessary other than that required for good health maintenance.

For the more aggressive skin cancer and particularly for melanomas, a more intensive follow-up is recommended. Table II is a suggested schedule for such a follow-up.

C. Rehabilitation

Physical rehabilitation of the patient with skin cancer is rarely necessary for the more common basal or squamous cell cancers. Patients with extensive resections will at times require one of many rehabilitative measures.

1. Functional Rehabilitation

When appropriate, joints must be mobilized early to prevent stiffness. Early ambulation is essential, and limb elevation is often necessary to reduce lymphedema. The use of elastic support is often very useful to expedite functional rehabilitation, and physiotherapy should be utilized whenever appropriate, including whirlpool, heat, exercises, etc.

2. Cosmetic Rehabilitation

Cosmetic rehabilitation may be required following extensive resections, particularly when the lesions were in the face. Prosthetic molds may be extremely useful, either temporarily or even on a permanent basis. Plastic surgery and revision of grafts or scars are often indicated to improve on the cosmetic

Table II

Long-Term Follow-Up Schedule for Aggressive Skin Cancer
(in Particular, Melanoma) Patients

Management	First 3 months			First and second year				Third year and thereafter	
	1	2	3	3 Months	6 Months	9 Months	12 Months	Every 6 months	Annually
History									
Symptoms related to operative site	X	X	X	X	X	X	X	X	
Abnormal pigmentation changes in any other nevi	X	X	X	X	X	X	X	X	
Other growths	X	X	X	X	X	X	X	X	
Any other symptoms	X	X	X	X	X	X	X	X	
Update on complete medical history					X		X		X
Physical									
Exam of operative site	X	X	X	X	X	X	X	X	
Exam of adjacent skin	X	X	X	X	X	X	X	X	
Exam of all integments					X		X	X	
Exam of regional nodes	X	X	X	X	X	X	X	X	
Complete physical evaluation (liver, lung, bones, etc.)					X		X		X
Investigations									
CBC, urine, SMA-12					X		X		X
Chest x-ray							X		X
Bone scan, x-rays					As indicated				
Liver, brain scan					As indicated				
Biopsy					As indicated				

result; contractures should be released; and keloid scars should be corrected.

3. Psychiatric Rehabilitation

It is essential that the treating physician be fully aware of the emotional impact of the cancer and its treatment on the patient. Social workers and nurse oncologists can offer significant support in that respect, and at times, psychiatric assistance should be sought if it appears as though the patient is having difficulties coping with his or her disease. Hygienic and preventive measures must be stressed to the patient: avoidance of sun exposure, use of sun screens and protection, etc.

VII. MANAGEMENT ALGORITHM FOR SKIN MELANOMA (see p. 125)

SUGGESTED READINGS

1. Albright, S. Treatment of skin cancer using multiple modalities. *J. Am. Acad. Dermatol.* **7,** 143–171 (1982).

2. Andrade, R., Gumport, S., Popkin, G., and Rees, T. "Cancer of the Skin." Saunders, Philadelphia, Pennsylvania, 1976.

3. Attie, J. A., and Khafif, A. "Melanotic Tumors, Bilogy, Pathology and Clinical Features" (monogr.). Thomas, Springfield, Illinois, 1964.

4. Balch, C. M., Murad, T. M., and Soong, S. J. Tumor thickness as a guide to surgical management of clinical stage I melanoma patients. *Cancer* **43,** 883–888 (1979).

5. Bennett. Communication at the Clinical Congress of the American College of Surgeons, 1982 (1982).

6. Bizer, L. S. Rhabdomyosarcoma. *Am. J. Surg.* **140,** 687–692 (1980).

6a. Breslow, A. Thickness, cross sectional area and depth of invasion in the prognosis of cutaneous melanoma. *Ann. Surg.* **172,** 902–908 (1970).

7. Breslow, A. Tumor thickness, level of invasion and node dissection in stage I cutaneous melanoma. *Ann. Surg.* **182,** 572–575 (1975).

8. Breslow, A. The surgical treatment of stage I cutaneous melanoma. *Cancer Treat. Rev.* **5,** 195–198 (1979).

9. Cascinelli, N., Morabito, A., and Bufalino, R. Prognosis of stage I melanoma of the skin. *Int. J. Cancer* **26,** 733–739 (1980).

9a. Clark, W. H. Jr., From, L., Bernardino, E. A., Mihm, M. C. The histogenesis and biologic behavior of human malignant melanomas of the skin. *Cancer Res.* **29,** 705–726 (1969).

10. Das Gupta, T. K. Results of treatment of 269 patients with primary cutaneous melanoma: A five-year prospective study. *Ann. Surg.* **186,** 201–209 (1977).

11. Davis, N. C. Cutaneous melanoma: The Queensland experience. *Curr. Probl. Surg.* **13,** 1–63 (1976).

12. Davis, N. C., and McLeod, G. R. Elective lymph node dissection for melanoma. *Br. J. Surg.* **58,** 820–823 (1971).
13. Epstein, E., and Epstein, E., Jr. "Skin Surgery." Thomas, Springfield, Illinois, 1979.
14. Goldsmith, H. S. The debate over immediate lymph node dissection in melanoma. *Surg., Gynecol. Obstet.* **148,** 403–405 (1979).
15. Helm, F. "Cancer Dermatology." Lea & Febiger, Philadelphia, Pennsylvania, 1979.
16. Kopf, A., Bart, R., Rodriguez-Sains, R., and Ackerman, A. "Malignant Melanoma." Masson, New York, 1979.
17. Roses, D. F., Harris, M. N., Grumberger, I., and Gumport, S. L. Selective surgical management of cutaneous melanoma of the head and neck. *Ann. Surg.* **192,** 629 (1980).
18. Snow, G. B., van der Esch, E. P., and van Slotten, E. A. Mucosal melanoma of the head and neck. *Head Neck Surg.* **1,** 24–31 (1978).
19. Stehlin, J. S. Communication at the Clinical Congress of the American College of Surgeons, *1982* (1982).
20. Veronesi, U., Adamus, J., and Bandiera, D. C. Inefficacy of immediate node dissection in stage I melanoma of the limbs. *N. Engl. J. Med.* **297,** 627–630 (1977).

ALGORITHM FOR SKIN MELANOMA

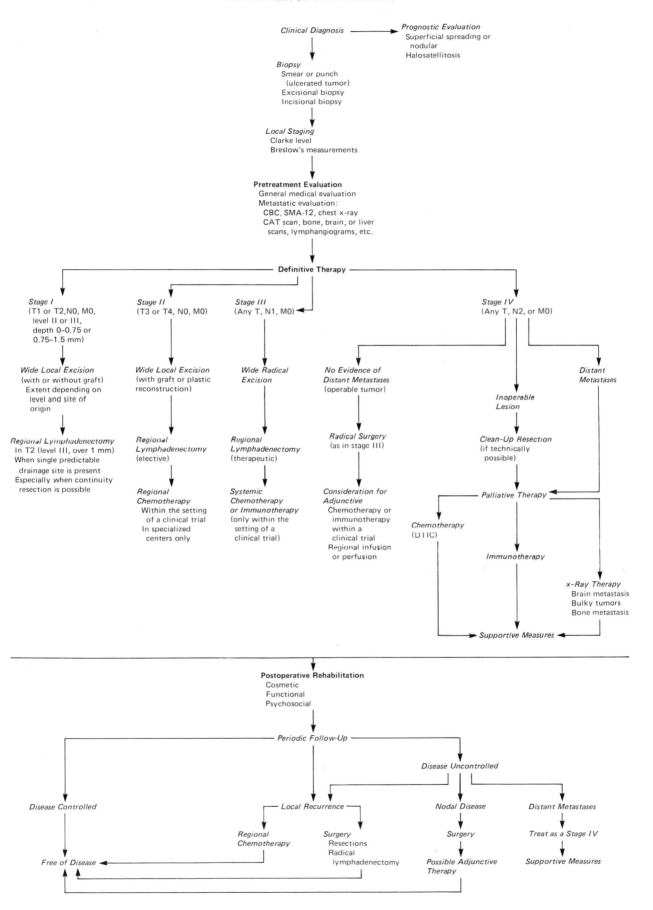

Section 4

Tumors of the Endocrine Glands

ROBERT LERNER

With Contributions by

Aizid Hashmat	Urology
Ramiro Requena	General Surgery
Rene A. Khafif	Surgical Oncology
Irvin Modlin	Surgery
Farida Khan	Endocrinology
Arnold Silverberg	Metabolic Diseases and Endocrinology
Burton Herz	General Surgery

127

Introduction

Tumors of the endocrine glands constitute a large, complex and disparate group of tumors that occur throughout the entire body and present with a multitude of symptoms dependent on the hormone secreted by the individual tumor. Although, the majority of the tumors are benign adenomas and, at times, the specific syndrome may even be the result of hyperplasia without any neoplasm; it seems appropriate to discuss the management of the syndromes themselves, since the finite diagnosis of the cause of the syndrome is often not available until after the treatment has been initiated. Furthermore, many of the tumors are multiple (e.g., pancreatic tumors); some are often not even identified at the time of surgery (e.g., gastrinomas or carcinoid tumors); and the majority of those that are malignant are not usually totally resectable. In addition, the morbidity and mortality of the disease is almost always the result of the physiological impact of the hormone produced, rather than the local spread of the tumor or its metastases. The management of a large number of these tumors is, therefore, primarily directed at the syndrome resulting from the tumor, rather than at eradication of the neoplasm itself.

By necessity, the discussion of endocrine tumors must be divided into separate sections according to the gland and the syndrome produced. The following separate sections will be presented:

- Tumors of the Adrenal Gland
- Pancreatic Tumors
- Parathyroid Tumors
- Paraneoplastic Endocrine Syndromes
- Multiple Endocrine Neoplasia
- Apudomas
- Carcinoid Tumors

Other endocrine tumors are presented in various specific sections of these volumes: thyroid tumors in §1 and pituitary tumors in §7.

Section 4. Tumors of the Endocrine Glands

Part A: Tumors of the Adrenal Gland

I. Primary Hyperaldosteronism   133
 A. Early Detection and Screening
 B. Pretreatment Evaluation and Work-Up
  1. History and Physical Evaluation
   a. History
   b. Physical Findings
  2. Laboratory Findings
  3. Confirmation of the Diagnosis
   a. Serum and Urine Aldosterone
   b. Plasma Renin
  4. Localization of the Tumor
   a. IV Urogram, CAT Scan, and Sonogram
   b. Adrenal Scan
   c. Bilateral Adrenal Venography
    and Venous Sampling
  5. General Medical Evaluation
  6. Multidisciplinary Evaluation
 C. Preoperative Preparation
 D. Therapeutic Management
  1. Glucocorticoid-Suppressible Hyperaldosteronism
  2. Bilateral Adrenal Hyperplasia
  3. Aldosterone-Producing Adenoma
 E. Postoperative Care, Evaluation, and Follow-Up
  1. Postoperative Care
  2. Follow-Up Evaluation
 F. Management Algorithm for Hyperaldosteronism
II. Cushing's Syndrome   136
 A. Early Detection and Screening
 B. Pretreatment Evaluation and Work-Up
  1. Laboratory Findings
  2. Diagnostic Testing
   a. Dexamethasone Suppression Test
   b. ACTH Stimulation Test
   c. Metyrapone Test
   d. Plasma ACTH Levels
   e. 24-Hour Urinary Ketosteroids
   f. 24-Hour Urinary 5 HIAA
  3. Localizing Investigations of the Cause
   of Cushing's Syndrome
   a. Intravenous Urogram
   b. Abdominal Sonogram
   c. CAT Scan
   d. Adrenal Angiography
   e. Selective Adrenal Vein Sampling
   f. ^{131}I Labeled Cholesterol Adrenal Scan
   g. Surgery
 C. Preoperative Preparation
  1. Cardiopulmonary Considerations
  2. Antibiotics
  3. Preoperative Steroid Coverage

  4. Psychiatric Evaluation
  5. Multidisciplinary Evaluation
 D. Therapeutic Management
  1. Adrenal Tumors
   a. Nonfunctioning Tumors
   b. Functional Tumors
  2. Adrenocortical Hyperplasias
   a. Patients with Enlarged Sella Turcica
   b. Patients without Sellar Enlargement
  3. Para-endocrine Tumors
 E. Postoperative Care, Evaluation, and Follow-Up
 F. Management Algorithm for Cushing's Syndrome
III. Pheochromocytoma   142
 A. Early Detection and Screening
  1. Early Detection
  2. Clinical Considerations
   a. Paroxysmal Hypertension
   b. Sustained Hypertension
   c. Vascular Complications
  3. Pathological Findings
 B. Pretreatment Evaluation and Work-Up
  1. Catecholamines
   a. Urinary Free Catecholamines
   b. Urinary VMA
   c. Urinary NM and M
   d. Plasma Catecholamines
  2. Provocative Tests
  3. Suppressive Tests
  4. Localization
   a. Chest X-ray
   b. IVP and Nephrotomogram
   c. CAT Scan of the Abdomen
   d. Angiography of the Adrenal Gland
   e. Selective Venous Catheterization
    with Catecholamine Samplings
  5. General Medical and Metastatic Evaluation
 C. Preoperative Preparation
  1. General Considerations
  2. Drug Preparation
   a. Alpha-Adrenergic Blockers
   b. Beta-Adrenergic Blockers
   c. Nonspecific Peripheral Vasodilators
  3. Intraoperative Drug Therapy and Preparation
   for Induction
 D. Therapeutic Management
  1. Surgery
  2. Nonoperative Treatment
   a. Phenoxybenzamine
   b. Alpha-methyl-*p*-tyrosine (MPT)
   c. Chemotherapy

      d. Radiotherapy
   E. Postoperative Care, Evaluation, and Follow-Up
     1. Immediate Postoperative Care
     2. Long-Term Postoperative Care
     3. Follow-Up Plan and Evaluation
   F. Management Algorithm for Pheochromacytomas
IV. Neuroblastoma 148
   A. Early Detection and Screening
     1. General Considerations
     2. Suggestive Signs and Symptoms
   B. Pretreatment Evaluation
     1. Physical Evaluation
     2. Laboratory Findings

     3. Confirmation of the Diagnosis
     4. Staging of Neuroblastoma
   C. Preoperative Preparation
   D. Therapeutic Management
     1. Stage I
     2. Stage II
     3. Stage III
     4. Stage IV
     5. Stage IVS
   E. Postoperative Care and Follow-Up
   F. Management Algorithm for Neuroblastoma

Suggested Readings 153

I. PRIMARY HYPERALDOSTERONISM

A. Early Detection and Screening

Primary aldosteronism is a disease characterized by hypertension due to an excessive discharge of aldosterone with suppression of renin production. The result is an increase in distal renal tubular reabsorption of sodium with resultant hypernatremia and hypervolemia. Simultaneously, there is an increase in tubular excretion of potassium, hydrogen, ammonia, and magnesium, leading to hypokalemic alkalosis. Longstanding hypokalemia will result in hypokalemic nephropathy characterized by vacuolation of the renal tubular cells and loss of concentrating ability.

The most common cause (70–80% of cases) of primary aldosteronism is a benign adenoma arising from the zona glomerulosa of the adrenal gland. Sometimes the cells resemble those of the zona fasciculata or suggest a mixture of the two zones. In some patients, there may be more than one adenoma, and at times, multiple microadenomatous changes of the ipsilateral adrenal gland will be found. In 15–25% of patients the cause will be nonneoplastic, resulting from bilateral adrenal hyperplasia. Indeterminate hyperaldosteronism and glucocorticoid remediable hyperaldosteronism unrelated to pathology in the adrenal glands are found only on rare occasions.

The usual age of the patient ranges between 30 and 50 years, although cases have been reported in children as well as in elderly people. The presenting symptom is usually muscle weakness, hypertension with headaches, and an antidiuretic hormone (ADH)–resistant polyuria.

Any young patient who is found to be hypertensive on routine physical examination requires investigation in order to identify the cause of the hypertension. Of patients with hypertension, 1–2% will be found to have hyperaldosteronism.

The most commonly used screening test for hyperaldosteronism is the detection of hypokalemic alkalosis, especially in an untreated hypertensive patient. The hypokalemia is often found to develop shortly after diuretic treatment has been started for mild hypertension. Some of these patients, however, are simultaneously being treated with a low-sodium diet. Sodium restriction decreases the sodium load in the distal tubule, and there is reduced tubular secretion and excretion of potassium so that the patient may thus be found to be normokalemic. In these patients, a normal salt diet should be reordered to reveal the tendency to hypokalemia. In reality, no practical screening is sensible to detect hyperaldosteronism beyond the screening of patients for hypertension in general; there are no other early signs, and only a keen sense of awareness is important in order to identify the disease and correct it at an early stage.

B. Pretreatment Evaluation and Work-Up

1. History and Physical Evaluation

a. History

The female/male ratio is about 2 : 1, and most of the patients are between 30 and 60 years of age. There are no real specific symptoms or signs as a clue to the diagnosis. The most common symptoms are:

- Muscular weakness, involving mainly the trunk and lower extremities; in severe and untreated cases, transient paralysis may even occur.
- Paresthesia of the face, hands, and feet or even tetany.
- Polyuria, polydypsia, and sometimes marked nocturia may develop.

b. Physical Findings

On physical examination, the most important finding is "hypertension." Almost all of the patients are hypertensive; this is usually benign in nature, and about half of the patients have a mild-to-moderate degree of retinopathy. Other findings might include:

- Cardiomegaly, cardiac arrhythmia, and premature contractions.
- Loss of deep-tendon reflexes.
- Positive Chvostek and Trousseau signs in advanced cases.
- Pitting edema of the extremities; not present until longstanding heart failure or renal failure has occurred.

133

2. Laboratory Findings

- Hypokalemic alkalosis.
- Hypernatremia. Although total body sodium is increased, serum sodium levels are usually borderline high.
- Decreased serum magnesium.
- Urinalysis.
  - Decreased specific gravity (less than 1015) because of the associated nephropathy.
  - Elevated urinary potassium (50 meq per day) as compared with a normal of 10–20 meq per day.
  - Abnormal glucose tolerance in about 50% of the cases.

3. Confirmation of the Diagnosis

When suspected, the diagnosis of hyperaldosteronism needs to be confirmed by identifying an elevation of the urinary and plasma aldosterone in association with unprovoked hypokalemia and a depressed renin level. Prior to any testing, the patient must be taken off all hypertensive medication.

a. Serum and Urine Aldosterone

In normal subjects in a supine position, the plasma aldosterone level is around 0.015 μg %; the 24-hours urine aldosterone level is 3–32 μg per day.

Because of the variable nature of blood levels, some authors stress the importance of documenting that the aldosterone levels are nonsuppressible. This can be accomplished by one of two tests:

i. Salt-Loading Test. The salt-loading test may be done in one of two ways:

- Administration of Na (200 meq) and K (60–90 meq) each day for 3–5 days.
- Institution of a low-salt diet (Na 10 meq and K 60 meq per day) for 5 days, followed by an IV infusion of normal saline (2000 cc in 2 hours) for 2 days.

Blood aldosterone levels are measured on the day before and the day after salt-loading procedures. In a normal individual, the aldosterone level will drop to about one-fourth of the control value, or less; in patients with primary aldosteronism, the levels cannot be suppressed.

ii. DOC Test. In 1967 Biglieri suggested an alternative test of aldosterone secretion; the patient is given a high-sodium diet for 4 days, followed by the administration of either deoxycorticosterone (DOC) (10 mg IM q. 12 h. for 3 days) or the ingestion of fluorocortisone (Florinef) 400 μg p.o. t.i.d. for 3 days).

The serum aldosterone level is measured before and on the third day of the DOC or Florinef administration. The level of serum aldosterone will decline by more than 70% in normal subjects, in patients with essential hypertension, and in some patients with primary aldosteronism who do not have aldosterone-producing adenomas. In patients with an aldosterone-producing adenoma, the levels are not suppressed.

b. Plasma Renin

The second criterion of primary hyperaldosteronism is the finding of a low plasma renin in spite of salt deprivation. One must be familiar with the conditions and drugs that normally result in low renin levels:

- Supine position.
- High sodium or potassium intake.
- Medicines such as propranolol, methyldopa, ganglionic blockers, reserpine, etc.

The blood renin levels should be measured after a direct stimulation with diuretics. Furosemide (Lasix) can be used in one of three possible schedules:

- Lasix, 40–80 mg p.o., then upright position for 3–4 hours.
- Lasix, 60 mg IV, then upright position for 30 min.
- Lasix, 40 mg, p.o., at 6 P.M., 10 P.M., and 6 A.M., followed by 3 hours of ambulation.

For those patients who cannot tolerate furosemide or when diuretics are contraindicated, the following regimen is suggested: low-salt diet (10–20 meq Na per day) for 3–4 days, followed by 3–4 hours of upright position on the fourth day before the blood test. In patients with primary aldosteronism, persistently low plasma renin will be found before and after the diuretic stimulation

4. Localization of the Tumor

Few patients with glucocorticoid-suppressible hyperaldosteronism have been reported, and most of these were familial and easily controlled with dexamethasone. Adrenocortical carcinoma is usually associated with other evidence of excessive glucocorticoids, and the diagnosis can be made with relative ease. The most important problem is actually to distinguish between primary aldosterone-producing adenomas and idiopathic bilateral adrenocortical hyperplasia. Once the diagnosis of primary aldosteronism is made, the next step is to localize the lesion. The following procedures are used to localize the disease:

- Intravenous urogram.
- Sonography.
- Computerized axial tomography (CAT) scan.
- Scanning of the adrenals.
- Adrenal venography.
- Differential adrenal vein sampling for aldosterone levels.

a. IV Urogram, CAT Scan, and Sonography

These routine procedures may be helpful in localizing the lesion, if a sizable tumor is present.

b. Adrenal Scan

Adrenal scanning using [131I]19-iodocholesterol has produced a high success rate in localization of aldosterone-producing adenomas. They have been detected as areas of increased radioactivity on the scan. Increased activity has also occurred in glucocorticoid-producing adenomas and adrenal remnants after radical surgery. In the adrenocortical carcinoma and pheochromocytoma, however, the lesions have appeared as cold areas. Some centers use dexamethasone in conjunction with the adrenal scanning to suppress the remaining normal tissue and report a 77% accuracy. The main drawback of [131I]19-iodocholesterol is that the radioactive agent is being taken up by the gland at a very slow rate (7–14 days); a newer agent, 59Np, has been used with a peak uptake in 24 hours, and it may become the agent of choice.

c. Bilateral Adrenal Venography and Venous Sampling

Bilateral adrenal venography and simultaneous aldosterone assay of the venous blood is the most diagnostic and reliable of all tests. The size of most tumors is between 5 and 15 mm, and aldosteronomas are relatively avascular; arteriography will therefore not demonstrate the lesion in most cases. Selective venogram will show distortion and stretching of the vessels that drape around the lesion, and several reports have been cited with a 95–100% accuracy using this method.

A greater-than-twofold difference between two simultaneously obtained venous blood samples strongly suggests a unilateral adenoma; if the values of both sides are elevated with almost identical levels, bilateral adrenal hyperplasia is likely. The procedure has a complication rate of about 5–10%, the most serious complications being adrenal hemorrhage and adrenal vein perforation.

5. General Medical Evaluation

A thorough, comprehensive evaluation of patients with hyperaldosteronism is most important. Most patients suffer from significant electrolyte disturbances that must be elicited and corrected before surgery. Those patients with long-standing disease will also have renal damage and cardiac changes that need to be compensated.

A metastatic evaluation is uncalled for since almost all aldosterone-producing tumors are benign.

6. Multidisciplinary Evaluation

There is an obvious need for a multidisciplinary dialogue in the approach to the patient with an adrenal tumor. The resources of several types of practitioners need to be tapped to offer the patient the best possible care. Most of the patients will first be seen by their primary physician. If hyperaldosteronism is suspected, the internist and/or endocrinologist should be involved in the evaluation of the patient. Once a definitive diagnosis has been arrived at, the radiologist is then consulted to assist in the localization of the tumor. Only then can a decision be made regarding the best form of treatment. The urologist, endocrinologist, and general surgeon can then plan on a therapeutic approach, both for the short and long term.

C. Preoperative Preparation

As soon as the diagnosis is established, a low-salt diet must be instituted. This will reduce the distal tubular Na load and consequently decrease the K exchange. The hypokalemic alkalosis should be corrected with supplemental oral KCl. The usual regimen is to administer 60–90 meq of KCl per day, although as much as 120 meq per day may be necessary.

In severe hypokalemic alkalosis, especially if associated with marked hypertension, spironolactone should be given. In a study of 32 patients treated with oral spironolactone (50–400 mg per day for 4 weeks), Brown and his associates found a good correlation between the preoperative hypotensive response to spironolactone and the decrease in blood pressure following adrenalectomy.

D. Therapeutic Management

The treatment of primary aldosteronism depends primarily on the cause of the disease.

1. Glucocorticoid-Suppressible Hyperaldosteronism

As mentioned previously, glucocorticoid-suppressible hyperaldosteronism is treated with dexamethasone 0.5 mg orally, twice daily.

2. Bilateral Adrenal Hyperplasia

Adrenal hyperplasia with hyperaldosteronism is treated medically; the drug of choice is spironolactone in doses ranging from 100 to 500 mg per day, the lower dosages being sufficient in patients receiving diuretics (e.g., thiazide). It takes about 8 weeks for a maximal effect. Side effects, however, may be significant and include:

- Gastrointestinal symptoms of anorexia, nausea, and vomiting.
- Impotence.
- Gynecomastia in male patients.
- Hirsutism in female patients.
- Intramenstrual bleeding.
- Sweating and skin pigmentation.

If the patient cannot tolerate spironolactone or has severe side effects, the potassium-retaining amiloride is the next choice. The role of surgery in these patients is still controversial.

3. Aldosterone-Producing Adenomas

These patients are generally treated surgically. Surgery is usually reserved, however, for those patients who have been diagnosed as having unilateral disease. The exposure is preferably obtained via a posterior flank approach through the eleventh rib if the tumor has been preoperatively localized. The adrenal gland is exposed, meticulously dissected, and removed. Of patients in this category, 80% become normotensive following surgery, whereas about 20% of them will require supplemental therapy with spironolactone (Aldactone).

In the absence of definitive localization, a transabdominal approach is recommended, and the left adrenal gland is exposed first, followed by examination of the right gland. If still no definite tumor can be identified, a left adrenalectomy with or without partial right adrenalectomy is recommended.

E. Postoperative Care, Evaluation, and Follow-Up

1. Postoperative Care

Immediately after the surgery, some patients will develop transient adrenal insufficiency and present with fever, headache, anorexia, nausea, vomiting, diarrhea, hypotension, and dehydration. Blood chemistries may identify azotemia, hyponatremia, and hyperkalemia.

Replacement treatment should be initiated with the IV administration of a soluble cortisol preparation (75–100 mg stat., then 100–200 mg IV infusion in 12–24 hours) followed by 50–100 mg IM q. 8 h. until the patient is fully recovered and can tolerate food. Fluorocortisone can then be administered orally and tapered off gradually.

Other postoperative measures include:

- Symptomatic relief of any postoperative symptoms (nausea, vomiting, diarrhea, etc.).

- Fluid and electrolyte monitoring and careful correction of aberrant findings, initiated slowly.
- The usual postoperative care described in §9 and 12, which also applies to these patients.
- Spironolactone, for patients with persistent hypertension after 4 weeks.

2. Follow-Up Evaluation

All patients should be followed up indefinitely at 3- to 6-month intervals, and serum electrolytes must be monitored regularly. If possible, serum aldosterone levels and urinary potassium excretions should be measured every 6 months. Table I is a suggested schedule of such an evaluation.

F. Management Algorithm for Hyperaldosteronism (see p. 137)

II. CUSHING'S SYNDROME

Cushing's syndrome was described by Harvey Cushing in 1932. It is a rare condition that affects mainly young adults; the female/male ratio is 5 : 1, and the 5-year mortality of undiagnosed, untreated Cushing's syndrome is 50%. In its typical form, the clinical presentation of the patient is characteristic, with truncal obesity, moon facies, hirsutism, osteoporosis, and an impaired glucose tolerance curve. There are three main causes of Cushing's syndrome:

- Adrenocortical tumors that secrete cortisol autonomously. These may be solitary or multiple, benign or malignant.
- Pituitary dysfunction with excessive ACTH secretion from a chromophobe or basophilic adenoma. True Cushing's disease actually results from pituitary hypersecretion of ACTH.
- Paraendocrine tumors synthesizing ACTH immunologically indistinguishable from pituitary ACTH, (e.g., oat cell carcinoma of the lung, bronchial carcinoid, etc.).

Adrenal carcinoma is the most common cause of Cushing's disease in children, while adults suffer more often from hyperplasia.

A. Early Detection and Screening

Early detection is dependent on identification of the following classical signs and symptoms of Cushing's syndrome:

- Truncal obesity.
- Moon facies, buffalo hump.

ALGORITHM FOR HYPERALDOSTERONISM

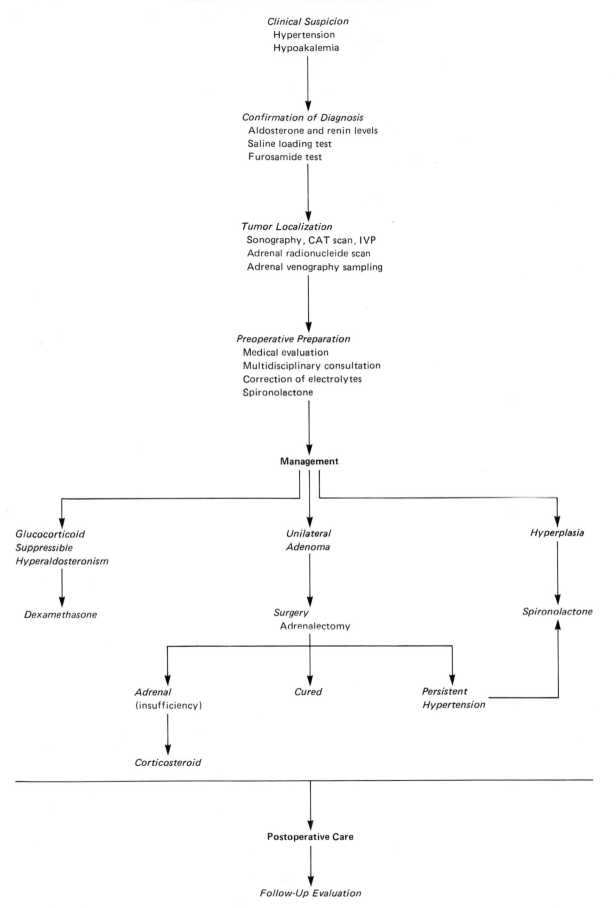

Table I

Long-Term Follow-Up Schedule for Primary Aldosteronism

Management	First and second year				Third-to-fifth year		Thereafter, annually
	3 Months	6 Months	9 Months	12 Months	6 Months	12 Months	
History							
General malaise	X	X	X	X	X	X	X
Muscular weakness	X	X	X	X	X	X	X
Headache	X	X	X	X	X	X	X
Paresthesia	X	X	X	X	X	X	X
Palpitations	X	X	X	X	X	X	X
Physical							
Blood pressure	X	X	X	X	X	X	X
Cardiac arrhythmia	X	X	X	X	X	X	X
Deep tendon reflex	X	X	X	X	X	X	X
Chvostek and trousseau signs	X	X	X	X	X	X	X
Fundoscopy	X	X	X	X	X	X	X
Investigations							
CBC	X	X	X	X	X	X	X
SMA-6	X	X	X	X	X	X	X
SMA-12	X	X	X	X	X	X	X
EKG	X	X	X	X	X	X	X
24-hour urinary chemistry (including K$^+$ excretion)		X		X	X	X	X
Serum aldosterone		X		X	X	X	X

- Hirsutism in females.
- Purplish striae, plethora.
- Amenorrhea in females.
- Impotence in males.
- Muscle weakness.
- Easy bruisability.
- Mental disturbances.
- Visual disturbances and headaches in cases of pituitary adenomas.
- Hypertension.

Although no screening is indicated because of the rarity of the disease and the obvious nature of the symptoms, education of the public, as well as physicians, is likely to yield earlier reporting of cases.

B. Pretreatment Evaluation and Work-Up

If the diagnosis is suspected from the physical findings described above, evaluation of the patient will follow three directions.

- Establishment and confirmation of the diagnosis of Cushing's syndrome.
- Identification of the cause.
- Localization of the actual offending lesion.

1. Laboratory Findings

- Complete blood count (CBC). There is moderate neutrophilic leukocytosis with eosinophils below 100 cells per cubic millimeter in more than 90% of the patients.
- Metabolic alkalosis with hypokalemia and hypochloremia is usually present in patients with markedly elevated cortisol levels (most typically in ectopic ACTH syndromes).
- Abnormal glucose tolerance curve is seen in 60–70% of patients. Diabetic ketoacidosis is rare.
- Increased urinary excretion of calcium resulting in nephrolithiasis.
- Osteoporosis, most marked in the spine and pelvic area. Pathological fractures are a common occurrence.
- Free urinary cortisol will be elevated to levels of 100 μg per day or more.

2. Diagnostic Testing

The basis of all tests performed to establish the diagnosis of hyperfunction of the adrenal gland is an elevation of cortisol secretion and the loss of normal diurnal rhythm. The following investigations are helpful in arriving at a diagnosis:

a. Dexamethasone Suppression Test

i. Overnight Dexamethasone Suppression. This test is used for initial screening in a patient where the diagnosis is clinically suspicious.

- A baseline plasma cortisol is drawn between 8 and 9 A.M.
- 1 mg dexamethasone is administered at 11 P.M.
- Repeat cortisol level is determined at 8 A.M. the next morning.

Patients with no Cushing's syndrome will not suppress and will maintain a serum cortisol level around 12 μg. Some patients (e.g., with severe obesity) may drop to 6 μg, whereas patients with Cushing's Syndrome will drop lower. A normal test precludes any further testing.

ii. Low-Dose Dexamethasone Test.   This is performed if the overnight test is positive.

- 0.5 mg of dexamethasone is administered q. 6 h. × 12.
- 24-hour urine specimens are collected for 17-hydroxycorticosteroids (17-OHCS) and free cortisol.

A normal response is suppression of the 17-OHCS to less than 4 mg per 24 hours and the free cortisol to less than 20 μg. Failure to suppress establishes the diagnosis of Cushing's syndrome.

iii. High-dose Dexamethasone Test.   This is used to identify the cause of the syndrome.

- 2 mg of dexamethasone is given q. 6 h. × 8.
- Urine collected as above.

A suppression of 50% or more establishes a diagnosis of adrenal hyperplasia from pituitary-origin ACTH (Cushing's disease). One third of such patients however may not show suppression, though some of these may respond to higher doses (32 mg per 24 hours), and some patients with ectopic ACTH syndromes may also suppress. Patients with adrenal tumors do not suppress.

b. ACTH Stimulation Test

Continuous IV infusion of corticotrophin is given for 8 hours and cortisol levels are measured.

An increased secretion of cortisol is found in patients with hyperplasia. This is sometimes so in adenomas but never in carcinomas of the adrenal gland.

c. Metyrapone Test

The hypothalamic pituitary system is not suppressed in patients with adrenal hyperplasia but is functioning at a higher level. Patients with adrenal hyperplasia demonstrate a hyperactive response to metyrapone, and there is an excessive rise in urinary 17-hydroxycorticoids.

In patients with adrenal tumors (i.e., adenoma, carcinoma, or para-endocrine tumors), the pituitary gland is inhibited, and metyrapone administration fails to release corticotrophin in the normal manner; the usual rise in urinary steroids, therefore, is not seen. The test, when positive, is more specific than the dexamethasone suppression test.

d. Plasma ACTH Levels

The measurement of plasma ACTH by radioimmunoassay will help distinguish Cushing's syndrome of adrenal etiology (which suppresses ACTH) from pituitary-origin Cushing's disease, where the levels are usually high, normal, or slightly elevated. Markedly elevated levels (>200 pg per milliliter) are strongly suggestive of ectopic ACTH syndrome.

*e. 24-Hour Urinary 17-Ketosteroids
(17-KS) (or Plasma
Dehydroepiandrosterone (DHEA)
Sulfate)*

Extremely elevated levels (17-KS > 40 mg or DHEA > 8000 mg) are strongly suggestive of carcinoma.

*f. 24-Hour Urinary 5-Hydroxyindoleacetic
Acid (5-HIAA)*

This test is useful in the identification of Cushing's syndrome resulting from otherwise indistinguishable carcinoid tumors producing ACTH.

3. Localizing Investigations of the Cause of Cushing's Syndrome

After having established the diagnosis of Cushing's syndrome, other studies need to be carried out, together with the chemical assays, to determine the cause of the disease and to localize it. The following sequential procedures may be performed to achieve that goal.

a. Intravenous Urogram

In a majority of the patients the intravenous urogram is perfectly normal; it may, on occasion, reveal a large mass above the kidney, displacing it and altering its axis or there may be extrinsic compression of the pelvicalyceal system.

b. Abdominal Sonogram

Properly conducted, this noninvasive study may be invaluable in the diagnosis of tumors of the adrenal glands. It is of little help in patients with bilateral hyperplasia.

c. CAT Scan

This relatively recent modality is fairly sensitive in delineating space occupying lesions of the adrenal gland as small as 1–2 cm and surpasses the intravenous pyelogram (IVP) or sonogram in accuracy and specificity. It is most valuable not only in identifying a normally situated organ, but also in outlining the retroperitoneal area and any adjacent metastatic disease. When other testing suggests a pituitary origin, CAT scanning can readily detect those cases with macroadenomas (10% of cases), and with the most modern equipment, even the microadenomas can be seen on coronal views.

d. Adrenal Angiography

Adrenal angiography, frequently used in the past, may adequately outline the tumor; it is not performed as frequently today because of the marked improvement in the noninvasive imaging techniques.

e. Selective Adrenal Vein Sampling

f. ^{131}I-Labeled Cholesterol Adrenal Scan

This test will identify bilateral uptake in patients with hyperplasia, as opposed to unilateral in cases of adrenal tumors.

g. Surgery

The last method of identification of the exact nature of the pathology is by surgical exploration, and often the final diagnosis will not be absolutely certain until the time of surgery. When the studies point to an adenoma of the adrenals, surgery is indicated.

C. Preoperative Preparation

1. Cardiopulmonary Considerations

Any type of cardiopulmonary decompensation should be corrected preoperatively. Severe potassium depletion should also be corrected prior to surgery. It is important to recognize that small decreases in the level of serum potassium indicate much greater depletion of the total body potassium, and a drop in serum K to 3 meq per liter suggests a total body deficit of over 450 meq of potassium.

2. Antibiotics

Patients with Cushing's syndrome are prone to infections and have lowered resistance; therefore, the use of prophylactic pre- and postoperative broad-spectrum antibiotics is strongly recommended and is usually continued well into the postoperative period.

3. Preoperative Steroid Coverage

Patients undergoing bilateral adrenalectomy are started on an IV infusion of steroids the night before the surgery and con-

tinued during, and indefinitely after, the surgery. Likewise, patients who have tumors of the adrenal gland or para-endocrine tumors resulting in Cushing's syndrome should also be prophylactically covered by IV steroids.

Water-soluble preparations of cortisol (e.g., hemisuccinate or phosphate) are given preoperatively. An IV infusion of 10 mg per hour is administered during the operation and continued for 24 hours during the postoperative period; the dosage is then reduced over the next 5–7 days. Once the patient is able to tolerate oral fluids, the IV injection is replaced by oral steroid supplements, which, in patients who had resection of only one gland, can be gradually weaned off depending upon the symptoms (e.g., aching muscles, weakness, anorexia). The first step in the withdrawal schedule, which is designed to reactivate the patient's own adrenal function gradually, is to administer a single morning dose. A gradual reduction in this dose (by increments of 5 mg at a time every 2–4 weeks) is pursued until the patient is stabilized. Ordinarily, all hormone treatment is withdrawn at approximately 3–6 months. If a major illness occurs within the next year, however, supplemental cortisol therapy should be administered; it is started the same way, is continued during the period of illness and for 48 hours afterward, and then weaned off.

Patients undergoing bilateral adrenalectomy for hyperplasia will require steroids indefinitely.

4. Psychiatric Evaluation

Mental disturbances are fairly common in patients with Cushing's syndrome. Psychosis of a depressive or paranoid nature may occur. Psychiatric evaluation is, therefore, necessary in these patients and must be part of the preoperative preparation of the patient.

5. Multidisciplinary Evaluation

Cushing's syndrome is a rare condition. In consequence, it is necessary to stress that proper treatment requires cooperation between the primary physician, the endocrinologist, the radiologist, the urologist, as well as the surgeons (neurosurgeon or general surgeon), and on rare occasions the medical oncologist.

D. Therapeutic Management

The treatment of Cushing's syndrome usually involves procedures of considerable magnitude. Once the diagnosis is established, treatment should be instituted at once since the mortality of the disease is otherwise quite high and increases with the duration of the illness. The results of treatment are usually quite satisfactory. The signs and symptoms gradually regress; mental status shows great improvement, but the most resistant disturbance is osteoporosis, which does not result in significant healing.

Treatment will vary according to the cause and location of the pathology.

1. Adrenal Tumors

Tumors of the adrenal gland can be of several varieties:

a. Nonfunctioning Tumors

- Adrenocortical nodules. These lesions, often found at autopsy, are extremely common, asymptomatic, and of no clinical significance. There is no evidence that they ever develop into true neoplasms.
- Myelolipomas. These lesions affect mainly the medulla and appear to represent a type of metaplasia.
- Adrenal cysts. These lesions, sometimes huge in size, are usually accidentally discovered during sonography or laparotomy for other causes. Intervention is rarely indicated.
- True cortical adenomas are usually single and small in size.
- Carcinomas of the adrenal gland. Larger tumors are usually malignant, and most nonfunctioning tumors large enough to produce signs are malignant. These nonfunctioning carcinomas are excessively rare tumors that are usually discovered after they have metastasized. The most common sites of metastases are the lungs, liver, and lymph nodes. The tumor itself may invade the adjacent structures, especially the kidney. Metastases to the bones and brain are unusual. The prognosis in these patients is dismal (50% dead in 2 years).

b. Functional Tumors

Functional tumors of the adrenal glands are very rare indeed in relation to the general population (1.1 per million). A significant number of cases occur in children before age 10, and about 80% of patients are women. Less than 20% of functional tumors are actually malignant. The tumor may produce any of the following syndromes, either alone or in combinations:

- Cushing's syndrome.
- Isosexual precocity in male children.
- Aldosteronism.
- Hypoglycemia (rarely).

The combination of Cushing's syndrome and virilization in the female is the most common combination. Feminizing tumors may also occur in the male between 25 and 50 years of age with gynecomastia as the most frequent presenting sign; testicular atrophy, decrease in libido, oligospermia, as well as penile atrophy occur in about 50% of patients. The tumor in these patients excretes androstenedione, which is converted peripherally into estrogen.

The treatment of adrenal tumors is complete surgical re-moval of the tumor, which, in most cases, is unilateral. Malignant tumors can often be completely removed, but if complete removal is not possible, postoperative chemotherapy should be administered. Although a large number of drugs are presently on trial (adriamycin, 5-fluorouracil, vinblastine, Cytoxan, methyl chloroethyl cyclohexyl nitrosourea (CCNU), etc.), the one specific cytotoxic agent for adrenal tissue is $o'p'$DDD (mitotane), which blocks the response to ACTH and causes focal degeneration of the zona fasciculata and reticularis of the gland. Long-term results, however, with $o'p'$DDD are disappointing. Radiation therapy has not been employed widely enough to allow for proper evaluation, although sporadic case reports seem to show some response in residual local disease.

2. Adrenocortical Hyperplasia

In most instances, the hyperplasia is due to hypersecretion of ACTH without a grossly detectable tumor in the pituitary. In 5% of patients, the sella turcica is enlarged, and a chromophobe adenoma can be identified. Bilateral adrenalectomy as a primary approach in these cases has been generally de-emphasized as a result of the success reported with transsphenoidal hypophysectomy and of the risk of aggressive postoperative pituitary tumors (Nelson's syndrome) that occur in over 10% of these patients after bilateral adrenalectomy.

a. Patients with Enlarged Sella Turcica

The recommended treatment of most tumors of the pituitary gland has, in the past, been radiotherapy; ^{90}Yttrium implanted through a transsphenoidal route was commonly used before the advent of electron beam therapy. In adults, however, the preferred treatment today is transsphenoidal hypophysectomy; although favorable results have been reported with photon beam therapy, the results of surgery in the adult approach 80% cure rates as compared with 20% for radiotherapy.

Tumors exhibiting progressive expansion and producing visual field defects or ophthalmoplegia should be removed surgically. When the sella is moderately enlarged, a transsphenoidal approach can be used; with considerable enlargement or lateral extension, a transfrontal approach becomes necessary. Postoperatively, these patients will not only need steroid replacement, but also thyroid and gonadal hormone replacement.

b. Patients without Sellar Enlargement

If a diagnosis of Cushing's disease of pituitary origin can be established, the preferred treatment is by surgery (transsphenoidal hypophysectomy).

Bilateral total adrenalectomy with replacement therapy is, however, sometimes indicated in patients with severe symptoms and is preferably carried out through a posterior approach. Alternative methods of treatment are also available for those patients where surgery is either contraindicated or otherwise rejected. These include

- Daily administration of a serotonin antagonist such as cyprohepatadine; the disadvantage of such therapy is that it has to be continued indefinitely; it may be extremely useful, however, as a stopgap measure while awaiting more definitive therapy.
- The adrenal antagonist aminoglutethimide could be useful in the symptomatic control of the disease.
- Irradiation of the pituitary fossa to decrease the production of ACTH has also been useful in selected cases.

Of patients who have had bilateral adrenalectomy, 10% will develop a secondary pituitary adenoma and Nelson's syndrome. The latter syndrome is marked by aggressive behavior of the adenoma, the presence of chromophobe granulations, and, possibly, by the secretion of ACTH and beta melanocyte-stimulating hormone (β-MSH) with dermal pigmentation. Such tumors may appear 10–15 years after adrenalectomy, and the patients should, therefore, be monitored with a yearly check-up of the sella and of ACTH level determinations following the adrenalectomy. These patients should also be monitored for increased levels of MSH. Radiotherapy may be effective in the treatment of Nelson's syndrome, but surgery is required if the tumor is large. Prophylactic pituitary irradiation should be considered following bilateral adrenalectomy, though it does not confer absolute protection against Nelson's syndrome.

3. Para-endocrine Tumors

Para-endocrine tumors are peripheral tumors, benign or malignant, that produce ACTH. In most cases, these tumors have already metastasized before the diagnosis is made. Most of them are highly malignant, and a majority arise from the lungs (50% are oat cell cancers of the lung). Usually other symptoms will overshadow the symptoms of hypercortisolism (wasting weakness and hyperpigmentation); metyrapone or $o'p'$DDD can be administered to reduce cortisol production and associated metabolic abnormalities (hypokalemia and hyperglycemia). Bilateral total adrenalectomy may, at times, be indicated for palliation.

E. Postoperative Care, Evaluation, and Follow-Up

The immediate treatment following adrenalectomy has been mentioned in §4A.I.D. Once stabilized, the patient is started on a moderate dose of hydrocortisone hemisuccinate (25 mg daily), which needs to be increased in any stressful situation

(e.g., infection, surgery, or other stress). These patients should be followed for an indefinite period; Table II is a schedule of check-ups for the evaluation of the patients with treated Cushing's syndrome.

F. Management Algorithm for Cushing's Syndrome (see p. 143)

III. PHEOCHROMOCYTOMA

A. Early Detection and Screening

1. Early Detection

Pheochromoyctoma is a rare tumor arising from catecholamine-producing cells of the adrenergic nervous sytem. It constitutes the most common tumor of the adrenal medulla and yet accounts for less than 1% of all hypertensive patients. The disease is characterized by dramatic clinical symptoms that result from excessive catecholamine release and, when undiagnosed, may lead to cardiovascular and renal failure and eventually death; nearly 800 people die yearly of pheochromocytoma in the United States, yet the disease often goes unrecognized. In a large series of autopsy reports, a frequency of discovery of 1 in 1000 autopsies is far greater than the clinical rate of detection of pheochromocytoma. It is imperative that the lesion be recognized and diagnosed early to avoid the serious complications that may result from the untreated disease. The tumor can occur at any age, and the presenting feature is usually paroxysmal hypertension; a hypertensive crisis following anesthesia or unexplained shock following minor surgery may be the initial clinical feature. Deaths are attributed to the complications of unrecognized disease rather than to the therapy, further stressing the importance of early detection.

No screening is available other than the usual identification of hypertension on routine physical examinations or on mass screening. Just as in hyperaldosteronism, a keen degree of awareness and a high index of suspicion are the only attributes that need be prompted in order to detect a pheochromocytoma in patients with hypertension, before a catastrophic crisis occurs. The following clues will suggest a pheochromocytoma as the cause of the hypertension:

- Patients with a history of paroxysmal attacks of severe headache, profound sweating, and palpitation, etc.
- Patients with early onset of hypertension.
- Severe hypertension in children, especially associated with headache, excessive sweating, and weight loss.

ALGORIYHM FOR CUSHING'S SYNDROME

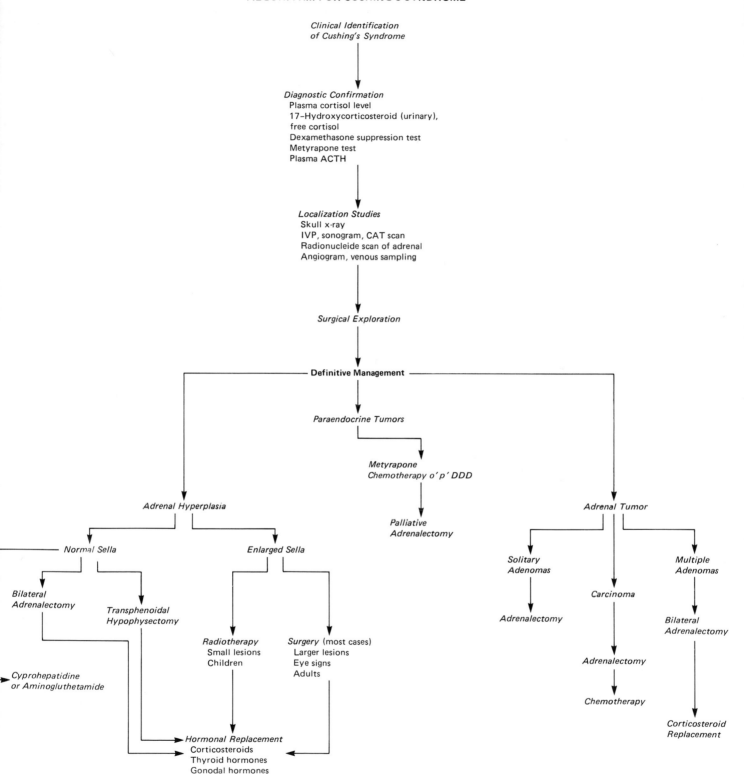

*Clinical Identification
of Cushing's Syndrome*

Diagnostic Confirmation
Plasma cortisol level
17–Hydroxycorticosteroid (urinary),
free cortisol
Dexamethasone suppression test
Metyrapone test
Plasma ACTH

Localization Studies
Skull x-ray
IVP, sonogram, CAT scan
Radionucleide scan of adrenal
Angiogram, venous sampling

Surgical Exploration

Definitive Management

Paraendocrine Tumors

*Metyrapone
Chemotherapy o' p' DDD*

*Palliative
Adrenalectomy*

Adrenal Hyperplasia

Adrenal Tumor

Normal Sella

Enlarged Sella

*Solitary
Adenomas*

*Multiple
Adenomas*

*Bilateral
Adrenalectomy*

*Transphenoidal
Hypophysectomy*

Carcinoma

Adrenalectomy

*Bilateral
Adrenalectomy*

Radiotherapy
Small lesions
Children

Surgery (most cases)
Larger lesions
Eye signs
Adults

Adrenalectomy

*Cyprohepatidine
or Aminogluthetamide*

Chemotherapy

*Corticosteroid
Replacement*

Hormonal Replacement
Corticosteroids
Thyroid hormones
Gonodal hormones

Table II

Long-Term Follow-Up Schedule for Cushing's Syndrome

Management	First and second year				Third-to-fifth year		Thereafter, annually
	3 Months	6 Months	9 Months	12 Months	6 Months	12 Months	
History							
Muscle weakness	X	X	X	X	X	X	X
Amenorrhea in females	X	X	X	X	X	X	X
Impotence in males	X	X	X	X	X	X	X
Easy bruisability	X	X	X	X	X	X	X
Headache	X	X	X	X	X	X	X
Physical							
Moon facies	X	X	X	X	X	X	X
Truncal obesity	X	X	X	X	X	X	X
Buffalo hump	X	X	X	X	X	X	X
Hirsutism in females	X	X	X	X	X	X	X
Visual-field defect	X	X	X	X	X	X	X
Investigations							
CBC with differential count	X	X	X	X	X	X	X
SMA-6	X	X	X	X	X	X	X
Fasting blood sugar	X	X	X	X	X	X	X
X-ray of the skull		X		X	X	X	X
24th urinary 17-OHCS and free cortisol		X		X	X	X	X
ACTH levels		X		X	X	X	X
Diagnostic tests				As indicated			
IVP				As indicated			
CAT scan				As indicated			
Adrenal angiogram				As indicated			

- Hypertensive patients with positive family history and evidence of tumors of other endocrine systems (i.e., thyroid tumor, neurofibroma, café-au-lait lesions, retinal angiomas, etc.).

2. Clinical Considerations

The disease occurs at any age, with a peak in the fourth and fifth decades; 5–10% are familial, and some of these patients have associated tumors of other endocrine systems (e.g., medullary carcinoma of the thyroid and hyperparathyroidism as in Sipple's syndrome). About 35–45% of patients present with paroxysmal hypertensive attacks; the remainder either suffer from sustained hypertension or present with brief paroxysmal episodes.

a. Paroxysmal Hypertension

The most common symptoms are:

- A sudden onset of headache.
- Palpitation, excessive sweating, and severe anxiety.
- Tremor.
- Chest or epigastric pain associated with nausea and vomiting.

Usually, the headaches are severe, throbbing, and generalized. They are always abrupt in onset and last for a few minutes to 2 hours. Excessive sweating can be either paroxysmal or continuous and is especially prominent in children. During the attack, the blood pressure may be increased up to 180 diastolic. Characteristically, chest pain develops at the peak of the attack, which can be helpful in differentiating it from that of myocardial infarction.

The frequency and duration of the attacks vary a great deal, and usually the patient is quite normal between attacks. The following are some of the known trigger factors for the attacks:

- Certain position or posture of the body.
- Emotional changes.
- Body or environmental temperature changes.
- Sexual activity.
- Pressure over certain parts of the body, e.g., abdomen.
- Smoking or alcohol.
- Eating, coughing, laughing, etc.

b. Sustained Hypertension

Patients who suffer from a sustained, stable hypertension may present a clinical picture indistinguishable from that of essential hypertension but are prone to persistent tachycardia, nervousness, recurrent headache, and perspiration. These patients are likely to lose weight with a high incidence of hypermetabolism and vascular complications. Elevated basal metabolic rate with normal thyroid function, glycosuria, hyperglycemia, and elevated serum free fatty acid are common laboratory findings.

c. Vascular Complications

Patients of sustained hypertensive type have a high incidence of vascular complications, which include

- Retinopathy.
- Cerebrovascular hemorrhage.
- Myocardial ischemia, cardiac arrhythmia, and cardiac failure.
- Malignant hypertension.

A specific myocarditis is found in this group of patients, with focal degeneration and necrosis of myocardial fibers around small blood vessels; it should be suspected whenever a patient develops profound myocardial failure or arrhythmia. Most of these patients will show healing of the myocarditis following removal of the pheochromocytoma.

3. Pathological Findings

The majority of the tumors occur as a single unilateral adrenal medullary tumor; 10% occur as multiple adrenal tumors, especially in patients with familial disease; and 10–15% occur as extra-adrenal paragangliomas. More than 90% of these ectopic tumors are located beneath the diaphragm and situated around the superior para-aortic region, the renal pedicle, the inferior mesenteric artery, or the aortic bifurcation.

Grossly, the tumors are round, lobulated, and highly vascular. On cut surface areas of calcification, hemorrhagic degeneration and cyst formation can be identified. About 10% are malignant, although histologically the malignant tumor cells are often identical to those in benign tumors; the only criterion of malignancy is the development of metastases, which can occur in bones, lungs, liver, spleen, lymph nodes, and bone marrow.

B. Pretreatment Evaluation and Work-Up

The diagnosis of pheochromocytoma is suggested by the clinical symptoms and signs; confirmation of the diagnosis must be done by appropriate tests. These include

- Measurement of urinary or plasma catecholamine and its metabolites.
- Provocative test (with histamine, glucagon, or tyramine).
- Suppressive test (with phentolamine).
- Localization of the offending tumor.

1. Catecholamines

The tests available for measurement of urinary catecholamine and its metabolites are: free catecholamines, vanillylmandelic acid (VMA), and metanephrines. After metabolism, only a small portion of catecholamine is excreted as free catecholamine; a larger portion is excreted as an o-methylated product—normetanephrine (NM) and metanephrine (M); an even larger portion is excreted after further oxidation to VMA.

a. Urinary Free Catecholamines

This can be further separated into epinephrine and norepinephrine. A proportionately high epinephrine level is suggestive of a tumor in the adrenal gland or around it. Free catecholamine values are elevated in 80–100% of cases, but one should be aware of false positive results from exogenous catecholamines in nasal drops, eye drops, etc.

b. Urinary VMA

Urinary VMA is the most widely used test for pheochromocytoma. It is affected, however, by many drugs and chemicals such as nalidixic acid, levodopa, lithium, lecithin, and nitroglycerine, all of which will increase the VMA levels, or monoamine oxidase inhibitors and ethanol, both of which may decrease it.

c. Urinary NM and M

Normetanephrine and metanephrine are not readily separated, and few factors affect their value. Total metanephrine excretion is elevated in 85–100% of cases of pheochromocytoma. Since metanephrine excretion is relatively constant and its measurement is easy to perform, spot urinary metanephrine determination is the most useful screening test in patients suspected of having pheochromocytoma. The test is especially sensitive when the urine specimen is collected during or immediately after an attack.

d. Plasma Catecholamines

These are elevated in pheochromocytoma, especially during an attack, but because it is more expensive and difficult to measure plasma catecholamines than to carry out the various urine tests, it is only performed on blood samples obtained during adrenal venography for localization of the tumors.

It is advisable that all three urinary tests be performed on the suspected patients. There are several cases with normal values in one or two of the three urinary tests, but at least one of the three tests is abnormal in all cases.

2. Provocative Tests

Provocative tests with histamine, glucagon, or tyramine may induce severe hypertensive crisis and are therefore dangerous.

They are only indicated in those rare instances where patients present with an unwitnessed history of severe life-threatening paroxysmal attacks but are completely normal in between; early diagnosis with these tests may be advisable in such cases.

3. Suppressive Tests

Suppressive tests with phentolamines are also risky, as they sometimes induce hypotensive shock. They are, however, indicated, on rare occasions, in those patients with sustained, stable hypertensive disease; a drop in blood pressure of greater than 35/25 mm Hg is considered as a positive result. False positive reactions occur in approximately 25% of the cases, and extensive further laboratory evaluation is mandatory.

4. Localization

a. Chest X-ray

A chest x-ray should be the first test obtained to check for any lesion in the lung or paravertebral area.

b. IVP and Nephrotomogram

Positive findings include enlargement of the adrenal glands, and about 10% will show calcification. The overall accuracy is about 30–40%.

c. CAT Scan of the Abdomen

This is a noninvasive method of great value, which should always be performed. Special attention should be paid to the presence of paraganglionic tumors at different levels around the aorta.

d. Angiography of the Adrenal Gland

Angiography with selective arteriograms has a rather high success rate in localizing the tumor, especially in cases of multiple tumors or in those of ectopic locations. The findings include

- Enlarged adrenal gland.
- Distorted vessels and neovascularity with dense vascular staining.
- Presence of thoracic and pelvic branches.

During angiography, cases of paroxysmal life-threatening hypertensive attacks have been reported, and it has been suggested that routine Dibenzyline (or Regitine) treatment be given before the procedure. The elevation of the blood pressure during the procedure, however, could be considered diagnostic, and some have suggested careful vital-sign monitoring with Dibenzyline standby, rather than routine treatment, in order to identify this elevation of the blood pressure.

e. Selective Venous Catheterization with Catecholamine Samplings

Among pheochromocytomas, 15–20% are hypovascular lesions, and sometimes multiple or ectopic lesions will not show on arteriograms. Adrenal venography is an additional modality that may be used, especially with simultaneous venous samplings and assay of catecholamines at different levels of the inferior vena cava.

5. General Medical and Metastatic Evaluation

A thorough multisystem medical evaluation must always be carried out in these patients prior to instituting any therapy. Any coexisting medical illness, particularly cardiac, renal, or pulmonary, must be recognized, assessed, and treated.

An extensive work-up may be indicated in cases of extra-adrenal paraneoplastic tumors to identify the exact location of the tumor. Furthermore, in cases of suspected malignant tumors, a standard metastatic survey is necessary (chest x-ray, SMA-12), with extended studies (bone scan, liver scan, chest CAT scan, etc.) carried out as indicated.

A multidisciplinary approach is most useful in these patients because of the rarity of the disease and the complexity of its ramifications; this should include the primary physician, endocrinologist, surgeon, radiotherapist, and chemotherapist.

C. Preoperative Preparation

1. General Considerations

Because of the hypermetabolic state often associated with pheochromocytoma, most of the patients are underweight and dehydrated. General nutritional support and hydration are therefore equally as important as pharmacological preparation. In addition, 1–2 units of blood are recommended preoperatively in most patients.

2. Drug Preparation

Once the diagnosis of pheochromocytoma is established, the patient should be medically treated, and his general condition stabilized for a period of time (usually about 10–14 days) prior to surgery. The mortality and morbidity during the surgery are related to hypertensive crisis, severe cardiac arrhythmia, and hypotensive vascular shock. The following agents should be judiciously used in the preparation of the patient.

a. Alpha-Adrenergic Blockers

Either one of the following drugs may be administered to control blood pressure: phentolamine, 25–50 mg, p.o., q. 4–6 h., or Phenoxybenzamine, 5–10 mg, p.o., b.i.d. The amount of the drug can then be increased until the patient's hypertension is under control. The patient is then kept on a maintenance dose of 40–100 mg per day of phentolamine in divided doses.

b. Beta-Adrenergic Blockers

Propranolol (Inderal) 10–40 mg, p.o., q. 6–8 h. is indicated in patients with persistent tachycardia or arrhythmia after adequate alpha-blocker treatment; it is contraindicated in patients with bronchial asthma, heart block, or untreated heart failure.

c. Nonspecific Peripheral Vasodilators

These agents (e.g., nitroprusside, 50–100 mg per liter of IV fluid) may be administered and titrated to maintain a normal blood pressure. This is particularly useful in the patient under anesthesia and during surgery.

3. Intraoperative Drug Therapy and Preparation for Induction

Scopolamine is given as a preanesthetic agent, and induction is performed with sodium pentothal and maintained by halothane. Continuous monitoring of the patient is performed with an arterial line, central venous pressure, and electrocardiogram. The patient must be watched very closely, and the blood pressure is maintained in the normal range. A preoperative hypertensive crisis can be dealt with by using either phentolamine or nitroprusside (Nipride) infusion; hypotension following removal of the tumor, on the other hand, must be treated with copious IV fluids and, if necessary, with dopamine infusions. Propranolol or lidocaine may be necessary to reverse any arrythmias during the procedure, and if a bilateral adrenalectomy is performed, an IV infusion of hydrocortisone phosphate is given at a rate of 15 mg per hour.

D. Therapeutic Management

1. Surgery

Pheochromocytomas are usually exposed through a transperitoneal approach because of their multiplicity and the need to explore both sides; large tumors in adults may require a thoracoabdominal approach. Ectopic tumors should be identified and localized preoperatively to allow for the most appropriate surgical approach; careful inspection of the entire retroperitoneal area with exploration of both adrenals and the para-aortic tissues is highly recommended. Gentle massage of the suspected area, with continuous monitoring of the blood pressure, is usually helpful in locating ectopic or multiple tumors.

2. Nonoperative Treatment

a. Phenoxybenzamine

This medical agent can be used when surgery is refused or deferred due to a recent myocardial infarction or other serious medical contraindications and for unresectable tumors or metastatic disease.

b. Alpha-methyl-p-tyrosine (MPT)

This drug interferes with catecholamine synthesis by inhibiting the enzyme tyrosine hydroxylase. Its use, however, has marked side effects, sometimes causing severe renal damage and a Parkinson's-like syndrome.

c. Chemotherapy

A few remissions have been reported with chemotherapy, but overall results are discouraging. A large variety of drugs have been used, and favorable responses have been anecdotally reported. The drugs used are

- o'p'DDD (mitotane).
- Cyclophosphamide and vincristine.
- Bichloroethyl nitrosourea (BCNU) and vincristine.
- Adriamycin.
- Streptozotocin.

d. Radiotherapy

Radiation therapy has been reported to yield favorable responses in metastatic pheochromocytoma, particularly in bone.

E. Postoperative Care, Evaluation, and Follow-Up

1. Immediate Postoperative Care

Continuous monitoring with EKG and continuous arterial-line recording of intra-arterial blood pressure should be carried out in the recovery room. Hourly intake and output, central venous pressure, and temperature measurements are also mandatory. After full recovery from anesthesia, the patient should be moved and turned very carefully to avoid hypotension; the blood pressure must be maintained with IV dopamine, but after the vital signs are stabilized for 24–48 hours, these vasopressors should be tapered off gradually and discontinued as soon as possible.

2. Long-Term Postoperative Care

Following bilateral total adrenalectomy, it is very important that replacement therapy with hydrocortisone be given immediately after the removal of the adrenal glands. The proposed schedules are:

- Intraoperatively and during the day of surgery, as well as during the next 2 days: hydrocortisone, 100 mg IV drip, q. 8 h.
- Postoperative day 3 and day 4: hydrocortisone, 50 mg IV/IM, q. 12 h.
- Postoperative day 5: hydrocortisone 20 mg IV/IM, q. 12 h.
- Postoperative day 6: hydrocortisone 20 mg IM/p.o., q. 8 h.

Thereafter, if the patient can tolerate a normal diet and oral medication, cortisone acetate may be administered in a dose of 25 mg p.o. in the A.M. and 12.5 mg p.o. in the P.M.

Mineralocorticoid requirements are variable and dependent on the type and amount of corticosteroid preparation used. With cortisol acetate treatment, 0.1 mg fluorocortisone p.o. daily will be sufficient; if the patient is having a good fluid and electrolyte supply, mineralocorticoid treatment may not be necessary.

3. Follow-Up Plan and Evaluation

Before discharge from the hospital, a repeat urinary catecholamine measurement should be taken. Some of these patients may have persistently high catecholamine levels for a few weeks, and a few might even have sustained hypertension even with normal catecholamine levels. Essential hypertension or hypertension secondary to renal damage must be suspected in this case and treated accordingly.

Following discharge, the patient should be followed in the office regularly for the possibility of recurrent pheochromocytoma or metastatic malignant tumors. The suggested plan of follow-up is shown in Table III.

F. Management Algorithm for Pheochromocytomas (see p. 149)

IV. NEUROBLASTOMA

A. Early Detection and Screening

1. General Considerations

Neuroblastoma is the commonest solid tumor of infancy and childhood; most of the cases are diagnosed between the ages of 1 and 1.5 years. There are no specific symptoms and signs for

Table III

Long-Term Follow-Up Schedule for Pheochromocytoma

Management	First and second year				Third-to-fifth year		Thereafter, annually
	3 Months	6 Months	9 Months	12 Months	6 Months	12 Months	
History							
Palpitation	X	X	X	X	X	X	X
Anxiety	X	X	X	X	X	X	X
Perspiration	X	X	X	X	X	X	X
Chest pain and/or epigastric pain	X	X	X	X	X	X	X
Pallor or flushing	X	X	X	X	X	X	X
Physical							
Blood pressure	X	X	X	X	X	X	X
Tremors	X	X	X	X	X	X	X
Cardiac arrhythmia	X	X	X	X	X	X	X
Pupil dilatation	X	X	X	X	X	X	X
Pitting edema	X	X	X	X	X	X	X
Investigations							
EKG	X	X	X	X	X	X	X
SMA-6 and creatinine	X	X	X	X	X	X	X
SMA-12	X	X	X	X	X	X	X
Urine catecholamine		X		X	X	X	X
Serum catecholamine				As indicated			
Urinary chemistry				As indicated			
Other tests				As indicated			
CAT scan and IVP				As indicated			

ALGORITHM FOR PHEOCHROMOCYTOMAS

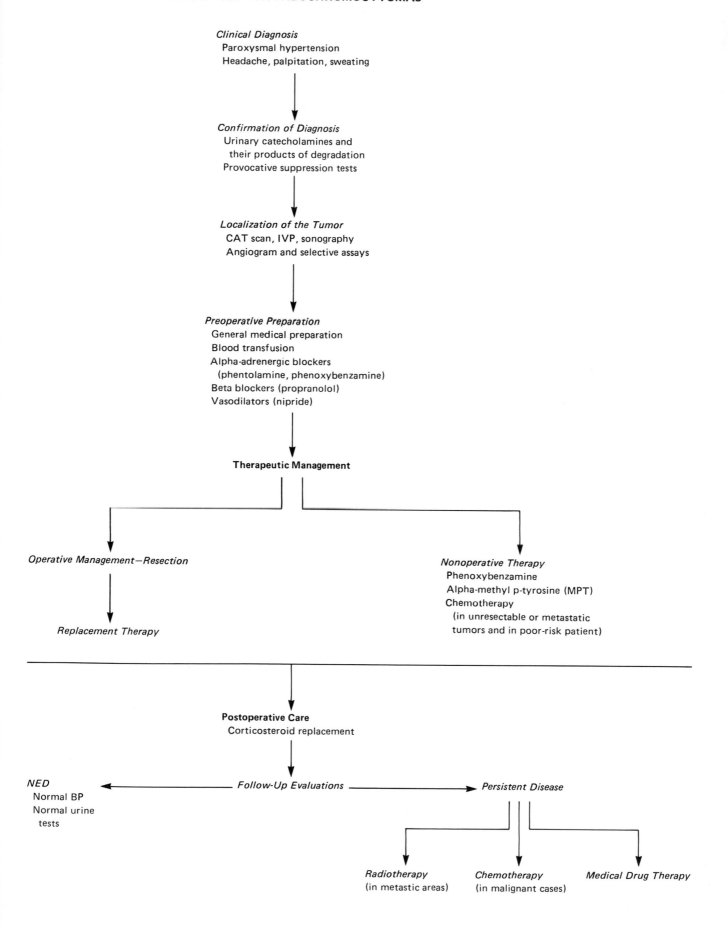

Clinical Diagnosis
  Paroxysmal hypertension
  Headache, palpitation, sweating

Confirmation of Diagnosis
  Urinary catecholamines and
    their products of degradation
  Provocative suppression tests

Localization of the Tumor
  CAT scan, IVP, sonography
  Angiogram and selective assays

Preoperative Preparation
  General medical preparation
  Blood transfusion
  Alpha-adrenergic blockers
    (phentolamine, phenoxybenzamine)
  Beta blockers (propranolol)
  Vasodilators (nipride)

Therapeutic Management

Operative Management—Resection

Replacement Therapy

Nonoperative Therapy
  Phenoxybenzamine
  Alpha-methyl p-tyrosine (MPT)
  Chemotherapy
    (in unresectable or metastatic
    tumors and in poor-risk patient)

Postoperative Care
Corticosteroid replacement

NED
Normal BP
Normal urine
  tests

Follow-Up Evaluations

Persistent Disease

Radiotherapy
(in metastic areas)

Chemotherapy
(in malignant cases)

Medical Drug Therapy

early detection and diagnosis; the most common presentation is an abdominal mass found incidentally by the mother.

Neuroblastomas are highly malignant tumors with metastases found in 50% of patients at the time of diagnosis; these particularly affect bone. Early diagnosis and management is mandatory, as the prognosis is better if surgery is performed before age 1.

2. Suggestive Signs and Symptoms

Parents and pediatricians should be aware of the following presentations:

- Abdominal or flank mass.
- Pallor associated with fever and progressive weight loss.
- Bone pain or backache.
- Ptosis and palpable orbital mass.
- Young children with failure to thrive.
- Chronic diarrhea without definite pathogens.

B. Pretreatment Evaluation

1. Physical Evaluation

On physical examination, a nontender abdominal mass can be felt in the majority of cases. About 40% will have hypertension, and most patients are usually slim, emaciated, and pale.

2. Laboratory Findings

Hematologic findings include

- Anemia, thrombocytopenia, and leukocytosis.
- Urinary catecholamine and its metabolites and precursors are elevated (i.e., dopamine, dopa, norepinephrine, and VMA).

3. Confirmation of the Diagnosis

Definitive diagnosis is only made at surgery; a presumptive diagnosis of neuroblastoma, however, can be made by careful history taking, physical examination, and laboratory data. The mass is confirmed by x-ray techniques:

- Flat plate of the abdomen (KUB).
- IV urogram.
- CAT scan.
- Angiography.

About 40% of the patients will have punctate calcification in the tumor mass on plain KUB film. Excretory urography may show an inferiorly displaced kidney and deviation of the upper pole; there is usually no intrinsic distortion of the pelvicalyceal

system. CAT scan can be used to determine the extent of the tumor and to identify involvement of adjacent tissues and the retroperitoneum. The role of angiography in the diagnosis of neuroblastoma is controversial. A characteristic appearance of "puddling" may at times be seen.

Although most neuroblastomas are in the adrenal gland, slightly less than half are extra-adrenal. They may present as a retroperitoneal tumor, a posterior mediastinal mass, an orbital tumor, or a head and neck tumor.

4. Staging of the Neuroblastoma

- Stage I. Tumor confined to the adrenal gland.
- Stage II. Tumor extends in continuity beyond the organ of origin. Ipsilateral nodes may be positive.
- Stage III. Tumor extends in continuity across the midline. Regional lymph nodes may be involved bilaterally.
- Stage IV. Remote disease in bone marrow, lungs, soft tissues.
- Stage IVS. This stage denotes the absence of bony metastases in a very specific subset of patients.

C. Preoperative Preparation

- General supportive treatment with a high-nutrient diet is especially important for the very young and for emaciated patients. IV fluid with supplemental calories is indicated in patients who cannot tolerate oral diet.
- Blood transfusions should be given whenever indicated.
- Fluid, electrolytes, and acid/base balance should be monitored daily and stabilized for several days before surgery can be undertaken.

D. Therapeutic Management

1. Stage I

Excision of the lesion with lymphadenectomy of the regional lymph nodes is the treatment of choice.

2. Stage II

Local excision and lymph node dissection, and if the patient has residual disease, radiation plus chemotherapy, as described in Stage III, is the treatment of choice.

3. Stage III

Total surgical extirpation at this stage is usually not feasible. Cytoreductive surgery has been tried but does not seem to improve the prognosis. Radiotherapy plus chemotherapy as described for Stage IV disease is, therefore, the treatment of choice. Patients less than 18 months old can tolerate 1800–2400 rads; those over 30 months old can be treated with 3000–4000 rads.

4. Stage IV

Radiation therapy may play a part in the symptomatic relief of the patient with Stage IV disease, especially in bone and brain metastases; otherwise, chemotherapy is the treatment of choice. Combination chemotherapy with vincristine, cyclophosphamide, and dimethyl triazens imidazole carboxamide (DTIC) seems to be the best regimen. There have been 30% complete remission and 40% partial remission for as long as 11 months reported. Adriamycin may be used in patients who relapse after the above treatment.

5. Stage IVS

These patients are managed in a unique manner; they require little, if any, treatment. The primary lesion may be very small, and the metastatic disease may, at times, spontaneously regress. Patients will require small doses of radiation therapy or chemotherapy, and total regression of the disease may be initiated by the above treatment.

E. Postoperative Care and Follow-Up

The immediate postoperative care is just like that for any other major intra-abdominal surgery in children and includes close monitoring of vital signs, hourly intake and output, CBC, electrolytes, and, if necessary, blood transfusions. In an infant, especially an emaciated one, respiratory care can be maintained with an endotracheal tube in place, and the child can then be weaned off it gradually.

Long-term postoperative care is also very important, and those patients should be followed up at regular intervals. The management of patients with neuroblastomas is discussed in more detail in §8, and the reader is referred there for further information.

Table IV is a follow-up plan for patients with neuroblastoma.

F. Management Algorithm
for Neuroblastoma (see p. 152)

Table IV

Long-Term Follow-Up Schedule for Neuroblastoma

Management	First and second year				Third-to-fifth year		Thereafter, annually
	3 Months	6 Months	9 Months	12 Months	6 Months	12 Months	
History							
History	X	X	X	X	X	X	X
Malaise	X	X	X	X	X	X	X
Anorexia	X	X	X	X	X	X	X
Weight loss	X	X	X	X	X	X	X
Bone pain	X	X	X	X	X	X	X
Back ache	X	X	X	X	X	X	X
Diarrhea	X	X	X	X	X	X	X
Physical							
Body temperature	X	X	X	X	X	X	X
Pallor	X	X	X	X	X	X	X
Abdominal mass	X	X	X	X	X	X	X
Hepatomegaly	X	X	X	X	X	X	X
Rectal mass	X	X	X	X	X	X	X
Inspection and palpation of the operative site	X	X	X	X	X	X	X
Investigations							
CBC including hematocrit, platelet, WBC	X	X	X	X	X	X	X
Urinary catecholamines		X	X	X	X		X
IVP		x	x	x	x		x
Liver and bone scan		X			X		X
CAT scan				As indicated			

ALGORITHM FOR NEUROBLASTOMA

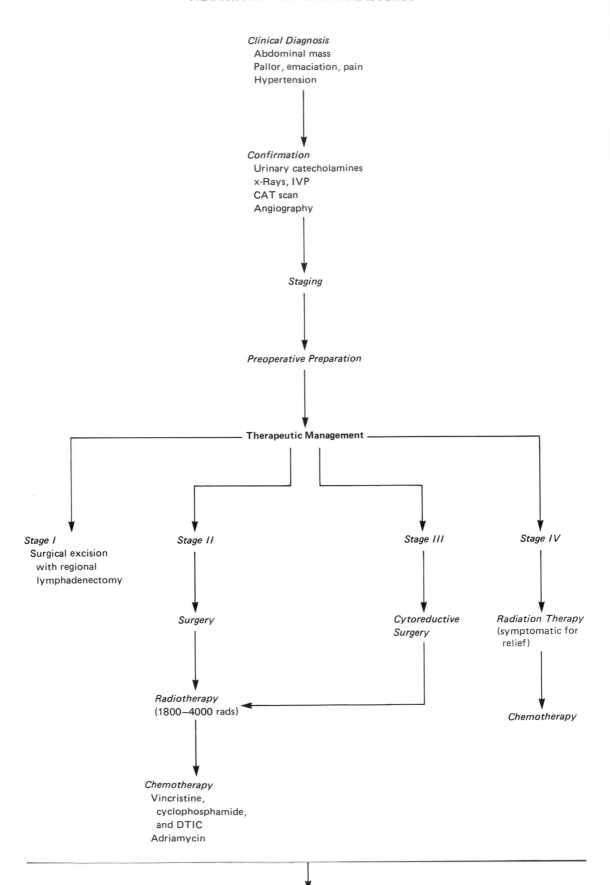

Clinical Diagnosis
Abdominal mass
Pallor, emaciation, pain
Hypertension

Confirmation
Urinary catecholamines
x-Rays, IVP
CAT scan
Angiography

Staging

Preoperative Preparation

Therapeutic Management

Stage I
Surgical excision
with regional
lymphadenectomy

Stage II

Surgery

Radiotherapy
(1800—4000 rads)

Chemotherapy
Vincristine,
cyclophosphamide,
and DTIC
Adriamycin

Stage III

*Cytoreductive
Surgery*

Stage IV

Radiation Therapy
(symptomatic for
relief)

Chemotherapy

Follow-Up Evaluation

SUGGESTED READINGS

1. Axelrod, J., and Weinshilboum, R. Catecholamines. *N. Engl. J. Med.* **287,** 237 (1972).
2. Bennett, A. J., Cain, J. P., Dluhy, R. G., Tynes, W. V., Harrison, J. H., and Thorn, G. W. Surgical treatment of adrenocortical hyperplasia: 20-year experience. *Trans. Am. Assoc. Genito-Urin. Surg.* **64,** 90 (1972).
3. Biglieri, E. G., and Forsham, P. H. Studies on the expanded extracellular volume and responses to various stimuli in primary aldosteronism. *Am. J. Med.* **30,** 564 (1960).
4. Biglieri, E. G., Slaton, P. E., Jr., Kronfield, S. J., and Schambelan, M. Diagnosis of an aldosterone-producing adenoma. *JAMA, J. Am. Med. Assoc.* **201,** 510 (1967).
5. Biglieri, E. G., Slaton, P. E., Schambelan, M., and Kronfield, S. J. Hypermineralocorticoidism. *Am. J. Med.* **45,** 170 (1968).
6. Brown, J. J., Chinn, R. H., Davies, D. L., Dusterdieck, G., Fraser, R., Lever, A. F., Robertson, J. I. S., Tree, M., and Wiseman, A. Plasma electrolytes, renin and aldosterone in the diagnosis of primary aldosteronism. *Lancet* **2,** 55 (1968).
7. Brunjes, S., Johns, V. J., Jr., and Crance, N. G. Pheochromocytoma: Postoperative shock and blood volume. *N. Engl. J. Med.* 262:393 (1960).
8. Campbell, M. F. Anomalies of the genital tract. *In* "Urology" M. F. Campbell and J. H. Harrison, eds. 3rd ed., Saunders, Philadelphia, Pennsylvania, 1970.
9. Conn, J. W. Plasma renin activity in primary aldosteronism. Importance in differential diagnosis and in research of essential hypertension. *JAMA, J. Am. Med. Assoc.* **190,** 222 (1964).
10. Conn, J. W. Presidential address. Primary aldosteronism, a new clinical entity. *J. Lab. Clin. Med.* **45,** 3 (1955).
11. Conn, J. W., Cohen, E. L., and Rovner, D. R. Suppression of plasma renin activity in primary aldosteronism. Distinguishing primary from secondary aldosteronism in hypertensive disease. *JAMA, J. Am. Med. Assoc.* **190,** 213 (1964).
12. Conn, J. W., Knopf, R. F., and Nesbit, R. Primary aldosteronism: Present evaluation of its clinical characteristics and of the results of surgery. *In* "Aldosterone" (E. E. Balieu and P. Robel, eds.), p. 327. Davis, Philadelphia, Pennsylvania, 1964.
13. Cushing, H. "Pituitary Body, Hypothalamus, and Parasympathetic Nervous System." Thomas, Springfield, Illinois, 1932.
14. Dluhy, R. G.,Himathongkam, T., and Greenfield, M. Rapid ACTH test with plasma aldosterone levels. *Ann. Intern. Med.* **80,** 693 (1974).
15. Dluhy, R. G., Lauler, D. P., and Thorn, G. W. Pharmacology and chemistry of adrenal glucocorticoids. *Med. Clin. North Am.* **57,** 1155 (1973).
16. Eberlein, W. R., and Bongiovanni, A. M. Congenital adrenal hyperplasia with hypertension: Unusual steroid pattern in blood and urine. *J. Clin. Endocrinol. Metab.* **15,** 1531 (1955).
17. Engleman, K., and Sjoerdsma, A. Chronic medical therapy for pheochromocytoma; a report of four cases. *Ann. Intern. Med.* **61,** 229 (1964).
18. Harrison, J. H. The adrenals. *In* "Reoperative Surgery" (R. E. Rothenberg, ed.). McGraw-Hill, New York, 1964.
19. Harrison, J. H., Thorn, G. W., and Jenkins, D. Further observations of bilateral adrenalectomy in man. *Trans. Am. Assoc. Genito-Urin. Surg.* **44,** 85 (1952).
20. Hutter, A. M., and Kayhoe, D. E. Adrenal cortical carcinoma. Results of treatment with o,p'DDD in 138 patients. *Am. J. Med.* **41,** 581 (1966).
21. Koop, C. E., and Hernandez, J. R. Neuroblastoma: Experience with 100 cases in children. *Surgery (St. Louis)* **56,** 726 (1964).
22. Laragh, J. H., Sealey, J. E., and Sommers, S. C. Patterns of adrenal secretion and urinary excretion of aldosterone and plasma renin activity in normal and hypersensitive subjects. *Circ. Res.* **18,** Suppl., 158 (1966).
23. Liddle, G. W. Cushing's syndrome. *In* "The Adrenal Cortex" (A. B. Eisenstein, ed.), p. 523. Little, Brown, Massachusetts, 1967.
24. Liddle, G. W. Test of pituitary-adrenal suppressibility in the diagnosis of Cushing's syndrome. *J. Clin. Endocrinol. Metab.* **20,** 1539 (1960).
25. Lubitz, J. A., Freeman, L., and Okun, R. Mitotane use in inoperable adrenal cortical carcinoma. *JAMA, J. Am. Med. Assoc.* **223,** 1109 (1973).
26. Moore, T. J., Dluhy, R. G., Williams, G. H., and Cain, J. P. Nelson's syndrome: Frequency, prognosis and effect of prior pituitary irradiation. *Ann. Intern. Med.* **85,** 731 (1976).
27. Nugent, C. A., Nichols, T., and Tyler, F. H. Diagnosis of Cushing's syndrome: Single dose of dexamethasone suppression test. *Arch. Intern. Med.* **116,** 172 (1965).
28. Paloyan, E. Familial pheochromocytoma, medullary thyroid carcinoma, and parathyroid adenomas. *JAMA, J. Am. Med. Assoc.* **214,** 1443 (1970).
29. Pisano, J. J. A simple analysis for normetanephrine and metanephrine in urine. *Clin. Chim. Acta* **5,** 406 (1960).
30. Plotz, C. M., Knowlton, A. I., and Ragan, C. The natural history of Cushing's syndrome. *Am. J. Med.* **13,** 597 (1952).
31. Rapaport, E., Goldberg, M. B., Gordan, G. S., and Hinman, F., Jr. Mortality in surgically treated adrenocortical tumors. *Postgrad. Med.* **11,** 325 (1956).
32. Schambelan, M., Stockigt, J. R., and Biglieri, E. G. Isolated hypoaldosteronism in adults, a renin deficiency syndrome. *N. Engl. J. Med.* **287,** 573 (1972).
33. Sinks, L. F., and Woodruff, M. W. Chemotherapy of neuroblastoma. *JAMA, J. Am. Med. Assoc.* **205,** 161 (1968).
34. Tefft, M., and Wittenborg, M. H. Radiotherapy and neuroblastoma in childhood. *JAMA, J. Am. Med. Assoc.* **205,** 159 (1968).
35. Tyrrell, J. B., Brooks, R. M., Fitzgerald, P. A., Cofoid, P. B., Forsham, P. H., and Wilson, C. B. Cushing's disease: Selected trans-sphenoidal resection of pituitary microadenomas. *N. Engl. J. Med.* **298,** 753 (1978).

Section 4. Tumors of the Endocrine Glands

Part B: Pancreatic Tumors

I. Insulinoma   157
   A. Early Detection and Screening
   B. Pretreatment Evaluation and Work-Up
      1. History and Physical Examination
      2. Laboratory Findings
         a. Fasting Blood Sugar
         b. Immunoreactive Insulin (IRI) Glucose Ratio
         c. Diazoxide Test
         d. Serum Proinsulin
         e. Insuline Suppression Test
         f. Tolbutamide Test
      3. Localization of the Tumor
      4. Multidisciplinary Evaluation
   C. Therapeutic Management
      1. Medical Treatment
         a. Diazoxide
         b. Chemotherapy
      2. Surgical Treatment
      3. Radiotherapy
   D. Postoperative Care, Evaluation, and Follow-Up
   E. Management Algorithm for Insulinomas
II. Gastrinoma (Zollinger-Ellison Syndrome)   160
   A. Early Detection and Screening
   B. Pretreatment Evaluation and Work-Up
      1. History and Physical Examination
      2. Specific Laboratory Tests
         a. Gastric Secretion Studies
         b. Serum Gestrin Levels
         c. Differential Diagnostic Tests

      3. Radiological Studies
         a. Upper GI Series
         b. CAT Scan and Angiography
         c. Percutaneous Transhepatic Portal
            Splenogrophy (PTPS)
      4. General Medical Evaluation
      5. Multidisciplinary Evaluation
   C. Preoperative Preparation
   D. Therapeutic Management
      1. Surgical Treatment
      2. Medical Treatment
         a. Cimetidine
         b. Chemotherapy
   E. Postoperative Care, Evaluation, and Follow-Up
   F. Management Algorithm for Gastrinomas
III. Glucagonoma (Hyperglycemic Syndrome)   163
   A. Early Detection and Screening
   B. Pretreatment Evaluation and Work-Up
   C. Therapeutic Management
   D. Postoperative Care and Follow-Up
   E. Management Algorithm for Glucagonomas
IV. Vipoma (Pancreatic Cholera, the WDHA Syndrome,
    or Verner-Morrison Syndrome)   166
   A. Early Detection and Screening
   B. Therapeutic Management and Postoperative Care
   C. Management Algorithm for Vipomas

Suggested Readings   169

The pancreatic islets are composed of different types of cells, each synthesizing and secreting a specific polypeptide. Benign or malignant neoplasms may arise from each type of cell. These tumors are usually functional, producing specific peptide substances that result in one of several major clinical syndromes according to the cell type involved. Table I summarizes the various clinical syndromes that result from the various tumors of the pancreatic islets. These syndromes and the tumors that produce them will be discussed individually.

Table I

Syndromes Resulting from Pancreatic Tumors

Cell type	Hormone produced	Tumor	Resulting syndrome
β Cell (B)	Insulin	Insulinoma	Hypoglycemic syndrome
δ Cell (D)	Gastrin	Gastrinoma	Ulcerogenic (Zollinger-Ellison) syndrome
α Cell (A)	Glucagon	Glucagonoma	Hyperglycemia syndrome
ζ Cell (D1)	Vasoactive intestinal polypeptide (VIP)	Vipoma	WDHA or Verner-Morrison syndrome
F Cell	Pancreatic polypeptide	Ppoma	Diarrhea
δ Cell (D)	Somatostatin	Somatostatinoma	Diabetogenic and malabsorption syndromes

I. INSULINOMA

This is a relatively rare tumor, which may go undiagnosed for several years.

A. Early Detection and Screening

Because of the rarity of this disease and the striking clinical picture, which rapidly brings the patient for professional care when the disease becomes symptomatic, a screening method for early detection is not necessary. Routine blood chemistries that are ordered for a variety of reasons will, however, identify a decreased blood sugar and should alert the physician to pursue an investigation for the presence of an islet cell tumor.

Early detection depends on a keen sense of awareness in recognizing some of the less specific symptoms of insulinomas. The presenting symptoms are those of hypoglycemia; the brain is mainly dependent on glucose for its energy supply; thus when it is deprived of this energy source, neurological manifestations may develop

- Dizziness.
- Clouded sensorium.
- Behavioral changes.
- Neurological deficits such as paresis, sensory losses, and paralysis.
- Diplopia.
- Seizures.
- Coma.

In some cases, when the hypoglycemia is abrupt and profound, an adrenergic response secondary to the discharge of epinephrine will occur. The clinical picture then includes

- Nervousness.
- Tremulousness.
- Sweating and pallor.
- Palpitations.

Severe hypoglycemia can also cause certain GI symptoms such as hunger, nausea, and vomiting.

B. Pretreatment Evaluation and Work-Up

In clinical medicine, a varied number of disorders may produce hypoglycemia. Consequently, an organized approach to the diagnostic possibilities is essential. In the differential diagnosis, one must exclude:

- Liver disease.
- Alcoholism.
- Hypopituitarism.
- Neoplastic hypoglycemia.

1. History and Physical Examination

The symptoms presented above should be sought. Since the illness may present as an intermittent condition, thorough questioning is important.

The physical examination will not ordinarily identify any specific findings, but a complete examination is essential. A search for other endocrinopathies is most important since insulinoma may be part of the multiple endocrine adenomatosis (MEA) syndrome Type I.

2. Laboratory Findings

The single most important step in making the diagnosis of an insulinoma is the demonstration of a high level of endogenous insulin in the face of fasting hypoglycemia.

a. Fasting Blood Sugar

Fasting blood sugar determinations may not identify the condition unless blood samples are obtained during a hypoglycemic crisis. The 6-hour glucose tolerance test, on the other hand, is useful in ruling out other causes of hypoglycemia:

- Immediate hypoglycemia suggests a dumping syndrome.
- Hypoglycemia at 2 hours is usually functional hypoglycemia.
- Hypoglycemia at 4 hours indicates a prediabetic state.
- Hypoglycemia at 6 hours is suspicious for an insulinoma.

Actually, the diagnosis of insulinoma depends on the identification of an inappropriately elevated level of insulin for a given level of glucose. The usual overnight 8–12 hours of fasting may not be long enough to provoke hypoglycemia. It may, at times, be necessary to fast the patient for 48–72 hours and follow this by a period of vigorous exercise to induce the hypoglycemia in a patient with an insulinoma. One looks to induce a blood sugar of 50 mg % in men and 35 mg % in women.

b. Immunoreactive Insulin (IRI)/Serum Glucose Ratio

The fasting IRI/glucose ratio is over 0.3 in patients with islet cell pathology.

c. Diazoxide Test

The diazoxide test may be used in those patients in whom a high IRI has been demonstrated; it inhibits insulin release by its direct action on the beta cells and by stimulating epinephrine release. The dose of diazoxide is usually between 300 and 800 mg.

d. Serum Proinsulin

Proinsulin, the single-chain intracellular precursor of insulin, normally constitutes 5–22% of circulating IRI. A higher proportion is often an indication of insulinoma.

e. Insulin Suppression Test

Hypoglycemia is normally induced by infusion of proinsulin and C-peptide (which connects the alpha and beta chains of insulin in proinsulin). Patients with insulinomas have endogenous insulin secretion and fail to suppress with C-peptide.

f. Tolbutamide Stimulation Test

This test may provoke dramatic bursts of insulin in patients with insulinoma.

3. Localization of the Tumor

The tumor may at times be identified and localized preoperatively by one of several techniques:

- CAT scanning and sonography of the pancreas.
- Selective angiography (success rate about 45%).
- Venous catheterization with selective pancreatic blood sampling.

Other methods to identify pancreatic tumors such as endoscopic retrograde canulation of the pancreatic ducts and upper GI series are less likely to be helpful because of the small size of these tumors.

4. Multidisciplinary Evaluation

Early diagnosis and proper management of patients with functioning tumors of the pancreatic islets requires the participation and cooperation of the endocrinologist, the radiologist, the surgeon, and the medical and radiation oncologists. Autonomous hyperinsulinism is a frequent occurrence in patients with MEA Type I. Therefore, patients diagnosed as having an insulinoma should undergo extensive medical and endocrinologic investigation. Medical preparation of the patient before surgery is most important, and alternate medical, chemotherapeutic, and radiotherapeutic modalities of treatment must be considered.

C. Therapeutic Management

The treatment of insulinomas may be medical or surgical.

1. Medical Treatment

Medical treatment is reserved for patients who are poor surgical candidates as a result of other medical conditions, for those who refuse surgery, and for patients with documented widespread metastases.

a. Diazoxide

The drug of choice for the medical control of hypoglycemia is diazoxide; this can be administered orally or intravenously in doses of 300–1200 mg per day. The side effects are numerous and must be kept in mind; the salt-retaining property of diazoxide may be overcome by the use of diuretics. Other side effects of the drug, however, include

- Dermatologic disturbances.
- GI symptoms.
- Tachycardia and postural hypotension.
- Hirsutism.
- Immunoglobulin depression.
- Hyperuricemia.
- Lymphadenitis, gingival hyperplasia, and muscle wasting.

b. Chemotherapy

Streptozotocin has been used in patients with islet cell carcinomas that are either not totally resectable or have already metastasized. The usual dose is 2–4 g per square meter of body surface, administered over a period of several weeks. Side effects include nausea, vomiting, and renal and hepatic toxicity, but it has been demonstrated to result in some remissions in patients with advanced disease, and palliation has been reported in about 60% of cases. 5-Fluorouracil (5-FU) singly or in combination with streptozotocin has also been used. The effectiveness of various chemotherapeutic agents or combinations has not been adequately evaluated because of the rarity of the disease.

2. Surgical Treatment

The treatment of choice for insulinoma is surgical. Unlike the prevailing situation in patients with gastrinomas, the majority (84%) of these tumors are benign, solitary, and small; and almost all are found in the pancreas, with equal frequency in the head, body, and tail of the gland. Of all insulinomas, 1 or 2% may be found outside the pancreas, usually in the peripancreatic or periduodenal regions.

In the patient with a labile blood sugar and severe symptoms of hypoglycemia, preoperative preparation with diazoxide is sometimes desirable. Preoperative dextrose infusions can also be used but should be discontinued 2 hours before the procedure so that the glucose concentration is low enough to be able to detect any rebound increase when the insulinoma is removed.

Either a bilateral subcostal or a long midline incision is adequate for exploration of the pancreas. The liver should be carefully examined for metastases, and any enlarged lymph node in the region of the porta hepatis must be biopsied for a frozen-section study. If localization of the lesion has been accomplished preoperatively, one can attack the tumor directly; thorough exploration of the pancreas, duodenum, and peripancreatic and periduodenal areas is mandatory, however, since 10% of patients will have multiple lesions. The duodenum must be fully kocherized and the lesser sac opened to expose all surfaces of the pancreas. During the surgery:

- Superficial tumors are seen as reddish-brown lesions, firmer than the rest of the pancreatic parenchyma, and can often be enucleated with care, avoiding injury to the pancreatic ducts.
- If the lesion is located deeply in the tail of the pancreas, a distal pancreatectomy should be performed.
- In cases of deep lesions of the pancreatic head, a pancreaticoduodenectomy is necessary to eradicate the tumor.
- A malignant tumor will require a total pancreatectomy with regional lymphadenectomy. Even when the tumor seems to be inoperable, an effort should be made to resect as much of it as possible; this debulking procedure will often help to alleviate the hypoglycemic symptoms and facilitate postoperative chemotherapy.
- In 20–30% of the cases, surgical exploration will not identify the tumor; there, digital exploration of the duodenal mucosa through a duodenotomy may be helpful. If, after a complete exploration, however, one is unable to find the lesion, a wide distal pancreatectomy should be performed with intraoperative examination and biopsy of the specimen. This carries a 50% chance of including the offending lesion in the resected specimen or of identifying hyperplasia; in these cases, a rebound hyperglycemia can be demonstrated within 30–60 minutes after the extirpation of the pancreas. If the resected specimen does not contain the tumor and the blood glucose does not exhibit a rebound, a 90% pancreatic resection must then be carried out. Total pancreatectomy should only be considered as a secondary procedure after treatment with diazoxide has been unsuccessful to control the hypoglycemia in a patient who underwent 90% pancreatectomy.
- Blood glucose concentration should be monitored during the induction of anesthesia and every 15 min during the procedure. A significant rebound increase of glycemia is usually observed 30–60 min after excision of the tumor, and it may be used as an indication of adequacy of the operation.

Disappearance of the hypoglycemic syndrome can be expected in about 60% of patients who are treated surgically.

About 25% of cases will become diabetic, and the operative mortality varies according to the extent of the resection but has been reported around 10%. Debulking procedures in large, invasive malignant tumors may achieve considerable palliation in some patients and will facilitate the use of postoperative adjuvant therapy by radiation or by the use of cytotoxic drugs (streptozotocin).

3. Radiotherapy

There is no clear data as to the value of radiotherapy in the treatment of islet cell tumors of the pancreas. It has been used when residual disease is left after surgery, and at least one report seems to indicate a beneficial effect.

D. Postoperative Care, Evaluation, and Follow-Up

The postoperative care of the patient following surgery for insulinoma is similar to that of any patient undergoing pancreatic surgery (see §10). The same complications may be seen, particularly pancreatic fistulas, pseudocyst formation, pancreatitis, abscess, etc. In addition, the patient has to be checked for the occurrence of diabetes or the recurrence of hypoglycemia. Serial determinations of the IRI level and IRI/glucose ratio, as well as regular blood sugar levels, must be done at regular intervals; a complete history should be taken during such follow-up evaluations, and any suggestive symptom must be pursued with an appropriate investigation (IRI/glucose ratio, diazoxide test, etc.). A metastatic survey must be repeated yearly in cases of malignant insulinomas or as often as symptoms warrant. Endocrine evaluation to rule out multiple endocrinopathy should also be carried out as needed.

E. Management Algorithm for Insulinomas
(see p. 161)

II. GASTRINOMA (ZOLLINGER-ELLISON SYNDROME)

In this syndrome, hyperplasia or tumors arising from the D cells of the pancreas result in increased levels of the hormone gastrin, which in turn produces an ulcerogenic syndrome known as the Zollinger-Ellison (Z-E) syndrome. This clinical entity is rare, but its implications are serious, and the clinician must be aware of its possible existence in any patient with severe peptic ulcer diathesis.

A. Early Detection and Screening

The clinical presentation is that of an intense peptic ulcer diathesis characterized by

- Epigastric pain (in over 90%).
- Vomiting and diarrhea.
- Weight loss and weakness.

The diagnosis should be suspected in patients with intractable peptic ulcer and especially in those who develop recurrent ulceration after apparently adequate surgical treatment of their ulcer, or those with extremely high gastrin acid levels. Serum gastrin levels should be determined in these patients to rule out or confirm the presence of a Z-E syndrome.

B. Pretreatment Evaluation and Work-Up

1. History and Physical Examination

Symptoms and physical findings are not different from those of any other patient with severe peptic ulcer diathesis. They include

- Epigastric pain and dyspepsia.
- Upper GI bleeding.
- Signs of duodenal obstruction.
- Vomiting and diarrhea.
- Weight loss, etc.

2. Specific Laboratory Investigations

a. Gastric Secretion Studies

Basal hydrochloric acid secretion greater than 100 meq overnight (12 hours) or 15 meq in 1 hour suggests the presence of a Z-E syndrome. Since the parietal cells are under maximal stimulation, little or no increase in acid output will be observed after stimulation with Histalog.

b. Serum Gastrin Levels

Fasting serum gastrin levels of 200 pg per milliliter to 1000 pg per milliliter or greater are very suggestive of gastrinoma.

c. Differential Diagnostic Tests

Other causes of elevated serum gastrin must be ruled out in borderline cases. These include

- Retained antrum after a Billroth II gastrectomy.
- Gastric outlet obstruction.
- Pernicious anemia.
- G-cell hyperplasia.

ALGORITHM FOR INSULINOMAS

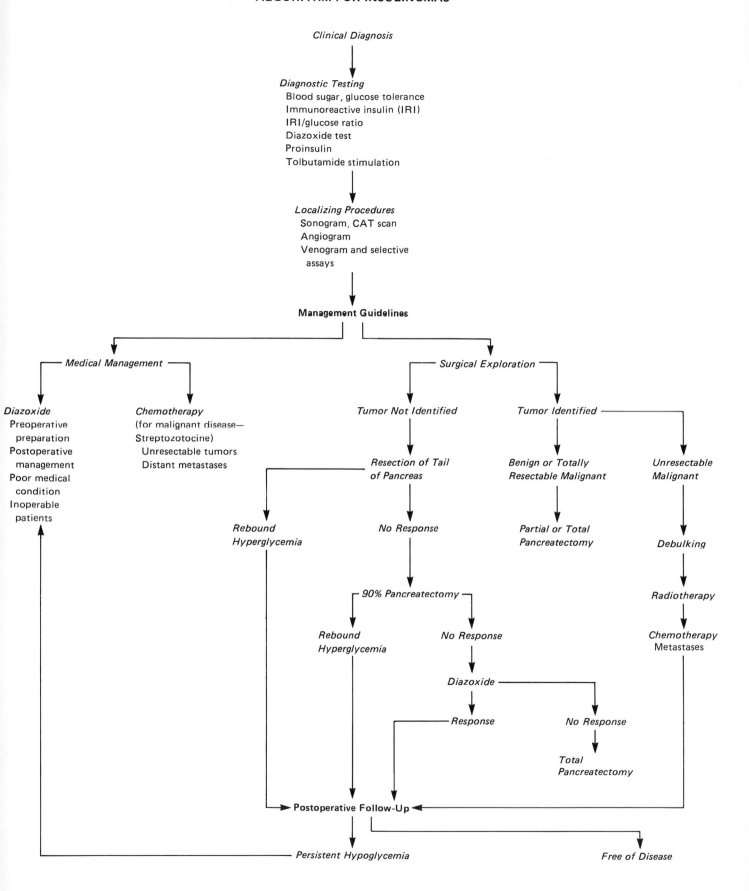

- Atrophic gastritis.
- Gastric cancer.

These must be ruled out by the appropriate studies, and provocative tests such as feeding, calcium infusion, and secretin infusion tests might be necessary.

i. Feeding Test. In the feeding test, a 50–300% increase in serum gastrin is observed during the first hour after a protein meal in normal individuals; this increase is even greater in patients with G-cell hyperplasia. In patients with Z-E syndrome, a protein meal does not stimulate the release of additional gastrin from the tumor.

ii. Calcium Test. The infusion of 4 mg of calcium gluconate per kilogram of body weight in 3 hours stimulates the release of gastrin. In normal individuals and in duodenal ulcer patients, a small rise (15 pg per milliliter average) in gastrin levels is observed. In patients with the Z-E syndrome, the increase is much greater (395 pg per milliliter in 98% of the cases).

iii. Secretin Test. The infusion of secretin (2 units per kilogram of body weight) will produce a small rise or fall in the serum gastrin levels in normal individuals or in duodenal ulcer patients; a clear-cut rise (110 pg per milliliter) characterizes gastrinoma patients.

3. Radiological Studies

a. Upper GI Series

Routine GI series may reveal large gastric folds, a large atonic stomach, and multiple ulcerations of the stomach and duodenum.

b. CAT Scanning and Selective Angiography

These modalities may be useful in localizing the tumor and/or its metastases, much as in the evaluation of patients with insulinomas.

c. Percutaneous Transhepatic Portal Splenography (PTPS)

This procedure is a complex procedure performed only by highly skilled radiologists in selected centers. When combined with selective sampling of blood drawn from various portions of the portal vein system, it can localize the offending tumor in a rather exquisite manner.

4. General Medical Evaluation

A complete evaluation of the patient is necessary to

- Identify the general condition of the patient and his or her suitability for major surgery (assess cardiac, renal, pulmonary, and other functions).
- Identify any other endocrinopathy to determine whether a multiple endocrine adenopathy exists such as in the MEA Type I (adrenal tumor, parathyroid tumor, pituitary tumor, etc.).
- Identify any fluid and electrolyte disturbance, which will often result from gastric obstruction, vomiting, and diarrhea (serum electrolytes, blood gases, etc.).
- Identify any blood volume deficit from past or present upper GI bleeding (hemoglobin and hematocrit, blood volume, etc.).
- Identify any metastatic disease (x-rays, a multichannel biochemical profile (SMA-12), and scans as indicated).

5. Multidisciplinary Evaluation

This is most important in all patients with islet cell tumors (see §4B.I.B.4).

C. Preoperative Preparation

- Intensive antacid therapy may be required in combination with nasogastric suction to combat severe diarrhea.
- Accurate fluid with electrolyte replacement.
- Cimetidine (an H_2-receptor blocker) administered intravenously is extremely useful for the control of symptoms and preparation of these patients for surgery.
- Blood transfusions may be necessary in those patients with GI hemorrhage.
- Correction of any coexisting medical or endocrinologic condition.

D. Therapeutic Management

Gastrinomas are multicentric in 35% of the cases, and approximately 60% are malignant; occult metastases are present at the time of diagnosis in over 80% of this group. The tumors are usually small lesions, difficult to detect, and actually grow quite slowly. As a result of this, direct attack on the pancreas is difficult and rarely effective; complete removal of the target organ (total gastrectomy) is recognized as the treatment of choice for the Z-E syndrome.

1. Surgical Treatment

An upper midline incision is used. The liver is inspected and palpated for the presence of metastases. The stomach should be carefully inspected and is usually hyperemic and hypertrophic and usually contains large amounts of gastric secretion.

The duodenum, which is usually enlarged, should be kocherized and carefully palpated; it may show ulcerations as far down as its second part, and on occasion, a submucosal gastrinoma may be identified within it. Ulceration distal to the ligament of Treitz is pathognomonic of Z-E syndrome. The lesser sac should then be opened and the pancreas carefully inspected and palpated in its entirety; the body and tail of the pancreas are better examined after mobilization of the spleen. Any tumors or enlarged lymph nodes should be biopsied and sent for frozen-section tissue diagnosis. Once the diagnosis of Z-E syndrome has been established, a total gastrectomy followed by Roux-en-Y esophagojejunostomy reconstruction is performed; a total gastrectomy should be performed even if a thorough exploration proves negative in patients with elevated gastrin levels and positive responses to calcium and secretin infusions. Total gastrectomy is also indicated as a palliative procedure in those patients in whom an unresectable tumor is identified. In those rare instances where a tumor is identified in the pancreas and is apparently localized and easily accessible, resection of the tumor should be carried out. However, because of the high incidence of multicentricity and occult metastases, cure is rarely (<10%) achieved by resection of the tumor alone, and a total gastrectomy should still be performed.

The best results are obtained in those patients in whom a definitive preoperative diagnosis is made and a total gastrectomy is performed as the initial procedure. The 5-year survival after this procedure is 60%, but only 25% of these patients are alive at 10 years. Death may be the result of the ulcer diathesis and its complications, postoperative complication, or tumor spread. Control of acid secretion is the most important factor influencing the outcome.

2. Medical Treatment

a. Cimetidine

Cimetidine (Tagamet), an H_2 receptor antagonist, is a useful agent in the management of Z-E patients, particularly in the elderly and other poor surgical risk patients, or in those who refuse surgery. Treatment with cimetidine markedly reduces acid secretion and improves the appetite. It helps in the control of diarrhea and steatorrhea, and it leads to better nutrition. The long-term effects of cimetidine therapy, however, have not as yet been totally assessed. More recently, the combination of cimetidine with a transparietal vagotomy has been found to be an effective alternate to a total gastrectomy and has permitted the use of much lower doses of cimetidine.

b. Chemotherapy

Streptozotocin has been tried in a limited number of Z-E patients. The results have not been encouraging, and major toxic side effects have been observed. Therefore, this form of therapy cannot be recommended as a desirable alternative but may be tried in patients with advanced metastatic tumors.

E. Postoperative Care, Evaluation, and Follow-Up

Postoperative care includes the following:

- Maintenance of fluid and electrolyte balance is mandatory.
- Nasogastric suction should be maintained until return of normal bowel function.
- Nutrition and diet must be regulated. A dietician should be called to advise the patient about diet and caloric needs; feedings should be gradually increased to six small feedings a day.
- Avoidance of smoking and drinking of alcoholic beverages is advised.
- B_{12} injections must be administered monthly.
- The usual postoperative care of patients undergoing major abdominal surgery applies to these patients as well.

A follow-up schedule of evaluation is most important to achieve optimum results in survival and quality of life; a history of ulcer symptoms should be elicited, and further tests need to be ordered at regular intervals (see Table II). Gastrin levels remain elevated after surgery in almost all patients; this is an indication of multicentricity of the tumors or of the presence of occult metastases. Recurrence of symptoms or detection of an elevated fasting or postprovocative gastrin level (greater than 1000 pg per milliliter) is often an indication of metastases to the liver, and a hepatic angiogram may be performed to confirm the diagnosis. Chemotherapy should be considered when diffuse metastases are found; interestingly enough, however, patients with multiple metastases in their livers may survive many years without clinical evidence of serious disease.

Table II presents a follow-up schedule for gastrinoma patients.

F. Management Algorithm for Gastrinomas (see p. 164)

III. GLUCAGONOMA (HYPERGLYCEMIA SYNDROME)

This rare entity, which results from tumors arising from the A cells of the pancreas, is characterized by diabetes melitus, skin rash, and hyperglucagonemia.

A. Early Detection and Screening

Patients harboring this tumor are usually first seen in dermatologic or diabetic clinics. The syndrome may fall in one of the following three categories:

ALGORITHM FOR GASTRINOMAS

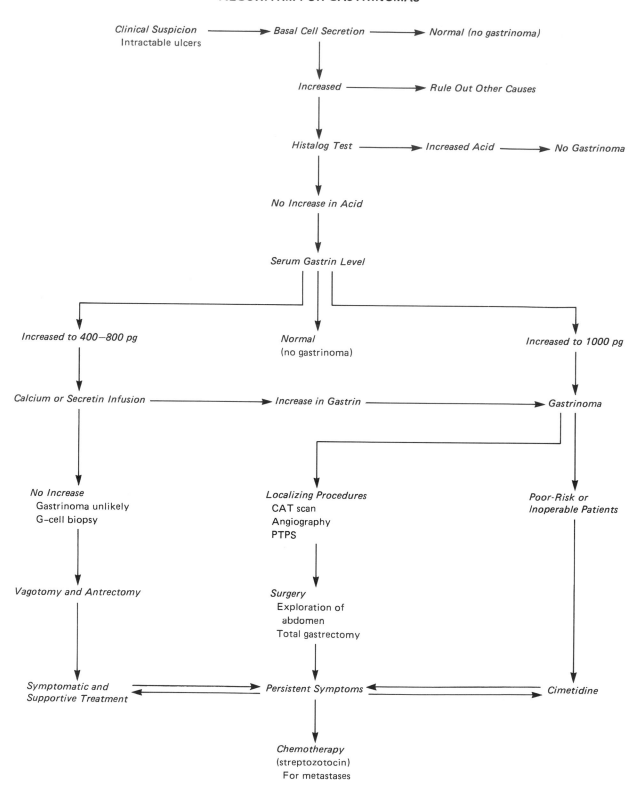

Table II

Long-Term Follow-Up for Gastrinomas

Management	First year				Second-to-third year		Thereafter	
	3 Months	6 Months	9 Months	12 Months	6 Months	12 Months	6 Months	12 Months
History								
Complete history		X		X	X	X		X
Epigastric pain	X	X	X	X	X	X		X
Diarrhea, vomiting	X	X	X	X	X	X		X
GI bleeding	X	X	X	X	X	X		X
Weight loss	X	X	X	X	X	X		X
Other	X	X	X	X	X	X		X
Physical								
Complete physical		X		X	X	X		X
Exam of surgical site	X	X	X	X	X	X		X
Liver	X	X	X	X	X	X		X
Rectal exam (stool guaiac)	X	X	X	X	X	X		X
Investigations								
CBC, HCT	X	X	X	X	X	X		X
SMA-6	X	X	X	X	X	X		X
SMA-12		X	X	X	X	X		X
Chest x-ray				X	X	X		X
Serum calcium		X		X		X	X	
Glucose level		X		X	X	X		X
Provocative tests				As indicated				
Other endocrine tests				As indicated				
Metastatic survey				As indicated				

- Glucagonoma with cutaneous syndrome.
- Glucagonoma without cutaneous manifestations.
- Glucagonoma as part of a multiple endocrine neoplasia (MEN) Type I.

The cutaneous syndrome is made of necrolytic migratory erythema (NME), which is present in 80% of all cases; glossitis and or cheilitis are frequent (over 90% of cases). Diabetes mellitus, diarrhea, anemia, and weight loss may also be part of this syndrome. The skin rash is usually migratory, and it involves the lower abdomen and perineum. The lower extremities (especially the feet), the peribuccal skin, and the upper limbs are sometimes affected. When the diagnosis is suspected, skin biopsy should be done. The pathognomonic finding is necrosis of the upper epidermal layer of the stratum malpighii with liquefaction necrosis of the granular layer and blister formation without acantholysis.

In cases without skin manifestations, the disease is characterized by diabetes mellitus and hyperglucagonemia.

In the MEA syndrome, the picture is usually dominated by the other endocrine manifestations of the MEA I type.

B. Pretreatment Evaluation and Work-Up

The diagnosis is usually suspected in a diabetic patient with a persistent skin rash. However, these manifestations may not be present, and neither is particularly specific. Hyperglycemia can be identified, which does not rise sharply with glucagon provocative testing. The diagnosis of glucagonoma is confirmed by the finding of grossly elevated levels of plasma glucagon in the range of 1000–7000 pg per milliliter (normal: 50–150 pg per milliliter).

Isotope scanning of the pancreas and liver, CAT scanning, and selective angiography are indicated for the localization of the tumor and its metastases. Additional medical, cardiovascular, and metastatic evaluations are sometimes necessary as for other pancreatic tumors.

C. Therapeutic Management

- The treatment of choice of glucagonomas is complete surgical extirpation of the tumor with a surgical approach similar to that described in §4B.I.C.2.
- In patients with extensive metastases or contraindications for surgery, chemotherapy with streptozotocin may be effective; 5-FU and DTIC have also been used in this disease with some degree of success.
- The skin rash may be treated with topical corticosteroids or zinc sulfate.
- Diabetes mellitus is controlled with insulin.

D. Postoperative Follow-Up

Glucagonomas are slow-growing tumors, and recurrence may appear at a later date; these patients must, therefore, be followed for many years.

E. Management Algorithm for
Glucagonomas (see p. 167)

IV. VIPOMA (PANCREATIC CHOLERA, THE WDHA SYNDROME, OR VERNER-MORRISON SYNDROME)

This is an extremely rare entity characterized by profuse choleralike diarrhea associated with a non-beta-cell tumor of the pancreas that produces vasoactive intestinal polypeptides (VIPs).

A. Early Detection and Screening

This syndrome should be suspected in patients with severe diarrhea accompanied by hypokalemia and achlorhydria. The fecal loss of electrolytes is responsible for the biochemical disturbances, the most prominent of which are hypokalemia and metabolic acidosis resulting from the loss of bicarbonate. The VIPs secreted by this pancreatic tumor seem to be responsible for the hypochlorhydria or achlorhydria and for the hyposecretion of pepsin observed in these patients. In addition, hypercalcemia and hyperglycemia have been reported in some cases.

In the differential diagnosis, other conditions producing severe diarrhea and dehydration should be excluded:

- The Z-E syndrome is easily differentiated since it is accompanied by gastric hyperacidity rather than hypochlorhydria or achlorhydria.
- Hyperthyroidism when accompanied by severe diarrhea can be readily diagnosed by the presence of an enlarged thyroid gland and elevated levels of tri- and tetraiodothyronine (T3–T4 levels) in the blood.
- The carcinoid syndrome, which also presents with diarrhea, is characterized by flushing of the skin.
- Glucagonoma, discussed earlier, usually presents with characteristic skin lesions.
- Medullary carcinoma of the thyroid may also present with diarrhea.

Elevated plasma levels of VIPs and prostaglandin E are diagnostic of this pancreatic tumor, and an attempt at preoperative localization of the tumor can be pursued by the use of CAT scan and selective angiography.

B. Therapeutic Management and Postoperative Care

Correction of water and electrolyte abnormalities is essential and must precede any surgical intervention. At the time of surgical exploration, complete resection of the diarrheogenic tumor is the only effective modality to achieve a cure or long-lasting remission. Complete exploration of the entire pancreas, peripancreatic areas, and liver is necessary; if a tumor is identified, a wide resection should be carried out; the majority of these tumors are located in the body or tail of the pancreas. In the event of a negative exploration, the syndrome may be due to hyperplasia, and a subtotal pancreatectomy is indicated as the initial procedure. If these operations fail to relieve the diarrhea, reexploration with a total pancreatoduodenectomy may even become necessary.

In those patients on whom surgery cannot be performed or where only partial excision is possible and when multiple metastases are present, streptozotocin may be useful for the alleviation of the diarrhea. Indomethacin has also been reported to offer some symptomatic relief.

Complete resection of the tumor often results in a rebound acid hypersecretion. Patients must be carefully followed after surgery to identify such an occurrence, and the administration of cimetidine may become necessary to control this complication.

C. Management Algorithm for Vipomas
(see p. 168)

ALORITHM FOR GLUCAGONOMAS

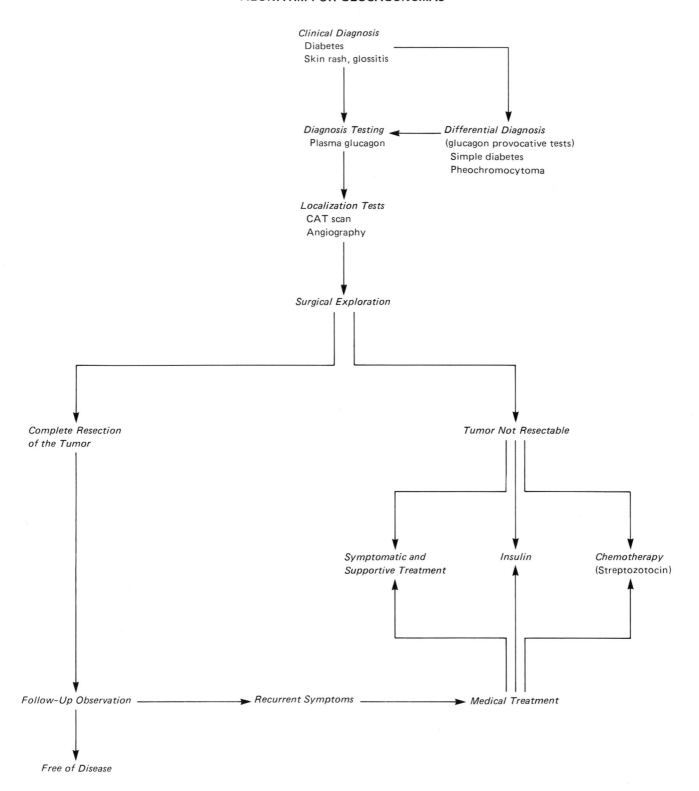

ALGORITHM FOR VIPOMAS

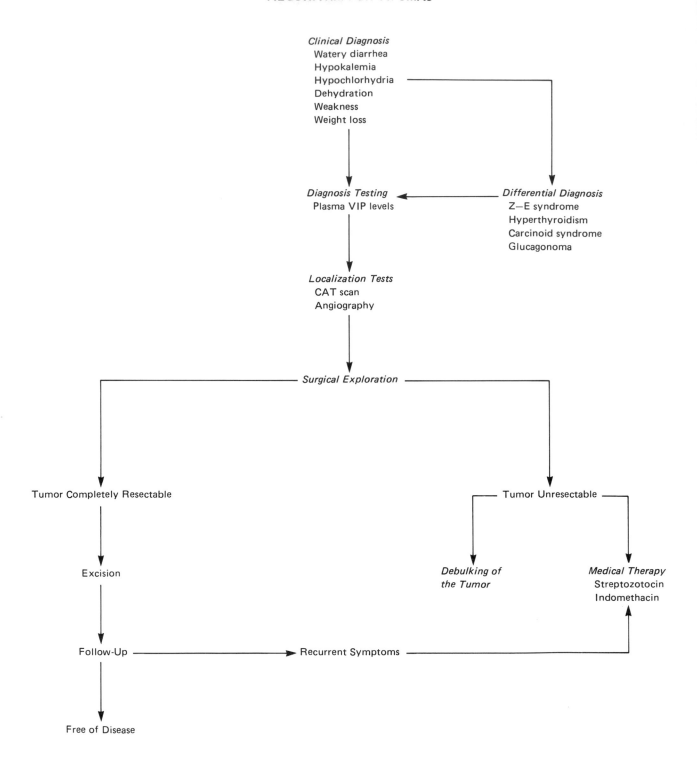

Clinical Diagnosis
Watery diarrhea
Hypokalemia
Hypochlorhydria
Dehydration
Weakness
Weight loss

Diagnosis Testing
Plasma VIP levels

Differential Diagnosis
Z—E syndrome
Hyperthyroidism
Carcinoid syndrome
Glucagonoma

Localization Tests
CAT scan
Angiography

Surgical Exploration

Tumor Completely Resectable

Tumor Unresectable

Excision

*Debulking of
the Tumor*

Medical Therapy
Streptozotocin
Indomethacin

Follow-Up

Recurrent Symptoms

Free of Disease

SUGGESTED READINGS

1. Brooks, J. R. ''Surgery of the Pancreas.'' Saunders, Philadelphia, Pennsylvania, 1983.
2. Dent, T. L. ''Pancreatic Disease, Diagnosis and Therapy.'' Grune & Stratton, New York, 1981.
3. Moosa, A. R. ''Tumors of the Pancreas.'' Williams & Wilkins, Baltimore, Maryland, 1980.
4. Najarian, J. ''Hepatic, Biliary & Pancreatic Surgery.'' Year Book Medical Publications, Chicago, Illinois, 1980.

Section 4. Tumors of the Endocrine Glands

Part C: Parathyroid Tumors

  I. Early Detection and Screening   173
   A. Detection of Hyperparathyroidism
   B. Early Signs of Hyperparathyroidism
   C. Screening
 II. Pretreatment Evaluation and Work-Up   174
   A. Symptoms
   B. Physical Examination
     1. Local Examination
     2. General Evaluation
   C. Laboratory Findings
     1. Serum Calcium and Phosphorus
     2. Other Laboratory Tests
     3. Parathyroid Hormone Assays
   D. Radiological Evaluation
   E. Differential Diagnosis of Hypercalcemia
   F. Localization of a Parathyroid Tumor

   G. Systemic Evaluation of the Patient
   H. Multidisciplinary Evaluation
   I. Site-Specific Data Form for Parathyroid Tumors
III. Preoperative Preparation   175
   A. General Medical Preparation
   B. Renal Preparation
   C. Acute Hypercalcemia
IV. Therapeutic Management   176
   A. Benign Hyperparathyroidism
   B. Carcinoma of the Parathyroid Gland
 V. Postoperative Care, Evaluation, and Follow-Up   178
   A. Postoperative Care
   B. Follow-Up Evaluation
VI. Management Algorithm for Parathyroid Tumors   178

   Suggested Readings   180

The parathyroid glands, generally numbering four, are situated in the tracheoesophageal grooves in the vicinity of the thyroid and are primarily responsible for maintaining the level of serum calcium in the blood within a narrow range (9–10.5 mg %) considered to be normal. Any increase or decrease in the serum calcium level will result in a feedback mechanism that will respectively decrease or increase the amount of parathyroid hormone secreted, thus rapidly correcting the blood calcium. The mechanisms through which the parathyroid hormone affects the serum calcium are multiple: it increases absorption through the GI tract by virtue of its stimulation of vitamin D_1 hydroxylation in the kidney, increases mobilization from the bone, and increases calcium reabsorption and tubular loss of phosphates through the kidneys. These mechanisms explain the wide range of clinical presentations and complications that can be seen with parathyroid tumors.

Parathyroid tumors are usually functioning tumors that cause an increase in parathormone production that is no longer responsive to the consequent increase in serum calcium. Hyperparathyroidism can result from diffuse hyperplasia of all parathyroid glands (3–5%), a solitary adenoma of one gland (90–92%), multiple adenomas (1–2%), or functioning carcinomas (1–2%). Very few cases of nonfunctioning parathyroid cancers have been reported. In approximately 10% of cases, more than four parathyroid glands are present and must be duly recognized by the surgeon carrying out parathyroid surgery.

I. EARLY DETECTION AND SCREENING

A. Detection of Hyperparathyroidism

The early detection of hyperparathyroidism has been markedly enhanced by the routine total biochemical blood profile (SMA-12 or SMA-18) that is, today, almost always part of a complete patient evaluation, whether done upon admission in the hospital or as part of a comprehensive physical evaluation in an outpatient setting. An elevated serum calcium is the alert that should be immediately followed by a more comprehensive assessment of the patient to establish or rule out the diagnosis of hyperparathyroidism. Although less than 2% of cases of hyperparathyroidism are caused by carcinoma of the parathyroid glands, early treatment of all cases of hyperparathyroidism will result in the earlier detection and treatment of carcinomas of the parathyroid. Furthermore, early investigation of hypercalcemia may uncover other peripheral tumors that are parathyroid hormone–producing (lung, kidney, gallbladder, etc.) and thus be instrumental in earlier detection of those specific tumors.

B. Early Signs of Hyperparathyroidism

The usual symptoms of advanced hyperparathyroidism, namely, renal stones and osteitis fibrosa cystica, are becoming less common since the advent of early detection resulting from the multichannel automated blood tests. There are, however, several less specific symptoms that may be related to hypercalcemia that should be recognized and lead to a blood calcium determination:

- Vague GI symptoms, anorexia, dyspepsia, or constipation.
- Peptic ulcer disease.
- Dysurias or polyurias.
- Pancreatitis.
- Fatigue or mental sluggishness.
- Mild psychiatric disturbances: agitation, depression, or just personality or behavioral changes.
- Osteoporosis.
- Chondrocalcinosis (pseudogout).

C. Screening

No systematic screening beyond the routine performance of blood chemistry determinations in a broad spectrum of circumstances is necessary or available. There are no selected groups that are at a high risk and no occupational or environmental predispositions; it must be stressed, however, that all patients with calculus disease of the kidneys should be investigated for hyperparathyroidism.

II. PRETREATMENT EVALUATION AND WORK-UP

A. Symptoms

Most patients with hyperparathyroidism are asymptomatic. In evaluating a patient, however, the more subtle symptoms previously mentioned should be sought: dysuria, fatigue, mental sluggishness, personality change, constipation, bone pains, or past history of urinary calculi. Patients who present with symptoms of pancreatitis or a past history of pancreatitis or peptic ulcer may also have a link between the two conditions.

B. Physical Examination

The physical examination is usually unremarkable. Occasionally, the patient will have, in the anterior neck in the vicinity of the thyroid, a tumor mass usually believed to be a thyroid nodule. Hypertrophied parathyroid glands are usually soft, collapsible, and difficult to feel because of their deep location. Large carcinomas, however, can be palpable and sometimes cause vocal cord paralysis and/or dysphagia. The following evaluation should be done:

1. Local Examination

- Examination of the neck and thyroid.
- Evaluation of any mass for location, size, consistency, mobility, fixation, etc.
- Presence or absence of nodes.
- Indirect laryngoscopy; evaluation of vocal cords.
- Examination of the mouth, teeth, etc.

2. General Evaluation

- Full physical examination.
- Evaluation of bones and kidneys.
- Search for evidence of any other tumors (identification of an MEA syndrome).

C. Laboratory Findings

1. Serum Calcium and Phosphorus

The most important laboratory findings are an elevated serum calcium and, less consistently, a decreased serum phosphorus. If these tests are positive on routine screening, the possibility of hyperparathyroidism should be considered. The serum calcium and phosphorus tests should be repeated to rule out laboratory error, and if consistently positive, further blood tests are in order.

2. Other Laboratory Tests

- Urinary calcium (elevated).
- Urinary phosphorus (elevated).
- 1,25-dihyroxyvitamin D (elevated).
- Urinary cyclic AMP (elevated).
- Alkaline phosphatase (normal in the absence of bone changes).

Several other tests of some importance prior to the advent of the parathyroid hormone assays are of limited usefulness today except in rare circumstances:

- Creatine and phosphorus clearance and tubular reabsorption of phosphate (decreased below 80% in hyperparathyroidism).
- Phosphate restriction test (used to induce an identifiable hypercalcemia in the normocalcemic hyperparathyroidism).
- Calcium infusion test.
- Cortisone infusion test (will only decrease serum calcium in nonparathyroid-related hypercalcemias: sarcoid, hypervitaminosis D, metastatic carcinoma, adrenal insufficiency).

3. Parathyroid Hormone Assays

Identification of an elevated serum parathyroid hormone (PTH) by immunoreactive assays is, today, the mainstay of the diagnosis of hyperparathyroidism. The level of the PTH, however, must be correlated with the level of serum calcium; in normal individuals, hypercalcemia (not caused by hyperparathyroidism) will result in a decrease of the PTH level; thus a normal PTH in the face of hypercalcemia is also strongly suggestive of hyperparathyroidism, though not as diagnostic as an elevated level. A decreased PTH, however, rules out hyperparathyroidism as the cause of the hypercalcemia.

D. Radiological Evaluation

The following x-ray findings identified on skeletal survey may be helpful:

- Minor changes, present in the form of decreased bone density.
- Moderate changes, including subperiosteal bone resorption best seen in the fingers and outer portions of the clavicles.
- More advanced changes, cyst formation, particularly in the mandible or maxilla.
- Changes of osteitis fibrosa cystica.

E. Differential Diagnosis of Hypercalcemia

Prior to any treatment, primary hyperparathyroidism must be separated from many other conditions associated with elevated serum calcium levels:

- Metastatic cancer (lung, kidney, or other).
- Sarcoidosis.
- Multiple myeloma.
- Hyperthyroidism.
- Milk-alkali syndrome.
- Hypervitaminoses A and D.
- Immobilization of long duration.
- Addison's disease.
- Benign familial hypocalciuric hypercalcemia.

The most difficult condition to rule out when establishing a diagnosis of hyperparathyroidism is the pseudohyperparathyroidism that results from peripheral PTH–producing tumors. These tumors often cause an increase in alkaline phosphatase in the absence of bone changes and may respond to a cortisone infusion test. It may be necessary, at times, to carry out an extensive work-up to rule out tumors at the various sites:

- chest x-ray or lung scan.
- IVP.
- GI series.
- Barium enema.
- Bone survey.

The PTH level is usually of little value in these cases, since it may be high normal or even elevated and cannot be distinguished from the PTH produced by a true parathyroid tumor.

F. Localization of a Parathyroid Tumor

Although several methods have been described to identify the location of a parathyroid tumor in a hypercalcemic patient, most are not entirely reliable, and some are extremely complex and available only in some highly specialized centers, making them of use only in cases of failures of a primary surgical exploration. Surgical exploration is the mainstay of diagnosis and treatment in the large majority of cases of hypercalcemias presumed to be due to hyperparathyroidism. Other preliminary tests that may prove useful include

- Barium swallow and upper esophagogram.
- Sonography.
- Selenomethionine scan. More recently, digital subtraction scans of the thyroid and parathyroid using thallium 201 and technitium 99 *M* pertechnatate have been effective in identifying parathyroid glands.

- CAT scan of the neck and mediastinum.
- Digital subtraction angiography.

Following unsuccessful exploration, the following localizing procedures should be carried out prior to reexploration:

- CAT scan of neck and mediastinum.
- Venous catheterization with selective venous sampling and parathormone assays.
- Arteriography.

G. Systemic Evaluation of the Patient

Prior to any surgery for hyperparathyroidism, the patient must be fully evaluated to assess the following parameters:

- General medical evaluation, cardiopulmonary, etc.
- Renal evaluation, especially when calculous disease is present or when renal damage is suspected.
- Metastatic evaluation, when carcinoma is suspected.

H. Multidisciplinary Evaluation

The primary physician, endocrinologist, and surgeon will be needed to treat the patient with parathyroid tumors or cancer. A radiation therapist and medical oncologist will sometimes be required to help in selected cases with carcinoma of the parathyroid.

The primary physician is the person who will make the presumptive diagnosis of hyperparathyroidism on the basis of an abnormal blood test. The endocrinologist will assist in the work-up and is required to rule out the many other significant conditions that cause hypercalcemia. The surgeon with expertise in head and neck surgery will be needed to explore the neck and find and excise the tumor with a minimum mortality and morbidity. In addition, an excellent pathologist is a *sine qua non* for the proper microscopic diagnosis of parathyroid tumors.

I. Site-Specific Data Form for Parathyroid Tumors (see pp. 177–178)

III. PREOPERATIVE PREPARATION

In the routine, uncomplicated cases of hyperparathyroidism, no specific preoperative preparation is required. The patient should be prepared for neck exploration and should be told that the operation may possibly be extended into the mediastinum.

A. General Medical Preparation

Patients with any type of medical disability may need to have some preparation to achieve optimum compensation of their cardiopulmonary and hematologic status prior to surgery.

B. Renal Preparation

Likewise, those patients with advanced renal disease may require some precautionary measures to improve renal function and decrease the blood urea nitrogen (BUN) and creatinine. These measures include the following steps:

- The state of hydration and electrolyte balance must be corrected.
- Small obstructive stones may be treated endoscopically to relieve obstruction.
- Urinary infections may require antibiotic treatment.

Removal of large stones or nephrectomy for irreversibly destroyed kidneys should be deferred until the hypercalcemia is corrected.

C. Acute Hypercalcemia

The preparation of the patient with acute hypercalcemic crisis is more demanding. These patients are often disoriented, confused, or comatose and constitute real emergencies. One or more of the following measures must be instituted immediately:

- Active hydration (with central venous pressure control) and use of diuretics (furosemide).
- Phosphate infusions (rarely employed today).
- Mithramycin (5–25 mg per 1 kg weight, repeated every 48–72 hours).
- Calcitonin, with or without steroids.
- Dialysis, peritoneal or hemodialysis.

These measures may be effective in decreasing the levels of serum calcium temporarily and may allow the physician a certain amount of time to assess and prepare the patient for surgery. It must be understood, however, that these are temporary measures and the patient must be submitted to a cervical exploration as soon as the diagnosis is confirmed and his or her condition allows. This can even be carried out under local anesthesia when necessary.

IV. THERAPEUTIC MANAGEMENT

A. Benign Hyperparathyroidism

The definitive treatment of any patient with hyperparathyroidism, whether resulting from hyperplasia, adenoma, or carcinoma, is surgical. The following guidelines must be adhered to in order to achieve the best results:

- Cervical exploration should be carried out by an operator experienced in identifying the normal and pathological parathyroid glands.
- Meticulous bloodless dissection is essential.
- A systematic, routine search of the parathyroids should be carried out; the recurrent laryngeal nerves must be carefully dissected in order to identify the anterior (inferior parathyroid) and posterior (superior parathyroid) paratracheal compartments. Thorough search in the following areas is mandatory:
  For the inferior parathyroids: anterior surface of the lower pole of the thyroid, space medial and below the recurrent laryngeal nerve, in the tracheoesophageal groove, in the pretracheal and superior mediastinal fat pad, and within the capsule of the thymus.
  For the superior parathyroids: on the posterior surface of the upper pole of the thyroid; along the constrictor muscles of the pharynx, retropharyngeal, retroesophageal, posterior mediastinal; and within the cartoid sheath.
- No excision should be carried out until all parathyroids have been identified.
- Small biopsies (1–2 mm) of the parathyroids may be desirable in the case of a questionably enlarged parathyroid gland to identify the nature of the structure and whether the gland is normal (large amounts of fat content) or pathological.
- In the case of benign parathyroid adenomas, single or multiple, it is recommended that only the grossly diseased gland be removed. Normal-looking glands should be left undisturbed. Questionably enlarged glands should be biopsied to rule out hyperplasia or multiple adenomas.
- Hyperplasias should be treated by subtotal parathyroidectomy in the form of resection of: all of three glands and one-half of the fourth *or* two full glands and two-thirds of each of the other two glands *or* all four glands with reimplantation of one gland in the forearm.
- If no tumor or hyperplasia is identified after an exhaustive search of the neck, the procedure should be stopped. If a parathyroid is missing, that lobe of the thyroid and the thymus should be removed and the wound closed. The patient must then be reevaluated to confirm the diagnosis of hyperparathyroidism, and a complete gamut of localizing tests should then be carried out to try and identify the exact location of the tumor prior to reexploration. It is not recommended that sternal splitting and chest exploration be carried out at the time of the first operation.
- The surgeon must bear in mind the fact that there may be more than four parathyroids and that there may be more than one adenoma.

SITE-SPECIFIC DATA FORM—PARATHYROID TUMORS

HISTORY

Age: _____

Symptoms
_____ Dysuria
_____ Dyspepsia
_____ General malaise
_____ Mental sluggishness
_____ Bone pains
_____ Dysphagia
_____ Renal calculi
_____ Bone cysts or fractures
_____ Past pancreatitis
_____ Past ulcer
_____ Psychoses
Duration: _____

Social history
  Occupation: _____
  Race: _____ White _____ Black _____ Oriental _____ Other
  Marital status: _____ Single _____ Married _____ Other

Family history of carcinoma
  Relation: _____ Site: _____

Previous history of carcinoma
_____ No _____ Yes   Site: _____

Previous treatment (describe): _____
_____
_____

PHYSICAL EXAMINATION

	Negative	Positive	Suspicious
Neck and thyroid area	_____	_____	_____
Nodes	_____	_____	_____
Evaluation of bones	_____	_____	_____

Other positive findings (describe): _____
_____

PREOPERATIVE EVALUATION (Check, if done)

	Neg.	Pos.	Suspicious		Neg.	Pos.	Suspicious
Serum calcium	___	___	___	IVP	___	___	___
Serum phosphorus	___	___	___	GI series	___	___	___
Urinary calcium	___	___	___	Barium enema	___	___	___
and phosphate	___	___	___	Sonography	___	___	___
TRP	___	___	___	CAT scan of neck			
Parathormone level	___	___	___	and medastinum	___	___	___
Calcium infusion test	___	___	___	Selenomethionine			
Phosphate withdrawal				scan	___	___	___
test	___	___	___	Digital subtraction			
Alkaline phosphatase	___	___	___	thyroid and			
x-Rays of bone	___	___	___	parathyroid scan	___	___	___
x-Rays of chest	___	___	___				

Localization procedures: _____ No _____ Yes _____ Arteriography _____ Venography
_____ Selective PTH samplings

Signature: _____
Countersignature: _____
Date: _____

B. Carcinoma of the Parathyroid Gland

In the case of parathyroid carcinoma, whether recognized grossly or on frozen section, the optimal result will be achieved if the surgeon removes it widely and completely. Frozen sections are always in order, but most carcinomas of the parathyroid are hard, encased by dense fibrous tissue, and usually invade surrounding tissue. Optimal treatment is achieved by wide excision of the tumor and surrounding tissues including the ipsilateral thyroid lobe and an ipsilateral neck dissection in the case of large infiltrating carcinomas or when nodes are grossly involved.

Erroneous diagnoses of parathyroid cancer have often been made in the past, particularly when a metastatic cancer is found in the thyroid area (e.g., clear-cell carcinomas of the kidney). To be certain that a parathyroid tumor is malignant, the pathologist should demonstrate invasion of contiguous structures or metastatic cancer in regional nodes or in distant structures.

In one large series of parathyroid cancers [Schantz and Castleman (4)], follow up showed that 41% of patients died of disease and 13% were alive but with residual disease. Another earlier series (Holmes, et al.) showed that one-third of 46 cases of parathyroid carcinomas had cervical node metastases and one-fourth had pulmonary metastases. In addition, in this latter series, three-fourths of the patients presented with symptoms of skeletal disease, while one-third had renal disease. When this group of cases was followed, it was found that less then one-fifth of the patients were living without evidence of disease.

Little is known about the value of radiation or chemotherapy for this malignancy. Response to irradiation, however, should be expected to be similar to that of other adenocarcinomas (e.g., thyroid or salivary glands), and high doses are necessary to achieve any worthwhile results.

V. POSTOPERATIVE CARE, EVALUATION, AND FOLLOW-UP

A. Postoperative Care

The usual postoperative care of the patient following cervical exploration with resection of a parathyroid tumor is much like that for thyroid surgery:

- Early ambulation.
- Drains for 24–48 hours.
- Skin sutures for 3–4 days only.
- Observation for respiratory distress, which may result from laryngeal edema, vocal cord paralysis, postoperative bleeding, or tracheal compression.

Following parathyroidectomy, the serum calcium level must be closely monitored, and symptoms of hypocalcemia should be identified early: parathesia of hands, feet, and lips; cramps; and positive Chvostek's sign. Later symptoms of carpopedal spasm or tetany must be avoided by early detection and treatment. The following guidelines for therapy of hypocalcemia are recommended:

- Do not administer calcium preventatively.
- Avoid utilizing calcium for serum levels above 7 mg %, unless the patient is symptomatic.
- In cases of severe symptoms (tetany or spasm), use calcium gluconate intravenously until symptoms abate; then institute oral medication.
- In all other cases, calcium may be administered orally but must be given in large quantities and combined with vitamin D_2, dihydrotachysterol, or calciferol.
- In the presence of osteitis fibrosa cystica, a much longer period of calcium administration may be required to stabilize the patient. The depleted bones will rapidly remove large quantities of calcium from the serum until they are reconstituted.

B. Follow-Up Evaluation

The long-term follow-up of the hyperparathyroid patient following surgery will include:

- Regular serum calcium determinations as often as necessary until the serum calcium stabilizes (daily, if wide fluctuations are noted or if the patient has severe bone depletion). Once stabilized and off any oral calcium medication, a serum calcium must be obtained every 3 months the first year and yearly thereafter. The slightest elevation of serum calcium needs to be followed up by a PTH determination.
- In addition the patient with carcinoma should be followed according to the schedule of follow-up detailed for head and neck cancers other than aerodigestive (see §1, Table IV). Most patients who develop metastatic or recurrent disease do so in the first 2 years. Recurrences are often in the neck, and pulmonary metastases are frequent.

VI. MANAGEMENT ALGORITHM FOR PARATHYROID TUMORS

(see p. 179)

ALGORITHM FOR PARATHYROID TUMORS

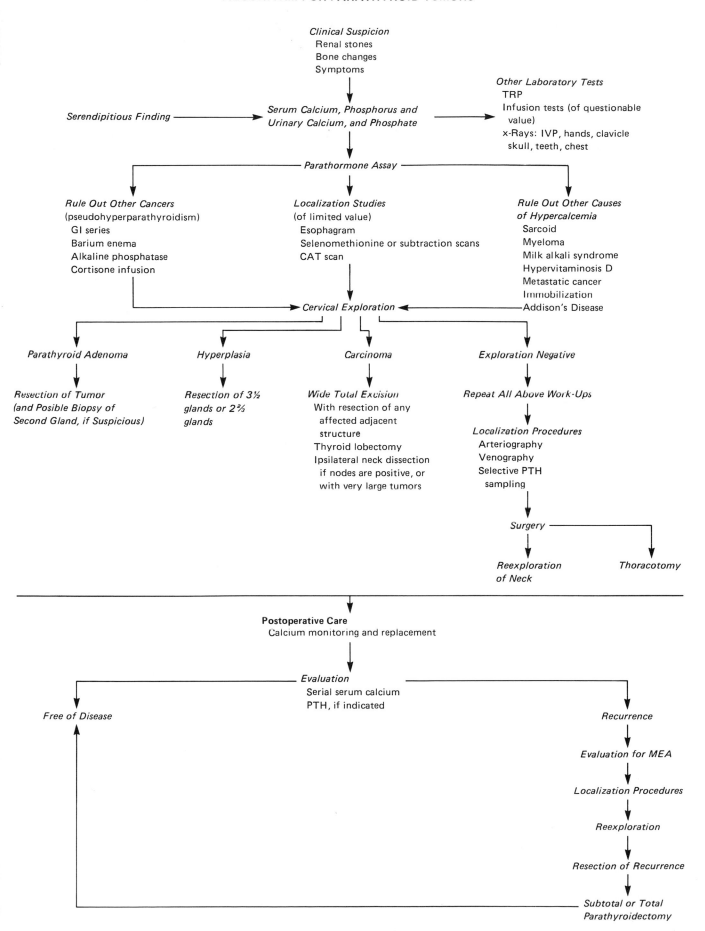

SUGGESTED READINGS

1. Friesen, S. T. ''Surgical Endocrinology, Clinical Syndromes.'' Lippincott, Philadelphia, Pennsylvania, 1978.
2. Geelhoed, G. W. ''Problem Management In Endocrine Surgery.'' Year-book Medical Publishers, Chicago, Illinois, 1983.
3. Holmes, E. C., Morton, D. L., and Ketcham, A. S. Parathyroid carcinoma: A collective review. *Ann. Surg.* **169;** 631–640 (1969).
4. Schantz, A., and Castleman, B. Parathyroid carcinoma. *Cancer* **31;** 600–605 (1973).

Section 4. Tumors of the Endocrine Glands

Part D: Paraneoplastic Endocrine Syndromes
(Ectopic Hormone Producing Tumors)

I. Evaluation of the Patient   184
  A. Physical Evaluation
    1. History
    2. Clinical Examination
      a. General Physical
      b. Systemic Examination
  B. Diagnostic Testing
    1. Hypercalcemia
    2. Ectopic ACTH Production
    3. Hypoglycemia-Associated Tumors
    4. Hyponatremia with Ectopic ADH Production
  C. Radiological Localization of the Tumor
  D. General Medical Evaluation
  E. Multidisciplinary Evaluation

II. Preoperative Preparation   185
III. Therapeutic Management   186
  A. Pseudohyperparathyroidism
    1. Acute Hypercalcemia
      a. Hydration and Diuretics
      b. Calcitonin
      c. Mithramycin
    2. Chronic Hypercalcemia
  B. Ectopic ACTH Syndrome
  C. Tumor Hypoglycemia
  D. Ectopic ADH Syndrome
  E. Gonadotrophin-Secreting Tumors
IV. Postoperative Care and Follow-Up   188

Suggested Readings   188

The paraneoplastic endocrine syndromes are a group of endocrine disorders produced by a variety of tumors that ordinarily do not produce the responsible hormone. Five such syndromes are recognized:

- Pseudohyperparathyroidism with hypercalcemia due to a parathormonelike substance secreted by a variety of tumors.
- Ectopic ACTH syndrome.
- Hypoglycemia, nonpancreatic in nature.
- Ectopic ADH production.
- Ectopic gonadotrophin production.

Tables I through V list the more common locations of these ectopic hormone-producing tumors that present with a paraneoplastic endocrine syndrome. In addition, a small number of patients have been reported as having acromegaly resulting from ectopic secretion of growth hormone or its releasing factor by bronchial carcinoid and islet cell tumors of the pancreas.

Table I

Neoplasms Associated with Hypercalcemia

Tumor type	Approximate frequency (%)
Carcinoma of lung	35
Carcinoma of kidney	24
Carcinoma of ovary	8
Miscellaneous (gallbladder, genitals, etc.)	Each less than 3

Table II

Neoplasms Associated with Ectopic ACTH Production

Tumor type	Approximate frequency (%)
Lung carcinoma	50
Thymic carcinoma	10
Pancreatic carcinoma (including islet cell carcinoma)	10
Neoplasms from neural crest tissue (pheochromocytoma, neuroblastoma, paraganglioma, ganglioma)	5
Bronchial adenoma (including carcinoid)	2
Medullary carcinoma of the thyroid	5
Miscellaneous (carcinoma of the ovary, prostate, breast, thyroid, kidney, salivary glands, testis, stomach, colon, gallbladder, esophagus, appendix, etc.)	Less than 2 each

Table III

Non-Islet Cell Tumors Associated with Hypoglycemia

Tumor type	Approximate frequency (%)
Mesenchymal tumors	45
Hepatoma	23
Adrenocortical carcinoma	10
Gastrointestinal tumors	8
Lymphomas and leukemia	6
Others	8

Table IV

Neoplasms Associated with Ectopic ADH Production

Tumor type	Number of cases reported
Lung	22
Oat cell	8
Small-cell undifferentiated	11
Large-cell undifferentiated	1
Squamous cell	1
Thyroid	1
Stomach	1

Table V

Neoplasms Associated with Ectopic Gonadotrophin Production

Bronchogenic carcinoma (large, undifferentiated type)
Hepatoblastoma
Renal cell carcinoma
Adrenal carcinoma

Identification of these syndromes is solely on the basis of identification of the responsible tumor in a patient who presents with the endocrine syndrome in the absence of the endocrine tumor usually responsible for such a syndrome (parathyroid, adrenal, pancreatic, or pituitary). At times, the diagnosis is serendipitous during evaluation of a patient with a primary tumor in the lung, kidney, ovary, thyroid, liver, or GI tract, in whom the endocrine signs are identified during such evaluation.

The early detection and screening of these syndromes is almost impossible, and only a sharp awareness of the existence of these entities would enhance early recognition.

I. EVALUATION OF THE PATIENT

A. Physical Evaluation

1. History

The early signs of the various paraneoplastic syndromes are based on the type of tumor, its size, and the specific hormone secreted by the tumor. The presenting symptoms may be related directly to the location of the tumor (lung cancer, kidney cancer, ovarian cancer, etc.) or to the hormone it produces. In the latter case, the signs and symptoms will be similar to those found in patients with the ordinary endocrine tumor that usually produces that specific substance:

- Signs and symptoms of hyperparathyroidism, particularly vague dyspepsia, dysuria, tiredness, disorientation, and lethargy.
- Signs of hypoglycemia: dizziness, fainting, hunger, tremulousness, sweating, and palpitation.
- Signs and symptoms suggestive of Cushing's disease, with muscle weakness, polyuria, hypokalemia, skin changes, and truncal obesity.
- Precocious puberty and gynecomastia.

Since carcinoma of the lung is the most common hormone-producing ectopic tumor, the signs and symptoms of lung cancer may often be early signs of the disease. These symptoms include chest pain, cough, hemoptysis, and weight loss.

2. Clinical Examination

A complete physical examination is required, including a general and system-oriented examination.

a. General Physical

Bilateral proptosis, plethora of the face, hirsutism in the female, buffalo hump, centripetal obesity, and mild hypertension are all suggestive of Cushing's syndrome. Increase in pigmentation of the skin or mucus membrane, dehydration, any lymph node enlargement, edema, etc. may also be identified.

b. Systemic Examination

This examination must be exhaustive to identify the following:

- Any swelling or mass.
- Deformity or decreased movements of the chest wall, wasting of localized areas of chest wall; tenderness of chest wall, shift of trachea; abnormal area of dullness; bronchial breath sounds, decreased areas of breathing, abnormal sounds like crepitations or rhonchi.
- Abdominal inspection: abnormal areas of fullness, scars of previous surgery; palpable masses, liver size, kidney size; presence or absence of free fluid in the peritoneal cavity.
- Cardiovascular: routine examination; look for any shift of cardiac impulse or presence of pericardial effusion.
- Central nervous system examination: higher functions like memory, consciousness, sleep, and cranial nerves; muscle weakness; loss of sensations in the distribution of peripheral nerves; evidence of peripheral neuropathy.
- Tenderness or deformity of bones.

B. Diagnostic Testing

The routine laboratory tests needed include CBC, SMA-12, Urinalysis, EKG and chest x-ray. Further laboratory testing in paraneoplastic syndromes depends on the individual clinical syndrome. The following guidelines are recommended for each individual syndrome. A more detailed review of the diagnostic tests available for the various endocrinopathies may be found in the previous specific parts of this section.

1. Hypercalcemia

- Serum calcium and phosphate, urinary calcium and phosphorous, and tubular reabsorption of phosphate (TRP).
- Measurement of PTH. Not usually helpful. A low-normal value is strongly suggestive of some other humoral substance causing hypercalcemia. The level, however, cannot distinguish true primary hyperparathyroidism from an ectopic PTH-producing tumor.

- Metastatic survey of the bone for any skeletal metastases.
- Alkaline phosphatase. An elevated level in the absence of bone changes is suggestive of an ectopic tumor.
- Radioimmunoassays of prostaglandin and prostaglandin metabolites in the urine. Not usually available but may be of help; when elevated they may be indicative of an ectopic PTH-producing tumor.
- A therapeutic test using indomethacin can be done. A response showing decreased calcium values is suggestive of prostaglandin mediation and an ectopic tumor.

2. Ectopic ACTH Production

To confirm the presence of Cushing's syndrome, the following laboratory tests are recommended:

- Serum cortisol higher than 25 μg per 100 ml with loss of diurnal variation.
- Plasma ACTH higher than 150 pg per milliliter.
- Dexamethasone suppression, failure to show any lowering of plasma cortisol or urinary 17-OHCS.
- Venous catheterization and collection of blood at different sites for measurement of ACTH may give a high plasma ACTH level near the tumor and is very useful for diagnostic localization of the tumor.

3. Hypoglycemia-Associated Tumors

- Plasma glucose measurements in fasting and fed state.
- Elevated levels of free fatty acids and lactate.
- Measurement of more specific humoral substances like NSILA (nonsuppressible insulinlike activity) and somatomedins that have been found to be elevated by some investigators, although the latter is controversial.
- Measurement of IRI, normal in most of the cases.

4. Hyponatremia with Ectopic ADH Production

- Urinary osmolarity: greater than serum osmolarity (reflecting urinary solutes in excess of plasma concentration).
- Urinary sodium: greater than 20 meq with hyponatremia.
- Plasma renin activity: suppressed despite hyponatremia.
- Measurement of plasma arginine vasopressin (AVP): a recently developed radioimmunoassay; shows a high serum value and is confirmatory for the diagnosis.

C. Radiological Localization of the Tumor

In all patients with paraneoplastic syndromes, it is most important to recognize the site of the primary tumor. The lung is a very common site of tumors secreting ectopic hormones. The following radiological procedures are used:

- X-ray of the chest with tomography and CAT scanning.
- Routine radiographic studies (GI series, IVP, barium enema, etc.)
- CAT scan of the abdomen and pelvis for pancreatic carcinoma, pheochromocytoma, renal cell carcinoma, hepatoma, and carcinoma of the ovary.
- Specialized radiological procedures, such as venous catheterization and selective measurements of hormones in difficult cases, are sometimes advocated. The site of catheterization depends upon the tumor and system involved.
- Arteriography may be useful to localize the specific tumor.

D. General Medical Evaluation

A general evaluation of the patient is most important to identify any aberration in physiological functions resulting from the endocrinopathy (particularly electrolyte changes, hypoglycemia and acidosis, renal function changes, etc.). In addition, a complete assessment of the patient's medical status (cardiac evaluation, pulmonary evaluation, etc.) in order to determine his or her ability to withstand any major surgical procedures needs to be done.

A metastatic survey should be carried out if one is contemplating definitive curative surgery since, unlike patients with primary endocrine tumors, these patients almost always have malignant tumors.

E. Multidisciplinary Evaluation

Patients with paraneoplastic syndromes need involvement and consultations by a radiologist, an endocrinologist, a radiotherapist, an oncologist, and a surgeon. A team approach to the problem is the best approach. A number of these tumors may be inoperable by the time the diagnosis is made, and hence, symptomatic relief by radiotherapy and correction of hormonal effects by antihormone therapy may be the best that we can offer. A team consultation should be requested before making a final decision regarding treatment.

II. PREOPERATIVE PREPARATION

Patients with paraneoplastic syndromes must have the following electrolyte imbalances corrected if they are present:

- Hypercalcemia. Patients with ectopic production of parathormone or parathormonelike substance can have severe hypercalcemia. Patients with a very high serum calcium threatening an acute hypercalcemic crisis should have an attempt at lowering of the serum calcium to a range of 10–11mg %. Normal saline in large quantities with central venous pressure (CVP) monitoring and furosemide is the simplest method of reducing the serum calcium; phosphate infusion may be attempted if the serum phosphorus is low; calcitonin and mithramycin are also very useful. In the final analysis, however, dialysis (peritoneal or hemodialysis) is the most effective method of reducing the serum calcium.

- Hypokalemia. In cases of ectopic ACTH syndrome, the patient must have proper potassium replacement before undergoing any surgical intervention.
- Hypoglycemia. Hypoglycemia in tumors that secrete insulin or insulinlike substances must be corrected by intermittent or continuous infusion of dextrose solution.
- Hyponatremia. A patient with ectopic ADH production can present with hyponatremia, and it should be corrected by restricting the volume or giving 3% hypertonic saline before the patient goes for surgery. This may be given in combination with furosemide.

Anemia should be corrected by blood transfusions; nutritional support, pulmonary physiotherapy, cardiac compensation, etc. may also be required.

III. THERAPEUTIC MANAGEMENT

Definitive therapy for all the various paraneoplastic syndromes should, whenever possible, be directed toward the removal of the tumor that is the source of hormone production. Tables I through V summarize the sites of the various tumors that produce hormones in relation to the respective syndrome. An attempt should always be made to identify and resect the primary tumor. In general, however, by the time the patient presents with a paraneoplastic syndrome, the underlying malignant lesion, which is the source of hormone production, has already metastasized, and surgical resection may no longer be indicated.

A. Pseudohyperparathyroidism

The two most common tumors associated with hypercalcemia are carcinoma of the lung and carcinoma of the kidney. An attempt to localize the tumor should diligently be made, and specific therapy by surgical removal is desirable depending on the extent of the tumor and the tissue type. The use of chemotherapy and/or radiation therapy also depends on the site, type, and stage of the tumor. If the tumor does not respond to the specific therapy, correction of the acute or chronic hypercalcemia then becomes the goal of therapeutic management.

1. Acute Hypercalcemia

a. Hydration and Diuretics

Acute hypercalcemia can be treated to a great extent just by fluid replacement and diuretics. After dehydration is corrected, 1 liter of normal saline with IV or IM furosemide (20–80 mg) is recommended and can be repeated every 3–4 hours. Strict attention must be paid to the patient's cardiopulmonary status.

b. Calcitonin

If saline and diuretics alone are not effective in bringing down the calcium to a range of 10–11 mg % and keeping it in that range, the next drug of choice is calcitonin. It is administered subcutaneously or by IM injections in dosages that range from 4 IU (MRC unit) per kilogram every 12 hours to a maximum of 8 IU (MRC unit) per kilogram every 6 hours. Steroids (40–60 mg of prednisone) administered concomitantly will potentiate the effect of calcitonin and prevent escape.

c. Mithramycin

If these modalities are not effective and the patient continues to have serum calcium levels over 12 mg %, the use of mithramycin is recommended. Mithramycin is a cytotoxic antibiotic that inhibits RNA synthesis and may have a direct effect on normal bone-resorbing cells. It is given intravenously in a dose of 25 μg per kilogram body weight and can be repeated every 48–72 hours. Responses may be obtained within 24–48 hours and may last several days, but severe complications from the drug may be seen with as little as two injections.

2. Chronic Hypercalcemia

Other therapeutic modalities can inhibit bone resorption and can be effective in lowering the serum calcium on a chronic basis. These agents and their probable mechanisms are summarized as follows:

- Phosphates. Oral phosphates are given in a dose of 1.5–3.0 g over 24 hours in divided dosages. These compounds inhibit bone resorption and form insoluble calcium salts.
- Indomethacin inhibits prostaglandin synthesis, thereby lowering prostaglandin levels. This has only proven effective in individual patients with ectopic hyperparathyroidism.
- Corticosteroids: cortisone, prednisone, and dexamethasone. These agents act in various ways. They stabilize the lysosomal membranes, thereby blocking enzyme release; block prostaglandin synthesis; and are cytotoxic for lymphocytes, thereby presumably decreasing osteoclast activator factor (OAF) release. OAF is a protein normally produced

by white blood cells, which has been associated with the hypercalcemia of multiple myeloma and leukemias.

All are given as oral medications, and the doses are titrated against the serum calcium and the toxic effects of the drug.

B. Ectopic ACTH Syndrome

The most common cause of ectopic ACTH syndrome is oat cell carcinoma of the lung; the prognosis of this disease is extremely poor. The prognosis of the syndrome is considerably better if it is associated with a pheochromocytoma, paraganglioma, thymoma, or bronchial carcinoid. All preoperative preparation, precautions, and postoperative suggestions discussed in §4A apply to the surgical therapy of ectopic ACTH-producing tumors.

Only 10% of ectopic ACTH syndrome patients are cured by the surgical removal of the primary tumor. If the course of the neoplastic disease is favorable enough to anticipate a survival of 1 year or more, bilateral adrenalectomy or its medical equivalent might be considered to relieve the symptoms of Cushing's syndrome.

This can be accomplished with aminoglutethimide (which blocks the synthesis of corticosteroid hormones by interfering with the conversion of cholesterol into 5-pregnenolone) or with *o'p'*DDD (mitotane), which has a dual action of ACTH blockage and selective cytotoxic effect on the adrenal gland, causing focal degeneration of the zona fasciculata and reticularis. Thus, if surgical cure is not possible for a patient with an ectopic ACTH syndrome, adrenal inhibitors (i.e., metyrapone or aminoglutethimide) can be used to relieve the symptoms of Cushing's syndrome. During this therapy, patients must be placed on replacement doses of corticosteroids.

C. Tumor Hypoglycemia

For tumors associated with hypoglycemia, a search for the site of the tumor is the first management goal. The most common among these tumors are mesenchymal tumors and hepatomas. Other causes are adrenocortical carcinoma and GI tumors. Specific therapy is related to surgical excision whenever possible. A decision has to be reached in conjunction with the surgeon and the oncology team. Radiation therapy, with or without chemotherapy, may also be selected as an alternative modality. Hypoglycemic symptoms may ameliorate with surgical resection or with radiation or chemotherapy. Even palliative surgery to reduce the tumor mass may be extremely helpful in prolonging life and ameliorating the symptoms in certain cases (e.g., mesotheliomas).

In patients where hypoglycemic symptoms continue or in patients where surgery or radiotherapy is ineffective, medical management of the hypoglycemia is advocated:

- Primary therapy for the symptoms of hypoglycemia is dietary. Frequent feedings between meals, at bedtime, and even throughout the night can often ameliorate the attacks of hypoglycemia during the early stages of the disease.
- The use of diazoxide, which inhibits insulin secretion from the pancreatic insulin-secreting tumors, has been found to be ineffective in these cases and is not recommended in the therapy of ectopic hypoglycemia.
- In some cases, the use of specific cytotoxic chemotherapy (Streptozotocin) may be indicated.

D. Ectopic ADH Syndrome

The most common site of tumors associated with ADH secretion is the lung. In the majority of cases, the tumor is inoperable by the time the patient presents with the syndrome; surgical removal of the source of ADH, which is the only specific therapy, is, therefore, not possible in the majority of cases. Some tumors may respond to external radiation therapy, while others may respond to some combination of chemotherapeutic drugs or combined modalities of radiotherapy and chemotherapy. These are temporary measures that might, however, stabilize the patient for a reasonable amount of time.

Adjuvant medical therapy to treat the electrolyte disturbances of ectopic ADH syndrome should be started as soon as the diagnosis is established. The following measures are recommended:

- If the serum sodium is 120 meq per liter or if the patient has clinical manifestations of hyponatremia, an attempt to raise the serum sodium quickly should be made. Intravenous administration of hypertonic saline with simultaneous use of furosemide injection is recommended. The amount and duration of therapy is dependent on frequent determinations of the serum electrolytes and on the cardiac status of the patient.
- In patients with mild disturbances of serum sodium, water restrictions may suffice. Water intake of not more than 1000 ml in 24 hours may improve the hyponatremia.
- In some cases where water restriction alone is not effective and chronic medical management is desirable to keep the serum sodium normal, the use of a tetracycline derivative, i.e., demeclocycline, is recommended. This drug counteracts the action of ADH at the renal tubular level and can be used for correction of antidiuresis; it is administered in doses of 300 mg b.i.d. Lithium is also known to have the same effect, but to a lesser extent.

E. Gonadotrophin-Secreting Tumors

Those tumors are summarized in Table V. Localization of the primary tumor and specific surgery, radiation, or chemotherapy is recommended whenever possible. No specific blockers are available to block the effects of gonadotrophin, and no medical treatment is available for tumors secreting it.

IV. POSTOPERATIVE CARE
AND FOLLOW-UP

The actual postoperative care of the patient is very much the same as that of patients treated for the same tumor when not producing hormones. In addition, attention must be paid to the endocrine changes produced by the tumor and its resection; all the measures described in other parts of §4 on endocrine tumors applies to these patients as well.

Patients with paraneoplastic syndromes should be followed postoperatively to recognize the reappearance of the clinical syndrome related to the above-mentioned hormones. Sometimes this could be the earliest manifestation of a regrowth or a metastatic lesion. Patients must be screened periodically in their respective syndromes for chemical abnormalities such as hypokalemia, hypercalcemia, hyponatremia, or hypoglycemia. Further investigations should be pursued as indicated, to recognize metastases or regrowth of the tumor, if the above abnormalities are recognized.

SUGGESTED READINGS

1. Beckman, S. R. Hypercalcemia in malignancy. *Clin. Endocrinol. Meta.* **9**(2), 317–330 (1980).
2. Blackman, M. R., Rosen, S. W., and Weintraub, B. D. Ectopic hormones. *Adv. Intern. Med.* **23**, 85–113 (1978).
3. Hiru, I. Ectopic hormone syndromes. *Clin. Endocrinol. Metab.* **9**(2), 235–260 (1980).
4. Odell, D. W. Humoral manifestations of cancer. *In* "Textbook of Endocrinology" (R. H. Williams, ed.), 6th ed., pp. 1228–1241. Saunders, Philadelphia, Pennsylvania, 1981.
5. Pearse, A. G. APUD concept and hormone production. *Clin. Endocrinol. Metab.* **9**(2), 211–222 (1980).

Section 4. Tumors of the Endocrine Glands

Part E: Multiple Endocrine Neoplasia

I. Multiple Endocrine Neoplasia, Type I
   (MEN-I or Wermer's Syndrome) 191
   A. Clinical Presentation
      1. Hyperparathyroidism
      2. Pancreatic Islet Cell Tumors
      3. Pituitary Gland Tumors
      4. Adrenal Tumors
      5. Thyroid Lesions
      6. Other Lesions
   B. Pretreatment Evaluation
   C. Therapeutic Management
II. Multiple Endocrine Neoplasia, Type II
   (Sipple's Syndrome) 193
   A. Pathogenesis

   B. Clinical Presentation
      1. Medullary Carcinoma of the Thyroid
      2. Pheochromocytoma
      3. Hyperparathyroidism
   C. Diagnosis and Treatment
      1. Medullary Carcinoma of the Thyroid
      2. Pheochromocytoma
      3. Hyperparathyroidism
   D. Prognosis

Suggested Readings 194

Multiple endocrine neoplasia [MEN, also called multiple endocrine adenomatosis (MEA)] syndromes are familial disorders inherited as autosomal dominant traits whereby tumors or hyperplasia occur in two or more endocrine organs either synchronously or metachronously. Characteristically, there is bilaterality of involvement of the affected glands. The MEN syndromes are divided into two types: MEN-I, or Wermer's syndrome, and MEN-II, or Sipple's syndrome. The latter syndrome has two versions: MEN-IIa and MEN-IIb, sometimes called MEN-III. Table I indicates the primary neoplasia combinations in each type.

Table I

Variants of Multiple Endocrine Neoplasia: Primary Presentation

MEN-I	MEN-IIa	MEN-IIb (or MEN-III)
Parathyroid tumors	Medullary thyroid carcinoma	Medullary thyroid carcinoma
Pancreatic islet tumors	Pheochromocytoma	Pheochromocytoma
Pituitary tumors	Parathyroid disease	Ganglioneuroma, marfanoid habitus

I. MULTIPLE ENDOCRINE NEOPLASIA, TYPE I (MEN-I OR WERMER'S SYNDROME)

MEN-I is inherited as a mendelian autosomal dominant trait with a high degree of penetrance. Some patients with MEN-I have no family history of endocrine disorders; these cases are considered either to represent a first mutant of a line or to be a familial case with an inadequate search for other relatives with the disorder. The significance of this fact is that even when patients with MEN-I do not have a positive family history, they must be managed as a carrier of the affected gene.

The pathogenesis of MEN-I is still not understood. According to Wermer's hypothesis, a single, defective, dominant pleiotropic (affecting change in more than one character) gene is responsible for the syndrome. The other hypothesis, proposed by Vance et al., states that oversecretion from one MEN-I lesion causes the other lesions; they hypothesize that the primary genetic defect lies in the nesidioblast or a stem cell in the pancreas. It has also been proposed that the fundamental defect in MEN-I is an abnormal differentiation of neural crest tissue (according to the APUD concept of Pearse). It is obvious that these theories are speculative, and further investigation is needed to elucidate the pathogenesis of this syndrome.

A. Clinical Presentation

The incidence of this syndrome is unknown. The disease has been described in all age groups subsequent to the first decade. The peak incidence for males is in the fourth decade, whereas the majority of women develop disease in the third decade.

The clinical manifestations of MEN-I are protean, depending on the endocrine glands involved and the hormones that are predominantly elevated. In Ballard's series of 85 patients, the most frequent form of clinical presentation was peptic ulcer disease and its complications. Manifestations of hypoglycemia represented the second most common presenting feature, while symptoms due to altered parathyroid function, generally reported as the most resistent part of the MEN-I, and complaints referable to pituitary dysfunction were the least frequent.

More than half of patients with MEN-I have adenomas of two or more different endocrine glands, and the involvement of three or more glands is seen in up to 20% of affected individuals. The frequency of glandular involvement, in descending order, is approximately as follows: parathyroids (90%), pancreatic islet cells (75%), pituitary (65%), adrenal cortex (40%), and thyroid (10–15%).

1. Hyperparathyroidism

Evidence of hyperparathyroidism is the most common endocrine abnormality. Chief-cell hyperplasia is the characteristic pathological lesion. The hyperparathyroidism is often mild and the patient asymptomatic. Patients may present with a history of kidney stones or with progressive renal failure as a first manifestation, or more commonly, hypercalcemia may be detected incidentally upon routine screening.

2. Pancreatic Islet Cell Tumors

It has been demonstrated that pancreatic islet cell tumors occur in almost 80% of patients with MEN-I and take the form of gastrinomas, insulinomas, and vipomas, in that order of frequency. Histologically, the lesions consist of hyperplasia, adenoma, or carcinoma of the islet cells. The lesions are almost invariably multicentric and may often produce more than one hormone during the clinical course of the disease.

The production of gastrin by islet cell tumors results in gastric acid hypersecretion with associated peptic ulcer diathesis. More than one-third of patients complain of diarrhea, which is due to the large amount of hydrochloric acid pouring into the upper GI tract. When islet cell tumors produce insulin, the syndrome characterized by fasting hypoglycemia develops. A VIP-secreting islet cell tumor produces a syndrome characterized by severe watery diarrhea, hypoakalemia, achlorhydria or hypochlorhydria, hypercalcemia, and abnormal glucose tolerance. Tumors producing glucagon result in a clinical picture characterized by diabetes mellitus and the distinct skin eruption NME (see §4.B.III.A).

3. Pituitary Gland Tumors

Pituitary tumors occur in 60–70% of cases, but only less than 30% of patients have evidence of a pituitary lesion clinically. Of the tumors present, about 45% are chromophobe adenomas and present with signs and symptoms of hypopituitarism; about 30% are eosinophilic with associated acromegaly; and the remainder are mixed basophylic, chromophobe, and eosinophilic. Secondary amenorrhea in women and hypogonadism in men are the most common manifestations of altered pituitary function, while less often, headaches or visual-field defects due to pressure on the optic chiasm are observed. Pituitary tumors that secrete excessive amounts of hormones may result in some dramatic syndromes: acromegaly or gigantism due to growth hormone excess, galactorrhea (rarely) or impotence in men, Forbes-Albright syndrome (amenorrhea and/or galactorrhea) due to hyperprolactinemia in women, and Cushing's syndrome due to ACTH excess (in 5% of patients). Pituitary tumors that secrete excessive amounts of FSH, TSH, and MSH have been reported, but these are rare and when present are usually associated with GH-, prolactin (PRL)-, or ACTH-secreting tumors.

4. Adrenal Tumors

Adrenocortical involvement, including adenoma, multiple adenomas, cortical hyperplasia, and nodular hyperplasia, occurs in 40% of patients. However, adrenocortical hyperfunction is rarely manifested clinically.

5. Thyroid Lesions

Thyroid diseases occur in about 10–15% of patients with MEN-I. While the spectrum of lesions includes adenoma or adenomata, colloid goiter, thyroid carcinoma (other than medullary thyroid carcinoma), Hashimoto's disease, and thyrotoxycosis, the most common lesions are functioning thyroid adenomas and colloid goiters.

6. Other Lesions

Other tumors that can form a part of the clinical picture of MEN-I include schwannomas, multiple cutaneous lipomas, thymomas, and both bronchial and small intestinal carcinoids.

B. Pretreatment Evaluation

The management of the individual components of the MEN-I is no different than that of patients with sporadic endocrinopathy. The most important consideration is for the physician to be aware, in dealing with apparently sporadic cases of hyperparathyroidism, pancreatic islet cell tumors, or pituitary tumors, of the possibility of second- or third-gland involvement. For example, in patients with established pancreatic islet cell lesions, serum calcium, phosphate, and PTH should be evaluated. Similarly, documented hyperparathyroidism of chief-cell hyperplasia or of a multiple adenomatosis etiology in the patient with peptic ulcer disease should be followed up with an MEN-I screening. This includes

- Upper GI series, gastric acid secretory studies, and fasting serum gastrin determination.
- Fasting blood sugar and serum insulin.
- Visual-field examination and skull x-rays.
- Serum GH, PRL, ACTH, gonadal steroid, thyroxine determinations (T3 and T4), etc.

Diagnosis of further endocrine involvement can only be made by regular and constant screening with appropriate tests, as all the tumors do not manifest themselves synchronously. Furthermore, it is incumbent upon the physician taking care of patients with MEN-I to offer other family members screening tests for the identification of those that may be afflicted by the disease.

C. Therapeutic Management

The sequence of treatment of the various endocrinopathies will depend on the predominant lesion and the most severe clinical syndrome present. The same principles of therapy detailed in the management of each individual endocrine tumor apply to the treatment of patients with MEN-I. The overall prognosis of the patients with MEN-I seems worse, however, than the prognosis in those patients with isolated glandular involvement; this is due to the higher incidence of malignancy and involvement of other endocrine glands, especially the pituitary gland.

II. MULTIPLE ENDOCRINE NEOPLASIA, TYPE II (SIPPLE'S SYNDROME)

In 1961 Sipple (6) (for whom the syndrome was named), after an extensive review of the literature, discovered that thyroid carcinoma was 14 times more prevalent in patients with pheochromocytoma than in the normal population. Later on, in 1963, Manning et al. appreciated that hyperparathyroidism was an integral part of this syndrome. It was subsequently noted that the particular thyroid carcinoma involved was of the medullary type and that it was of a familial nature, it being transmitted in a mendelian autosomal dominant pattern with a high degree of penetrance. Steiner and associates (1968) termed this disease constellation—medullary carcinoma of the thyroid (MCT), pheochromocytoma, and hyperparathyroidism—multiple endocrine neoplasia, Type II.

Two variants of MEN-II have been recognized, MEN-IIa and MEN-IIb. The term MEN-IIa is used to describe affected patients who have a normal physical appearance. The second variant, for which the term MEN-IIb is used, includes patients who have a striking appearance due to labial and mucosal ganglioneuromas, a marfanoid habitus, and other somatic abnormalities primarily consisting of diverticulosis and ganglioneuromatosis. Those patients rarely have parathyroid disease. In contrast to MEN-IIa, MEN-IIb most commonly occurs sporadically without familial involvement.

A. Pathogenesis

Both the parafollicular cells of the thyroid, which give rise to MCT, and the adrenal medullary cells originate from the neural crest and have APUD (amine precursor uptake and decarboxylation) cell characteristics. The inheritance of simultaneous pheochromocytomas and MCT may result from a single or combined genetic aberration in the neural crest tissue. The parathyroid disorder, however, is not easy to explain; although the parathyroids produce a polypeptide hormone, they are derived from the pharyngeal endoderm and not the neural crest and do not have the biochemical features of APUD cells. It is possible that abnormalities of the non-APUD parathyroid gland are perhaps secondarily related to the induced hypocalcemic state of hypercalcitonemia with resultant glandular hyperplasia. However, patients with nonfamilial MCT and MEN-IIb rarely have hyperparathyroidism, thereby raising the possibility that the parathyroid lesions could be a primary rather than a secondary feature in MEN-II.

B. Clinical Presentation

The syndrome of MEN-II affects the two sexes equally and is most common between ages 20 and 40.

1. Medullary Carcinoma of the Thyroid

The earliest recognizable manifestation of these syndromes is MCT. It is the constant feature in MEN-II, being present in virtually 100% of the affected individuals. The tumors are bilateral and multifocal in 70–80% of cases of MEN-II, whereas in sporadic cases they are bilateral in only 30%. The biochemical hallmark of MCT is the production of calcitonin. In addition to calcitonin, MCT cells have been shown to produce ACTH, MSH, serotonin, VIP, histaminase (elevated plasma levels in 50% of patients), and a number of prostaglandins. The most common type of presentation of MCT in patients with MEN-II is a multinodular thyroid gland, although occasionally only a single nodule is felt. Cervical lymphadenopathy is present in 15–20% of patients at initial evaluation. More recently, patients with no symptoms or findings are being seen and studied because of the known family history of the disease. Approximately 30% of patients with MCT develop clinically significant diarrhea. Rarely, MCT could also produce Cushing's syndrome. It should be stated that when these paraendocrine syndromes occur in patients with MCT, a relatively advanced disease state is indicated, and the patient is often incurable.

2. Pheochromocytoma

In approximately 50–70% of the MEN-II cases, pheochromocytoma occurs; it is bilateral in about two-thirds of these patients. Nearly all these pheochromocytomas are in the adrenal gland and are benign. Histologically, pheochromocytomas in the MEN-II are indistinguishable from those occurring sporadically in a nonfamilial setting. The pheochromocytoma in MEN-II usually appears in the second or third decades of life and may either be clinically silent or produce dramatic clinical symptoms. Hypertension (episodic rather than sustained), sweating, palpitation, and headaches may be found in patients with active pheochromocytoma. Recognition of the associated adrenal neoplasm in patients with MEN-II is mandatory, even in the absence of symptoms, since general anesthesia induction in the unprepared patient with pheochromocytoma may provoke a hypertensive crises with high morbidity and mortality.

3. Hyperparathyroidism

Even though the incidence of histological parathyroid abnormalities (mostly chief-cell hyperplasia) ranges from 45 to 90% in patients with MEN-II, hypercalcemia is present in only about 10–30% of cases. The most common manifestation of altered calcium metabolism in patients with MEN-II is asymptomatic or symptomatic nephrolithiasis.

C. Diagnosis and Treatment

1. Medullary Carcinoma of the Thyroid

The demonstration of an elevated serum calcitonin level, either under basal conditions or in response to provocative stimuli of calcium or pentagastrin infusion, is the most important step in the diagnosis of MCT. The radioimmunoassay (RIA)-detectable polypeptide is increased in virtually all patients with MCT. Measurement of calcitonin in the plasma is more sensitive than either thyroid palpation or scan. Its use results in early diagnosis and treatment of asymptomatic patients. Hypercalcitonemia is not absolutely specific for MCT. Elevated blood levels of this hormone have been reported in patients with other tumors such as small-cell carcinoma of the lung, carcinoid, breast cancer, and pheochromocytoma. Despite this, in the proper clinical setting, hypercalcitonemia has a high degree of specificity for MCT.

Once the diagnosis is made and after the exclusion or treatment of pheochromocytoma, total thyroidectomy is mandatory because MCT is usually bilateral and multicentric. As part of the procedure, lymph nodes in the midline compartment should be removed, and those in both internal jugular chains must be sampled. Should obvious metastatic disease exist in the jugular nodes, then a radical neck dissection should be performed. Postoperatively, all patients should be evaluated with calcitonin determination tests and receive thyroid hormone replacement.

2. Pheochromocytoma

The establishment of the diagnosis of pheochromocytoma in patients with suspected MEN-II is no different from that of sporadic cases and depends upon the measurements of urinary

catecholamines, VMA, or metanephrines. Radiologically, CAT scan, angiography, venous catheterization, ultrasound, and scans are valuable for localization of tumors. After the diagnosis of pheochromocytoma is made and following appropriate alpha- and beta-adrenergic blockade, bilateral total adrenalectomy is indicated because of the high incidence of bilateral disease. This should precede the treatment of any other endocrinopathy.

3. Hyperparathyroidism

The diagnosis of hyperparathyroidism is largely dependent on the finding of an elevated serum calcium determination. Determination of serum PTH can be misleading since increased values have been reported in members of involved kindreds despite normocalcemia and absence of MCT. The preferred method of treatment is subtotal parathyroidectomy (resection of 3.5 glands). Total parathyroidectomy and autotransplantation is an alternative approach.

D. Prognosis

Of patients with MTC and MEN-IIa, 50% live for at least 10 years. The outlook for patients with MEN-IIb is worse because the MCT develops at a younger age, progresses relentlessly, metastasizes earlier, and is rarely cured by surgical or medical intervention.

SUGGESTED READINGS

1. Ballard, H. S., Frame, B., and Hartsock, R. J. Familial Multiple endocrine adenoma, peptic ulcer complex. *Medicine (Baltimore)* **43,** 481 (1964).
2. Khairi, M. R. A., Dexter, R. N., Burzynski, N. J., *et al.* Multiple endocrine neoplasia, type 3. *Medicine (Baltimore)* **45,** 89 (1975).
3. Melvin, K. E. W., Tashjian, A. H., Jr., and Miller, H. H. Studies in familial (medullary) thyroid carcinoma of the thyroid gland. *N. Engl. J. Med.* **278,** 523 (1968).
4. Norton, J. A., Froome, L. C., Farrel, R. D. *et al.* Multiple endocrine neoplasia, type IIB. The most aggressive form of medullary thyroid carcinoma. *Surg. Clin. North Am.* **59**(1), 109 (1979).
5. Pearse, A. G. E. The APUD cell concept and its implications in pathology. *In* "Pathology Annual" (S. C. Somers, ed.), pp. 27–41. Appleton, New York, 1974.
6. Sipple, J. H. The association of pheochromocytoma with carcinoma of the thyroid gland. *Am. J. Med.* **31,** 163 (1961).
7. Vance, J. E., Stoll, R. W., Kitabchi, A. E. *et al.* Familial nesidioblastosis as the predominant manifestation of multiple endocrine adenomatosis. *Am. J. Med.* **52,** 211 (1972).
8. Wermer, P. Endocrine adenomatosis: Peptic ulcer in a large kindred. *Am. J. Med.* **35,** 205 (1963).

Section 4. Tumors of the Endocrine Glands

Part F: Apudomas

 I. APUD Cell Characteristics   197
   A. Cytochemical Properties
   B. Ultrastructural Properties
II. Classification   197
   A. Orthoendocrine Group

   B. Para-endocrine Group
   C. Multiple Endocrine Adenopathy

Suggested Readings   199

The term *APUD* is an acronym taken from the initial letters of the most constant cytochemical properties of a series of cells whose apparent common function is the synthesis and secretion of amine or peptide hormones. Apudomas include all proliferative lesions (hyperplastic and neoplastic) of these APUD cells.

The letter *A* refers, first, to their (inconstant) content of the endogenous *a*mines and, second, together with the letters *P* and *U,* to their ability for *p*referential *u*ptake of the *a*mino acid precursors of the two amines, dopamine and 5-hydroxytryptamine (serotonin). The letter *D* stands for the ability of these cells to *d*ecarboxylate the relevant precursors 3,4-dihydroxyphenylalanine and 5-hydroxytryptophan (5-HTP) to dopamine and serotonin.

The working hypothesis regarding the histogenesis and embryogensis of the APUD cell was formulated by A. G. E. Pearse of the Royal Postgraduate Hospital in London in 1966. He proposed the existence of a group of apparently unrelated endocrine cells—some in endocrine glands, others in nonendocrine tissues—that shared common secretory as well as cytochemical and ultrastructural characteristics. All these cells he regarded as neuroendocrine, with some derived from neuroectoderm, others from neural crest cells, and still others from more primitive cells of the ectoblast before migrating into their definitive positions (like primitive gut and derivatives). However, conflicting data have been reported in this regard, and the controversy is far from resolved.

The charter members of the APUD cell system are:

- The peptide-secreting gastric and intestinal cells.
- All pancreatic islet cells.
- The cells of the adrenal medulla and all the extra adrenal paraganglia.
- The parafollicular thyroid cells.
- The hypophyseal ACTH-, MSH-, FSH-, LH-, and TSH-producing cells.
- The melanoblasts.
- The carotid body Type I cells.

Additional cells with APUD characteristics may be found in the respiratory and urogenital tracts, although their possible secretory materials and their function remains speculative. The inclusion of parathyroid glands within the APUD cell system is controversial; they produce a peptide hormone and have secretory granules, but their cytochemical charactertics differ from those of the APUD cells.

I. APUD CELL CHARACTERISTICS

A. Cytochemical Properties

- Amine-precursor (5-HTP, dopa) uptake.
- Amine-precursor decarboxylation to biogenic amines (serotonin, dopamine).
- High level of alpha-glycerophosphate dehydrogenase.
- High levels of nonspecific esterases and/or cholinesterase.
- Argyrophilia and/or chromaffinity.
- Marked metachromasia.

B. Ultrastructural Properties

- Abundant smooth endoplasmic reticulum and free ribosomes.
- Lower levels of rough endoplasmic reticulum.
- Abundant electron-dense mitochondria.
- Prominent microfibrils and membrane-bound neurosecretory granules (average size 100–200 nm).

II. CLASSIFICATION

Welbourn has conveniently divided apudomas into three groups with regard to the amine or peptide secretion from the parent cell: orthoendocrine, para-endocrine, and MEA.

A. Orthoendocrine Group

Orthoendocrine apudomas secrete the normal amines or peptides of the cells of origin. Examples of orthoendocrine apudomas arising outside of the digestive tract are:

Table I

APUDOMAS

Organ	APUD cell	Hormone (amine/peptide)	Specific clinical tumor	Clinical syndrome(s)	
				Orthoendocrine	Para-endocrine
Pituitary	C	ACTH	Pituitary adenoma	Cushing's disease	
	M	MSH		Hyperpigmentation	
	S	STH (somato-trophin)		Acromegaly or gigantism	
	1	PRL		Hypogonadism or Forbes-albright syndrome; impotence in men	
Thyroid	"C" (parafollicular cell)	Calcitonin	Medullary carcinoma	Hypercalcitonemia	
		ACTH			Cushing's syndrome
		Serotonin			
		Prostaglandins			
		VIP			Watery diarrhea
Skin	Melanocyte		Melanoma		Cushing's syndrome (ACTH)
Adrenal	E	Epinephrine ACTH	Pheochromocytoma	Hypertension	WDHA (VIP), Cushing's syndrome
Stomach	G	Gastrin	Gastrinoma	Z-E syndrome	
Duodenum and small bowel	EC	5-HT (5-Hydroxy-tryptamine) 5-HTP (5-hydroxy-tryptophan, motilin)	Carcinoid	Atypical carcinoid syndrome	
Pancreas	A (α1, α2)	Glucagon	Glucagonoma	Diabetes, NME	
	B (β)	Insulin	Insulinoma	Hypoglycemia	
	D (δ)	Gastrin	Gastrinoma		Z-E syndroma
		Somatostatin	Somatostatinoma	Diabetes, cholelithiasis, malabsorption syndrome	
	D1	VIP	Vipoma	WDHA syndrome	
	F	PP (pancreatic polypeptide)	Ppoma	Diarrhea	
Lung	P (Feyrter)	ACTH, ADH, VLP (vasoactive lung peptide)	Oat cell carcinoma		Schwartz-Bartter syndrome (ADH) Cushing's syndrome (ACTH)
	EC	5-HT, 5-HTP GH	Carcinoid		Carcinoid Acromegaly
Carotid body	Glomus cell	Catecholamine, 5-HT	Chemodectoma	Hypertension	

- Medullary carcinoma of the thyroid.
- Pheochromocytoma.
- Apudomas arising from the APUD cells of the pituitary gland.

Orthoendocrine apudomas originating from the GI tract are rare. They include

- Carcinoid tumors, which are the best known apudomas.
- Gastrinomas arising from the stomach and duodenum; these are rare variants of the Z-E syndrome and could be classified as orthoendocrine apudomas.
- Tumors of pancreatic origin. Five types of orthoendocrine apudoma may arise from the five types of APUD cells present in the adult pancreas (see §4B, Table I); these apudoma

types are insulinomas, vipomas, glucagonomas, somatostatinomas, and Ppoma (pancreatic polypeptide).

B. Para-endocrine Group

Para-endocrine apudomas may arise from endocrine glands or from tissues not normally regarded as endocrine in nature. They are characterized by the fact that the secretory peptide or amine is not normally produced by the endocrine organ or tissue involved. Inappropriate ACTH secretion by a medullary carcinoma of the thyroid or pheochromocytoma and secretion of ADH by an oat cell tumor of the bronchus are examples of this type of apudoma. The presence of neurosecretory granules in the cells of oat cell tumors of the bronchus and the ability of some of these tumors to secrete a variety of polypeptide hormones are characteristics that these tumors share with cell groups belonging to the APUD system. Some oat cell carcinomas, however, coexist with squamous carcinomas, which clearly do not belong to the APUD system; hence, the precise histogenesis of oat cell carcinoma remains unsettled. Gastrinomas arising from the pancreas, that are the usual cause for the Z-E syndrome, provide an excellent example of a paraendocrine apudoma since gastrin-producing G cells are not a normal constituent of the adult pancreas.

C. Multiple Endocrine Adenopathy

Multiple endocrine adenopathies occur when neoplastic lesions are present in two or more endocrine glands (often as apudomas) in the same individual (e.g., MEA I: pancreas, parathyroids, and pituitary are commonly involved; in MEA II, the involved glands are thyroid—the parafollicular cells—, adrenal medulla, and parathyroids.)

All APUD cells have the ability to elaborate a variety of amine and peptide hormones, and some of the cells can even produce more than one hormone. Thus apudomas may be associated with multiple hormone production. The clinical manifestations of apudomas depend mainly upon the functional status of the tumor and the biologic activity of the hormone produced. If the tumor secretes a large amount of hormone, symptoms resulting from the physiological effects of the hormone will occur. When, however, the hormone produced by the tumor does not reach a high enough concentration in the plasma to produce a clinical syndrome, it is considered to be clinically nonfunctioning. In certain specific instances, the tumor produces large amounts of hormones without clear biologic activity; here again, it is considered clinically nonfunctioning (e.g., calcitonin production by the medullary carcinoma of the thyroid, and prolactin production in pituitary tumors in children). These nonfunctioning tumors present as a nodule (e.g., in the thyroid) or may give symptoms as a result of destruction of the adjacent normal tissues (e.g., pituitary tissue). The determination of the plasma hormone level in these cases, however, is very helpful as a tumor marker.

The various apudomas, their cell of origin, the hormones produced, and the associated clinical syndromes that result from them are listed in Table I. These specific tumors and the syndromes that result from them are discussed individually in other parts of this section.

SUGGESTED READINGS

1. LeDouarin, N. The embryonical origin of the endocrine cells associated with the digestive tract. *In* "Gut Hormones" (S. R. Bloom, ed.), Chapter 6. Churchill-Livingstone, Edinburgh and London, 1978.
2. Pearse, A. G. E. The cytochemical and ultrastructure of polypeptide-hormone producing cells of the APUD series and the embryologic, physiologic, and pathologic implications of the concept. *J. Histochem. Cytochem.* **17**, 303 (1969).
3. Pearse, A. G. E. The APUD cell concept and its implications in pathology. *Pathol. Annu.* **9**, 27 (1974).
4. Pearse, A. G. E., and Polak, J. M. The diffuse neuroendocrine system and the APUD concept. *In* "Gut Hormones" (S. R. Bloom, ed.), Chapter 4. Churchill-Livingstone, Edinburgh and London, 1978.
5. Pictet, R. L., Rall, L. R., *et al.* The neural crest and the origin of the insulin producing and other gastrointestinal hormone producing cells. *Science* **191**, 191 (1976).
6. Welbourn, R. B. Current status of the apudomas. *Ann. Surg.* **185** (1), 1 (1977).

Section 4. Tumors of the Endocrine Glands

Part G: Carcinoid Tumors

BY: IRVIN MODLIN

I. Clinical Considerations   203
  A. Organ-Related Symptoms
  B. Carcinoid Syndrome
    1. Flushing and Sweating
    2. Diarrhea and Abdominal Colic
    3. Wheezing
    4. Cardiac Lesions
    5. Edema
    6. Skin Lesions
II. Pathological Considerations   204
III. Early Detection and Screening   204
  A. Signs of Carcinoid Tumors
    1. Intestinal Carcinoids
    2. Gastric Carcinoids
    3. Bronchial Carcinoids
  B. Detection
    1. Previous Appendectomy
    2. Previous History of Bronchial Adenoma
IV. Pretreatment Evaluation and Work-Up   205
  A. Establishment of the Diagnosis
    1. Physical Evaluation
      a. History
      b. Physical Examination
    2. Routine Clinical Laboratory Tests
    3. Biochemical Assessment
    4. Provocative Tests
      a. Calcium Infusion
      b. Alcohol Ingestion
      c. Secretin IV
      d. Catecholamine Infusions
  B. Topographical Localization
    1. Chest X-ray and CAT Scan

    2. Upper GI Series
    3. Gastroscopy
    4. Proctosigmoidoscopy
    5. Bronchoscopy
    6. Selective Celiac and Superior Mesenteric
      Arteriography
    7. CAT Scan
  C. General Medical Evaluation
  D. Metastatic Evaluation
  E. Multidisciplinary Approach
  F. Site-Specific Data Form for Carcinoid Tumors
V. Therapeutic Management   207
  A. Pharmacological Therapy
  B. Surgical Therapy
    1. Small-Bowel Carcinoid
    2. Appendix Carcinoid
    3. Rectal Carcinoid
    4. Gastric Carcinoid
    5. Bronchial Carcinoid
    6. Hepatic Carcinoid Metastases
  C. Adjunctive Therapy
    1. Radiation Therapy
    2. Cytotoxic Therapy
    3. Pharmacological Therapy
VI. Postoperative Care, Evaluation, and Follow-Up   210
  A. Postoperative Care
    1. Gastrointestinal Tumors
    2. Bronchial Tumors
  B. Nutritional Support
  C. Psychological Support
  D. Follow-Up Evaluation
VII. Management Algorithm for Carcinoid Tumors   211

Although not clearly recognized as a clinical or pathological entity until 25 years ago, carcinoid tumors and their syndromes are now evoking considerable attention, partly as a result of the increasing recognition of their protean manifestations. The endocrine nature of the neoplasm and its ability to secrete various amines and peptides has led to considerable interest in the cells of origin of these tumors and their biologically active products. Since many of these products can now be measured in the plasma by radioimmunoassay (RIA), their relation to the clinical manifestations of the syndromes is being carefully examined.

Carcinoid tumors are probably a heterogeneous group of endocrine neoplasms producing many different amines and peptides. The following are those substances that have been, to date, identified as being produced by carcinoid tumors:

- Serotonin.
- 5-HTP.
- Histamine.
- Substance P.
- Motilin.
- Other substances that are possibly produced by carcinoid tumors (prostaglandin, VIP, bradykinin).

Some of these substances are believed to be of fundamental importance for the control of cell multiplication; there is a frequent association of other neoplasias in patients with carcinoid tumors: 26% of patients with carcinoid tumors have an associated independent neoplasm.

I. CLINICAL CONSIDERATIONS

The tumors may be found wherever APUD cells are present and have been identified throughout the GI tract (except in the esophagus), lungs, ovaries, testes, and thymus. The overall incidence of carcinoid tumors in the population appears to be between 1 and 2%. Although the most common site is the appendix, this particular location is associated with a very low incidence (2.9%) of metastatic spread. Metastases occur in about 35% of all cases; in addition, it is important in the

evaluation of the patient, for both management and prognosis, to be aware that another noncarcinoid neoplasm may coexist.

The manifestations of carcinoid tumors will fall into two categories:

A. Organ-Related Symptoms

The most common manifestations are related to the sequelae of the tumor:

- Bowel obstruction.
- Anemia.
- Hemoptysis.
- Rectal bleeding.
- Abdominal pain.

All these symptoms indicate the site of the primary tumor, and indeed, the florid and complete picture of the carcinoid syndrome will appear in only a small percentage of these patients.

B. Carcinoid Syndrome

The second category of manifestations is related to the carcinoid syndrome itself. Initially, the symptoms consist of episodic attacks that may be brought on by alcohol, food, emotional strain, exercise, or straining during defecation. Pharmacological provocation can be produced by alcohol, catecholamines, and calcium and pentagastrin infusions. Unless the tumor is in the lung, ovary, liver, testis, or retroperitoneal tissues, the humoral manifestations of the carcinoid syndrome are absent; humoral agents produced by the tumor are metabolized by the liver so that systemic effects do not occur while those agents are confined to the portal venous drainage area. Most carcinoid tumors occur in the gut, and their bioactive products are liberated into the portal venous system and deactivated by the liver; in those instances, therefore, the carcinoid syndrome will only become apparent when the tumor is large enough and has developed a systemic venous drainage, or if the liver is overwhelmed by metastases. Metastases are most often found within the abdominal cavity, especially in the liver; pulmonary spread is relatively common, whereas bony metastases occur more frequently with ileal carcinoids. Rectal carcinoids are very infrequently functional, whereas those from the midgut area are usually associated with the typical carcinoid syndrome.

Initially, 5-hydroxytroptamine and bradykinin were thought to be responsible for all the symptoms of the carcinoid syndrome, and in fact, many can be explained by the pharmacological actions of these substances. Often however, plasma values do not correlate with the symptoms, and it is probable that many other peptide and vasoactive substances are implicated in the genesis of the syndrome.

The following symptoms make up the carcinoid syndrome:

1. Flushing and Sweating

This is most characteristic and varies from a short-lived facial erythema to prolonged periods of violaceous and wheeled flushes, sometimes lasting for days. The clinical types described represent the action of different vasoactive peptides.

2. Diarrhea and Abdominal Colic

These may be caused either by hypermotility induced by the biologically active agents secreted by the tumors or by stimulation of intestinal secretion. Vasoactive intestinal peptides have been demonstrated to increase local small-bowel mucosal cyclic AMP levels and to produce watery diarrhea experimentally. Prostaglandins and serotonin also stimulate the fluid and electrolyte secretion of the small intestine. Somatostatin, which inhibits the actions of many peptide hormones, has been used to control this diarrhea.

3. Wheezing

This occurs in 25% of patients with the syndrome and is often associated with flushing attacks.

4. Cardiac Lesions

These primarily involve the right heart, producing tricuspid and pulmonic valve fibrosis associated with subendocardial fibrosis. In the case of bronchial carcinoids, the left side of the heart may be involved. High-output failure is the usual end result unless valvular surgery is undertaken.

5. Edema

This may be on the basis of either cardiac failure or albumin depletion from gross hepatic metastases.

6. Skin Lesions

Lesions resembling those in pellagra may be seen and are probably the result of nicotinamide deficiencies produced when dietary tryptophan is diverted to serotonin production.

II. PATHOLOGICAL CONSIDERATIONS

The morphological appearance of carcinoid tumors evident in light microscopy allows division of the tumors into five groups.

- Solid nodular nests and peripheral invading cords (22.6%).
- Trabecular or ribbon structure with frequent anastomosing pattern (21%).
- Tubular and acinar or rosettelike structure (3.2%).
- Lower or atypical differentiation (9.2%).
- Mixed tumors with combinations of any of the foregoing (43.5%).

With electron microscopy to delineate the ultrastructure, specific secretory granules can be identified in the majority of endocrine tumors. In some, the granule type can be correlated with the histological classification; in others, the secretory granules are actually identifiable as those of the presumptive parent cell, (e.g., enteroglucagonoma, gastrinoma, corticotrophinoma, and so forth). In carcinoid tumors, the secretory granules are not identifiable as such, nor is the actual product secreted known in most instances.

Most carcinoid tumors arise from the enterochromaffin (EC) or enterochromaffinlike (ECL) cells. These are known to produce serotonin, substance P, and motilin. Most bronchial and gastric carcinoids secrete 5-HTP and histamine. Bronchial carcinoids in particular may produce other peptides (especially ACTH) and can form part of the MEN-I syndrome.

III. EARLY DETECTION AND SCREENING

A. Signs of Carcinoid Tumors

Unfortunately, early signs of carcinoid tumors are not often present since the humoral substances produced by the tumor are rapidly metabolized in the normal liver; therefore, in most cases, hepatic spread will have usually taken place before symptoms of the carcinoid syndrome appear. In carcinoid tumors of the stomach, the early symptoms are often the result of the mechanical effect of the mass. Bronchial or gonadal carcinoids often manifest themselves earlier since their venous drainage is directly into the systemic circulation. The most common symptoms and signs of the various carcinoid tumors are

- Intestinal carcinoids.
  - Diarrhea, borborygmi, abdominal cramps.
  - Episodic flushing, cyanosis.
  - Pellagralike skin lesions, telangiectasia.
  - Bronchospasm.
  - Mass.
  - Clinical picture of appendicits.
- Gastric carcinoids.
  - Increased gastric acid secretion and peptic ulcers.
  - Paroxysm precipitated by spicy food or cheese.
  - Histamine production.
- Bronchial carcinoids.
  - Livid red flushing (prolonged attacks).
  - Tremulousness, anxiety, headache, and disorientation.
  - Facial and periorbital edema and sweating.
  - Salivation and lacrimation.
  - Nausea, vomiting, and explosive diarrhea.
  - Wheezing.
  - Left-sided cardiac lesions.
  - Pulmonary coin lesions.

B. Detection

Since the tumors are rare and their manifestations often bizarre and occult, it is not often feasible to screen for these lesions. Early detection, on the other hand, is dependent on a high index of suspicion and an awareness of the possibility of the condition in patients who present with unusual combinations of symptoms, particularly flushing and diarrhea. Workup and evaluation should be promptly carried out whenever suspicion is aroused. Furthermore, certain circumstances must alert the physician in any patient with symptoms suggestive of a carcinoid.

1. Previous Appendectomy

The highest incidence of carcinoid tumors is in the appendix, and often appendiceal carcinoids are inadvertently discovered at routine operation. A small but significant percentage of these may in fact have already undergone micrometastasis.

2. Previous History of Bronchial Adenoma

These tumors may be multiple and, if malignant, may metastasize. If the nature of the adenoma was originally not recog-

nized, subsequent growth of the tumor will result in the appearance of the syndrome.

IV. PRETREATMENT EVALUATION AND WORK-UP

A. Establishment of the Diagnosis

The diagnosis of carcinoid tumors is often difficult to establish and requires a combination of biochemical investigations and topographical studies. Of primary relevance is the establishment of the presence of a carcinoid lesion; thereafter, the site of the lesion should be identified. Once this has been ascertained, the presence of metastatic disease must be evaluated.

1. Physical Evaluation

Often the diagnosis is made only by serendipidity, although specific symptoms such as colicky abdominal pain, hemoptysis, rectal bleeding, diarrhea, or the development of the classical clinical syndrome may focus attention on the pathology.

a. History

- Diarrhea, abdominal cramps, borborygmus.
- Episodic flushing, cyanosis, facial edema, sweating.
- Pellagralike skin rashes, telegiectasia, patchy erythema.
- Salivation, lacrimation.
- Wheezing, hemoptysis.
- Peptic ulcer symptoms, paroxysms precipitated by spicy food.
- Nausea, vomiting, rectal bleeding.
- Tremulousness, anxiety, disorientation, headaches.

b. Physical Examination

- Abdominal examination: masses, liver enlargement, ascites.
- Chest examination: bronchospasm.
- Cardiac examination: valvular lesions, failure.

2. Routine Clinical Laboratory Tests

Routine clinical laboratory tests are rarely helpful:

- CBC may show leukocytosis and thrombocytosis.
- SMA-12 and liver function tests may reveal only a modest elevation of the alkaline phosphatase with a normal serum bilirubin.

- Hypoproteinemia and hypoalbuminemia indicate advanced disease.
- Chest x-ray may indentify a coin lesion or cardiomegaly.
- Liver scan may indicate multiple filling defects suggestive of hepatic metastases, and a liver biopsy in such cases is useful in confirming the nature of the tumor.
- Stool examination for occult blood. Bleeding from the gut may result from mucosal ulceration occasionally indicating the presence of an ileal tumor.

3. Biochemical Assessment

Many carcinoid tumors secrete one or several substances, other than serotonin, that can be identified in the plasma of many patients:

- Urinary 5-HIAA, the final degradation product of serotonin.
- Plasma and urinary serotonin.
- Plasma pancreatic polypeptide.
- Plasma substance P.
- Plasma histamine.
- Plasma 5-HTP.
- Plasma prostaglandins.

4. Provocative Tests

In certain individuals, the tumor may be biochemically covert and can be more easily diagnosed by the use of provocative tests. These stimulate the liberation of serotonin and other amines or peptides into the plasma in larger amounts and thus facilitate the diagnosis.

a. Calcium Infusion

A 3-hour IV infusion of 2 mg per kilogram of calcium gluconate raises the serum calcium to about 14 mg % and releases tumor substances into the blood. Side effects include tingling sensations, muscle cramps, nausea, and on rare occasions, EKG changes.

b. Alcohol Ingestion

A dose of 30–40 ml of whiskey releases tumor secretions into the blood and provokes symptoms, especially flushing.

c. Secretin (IV Bolus)

This is usually effective only in gastrin-secreting tumors.

d. Catecholamine Infusions

This may produce unpleasant side effects by evoking a carcinoid paroxysm.

B. Topographical Localization

1. Chest X-ray and CAT Scan of the Chest

This is useful in the detection of bronchial adenomas or identification of pulmonary metastases.

2. Upper GI Series

This may reveal

- Polypoid lesions of the stomach, duodenum, and jejunum.
- Multiple lesions in the ileum.
- Narrowing of the intestinal lumen secondary to a tumor mass.
- Adjacent fibrous tissue reaction with kinking.

3. Gastroscopy

This may demonstrate lesions in the stomach or duodenum, and a biopsy under direct vision will then establish the diagnosis.

4. Proctosigmoidoscopy

Rectal carcinoid can be identified by proctosigmoidoscopy; these tumors are, however, generally nonfunctional, and identification is often serendipitous.

5. Bronchoscopy

Flexible fiberoptic bronchoscopy will allow visualization and even biopsy of proximal adenomas in the bronchus.

6. Selective Celiac and Superior Mesenteric Arteriography

The following characteristics may be indentifiable:

- A satellite arterial pattern.
- Narrowing of the mesenteric vessels.
- Poor-to-moderate accumulation of the contrast medium.
- Nonvisualization of veins.
- Hepatic metastases are highly vascular, and the simultaneous injection of epinephrine markedly enhances tumor staining by contrast.

7. CAT Scan

CAT Scan of the abdomen and pelvis may locate the primary tumor and identify any liver or local metastases.

C. General Medical Evaluation

The complex nature of the disease, the serious complications (pulmonary, cardiac, fibrosis, etc.) that may result, and the delicate nature of the therapy make it mandatory that the patient be thoroughly evaluated prior to therapy. This evaluation must include

- Pulmonary assessment and pulmonary function tests.
- Cardiac evaluation.
- Endocrine evaluation to rule out MEA.
- Gastroenterologic evaluation, etc.

D. Metastatic Evaluation

Because of the high incidence of metastatic spread in patients with carcinoid tumors, a full metastatic survey is indicated:

- Chest x-ray, with CAT scan if indicated.
- SMA-12.
- Liver scan.
- Bone scan.

In addition, because of the high incidence ($> 25\%$) of concomitant neoplasms, one should be attuned to the possibility of other tumors, and further investigations should be pursued as indicated by any symptom or physical finding.

E. Multidisciplinary Approach

Since carcinoid tumors can occur in one of several organs and affect a number of different systems and physiological mechanisms, a group approach is advisable. The tumors can alter different physiological parameters not only by their spread into different systems but also by the bioactive nature of their secretions. Thus, a bronchial carcinoid may present as a pulmonary problem, yet the associated cardiac valvular lesions and diarrhea require the expertise of a cardiologist, cardiac surgeon, and gastroenterologist. Furthermore these tumors are often particularly show growing and reasonably amenable to cytotoxics; thus, the participation of personnel skilled in chemotherapy is mandatory in choosing the appropriate therapy. The cooperation of surgeons, internists, and oncologists is probably more intensely required in the management of these tumors than in any other condition. Furthermore, the diffuse nature of the spread of the disease, the wide systemic biologic effects of the tumor, and the often prolonged clinical course of the disease necessitates a long-term multidisciplinary interaction of physicians and other professionals.

F. Site-Specific Data Form for Carcinoid Tumors (see p. 209)

V. THERAPEUTIC MANAGEMENT

A. Pharmacological Therapy

A significant percentage of patients with carcinoid tumors may not be amenable to curative surgery since the tumor often presents at a late stage in the disease process when metastases have already occurred. Even in the resectable tumor, anesthesia or surgery itself carry a significant risk and may provoke a carcinoid paroxysm. Thus, careful pharmacological blockade of the tumor should be instituted preoperatively to minimize the risk of a crisis. Furthermore, long-term postoperative pharmacological therapy may be necessary in patients with residual or recurrent disease after surgery. Applicable pharmacological agents and their uses follow:

- Parachlorophenylalanine. This drug is a competitive inhibitor of serotonin synthesis. It is useful in the relief of nausea, vomiting and diarrhea but less effective in the control of flushing. Side effects include altered central nervous system function.
- Methysergide maleate. This is a serotonin anatagonist and can be used as an IV bolus dose to control acute attacks. It is particularly effective in the control of diarrhea, but patients can develop hypotension, weakness, and tachyphylaxis. Serious side effects can occur, including fluid retention and fibrotic lesions of the retroperitoneum and cardiac valves.
- Cyproheptadine. This agent is also a serotonin antagonist and can be used for the control of acute attacks or for long-term relief. It is particularly effective in the control of flushing and lacks the fibroproliferative propensities of methysergide.
- Antihistamines. These are of occasional value.
- Corticosteroids. These may be of some value in bronchial carcinoids (15–40 mg per day).
- Prochlorperazine. This agent is helpful in some cases of flushing (10 mg 3–4 times per day).
- Phenoxybenzamine. Phenoxybenzamine (10–30 mg per day) is also useful in the treatment of flushing.
- Methyldopa. Methyldopa (250–500 mg 4 times per day) may be of occasional value in the control of diarrhea.
- Cholestyramine. This agent is used if diarrhea is secondary to ileal resection (4–8 mg 4 times per day).

B. Surgical Therapy

The primary treatment of carcinoid tumors is surgical excision. The extent of the ablative procedure is dependent upon the tumor location, its size, and the absence or presence of metastatic disease. When the tumors are small and localized, the results are excellent, with 5-year survival rates in excess of 90%. Even when the regional lymph nodes are involved with metastatic disease, the 5-year survival rate still tends to be quite good. Furthermore, even in unresectable tumors or in patients with metastatic disease, the removal of as much tumor bulk as possible has been shown to improve the symptoms of the carcinoid syndrome and to have a beneficial effect on survival, since most carcinoids are slow-growing tumors. In patients with residual or recurrent tumor after resection and in those in whom surgery is precluded due to extensive metastatic disease, poor general condition, or medical contraindications, two approaches to treatment are available: pharmacological therapy to ameliorate those unpleasant symptoms caused by the elaboration of biologically active mediators by the carcinoid tumor, and cytotoxic chemotherapy aimed at killing the tumor cells.

The primary aim of surgery is to remove the tumor and as much metastatic tissue as is feasible. Once the carcinoid syndrome is present, cure is not often possible, since this usually implies the presence of hepatic metastases. On rare ocasions, however, when the tumor is ovarian or bronchial in origin, complete cure may be achieved.

Before subjecting the patient with carcinoid syndrome to surgery, the diarrhea and other symptoms of the syndrome should be controlled, if possible. Any fluid deficits and electrolyte abnormalities must be rectified. Consideration must be given to the correction of niacin deficiency and any other nutritional deficits such as hypoproteinemia consequent to prolonged diarrhea and malabsorption. The importance of closely monitoring the EKG, blood pressure, CVP, serum electrolytes, and arterial blood gases during induction and maintenance of anesthesia cannot be over emphasized. Physiological monitoring should be continued through the early postoperative period.

In the absence of clinical features of the syndrome, anesthesia presents no extraordinary difficulty, since no humoral products are involved. In the presence of the carcinoid syndrome, however, anesthesia and its concomitant physiological stimuli (such as release of catecholamines) may initiate the release of serotonin, bradykinin, or other substances secreted by the carcinoid tumor. Administration of beta-adrenergic receptor agonists and anesthetic agents known to release endogenous catecholamines should be avoided (beta-adrenergic agonists stimulate tumor kallikrein, an enzyme that catalyzes the formation of bradykinin from a serum, alpha-2-globulin). Likewise, anesthetic agents known to release endogenous catecholamines

should not be used. Such agents may result in profound flushing, hypotension, and bronchospasm, sometimes referred to as "bradykinin shock."

The preferred anesthetic technique includes preoperative administration of an antiserotinin (methysergide or cyproheptadine) and an antibradykinin (trasylol or epsilon-aminocaproic acid), as well as a sedative. Smooth induction with avoidance of hypotension and gentle intubation after local and topical anesthetic administration to the larynx, are extremely important. Pancuronium bromide is the muscle relaxant of choice, and nitrous oxide and oxygen are best supplemented with phenoperidine or fentanyl.

If hypotension occurs during anesthesia, colloids and crystalloids must be rapidly administered to fill the vascular space, since vasodilation is the most likely cause. If a vasoconstrictor agent is required, alpha-receptor agonists such as phenylephrine or methoxamine should be used since they will not cause flushing.

Tumors should be resected using the same principles as govern the resection of any malignant neoplasm; the fibrosis present may render this difficult in some cases and may, at times, even threaten the anastomoses with ischemia in the case of bowel neoplasms.

1. Small-Bowel Carcinoid

Wide radical excision of the lesion is necessary. Of particular importance is the necessity to excise adequately the lymphatic drainage area of the mesentery.

2. Appendix Carcinoid

Most appendiceal carcinoids are discovered incidentally by the pathologist after a standard appendectomy has been performed. If a carcinoid tumor of the appendix is recognized at operation, serious consideration of a right hemicolectomy is appropriate. This is mandatory if serosal extension of the tumor or lymph node involvement is evident.

3. Rectal Carcinoid

Carcinoids of the rectum are nonfunctional tumors in the vast majority of cases. They are, therefore, usually discovered at biopsy of what is often thought to be an adenocarcinoma of the rectum. Surgical management is therefore the same as that of rectal carcinoma.

4. Gastric Carcinoid

These tumors usually present late and are often not amenable to curative resection. Occasionally, a palliative gastrectomy will be indicated to prevent bleeding from ulcerating tumor masses.

SITE-SPECIFIC DATA FORM—CARCINOID TUMORS

HISTORY

Age: _____ Sex: _____

Symptoms
- _____ Flushing
- _____ Cyanosis
- _____ Edema
- _____ Sweating
- _____ Wheezing
- _____ Hemoptysis
- _____ Paroxysmal attacks
- _____ Skin lesions
- _____ Telangiectasia
- _____ Borborygmi
- _____ Diarrhea
- _____ Abdominal cramps
- _____ Nausea, vomiting
- _____ Peptic ulcer symptoms
- _____ Rectal bleeding
- _____ Weight loss _____ lbs.

Duration of symptoms: _____

Social history
  Occupation: _____
  Race: ____ White ____ Black ____ Oriental ____ Other
  Smoker: ____ Yes ____ No   How much? _____
  Drinker: ____ Yes ____ No   How often? _____

Family history of carcinoma
  Relation: _____ Site: _____
Previous history of carcinoma
  ____ No ____ Yes   Site: _____
  Rx: _____
Previous treatment (describe):
(Surgery, radiation, chemotherapy,
tracheostomy, etc.)
_____
_____

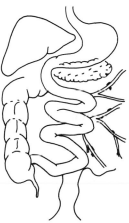

PHYSICAL EXAMINATION

General: _____
Cardiopulmonary: _____
Abdomen: _____

	Yes	No
Mass:	_____	_____
Visceromegaly	_____	_____
which organ: _____		
Ascites	_____	_____
Tenderness	_____	_____
Rectal mass	_____	_____

Site of tumor (describe): _____
Size of tumor: _____

PREOPERATIVE EVALUATION (Check, if done)

	Neg.	Pos.	Suspicious			Neg.	Pos.	Suspicious
CBC	_____	_____	_____		Gastroscopy	_____	_____	_____
SMA-12	_____	_____	_____		Bronchoscopy	_____	_____	_____
Chest x-ray	_____	_____	_____		Arteriography	_____	_____	_____
Liver scan	_____	_____	_____		CAT scan	_____	_____	_____
Serotonin	_____	_____	_____		Other	_____		
5 HIAA	_____	_____	_____					
Provocative tests	_____	_____	_____					
UGI series	_____	_____	_____					

Operative staging
  Site: _____
  Size: _____
  Character: _____

	Yes	No
Mesenteric involvement	_____	_____
Lymph node involvement	_____	_____
Ascites	_____	_____
Hepatic	_____	_____
Pulmonary	_____	_____

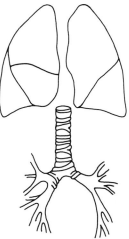

Signature: _____
Countersignature: _____
Date: _____

5. Bronchial Carcinoid

It is desirable to obtain histological confirmation of the lesion prior to definitive surgery; great care should be exercised at the time of biopsy since the tumors are often extremely vascular. The majority of carcinoids of the bronchus are resectable at the time of diagnosis; even in patients with carcinoid syndrome, removal of as much as possible of the tumor will facilitate further treatment. Because of the malignant potential of these neoplasms, the occurrence of irreversible bronchiectasis distal to the obstructing lesion, and the frequent delay concerning the histological interpretation of its malignancy, lobectomy is the advocated procedure of choice in those bronchial adenomas that are confined to a lobar or segmental bronchus. Pneumonectomy and hilar lymphadenectomy are required for neoplasms of the proximal main bronchus with extrabronchial extension or hilar invasion.

6. Hepatic Carcinoid Metastases

Carcinoid tumors are relatively slow growing, and patients can survive many years in spite of evidence of metastatic spread. Since many of the unpleasant symptoms are due to the bioactive agents secreted by the tumor and its secondaries, the ablation of as much tumor as possible is often of great benefit to the patient, even in the case of overt metastases. There are a number of different methods available for such a palliative approach:

- Tumor enucleation.
- Hepatic lobectomy.
- Hepatic arterial ligation.
- Hepatic arterial perfusion with cytotoxics.
- Tumor embolization (via a percutaneous transfemoral route).
- Delivery of radioactive spheres via the hepatic artery.

C. Adjunctive Therapy

In most patients, there will be residual neoplasm left after surgery, and the symptoms of the carcinoid syndrome will eventually return. Amelioration of this problem can be achieved by a number of different methods.

1. Radiation Therapy

Large-field irradiation has been reported to be of little value in the management of carcinoid tumors since a substantial dose (5500–6000 rads) is needed for effective control. On the other hand, the local delivery of radioactive microspheres to the liver via the hepatic artery has met with some encouraging results, and some tumors may prove to be unusually radiosensitive.

2. Cytotoxic Therapy

Since the disease is indolent in its course in a large number of cases, it seems prudent to withhold the initiation of chemotherapy in early metastatic disease; it should probably only be used when the standard pharmacological measures described above have failed. Furthermore, extreme caution should be exercised; if the cytotoxic agents are rapidly effective, massive tumor lysis may occur, with the onset of an acute carcinoid crisis. No predictably effective or specific chemotherapeutic agent exists for carcinoid tumors; there are a few reports of effective therapy using either methotrexate, 5-FU, cyclophosphamide, or cytosine arabinoside. The combination of streptozotocin and 5-FU seems so far to have produced the best results.

The indications for cytotoxic chemotherapy are rapidly progressive metastatic disease and failure to control the symptoms of carcinoid syndrome with surgery or pharmocological agents.

3. Pharmacological Therapy

The various pharmacological agents described in the preoperative preparation of the patient with a carcinoid tumor can also be used as an adjuvant modality for the control of symptoms in two settings: residual of recurrent disease following surgery and patients in whom surgery is precluded because of advanced metastatic disease or other medical contraindications to surgery.

VI. POSTOPERATIVE CARE, EVALUATION, AND FOLLOW-UP

A. Postoperative Care

The usual postoperative care required for any surgery in the abdomen or chest is indicated in these cases as well. The care will vary depending on the location of the tumor.

1. Gastrointestinal Tumors

The use of nasogastric drainage as indicated, IV fluids and electrolytes, drainage and wound care, etc. must be observed. Monitoring of vital signs, intake and output, blood gas determinations, etc. is most important. Pulmonary toilet, analgesics, and antibiotics are administered as needed.

2. Bronchial Tumors

Pulmonary toilet and inhalation therapy, chest tube drainage, antibiotics, and analgesics must be attended to as in all thoracic operations.

Table I

Long-Term Follow-Up Schedule for Carcinoid Tumors

Management	First three months monthly	First-to-third year				Fourth year and thereafter	
		3 Months	6 Months	9 Months	12 Months	Every 6 months	Annually
History							
Appetite	X	X	X	X	X	X	X
Weight	X	X	X	X	X	X	X
Diarrhea	X	X	X	X	X	X	X
Abdominal colic	X	X	X	X	X	X	X
Flushing	X	X	X	X	X	X	X
Wheezing	X	X	X	X	X	X	X
Shortness of breath	X	X	X	X	X	X	X
Bleeding	X	X	X	X	X	X	X
Headache	X	X	X	X	X	X	X
Anxiety	X	X	X	X	X	X	X
Physical							
Weight	X	X	X	X	X	X	X
Telangiectasia	X	X	X	X	X	X	X
Flushing	X	X	X	X	X	X	X
Ascites	X	X	X	X	X	X	X
Abdominal mass	X	X	X	X	X	X	X
Liver	X	X	X	X	X	X	X
Lymph nodes	X	X	X	X	X	X	X
Chest	X	X	X	X	X	X	X
Investigations							
Urinary 5-HIAA	X	X	X	X	X	X	X
Serotonin (plasma and urine)	X	X	X	X	X	X	X
Other markers (specific cases)	X	X	X	X	X	X	X
CBC		X	X	X	X	X	X
SMA-12		X	X	X	X	X	X
Chest x-ray		X		X			X
Liver scan				As indicated			
CAT scan				As indicated			

B. Nutritional Support

A nutritious diet containing at least 70 g of protein is important. Fat content may need to be limited, especially in patients with ileal resection, but adequate caloric and vitamin intake is paramount. Niacin is particularly necessary to avoid the development of pellagralike symptoms. In addition, the patient should be instructed to avoid foods that initiate carcinoid paroxysms: alcohol, milk products, eggs, and citrus fruits may need to be eliminated from the diet. Intractable diarrhea may need to be treated with diphenoxylate (Lomotil) or loperamide (Imodium).

C. Psychosocial Support

The same psychosocial support recommended in the management of other malignancies should be offered to patients with carcinoid tumors, particularly so if they suffer from the carcinoid syndrome with all its symptomatic effects.

D. Follow-Up Evaluation

Patients treated for carcinoid tumors must remain under observation and treatment for an indefinite time. Pharmacological therapy must be professionally controlled and the progression of the disease regularly evaluated. Those patients that are rendered free of disease should also be evaluated at regular intervals. Table I recommends a schedule for such an evaluation.

VII. MANAGEMENT ALGORITHM FOR CARCINOID TUMORS

(see p. 212)

ALGORITHM FOR CARCINOID TUMORS

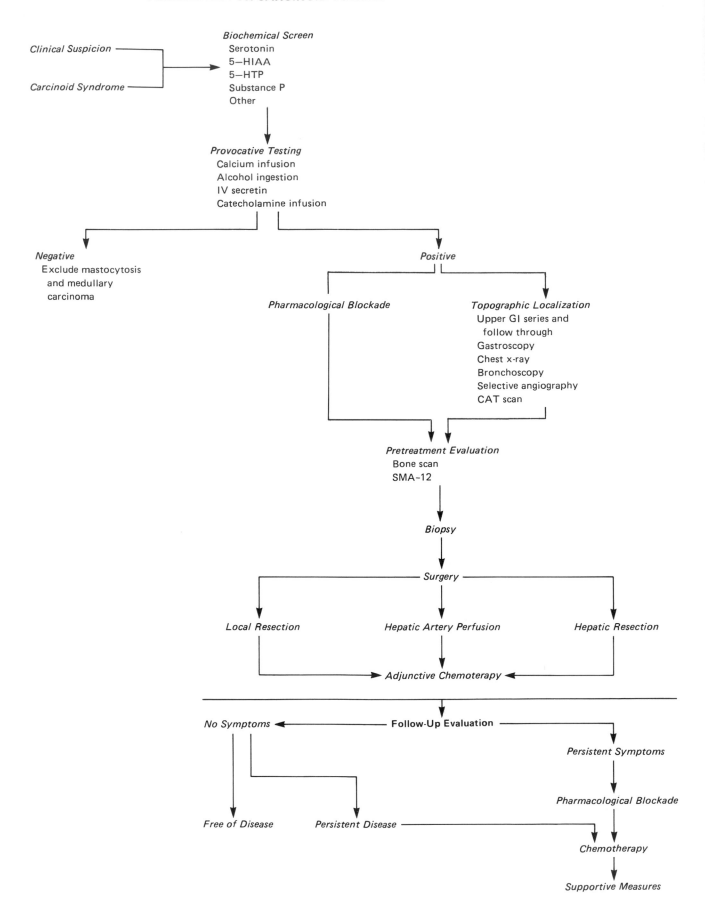

Section 5

Tumors of the Skeletal System

HUBERT S. PEARLMAN

With Contributions By

Mukund R. Patel	Orthopedic Surgery
Alan M. Crystal	Orthopedic Surgery
Rene A. Khafif	Surgical Oncology
Sameer Rafla	Radiotherapy
Samuel Kopel	Medical Oncology
Ari Feibel	Rehabilitation
Mario Anselmo	Pathology
Margaret Amato	Nursing Oncology

Section 5. Tumors of the Skeletal System

I. Introduction   217
  A. Definition and Nomenclature
  B. Characteristics
    1. General Characteristics, Radiology, and Pathology
    2. Anatomic Location of the Lesion
    3. Age Predilection of Bone Tumors
  C. Behavior of Bone Tumors
  D. Differential Diagnosis of Bone Tumors

II. Early Detection and Screening   226
  A. Patient Education
  B. Early Signs and Symptoms
  C. Preventive Measures

III. Pretreatment Evaluation and Work-Up   227
  A. History and Physical Examination
    1. History
    2. Physical Examination
  B. Laboratory Findings
    1. Serum Calcium and Phosphorus
    2. Serum Proteins and Electrophoresis
    3. Alkaline and Acid Phosphatase
    4. Routine Laboratory Studies
  C. Radiological Evaluation
    1. General Considerations
      a. Detection and Screening
      b. Documentation and Histologic Identification
      c. Differential Diagnosis
      d. Metastatic Evaluation
      e. Therapeutic Considerations
      f. Follow-Up Evaluation
    2. Specific Procedures
      a. Routine X-ray Studies
      b. Additional Techniques
    3. Diagnostic Clues
      a. Patterns of Destruction
      b. Indications of Aggressiveness
  D. Bone Scan
  E. Staging
  F. Diagnostic Clues
  G. Biopsy
  H. General Medical Evaluation
  I. Site-Specific Data Form for Bone Tumors
  J. Multidisciplinary Consultation

IV. Therapeutic Management   234
  A. Surgical Management
    1. Selection of the Extent of Surgery

    2. Operative Procedures Available
      a. Curettage
      b. Marginal Resection
      c. Wide Excision
      d. Radical Excision
      e. Amputation
      f. Conservation Resection with Reconstruction
      g. Palliative Procedures
    3. Therapeutic Approach by Type of Tumor
      a. Self-Healing Lesions
      b. Benign Locally Aggressive Lesions
      c. Low-Grade Malignancy
      d. High-Grade Malignancy
      e. Metastatic Carcinoma
  B. Radiotherapy
    1. Primary Bone Tumors
      a. Osteosarcoma
      b. Ewing's Sarcoma
      c. Giant-Cell Tumors
      d. Other Primary Tumors
    2. Metastatic Bone Disease
  C. Chemotherapy
    1. Adjuvant Chemotherapy in Osteogenic Sarcoma
    2. Palliative Chemotherapy in Metastatic Disease
    3. Chemotherapy in Ewing's Sarcoma

V. Postoperative Care, Evaluation, and Rehabilitation   243
  A. Postoperative Care
    1. Immobilization
    2. Care of Amputation
    3. Precautions for Internal Prosthesis
  B. Follow-up Evaluation
  C. Rehabilitation
    1. The Amputee
      a. Preoperative Preparation
      b. The Prosthesis
      c. Conditioning and Training
      d. Educational and Vocational Rehabilitation
    2. The Patient with Metastatic Disease
    3. Pain Management
  D. Nursing and Psychosocial Aspects of Aftercare
    1. Body Image Disturbance
    2. Coping with the Loss of a Body Part
    3. Age of the Patient
    4. Physical Care of the Patient

VI. Management Algorithm for Bone Tumors   248

Suggested Readings   248

I. INTRODUCTION

A. Definition and Nomenclature

Bone tumors can be subdivided according to their cell of origin; these cells may be cartilaginous, osseous, mesenchymal, fibrous, hematopoietic, embryonal, neurogenic, or, simply, collagen (see Fig. 1).

Benign bone tumors include:

- Nonmalignant osseous tumors: osteoid osteomas or osteoblastomas.
- Cartilaginous tumors: benign osteochondromas that become exostoses and primary cartilaginous tumors, namely, endochondromas and chrondroblastomas.
- Mesenchymal tumors and those of somewhat mixed stromal origin. These are the commonest and include the simple bone cyst, benign chrondromyxofibroma, aneurysmal bone cyst, and fibrous dysplasia. The giant-cell bone tumor is essentially a benign lesion, but it displays characteristics of local malignant behavior (invasion, recurrence, etc.).
- Tumors within bones and hematopoietic origin that are benign may be hemangiomas, hemangiopericytomas, or eosinophilic granulomas.
- Fibrous benign lesions: fibrous dysplasia and nonossifying fibroma.
- Neurilemmoma is the benign tumor of neural origin.

The great majority of malignant tumors of bone are metastatic. The most common tumors of osseous origin are:

- The highly malignant osteogenic sarcoma with its slightly less aggressive form, the juxtacortical osteogenic sarcoma.
- Chondrosarcoma is the malignant counterpart of cartilage cell tumors and is much less aggressive than osteogenic sarcoma.
- Giant-cell tumors may be considered mesenchymal and are often locally malignant, although extremely slow growing.
- Ewing's sarcoma, reticulum cell sarcoma.
- Histiocytic Lymphoma may present with osseous lesion.
- Plasmacytoma arising in a bone.
- Fibrosarcomas are malignant tumors of fibrous origin.

- Embryonal notochord tumors present in the spine as malignant chordomas.
- Neuroblastomas are neurogenic tumors within bone, often metastatic.

Table I summarizes the above classification of primary bone tumors.

A simpler classification of bone tumors was devised by Jaffe and is based on the site of the tumor:

- Tumors that are primary in bone (e.g., osteochondroma, chondrosarcoma).
- Tumors that arise adjacent to bone (e.g., juxtacortical osteogenic sarcoma).
- Tumors originating from hematopoietic tissue within bone (e.g., Ewing's sarcoma, multiple myeloma).
- Metastatic tumors to bone (arising primarily from breast, prostate, lung, kidney, or thyroid).
- Tumors that arise in bone secondary to noxious agents (e.g., osteogenic sarcoma in radium-dial watch painters).

B. Characteristics

Since biopsy of bone tumors is not always simple and can often only be done operatively, and since biopsy reports are often delayed because of the need to decalcify the specimen, it is most important to try to recognize and distinguish the various bone tumors on the basis of their clinical and radiologic characteristics, as well as their gross appearance at the time of surgery.

1. General Characteristics, Radiology, and Pathology

The general characteristics of bone tumors are summarized in Table II.

It is important to point out that the two most important factors, next to the radiologic appearance of the lesion, are the site of involvement within the bony framework and the age of the patient at the time of presentation.

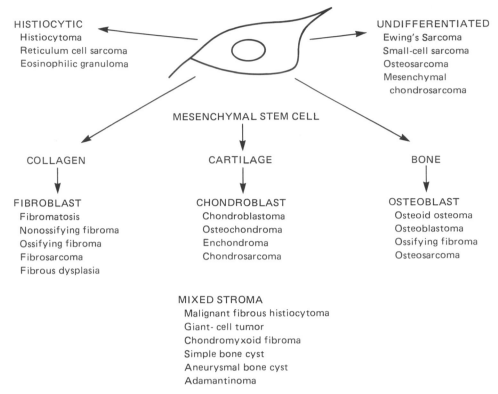

Fig. 1.   Histogenesis of mesenchymal tumors. See text for discussion.

2. Anatomic Location of the Lesion

The following general site guidelines are useful in assessing a bone tumor.

- Upper humerus. Benign bone cysts frequently involve the upper humerus. They may be quite large, and as much as half the shaft may be thinned out by the lesion; this will amost inevitably produce a pathologic fracture. Aneurysmal bone cysts also involve this area but may be found anywhere, which is also true of osteoid osteomas and Codman's tumor, or benign chondroblastoma. Benign bone cysts can grow through the shaft distal to the proximal epiphyseal line. Chondroblastomas, on the other hand, arise in the area just proximal to the epiphyseal plate and can be confused with a Brodie's abscess. All these entities are peculiar to children and young adults.
- Elbow. The elbow itself is usually spared tumor involvement, but the proximal radius is often the site of various cystic lesions that will affect the elbow with the attendant risk of radial-nerve injury.
- Distal radius. The distal radius is a frequent site of giant-cell tumors occurring in patients between the ages of 20 and 50.
- Hand. The hand is more frequently the site of endochondromas and hemangioendotheliomas and their malig-

nant counterparts, with pain and enlargement as the usual presenting symptoms.
- Spine. The spine is the site of predilection for chordomas; these are specifically found in the sacrum or in the clivus of the skull. In addition, metastatic carcinoma, multiple myeloma, and Paget's disease present in the spine and are frequent causes of low back pain.
- Shoulder girdle. The clavicle and scapula are common sites of several difficult-to-diagnose painful conditions.
- Pelvis. The pelvis can be a confusing site of pathology. Paget's disease and metastatic prostatic cancer frequently present in this site and are often difficult to differentiate. Appropriate laboratory tests are useful here, the alkaline phosphatase usually being elevated in the former and the acid phosphatase in the latter. Bone biopsy is sometimes necessary to establish a definitive diagnosis.
- Lower extremities. The lower extremities are the most frequent site of osteogenic sarcoma, particularly around the knee. This tumor has its peak incidence at the age of 16 and is seldom seen before 12 or after 19 years of age. Unexplained swelling or pain prompting an x-ray examination will usually reveal the diagnosis. Peculiar to the tibia is the adamantinoma, a tumor that also appears in the skull and in the mandible. Ewing's sarcoma can involve any bone but is also most often seen in the femur and tibia; when it starts

Table I

Classification of Primary Bone Tumors

	Benign	Malignant
Cartilaginous	Osteochondroma Chondroma Chondroblastoma	Chondrosarcoma
Osseous	Osteoma Osteoid osteoma Osteoblastoma Callus	Paget's disease degenerating into osteosarcoma Telangiectatic osteosarcoma Periosteal osteosarcoma Parosteal osteosarcoma Multicentric osteosarcoma Post irradiation osteosarcoma Dedifferentiated chondrosarcoma Low-grade central osteosarcoma Juxtacortical osteosarcoma
Mesenchymal	Giant-cell tumor Chondromyxoid fibroma Simple cysts Aneurysmal bone cysts Adamantinoma	Giant-cell tumor Mesenchymal chondrosarcoma
Hematopoietic	Hemangioma Hemangiopericytoma Eosinophilic granuloma	Myeloma Lymphoma Ewing's sarcoma Angiosarcoma
Fibrous	Nonossifying fibroma Fibrous dysplasia	Fibrosarcoma
Synovial	Synovial chondromatosis	Synovial sarcoma
Neural	Neurilemmoma	Chordoma

with elevated temperature, swelling, and pain, it mimics osteomyelitis.

Examination of the literature shows that no bone, not even the sesamoid bones, is immune from tumor involvement. Certain anatomic sites are, however, at greater risk. Tables III and IV identify such predilections.

3. Age Predilection of Bone Tumors

Table V lists the age predilection of the various bone tumors.

a. Young Children (Under 6 Years of Age)

Neuroblastoma is probably the most common malignant bone tumor at this age; it usually presents as a round-cell metastatic tumor. Fibrous dysplasia, eosinophilic granulomas, and unicameral bone cysts can also be seen at this age. Ewing's sarcoma is also a tumor of the very young.

b. Teen Years

Chondroblastoma, eosinophilic granuloma, osteochondroma, osteoid osteoma, as well as the previously mentioned fibrous

cortical defect and fibrous dysplasia are benign diseases of the young (i.e., usually under the age of 20); this helps in the differential diagnosis. Chondrosarcoma, except in malignant degeneration of an endochondroma, osteogenic sarcoma, Ewing's sarcoma, and occasionally chordoma are the malignant bone tumors of the young (usually under age 18).

c. The Young Adult

The most common bone tumors seen between the ages of 20 and 40 are benign giant-cell tumors and endochondromas. Occasionally an eosinophilic granuloma, neurilemmoma, chondromyxofibroma, osteoblastoma, adamantinoma, hemangioma, or hemangioendothelioma can present at this age. Malignant tumors of any type are also found at this age, particularly parosteal osteosarcomas, fibrosarcomas, and malignant histiocytomas.

d. Adult Years

The commonest malignant bone tumor in the adult is metastatic carcinoma of bone. Prostate cancer in the older male and breat cancer in the middle-aged and older female constitute the majority of these cases. Renal cancer and lung cancer will also metastasize to bone and even to remote bony sites such as the terminal phalanges; it is not uncommon to have the bone metastasis clinically apparent well before the primary tumor is recognized. Metastatic thyroid tumors often affect bones and may, at times, be identifiable by radioactive iodine uptake. Other carcinomas seldom invade bone, although back pain is often a presenting sign of a malignant tumor. This is particularly so in the gastrointestinal tract and pancreas where the backache is frequently not related to actual bone metastases but rather to pressure effects.

Other malignant tumors of the adult and elderly that involve the bones include myelomas, leukemias, and melanomas.

C. Behavior of Bone Tumors

Another method of classifying bone tumors pertains to their behavior and natural history, as well as to the host response they elicit. Tumors of bone can thus be subdivided into three categories:

- Self-healing lesions
  - Eosinophilic granuloma.
  - Cortical desmoid.
  - Unifocal fibrous dysplasia.
  - Osteoid osteoma.
  - Unicameral cysts.
  - Ossifying fibroma (Companacci's disease)
- Benign, aggressive lesions
  - Fibrous dysplasia.

Table II

General Characteristics of Bone Tumors

Tumor	Sex/age prevalence	Most common site	Radiologic characteristics	Gross features	Microscopic features	Miscellaneous characteristics
Osteochondroma	M > F Second-to-third decade	Metaphyseal, long bones 50% in the femur and humerus		Bony protuberance with thick cartilaginous capsule Pedunculated or sessile, arises at tendon insertion 2–3 mm to 1 cm in size (> 3 cm indicates a sarcomatous change)	Trabecular bone capped by hyaline cartilage	Most common tumor in bone May be multiple: osteochondromatosis (10% of these are malignant)
Chondroma (enchondroma)	Even distribution	Diaphyseal, rarely in the pelvis 40% in the hands and feet	Rarefaction with stippled calcification (to be differentiated from the peripheral calcification of bone infarction)	Lobular, bluish and semitranslucent; may be mucinous	Proliferation of cartilaginous cells with small, uniform nuclei	Usually curable by curettage Ollier's disease: multiple unilateral chondromas, 30% → chondrosarcoma Mafucci's syndrome: multiple lesions associated with soft-tissue angiomas
Chondroblastoma	M > F = 3 : 2 50% in the second decade	Epiphyseal (may extend to the metaphysis) Knee and proximal femur In the older patients, long bones spared	Lucent, sharply demarcated, lobulated Thin margin of increased density No periosteal reaction 25% calcification Differentiated from chondromas, chondrosarcomas and chondromyxoid fibromas	Lobulated and sharply demarcated 1–7 cm in size Thin rim of sclerotic bone Sometimes cystic	Polygonal or round cells Giant cells common Chondroid material may be present Lacy cacification	Is rarely aggressive, with occasional large recurrences May rarely become a sarcoma Rarely spreads to lung Will rarely recur after curretage
Chondromyxoid fibroma	M > F Second-to third decade	Metaphyseal (may extend to the epiphysis) 65% in long bones 33% in the tibias	Sharply circumscribed Eccentric, may result in expansion of the bone Trabecular Occasional peripheral sclerosis	Lobular, sharply demarcated Resembles hyaline cartilage Corrugations of the inner surface of the cavity	Chondroid, myxoid, and fibroid areas Lobular pattern, cells may be large multinucleated, or present with irregular nuclei Small focuses of calcification may be present Occasional fields of chondroblasts	Rare tumor

Table II (*Continued*)

Tumor	Sex/age prevalence	Most common site	Radiologic characteristics	Gross features	Microscopic features	Miscellaneous characteristics
Osteoma	F > M	Circumscribed area in the skull and facial bones: Outer table of skull Paranasal sinus		Circumscribed area of hard bone, nodular, ivory in appearance	Dense, bony tissue	Variants: Gardner's syndrome with intestinal polyposis, multiple fibromas, and inclusion cysts; juxtacortical osteomas; medullary osteoma; endostosis (bone islands)
Osteoid osteoma	M > F Almost all in the first three decades Predominates in the second	Diaphyseal or metaphyseal 50% in the femur or tibia	Lucent nidus surrounded by sclerotic bone Rarely → periosteal lamination simulating Ewing's sarcoma	Discrete round or oval nidus Reddish 1 cm, if larger overlaps with osteoblastoma	Complex network of osteoid and bony trabeculae with osteoblasts line up along the trabeculae and fibrovascular tissue and giant cells in the intertrabecular spaces. No cartilage	Severe pain, relieved by ASA
Osteoblastoma	M > F First three decades, peaks in the second	50% in vertebrae or sacrum 50% in long-bone diaphyses Mostly in the medulla, but may be cortical or subperiosteal	Variable calcification Lucent, often not well circumscribed May appear malignant Medullary lesion, no sclerosis	2–10 cm, reddish, well-circumscribed	Osteoblasts and osteoclasts with osteoid and trabeculae of woven bone; more osteoid and organized than in osteoid osteomas Highly vascular	Rare, 43 cases reported by Dahlin; 51 cases reported by Schajowicz May recur and are sometimes aggressive but rarely metastasize
Giant-cell tumor	F : M = 3 : 2 85% > 19 years, peaks in third decade	Epiphyseal, may extend to the metaphysis, even through the cortex 50% around the knee Distal radius, ulna, and sacrum Rarely, in the vertebrae, and feet	Radiolucent No sclerosis	Grayish-red tissue with areas of necrosis Partly cystic	Giant mononuclear cells, almost no stroma Mitoses infrequent; foam cells seen 30% have osteoid and, rarely, cartilaginous components May be aggressive and behave in a malignant fashion if not totally and widely resected Graded from 1–3	Recurs after curettage in 50% of cases Rarely becomes malignant; such a change may occur after radiation Few reported cases of "benign" metastases Block excision recommended Differential diagnosis: hyperparathyroidism with brown tumor, aneurysmal bone cyst, nonossifying fibroma, chondroblastoma, eosinophylic granuloma

(*continued*)

Table II (*Continued*)

Tumor	Sex/age prevalence	Most common site	Radiologic characteristics	Gross features	Microscopic features	Miscellaneous characteristics
Aneurysmal bone cyst	Second and thrid decade	Metaphyseal	Lucent, eccentric, well-circumscribed Soft-tissue extension	Cystic spaces filled with clotted blood	Trabculae of woven bone or fibrous tissue Solid areas may be seen Giant cells	
Unicameral bone cyst	M : F = 3 : 1 First and second decades	Metaphyseal Diaphyseal in older patients 60% in the humerus and femur	Fusiform Cystic appearance	Cystic lesion with yellowish blood-tinged fluid	Layers of fibrous tissue with some woven bone Occasional giant cells, mononuclear cells, and hemosiderin	
Myositis ossificans	Young adults and teenagers	Around the arm and thigh	Calcifications prominent around the periphery of a spherical lesion	Ill-defined hard mass in muscle	Resembles a callus Goes through three phases of maturation with, at times, chondroid material and fibrous trabeculae.	Not truly a bone tumor History of trauma
Ganglion (synovial) cyst		End of long bone	Cyst	Filled with mucoid fluid		Rare Associated with nondegenerative joint disease
Eosinophylic granuloma	Second and third decade	Any bone Mostly skull	Discrete lytic lesion May be poorly defined (suggesting malignancy)	Soft Faintly yellowish	Mixture of histiocytes (grooved nuclei) with eosinophils, lymphocytes, and neutrophils, and occasional giant cells	Solitary Arises from the reticuloendothelial system
Synovial chondromatosis	M : F = 2 : 1 Fourth and fifth decade	Knee		Multiple nodules Grayish-white	Lobules of hyaline cartilage, multinucleated cells, and nuclear abnormalities	Benign lesion History of trauma
Fibroma of bone	M > F Second decade	Metaphyseal Long bones	Eccentric and bulging, cortical Scalloped line of sclerosis	Tan, yellowish or brown (fat and hemosiderin)	Whorled fibrous tissue with scattered giant cells; foam cells and hemosiderin are seen; occasional osseous metaplasia	May resove spontaneously Curettege is curative Do not irradiate
Adamantinoma	M > F Second-to-fifth decade	90% in the tibia Occasionally other long bones	Lucent lesion with areas of sclerosis	Firm, rubbery Grayish	Nests and strands of cells of epithelial appearance resembling basal cell carcinoma of skin May be associated with areas of fibrous dysplasia	Rare Slow-growing tumor that may metastasize

Table II (*Continued*)

Tumor	Sex/age prevalence	Most common site	Radiologic characteristics	Gross features	Microscopic features	Miscellaneous characteristics
Fibrosarcoma	Even distribution Adults	Metaphyseal Long bones Mostly about the knee	Indistinguishable from osteosarcoma No characteristic features of malignant tumor	Irregular, well-circumscribed Grayish pink	Spindle cell tumor of various grades	25% 5-year survival Better prognosis if well differentiated
Angiosarcoma				Dark red Friable	Highly vascular with marked endothelial proliferation	Rare Highly malignant, bleak prognosis
Chondrosarcoma	M > F Adult age and older	75% in the trunk (including upper humerus and femur) Rare in the distal extremities [14 of 470 cases distal to the wrist per Dahlin (4)]	Destruction and calcification with stippling effect (characteristic)	Lobular Cartilaginous appearance	Cartilaginous cells with abnormal nuclei 90% are Grade 1 or 2 10% are equivocal for malignancy 10% recurrences, have an increased degree of malignancy Mesenchymal chondrosarcoma have a dimorphic pattern of cartilage and small cells	May arise from benign osteochondromas, especially when they are multiple Poor prognosis when high grade Variants: clear-cell chondrosarcomas, mesenchymal chondrosarcomas (rare) May arise from soft tissues; poor prognosis
Osteogenic sarcoma	M : F = 3 : 2 Second decade	Metaphyseal 50% around the knee Rare in the hand or feet	Highly destructive, sclerotic or mixed Ill-defined margins Breaking through the cortex and extending in soft tissues Sunburst pattern Codman's triangle	Bulky tumor of bone extending into soft tissues Intramedullary portion is more sclerotic than that in soft tissues Contiguous and grossly apparent spread May spread along the marrow cavity "Skip" areas seen occasionally	Cytologically highly malignant osteoid bone cells with multiple mitosis, large irregular nuclei, frequent giant cells, all in a predominantly spindle cell stroma. May be divided into: Fibroblastic osteosarcoma Chondroblastic osteosarcoma Osteoblastic osteosarcoma (worst prognosis)	20–35%, 5-year survival when distal to the elbow or knee Variants: de-differentiated chondrosarcoma; malignant fibrous histiocytoma; telangiectatic osteogenic sarcoma; intraosseous low-grade osteosarcoma; parosteal osteogenic sarcoma (mostly in the femur and in the older age group); osteogenic sarcoma, secondary to Paget's disease or radiation; periosteal osteogenic sarcoma

(*continued*)

Table II (*Continued*)

Tumor	Sex/age prevalence	Most common site	Radiologic characteristics	Gross features	Microscopic features	Miscellaneous characteristics
Ewing's sarcoma	M > F First and second decade	Bone of upper and lower extremities Occasionally in flat bones (e.g., ribs)	Lytic destruction, with extension through the cortex Multiple layers of subperiosteal reactive new bone (onion-skin appearance)	Soft and necrotic components	Sheets of small, uniform cells with inconspicuous nucleoli and scant stroma Periodic acid-Schiff positive cytoplasm	Elevated sediment rate and fever Classic 15% 5-year survival is better with chemotherapy and high-dose radiation Differential diagnosis: cell tumors; neuroblastoma (infants); lymphoma (adolescents); myeloma or metastatic oat cell carcinoma (adults)
Paget's disease	Adults and older	Pelvis, femur, skull, tibia, vertebrae	Osteoclastic activity Intertrabecular fibrous tissue	Thickening of affected bone	Irregular cement lines with osteoclastic activity and intertrabecular fibrous tissue; mosaic pattern in bone	
Chordoma	M : F = 2 : 1 Later decades	Occiput and sacro-coccygeal area (notochord origin)	Destructive midline lesion, usually soft-tissue mass with occasional calcifications	Lobulated, mucoid Gray, translucent	Lobulated, mucinous tumor, physaliphorous cells, PAS- and mucin- carmine–positive cytoplasm	Poor long-term prognosis, slightly better in the occipital lesions and when there is chondroid differentiation

Table III

Site Predilection of Specific Bone Tumors

Axila skeleton	Flat bones	Proximal humerus	Distal femur	Tibia
Osteoblastoma Aneurysmal bone cyst Eosinophilic granuloma Multiple myeloma Metastases	Chondrosarcoma Osteochondroma Metastases	Periosteal chondroma	Parosteal osteosarcoma Osteosarcoma Chondrosarcoma	Adamantinoma Ossifying fibroma Chondromyxoid fibroma

Table IV

Regional Predilection of Specific Bone Tumors

Epiphysis	Metaphysis	Diaphysis
Chondroblastoma	Aneurysmal bone cyst	Ewing's sarcoma
Giant-cell tumor	Simple cyst	Eosinophilic granuloma
Brodie's abscess	Fibrous dysplasia	Osteomyelitis
	Osteoblastoma	Osteoid osteoma
	Chondromyxoid fibroma	
	Osteosarcoma	
	Paget's disease	

- Desmoid (medullary).
- Aneurysmal bone cyst.
- Giant-cell tumor.
- Osteoblastoma.
- Enchondroma.
- Ossifying fibroma.
- Chondromyxoid fibroma.
- Fibroma.
- Malignant lesions (low- and high-grade)
  - Osteosarcoma.
  - Chondrosarcoma.
  - Fibrosarcoma.
  - Ewing's sarcoma.

Table V

Age Incidence of Bone Tumors

Age (years)	Benign	Malignant
0–10	Unicameral bone cyst Eosinophilic granuloma Osteoid osteoma Fibrous dysplasia	All rare: osteosarcoma, Ewing's sarcoma, leukemia
10–20	Fibrous dysplasia Osteoid osteoma Fibroma Aneurysmal bone cyst Osteochondroma Chondroma Chondroblastoma Chondromyxoid fibroma	Osteosarcoma Ewing's sarcoma
20–40	Aneurysmal bone cyst Giant-cell tumor Osteoblastoma Chondromyxoid fibroma Adamantinoma	Parosteal osteosarcoma Fibrosarcoma Lymphoma Malignant fibrous histiocytoma
40–80	Paget's disease Hemangioma	Metastatic disease of bone Multiple myeloma Chondrosarcoma Fibrosarcoma Malignant fibrous histiocytoma Dedifferentiated malignant tumor Lymphoma

- Malignant fibrous histiocytoma.
- Lymphomas (Hodgkin's or non-Hodgkin's).
- Multiple myeloma.

The host reaction to these lesions is usually characteristic and serves as an alert to the type of lesion present (see Fig. 2). Basically, the reaction ignited by the lesion as it grows establishes the local natural history of the lesion.

Benign self-healing lesions usually evoke a reactive border capable of walling off the tumor; since this "sequestration" involves the bony mesenchyme, the involucrum will form bone that is generally referred to as the reactive margination, or "sclerotic rim" (Fig. 2B). Often the differentiation between the self-healing and the benign-aggressive lesion is based on the ability of this reactive process to keep up with the lesion's growth. The term *self-healing* refers to the natural history of the lesion: ablation or permanent containment; in most instances, the tumors, or tumorlike conditions, will become quiescent once adolescence is past. It is believed that the mesenchymal milieu is contingent upon hormonal influence and the duration of the host reaction. Soft-tissue tumors evoke the same kind of reaction in the soft parts as do the benign bone

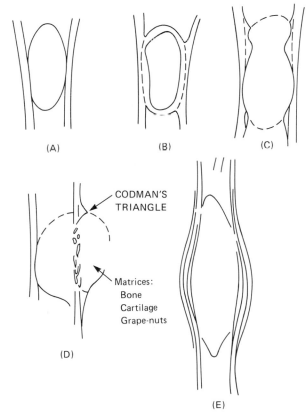

Fig. 2. Host reaction to various bone tumors. (A) *In situ* lesion. (B) Sclerotic reactive rim. (C) Partial breakthrough. (D) Permeative reaction. (E) Onion-skin reaction.

tumors, but since bone-forming mesenchyme is rarely involved, the involucrum formed is usually fibrovascular. The importance of this reactive zone (or pseudocapsule) will be stressed when discussing surgical margins and the predictable local cure rates of the various lesions.

Benign-aggressive and low-grade malignant lesions will often appear to "break through" their bony confinement. However, when examined microscopically, the mesenchymal reaction to the lesion can still be identified, and this reaction separates the tumor from the surrounding tissue (Fig. 2C). Pathologic fractures in these instances may be allowed to heal *in situ* since callus will "contain" the lesion; the fracture will heal in 6–8 weeks, and the lesion and its "containment" can then be resected en bloc, a procedure that often saves the extremity inasmuch as resection of an unstable pathologic fracture without local contamination is very difficult.

The high-grade lesions are more aggressive than their reaction and are thus not screened from the surrounding tissues: Although the host tries to wall them off, the effort is in vain. Codman's triangle (an attempted periosteal involucrum) characteristically ends abruptly as it lifts off the peripheral cortex, since the tumor advances through this reaction (Fig. 2D). The onionskin appearance seen in Ewing's sarcoma and in osteomyelitis represents the same kind of phenomenon; the "scalloping" of the low-grade intraosseous lesion (primarily cartilaginous) is an internal Codman's triangle, re-forming itself more distally with each tumor migration (Fig. 2E).

D. Differential Diagnosis of Bone Tumors

A large number of bone and joint conditions can simulate bone tumors both clinically and radiologically.

Melorheostosis, Engelmann's progressive diaphyseal dysplasia, and calcinosis circumscripta can produce x-ray changes that mimic bone tumors. The extent of involvement and reference to standard radiology and orthopedic texts should help interpret the x-rays correctly.

Arthritic involvement of the spine can be misleading, and confusion is often increased by the presence of positive finding on bone scan. A positive bone scan generally means increased bone activity in the bone metabolic unit and is not pathognomonic of malignancy.

Infections or myositis ossificans are frequently confused with bone tumors. The differential diagnosis is helped by the use of technitium and gallium bone scans, the latter being more sensitive in infections; in the absence of high fever, elevated white count, and increased sedimentation rate, a positive bone scan can add confusion to the diagnosis. Clinical judgment, as well as biopsy when indicated, is the appropriate course of management. For example, we have seen several hundred benign fibrous cortical defects and have biopsied only a few;

biopsy is not always necessary when the location of the lesion, its size, and its associated history make one suspect a benign lesion.

The lesions that often mimic malignant bone tumors in the young include

- Eosinophilic granulomas.
- Aneurysmal bone cysts.
- Chondroblastoma (the so-called Codman's tumor).

In the adult, the benign lesions that may be confused with malignant ones include

- Giant-cell tumors.
- Adamantinomas.
- Chondromyxofibromas.

II. EARLY DETECTION
AND SCREENING

Bone tumors are usually identified by means of serendipitous x-rays taken for unrelated causes (e.g., minor trauma) or because of the presenting features of pain or swelling. Although no systematic screening is recommended for bone tumors, a high degree of awareness by the general physician, as well as meaningful patient education, would be of value in early detection.

A. Patient Education

Patient education should be directed toward seeking early medical attention for unexplained pain and swelling, much as in other tumors. Unlike soft-tissue tumors, rather simple x-ray studies will quickly identify a bone lesion. Nevertheless, in clinical practice, the wary public will sometimes refuse a diagnostic x-ray as being hazardous; the infinitesimal radiation required to determine the presence of a tumor in an extremity, particularly in a young teenager, is associated with no ill effects whatsoever. Public education should, therefore, also address itself to judiciously explaining the dangers and advantages of radiological studies as well as the need for such studies for early detection in indicated situations.

Mass screening would require routine total body x-rays or scans and thus is not practical or desirable.

B. Early Signs and Symptoms

Unfortunately, there are few symptoms related to bone tumors, and these are often late occurring. The following symptoms should immediately arouse suspicion:

- Pain—any persistent skeletal or joint pain—especially in young patients.
- Swelling or mass in or about any bone.
- Fever associated with either of the above.

Pathological fractures, though often a late sign of bone tumors, may constitute the presenting symptom in many cases (e.g., various benign cystic lesions are discovered because the cystic area acts as a stress riser and a fracture occurs at the site of the cyst).

C. Preventive Measures

Three recognized factors are suspected of being associated with malignant bone tumors: the presence of certain benign tumors, Paget's disease, or a history of intense radiation. The extent to which industrial or medical use of radiation has resulted in bone tumors is unclear, but hazards associated with radium-dial watch paints and radiotherapy to the mandible are well documented. The potential of industrial wastes other than radioactive substances to cause tumors is problematic and very difficult to substantiate.

Dietary factors do not seem to influence bone tumors, in contrast to nonmalignant lesions such as osteomalacia, rickets, and scurvy, where dietary deficiencies play a pivotal role. Other socioeconomic factors appear to have no bearing on bone tumors.

III. PRETREATMENT EVALUATION AND WORK-UP

The evaluation of the patient prior to biopsy and therapy in order to come as close to a definitive diagnosis as possible is most important for the psychological well-being of the patient as well as for planning a therapeutic program. In addition, ruling out tumor-simulating entities is desirable before any therapeutic planning is undertaken.

A. History and Physical Examination

1. History

- Social and occupational history.
- The family history might help differentiate such genetic disorders as hereditary multiple exostoses, Gaucher's disease, sickle cell anemia, thalassemia, Fanconi's syndrome, etc.
- Age. One of the most important clues to bone tumor identification is the age of the patient. Table V, lists the age incidence of various bone tumors.

- A history of trauma might suggest myositis ossificans rather than a juxtacortical osteogenic sarcoma; the two conditions may look uncomfortably alike clinically early in the course of the disease.
- Pain and its character, duration, type (backache, arthralgia, neuralgia, etc.).
- Swelling or mass.
- Site of the lesion. Specific bone tumors have a definite predilection for certain bones and for certain regions within the bones. Tables III and IV, list the regional and site predilection of the various bone tumors.
- Fever. Frequent in Ewing's sarcoma, pseudomalignant ossifying soft-tissue tumor, and myositis ossificans.
- Pathological fracture (in cysts, fibrous dysplasia, giant-cell tumors, malignant fibrous histicytoma, and metastatic foci).
- Presence of associated lesions: café au lait spots, fibromas, familial polyps, hemangiomas, clubbing, etc.
- History of other diseases: renal failure, hyperparathyroidism, previous lesions treated by radiotherapy, etc.

2. Physical Examination

- Careful assessment of the site of pain or swelling by palpation and inspection.
- Examination of adjacent soft tissues.
- Range-of-motion and joint assessment.
- Limb-length measurements.
- Neurological evaluation.
- Vascular assessment of the limb.

B. Laboratory Findings

1. Serum Calcium and Phosphorus

A determination of the serum calcium will help differentiate cystic bone lesions due to hyperparathyroidism or renal disease with secondary hyperparathyroidism or pseudohyperparathyroidism such as the Seabright Bantam syndrome. An elevated serum calcium corrected for serum protein, a depressed serum phosphorus, or an increased parathormone level indicates excessive parathyroid activity. Primary bone changes identified in earlier years as the so-called brown tumor are almost unknown in today's milk-drinking societies.

2. Serum and Urine Protein Electrophoresis

These are particularly useful in identifying hematopoietic tumors, (e.g., multiple myeloma). The abnormalities of serum proteins, elevated sedimentation rate, and Bence Jones protein in the urine are dealt with in the section on hematologic tumors.

3. Alkaline and Acid Phosphatase

An elevated alkaline phosphatase is seen in highly active sarcomas and in metastatic bone tumors. Acid phosphatase elevation indicates a metastatic prostatic carcinoma but may be misleading since the test may revert to normal after treatment and may continue to remain so, even when the patient is no longer in remission. Moreover, the serum acid phosphatase may be normal in patients with untreated metastatic prostatic carcinoma. The biopsied bone of a metastatic deposit suspected to be of prostatic origin should be biochemically examined for the presence of acid phosphatase in the tissue; this may be found to be quite elevated even when serum values are uninformative.

4. Routine Laboratory Studies

The following determinations should be carried out as part of a general evaluation of the patient prior to surgery:

- Complete blood count (CBC).
- Automated multichannel chemistries (SMA-12 or SMA-18).

C. Radiological Evaluation

1. General Considerations

Diagnostic radiologic studies play a critical role in every phase of the evaluation and management of bone tumors.

a. Detection and Screening

It is not unusual for bone tumors to be discovered incidentally on x-ray studies, though most are uncovered after the onset of pain or following insignificant trauma.

b. Documentation and Histologic Identification

In the pretreatment evaluation of a patient with a suspected bone tumor, one should seek to establish a histological diagnosis. Radiologic studies play an important role in revealing an image that reflects the actual gross pathological findings of the bone tumor. It is important to correlate the pathologist's opinion of a biopsy specimen with that of the radiologist, especially when the microscopic or radiologic findings are inconclusive. For example, in cases of neuropathic joints and synovial chondromatosis, histological findings are usually inconclusive, whereas the radiologic diagnosis is simple and definitive. The collaboration of these two disciplines should be further extended to the selection of the most appropriate site for biopsy, based on the roentgenographic studies.

With the advent of radionuclide scanning and computerized axial tomography (CAT), the accuracy of diagnosis of bone tumors by radiologic methods has increased significantly. Conventional radiologic techniques with linear tomography and magnification are still the methods of choice but must be supplemented by computerized tomography, particularly in the examination of the spine, shoulder, and pelvic areas, where conventional methods are not usually adequate.

c. Differential Diagnosis

While bone tumors are rare, tumorlike bone lesions and normal variants are a common occurrence. X-ray findings are usually definitive in these cases (cortical defects, Paget's disease of bone, fibrous dysplasia, etc.), and often no microscopic examination is needed.

d. Metastatic Evaluation

With few notable exceptions such as Ewing's sarcoma and osteogenic sarcoma, the search for bone metastases is not a routine procedure for primary bone tumors. If such a search is warranted, radionuclide scanning is favored over routine x-rays. Computerized tomography can be used when there is a positive radionuclide scan or when there is a high index of suspicion of bone metastases, even though conventional films are not revealing; this is particularly important in such regions as the spine, pelvis, and shoulder.

e. Therapeutic Considerations

In the assessment of the extent of the lesion; the soft-tissue involvement; and the relationship of the lesion to vital structures such as vessels, nerves, and muscles; CAT has a distinct advantage over conventional x-ray and may be supplemented by arteriography, venography, and/or lymphangiography. Such information permits a complete assessment of the tumor, a more definite determination of operability, better radiotherapy planning, and a more solid basis to evaluate the results of preoperative chemotherapy used in an attempt to reduce the size of the tumor. The radiologic studies may also influence the surgeon's decision as to whether amputation or en-bloc resection is necessary in treating certain bone tumors.

f. Follow-Up Evaluation

Conventional radiological methods, as well as CAT scans, are also used to evaluate tumor response. Such an evaluation may even serve the purpose of ascertaining the validity of the original histological diagnosis. A case in point is the notable difference in roentgen appearance following appropriate therapy for giant-cell tumor and aneurysmal bone cysts.

Conventional methods are inadequate for detecting recurrences following previous surgery because such recurrences usually take place in the soft tissues. Computerized tomography is very useful in such instances.

2. Specific Procedures

a. Routine X-ray Studies

Such radiological studies must include:

- Anteroposterior, lateral, and oblique views of the involved area. This will demonstrate the destruction and replacement of bone, as well as the host reaction. The technique of a preliminary bone scan followed by x-ray studies of "hot" areas is not recommended, since it will fail to detect certain benign lesions such as multiple exostoses.
- A routine anteroposterior and lateral views of the chest as well as tomograms or CAT scans of the chest are indicated in selected cases to ascertain the presence or absence of metastatic disease to the lungs. Identification of pulmonary metastases is not necessarily a deterrent to local treatment but must be taken into account in the total management of the patient.

b. Additional Techniques

For further diagnostic clues or for planning a surgical approach, several other x-ray studies are needed:

i. Tomography. Tomography is of particular importance in osteoid osteoma and in planning a biopsy portal in cystic lesions. Tomography will also better demonstrate reactive border characteristics and matrix patterns.

ii. Computerized Axial Tomography. The introduction of the more recent generations of CAT scanners has nearly replaced the use of tomography, especially in certain sites (e.g., spine and pelvis). Computerized axial tomography also provides three-dimensional information in addition to a detailed study of the adjacent soft tissues.

iii. Arteriography. Prior to the advent of the CAT scan, arteriography was a key modality in studying and staging lesions suspected of malignancy and in evaluating their relation to major neurovascular bundles. At present, it is still used in the analysis of soft-tissue tumors and in the delineation of their major "feeder" vessels (e.g., lesions that might be amenable to embolization). It is extremely valuable in the preoperative evaluation of the vasculature of a tumor in order to select a safer portal of surgical approach and to facilitate early ligation of the tumor's blood supply during resection. In areas where there is a questionable penetration of the cortex near a neurovascular bundle (e.g., in the posterodistal femur) or in large, juxtacortical lesions (e.g., parosteal osteosarcoma or low-

grade chondrosarcoma), arteriography is still essential in evaluating the extent of the disease.

iv. Venography. Venography and computer-enhanced venography may permit one to anticipate some of the vascular problems that might occur during surgery.

v. Xerography. Soft-tissue techniques such as xerography have been superseded by CAT scan studies.

vi. Growth Potential. If the tumor under treatment is in a growing child, a baseline leg-length study and an estimate of potential growth is needed. Although the Todd *Atlas* may be referred to in comparing hand x-rays, counting the number of carpal bones that have made their appearance and an updated Green-Anderson growth prediction chart is of more value.

vii. Lymphangiography. Lymphangiograms are used only in special circumstances.

viii. Myelography. Myelography is specific for tumors of the spine.

ix. Sonography. Sonography is used occasionally in certain soft-tissue tumors.

3. Diagnostic Clues

a. Patterns of Destruction

Three basic patterns of bone destruction continue to be useful in identifying bone lesions.

i. Geographic. This presents as a uniformly destroyed area in bone with sharply defined edges, and it generally has a slow growth rate. This type of bone destruction is further divided into three classes, IA, IB, or IC, depending on whether the sharply marginated lesion is bordered by a sclerotic line, has no sclerotic line, or has a partially distinct margin, respectively. The IA pattern is seen in nonossifying fibroma. Eosinophilic granuloma in the skull illustrates the IB pattern.

ii. Moth-Eaten. This type of bone destruction indicates a moderately rapid growth process and has the appearance of a piece of cloth partially eaten by moths. Islands of partially destroyed bone lie within the lucent area. The pattern is characteristic of osteomyelitis and fibrosarcoma.

iii. Permeated. This is the most rapidly progressing pattern of bone destruction, is frequently associated with small round-cell tumors such as Ewing's sarcoma and reticulum cell sarcoma, and may also be seen in osteosarcoma. At first glance, this type of bone destruction may be mistaken for normal bone. The growing malignant tissue has flowed into the interstices of bone, enlarging the haversian canal system, and finally allowing a subtle abnormality to be visualized. With this type of bone destruction, the growing lesion usually lies far ahead of the apparent bone destruction.

b. Indications of Aggressiveness

Certain observations identified on x-rays are helpful in detecting the aggressiveness of a bone lesion.

Periosteal response would occur in one of the following patterns:

- Single line.
- Thick, homogeneous strip.
- Laminated (onion peel).
- Sunburst.
- Hair-on-end.
- Velvet.

The so-called Codman's sign (elevation of the periosteum along the cortex) is quite typical of bone malignancy and is usually regarded as a periosteal reaction. It does, however, also occur in response to fractures.

Other observations from x-rays helpful in detecting bone lesion aggresiveness are

- Cortical destruction.
- Calcium in malignant tissue.
- Soft-tissue mass.
- Buttressing.
- Saucerization.

D. Bone Scan

This is a critical modality in orthopedics and very helpful in evaluating the extent of the lesion, tumor spread by skips in the bone, extraosseous extent, occult metastases, etc.

Findings on bone scan impact staging as well as therapy. For example, in osteosarcomas the resection margin is recommended to be 7 cm above the *scan margin* if feasible. The ratio of the image to the "hot" area is translated to the scanogram of the bone involved (see Fig. 3).

The scan thus not only alerts to occult extension (e.g., skip lesions in osteosarcoma—a serious prognostic sign akin to bone metastases) but permits a more rational decision whether to conserve or amputate and also helps to establish realistic reconstruction goals.

Another important use of the scan is the evaluation of soft-tissue tumors near or juxtaposed to bone. If the reactive zone of the lesion involves the periosteum, the bone scan will show increased activity in this area. Often tangential views must be taken to assess this reaction properly if the soft-tissue lesion happens to hyperconcentrate the radioactive substance, as in liposarcoma, osteosarcoma, and hypervascular lesions, for example, or if there has been recent surgery in the area.

E. Staging

The term *staging* in the classification of bone tumors integrates the anatomic localization (surgical site) with the histologic diagnosis (surgical grade) of the tumor, i.e., compartmentalization with histologic grade. Table VI lists the com-

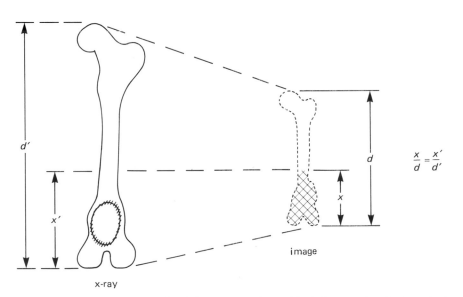

Fig. 3. Diagram of a bone scan in relation to an x-ray image. The lesion area x' can be determined from the ratio $x'/d' = x/d$, where d' and d are the lengths of the bone on the x-ray and on the scanogram, respectively, and x is the scan margin.

Table VI

Compartmentalization of Bone Tumors According to T Category
(Surgical Sites)

Intracompartmental (T1)	Extracompartmental (T2)
Introsseous	Intraosseous with soft-tissue extension
Intra-articular	Intra-articular with soft-tissue extension
Superficial to deep fascia	Superficial to deep fascia with deep fascial extension
Paraosseous	Paraosseous with intraosseous or extrafascial extension
Intrafascial compartments	Extrafascial planes or spaces
Ray of hand or foot	Mid and hind foot
Posterior calf	Popliteal space
Anterolateral leg	Groin–femoral triangle
Anterior thigh	Intrapelvic space
Medial thigh	Midhand
Posterior thigh	Antecubital fossae
Buttocks	Axilla
Volar forearm	Periclavicular
Dorsal forearm	Paraspinal
Anterior arm	Head and neck
Periscapular	

Table VII

Histological Types of Bone Tumors According to Histologic Grades (G)

Low (G1)	High (G2)
Parosteal osteosarcoma	Classic osteosarcoma
Endosteal osteosarcoma	Radiation sarcoma
	Paget's sarcoma
Secondary chondrosarcoma	Primary chondrosarcoma
Fibrosarcoma, Kaposi's sarcoma	Fibrosarcoma, undifferentiated primary
Atypical malignant fibrous histiocytoma	Malignant fibrous histiocytoma
Giant-cell tumor, bone	Giant-cell sarcoma, bone
Hemangioendothelioma	Angiosarcoma
Hemangiopericytoma	Hemangiopericytoma, malignant
Myxoid liposarcoma	Pleomorphic liposarcoma
	Neurofibrosarcoma (schwannoma)
	Rhabdomyosarcoma
Clear-cell sarcoma of tendon sheath	Malignant synovioma
Epithelioid sarcoma	
Chordoma	
Adamantinoma	
Alveolar cell sarcoma	Alveolar cell sarcoma
Other and undifferentiated	Other and undifferentiated

partments and illustrates the T categories. Table VII classifies the various histologic types according to grades. Table VIII groups the various parameters into stages.

Accurate surgical staging is essential prior to biopsy and requires careful physical examination, various x-ray studies, and CAT scans as previously described. Using these modalities, the surgeon should be able to compartmentalize the lesion, visualize the extent and location of the reactive zone, recognize characteristic matrix patterns, and plan definitive treatment.

F. Diagnostic Clues

After objective observations of the destructive bone pattern at hand are considered together with the patient's age, the clinical setting, and the laboratory data available, one can arrive at a reasonable conclusion supporting a likely diagnosis.

The following remarks are practical guidelines useful in the evaluation of difficult cases:

- Metastases to bone tend to have small or no soft-tissue mass.
- Malignant primary bone tumors tend to have large soft-tissue masses.
- The largest soft-tissue masses are seen with Ewing's sarcoma and chondrosarcoma.
- Aggressive bone destruction in the metaphysis of a child or teenager is most likely an osteosarcoma or Ewing's sarcoma, provided infection is ruled out.
- Lytic bone lesions in adults are most often metastases, myelomas (plasmacytomas or multiple myelomas), or infection.

- Pulmonary metastases from osteosarcoma and periosteal sarcoma may form bone and have a radiographic density greater than soft tissue.
- Ewing's tumors rarely metastasize from one bone to another; they generally spread to the lung.
- A destructive lesion of the sternum is malignant whether in a child or an adult.

Table VIII

Surgical Stages of Bone Tumors

Stage	Grade	Site
I	G1, without metastases	—
IA	G1, without metastases	T1
IB	G1, without metastases	T2
II	G2, without metastases	—
IIA	G2, without metastases	T1
IIB	G2, without metastases	T2
III	Any G, with metastasis	Any T, with metastasis

- "Benign" lesions that may have an aggressive radiographic appearance include osteomyelitis, aneurysmal bone cyst, eosinophilic granuloma, hemophilic pseudotumor, and brown tumor (hyperparathyroidism).
- Metastases to lung from osteosarcoma may cause spontaneous pneumothorax.
- Prior fracture or recent pathological fracture, prior irradiation therapy, prior biopsy, or surgery with placement of bone chips may alter the usual appearance of a lesion.

Given a solitary destructive bone lesion, the most important decision to be made is to choose one of two courses:

- The lesion is definitely benign and may be ignored or merely followed.
- The lesion has an aggressive or ambiguous appearance that necessitates biopsy.

G. Biopsy

The importance of early biopsy in the more aggressive bone tumors has been appropriately stressed. After all the above work-up, as well as the usual medical evaluation, has been completed, a decision must be judiciously made regarding the need for a biopsy. The surgeon doing the biopsy should be prepared to carry out the definitive procedure as well. The procedure might include local extirpative, radical extirpative, and/or rehabilitative surgery. It might include total joint replacement or the still-experimental use of partial limb and joint homografts from fresh cadavers.

Needle biopsy has many pitfalls, mechanical as well as interpretive. It is feasible in lesions of the vertebral bodies, using the calculation of Ottolhengi and the special table that enables the surgeon to use an image intensifier. The technique, using a trochar and guide, may be carried out with the Craig instrumentation with minimal morbidity. The cylinder of tissue obtained by needle biopsy compressed in a narrow tube may, however, result in either a misinterpretation or a false negative, so the pathologist generally prefers a more adequate portion of tissue. Craig needle biopsy is generally sufficient to diagnose metastatic lesions. Modified open techniques have, therefore, been preferred for primary bone tumors and are considered feasible even in difficult areas such as the spine.

Open biopsy with adequate tissue sampling for selective staining and microscopic evaluation, including electron microscopy, is, in most cases, the recommended approach. The surgical incision and exposure should take into account the needs of the definitive second procedure and need not be extensive. The best tissue for microscopic diagnosis can be found in the peripheral tumor area rather than the central portion, and it should, if possible, include the adjacent capsule and normal tissue.

Excisional biopsies as a primary procedure in malignant bone tumors are not usually indicated. Suspicious malignant lesions require histologic confirmation prior to therapy, and an excisional biopsy can seldom be definitive on bony tumors. Furthermore, frozen sections on tissues that require decalcification cannot be relied upon. The long-term survival of patients receiving planned, staged biopsy with delayed resection (5–7 days later) is not statistically different from the survival of those having immediate definitive surgery. When a malignancy is confirmed, the definitive procedure should include the entire area of prior biopsy, and a prior excisional biopsy would thus result in a need for an even more extensive definitive operation.

A few exceptions exist however; cartilaginous lesions usually do not require biopsy unless high-grade dedifferentiation is suspected; a wide excision is carried out initially and is generally sufficient for biopsy and definitive treatment. Other lesions such as osteoid osteomas or bone cysts also do not require preliminary biopsy and can be treated in one stage.

There are obvious advantages and disadvantages to incisional and needle biopsies. The interpretation and reliability is more risky with the needle. As there is a reactive rim to both soft- and hard-tissue tumors, and the biopsy must penetrate this zone to be accurate, multiple needle biopsies through tough, reactive bone can be frustrating and time consuming, as well as painful. On the other hand, if compartment location necessitates a biopsy in a more difficult area, a cortical window may be necessary for open biopsy, and an Avitene or a Gelfoam plug is often necessary to control hemorrhage from the defect. Needle biopsy can therefore be effectively used in such cases. Needle biopsy is also particularly desirable where there is soft-tissue disease; the amount of tissue obtained is often enough, and the exact diagnosis is, in many cases, not quite as important as the grade of differentiation of the tumor. Sharp, efficient instrumentation is essential.

Whether a needle biopsy or an open incisional biopsy is chosen, one must avoid entry into uninvolved joints, undermining soft tissues, deep or sharp retractors, self-retainers, and jet lavage. Open (incisional) or needle biopsy tracts should be placed through the compartment containing the lesion or via a compartment to be excised at the time of the definitive surgery. Extracompartmental lesions should be approached through a convenient involved compartment if they began as Stage IA or IIA lesions. Primary, low-grade extracompartmental tumors (osteochondromas, low-grade chondrosarcomas, juxtacortical or periosteal osteosarcomas, or soft-tissue tumors) either should not be biopsied or the biopsy should be placed through the overlying compartment. Removable drains inserted at the time of biopsy may result in direct tumor spread and should not be used in suspected malignant tumors.

The biopsy should be considered as part of the total therapeutic plan, and the surgical team must be prepared for surgery. Four options are available:

- If the lesion is benign, marginal or wide excision can be done.
- If the lesion is malignant, one can elect to close up and consider all the alternatives before proceeding to definitive therapy. Occasionally wide or radical excision may be performed.
- If the area is infected, one should excise, debride, and drain.
- If the diagnosis is uncertain, obtain a generous biopsy and close up. Therapy is determined after a definitive diagnosis is established, based on the study of permanent slides.

H. General Medical Evaluation

Most patients with primary tumors are otherwise in good general health; most are of a young age and without reason for nutritional or physiological aberrations. It is necessary, however, to carry out a complete medical evaluation of the patient including cardiopulmonary, hematologic, and renal evaluation. Correction of any medical problem and, more specifically, correction of anemia and nutritional depletion (particularly in patients who have received chemotherapy preoperatively) is essential prior to surgery.

In addition, a metastatic evaluation should include

- Complete biochemical profile and liver function tests.
- Liver scan, if indicated by liver profile tests.
- Chest x-ray and CAT scan as necessary.
- Bone scan.
- Other tests as indicated: brain scan, spinal fluid studies, etc.

Upon admission to the hospital and prior to therapy, it is useful to complete a site-specific data sheet with all the pertinent information for the individual patient as well as appropriate diagnostic mapping of the tumors and staging of the disease. This is not only essential in accurately assessing the patient prior to therapy but is invaluable for subsequent data collection and evaluation. Instructions for staging should be readily available with the site-specific data sheet to insure accurate staging.

I. Site-Specific Data Form
for Bone Tumors
(see pp. 234a–234b)

J. Multidisciplinary Consultation

A multidisciplinary approach to a patient with bone tumor is essential at every phase of the management: evaluation, diagnostic investigations, therapy, and rehabilitation.

The radiologist is usually the first team member solicited by the orthopedic surgeon to aid in establishing the diagnosis by performing and interpreting the many radiodiagnostic tests necessary (sonography, arteriography, venography, myelograms, lymphangiograms, bone scans, CAT scans, etc.).

A multidisciplinary consultation with the radiotherapist, pathologist, chemotherapist, and physical therapist should be obtained prior to setting out on a course of therapy. The inherent dangers of radiotherapy for benign disease (poor healing after a surgical procedure and malignant change), particularly in infants (with angiomas, eosinophilic granulomas, giant-cell tumors, and fibrous dysplasia), will then be properly evaluated. The expected radiation response of a particular tumor will also be adequately appreciated. Generally, sarcomas are radioresistant, whereas bone marrow lesions (e.g., myelomas and lymphomas) and small-cell lesions (Ewing's sarcoma) are highly radiosensitive. Metastatic carcinoma to bone, however, is where radiotherapy has its greatest use.

The pathologist must be included in the team. A forewarned pathologist is forearmed and, when presented with the biopsy specimen, is better able to make a cogent analysis.

When a malignant lesion is suspected, a medical oncologist is added to the team because chemotherapy may be required and must be tailored to the stage, location, and histologic picture of the disease. An informed interplay is required in planning preoperative versus postoperative chemotherapy. The lack of host response to the shock of surgery after some chemotherapeutic agents (e.g., Adriamycin and vincristine) are used may increase the likelihood of infected wounds when aggressive chemotherapy is used preoperatively. The induced anemia must also be considered in the group discussion of the planned attack.

A nurse oncologist and social worker should be added to the team. They are responsible for supportive therapy (e.g., for problems of daily living after a mutilating procedure or when undergoing chemotherapy) and can help prevent abject depression. Many a patient perceives the relegation of his or her life to "chemo" sessions, with hair loss, libido loss, job loss, and limb loss, as an intolerable assault on ego, independence, and self-image. Couple this with the fear of imminent death, and the patient may develop withdrawal and, often, antagonism. The use of persiflage in stating the more painful truths and the use of encouragement and the team approach can forestall and even eliminate some of the grim aspects of this period. Psychiatry; clergy; and caring, optimistic paraprofessionals are an essential help. But people vary. Some patients have amazing inner resources that allow them to cope; others don't. It is important for the clinician to differentiate patients' personality types and not to follow a rigid regimen for delegating the adjustment problems to others prior to his or her own attempt to work with the patient.

Usually, the physiotherapist, under the guidance of a rehabilitation expert, offers the most positive experience to the amputee. The daily contact, the staged program, the laying on of hand, and the critique of the prosthetist's handiwork often make the physiotherapist the link with hope and the ambition to function within the newly acquired handicap. The surgeon must recognize the resentment the patient unconsciously feels for his or her role as maimer rather than just healer. The clever designs of various devices, both prosthetic and orthotic, and the vital importance of an attentive, informed, and skilled prosthetist are also essential.

IV. THERAPEUTIC MANAGEMENT

Current principles of tumor surgery are based on an understanding of the biologic behavior of the various tumors. Tumors of the same histology may behave differently in different patients and in different sites, thus necessitating a customized treatment of each case.

The management of bone tumors is further complicated by a number of factors that will alter the therapeutic approach and, at times, render it arbitrary:

- A histological diagnosis is not always available at the time of therapy planning. One often has to plan the therapy on the basis of the behavior of the lesion as identified by its clinical and radiological presentation.
- Definitive therapy must often be instituted at the time of biopsy, in spite of the fact that frozen sections are not always possible or diagnostic.
- Therapy will often be dictated by the location of the lesion in the skeleton and by its effect on the function of the affected site.
- Further treatment should, whenever possible, be guided by the compartmentalization of the tumor (its T classification) as well as by its histologic type and grade (its G classification): in other words, by its stage.
- The response of a particular tumor to chemotherapy or radiotherapy is often difficult to anticipate, a fact that adds to the difficulties of designing a successful course of management.

The generally dismal cure rates historically reported in the literature for the treatment of malignant bone tumors have prompted intensive clinical investigation of combined-modality management utilizing radiotherapy and/or chemotherapy, thus increasing their role in the management of the above tumors. However, the mainstay of definitive therapy for bone tumors remains surgical.

A. Surgical Management

The question of biopsy has already been addressed. In summary, for lesions that are obviously benign (mobile, non-

enlarging, painless, etc.), primary excision will serve as biopsy and definitive therapy. If a lesion is obviously malignant (fixed, growing, painful, solid), it is desirable first to stage it with the various diagnostic tools available and then to do an incisional biopsy (or, if possible, a needle biopsy). When the diagnosis is equivocal, one must assume that the lesion may be a sarcoma and manage it as such until proven otherwise. Physicians should only biopsy what they are prepared to treat definitively and should not biopsy with a plan to treat if benign and refer if malignant. The disastrous results of injudicious biopsy have cost many patients their limbs or lives unnecessarily.

1. Selection of the Extent of Surgery

Four general types of procedures are defined for the resections of bone tumors, each specific in nature and indicated for specific types of lesions:

- Intralesional excision.
- Marginal excision.
- Wide (compartmental) excision.
- Radical (extracompartmental) excision.

Table IX lists these procedures, their margins, planes of dissection, local results, and equivalent amputation, should that be necessary. The extent of resection and surgical margin is primarily indicated by the stage of the disease, the site of the tumor, its extent, its histology, and its grade. Table X lists the indications for the various procedures in relation to the stage of the disease.

2. Operative Procedures Available

A large variety of procedures is available and selectively indicated in the treatment of bone tumors.

a. Curettage

This is an intralesional method of treatment indicated mostly in benign self-healing lesions. The procedure is usually associated with bone grafting of cancellous bone or, in selected cases, cortical bone.

b. Marginal Resection

Excision is carried out within the pseudocapsule of the tumor. The extended marginal resection includes cryo-, thermal, or chemical (phenolization) cauterization of the lesion following the conservative local excision. This procedure is usually recommended in the benign aggressive tumors of bone and also as an adjunctive modality in some tumors primarily treated by chemotherapy and radiotherapy (e.g., Ewing's sarcoma).

SITE-SPECIFIC DATA FORM—BONE CANCER

HISTORY

Age: _____ Sex: _____

Symptoms
_____ Pain
_____ Swelling
_____ Fever
_____ Pathologic fracture
_____ Weight loss _____ lbs.
_____ Functional impairment
_____ Malaise
_____ Other
Duration of symptoms _____

Social history
   Race: _____ White _____ Black _____ Oriental _____ Other
   Occupation: _____
   Smoker: _____ Yes _____ No How much? _____
   Drinker: _____ Yes _____ No How often? _____

Family history of carcinoma
   Relation: _____ Site: _____
Previous history of carcinoma
   _____ No _____ Yes Site: _____
Rx: _____
Previous treatment (describe):
(Surgery, radiation, chemotherapy, etc.)
_____
_____
_____

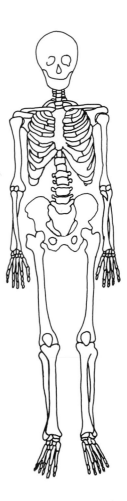

PHYSICAL EXAMINATION

Site of tumor: _____ Axial skeleton _____ Skull _____ Flat bone _____ Long bone
Precise bone: _____ Right _____ Left _____
Precise region: _____ Epiphysis _____ Metaphysis _____ Diaphysis _____ Proximal _____ Distal
Description of tumor: _____
Size: _____   _____
_____ Lymphedema _____ Muscle atrophy   Nodes: _____ Yes _____ No
Involvement of: _____ Adjacent soft tissue
           _____ Limb length
           _____ Range of motion
           _____ Major vessel. Describe: _____
           _____ Major nerve. Describe: _____

PREOPERATIVE EVALUATION (Check, if done)

	Neg.	Pos.	Suspicious		Neg.	Pos.	Suspicious
Serum calcium and phosphorus	_____	_____	_____	Routine x-ray of part	_____	_____	_____
Acid phosphatase	_____	_____	_____	Tomography	_____	_____	_____
Alkaline phosphatase	_____	_____	_____	CAT scan of part	_____	_____	_____
Serum proteins and electrophoresis	_____	_____	_____	Venography	_____	_____	_____
Bence Jones urine	_____	_____	_____	Arteriography	_____	_____	_____
Bone scan	_____	_____	_____	Xerography	_____	_____	_____
Chest x-ray	_____	_____	_____	Myelogram	_____	_____	_____
				Lymphangiogram	_____	_____	_____

CHARACTER OF BONE INVOLVEMENT ON X-RAYS

_____ Single tumor _____ Multiple in one bone _____ More than one bone
Size: _____

Intraosseous: _____ Yes _____ No. Extraosseous: _____ Yes _____ No
Edges: _____ Sharp with sclerosis _____ No sclerosis _____ Ill-defined
Character: _____ Sclerotic _____ Lytic
Cortical: _____ Thickening _____ Thinning _____ Perforation
Periosteal reaction: _____ Lamination _____ Sclerosis _____ Spiculation

Biopsy: _____ Needle _____ Incision _____ Excision
Diagnosis: _____
Distant metastasis: _____ Yes _____ No. Site: _____

Classification
_____ Intracompartmental (T1)
_____ Extracompartmental (T2)
Date: _____

Grading: _____ G1 _____ G2
Stage: _____
Signature: _____
Countersignature: _____

234a

Classification of Bone Cancers

The standard TNM classification based on the size of the primary and presence or absence of nodes or distant metastases does not apply to bone tumors. Likewise, standard grading according to differentiation (G1–G4) is also not applicable. The following T and G classification (as described in the text) has been suggested in staging bone tumors.

Grade

G1 (low-grade histologic types)
  Parosteal and endosteal osteosarcoma
  Well-differentiated and secondary chondrosarcoma
  Benign giant-cell tumor, adamantinoma
  Low-grade fibrosarcoma
  Hemangioendothelioma or pericytoma
  Myxoid liposarcoma
  Chordoma

G2 (high-grade histologic types)
  Osteogenic sarcoma, radiation sarcoma, Paget's disease
  Primary chondrosarcoma (spindle cell variety)
  Giant-cell sarcoma
  Fibrosarcoma—malignant histiocytoma, undifferentiated sarcoma
  Angiosarcoma
  Pleomorphic liposarcoma, neurofibrosarcoma, rhabdomyosarcoma
  Synovioma, alveolar cell sarcoma

Site

T1 (intracompartmental)
  Intraosseous or articular and paraosseous
  Deep to fascia
  Within intrafascial compartments (ray of hand, posterior calf,
    buttocks, anterior thigh, etc.)

T2 (extracompartmental)
  Soft-tissue extension
  Breaking through the fascia
  Intra- and paraosseous
  In extrafascial planes (popliteal space, axilla, groin, midhand,
    head and neck, paraspinal, etc.)

Stage

Stage I	All G1 without metastases
Stage IA	All G1 with T1
Stage IB	All G1 with T2
Stage II	All G2 without metastases
Stage IIA	All G2 with T1
Stage IIB	All G2 with T2
Stage III	All G or T with metastases

Table IX

General Procedures in the Resection of Bone Tumors

Type of procedure	Operation	Plane of dissection	Result	Equivalent amputation
Intralesion excision	Curettage Debulking	Inside the tumor Shelling out of the lesion Piecemeal removal	Leaves macroscopic disease	Debulking amputation
Marginal excision	Marginal excision	Shell out en bloc through the pseudocapsule or reactive zone	May leave microscopic disease, satellites, or skip areas	Marginal amputation
Wide excision	Wide local excision	Intracompartmental but en bloc with a cuff of normal tissue	May leave "skip" areas	Wide through-the-bone amputation
Radical excision	Radical excision	Extracompartmental en bloc resection of the entire compartment	No residual tumor	Radical disarticulation

c. Wide Excision

This is, in effect, a bloc resection of the tumor site with a margin of normal tissue, yet the procedure remains intracompartmental. Some benign tumors (giant-cell tumors, osteoid osteomas, and some fibrous dysplasias) and most low-grade malignant tumors can be effectively treated by wide-bloc resection.

d. Radical Excision

These procedures are primarily indicated for the high-grade malignancies and are characterized by an extracompartmental planned dissection. Their extent varies considerably from tumor to tumor and depends to a great extent on the availability of effective adjuvant therapy. In general, once a wide resection is planned and the reconstruction is organized, all adjoining tissues not needed for the reconstruction and/or function of the part should be excised with the tumor in an en-bloc resection. Local lymph node dissections are appropriate if included in this bloc but are not otherwise advised electively. Generally speaking, once the tumor has spread to nodes, survival depends more on systemic than on local therapy.

e. Amputation

Midthigh or arm amputations for peripheral extremity tumors, disarticulations for distal humeral or femoral tumors, or quarterectomies (forequarter amputation or hemipelvectomy) for proximal extremity tumors were the mainstay of surgery for the high-grade malignant bone tumors of the extremities. Chemotherapy and radiotherapy have managed to decrease the need for these amputations as a large variety of conservation procedures with reconstruction have been brought forth.

f. Conservation Resection with Reconstruction

These procedures are a challenge to the ingenuity of the surgeon; among them can be counted

- Large-bloc resection with cadaver bone graft for long-bone shaft tumors.
- Shaft prosthesis (e.g., femoral shaft prosthesis).
- Total joint resection with joint replacement (e.g., knee amputation for distal femur or proximal tibia sarcoma with knee joint replacement).
- Shoulder and hip replacements.

g. Palliative procedures

A large number of palliative surgical procedures are selectively indicated in certain specific circumstances:

- Spine decompression and stabilization whenever the cord is threatened.
- Prophylactic internal fixation for impending pathological fractures.
- Prosthetic replacement of severely diseased areas of long bones.
- Hip joint replacement.
- Use of methylmethacrylate in conjunction with the above procedures.

Table X

Indications for Surgical Procedures by Stage of Disease

Type of procedure	Purpose	Stages where indicated
Intralesional operation	Biopsy	For Stages I, II, and III
	Curettage	For benign self-healing lesions
	Palliative resection	For Stage III
	Ajunctive treatment	In Ewing's sarcoma
Marginal resection	Definitive resection	For benign, locally aggressive lesions
	Palliative resection	In Stage III
	With adjunctive treatment	In Stage I and II
Wide bloc excision	Definitive resection	For Stage IA
	Conservation resection (with adjunctive treatment)	For Stages IB–II
Radical excision	Definitive resection alone	In Stage IIA
	With adjunctive treatment	In Stage IIB
Amputation	Debulking-type operation (intralesional palliative)	For Stage III
	Marginal amputation:	
	As adjunctive treatment	In Stages I and II
	As palliative resection	In Stages I and II
	Wide amputation:	
	Curative resection alone	For Stage IB
	With adjunctive treatment	For Stage II
	Radical resection	For Stages IIB and III

3. Therapeutic Approach by Type of Tumor

There are several modes of treatment for bone tumors that can in general be grouped into five categories according to the tumor type and its behavior: self-healing lesions; benign, locally aggressive lesions; low-grade malignant lesions; high-grade sarcomas; and metastatic bone tumors.

a. Self-Healing Lesions

Eosinophilic granuloma, nonossifying fibroma, ossifying fibroma (Campanacci's disease), fibrous dysplasia, and unicameral bone cyst are all bone tumors of the self-healing variety. Observation or minimal treatment by one of the intralesional modalities is usually sufficient. Observation, injection, curettage, curettage and grafting, or at times, radiation therapy have all yielded 80–90% cure rates. The absence of these tumors in adults attests to the fact that these are indeed self-healing.

i. Fibrous Dysplasia. When located in safe anatomic sites (i.e., non-weight-bearing areas), observation is safe and may be the treatment of choice. Otherwise, treatment at the time of biopsy is indicated. Excision, marginal or wide, with cortical bone grafting is the procedure of choice. Cancellous bone grafts will rapidly convert into fibrous dysplasia as a result of the biologic behavior of graft incorporation, as stated by Enneking. Cancellous bone leads to immediate apposition, and thus the fibrous dysplastic mesenchyme will incorporate the graft into this disease process. Cortical bone requires haversian excavation prior to appositional bone formation; as new mesenchyme is required to excavate haversian systems of cortical bone, that fresh mesenchyme leads to the differentiation of osteoblasts and normal appositional bone. In spite of such measures, grafts are often eaten away by the disease process, and multiple grafts should be anticipated and the patients forewarned.

ii. Eosinophilic Granuloma. Observation or intralesional surgery such as grafting are the procedures of choice. Radiation for polyosseous aggressive lesions may be recommended.

iii. Unicameral Bone Cyst. The effect of treatment of unicameral cysts has not been adequately documented because the natural history and activities of these cysts has not been documented according to stage in large series (i.e., the active versus the latent cyst, the on–off cyst, etc.). Attempts at better histologic staging of these cysts must take into account factors such as the age of the patient, the site and distance from the plate, sequential film review, intralesional pressures and continuity, and escape time of radiopaque dyes. At the present time, most employ an injection technique using 80–200 mg of Depo-Medrol injected into the cyst once every 2 months for at least two and probably three sessions. Healing takes approximately 4–5 months to manifest itself on x-rays. An 80–90% success rate has been reported with these techniques. Fractures through the lesion have not been a reliable enough stimulus to healing as reported in most series.

iv. Nonossifying Fibroma. The indications for treatment of nonossifying fibromas are their size and location or the possibility of a pathological fracture occurring through the lesion. Curettage or curettage with grafting usually results in cure.

v. Campanacci's Disease (Ossifying Fibroma). Ossifying fibroma of bone requires diagnosis by biopsy; its similarity to the nonossifying fibroma histologically and to fibrous dysplasia anatomically makes the diagnosis confusing. The local reaction to trauma, coupled with the hormonal milieu of the young patient in whom these lesions present, leads to an aggressive recurrence of the lesion if operated on during the growth period. It seems desirable, therefore, to treat these lesions by observation or minimal treatment until the end of the growth period.

b. Benign Locally Aggressive Lesions

Benign locally aggressive lesions include giant-cell tumors, chondromyxoid fibromas, aneurysmal bone cysts, fibrous dysplasia, chondroblastomas, osteoid osteomas, osteoblastomas, desmoplastic fibromas, and hemangiomas. These lesions have all been reported to recur in as many as 30–50% of cases after curettage and grafting. Management is thus quite complex, and in general, observation is only recommended if a patient is managed in a tumor center where the complications of observation are diagnosed early and managed promptly.

Extended marginal excision is the preferred method of treatment in this group of tumors; the reactive callus is taken down with a burr or power drill; the tumor is excised or curetted; and cauterization is then carried out to reach all the nests of cells in the trabecular interspaces. Recurrence rate is somewhere in the neighborhood of 20% following "extended" subtotal excision when an aggressive approach and a "choice" operation is selected:

* A virginal lesion with good physis and subchondral bone can be managed by curettage, providing a failure will not jeopardize subsequent marginal or wide-excision surgery that might require reconstruction.
* A recurrent lesion, or one that is virginal but aggressive, requires a marginal or wide excision with reconstruction as a secondary, rather than a primary, goal.
* An aggressive approach is recommended for those lesions in the pubic and para-acetabular regions where observation and conservative procedures might lead to disaster.
* Radiation therapy is usually reserved and recommended only for those lesions in inoperable sites or where management requires early ablation. The risk of radiation-induced sarcoma in young patients (<30 years) must be taken into account.

Certain specific benign-aggressive lesions require specific comments:

i. Giant-Cell Tumors.

These are aggressive, slow-growing lesions with a high potential for recurrence. They are not always benign and can be aggressive, nor are they easily eradicated (cold or hot bath, liquid nitrogen, or methylmethacrylate often fail). Only total extirpation of the lesion can assure a high incidence of cure. The histological grading of the tumor from 1 to 4 depends on the mitochondrial activity of the ellipsoid stromal cell or the number of nuclei in one giant cell and may give an indication of the aggressiveness of the tumor. Recurrence may be seen even a decade later, and this is almost always a progression of a lesion that is not totally resected. Local resection seldom extirpates the tumor fully, whether it is or is not combined with a bone graft and even when it is associated with cryosurgery, methylmethacrylate, or phenolization of the tumor borders. This approach, however, may be acceptable in certain conditions with the recognition of both patient and surgeon of its limitations. Definitive extirpation is actually the treatment of choice and is preferable whenever possible. Radiotherapy is rarely used nowadays in the treatment of this tumor due to the many facts detailed earlier. It is only used under unusual circumstances (e.g., medical contraindication of surgery and a symptomatic lesion).

ii. Osteoid Osteoma.

The osteoid osteoma is a benign bone tumor characterized by extreme pain that is usually relieved by simple analgesics such as aspirin. Total excision of the entire nidus is mandatory to prevent recurrence. Multiple nidus sites have been reported; x-rays performed before and during the operation help in identifying them and insuring total resection. A recent scheme involves doing a bone scan preoperatively, performing a local en-bloc resection, and then rescanning to confirm the absence of the hot-spot nidus. The method may be impractical, however, as it requires the availability of a camera (scanner) in the operating room.

iii. Aggressive Fibrous Dysplasia.

Aggressive fibrous dysplasia is most often seen in children, frequently resulting in pathologic bone fractures. Wide excision and grafting is the procedure of choice in spite of the high rate of recurrence within the grafted bone. Radiotherapy should not be used in fibrous dysplasia.

c. Low-Grade Malignancy

The following malignant tumors could be considered low grade: adamantinoma, intraosseous fibrosarcoma, and G1 chondrosarcoma. These primary malignant lesions are often amenable to surgical cures. The slowly growing, locally invasive adamantinoma of bone usually seen in the jaw and the tibia can be successfully extirpated. The same is true of the low-grade chondrosarcoma. Usually, an incisional biopsy is necessary to establish the diagnosis, and definitive treatment is carried out by wide excision. Radiation therapy is rarely effective in this group of tumors.

d. High-Grade Malignancy

All other sarcomas will be included in the high-grade category except for round-cell bone marrow lesions (lymphoma and multiple myeloma). High-grade fibrosarcoma or chondrosarcoma, osteosarcoma, and Ewing's sarcoma constitute the bulk of this group of tumors.

i. Ewing's Sarcoma. This lesion is one where surgical therapy has been notoriously ineffective, and the treatment of choice today is multidisciplinary (see §8 on Pediatric tumors). A high incidence of local failure (35%) reported in the literature in patients who succumb to their disease, however, seems to suggest that the older method of low-dose radiotherapy alone is inadequate. It also suggests that there may be a place for conservative surgery. Current protocols recommend treating the disease with chemotherapy (vincristine, cyclophosphamide, and Adriamycin spanning 6 months to 2 years) and high-dose irradiation (5000–6000 rads), followed by excision of the lesion at 1 year following treatment, if the bone to be sacrificed is expendable. This would include parts of the pelvis (not including the acetabulum), the clavicle, and the proximal humerus. Such an approach may also be considered for the proximal and distal femur with present-day techniques of reconstruction. Preservation of the limb is an important objective if at all possible.

The complications of treatment include pathological fractures, loss of range of motion, leg-length discrepancies, etc. Each of these can be managed with insight and preventive measures:

• Exercises around the joints during radiation techniques will preserve motion.
• Bracing appropriate areas of ablations.
• Open reduction with internal fixation and bone grafting for impending pathological fractures. Pathological fracture at the time of diagnosis is a poor prognostic sign for limb salvage, and later pathological fractures through the area of prior tumor and irradiation have plagued physicians for years. Because of the altered biology of the tumor-bearing tissues, these pathological fractures need fixation and grafting to assure healing.

The 5-year survival rate of patients with Ewing's sarcoma in current series reported in the literature is somewhere in the neighborhood of 50–60%.

ii. Osteogenic Sarcoma. Osteogenic sarcomas are unkind at any age, attacking the teenager, but also occurring in the elderly in 5% of patients with Paget's disease. This reported figure of 5% is quite high and probably represents the severe cases of Paget's disease that come to the clinician's attention. It is often believed that almost everyone gets some Paget's disease if he or she lives long enough, and therefore the true incidence of osteosarcoma in Paget's disease is probably much lower than the reported 5%.

Treatment of osteosarcoma varies and is still controversial. In general, the introduction of effective chemotherapies has allowed a phased reduction in the surgical margin accepted as adequate for curative treatment; the extent of resection has changed from radical to wide margin for Stages IIA and IIB. A wide margin may be achieved either by a wide excision, amputation of a limb, or a salvage procedure (turn-up, total joint, etc.); the reconstruction depends on what is left after adequate resection has been accomplished. Most Stage IIB lesions, however, require amputation.

Prior to 1970 Marcove (16) reported a 17.4% 5-year survival rate for osteogenic sarcoma, with 80% of patients developing pulmonary metastases within 2 years of diagnosis. Likewise, Friedman and Carter in 1972 (9) reported a 20% 5-year survival in 1286 cases studied. With the advent of Adriamycin and high-dose methotrexate (MTX) with leucovorin rescue, the figures began to improve in the last decade; currently, a figure in the range of 50% or higher disease-free survival after 2 years can be expected in treated osteogenic sarcoma. At the Memorial Sloan-Kettering Cancer Center in New York, using protocols of preoperative chemotherapy with vincristine, high-dose MTX, Adriamycin and bleomycin, cyclophosphamide, and dactinomycin, an 82% 2-year survival was reported in a series of 61 selected patients. The Mayo Clinic in Rochester, Minnesota reported a 52% survival at 2 years in 37 patients treated with surgery, vincristine, and high-dose MTX. Others, however, are now reporting survival rates of around 40% with no chemotherapy, as opposed to the historical figure of 20%, and they question whether the above noted improved survivals are related solely to the use of adjuvant chemotherapy.

Utilizing chemotherapy pre- and postoperatively, a variety of conservation operations were described using femoral-shaft prostheses or knee replacements following knee amputations for distal femoral and proximal tibial osteogenic sarcomas; both of these procedures are limb sparing. Initial results are encouraging. Thus en-bloc resection with custom-made femoral shafts, hinged knee joints, and shoulder or humeral replacements can now be performed in conjunction with aggressive chemotherapy in order to avoid the standard mutilating ablative procedures previously carried out. Adjunctive radiotherapy is essential if one is to consider conservation surgery; local recurrence in high-grade osteosarcomas is in the range of 15–25%.

For a practical guide, the treating physician should consult Tables VI through X in considering staging by intracompartmental versus extracompartmental site and grading of the osteogenic sarcomas into low grade (or G1, parosteal and endosteal) versus high grade (or G2 for the more aggressive tumors) in estimating the specific patient's prognosis and in planning the type of resection or the amputation site.

Pulmonary metastases are extremely frequent in osteogenic sarcoma. Positive pulmonary CAT scans prior to surgery were present in 50% of patients in a recent series at the Mayo Clinic. Pulmonary CAT scans are superior to linear tomography or routine chest films in identifying pulmonary metastatic lesions. As previously stated, resection of solitary or limited metastatic lung lesions in osteogenic sarcoma yields a significant prolongation of survival in the range of 1–2 years from the time of wedge resections of the lung metatases. Resection of pulmonary metastases is also recommended in patients with giant-cell tumors or chondrosarcomas.

iii. Chondrosarcoma. In chondrosarcoma, local en-bloc resection and wide radical marginal procedures are adequate in G1 and G2 tumors when they are distal to the midfemur or the midhumerus. More proximal lesions have a worse prognosis, and no definitive guidelines can be enunciated at this time. We feel that hemipelvectomy in proximal femur and peripheral pelvic tumors is primarily the preferable surgical approach even in low-grade tumors. There are, however, advocates of local resection, cryosurgery, and repeat procedures, who report reasonable survival rates in low-grade tumors. Head and neck chondrosarcoma is a less aggressive tumor than the peripheral lesions; it affects the maxilla more often, whereas osteogenic sarcoma involves the mandible. Wide excision gives a 50% survival when resectable chondrosarcoma is encountered in the head and neck. Peripheral lesions, more frequent in adult life, are treated by local ablation; the survival rate as high as 50%. As the lesion moves proximally, however, the cure rate drops to about 25%.

Although adjuvant chemotherapy has been recommended for the high-grade tumors that might behave biologically as the more aggressive fibro- or osteosarcomas, no specific gain is established. In addition, radiotherapy is of questionable value in chondrosarcomas.

iv. Malignant Hemangioendothelioma. Malignant hemangioendothelioma accounts for less than 1% of all the malignant bone tumors. The term is used interchangeably with angiosarcoma or hemangiosarcoma. These tumors are recognized as being generally highly malignant. There have been, however, reports of a few genuine cases that pursued an indolent course with long survival after appropriate surgical therapy. These tumors are usually not identified clinically or roentgenographically prior to surgical biopsy. They present with the usual pain and swelling. Roentgenographically they display unifocal or multifocal areas of lytic lesions. Multiple lesions have a more favorable prognosis than solitary ones. Nearly all ages are affected by this tumor, but there is a better prognosis in younger age groups. Pathologically, the tissue is very vascular and bleeds profusely at biopsy. Silver staining for reticulum fibers accentuates the vascular nature of the tumor and helps in differentiating it from other malignant tumors. Furthermore, such stain determines whether the proliferating cells are inside the channels, as in true hemangioendothelioma, or outside, as in hemangiopericytoma.

Treatment of this tumor is surgical resection followed by radiation therapy. The value of each of these modalities is not strictly known.

v. Chordoma. Chordomas are rare, slow-growing malignant lesions that occur in the clivus in the skull, the sacrum, and on rare occasion, in the lower lumbar spine. In the skull the behavior of the tumor is not as aggressive as in the sacrum; the latter, however, is the more common location. Chordomas are believed to arise from notochordal arrest cells that become malignant, and they can be present for years without being detected. Low backache followed by constipation and urinary tract problems hail their onset; they usually present in young adults and have an equal sex distribution. Rectal exam will often identify a presacral mass.

The early lesions are usually midsacral, and only an excellent x-ray study will reveal the lytic lesion that could otherwise be obscured by rectal contents or be mistaken for a sacral foramina. X-ray studies should, therefore, be performed after a good cleansing enema. The destruction of the cortex is a later sign than the lytic lesion and must be differentiated from metastatic carcinoma, giant-cell tumor, or solitary plasma cell myeloma. Sometimes an anterior/posterior view shows the pathology only on retrospective scrutiny; however, a lateral view should demonstrate an expansile midsacral erosive lesion. Computerized axial tomography is invaluable for visualizing the usually large presacral soft-tissue expansion that is often present with this tumor.

Grossly, the tumor is lobulated, due to the fibrous septa that traverse it throughout. On histological examination, the myxomatous background with uniform epithelial-like cells in a homogeneous pattern is the characteristic appearance. The vacuolate or physaliphorous cells with peripherally displaced nuclei are the pervasive microscopic finding.

The treatment of malignant chordoma is surgical excision. Complete removal is often hard to accomplish without sacrificing the second sacral nerve roots, which controls the sphincteric musculature of urination, defecation, and ejaculation. A combined abdominoperineal approach, like that used for a rectosigmoid carcinoma that is locally invasive, can be used to assure total removal of the tumor. Some advocate a posterior approach alone as being less complicated, but only early lesions without extension are amenable to complete removal this way. Dissection of a large mass that extends to the bowel coverings anteriorly cannot be done blindly by the dissecting finger, and complete extirpation is difficult to achieve in this manner. If SII can be preserved, sexual, bowel, and bladder function can then also be preserved. An attempt to do this must be carried out even if it is possible only on one side; it will greatly improve detrusor function. Distant metastases occur infrequently, and a 50% overall cure rate can be expected following effective surgery.

Radiation therapy has been utilized in the treatment of chordomas (especially those arising in the skull), either exclusively for the inoperable patient, or as an adjunct to surgery. Results are indeterminate, and no data from large series is available to date.

e. Metastatic Carcinoma

The most frequent malignancy of bone is metastatic carcinoma. Patients may present with lesions after a long quiescent period, and to think of this situation as hopeless may be to deny someone a year or more of relatively pain-free living and limb function that could result from properly addressing the metastatic carcinoma in the bone. Needle biopsy is useful in establishing the diagnosis. Enzyme studies for alkaline and acid phosphatase or serum electrophoresis to detect gamma globulin spikes will distinguish Paget's disease and myeloma from metastatic disease in certain cases, specifically in the vertebral body.

Radiation therapy is traditionally the most universally used modality of treatment for symptomatic bone metastases. The combined use of chemotherapy and hormonal therapy in cases of hormone-dependent tumors such as breast, prostate, or thyroid tumors is also generally recommended in the treatment of bone metastases. In bone metastases from thyroid cancer, the use of radioactive iodine (^{131}I) may result in significant responses if the tumor picks up ^{131}I.

Surgery, however, plays a most important role in the treatment of selected patients with bone metastases. The patient with neurological deficit or cord deterioration is traditionally treated by decompression by laminectomy and then stablized surgically. The use of halo traction as an interim approach can be of great value, but stabilization of the spine to forestall cord compression and paralysis is extremely important. Using the newer techniques developed for stabilizing scoliosis (i.e., Harrington and Luque rods or Dwyer technique), this objective could be achieved successfully in many patients.

This surgical approach is justified, especially if the expected longevity is for 6 or more months of life. Several recent studies have shown that conservative management of cases of impending cord compression by a combination of radiotherapy and steroids could be equally effective.

A lytic lesion in a weight-bearing bone, even in the absence of pathological fracture, is a surgical indication. It should be prophylactically fixed, preferably by intramedullary nailing. If internal fixation, prosthetic replacement, or even external immobilization with expectation of healing is contemplated, radiation therapy must be properly timed to allow for early optimum results.

Hip joint replacements with long-stem prostheses have worked well in some limbs with metastatic disease. The methylmethacrylate reinforcement for such metastatic tumor surgery has been advocated, and it can be used for metallic fixation as well as joint replacement. Custom-made devices, shoulder replacements, and other ingenious apparatus have provided some patients with the ability to ambulate or utilize their upper extremities, thus greatly enhancing their quality of life and significantly relieving their pain.

Traction, splints, and bed rest are recommended as substitutes for major surgery in patients with a life expectancy under 3 months and in those high-risk patients with liver metastases, clotting deficiencies, and/or advanced lung metastases. Renal cell carcinomas bleed excessively with surgery, and major surgery at the site of renal tumor metastasis should be avoided. Even biopsy of renal cell carcinoma metastatic to bone could be associated with intense bleeding, and cross-matched blood, Gelfoam, and Avitene must thus be on hand during such procedures.

B. Radiotherapy

The place of radiotherapy in the treatment of primary bone tumors is in a state of flux. The whole management approach is undergoing great changes as a result of the continuing modification of various chemotherapeutic regimens. In addition, many innovations introduced by new surgical techniques aimed at saving limbs make it mandatory to introduce adjunctive radiation therapy in the definitive treatment of bone tumors.

1. Primary Bone Tumors

a. Osteosarcoma

In osteogenic sarcoma (the most common primary bone malignancy), radiotherapy may have an adjuvant role along with chemotherapy. Adequate surgical extirpation of the presenting tumor, however, remains the essential curative step. It seems that the treatment pendulum has swung from preoperative radiotherapy to preoperative intensive chemotherapy. Postoperative radiotherapy, however, along with systemic chemotherapy, is recommended by some authors to reduce the incidence of local recurrences, especially when surgery was marginal (e.g., when the tumor is too near to the resection margin or there were too many skip sites). The technique used is tailored to the surgical or stump site, and the dose delivered is kept at rather high levels (approximately 6000 rads). This dose should be modified, however, where extensive chemotherapy is used and myelosuppression is evident.

Recently, trials were designed to test the role of prophylactic lung irradiation (approximately 2000 rads delivered) in reducing the incidence of lung metastases after pilot studies showed a possible beneficial effect of such an approach. Furthermore, the palliative use of radiotherapy is often called for in recurrent or metastatic disease, but a higher dose should be aimed at (5000–6000 rads in 3–5 weeks).

b. Ewing's Sarcoma

Radiation therapy is used in conjunction with chemotherapy as the primary modality of treatment in Ewing's sarcoma; 5000–6000 rads are delivered together with one of several combinations of chemotherapy (see §5.IV.C.3). Surgery is not recommended until 6 months to 1 year after therapy.

c. Giant-Cell Tumors

The role of radiotherapy in giant-cell tumors continues to be controversial. It is generally agreed that it should only be used when surgery is inapplicable because of the tumor site (vertebra or pelvic bones) or the patient's general condition. While well-documented instances of radiation-induced sarcomatous changes are rather limited, such a possibility should persuade the treating physician to use radiation only when absolutely necessary. Moreover, for radiation to be successful in achieving its objective in tumor control and relieving symptoms, an effective dose (5000–6000 rads in about 5 weeks) should be used.

d. Other Primary Tumors

Although radiotherapy is often used as an adjuvant modality with surgery in chondrosarcomas, chordomas, and hemangio-endotheliomas, its value has not actually been documented.

2. Metastatic Bone Disease

Radiation therapy is probably the most important palliative modality in the treatment of bone metastases. Its primary role is in the management of the pain that so often accompanies bone metastases. That pain is usually deep-seated and persistent, with a progressive pattern that bears little relation to the size of the offending lesion, its origin, or its duration. The site of the bone metastasis may have a modifying effect on the nature of the ensuing symptoms; e.g., long-bone metastases may, in addition, be accompanied with bone disruption that threatens a pathologic fracture. Vertebral metastases are probably the most frequent symptomatic lesions, and pain may be accompanied with cord compression symptoms that result in neurological deficits (e.g., paraplegia). Metastatic bone pain is often unrelated to activity (walking versus resting) or posture (erect or horizontal at bed rest) and is sometimes felt most acutely during night rest.

While radiotherapy is successful in controlling bone pain in over 75% of cases, the pathogenesis of this effect, or of the pain itself, is poorly understood. The pattern of response is fairly consistent however, occurring after a lag period varying from 1 to 2 weeks and continuing until it reaches its zenith a few weeks later. One must bear in mind other factors that may have contributed to the pain. Pathological fractures or mechanical misalignments will have an impact on this pattern. A painful long-bone metastasis that has led to even a minor partial fracture will continue to be painful despite radiotherapy, until the fracture is stabilized either by fixation or effective splinting.

The great majority of metastases in bone appear on radiological examination as lytic lesions, but the presence of both lytic and sclerotic components is also common. Some lesions may look predominantly sclerotic, such as those originating from prostatic carcinoma. Lytic lesions in long bones may tend to fracture earlier than the sclerotic ones; no other major differences exist between the behavior of lytic and that of sclerotic lesions. The response of both lesions to radiotherapy is very similar, although sclerotic lesions may require a somewhat higher dose of radiation.

The technique of radiotherapy is rather simple, involving the use of a pair of parallel opposed fields (portals) in most cases, or a single field in the case of metastatic spine disease. Beams (^{60}Co units) are very often utilized, but linear accelerators and even, occasionally, orthovoltage (250 kV) units can be used. Special care must be exercised if orthovoltage is chosen, since bone has a significantly greater capacity for energy absorption, leading to substantial escalation of the normal dose. The dose used for control of bone metastases varies widely. Most metastatic lesions will be effectively controlled by 3000 rads given in 2 weeks (10 fractions). The treatment of metastases from some slow-responding tumors (e.g., prostatic carcinoma) necessitates a somewhat higher dose (4500 rads in 3.5 weeks). Other approaches, such as a single high dose, have been tried with apparent effectiveness, though perhaps of shorter duration compared with that noted with the standard setup. The single high dose is currently being evaluated in a clinical trial conducted by a cooperative national group.

C. Chemotherapy

1. Adjuvant Chemotherapy in Osteogenic Sarcoma

There has been major progress in the chemotherapy of osteogenic sarcoma in the past decade. For several decades, the 5-year survival rate for this disease did not exceed approximately 20%. Since 1970, however, it has been appreciated that several agents, notably Adriamycin and high-dose MTX, were active in the treatment of advanced disease, prompting a number of attempts to introduce these agents in the adjuvant setting. Initially, adjuvant chemotherapy was given shortly after definitive surgical removal of the primary tumor, which generally meant amputation. In some centers, effective presurgical chemotherapy was instituted, offering an opportunity to explore limb-salvage surgery with an end result equivalent to that of amputation. Available chemotherapy trials may be separated into single-agent and multiple-agent trials.

a. Single-Agent Trials

At least one large study reported the use of *Adriamycin* alone following surgery [cancer and leukemia Group B (CALGB)]. The drug was given at 30 mg per square meter of body surface area per day for 3 days every 28 days. The patients treated as per protocol, who did not require dose reductions, had a 5-year survival rate of only 32%, emphasizing the contention that in osteogenic sarcomas, as in soft-tissue sarcomas, Adriamycin, to be effective, must be used at full doses. A similar point is made when one considers that only those patients who experience leukopenia when treated with Adriamycin for metastatic disease obtain remissions.

Several uncontrolled series using *high-dose MTX* are available. The most impressive results are obtained when very high doses of MTX (8 g per square meter) were used in a very intensive schedule (i.e., weekly). It must be stressed that high-dose MTX requires very careful pharmacologic monitoring by an experienced and disciplined staff; careful attention must be paid to vigorous pre- and posthydration monitoring of serum creatinine *and* serial blood levels of MTX. Leucovorin reversal must be started promptly, and the patient must be instructed absolutely not to miss any doses of leucovorin. Intensive leucovorin reversal must be extended for any patient whose serum creatinine rises or whose serum MTX levels remain elevated. If all precautions are taken, it is possible to give very high dose MTX as often as once a week. Many series reported in the literature suggest a cure rate in excess of 40%. There is some evidence that even higher doses (12 g per square meter) of MTX are superior yet. A steep dose–response curve appears to be a feature of sarcomas in general.

b. Multiple-Agent Trials

Adjunctive chemotherapy using a combination—Conpadri 1—consisting of cyclophosphamide, vincristine, phenylalanine mustard, and Adriamycin was reported to produce a 55% disease-free survival rate. When high-dose MTX was added to this regimen, there was, surprisingly, no increase in the survival rate.

High-dose MTX and Adriamycin have been combined in several different trials. A recent study, from the Dana Farber Cancer Institute, reported a survival rate of 75% at 2 years. The Memorial Sloan-Kettering Cancer Center has also reported a very elaborate multidrug trial, which includes high-dose MTX, Adriamycin, and several other agents, with an 84% 2-year survival rate. It should be kept in mind that most patients destined to relapse in surgical series will have done so by 24 months after surgery.

At the present time, one cannot necessarily state that any one adjuvant program is superior to any other. Clearly, further investigation is necessary. The complexity of some of the regimens should make it obvious that these patients are best managed at centers equipped to carry out such programs.

c. Preoperative Chemotherapy and Conservation Surgery

An exciting by-product of the documented efficacy of chemotherapy when used early in this disease is the feasibility of limb-salvage surgery. Chemotherapy IV or IA is used as the initial treatment modality, sometimes accompanied by radiation, sometimes not. During the period of administration of chemotherapy, a custom-made endoprosthesis is fashioned. The tumor is then removed, and the prosthesis is inserted. Careful scrutiny of the pathological specimen removed at surgery allows one to judge the efficacy of the preoperative chemotherapy and then to apply this information in guiding postoperative adjuvant treatment. If massive necrosis is found, the same drugs are continued; otherwise an alternate regimen is employed. Several major national cancer centers have already accumulated a series of such patients, and the prospects seem promising indeed. In the experience of the Memorial Sloan-Kettering Cancer Center in New York, all subsequent relapses occurred in those patients who failed to show an excellent response to the preoperative chemotherapy. Yet another approach has been the use of intra-arterial Adriamycin and cisplatinum and radiotherapy preoperatively. Initial results for this approach are also quite promising.

Fairness dictates that we point out that the improvement in survival claimed for adjuvant chemotherapy of osteogenic sarcoma is not universally accepted. Investigators from the Mayo Clinic have pointed out that they have recently observed better-than-expected results in patients who did not receive adjuvant chemotherapy for a variety of reasons. Whether this improvement is a result of better surgical technique, more detailed staging (i.e., eliminating patients with positive chest CAT scans who may have been included in earlier series), or a change in the natural history of the disease is, at present, unknown. The Mayo Clinic has reported a prospectively randomized study, even though several other centers have challenged the premise of improved survivals in recent surgical series in their own hands. Their study shows no advantage to postoperative high-dose MTX plus vincristine, compared to surgery alone. Unfortunately, the number of patients entered into each arm of the study was small (osteogenic sarcoma remains rare), and many observers feel that one negative, albeit randomized and controlled, study does not definitively demonstrate that adjuvant chemotherapy is not beneficial. In addition, the question of postoperative adjuvant chemotherapy may well become moot because of the trend to adopt *preoperative* chemotherapy and institute conservation surgery. Indeed, it is difficult to challenge the recent results reported of up to 90% disease-free survival at 2 years in patients treated with this approach. Only time will tell whether the excellent early results will prove durable.

2. Palliative Chemotherapy in Metastatic Disease

Adriamycin and high-dose MTX remain the mainstays of treatment for metastatic osteosarcoma with chemotherapy. If the patient was not exposed to either or both of the agents previous to the development of metastases, a trial of one or both in combination is surely warranted. A careful search should be carried out for all sites of possible metastases. If all apparent metastatic lesions are confined to the lung, and if the disease responds to chemotherapy, surgical resection of remaining deposits should be entertained. A small percentage of patients has been cured by this approach! In an occasional patient, repetitive thoracotomy may even prove necessary and beneficial. It should be stressed that the apparent cure rate of resection of metastases from osteosarcoma, when combined with chemotherapy, exceeds the expected surgical cure rate of primary lung cancer.

Other active agents include cyclophosphamide, bleomycin, dimethyl triazeno imidazole carboxamide (DTIC), and more recently, *cis*-platinum. In general, combinations have not proven themselves to be substantially superior to single-agent Adriamycin, possibly as a result of the dose reduction of the latter when it is combined with other myelotoxic agents.

3. Chemotherapy in Ewing's Sarcoma

Despite the early presentation as localized disease, most patients with Ewing's Sarcoma develop hematogenous metastases within 6 months of diagnosis. Surgery and radiotherapy are applied to the primary tumor, but experience has taught that the use of combination chemotherapy at presentation, when no obvious metastases are demonstrable but micrometastases may be presumed to exist, has substantially improved the prospects of cure.

The "classic" regimen in this disease, devised more than a decade ago for the treatment of metastatic disease, consists of the combination of vincristine, dactinomycin, and cyclophosphamide (VAC). This combination was incorporated as an adjuvant modality into the initial management schema, which included radiotherapy and, where feasible, surgery. Improved cure rates resulted compared with historical controls. Subsequent studies have examined the addition of Adriamycin to the VAC regimen or to VAC with the further addition of pulmo-

nary irradiation. There seems to be an increased efficacy for the Adriamycin arm over both VAC alone or VAC with radiotherapy. Intensive chemotherapy has also proven effective in controlling the primary lesion, and it has been suggested that primary treatment be radiation therapy and chemotherapy, followed by surgery at a later date.

Final evaluation of chemotherapy protocols has to take into account various prognostic factors. For instance, the prognosis is worse for patients whose disease originates in pelvic bones (<40% local control compared with >80% in other sites). A better prognosis is also seen with disease in distal extremities and in patients with normal lactic dehydrogenase values. The outlook for patients who have failed initial chemotherapy trials is uniformly poor.

V. POSTOPERATIVE CARE, EVALUATION, AND REHABILITATION

A. Postoperative Care

1. Immobilization

Areas of benign tumors treated with curettage and bone packing must be protected from activity so as to prevent fractures at the weakened operative site. In the upper extremity, 6 weeks will usually suffice to protect the limb from a stress-riser fracture; in the lower extremity, 12 weeks is often required. Even in the case of a small open biopsy, when the pathologic report indicates a benign process, protection for a month is needed to allow cortical bone to heal enough to avoid a fracture.

More extensive resections, with or without reconstruction, will demand various periods of immobilization. One advantage of the use of prosthetic devices in joints or metallic fixation is early ambulation and mobilization.

2. Care of Amputation

Stump care begins at once with the use of compression dressings to allow for shrinking of the stump and early prosthetic fitting. There are mixed feelings about immediate prosthetic fitting; although the psychological advantage of having something to feel in bed and walk on postoperatively is desirable, wound healing is sometimes compromised, and flaps that are at all tenuous are less likely to survive. Open-air exposure and closed evacuation systems for wound drainage in the first several days are more salubrious to stump healing than a closed casted system. Stump fitting can start after a week has elapsed and the wound edges are securely healed. Discussion of prosthetic devices and fitting and adjusting of same is found in the rehabilitation section.

When a stump flap is devitalized, revision is needed. A plastic surgeon adept at the use of fluorescent injection and Wood's lamp can be of tremendous help in stump revision. Myocutaneous flaps and free pedicle grafts with microvascular reanastomosis can be utilized when proximal stumps about the shoulder and thigh require it. Correct stump planning can avoid troublesome dehiscence and must be carefully done preoperatively.

3. Precautions for Internal Prosthesis

The custom-made internal prostheses require warning to the patient that the metal, although strong, is not as elastic as human bone and the fixation to bone by methylmethacrylate is subject to loosening. It is not a total substitute for normal bone but an expedient one. The device can break or loosen or both.

B. Follow-Up Evaluation

Unlike tumors in other sites, bone tumors, even when benign, require long-term follow-up.

- Multiple exostoses or multiple enchondromas need to be followed through life with evaluation and possible x-ray studies because of the possibility of sarcomatous degeneration (10 and 35%, respectively).
- Bone cysts treated by packing or injection should be followed at progressively longer postoperative intervals, from monthly to yearly until growth ceases.
- Malignant lesions need constant, indefinite surveillance, particularly osteogenic sarcomas, fibrosarcomas, and aggressive or proximal chondrosarcomas. For Stage I tumors, visits at 6-month intervals are sufficient, whereas the Stage III or IV lesions should be followed every 6–12 weeks.
- Periodic chest x-rays are required in all aggressive bone malignancies, and CAT scans, which are more sensitive to early detection of lung metastases, must be liberally obtained if one contemplates successful treatment for pulmonary metastases. The frequency of these studies is dependent on the aggressiveness of the lesion.

Local recurrence can occur from seeding at the time of surgery, inadequate resection, or microscopic insidious extension of the tumor beyond the wide margins of an apparently adequately excised tumor. Close observation of the site of excision is therefore mandatory.

Table XI is a suggested schedule of follow-up that can be used for malignant bone tumors, with some adjustment being made according to the aggressiveness of the tumor.

C. Rehabilitation

The integration of rehabilitation medicine into the multidisciplinary team approach has favorably influenced the quality of care and the quality of life of many cancer patients. The goals of rehabilitation medicine are the prevention of secondary disabilities (e.g., deconditioning, contractures, decubiti) and the functional restoration of the individual. The increasing number of cancer patients whose disease is now cured or controlled or who are given a longer life expectancy by more aggressive therapeutic approaches or by conservation operation has led to a more optimistic and realistic management strategy in contrast to the old, fatalistic attitude. A conservative impetus in this direction followed the National Cancer Act of 1971, which has recognized the rehabilitation needs and potential of cancer patients.

This section deals with the specific problems of the patient with bone cancer, some of these problems being quite similar to those of the patient with cancer of the soft tissues. The role of the rehabilitation process is to evaluate the patient's capability of performing the activities of daily living and to plan, prescribe, and implement a realistic treatment program. This is aimed at optimal functional restoration: physical, emotional, and social. The rehabilitation team is a multidisciplinary group by itself comprised of a physiatrist, a physical therapist, an occupational therapist, a rehabilitation nurse, a prosthetist, an orthotist, a clinical psychologist, a social worker, and a vocational counselor.

1. The Amputee

Although progress in chemotherapy and radiation therapy has managed to reduce the number of limb amputations, this type of surgery is still widely used for many malignant bone tumors of the extremities. Patients with amputations for malignancies are of younger age (under 30) than those with amputations for peripheral vascular disease (over 55); furthermore, the level of amputation tends to be more proximal in cancer patients because of the necessary anatomic margin, resulting in a higher degree of disability. Cancer occurring in the foot may require a below-knee amputation; cancer of the tibia or fibula requires an above-knee or midthigh amputation; cancer of the femur, a hip disarticulartion; and pelvic bone involvement may require hemipelvectomy or hemicorporectomy. In general, the lower extremities are more frequently involved than the upper ones. If mentally competent, most patients with amputation of lower extremities should be considered potential candidates for prosthetic rehabilitation regardless of their life expectancy.

a. Preoperative Preparation

Preprosthetic training in the form of strengthening of the upper extremities, range-of-motion exercises, posture and bal-

Table XI

Schedule for Follow-Up of Bone Tumors

Management	First year			Second-to-third year				Thereafter	
	Monthly	6 months	12 months	3 months	6 months	9 months	12 months	6 months	12 months
History									
Pain	X			X	X	X	X	X	X
Swelling or mass	X			X	X	X	X	X	X
Stiffness	X			X	X	X	X	X	X
Restriction of use	X			X	X	X	X	X	X
Fever	X			X	X	X	X	X	X
Fracture	X			X	X	X	X	X	X
General review of symptoms		X	X		X		X		X
Physical									
Local exam of tumor site	X			X	X	X	X	X	X
Range of motion	X			X	X	X	X	X	X
Neurological assessment	X			X	X	X	X	X	X
Vascular assessment	X			X	X	X	X	X	X
Complete physical exam		X	X		X		X		X
Investigation									
CBC and SMA-12		X	X		X		X		X
Chest x-ray (and/or CAT scan)		X	X		X		X		X
X-ray of tumor site	X				X		X		X
CAT scan of site		X	X		X		X		X
Bone scan	As indicated by type of tumor or presenting symptoms								
Liver scan	As indicated by type of tumor or presenting symptoms								
Other x-ray modalities	As indicated by type of tumor or presenting symptoms								
Serum electrophoresis	As indicated by type of tumor or presenting symptoms								
Urinary Bence-Jones	As indicated by type of tumor or presenting symptoms								
Acid phosphatase	As indicated by type of tumor or presenting symptoms								

ance exercises, and use of walkers and crutches should be started in the preamputation period when the patient's general condition and mental outlook is better. A discussion with the patient about the likelihood of experiencing a phantom limb sensation postsurgery will help to alleviate anxiety and misinterpretation in the postoperative period. It has been recommended that a well-trained and well-adjusted amputee, preferably with a similar anatomic level, should be introduced to the patient as a resource for psychological support and positive reinforcement. Following surgery, the management of the amputee during all recovery steps from healing, shaping, and conditioning of the stump to prescribing and fabrication of the prosthesis, as well as training in its use, follows well-established guidelines with enough flexibility for individual adjustments.

b. The Prosthesis

- Below-knee amputation. The prosthesis of choice for a patient with below-knee amputation is the patellar tendon–bearing (PTB) type with a solid-ankle cushion-heel (SACH) foot. Such a prosthesis can be securely attached by a cuff-suspension strap or a thigh corset and side bars.

- Above-knee amputation. For the above-knee amputee, the prosthesis will have an ischial weight-bearing quadrilateral socket and a knee mechanism selected from a variety of available types (constant friction, hydraulic, etc.), each with its advantages and drawbacks. The above-knee prosthesis is heavier, and it is suspended by waist belts and pelvic bands or suction devices.

- Hip disarticulation. For the patient with hip disarticulation, the prosthesis of choice is the Canadian type, in which the socket encircles the pelvis and provides a weight-bearing area under the ischial tuberosity on the amputated side.

- Hemipelvectomy. Following hemipelvectomy, the loss of pelvic bones requires the addition of a cushioning segment in order to align the body vertically and to prevent scoliosis when sitting. This prosthesis is heavier, and its fitting and use is more cumbersome.

- Hemicorporectomy. In a few cases in which a translumbar amputation (hemicorporectomy) was performed, the patients were provided with a bucket type of prosthetic jacket serving as a sitting device mounted on a rotating platform on a wheelchair, which they could operate independently. Lower extremities' prostheses can be attached to the jacket, and successful rehabilitation with independent ambulation can sometimes be achieved. In motivated patients, rehabilitative solutions can be offered for even the most complex situations.

- Amputations of the upper extremity. Patients with amputations of upper extremities can be fitted and trained with prosthetic devices for any anatomic level from forequarter amputations and shoulder disarticulations to below-elbow amputation. According to a patient's capabilities and wishes, one can provide a cosmetic device with no functional use but a satisfactory appearance, or a functional prosthesis having a terminal device made in the shape of a hand or a variety of hooks. A system of cables activated by the proximal muscles can supply the mechanism and power to provide grasp and release. More complex myoelectrically activated hand prostheses can be obtained in rehabilitation centers with adequate bioengineering resources.

Successful prosthetic rehabilitation owes a great deal to the skill and experience of the prosthetist. Periodic reevaluation of the patient and of the prosthetic device are mandatory. In addition to the training of the limb bearing the prosthesis, all patients with an amputation of an upper extremity should receive training for one-hand activities, thus reinforcing the usefulness of the contralateral extremity.

c. Conditioning of the Stump and Prosthetic Training

Conditioning of the stump tissue is essential for a successful prosthetic fitting.

Control of edema, strengthening of the remaining muscles, and toughening of the skin are obtained by firm bandaging of the stump and conditioning exercises under the close supervision of a physical therapist. The ultimate shape of the stump will determine the degree of pressure tolerance at the stump socket interface. During the rehabilitation training, the prosthetic device can be modified and adjusted as needed.

The prosthetic training following stump healing for the below-knee amputee can take as little as 2–3 weeks and for the above-knee amputee from 4 to 6 weeks. The energy expenditure (measured in oxygen consumption) required to ambulate with a unilateral below-knee prosthesis is about 20% higher than that of a normal individual. It is up to 40% higher than normal in the case of a unilateral above-knee amputee. This should be taken into account in patients with cardiopulmonary problems, who thus need a slower and more gradual training program.

For patients with slowly healing stumps or with skin lesions secondary to radiation therapy, the temporary use of a by-pass, ischial weight-bearing prosthesis—one in which the stump hangs free with no contact to the prosthetic device—should be considered. This will allow ambulation, while healing continues, long before the definitive prosthesis can be properly fitted.

d. Educational and Vocational Rehabilitation

New vocational goals must be realistically assessed and pursued by most amputees. The rehabilitation process should also include the psychosocial adaptation of the patient to his amputation, to the prosthesis, and to his new environment. Some patients may require counseling and/or supportive psychotherapy.

2. The Patient with Metastatic Disease

Metastic bone lesions localized in weight bearing bones (vertebrae, femur, etc.) are known to have the potential of causing pathological fractures. Clinicians have been challenged for years by the dilemma of whether to curtail the physical activities of patients with bony metastases out of concern that this might increase the risk of fractures. On the other hand, there was the awareness that prolonged bed rest will enhance osteoporosis, muscle atrophy, and contractures without any assurance that pathological fractures will be prevented. Over the last decade, we have adopted the principle of progressive and protected mobilization using canes, walkers, splints, braces, and corsets in accordance with the patient's tolerance, while alerting the patient's family about the possibility of spontaneous pathological fractures. The more recent favorable reports following preventive surgical stabilization (nailing and cementing) of impending fracture sites of proximal femurs are offering new methods that will further enhance early active mobilization of these patients.

3. Pain Management

In the management of severe chronic pain and postoperative pain, the use of transcutaneous electrical nerve stimulation (TENS) is gaining an increased acceptance and is being used alone or in conjunction with analgesic drugs. Its noninvasive nature and lack of side effects makes it an ideal modality to be considered, although its effectiveness remains to be proven.

D. Nursing and Psychosocial Aspects of Aftercare

Caring for the patient with a primary bone malignancy offers many challenges to the nurse. Major factors that influence the care of these patients include patient's body image disturbance; patient's need to cope with loss of a body part; age of the patient (50% of the patients treated by amputation are under the age of 29); and physical care of the patient including preoperative and postoperative care, prosthesis care, and phantom pain.

1. Body Image Disturbance

''Body image'' relates to the individual's perception of his or her outward appearance. It results from internal feelings as well as influences from society, cultural practices, and previous experiences with the handicapped or infirm. The assessment of the patient undergoing amputation should include the knowledge of any behavioral changes that may be indicative of body image disturbance. These include

- Denial or refusal to look at the body area in question.
- Lack of self-care ability.
- Hostility and refusal to talk.
- Responses to the loss.

Both the patient and family members should be encouraged to express their feelings, whether positive or negative. No judgments should be made by the nurse, nor should hostile comments by the patient be taken personally. Furthermore, while providing physical care, it is important to be ready to prepare the patient to look at the affected body part. It might be helpful to arrange for the patient to speak with a peer who has previously had similar surgery and has properly adapted to his or her prosthesis. If the patient requests, referral to a member of the clergy is in order.

Many times, patients experiencing a change in body image will have fears related to sexuality and rejection. These fears may become apparent in the hospital even before the patient is ready to be discharged. The patient and partner should be encouraged to express their feelings. This may be a difficult topic to discuss, and it might be necessary for the nurse to refer the patient to another health professional if she or he feels uncomfortable with the subject.

2. Coping with the Loss of a Body Part

Adaptation to loss includes three stages: shock and disbelief, developing awareness to the loss, and restitution. During the first phase, it is important to accept the patient's behavior, unless he or she becomes physically destructive, and to encourage the expression of his or her feelings. In the second phase, it becomes easier to involve the patient in his or her own care and to encourage the family members to continue the support. The patient may be discharged prior to the restitution phase, but his or her efforts to accept the loss should be praised.

3. Age of the Patient

Osteogenic sarcoma occurs most often in adolescence—a difficult period of adjustment. Amputation is devastating at any age, but problems with identity and self-image compound the situation. Alopecia due to chemotherapy can further impact negatively on self-image.

4. Physical Care of the Patient

a. Pre- and Postoperative Nursing Care

Prior to any intervention, it is important to assess the patient's level of knowledge about the disease process and the contemplated treatment. This will enable the nursing staff to reinforce and explain the information given by the physician to correct any misconceptions and to relieve or diminish any anxiety. It is beyond the realm of this manual to discuss general preoperative nursing care, which can be found in any nursing text.

The aims of immediate postoperative care are to prevent infection and contractures and to minimize edema. Elevation of the stump, proper positioning, management of dressing changes, and keen observation are most important. A physical therapist should be consulted and his or her assistance sought to provide and teach full range-of-motion exercises to all limbs, upper extremity exercises, quadriceps-setting exercises of the unaffected leg, and crutch walking (if necessary).

As the patient progresses in his or her recovery, he or she should be taught stump care and preparation for the prosthesis.

b. Prosthesis

The patient will be fitted with an artificial limb by a prosthetist. Psychosocial support and reinforcement should be provided, especially since the temporary initial prosthesis is not attractive in appearance. Observance of the patient's technique in preparing the stump for prosthesis fitting is of utmost importance. The patient should be encouraged to report any problems with the prosthesis to the nurse or another health professional.

c. Phantom Pain

Phantom limb sensation is a group of feelings such as pain, itching, or cramping in the lost part. It often occurs in the immediate postoperative period and fades with time.

The patient should be informed that it is perfectly normal. Phantom limb ''pain'' does not usually appear until a few weeks after the surgery and frequently disappears after a few months.

Nursing interventions to relieve the problems of phantom limb include

- Encouragement of ambulation.
- Diversion.
- Encouragement of mental exercise of the lost limb.
- Administration of analgesics as prescribed.

VI. MANAGEMENT ALGORITHM FOR
BONE TUMORS

(see p. 249)

SUGGESTED READINGS

1. Abelson, H. T., and Goorin, A. M. Current controversies in oncology: Osteosarcoma. *Surg Rounds* **5,** 44–55 (1982).
2. Arlen, M., Tollefson, H. R., Huvos, A. G., and Marcove, R. C. Chondrosarcoma of the head and neck. *Am. J. Surg.* 120–456 (1970).
3. Bleyer, W. A., Haas, J. E., Feigel, P., Greenle, T. K., Schaller, R. T., Morgan, A., Tendergass, T. W., Johnson, F. L., Bernstein, I. O., Chard, R. L., and Hartmen, J. R. Improved three-year survival in osteogenic sarcoma. *J. Bone J. Surg., Br. Vol.* **64B,** 233–238 (1982).
4. Dahlin, D. C. "Bone Tumors, General Aspects and Data on 6,221 Cases," 3rd ed., pp. 329–343. Thomas, Springfield, Illinois, 1978.
5. DeLisa, J. A., Miller, R., Melnick, R. R., and Mikulic, M. A. Rehabilitation of the cancer patient. *In* "Cancer, Principles and Practice of Oncology" (V. T. DeVita, Jr., S. Hellman, and S. A. Rosenberg, eds.), Chapter 46. Lipincott, Philadelphia, Pennsylvania, 1982.
6. Dietz, J. H. Adaptive rehabilitation of the cancer patient. *Curr. Probl. Cancer* **5,** No. 5 (1980).
7. Enneking, W. F., Spanier, S. S., and Goodman, M. A. A system for the surgical staging of musculoskeletal sarcoma. *Clin. Orthopedics* **153,** 106–120 (1980).
8. Fried, E., III, Jaffe, N., *et al.* Adjuvant chemotherapy of osteogenic sarcoma: Progress and perspecties (Editorial). *J. Natl. Cancer Inst. (U.S.)* **60,** 3–10 (1978).
9. Friedman, M. A., and Carter, S. K. The therapy of osteogenic sarcoma: Current status and thoughts for the future. *J. Surg. Oncol.* **4,** 482–451 (1972).
10. Gitelis, S., Sheinkop, M., *et al.* The role of prophylactic surgery in metastatic hip disease. *Orthopedics* **5,** No. 8 (1982).
11. Heffelfinger, M. J., Dahlin, D. C., MacCarty, C. S. *et al.* Chordomas and cartilagenous tumors of the skull base. *Cancer (Philadelphia)* **32,** 410–420 (1973).
12. Henderson, E. D., and Dahlin, D. C. Chondrosarcoma of bone, 288 cases studied. *J. Bone J. Surg., Am. Vol.* **45A,** 1450 (1963).
13. Jaffe, H. L. "Tumors and Tumorous Condition of the Bones and Joints." Lea & Febiger, Philadelphia, Pennsylvania, 1958.
14. Jaffe, N. Progress report on high dose methotrexate with citrovorum rescue in the treatment of metastatic bone tumors. *Cancer Chemother. Rep.* **58,** 275 (1974).
15. Marcove, R. C. New trends in the treatment of osteogenic sarcoma. *Orthop. Dig.* **3,** 11 (1975).
16. Marcove, R. C. "The Surgery of Tumors of Bone and Cartilage." Grune & Stratton, New York, 1981.
17. Marcove, R. C., Hutter Mikev, R. V. P., Huvos, A. G., Shojo, H., Miller, T. R., and Kosloff, R. Chondrosarcoma of the pelvis and upper femur: An analysis of factors influencing survival time in 113 cases. *J. Bone J. Surg., Am. Vol.* **54A,** 561 (1972).
18. Patel, M. R., Sanchez, M. O., Silver, J. W. and Pearlman, H. S. Metastatic malignancy of the hand—a clinical manifestation of bronchogenic carcinoma. *N. Y. State J. Med.* **78,** No. 14, 2233–2236 (1978).
19. Patel, M. R., Silver, J. W., Lipton, D. E., and Pearlman, H. S. Lipofibroma of the median nerve, palm and digits of the hand. *J. Bone J. Surg., Am. Vol.* **61A,** 393–397 (1979).
20. Patel, M. R., Srinivasan, C. K., and Pearlman, H. S. Malignant hemangioendothelioma in the hand. *J. Hand Surg.* **3,** No. 6, 585–589 (1978).
21. Pearlman, H. S., Cuculo, G. F., and Ramachandran, R. S. Neurilemmonm of os calcis. *N. Y. State J. Med.* **64,** 3015–3016 (1964).
22. Pritchard, D. J., Cooper, K. L., and Unni, K. K. Chordoma of the sacrum. *Orthopedics* **5,** No. 5, 587–598 (1982).
23. Rosen, G., Marcove, R. C. *et al.* Primary osteogenic sarcoma: The rationale for preoperative chemotherapy and delayed surgery. *Cancer (Philadelphia)* **43,** 2163–2177 (1979).
24. Rosen, G., Wollner, N., Tan, C., Wu, S. J., Hadju, D. I., Cham, W., D'Angio, G. J., and Murphy, M. L. Disease-free survival in children with Ewing's sarcoma treated with radiation therapy and adjuvant four-drug sequential chemotherapy.
25. Srinivasan, C. K., Patel, M. R., and Pearlman, H. S. Malignant hemangioendothelioma of the bones. *J. Bone J. Surg., Am. Vol.* **60A** (5), 696–700 (1978).
26. Taylor, W. F., Irvins, J. C. *et al.* Trends and variability in survival from osteosarcoma. *Mayo Clin. Proc.* **53,** 695–700 (1978).

ALGORITHM FOR BONE CANCER

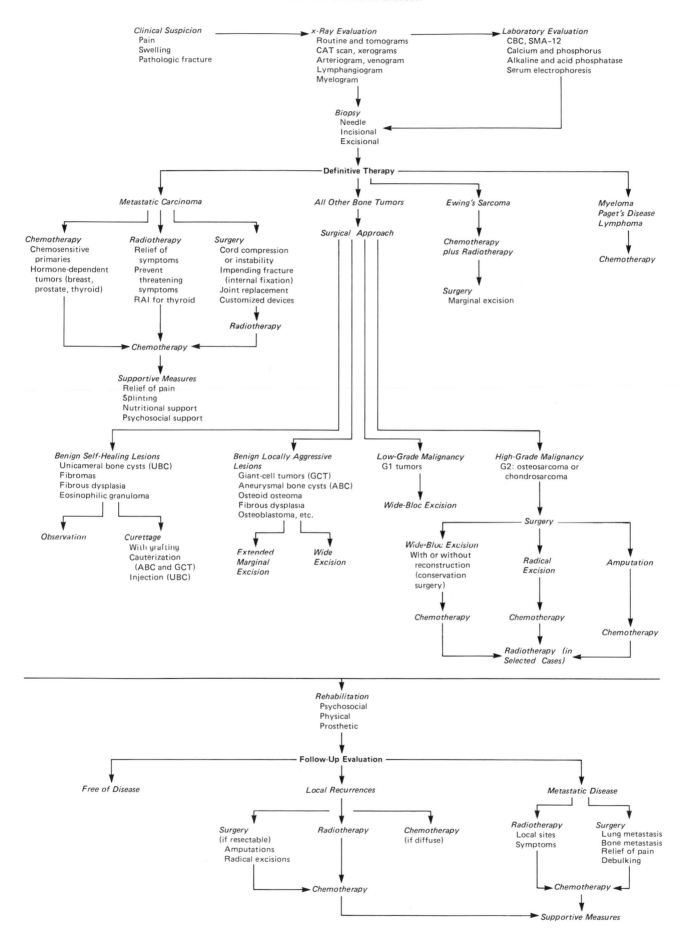

Section 6

Soft-Tissue Sarcomas

ROBERT LERNER

With Contributions By

Rene A. Khafif	Surgical Oncology
Payyalore Venkitachalam	Surgery
Sameer Rafla	Radiotherapy
Samuel Kopel	Medical Oncology
Carmencita Soriano	Pathology
Ari Feibel	Rehabilitation
Randi Moskowitz	Nursing Oncology
Helen McCarthy	Nursing Oncology

251

Section 6. Soft-Tissue Sarcomas

I. Early Detection and Screening   255
  A. Patient Education
  B. Risk Factors
  C. Early Detection

II. Pretreatment Evaluation and Work-Up   256
  A. Establishment of the Diagnosis
    1. Physical Evaluation
    2. Biopsy
      a. Aspiration Biopsy
      b. Needle Core Biopsy Using Vim Silverman or
        Tru-Cut Disposable Needles
      c. Excisional Biopsy
      d. Incisional Biopsy
  B. Evaluation of the Primary and Planning Therapy
    1. X-ray of the Affected Part of the Body
    2. Computerized Axial Tomography Scan of the
      Affected Part
    3. Angiogram
    4. Other
  C. Metastatic Evaluation
    1. Chest X-ray, Tomograms, and CAT Scan of
      Lungs
    2. Complete Blood Count, Serum Electrolytes, and
      Blood Chemistries
    3. Bone Scan
    4. Liver Scan
    5. Lymph Node Evaluation
    6. Intravenous Pyelogram
    7. Abdominal and Pelvic CAT Scan
  D. General Medical Evaluation
  E. Multidisciplinary Evaluation
  F. Site-Specific Data Form for Soft-Tissue Sarcoma

III. Preoperative Preparation   258

IV. General Management Guidelines   258
  A. Management Goals
    1. Highest Possible Cure Rates
    2. Lowest Degree of Disability
    3. Rapid Rehabilitation
    4. Psychosocial and Occupational Adjustment
  B. Common Pitfalls
  C. Surgical Modalities
    1. Radical Resection (muscle group excision or
      compartment resection)
    2. Amputation

    3. Wide Local Excision
    4. Local Excision
    5. Regional Lymph Node Dissection
  D. Variations of Surgical Approach by Site of Sarcoma
  E. Radiotherapy
    1. Adjunctive Radiotherapy
    2. Definitive Radiotherapy
    3. Palliative Radiotherapy
  F. Chemotherapy
  G. Management of Recurrent Disease

V. Therapeutic Guidelines: Type-Specific   266
  A. Pathological Considerations
  B. Types of Soft-Tissue Sarcoma
    1. Rhabdomyosarcoma
    2. Liposarcoma
    3. Fibrosarcoma
    4. Neurofibrosarcoma
    5. Synovial Sarcoma
    6. Leiomyosarcoma
    7. Malignant Fibrous Histiocytoma
    8. Tumors of Blood and Lymphatic Vessels
      a. Angiosarcoma
      b. Lymphangiosarcoma
      c. Malignant Hemangiopericytoma
      d. Kaposi's Sarcoma
    9. Tumors of Uncertain Origin
      a. Alveolar Soft-Part Sarcoma
      b. Epithelioid Sarcoma
      c. Clear-Cell Sarcoma
      d. Malignant Granular Cell Tumor
  C. Therapeutic Considerations

VI. Postoperative Care, Evaluation, and Rehabilitation   269
  A. Immediate Postoperative Care
  B. Psychological Support
  C. Coordination of Postoperative Radiotherapy and
    Chemotherapy
  D. Rehabilitation
    1. The Immediate Postoperative Period
    2. Amputations
    3. Soft-Tissue Resections
    4. Reconstructive Surgical Procedures
  E. Follow-Up Evaluations

VII. Management Algorithm for Soft-Tissue Sarcoma   271

Suggested Reading   271

Soft-tissue sarcomas constitute a large group of malignant neoplasms, most of which are extremely aggressive, that arise from various cells originating from the mesoderm. They are nonepithelial in nature and can develop from any mesodermal cell: fat cells, fibrocytes, muscle cells, synovial cells, histiocytes, etc.

The behavior of the tumors will depend on the cell of origin, and they may present as a mixed-cell-type variety. Furthermore, the clinical presentation will vary according to their location. The management of these tumors, however, is much the same regardless of the histological subtype or location; although aggressive tumors will require more radical treatment, and the therapy will, by necessity, have to vary slightly to accommodate the anatomic setting of the tumor.

The most important presenting clinical feature of soft-tissue sarcomas is the presence of a mass or lump. This may arise in any part of the body, and it is most often painless and asymptomatic until it attains a considerable size. At times it may not be identifiable for long periods because of its location (e.g., retroperitoneal, intra-abdominal, or intrathoracic). In the extremities and head and neck areas, on the other hand, the mass is readily visible much earlier.

Symptoms are generally the result of pressure, traction, or invasion of adjacent structures such as nerves, vessels, or muscles by the tumor. This may cause pain, limitation of movements or, at times, obstruction of adjacent hollow structures. Other symptoms vary widely depending on the histologic type of the tumor and on its anatomic location:

- A leiomyosarcoma arising from the smooth muscle of the GI tract may cause GI bleeding or intestinal obstruction, whereas one that arises from the uterus may cause uterine bleeding or pelvic congestion or simply present as a pelvic mass.
- A retroperitoneal liposarcoma may present as increasing abdominal girth or ureteral obstruction or just cause vague abdominal pain.
- Kaposi's sarcoma presents as raised, pigmented skin lesions of the lower extremities. Visceral Kaposi will present with symptoms peculiar to the site of involvement.
- Mesotheliomas present with respiratory symptoms, hemothorax, etc.

Symptoms such as weight loss, cough, malaise, anemia, jaundice, anorexia, etc., may also be related to metastatic disease.

I. EARLY DETECTION AND SCREENING

There are no specific screening procedures available at this time that will facilitate early detection of soft-tissue sarcomas. A large percentage of these tumors occurs in young adults, a population for which a routine yearly physical examination is rarely recommended. Patient education seems to be the only avenue open for early detection.

A. Patient Education

Education of the patient and the general public about cancer warning signs throughout the various organ systems of the body and about the necessity of reporting to the physician the least suspicion is of paramount importance. This should be accomplished through the various health education channels available today:

- Health-related seminars organized by professional and paraprofessional groups for members of the local community.
- High school health education programs.
- Various periodical publications.
- News media and particularly television, documentaries, etc.

Most of these avenues are currently in use in public education in the health fields; efforts should be focused, however, where such education would be most useful. The following three directions should be pursued in all educational efforts.

- The public should be informed about the risk factors that may play a role in the etiology of soft-tissue sarcomas.
- Warning signs and symptoms of soft-tissue sarcomas should be widely publicized, with special emphasis on any ''lump'' or ''bump'' even if not symptomatic.

- Routine annual physical examination of children and adolescents, as well as people over the age of 40, should be emphasized; and patients should be encouraged to seek professional help at the slightest suspicion of any irregularity.

B. Risk Factors

- Age. Children under the age of 15 are at highest risk for soft-tissue sarcomas, which constitute the fifth most common tumor in children (6.5% of all cancers in children, compared with only 0.7% of all cancers in adults).
- Family history of cancer, particularly in siblings.
- Past history of cancer.
- Radiation treatments in childhood.
- Trauma. Even though trauma by itself may not be a cause of neoplasms, it sometimes calls attention to a preexisting lesion.
- Possible exposure to some environmental toxic products such as phenoxyacetic acids (herbicides) or chlorophenols (wood preservatives).
- Homosexual habits or residence in Haiti or in Africa (Kaposi's sarcoma).
- The association between a highly malignant form of Kaposi's sarcoma and acquired immune deficiency syndrome (AIDS) in homosexuals, drug addicts (users of intravenous drugs), and hemophiliacs (or those who receive multiple blood transfusions) is a recently reported and intriguing phenomenon.

C. Early Detection

Early detection can only be promoted in three ways:

- Patient education.
- High index of suspicion by physicians.
- Early evaluation and biopsy.

The signs of soft-tissue sarcomas, with the exception of "a mass," are extremely varied and nonspecific and may include any one of a large number of symptoms, depending on the location of the tumor:

- Pain.
- Ulceration.
- Bleeding.
- Discoloration.
- Asymmetry (indicative of nerve damage or a deep-seated mass).
- Obstructive symptoms (GI, GU, airway, vascular).
- Pressure symptoms, etc.

II. PRETREATMENT EVALUATION AND WORK-UP

A. Establishment of the Diagnosis

1. Physical Evaluation

- A complete history with special reference to risk factors in the etiology of soft-tissue sarcomas and to the signs and symptoms of soft-tissue sarcomas as already mentioned.
- Complete physical examination with special emphasis on the nature and details of the mass and on possible damage caused to various adjacent structures and organs.
- Organ system evaluation in search of metastases.

2. Biopsy

The single most important diagnostic modality in establishing the diagnosis of a soft-tissue sarcoma is the histologic examination. All soft-tissue masses should be biopsied, even if they appear to be benign. The only exceptions are those that are easily identifiable as benign lesions (lipomas, meningiomas, etc.) and that have been present and unchanged for several years.

a. Aspiration Biopsy

This is usually inadequate in soft-tissue sarcomas. Although it might identify malignant cells, it is practically impossible to classify the tumors on the basis of cytology alone.

b. Needle Core Biopsy Using Vim Silverman or Tru-Cut Disposable Needles

The histologic diagnosis, typing, grading, and classification of soft-tissue sarcomas is, at best, extremely difficult because of the similarity of pattern and cells of various types and because of the mixed cellularity present in the majority of tumors. A needle core biopsy might provide adequate sampling but is often insufficient to give all the details required. It is a good preliminary procedure to identify the pathology and is particularly useful for deep-seated tumors that would be difficult to biopsy otherwise. At times, it is a sufficient basis for planning further therapy, and thus facilitates decisions regarding a definitive therapeutic approach.

c. Excisional Biopsy

An excisional biopsy should be considered only for masses less than about 3 cm in diameter. It is never satisfactory for definitive therapy, and to attempt a total removal of a larger tumor would only complicate the definitive operation and open up planes that one would prefer to leave undisturbed until then.

d. Incisional Biopsy

Masses more than 3 cm in diameter that cannot be clearly identified by needle core biopsy should have an incisional biopsy. Excisional biopsy of such masses may preclude the chance for a curative resection afterward. The placement and orientation of the incision of the biopsy must be carefully planned to avoid problems or compromises of subsequent radical surgery. The biopsy skin incision should be completely resected during the definitive procedure and should not become part of a skin flap for closure of the wound. Flaps should not be raised during the biopsy, and usual anatomic planes should not be entered. It is also important to achieve complete hemostasis after the biopsy; extension of hematomas from the biopsy incision will often necessitate wider radical resections than would otherwise be necessary and may allow tumor spread in the planes of dissection of the hematoma. In some instances, the biopsy confirmation and the definitive surgery may be done at the same sitting, if frozen section is used. More often, however, a thorough study of the biopsy is necessary, and definitive surgery is usually deferred.

On other occasions, visceral masses may be excised widely on the basis of a gross pathological diagnosis rather than waiting for histological confirmation of a malignant tumor. Such confirmation is usually obtained subsequently.

B. Evaluation of the Primary and Planning Therapy

1. X-ray of the Affected Part of the Body

This often helps to differentiate soft tissue from bony masses; identify periosteal involvement; note calcification, fractures, or foreign bodies; etc. It is of minimal help, however, in the final diagnosis or in defining the extent of a soft-tissue sarcoma.

2. Computerized Axial Tomography Scan of the Affected Part

The CAT scan is extremely valuable in delineating the local extent of the tumor as well as the distortion, invasion, or alteration of adjacent structures (vessels, nerves, organs, etc.). It is also important in planning the appropriate extent of surgery or radiation. A recently introduced diagnostic tool, nuclear magnetic resonance, that utilizes no radiation exposure whatsoever, is claimed to produce remarkably accurate pictures of soft-tissue tumors.

3. Angiogram

Selective catheterization and angiography of various accessible vessels is sometimes extremely useful in planning the surgery. One may identify the feeding vessels, the vascularity of the tumor, pressure effects, or involvement of the vessels. Since sarcomas contain large avascular areas, angiograms are not usually helpful in defining the actual extent of the tumor. Digital angiography is highly accurate, much less invasive, and easier to perform.

4. Other

Depending on the site of the lesion, various other x-rays might be valuable in assessing the tumor:

- GI series or barium enema.
- Intravenous pyelogram (IVP).
- Venacavagram.
- Lymphangiogram.

C. Metastatic Evaluation

Metastatic evaluation should include the following:

1. Chest X-ray, Tomograms, and CAT Scan of Lungs

The lungs are the most common site of distant metastases in all soft-tissue sarcomas. Hence, a complete chest evaluation is mandatory prior to any definitive therapy.

2. Complete Blood Count, Serum Electrolytes, and Blood Chemistries

3. Bone Scan

These studies are helpful in assessing periosteal involvement when the tumor is close to bone. It is also indicated in assessing and screening for osseous metastases, which are not unusual with soft-tissue sarcoma.

4. Liver Scan

Metastatic involvement of the liver is less common than that in the lungs. Furthermore, the reliability of liver scans is not great. This procedure is only indicated in patients whose liver chemistries are abnormal. The procedure is of some value in cases of visceral malignancies of the abdominal cavity.

5. Lymph Node Evaluation

Lymph node metastases are less common in soft-tissue sarcomas than in carcinomas, metastatic spread of sarcomas being usually hematogenous. Nevertheless, synovial sarcomas and rhabdomyosarcomas have a higher propensity of lymph node metastases. Careful physical examination of regional lymph nodes and biopsy of any node that is clinically palpable are both indicated before setting up a course of therapy.

6. Intravenous Pyelogram

This is indicated in all soft-tissue tumors of the abdomen to assess the status of the retroperitoneal space (ureters, nodes, etc.). However, IVP has been largely superseded by CAT scan.

7. Abdominal and Pelvic CAT Scan

D. General Medical Evaluation

The general condition of the patient must be assessed for intercurrent disorders, cardiorespiratory disease, renal disease, psychosocial illness, nutritional status, allergies, etc. This is essential for total management of the patient. Prior to any radical surgery, further evaluation of the patient by the anesthesiologist is useful in assessing the surgical risk.

E. Multidisciplinary Evaluation

The multimodality approach to the management of the patient with soft-tissue sarcoma cannot be overemphasized. Careful planning of therapy has to be made by the surgeon, the radiotherapist, and the medical oncologist. Input from the radiologist and the pathologist is also extremely useful to assess the type and extent of the tumor. Whether the affected extremity should be amputated or treated by a lesser procedure followed by adjuvant therapies must be decided jointly, on any individual case, by the above group of specialists.

The role of each treatment and modality—namely, surgery, radiation, or chemotherapy—is dependent on the planned, combined use and timing of the other types of treatment.

The social worker, psychiatric liaison, nurse oncologist, and physiotherapist are also of great value in the postoperative care and rehabilitation of the patient, and it is often desirable for them to evaluate the patient preoperatively, get to know him or her and develop a rapport with the patient and family.

F. Site-Specific Data Form for Soft-Tissue
Sarcoma (see pp. 259–260)

III. PREOPERATIVE PREPARATION

The majority of patients with soft-tissue sarcomas are young and relatively healthy individuals who require little or no physical preparation prior to surgery. The following measures may, at times, be necessary:

- Relief of obstruction by the tumor and correction of associated physiological alterations (e.g., GI obstruction, tracheal obstruction, ureteral obstruction, etc.).
- Nutritional support (if indicated) and restoration of blood volume.
- Treatment of local inflammation or infection.
- Correction of any intercurrent illness (cardiac, pulmonary, etc.).
- Psychosocial evaluation and counseling, particularly in younger patients and whenever mutilating surgery is contemplated.

IV. GENERAL MANAGEMENT
GUIDELINES

A. Management Goals

Because of the young age of most of these patients, the aggressive nature of the disease with its relatively poor prognosis, and the mutilating effects of therapy, a concerted effort must be made to utilize all available modalities to the maximum of their abilities. The following goals must be kept in mind at all times when planning therapy.

1. Highest Possible Cure Rates

Although surgery is invariably the primary modality of treatment of soft-tissue sarcomas, results of surgery alone have been disappointing in many types of tumors. A combined approach with various modalities of treatment may achieve better results.

Early diagnosis and biopsy is imperative. Treatment must be aggressive, yet measured against the disability in which it would result.

2. Lowest Degree of Disability

Procedures should be weighed against the infirmity that they might cause; whenever possible, conservation operations must be considered and amputations avoided. If amputation becomes necessary, it should be so selected as to permit effective rehabilitation.

SITE–SPECIFIC DATA FORM—SOFT-TISSUE SARCOMAS

HISTORY

Age: _____ Sex: _____

Symptoms

_____ Mass or lump

_____ Weight loss, anorexia, malaise

_____ Pain

_____ Paralysis

_____ Limitation of movements

_____ Abdominal discomfort

_____ Dyspnea

_____ Hemoptysis

Duration: _____

Social history

  Occupation: _____

  Race: _____ White _____ Black _____ Oriental _____ Other

  Marital status: _____ Single _____ Married _____ Other

  Travel habits: _____

Family history of carcinoma

  Relation: _____ Site: _____

Previous history of carcinoma:

  _____ No _____ Yes Site: _____

Previous treatment (describe): _____

_____

_____

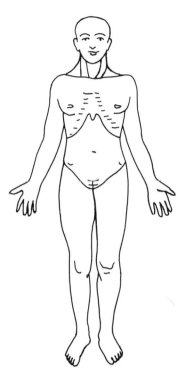

PHYSICAL EXAMINATION

Primary

  Size: _____ <5 cm _____ >5 cm _____ Massive   Consistency: _____ Fluctuant _____ Firm _____ Rock hard

  Shape: _____

Mobility	Yes	No	Location	Precise site
Fixation to muscles:	___	___	Head and neck	_____
Fixation to bone/periosteum	___	___	Trunk	_____
Fixation to skin/subcutaneous tissue	___	___	Upper extremity	_____
Tenderness	___	___	Lower extremity	_____
Skin changes	___	___	Retropertoneal	_____
Impaired nerve functions above or below the mass	___	___	Abdominal	_____
			Mediastinal	_____
Impaired joint functions above or below the mass	___	___		
Other bone involvement	___	___		

Pulses above/below the mass: _____ Normal _____ Impaired

REGIONAL LYMPH NODES

_____ Palpable _____ Nonpalpable

		Side		Size (cm)	
		R	L	0–5	>5
_____ Soft	Juguloomohyoid	___	___	___	___
_____ Rubbery	Upper deep cervical	___	___	___	___
_____ Hard	Lower deep cervical	___	___	___	___
_____ Fluctuant	Submaxillary	___	___	___	___
_____ Movable	Submental	___	___	___	___
_____ Fixed	Parotid	___	___	___	___
	Axilla	___	___	___	___
	Groin	___	___	___	___

Distant metastases: _____ No _____ Yes. Type: _____

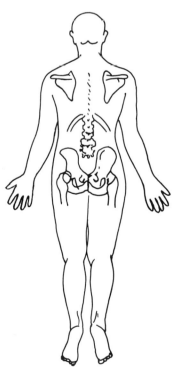

PRETREATMENT WORK-UP (Check, if done)

	Neg.	Pos.	Suspicious		Neg.	Pos.	Suspicious
CBC	___	___	___	Chest x-ray	___	___	___
Chemistry profile	___	___	___	Chest tomograms	___	___	___
x-Ray of the part	___	___	___	Bone scan	___	___	___
CAT scan of part	___	___	___	Liver scan	___	___	___
Angiogram	___	___	___	Biopsy of the mass	___	___	___
IVP	___	___	___	Biopsy of lymph nodes	___	___	___
GI series	___	___	___	Others (specify)	___	___	___
Barium enema	___	___	___				
Venograms	___	___	___				

Classification

  Histologic variety: _____

  Site of involvement: _____

Staging: _____ T _____ N _____ M

Stage: _____

Histologic grade: _____ G1 _____ G2 _____ G3

Signature: _____

Countersignature: _____

Date: _____

Staging of Soft-Tissue Sarcomas

The staging recommended by the Task Force on Soft-Tissue Sarcomas of the American Joint Committee for Cancer Staging and End Results published by Russell *et al.*(1977) is as follows.

TNM Classification

Primary tumor (T)

T1	Tumor less than 5 cm
T2	Tumor 5 cm or more
T3	Tumor that grossly invades bone, major vessel, or nerve

Regional lymph nodes (N)

N0	No histologically verified metastasis to regional lymph nodes
N1	Histologically verified regional lymph node metastases

Distant metastasis (M)

M0	No distant metastases
M1	Distant metastases

Grading of the Tumor

Histologic Grade of Malignancy

G1	Low grade, well differentiated
G2	Moderate
G3	High grade, undifferentiated

Stage I

G1, T1, N0, M0 (Ia) or G1, T2, N0, M0 (Ib)	Grade I histology (5 cm, stage Ia) or greater (stage Ib), no regional nodes and no distant metastases

Stage II

G2, T1, N0, M0 (IIa), or G2, T2, N0, M0 (IIb)	Grade 2 tumor less than 5 cm (IIa) or greater than 5 cm (IIb) with no regional nodes and no metastases distally

Stage III

G3, T1, N0, M0 (IIIa) or G3, T2, N0, M0 (IIIb)	Grade 3 tumor less than 5 cm (IIIa) or greater than 5 cm (IIIb) in diameter with no regional nodes or distant metastases
Any G, T, N1, M0 (IIIc)	Tumor of any grade or size (with no invasion) with involved regional lymph nodes, but with no distant metastasis

Stage IV

Any G or N, T3, M0 (IVa)	Tumor of any grade that grossly invades bone, major vessel or nerve, with or without regional nodes, but without distant metastases
Any GTN, M1 (IVb)	Any grade and size tumor, with or without metastatic lymph nodes, but having distant metastasis

As noted, the most important prognostic factor and the predominant factor in staging of soft-tissue sarcomas is the histologic grade of the malignancy. Other prognostic factors are the site of the tumor, size, and pattern of local extension and lymph node involvement.

3. Rapid Rehabilitation

Functional rehabilitation is paramount whenever mutilating resections must be done. This should be planned and discussed with the patient and his or her family preoperatively and should be started as soon as possible. Cosmetic rehabilitation is also important to permit the patient to return to a normal social existence.

4. Psychosocial and Occupational Adjustment

This must always be kept in mind as an important parameter of the patient's total care.

B. Common Pitfalls

The following are some pitfalls that should be avoided:

- Delay in treatment as a result of ignoring early signs and minimizing the significance of a lump.
- Improper biopsy
  - Accepting negative results of a biopsy in a suspicious lesion.
  - Inadequate biopsy.
  - Poor biopsy technique that complicates therapy and promotes spread.
  - Too extensive a biopsy (attempts at excisional biopsy of large tumors), which would also complicate definitive therapy.
- Failure to recognize distant metastases.
- Inadequate surgery
  - Insufficient resection.
  - Sacrificing cancer control for conservation.
  - Missing lymph node metastases.
- Failure to consider adjunctive modalities of treatment.
- Unnecessarily mutilating procedures and the inability to recognize the fact that some patients are beyond cure.

C. Surgical Modalities

A multidisciplinary approach to the management of soft-tissue sarcomas has become essential for achieving the best possible outcome. The three principal modalities of cancer therapy—surgery, radiation, and chemotherapy—are all of value in the treatment of soft-tissue sarcoma. The best results occur from the wise integration of all three treatments. Surgery, however, is generally the primary therapeutic modality for cure.

The essential principle of surgery is to remove all involved tissue and all tissues at significant risk for involvement. The various surgical procedures available are radical resection of the sarcoma (also called muscle group dissection or compartmental resection), amputation (standard or radical quarterectomies), wide excision of the sarcoma, local excision of the sarcoma (to be condemned), and lymph node dissections. The type and extent of the surgical procedure in any given case depends on the type of tumor, its stage, and its location and is often controversial.

1. Radical Resection (Muscle Group Excision or Compartment Resection)

This radical procedure is done for patients in whom one expects a cure. It involves complete excision of all the structures in the anatomic compartment occupied by the tumor. This type of resection is based on the propensity of the sarcoma to spread along the muscle bundles and other compartmental structures such as nerves, vessels, etc.; it also recognizes the fact that sarcomas do not usually transgress fascial boundaries. The dissection takes place at planes well beyond the palpable tumor, never visualizing or cutting through it. The muscles are completely excised from their point of origin to their insertion; and structures such as vessels, nerves, bones, and joints are sacrificed, if necessary, to accomplish this type of an en bloc resection. Some surgeons make a slight distinction between muscle group dissection and compartmental resection; although the difference is actually semantic, the principle is quite the same: the dissection is performed at one anatomic plane away from the tumor in all directions, and both procedures are radical procedures done for cure.

Radical resections can result in significant disability even if the limb is salvaged. Reconstruction is done by using rotational skin flaps where necessary; it may also be necessary to perform reconstruction of arteries and veins, to carry out muscle transfers to ensure stability, and at times, to substitute for bone (using cadaver bone transplant, customized internal devices, joint replacement, etc.).

Other principles to be observed during radical resection include

- Excision of all skin and subcutaneous tissues near the tumor.
- Resection of all scars and previous biopsy sites, including all the hematoma that may have resulted from a previous biopsy.
- Ligation of venous outflow to the body from the affected area as a first step, prior to manipulation of the tumor area (or application of tourniquets).
- Inclusion of all draining lymph nodes if they are involved by tumor or, in certain varieties of soft-tissue sarcoma (such as epithelioid sarcomas), if the tumor is in close proximity to the node-bearing areas.
- Application of metallic clips along the margins of resection as a guide for future radiation therapy.

Radical surgery done in this fashion can result in a local cure rate of up to 80%, only marginally lower than when amputations are done as the sole radical surgery in such cases. Anything less than a properly performed radical procedure has a still higher local recurrence rate and, if unavoidable, should be followed by radiation and, if indicated, by chemotherapy. In an otherwise early curable lesion, after properly performed radical surgery, one could justifiably withhold adjunctive treatment. The addition of prophylatic therapy (radiation or chemicals), however, is practiced in some centers today, although the final verdict as to its efficacy is not yet in.

2. Amputation

For certain extremity sarcomas, an amputation may be the only way to accomplish radical surgical excision; it is noted in many series that amputation is required in as many as 50% of extremity sarcomas. Some even believe that amputation is the procedure of choice for better local control in all cases. With increasing multimodality support, this approach is becoming discredited, and more emphasis is being placed on conservation and limb salvage.

Amputation may, in rare occasions, be necessary purely for palliation and is done in situations of uncontrollable ulceration or bleeding, simply to make the patient more comfortable.

When done for cure, all principles of oncologic surgery should be observed, and the amputation should be done at least one joint space above the tumor. The following are the various types of amputations required in selected cases.

- Below-knee amputation. For lesions of the forefoot distal to the ankle joint, amputation is done at a level about one-third of the distance between the knee and the ankle.
- Above-knee amputations. For lesions involving up to the lower half of the leg, the amputation is done through the midthigh or slightly above that level.
- Hip disarticulation. This involves complete removal of the femur and most muscles of the lower extremity. It is suitable for lesions around the knee joint, distal thigh, and on occasion, up to the midthigh.
- Hemipelvectomy. This involves removal of the entire lower extremity and half of the pelvic bones, with disarticulation taking place at the sacroiliac joint and pubic symphysis. This is necessary for lesions involving the upper thigh up to the buttocks. If the lesion is located posteriorly, an anterior skin and muscle flap may be used to cover the defect, and if it is located anteriorly, a posterior skin and muscle flap may be used.
- Modified hemipelvectomy. Preservation of the wings of the iliac bone with division of the bone over the acetabulum to the pubic symphysis may be used as an extended hip disarticulation.

- Extended hemipelvectomy. The hemipelvectomy may be extended to include division of the sacral ala up to the lateral vertebral bodies to gain additional clearance.
- Below-elbow amputation. For lesions distal to the wrist joint, the amputation is done at a level one-third of the distance from the elbow to the wrist.
- Below-shoulder or above-elbow amputation. For lesions of the forearm well below the elbow joint, amputation is done at one-third of the distance from the shoulder to the elbow joint.
- Disarticulation of the shoulder joint. For lesions involving the elbow joint or distal arm, the shoulder joint is disarticulated.
- Forequarter amputation. This procedure involves removal of the entire upper extremity including the scapula and clavicle, leaving only the chest wall at the base. This is necessary for lesions involving the proximal arm or shoulder region but not extending to the chest wall.

The level of the amputation is at a joint above the tumor but at the same time insuring that all the muscles and tendons from the tumor-bearing area are completely removed. An amputation done for cure in early cases has a minimum local recurrence rate (5–7%), and the patient may not need further adjuvant therapy.

3. Wide Local Excision

A true radical surgical resection as described above is technically not possible in certain anatomic locations such as the head and neck, trunk, peritoneum, chest, etc. There are no definable compartments in these locations, and radical procedures carry great risk without true anatomic designs. In such cases, wide local excision of the tumor is the treatment of choice for achieving local control. The entire tumor is excised with the widest possible margins around the tumor in all directions; the dissection is always done through uninvolved tissues; the edges of resection are marked with metallic clips to facilitate postoperative radiation therapy; and the generous use of frozen section is encouraged.

Even in the extremities, it has been suggested that a wide local excision followed by radiation therapy could be considered in lieu of a radical muscle group dissection or a compartmental resection. The benefits of such an approach are a marked reduction in postoperative morbidity and subsequent disability. The local recurrence rate after wide local excision alone, however, is about 50%, and such an excision of the tumor, if performed, should always be followed by radiation therapy to the area. Chemotherapy may be added as indicated under various protocol studies.

4. Local Excision

This is mentioned only to be condemned as an inadequate surgical procedure in the management of soft-tissue sarcomas. There is a tendency at times for surgeons to resort to local excisions of the tumors, either because the diagnosis was not appreciated at surgery or because of the ease with which the local excision can be carried out. Soft-tissue sarcomas often develop a pseudocapsule because of compression of the surrounding soft tissues. They have no true capsule, however, and the tumor tends to get "shelled out" along this plane. Shelling out or local excision of soft-tissue sarcomas results in a high recurrence rate (>90%), which is unacceptable.

5. Regional Lymph Node Dissection

Metastases to regional nodes are rare in soft-tissue sarcomas. Hematogenous spread to the lungs is the most common means of dissemination. In a review of over 30 reported series by Weingrad and Rosenberg (8) only 5.8% of almost 3000 patients developed lymph node metastases. Certain histological varieties, however, such as synovial sarcoma, rhabdomyosarcoma, and epithelioid sarcoma, have a greater propensity for lymph node metastases.

The indications for regional lymph node dissections may be as follows:

- When the nodes are clinically palpable, suspicious of metastases, and confirmed by biopsy. A radical surgical procedure in these patients may still be contemplated if there is no evidence of distant metastases and if the primary tumor is resectable.
- If the limits of a radical muscle group or compartmental resection encroach on a lymph node–bearing area; it then becomes more practical and reasonable to include such nodes in the resection.
- A prophylactic lymph node dissection in synovial sarcoma or epithelioid sarcoma should be considered electively, although its value is still controversial. Alternatively, the node-bearing area may be given postoperative radiation therapy.

D. Variations of Surgical Approach by Site of the Sarcoma

The anatomic location of the sarcoma has a great bearing on the clinical features, prognosis, and the type of surgery that can be done. It is next in importance only to the histologic grade of the malignancy, as a prognostic factor.

In general, it can be said that a difference exists between extremity sarcomas and truncal sarcomas. Extremity sarcomas are diagnosed earlier and treated with relative ease by surgery, including if necessary, amputation. The more proximal the lesion, however, the less effective is the margin, the greater the chance for local recurrence, and the greater the postoperative disability. In the head and neck region, a satisfactory radical resection may not always be effectively carried out because of technical considerations. Whatever surgery is done must, therefore, be followed by radiation therapy.

For truncal sarcomas, one has to differentiate between sarcomas arising from the parieties and those arising from the core. Parietal sarcomas are treated by radical local excision and reconstruction. Retroperitoneal sarcomas may become huge before a diagnosis is made, and often the patient will present with a protruberant abdomen as the first symptom. Special diagnostic investigations are always done to identify the extent of involvement. At surgery, adjacent organs such as kidney, spleen, colon, or small bowel may have to be resected in order to remove the primary, and resection is often incomplete. The diaphragm may also have to be resected and reconstructed with synthetic material, and it may be necessary to excise part of the parietal walls and reconstruct these too with synthetic materials. Therefore, prior to surgery the surgeon should be prepared for such extended procedures. These patients will often need postoperative radiation therapy, and metallic clips should be placed at the margins of resection.

Operative mortality varies with the type and extent of the surgery and can vary from less than 1% for an extremity amputation to almost 30% for a large retroperitoneal sarcoma.

E. Radiotherapy

The role of radiotherapy in the treatment of soft-tissue tumors is still controversial, with the battle being fueled by claims and results reported by various radiotherapists that contradict the old dogma of the radioresistence of these tumors.

1. Adjunctive Radiotherapy

The major benefit of radiotherapy is demonstrated when it is applied in an adjuvant setting, particularly postoperatively. The main indications for adjuvant therapy are

- Poorly differentiated tumors.
- Incomplete surgical excision by virtue of tumor size or tumor site (e.g., head and neck or pelvis).
- Certain specific tumor cells of origin. Although this factor does not seem to play a clear role in the contribution of postoperative radiotherapy, certain tumors are claimed to be more radiosensitive than others (e.g., certain types of liposarcomas, fibrosarcoma, and malignant fibrous histiocytoma).

Some authors such as Lindberg and others (4a) have advocated the use of radiotherapy to lessen the magnitude of surgery. They recommend that radical compartmental resections or amputations be avoided. Instead, they advocate performing wide local excisions followed by extensive radiation therapy as the treatment of choice in all cases. The benefits versus the risks of such an approach must be carefully evaluated. Benefits that might accrue from the use of radiotherapy combined with conservation surgery include less mutilating surgery and an improved quality of survival. Risks of failure to control the disease locally have been raised, however, as well as risks of complications (e.g., pain, edema) that may follow high-dose irradiation to a large segment of the limb. It must be emphasized that such a limb-sparing approach is only justified if a useful, functioning limb can be preserved, yet tumor excision must also be complete. No conclusive results are available to suggest whether such an approach is superior to radical surgery.

Preoperative radiation therapy has also been advocated by some, but there are no prospective, randomized control studies to compare this method with that utilizing postoperative radiation. Some individual groups suggest that better local control of the disease is achieved by this method, particularly when the lesion is locally advanced. The tumor mass becomes smaller in volume and is surrounded by a denser pseudocapsule, and often necrosis is noted on pathological examination. Preoperative radiotherapy can be recommended when the tumor is too large to allow safe excision or when immediate surgery is contraindicated. Tumor regression usually occurs only after a rather high dose and is better demonstrated after a lapse of several weeks following treatment. Such high-dose preoperative courses of radiotherapy must be planned and executed with great care to keep the treatment within tissue tolerance and to avoid jeopardizing healing following subsequent surgery. For the plan of treatment to be optimal, it must be outlined jointly by both the radiotherapist and the surgeon, taking into consideration future lines of incision (to limit radiation exposure of these sites and allow satisfactory, timely healing), the status of the organ's vascular and neurological supplies, as well as the future function of the organ. Necessary rehabilitative procedures should also be planned ahead.

The technique of radiotherapy in the adjuvant setting necessitates the use of high-quality beams, the ^{60}Co being the lowest useful beam on a priority list of available tools. Effectiveness is improved by the high-energy accelerator beams (6–24 MeV). The main advantage of the supervoltage beams is the sparing effect of this type of irradiation on the skin and superficial tissues while delivering a high dose to the tumor at a deeper plane. A well-collimated ^{60}Co beam, however, may be adequate in the treatment of limb lesions. Careful planning of the radiotherapy course is essential for a successful outcome. The use of various diagnostic modalities including sonograms

and CAT scanning of the region treated is very helpful in delineating the exact extent of the tumor and in outlining the adjacent radiosensitive tissues or organs that must be protected against radiation damage.

Radiation dose given to soft-tissue sarcoma must be of the order of 6000 rads (60 grays) or more if it is to be effective, since these tumors are of limited sensitivity. Such dosage cannot be safely given to a large volume of the limb, nor is it necessary in most cases. While the irradiated volume must be rather large at the beginning to include the whole compartment, it is decreased in a stepwise fashion as the dose delivered inches above 5000 rads; consequently the volume that receives the full dose is kept limited to the area of the original tumor. When irradiating a limb, every effort is made to avoid including the whole circumference. Instead, it is preferable to leave a sliver of unirradiated tissues to minimize the incidence of subsequent lymphatic obstruction and edema.

The use of adjuvant radiotherapy in the form of brachytherapy at the time of surgery is also being tried in various centers with encouraging results. Interstitial irradiation is used in the form of ^{192}Ir applied to the surgical bed immediately after the conservative total resection of the tumor. An afterload technique is used starting 72 hours after surgery and delivering 4000 rads in 4 days. A recent report from the Memorial Sloan-Kettering Cancer Center claims an 82% overall local control rate (with 100% local control in previously untreated cases) in 33 advanced lesions where nerves, vessels, and bone were spared and where margins were minimal. Wound complications were 35%, but loss of limb occurred in only 6% of the cases.

2. Definitive Radiotherapy

Occasionally, radiotherapy is called upon to play a definitive role in the treatment of certain tumors. This is done only when surgery is inapplicable because of either the patient's general condition or refusal of surgery, or because of the site of tumor (e.g., fixed retroperitoneal tumors). Except for the small or unusually sensitive tumors, the results of such trials are usually extremely frustrating. When radiation is used as the definitive therapy, it is necessary to boost the dose up to about 7000 rads. Since such doses skirt the margins of maximum soft-tissue tolerance, extreme care is indicated, and booster doses are usually given using either interstitial implants or specialized beams (e.g., high-electron beam) that possess the unique characteristic of controlled, limited penetration. Intraoperative radiotherapy is also being tried with promising results.

3. Palliative Radiotherapy

The palliative role of radiotherapy is universally accepted although not extremely effective. Its use is limited essentially to the relief of pain or alleviation of pressure symptoms. While the response is no different from that anticipated in other circumstances, high doses are needed, especially if symptoms are due to the effect of a bulky lesion (e.g., pressure).

In general, radiation therapy is added in the treatment of soft-tissue sarcomas in all circumstances except when a radical and curative operation has been satisfactorily accomplished. All cases of head and neck sarcomas and all cases of truncal and retroperitoneal sarcomas should be considered for postoperative radiation therapy.

F. Chemotherapy

The soft-tissue sarcomas are a bewildering group of neoplasms with many different histological subgroups and different stages. Because no one institution is able to gather sufficient statistics regarding chemotherapy in all the various types of sarcomas, it is necessary to group various reports together in order to reliably assess the response rates to chemotherapy. Yet, even after one combines many single-institution series and the results of multi-institutional clinical trial studies, sufficient information is still lacking as to the true response rate of the various types of sarcomas to the available agents. Although one report indicates response rates to be similar for all histological subtypes, it is not unreasonable to expect that, just as various soft-tissue sarcomas manifest different clinical behaviors, they may also exhibit different responsiveness to the same chemotherapeutic agent. It should be noted that most of the patients reported in the literature have had far-advanced disease; it may prove to be the case that if patients are treated earlier in their disease, higher response rates might be achieved.

The most effective single agent in soft-tissue sarcomas is Adriamycin (doxorubicin). Many studies have indicated its efficacy, and in general, response rates of between 20 and 35% have been obtained. Other agents of demonstrated clinical efficacy in sarcoma include cyclophosphamide, DTIC (dacarbazine), vinca alkaloids, and dactinomycin. In addition, several studies suggest efficacy for high-dose methotrexate. More recently, some data have become available suggesting that *cis*-platinum may also be a useful agent.

Several authors have stressed that in general, but especially in soft-tissue sarcomas, a steep dose-response relationship exists for Adriamycin. It seems that the relatively poor response rates seen in multiple small studies, as well as in some larger ones, are more likely a consequence of underdosing than of unresponsive disease. This contention is at least partially borne out by studies that compare Adriamycin alone to several different combination chemotherapy regimens. When cyclophosphamide or DTIC is added to Adriamycin, reported response rates have been slightly higher but by no means as high as the sum of the individual agents. Furthermore, the durations of response and survival were not substantially prolonged, suggesting that lowering the dose of Adriamycin in order to accommodate other agents reduces it efficacy. At 45 mg/m^2 of Adriamycin, the response rate is less than 20%, whereas at 75 mg/m^2, the response rate apparently doubles.

The CYVADIC regimen (consisting of cyclophosphamide, vincristine, Adriamycin, and DTIC) has been reported to have a response rate of 40–50%, with complete responses in the range of 10–15%. At present, it is an urgent goal of investigative chemotherapy to detect new, active agents for soft-tissue sarcomas; the demonstrated synergism between cyclophosphamide, *cis*-platinum, and Adriamycin is an avenue requiring further exploration.

Because of the relatively high cure rate that may be obtained with surgery alone in sarcomas in some anatomic sites, especially the limbs, and given the relative paucity of early cases available to the chemotherapist, adequately controlled adjuvant trials in sarcomas are few and far between. The National Cancer Institute (NCI) recently published a study comparing local treatment alone with local treatment plus a combination of Adriamycin and cyclophosphamide in patients with resectable sarcomas of the extremities. The results in favor of chemotherapy are statistically significant, but it is not yet clear whether longer follow-up will continue to show a statistically significant difference in favor of the adjuvant chemotherapy group. Furthermore, it should be pointed out that the NCI study had a relatively high incidence of late cardiotoxic effects resulting from Adriamycin, including serious toxicity in some patients who were likely to have been cured by local measures alone. A national intergroup sarcoma study is currently in the planning stages and is urgently needed to better define the potential value of chemotherapy after adequate local treatments have been completed. At present, adjuvant chemotherapy for soft-tissue sarcomas should still be considered investigational.

Notwithstanding all the above reservations about the value of radiotherapy and chemotherapy in the treatment of the potentially curable patient with a soft-tissue sarcoma, a multimodality therapeutic approach is being advocated as the ideal method of management of patients with soft-tissue sarcomas. Although radical procedures (and particularly amputations) achieve a higher rate of local control, conservation of function will at times encourage lesser operations in conjunction with one or more adjunctive thereapeutic modalities (radiotherapy, chemotherapy, or both). Anytime a procedure is selected that is less than an amputation or a radical compartmental excision, it should be followed by radiotherapy. The role of chemotherapy in the adjuvant setting remains unclear but seems to be the only potential method of improving long-term survival, particularly in patients with more advanced disease.

G. Management of Recurrent Disease

Patients who present with local or regional recurrent disease but with no evidence of distant metastases may still be salvageable in a significant percentage of cases. Surgery is still the preferred modality of treatment and should be aggressively pursued whenever possible; adjuvant therapy in these cases, however, is mandatory. One suggested regimen has been the use of preoperative chemotherapy (Adriamycin, 30 mg/m²/day, X3) and radiotherapy (3500 rads in 10 days) followed by radical resection of the recurrence and the previous operative field; the adequacy of resection must be ensured by frozen section since no patient in whom margins are involved will remain free of disease. Radiotherapy and chemotherapy may also be used postoperatively. A 5-year survival as high as 75% has been predicted in selected cases with such aggressive treatment of locally recurrent soft-tissue sarcoma.

Patients with systemic metastases do not fare as well. Treatment of these patients is primarily palliative (radiotherapy); systemic chemotherapy is used, but overall results are disappointing.

An occasional patient will prove amenable to resection of lung metastases.

V. THERAPEUTIC GUIDELINES: TYPE SPECIFIC

A. Pathological Considerations

Although the major groups and subgroups of soft-tissue sarcomas number no more than 40, over 300 synonyms exist in the medical literature that identify various soft-tissue tumors. This profusion of terms has created great confusion and difficulties in assessing the incidence, as well as the mortality rates, of each group.

Soft-tissue tumors arise from mesenchymal cells. These mesenchymal cells differentiate into several elements such as lipocytes, myocytes, fibrocytes, etc. The classification of soft-tissue tumors is based on the differentiated cells that predominate. In malignant neoplasms, these differentiated elements exhibit the ability to dedifferentiate into poorly differentiated or undifferentiated elements, which account for the cellular variations that may be seen within a single tumor. For some types of sarcoma, the exact cell of origin is sometimes impossible to identify.

The ability of a tumor to metastasize distinguishes a malignant tumor from its benign variant. Metastases may result from lymphatic and/or hematogenous spread. Some soft-tissue sarcomas are the source of great controversy as to their malignant potential, some (e.g., dermatofibrosarcoma protuberans) exhibit a very low risk of systemic metastases but are recognized as being locally extremely aggressive. The tendency for local recurrences, although common to malignant tumors, should not be construed as sole evidence of malignancy; this property is also shared by several benign lesions (e.g., fibromatosis and giant-cell tumors of bone).

To assess adequately the malignant potential of a soft-tissue tumor, consideration must be given to its histologic type and grade, as well as its size and site. Histologic typing is based on the predominant cell type within the tumor. The tumor tends to assume the morphologic characteristics of the cell of origin, and the presence of mature or well-differentiated cells simplifies histologic typing. In poorly differentiated tumors, classification becomes difficult, and often it is necessary to resort to a larger biopsy, electron microscopy, histochemical studies, and tissue culture to help distinguish the various types.

Histologic grading of the tumor has been shown to be the most useful parameter in assessing prognosis. High-grade tumors are characterized by hypercellularity, minimal stroma, marked necrosis, poor maturation, and high mitotic rate (more than 5–10 per high-power field). Hypocellularity, marked stroma, absence of necrosis, good maturation, and low mitotic rate indicate a low-grade tumor. Small biopsy specimens can limit grading accuracy because of the nonhomogeneity of many of these tumors. Some soft-tissue sarcomas (e.g., rhabdomyosarcoma), however, are considered highly malignant irrespective of histological grading criteria.

Regarding the size and site, tumors less than 5 cm in diameter have a better prognosis than those over 5 cm and superficially located tumors (not beyond the superficial fascia) have a better prognosis than deeply located tumors.

Table I lists the more common types of soft-tissue sarcomas and their presumed cell of origin. Table II identifies the low-grade and high-grade soft-tissue sarcomas.

Although the majority of soft tissue sarcomas present in the extremities, each type seems to have a site predilection. Table III indicates the most common site according to type.

The mode of spread of soft-tissue sarcomas is primarily hematogenous, although each type seems to have a predilection to spread to certain sites, and some even spread significantly via lymphatic channels. Table IV lists the most common metastatic sites for the various soft-tissue sarcomas.

B. Types of Soft-Tissue Sarcoma

1. Rhabdomyosarcoma

Rhabdomyosarcomas constitute the most common soft-tissue sarcoma occurring in childhood. Three major categories exist: embryonal, alveolar, and pleomorphic (or adult). The most frequently encountered type is the embryonal cell rhabdomyosarcoma, and when it occurs in subepithelial locations it tends to form polypoid masses, designated "sarcoma botryoids." The pleomorphic and alveolar types of rhabdomyosarcoma

Table I

Pathological Classification of Malignant Soft-Tissue Tumors

Presumed cell of origin	Tumor
Fibrocyte	Fibrosarcoma
	Desmoid tumor
Striated muscle cell	Rhabdomyosarcoma
Smooth muscle cell	Leiomyosarcoma
Synovial cell	Synovial sarcoma
Adipose cell	Liposarcoma
Histiocyte	Dermatofibrosarcoma protuberans
	Malignant fibrous histiocytoma
Neural cell	Neurofibrosarcoma (malignant schwannoma)
Vascular and lymphatic cell	Angiosarcoma
	Lymphangiosarcoma
	Hemangiopericytoma
	Kaposi's sarcoma
Pluripotential mesenchyme	Malignant mesenchymoma
Metaplastic mesenchyme	Extraskeletal chondrosarcoma
	Extraskeletal osteosarcoma
Uncertain origin	Malignant granular cell tumor
	Alveolar soft-part sarcoma
	Clear-cell sarcoma
	Epithelioid sarcoma

usually present as extremity tumors, whereas the embryonal rhabdomyosarcoma is more common in the head and neck region. Alveolar rhabdomyosarcoma carries the worst prognosis.

An extensive discussion of the management of rhabdomyosarcoma in children is presented in §8.VI.C, since this tumor constitutes a large percentage of tumors in the pediatric age group.

2. Liposarcoma

Liposarcomas are the most frequent soft-tissue sarcomas in adults. The site of greatest predilection is the lower extremity (especially in the popliteal fossa and the thigh), followed by the retroperitoneal space. Four histologic subtypes are recog-

Table II

Grade of Soft-Tissue Sarcoma according to Type

Low-grade sarcomas	High-grade sarcomas
Dermatofibrosarcoma protuberans (believed by some to be benign)	Pleomorphic fibrosarcoma
Desmoid tumor (believed by some to be benign)	Synovial sarcoma
Well-differentiated liposarcoma	Lipoblastic liposarcoma
Myxoid liposarcoma	Pleomorphic liposarcoma
Kaposi's sarcoma	Rhabdomyosarcoma
Malignant granular cell tumor	Lymphangiosarcoma
Alveolar soft-part sarcoma	

Table III

Most Common Sites of Malignant Soft-Tissue Tumors[a,b]

	Head and Neck	Extremities		Trunk
		Upper	Lower	
Dermatofibrosarcoma protuberans		+1		X
Malignant giant-cell tumor		+1	X2	
Malignant pleomorphic fibrous histiocytoma		+1	X2	
Desmoid tumor	+	X3	X3	+
Fibrosarcoma		+3	X3	
Tendosynovial sarcoma		+	X	
Liposarcoma		+	X4	
Embryonal rhabdomyosarcoma	+			
Pleomorphic rhabdomyosarcoma		+	X4	
Hemangiosarcoma	+	+		
Kaposi's sarcoma		+5	X5	X
Hemangiopericytoma			X	+
Lymphangiosarcoma	+	X		
Ostcogenic sarcoma		+	X	
Chondrosarcoma		+	X	
Ewing's sarcoma			4	+
Malignant granular cell tumor	+		X	+
Alveolar sort-part sarcoma		+	X4	

[a] By permission from Hajdu (4).
[b] Key: + = common   3 = proximal part
X = most common   4 = thigh
1 = shoulder   5 = distal part
2 = buttock

Table IV

Most Common Metastatic Sites of Soft-Tissue Sarcomas[a,b]

Histological type	Site of metastasis
Malignant fibrous tumors	Lung, bone, lymph node, intestine, liver
Tendosynovial sarcoma	Lung, chest wall, diaphragm, bone, lymph node
Liposarcoma	Lymph node, intestine, lung, liver, chest wall
Embryonal rhabdomyosarcoma	Bone, lymph node, lung, intestine, liver
Pleomorphic rhabdomyosarcoma	Lung, kidney, heart, lymph node, liver
Leiomyosarcoma	Intestine, lung, lymph node, liver, kidney
Angiosarcoma	Bone, skin, lymph node, intestine, liver
Malignant schwannoma	Skin, lymph node, intestine, retroperitoneum, chest wall

[a] By permission from Hajdu (4).
[b] Based on an analysis of 294 soft-tissue sarcomas at autopsy.

nized: well-differentiated, myxoid, pleomorphic, and round-cell. The first two subtypes carry a better prognosis than the latter two.

3. Fibrosarcoma

Fibrosarcomas occur in any age group but are seen more commonly in adults. Lesions occurring in children under 10 years of age have a markedly lower tendency for metastases than those seen in older individuals, and this is in spite of their alarming histological features. Fibrosarcomas tend to be well circumscribed with a misleading pseudocapsule. In contrast, lesions of the *fibromatosis* group usually have ill-defined margins and can have an aggressive clinical behavior, as shown by repeated local recurrences; unlike the fibrosarcomas, however, they do not metastasize. The distinction between these two lesions is not always easy but usually does not make much difference in terms of therapy since both require wide radical excision.

Desmoid tumors remain a controversial entity. They are included in this discussion as a type of low-grade fibrosarcoma because of a few reports of cases showing distant metastases; most pathologists, however, classify desmoid lesions as a type of fibromatosis.

4. Neurofibrosarcoma

This tumor is also designated as neurogenic sarcoma or malignant schwannoma. It is the malignant counterpart of the neurofibroma, not the benign schwannoma. The diagnosis should be strongly considered in tumors developing in patients with von Recklinghausen's disease arising in an anatomic compartment of a major nerve or in tumors showing direct continuity with an unquestionable neurofibroma. Outside of these situations, the diagnosis must be confirmed by electron microscopy.

5. Synovial Sarcoma

Synovial sarcomas are less common tumors, 80% of which arise about the knee and ankle joints in young adults; only rarely do they actually involve the synovial membrane. Two forms are recognized—monophasic and biphasic—based on the presence of one or the other of sarcomatous or epithelial elements, as opposed to both. Calcification and hyalinization may be seen within the tumor and are believed to indicate a more favorable prognostic connotation.

6. Leiomyosarcoma

These are relatively rare tumors, mostly arising from the smooth muscle of blood vessels and viscera. Tumor size and location are the two major prognostic factors, but they are usually aggressive tumors. Metastases sometimes appear 15–20 years after excision of the primary tumor.

7. Malignant Fibrous Histiocytoma

Fibrous histiocytoma was characterized by Stout in 1963. The precise histogenic derivation of these tumors is far from clear, but the currently favored theory holds that these are histiocytic neoplasms with histiocytes possessing the property of becoming facultative fibroblasts. Malignant fibrous histiocytoma tends to occur in deep locations and most commonly presents in the lower extremity.

Dermatofibrosarcoma protuberans is a clinicopathological entity that is currently classified in the general group of fibrous histiocytomas. It is a low-grade malignant neoplasm with a local recurrence rate of up to 55% but a low metastatic potential (less than 10%). It presents as a multinodular firm mass fixed to the skin and must be aggressively treated locally.

8. Tumors of Blood and Lymphatic Vessels

a. Angiosarcoma

The term *angiosarcoma* refers to the malignant neoplasm arising from the endothelium of blood vessels. It occurs at any age, and the soft tissue of the female breast is one of the commonest sites. Angiosarcomas arising in subcutaneous sites, especially in the head and neck region, are usually multiple and tend to affect elderly patients.

b. Lymphangiosarcoma

These are highly malignant neoplasms that usually develop in patients who have had long-standing lymphedema (e.g., following radical mastectomy). The 5-year survival rate is only about 6% in a reported series of 129 patients.

c. Malignant Hemangiopericytoma

This tumor is believed to arise from the smooth muscle cell that surrounds small blood vessels (pericyte). The 5-year survival rate is around 50%.

d. Kaposi's Sarcoma

This is a tumor believed to be of endothelial origin. It presents as multifocal purplish papular skin lesions, particularly frequent among Jewish and Italian males. Progression of the disease is slow and frequently associated with malignant lymphoreticular neoplasms. More recently, reports of Kaposi's sarcoma developing in homosexuals and in immune-deficient individuals have renewed interest in this disease (see §3.V.C, Vol. 1). However, the natural history of lesions developing as part of AIDS is distinctly different from the classical Kaposi's sarcoma.

9. Tumors of Uncertain Origin

a. Alveolar Soft-Part Sarcoma

The histogenesis of this tumor is not definitely established. At the present time, published data favors a myogenic origin. This tumor has distinct histological features. It most often involves the deep tissues of the thigh and leg of young adults, especially females, and its clinical course is slow and protracted.

b. Epithelioid Sarcoma

This tumor is believed to be a variant of synovial sarcomas that affect the skin; it is seen most frequently in the extremeties (hands) and has often been labeled "spindle cell carcinoma."
Local recurrence was seen in 85% of the patients and distant metastases in 30%. Lymph node metastases are relatively common and are an ominous prognostic sign.

c. Clear-Cell Sarcoma

These arise chiefly from large tendons and aponeuroses of the extremities, especially the feet. The clinical course is characterized by slow but relentless progression, with frequent local recurrences and, eventually, distant metastases.

d. Malignant Granular Cell Tumor

Most granular cell tumors are benign. There have been, however, rare cases with proven metastases documented in the literature, and these must, therefore, be classified as malignant granular cell tumors.

C. Therapeutic Considerations

Although the histologic type of the tumor often has little impact on the therapeutic considerations, some important distinctive features need to be identified.

- Diffuse multifocal sarcomas (e.g., lymphangiosarcomas, Kaposi's sarcoma, etc.) are not candidates for surgical therapy. These are better treated by other modalities.
- Some extremely aggressive lesions (e.g., hemangiosarcomas), or those with poorly identifiable limits, are also poor candidates for a surgical cure and require other modalities of therapy.
- Certain soft-tissue sarcomas (e.g., embryonal cell rhabdomyosarcoma) are particularly sensitive to both radiation and chemotherapy, and a combined-modality approach with surgery, radiotherapy, and chemotherapy is yielding extremely high cure rates.

- A large variety of soft-tissue tumors, often labeled sarcomas (e.g., fibromatosis, desmoid tumors, dermatofibrosarcoma protuberans, and some fibrous histiocytomas), are in reality aggressive local lesions, not even neoplastic in nature, that rarely metastasize but have a high rate of local recurrence. These tumors should be treated by wide local excision and close follow-up observation. The group of nodular fibromatoses and desmoid tumors have also been recognized as somewhat radiosensitive, and adjuvant radiotherapy has the advantage of limiting the extent of resection when applied preoperatively and the incidence of local recurrence when used postoperatively.
- Most often, soft-tissue sarcomas are primarily treated surgically, some (e.g., hemangiopericytomas, alveolar soft-part sarcomas, neurofibrosarcomas, and clear-cell sarcomas) by wide local excision and others (e.g., epithelioid sarcomas, liposarcomas, synovial sarcomas, and rhabdomyosarcomas) by more radical excision and regional lymphadenectomy.

VI. POSTOPERATIVE CARE, EVALUATION, AND REHABILITATION

A. Immediate Postoperative Care

This includes attention to hemodynamic monitoring, vital signs, respiratory and cardiac evaluations, monitoring of intake and output, correction of electrolyte abnormalities, and transfusion, if necessary. Any suction drains or tubes should be noted and their output assessed. Dressings and splints are to be used as needed. Usually there is no need for prophylactic antibiotics unless there was contamination during surgery. Adequate amounts of pain medication and sedatives are ordered. Deep breathing and coughing, as well as early ambulation, are encouraged.

B. Psychological Support

Knowledge of the existence of a malignancy and the need for prolonged treatments and follow-up is most traumatic for the patient. Surgery, especially amputation of an otherwise normal looking and asymptomatic extremity, or radical resection that leaves the extremity permanently disabled, is a shocking experience. It is important to have input from the oncologic nurse, a social worker, and a psychiatric nurse. The goal is to help the patient emotionally and also to establish a continuous educational program for the patient and the family.

C. Coordination of Postoperative Radiation and Chemotherapy

The appropriate time and actual techniques involved should be decided on an individual basis. Reevaluation of the patient's condition may be necessary from time to time, taking into consideration the patient's desires and reactions. All consultations and care should be channeled through the treating physician in order to maintain continuity of care, but multidisciplinary consultations are strongly urged.

D. Rehabilitation

The rehabilitation goals and management programs outlined in §§5.V.C and 7.VI.C overlap in many aspects with those for patients with sarcoma of soft tissue. Prevention of secondary complications and disabilities and functional restoration are essentially similar.

1. The Immediate Postoperative Period

Whenever amputations or radical extremity procedures requiring appliances are done, the physiatrist should be consulted at the outset. Early exercises to the parts, both passive and active, are necessary, and ambulation is encouraged. Appropriate exercises are also instituted for strengthening of the muscles. It is often desirable to apply splints or casts to prevent contractures. Fitting an early (temporary) prosthesis for the leg may even be more beneficial than waiting for complete wound healing.

2. Amputations

For patients in whom the sarcoma has lead to partial or total amputation of a limb, the rehabilitation process follows exactly the guidelines outlined for amputations in §5.V.C.1; the reader is referred to that section, which deals in detail with that subject. Early plans must be made to provide the patient with a well-fitting prosthetic device in order to permit recovery of maximum functional capacity as soon as possible. The exact type and material will depend on the individual circumstances, but the feeling of returning to normal, cosmetically and functionally, is of extreme importance to the patient and should be a primary goal.

3. Soft-Tissue Resections

Following resections of a given muscle mass, specific problems will result requiring a special rehabilitative solution.

- Resection of the quadriceps. Resection of the quadriceps will impair knee extension, which can result in difficulty in ambulation, tendency to knee buckling, and inability to run. Management will include the strengthening of the remaining muscles and a long leg brace with the capacity to lock the knee in extension.
- Resection of the gastrocnemius. This resection will impair the toe-off phase of gait, which can be partially corrected by ambulation retraining using a short leg brace with a dorsiflexion stop.
- Resection of the tibialis anterior. This results in a foot drop correctable with a short leg brace (plastic or metal).
- Resection of the hamstrings. This will interfere with a smooth gait pattern and is correctable in part through therapeutic exercises.
- Wide excision of the gluteus maximus. This type of excision will weaken the hip extension, and the patient will have difficulty getting up from a sitting position or climbing stairs. Using a cane and training the contralateral side as prime mover will improve the patient's level of functioning.

Table V

Follow-Up Evaluation of Soft-Tissue Sarcoma

Management	First-to-second year, every 3 months	Third-to-fifth year, every 6 months	Thereafter, annually
History			
Soft-tissue masses	X	X	X
Pain at surgical site	X	X	X
Cough, dyspnea	X	X	X
Chest pains	X	X	X
Hemoptysis	X	X	X
Bone pain	X	X	X
Weight loss	X	X	X
Headache, seizure	X	X	X
Function of extremity	X	X	X
Physical			
Complete[a]		Annually	
Surgery site	X	X	X
Soft-tissue nodules	X	X	X
Lymph nodes	X	X	X
Nerve function in the extremity	X	X	X
Functional status of the extremity	X	X	X
Abdomen: masses ascites, liver	X	X	X
Chest examination	X	X	X
Bones	X	X	X
Skin	X	X	X
Investigations			
CBC	X	X	X
SMA-12	X	X	X
Chest x-ray	X	X	X
Others:			
Bone scan		As indicated	
Liver scan		As indicated	
CAT scan of head		As indicated	

[a] For detection of other tumors.

• Weakness of the musculature of the wrist and fingers. For weakness of the musculature of the wrist and fingers, a variety of supportive and dynamic splints are available. The occupational therapist will select the proper type and train the patient in its proper use.

The active involvement of the patients in the process of functional rehabilitation has a considerable positive psychological impact. The realization by the patients that concrete solutions are available and within reach for improving the quality of their lives is of great therapeutic value and a powerful positive reinforcer.

4. Reconstructive Surgical Procedures

This will often depend upon the extent and type of surgery that was carried out. It may include grafts, rotational skin flaps, or pedicle flaps to cover defects; muscle and tendon transfers to correct nerve and motor deficits or to provide joint stability; and at times, nerve grafting. The timing and need for such procedures should be thoroughly discussed with the patients and must take into account the prognosis of the disease and the anticipated longevity of the patient.

E. Follow-Up Evaluations

The follow-up of the patient with soft-tissue sarcoma is most important to identify recurrences or distant metastasis. Table V is a suggested schedule for such follow-up.

VII. MANAGEMENT ALGORITHIM FOR SOFT-TISSUE SARCOMA
(see p. 272)

SUGGESTED READINGS

1. Deitz, J. H. Adaptive rehabilitation of the cancer patient. *Curr. Probl. Cancer* **5,** No. 5 (1980).
2. DeLisa, J. A., Miller, R., Melnick, R. R., and Mikulic, M. A. Rehabilitation of the cancer patient. *In* "Cancer, Principles and Practices of Oncology" (V. T. DeVita, Jr., S. Hellman, and S. A. Rosenberg, eds.), Chapter 46. Lippincott, Philadelphia, Pennsylvania, 1982.
3. DeVita, V. T., Jr., Hellman, S., and Rosenberg, S. A., eds. "Cancer, Principles and Practices of Oncology." Lippincott, Philadelphia, Pennsylvania, 1982.
4. Hajdu, S. "Pathology of Soft Tissue Tumors." Lea & Febiger, Philadelphia, Pennsylvania, 1979.
4a. Lindberg, R. D., Martin, R. G., Romsdahl, M. M. Surgery and postoperative radiotherapy in the treatment of soft tissue sarcoma in adults. *Am. J. Roentgenol. Rad. Ther. Nucl. Med.* **123,** 123–129 (1975).
5. Rossai, J. "Ackerman's Surgical Pathology." Mosby, St. Louis, Missouri, 1981.
6. Russell, W. *et al.* A clinical and pathological staging system for soft tissue sarcomas. *Cancer (Philadelphia)* **40,** 1562–1570 (1977).
7. Stout, A., and Lattes, R. Tumors of the soft tissues. *In* "Atlas of Tumor Pathology" (M. O. Dayhoff, ed.), 2nd Ser. Armed Forces Inst. Pathol., Washington, D.C., 1967.
8. Weingrad, D. W., Rosenberg, S. A. Early lymphatic spread of osteogenic and soft tissue sarcomas. *Surgery* **84,** 231–240 (1978).

ALGORITHM FOR SOFT-TISSUE SARCOMAS

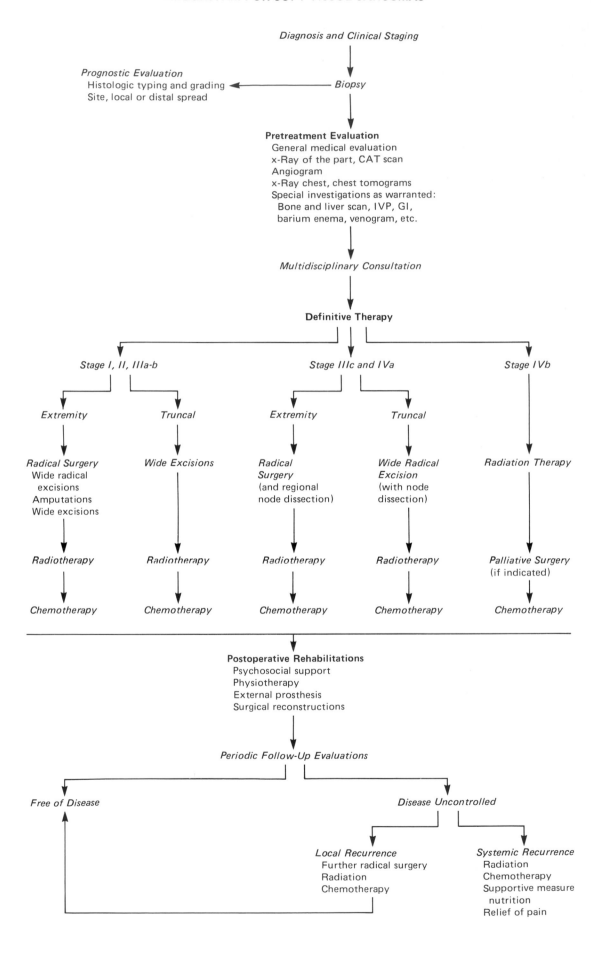

Diagnosis and Clinical Staging

Prognostic Evaluation
   Histologic typing and grading ◄——— *Biopsy*
   Site, local or distal spread

Pretreatment Evaluation
   General medical evaluation
   x-Ray of the part, CAT scan
   Angiogram
   x-Ray chest, chest tomograms
   Special investigations as warranted:
     Bone and liver scan, IVP, GI,
     barium enema, venogram, etc.

Multidisciplinary Consultation

Definitive Therapy

Stage I, II, IIIa-b   *Stage IIIc and IVa*   *Stage IVb*

Extremity   *Truncal*   *Extremity*   *Truncal*

Radical Surgery   *Wide Excisions*   *Radical Surgery* (and regional node dissection)   *Wide Radical Excision* (with node dissection)   *Radiation Therapy*
Wide radical excisions
Amputations
Wide excisions

Radiotherapy   *Radiotherapy*   *Radiotherapy*   *Radiotherapy*   *Palliative Surgery* (if indicated)

Chemotherapy   *Chemotherapy*   *Chemotherapy*   *Chemotherapy*   *Chemotherapy*

Postoperative Rehabilitations
   Psychosocial support
   Physiotherapy
   External prosthesis
   Surgical reconstructions

Periodic Follow-Up Evaluations

Free of Disease   *Disease Uncontrolled*

Local Recurrence
   Further radical surgery
   Radiation
   Chemotherapy

Systemic Recurrence
   Radiation
   Chemotherapy
   Supportive measure
     nutrition
   Relief of pain

Section 7

Tumors of the Central Nervous System

AARON MILLER

With Contributions By

Robert Holtzman	Neurosurgery
Marshall Keilson	Neurology
Jerome Tepperberg	Pediatric Neurology
Ezzat Youssef	Radiotherapy
Michael Bashevkin	Medical Oncology
Ari Feibel	Rehabilitation
Randi Moskowitz	Nursing Oncology

Section 7. Tumors of the Central Nervous System

I. Early Detection and Screening   277
   A. Early Signs of CNS Tumors
      1. Alterations in Mental Status
      2. Focal Symptoms
      3. Seizures
      4. Increased Intracranial Pressure
      5. Specific Syndromes Resulting from the Location
         of the Tumor
   B. Education
II. Pretreatment Evaluation and Work-Up   278
   A. Neurological Evaluation
      1. History and Physical Examination
         a. History
         b. Physical Examination
      2. Radiological Evaluation
         a. Plain Skull X-ray
         b. CAT Scan of the Head
         c. Tomography and Pneumoencephalography
         d. Angiography
         e. Myelography
         f. CAT Scan of the Spine
      3. Brain Scan
      4. Electroencephalography
      5. Spinal Tap and Study of the Cerebrospinal Fluid
      6. Electromyography
      7. Nuclear Magnetic Resonance
   B. Ophthalmologic Evaluation
   C. Endocrine Evaluation
   D. Metastatic Evaluation
   E. Other Evaluation
   F. Multidisciplinary Evaluation
   G. Site-Specific Data Form for CNS Tumors
III. Pretreatment Preparation   283
   A. General Systemic Preparation
      1. Correction of Preexisting Medical Diseases
      2. Nutritional Support
      3. Endocrine Disturbances
   B. Control of Increased Intracranial Pressure
      1. Corticosteroids
      2. Mannitol and Urea
   C. Anticonvulsants
IV. Therapeutic Management   283
   A. General Guidelines
      1. Establishment of the Diagnosis
      2. Biopsy
      3. The Curable Lesion
      4. The Incurable Lesion
      5. Nonintervention
      6. Rehabilitation

   B. Common Pitfalls
      1. Lack of Recognition of the Biologic Behavior of
         the Tumor
      2. Inadequate Evaluation of the Patient
      3. Unwarranted Delay in Treatment
      4. Inadequate Preoperative Preparation
      5. Unwarranted Aggressive Treatment
      6. Inadequate Intraoperative Management
      7. Inadequate Evaluation of the Available
         Histological Material
   C. Selection of Treatment Modality
      1. Brain Tumors
      2. Tumors of the Spine
   D. Surgical Therapy
      1. Goals of Surgical Management
      2. Urgent Situations
      3. Surgical Approach
         a. Preparation for Surgery
         b. Incisions and Flaps
         c. Method of Dissection
      4. Results
   E. Adjuvant Therapy
      1. Radiotherapy
         a. Tolerance of CNS Tissues to Radiation
         b. Indications for Radiation Therapy
         c. Contraindications to Radiation Therapy
      2. Chemotherapy
V. Specific Neurologic Tumors   291
   A. Astrocytic Tumors
      1. Glioblastoma Multiforme
         a. Clinical Presentation
         b. Diagnostic Evaluation
         c. Therapeutic Management
      2. Astrocytomas
         a. Clinical Presentation
         b. Diagnostic Workup
         c. Therapeutic Management
   B. Oligodendrogliomas
      1. Clinical Presentation
      2. Diagnostic Evaluation
      3. Therapeutic Management
   C. CNS Metastases
      1. Brain Metastases
         a. Clinical Presentation
         b. Diagnostic Evaluation
         c. Therapeutic Management
      2. Meningeal Carcinomatosis
      3. Spinal Epidural Metastases
         a. Clinical Presentation

b. Diagnostic Evaluation
c. Therapeutic Management
D. Meningiomas
1. Clinical Presentation
a. Parasaggital and Falx Meningiomas
b. Meningiomas of the Convexity
c. Sphenoid Wing Meningiomas
d. Olfactory Groove Meningiomas
e. Tuberculum and Suprasellar
Meningiomas
f. Posterior Fossa Tumors
g. Meckel's Cave and Tentorial Incisura
Dumbell Lesions
h. Intraventricular Lesions
i. Primary Intraorbital Meningiomas
j. Spinal Meningiomas
2. Diagnostic Evaluation
3. Therapeutic Management
E. Hemangioblastomas
F. Pituitary Tumors
1. Clinical Presentation
2. Diagnostic Evaluation
3. Therapeutic Management
a. Medical Treatment
b. Surgery
c. Radiotherapy
G. Pineal Region Tumors
H. Craniopharyngiomas
1. Clinical Presentation
a. Childhood Tumors
b. Adult Tumors
2. Diagnostic Evaluation
3. Therapeutic Management

I. Malignant Lymphomas
1. Clinical Presentation
2. Diagnostic Evaluation
3. Therapeutic Management
J. Neuromas and Neurofibromas
1. Acoustic Neuromas
2. Trigeminal Neuromas
3. Spinal Neuromas
4. Neuromas of Peripheral Nerves
5. Neurofibromas
K. Other Brain Tumors
1. Epidermoid and Dermoid Cysts
2. Colloid Cysts
L. Chordomas
M. Intracranial Neoplasms in Children
1. Cerebellar Astrocytomas
2. Medulloblastomas
3. Fourth-Ventricle Ependymomas
4. Brainstem Gliomas
VI. Postoperative Care, Evaluation, and Rehabilitation   304
A. Postoperative Care
B. Nursing Care and Psychosocial Aspects
1. Changes in Mental Status
2. Changes in Motor and Sensory Function
3. Changes in Appearance
4. Changes in Roles
5. Isolation
6. Side Effects and Complications of Treatment
C. Rehabilitation
D. Follow-Up Evaluation
VII. Management Algorithm for Brain Tumors   307

Suggested Readings   307

Tumors of the central nervous system defy the traditional means of distinguishing benign from malignant tumors, even after definitive therapy. Because of the highly specialized function of central nervous tissue and its tight confinement within a rigid, bony protecting vault (the cranial cavity or spinal canal), all tumors of the CNS may present with a severe clinical picture and may, for all practical purposes, be considered malignant as a result of their potential for causing serious morbidity or mortality. Furthermore, the usual criteria by which malignancy is established in other organ systems—particularly the properties of infiltrative growth and the capacity to metastasize to sites remote from the tumor—are often lacking with brain and spinal cord tumors. Finally, biopsies are not usually possible prior to therapy, and therapy is often instituted without knowledge of the exact histologic nature of the lesion. The guidelines in this section for the management of tumors of the CNS will, therefore, apply to all tumors.

The incidence of brain tumor for all ages is estimated to be between 4.2 and 5.4 per 100,000 population. The annual incidence of spinal cord tumors varies between 1.3 and 2.5 per 100,000. The ratio of intracranial neoplasms to spinal neoplasms has been given at approximately 4 : 1. The mortality from tumors of the CNS, including benign and malignant lesions, was reported in 1968 at 0.45% of all deaths, and these tumors accounted for 2.7% of deaths from all cancers. The mortality due to spinal cord tumors is close to 0.5 per 100,000 per year.

I. EARLY DETECTION AND SCREENING

There are, to date, no known specific factors or elements that have been identified as being instrumental in the causation of neurologic tumors. Prevention is, therefore, strictly speaking not possible. Furthermore, screening evaluation for CNS tumors is not a practical possibility. Unlike early clinical manifestations of cancer in some other sites, mild neurological symptoms are often ignored by the patients. The responsibility of early detection, therefore, rests with the primary physician, who must recognize important neurological symptoms and perform the initial triage of patients with neurological complaints. A very high proportion of patients seeking medical attention have symptoms attributable to the nervous system; but not all patients with headaches or dizziness, for example, require intensive neurological investigation. However, the physician must recognize those symptoms and signs that imply a reasonable possibility of structural neurological disease. When such symptoms or signs arouse concern in the primary physician, appropriate neurological consultation should be sought promptly.

In addition to the primary physician who might be consulted for a variety of complaints indicative of neurological tumors, other professionals who come in contact with the public may be instrumental in early tumor detection, particularly in children. These professionals include school teachers, psychologists, camp counselors, optometrists, ophthalmologists, and endocrinologists.

A. Early Signs of CNS Tumors

Brain tumors, no matter what their histology, may demonstrate one of the following presentations: nonspecific neurological symptoms and signs, alterations in mental status, focal motor or sensory abnormalities, seizures, symptoms and signs of increased intracranial pressure, or specific clinical syndromes (e.g., acoustic neurinomas or pituitary adenomas) resulting from the particular location of the tumor.

1. Alterations in Mental Status

Alterations in mental status often develop insidiously as subtle changes in personality, lassitude, irritability, or lack of initiative. Often such signs are noted only in retrospect, and the patient does not come to medical attention until more flagrant signs of confusion, psychoses, or even lethargy have appeared. At times, more localizing cortical dysfunction such as aphasia may be seen.

2. Focal Symptoms

Motor and/or sensory symptoms are among the most common presenting manifestations of both brain and spinal cord tumors. Typically, weakness or paresis develops gradually over a period of weeks, or even months, depending on the tumor type. A major exception to this slow, progressive onset of symptoms is epidural cord compression resulting from metastatic carcinoma, in which paraparesis progresses rapidly. Likewise, brain tumors may, at times, declare themselves with strokelike suddenness as a result of hemorrhage into a mass or rapid expansion of a fluid-filled cyst. Changes in sensation and paresthesias often accompany the paresis.

3. Seizures

Seizures, either focal or generalized, are among the most common declarations of cerebral tumors. The presentation of seizures for the first time during adult life always demands immediate and intensive investigation.

4. Increased Intracranial Pressure

The most frequent and prominent symptom of increased intracranial pressure is headache. The pain is often vague and poorly localized, although supratentorial tumors tend to project pain to anterior head regions, whereas posterior fossa tumors usually produce occipital pain. Headaches that are worse in the early morning and become less severe as the day progresses should alert the physician to the distinct possibility of increased intracranial pressure. On the other hand, the severity of the pain is not a good indicator; migraine, neuralgias, or muscle contraction (tension) headaches may be much more severe than those associated with brain tumors.

Nausea and vomiting may also be associated with the headaches of raised intracranial pressure, but these symptoms tend to be much more prominent in children than in adults. Another symptom of elevated pressure is visual obscuration, a transient "graying out" of vision, bilaterally, usually lasting a few seconds. Fundoscopic changes are, of course, the most reliable findings of increased intracranial pressure.

Symptoms and signs of increased intracranial pressure will eventually progress to lethargy, stupor, and coma and tend to develop particularly rapidly in patients with posterior fossa tumors that obstruct the egress of cerebrospinal fluid, producing hydrocephalus.

5. Specific Syndromes Resulting from the Location of the Tumor

The other general mode of presentation of CNS tumors, that of specific neurological syndromes, will be discussed individually with the relevant tumor. However, symptoms such as ataxia, gait difficulties, cranial nerve deficits, visual field and ocular motor aberrations, speech difficulties or aphasia, sphincteric dysfunction, hypothalamic and endocrine changes, etc. must alert the physician or paraprofessional who detects them to the potential presence of a brain tumor.

B. Education

The physician's vigilant attention to early neurological symptoms as well as timely referral for neurological consultation may spare the patient the devastating consequences of a major neurological deficit and is especially relevant for patients with tumors that are histologically benign and/or surgically resectable.

Proper education of physicians, particularly those involved in primary care, is paramount in order to increase their awareness. School teachers and psychologists also need to be alerted to the early signs of neurological tumors, especially in children and adolescents, and should be encouraged to make early referrals. No public education program, however, is available or advisable at this time.

II. PRETREATMENT EVALUATION AND WORK-UP

A. Neurological Evaluation

1. History and Physical Examination

Although history and neurological examination is only the initial step in evaluating a patient with a brain or spinal cord tumor, this will not only establish the groundwork for the diagnosis but will often locate the actual lesion.

a. History

The following symptoms should be elicited, and their intensity, onset and degree of progression should be ascertained.

- Pain: whether occipital, frontal, cervical, radicular, etc.; its nature, duration, irradiation, and other characteristics.
- Nausea and vomiting (especially in children).
- Seizures: localized or generalized convulsions.
- Sensorium and state of consciousness: degree of alertness, confusion.
- Mental symptoms: personality change, dementia, aphasia.
- Motor loss: weakness, atrophy, hemi- or paraparesis.
- Sensory deficits: paresthesias, numbness.
- Focal signs: changes in visual acuity, diplopia, hemianopsia, etc.; anosmia, hearing loss, vertigo, tinnitus; aphasia, slurred speech; loss of balance, gait changes, or ataxia.
- Cranial nerve deficits.

- Sphincteric dysfunction.
- Hypothalamic dysfunction: alteration of sleeping habits, eating habits, behavioral changes, etc.

b. Physical Examination

A thorough neurological examination must be carried out including assessment of sensorium and mental status, motor and sensory function, evaluation of extrapyramidal and cerebellar functions, cranial nerve function, peripheral nerve testing, and opthalmologic examination.

2. Radiological Evaluation

a. Plain Skull X-ray

- Calcifications, suggesting astrocytoma, oligodendroglioma, or craniopharyngioma.
- Hyperostosis (meningioma).
- Enlargement of the cranial foramina (e.g., optic nerve glioma).
- Enlargement of the sella turcica (pituitary tumors).
- Erosion of bone.
- Craniomegaly with hydrocephalus.

b. CAT Scan of the Head

Computerized axial tomography (CAT) is the most important early investigation to be carried out in patients suspected of harboring an intracranial mass lesion. It will show one or more of the following:

- Mixed-density lesion or increased attenuation.
- Mass effect, manifested by distortion of the ventricles and shift of the midline structures (particularly if the lesion is noninfiltrating).
- Decreased density surrounding the lesion, indicating cerebral edema.
- Contrast enhancement after IV infusion of contrast material.
- Multiplicity of lesions (pathognomonic of metastases).

c. Tomography and Pneumoencephalography

These procedures have been largely replaced by the CAT scan; they are rarely indicated, except in selected cases.

d. Angiography

Cerebral arteriography, usually performed by selective catheterization via the femoral artery, is still essential in the study of most brain tumors, particularly when surgery is contemplated. It may

- Confirm the presence of the mass by displacement of vessels in the vicinity of the tumor.
- Identify a characteristic pattern of small pathological blood

vessels (neovascularization) suggestive of malignant tumors.
- Provide detailed information about the vascular anatomy to guide the surgeon.
- Rule out an aneurysm.

e. Myelography

Lumbar or cisternal myelography is particularly useful in the study of epidural and spinal tumors (metastases, meningiomas, etc.).

f. CAT Scan of the Spine

A CAT scan of the spine may provide additional information in evaluating patients for spinal cord tumors.

3. Brain Scan

Radionuclide scanning has been largely replaced by computerized axial tomography, and flow studies are of little value in the study of tumors of the brain.

4. Electroencephalography

Brain tracings are of particular value in the study of patients with seizures. Changes will vary with the aggressiveness of the tumor.

5. Spinal Tap and Study of the Cerebrospinal Fluid

Lumbar puncture is usually contraindicated if there is any suspicion of increased intracranial pressure, lest herniation, with its potential risks, should occur. It should not be performed unless specific indications are present. It is of particular value whenever intracranial infection is suspected. Lumbar puncture may also be useful in establishing the diagnosis, if tumor cells can be identified on cytological studies; furthermore, an elevated CSF proteins level and a decreased glucose level are significant in the absence of infection. Lumbar puncture is particularly helpful in the diagnosis of lymphomas of the CNS and meningeal carcinomatosis.

6. Electromyography

This is only indicated in the case of spinal tumors or when peripheral nerve pathology is suspected.

7. Nuclear Magnetic Resonance

Nuclear magnetic resonance (NMR) is the newest and a most promising investigative modality for the evaluation of brain tumors. It is a method of brain imaging that uses magnetic bombardment of the cells to identify minute differences in water concentration within the brain cells. These differences are then analyzed by computers, which translate them into images similar to those seen by CAT. The procedure appears to be at least as sensitive as the CAT scan without exposing the patient to any radiation whatsoever. Today NMR is only available in certain specialized centers and is still undergoing considerable evaluation and assessment, but it does seem to have extraordinary potential.

B. Ophthalmologic Evaluation

Opthalmologic evaluation will include the following assessments.

- Fundoscopic examination. Evaluation of the fundi is most important in assessing a patient with a possible brain tumor. One sign of increased intracranial pressure is papilledema. Hyperemia of the optic discs is the first reliable fundoscopic finding; as the process continues, the disc margins become blurred, vessels are seen to dip as they exit the disc, and finally hemorrhages develop on and near the optic nerve heads.
- Visual fields. A variety of aberrations of the visual fields can be seen with tumors in the vicinity of the optic chiasm or optic nerves.
  - Most typically, bitemporal hemianopsia.
  - Unilateral blindness.
  - Homonymous hemianopsia.
- Oculomotor nerve testing.
- Visual Acuity.
- Other findings: exophthalmos (proptosis) and diplopia. Sixth-nerve palsies, causing diplopia, may also be seen as a nonspecific consequence of elevated pressure.

C. Endocrine Evaluation

A significant number of brain tumors will result in endocrine disorders as a result of alterations of pituitary function, either in the form of increased function (functioning tumors of the pituitary) or decreased function by compression (e.g., chromophobe adenoma of the pituitary and craniopharyngioma). In such cases, a complete evaluation of the endocrine system is warranted to identify such syndromes as:

- Gonadal dysfunction: amenorrhea, galactorrhea, impotence.
- Gigantism or acromegaly.
- Cushing's syndrome: truncal obesity, hypertension, hirsutism, striae, hyperglycemia.
- Addison's disease.
- Thyroid function aberrations.

D. Metastatic Evaluation

Tumors of the CNS are primarily morbid as a result of their location. Distant metastases are extremely rare, but a basic evaluation should be carried out, including chest x-ray and serum chemistries (SMA-12).

Metastatic evaluation could be important in identifying other sites of malignancy (primary or metastatic), thus suggesting that the brain lesion itself might be metastatic. In cases where a brain metastasis is suspected rather than a primary brain tumor, the evaluation should include an attempt to identify the primary:

- Pulmonary evaluation and CAT scan; sputum cytology, tomography.
- Breast examination.
- Intravenous pyelogram (IVP).
- Stool examination for occult blood loss.
- GI series and barium enema (reserved for patients who have other symptoms or signs of GI disease).
- Serologic studies for biologic markers (carcinoembryonic antigens (CEA), human chorionic gonadotrophins (HCG), alpha-fetoproteins (AFP).

E. Other Evaluation

A patient about to be treated for a CNS tumor must have a complete, comprehensive medical evaluation to include a thorough cardiac evaluation, hemotologic evaluation, pulmonary and renal evaluation, etc. Nutritional assessment is essential since some patients will require forced alimentation, enteral or parenteral.

Most patients with CNS tumors will require steroid therapy and must be evaluated as to the potential impact of this sort of therapy. Blood work should include a complete blood count (CBC), a multichannel profile (SMA-12), blood gases, a coagulation profile, etc.

F. Multidisciplinary Evaluation

A multidisciplinary approach to the evaluation of the patient with a CNS tumor is often necessary. The primary care physician, neurologist, radiologist, ophthalmologist, and endocrinologist have a valuable input in assisting to establish a diagnosis. Therapy should be planned jointly by the neurologist, neurosurgeon, radiotherapist, and chemotherapist, and input from all, at various phases of treatment, must be sought.

G. Site-Specific Data Form for CNS Tumors (see pp. 281–282)

SITE-SPECIFIC DATA FORM—CENTRAL NERVOUS SYSTEM TUMORS

HISTORY

Age: _____ Sex: _____

Symptoms
- _____ Headache
- _____ Nausea, vomiting
- _____ Stupor, lethargy
- _____ Mental changes
- _____ Motor weakness
- _____ Gait or incoordination
- _____ Sensory disturbances
- _____ Seizures
- _____ Speech disturbances
- _____ Visual disturbances

Other _____

Duration: _____

Social history

Race: _____White _____Black _____Oriental _____Other

Marital status: _____Single _____Married _____Other

Occupation: _____

Family history of carcinoma: _____No _____Yes

Relation _____ Site: _____

Previous history of carcinoma: _____No _____Yes

Site _____

Rx: _____

Previous treatment (describe):

_____

_____

PHYSICAL EXAMINATION

General condition: _____

	Right	Left
Signs		
Altered state of consciousness	_____	_____
Papilledema	_____	_____
Motor paresis	_____	_____
Sensory deficit	_____	_____
Cranial nerve deficit	_____	_____
Cerebellar deficit	_____	_____
Gait	_____	
Other	_____	

	Right	Left
Location of tumor		
Undetectable	_____	_____
Supratentorial	_____	_____
Infratentorial	_____	_____
Crossing midline	_____	_____
Crossing tentorium	_____	_____
Encroaching ventricle	_____	_____
Spine _____ Level _____		
Peripheral nerve _____		
Describe: _____		

Characteristics

Size: _____<3 cm _____3-5 cm _____ >5 cm
- _____ Encapsulated
- _____ Infiltrative
- _____ Cystic
- _____ Vascular
- _____ Obstructing CSF

PREOPERATIVE EVALUATION (Check, if done)

	Neg.	Pos.	Suspicious
CAT scan	_____	_____	_____
Radionucleide scan	_____	_____	_____
Angiogram	_____	_____	_____
EEG	_____	_____	_____

	Neg.	Pos.	Suspicious
CSF	_____	_____	_____
Myelogram	_____	_____	_____
x-Rays	_____	_____	_____
Other _____			
Biopsy: _____No _____Yes			

Histologic diagnosis: _____

_____

Classification: _____T _____N _____M

Stage: _____

Signature: _____

Countersignature: _____

Date: _____

Primary tumor

TX   Tumor cannot be assessed
T0   Primary tumor is undetectable
T1   Greatest diameter is 5 cm or less, confined to one side
        (3 cm or less, if infratentorial)
T2   Greatest diameter is more than 5 cm, confined to one side
        (greater than 3 cm, if infratentorial)
T3   Greatest diameter may be 3 cm or less, invades or encroaches
        upon the ventricular system
T4   Crosses the midline, invades the opposite hemisphere, or extends
        across the tentorium

Nodal involvement (N)
(Does not apply to this site)

Distant metastasis (M)

MX   Not assessed
M0   No evidence of distant metastases
M1   Distant metastases present. Specify according to the following notations:
      Subarachnoid space   CSF
      Pulmonary   PUL
      Lymph nodes   LYM
      Osseous   OSS
      Hepatic   HEP
      Bone marrow   MAR
      Occult   OCC
      Other   OTH

Add ''+'' to the abbreviated notation to indicate that the pathology is proved.

Grade

G1   Well-differentiated
G2   Moderately well differentiated, no mitosis
G3   Poorly differentiated, occasional mitosis
G4   Very poorly differentiated, frequent mitosis,
        and marked pleomorphism

Stage groupings

Stage I
Stage IA   G1, T1, M0
Stage IB   G1, T2, 3, M0

Stage II
Stage IIA   G2, T1, M0
Stage IIB   G2, T2, 3, M0

Stage III
Stage IIIA   G3, T1, M0
Stage IIIB   G3, T2, 3, M0

Stage IV   Any G with T4
              Any T with G4
              Any G, any T with M1

III. PRETREATMENT PREPARATION

The preoperative preparation of the patient with a CNS tumor is one that is primarily directed at controlling, or correcting in part, the secondary ill effects of the tumor.

A. General Systemic Preparation

Patients with neurological tumors are usually not affected systemically by the disease. Metastases are extremely rare, and physical debilitation is unusual at the time of first presentation of the disease.

1. Correction of Preexisting Medical Diseases

The patient with previous medical illnesses that require compensation must be actively treated to avoid unnecessary delay in dealing with the brain tumor itself.

- Hematologic and coagulation defects should be corrected.
- Cardiac status should be compensated as well as possible.
- Pulmonary function and reserve should be improved with respiratory therapy, inhalations, bronchodilators, etc.

2. Nutritional Support

Patients with long-standing disease, particularly when in coma, will require intensive and judicious nutritional support. This can usually be carried out by an oral feeding tube or gastrostomy, although intravenous hyperalimentation may, at times, be required.

It is not usual for a patient with an early brain tumor to require preoperative nutritional preparation.

3. Endocrine Disturbances

Tumors causing compression, destruction, or hyperactivity of the pituitary gland will result in a variety of endocrine disturbances. Most of these (e.g., gonadal deficiencies or excesses, gigantism or acromegaly, etc.) can only be corrected by treating the tumor directly; others, however, may result in severe physiological disturbances that must be corrected preoperatively:

- Adrenal insufficiency.
- Diabetes insipidus.
- Thyroid insufficiency or hyperactivity, etc.

Cooperation with a qualified endocrinologist is essential at this point to avoid serious operative or postoperative difficulties.

Furthermore, patients who have been previously treated with corticosteroids, should continue receiving them intravenously immediately prior to surgery, during the operation, and for a short period of time afterward.

B. Control of Increased Intracranial Pressure

The threat posed by increasing intracranial pressure is the most overwhelming, immediate concern of the physician treating a patient with a brain tumor. Although surgical decompression and/or resection or debulking of the tumor is, at times, the only way effectively to control the increased intracranial pressure, it is often essential to achieve some improvement of the situation by medical preparation prior to surgery.

1. Corticosteroids

Dexamethasone is the most effective and usually administered agent, and 16 mg per day are administered in divided doses. In urgent situations, or where the response to such dosage is unsatisfactory, the amount may be increased several fold, up to 120 mg per day. Methylprednisolone, in comparable dosage, is also commonly used.

Corticosteroids are extremely effective in controlling cerebral edema and achieving symptomatic relief. In addition to their preoperative use, they are often utilized for palliation in advanced disease.

2. Mannitol and Urea

These agents used intravenously are rapidly effective but should be reserved for preoperative or emergency use only.

C. Anticonvulsants

Phenytoin, phenobarbital, and/or Carbamazepine should be used in sufficient dosages to be effective in controlling convulsions; blood level concentrations should be monitored to achieve optimum results.

IV. THERAPEUTIC MANAGEMENT

Tumors of the CNS are either primary or secondary. Primary lesions may be intra-axial or extra-axial, the latter arising from bony and cartilaginous structures or embryonic cell rests. The leptomeninges provide a common source of neoplasm in the form of meningiomas (14% of all intracranial tumors). Intra-axial neoplasms usually arise from glia but may also have their source from nerve cells, neuroepithelium, peripheral and cranial nerves, vascular structures, paraganglia, the hypophysis, or the pineal gland. These tumors may consist of single or multiple discrete lesions or may be diffusely spread along the neuraxis by subarachnoid seeding or hematogenous spread. They may be cystic or solid or may exist in conjunction with cysts. They may be accompanied by endocrine disturbances or be reflected by polycythemia, urinary excretion of amino acids, and dermal lesions.

Central nervous system tumors may be benign or malignant; the benign lesions, however, may be as dangerous as the malignant ones by virtue of their proximity to vital structures.

Secondary lesions are considered under the heading of cerebral metastases; they may encroach upon the cranial cavity by direct extension (as in nasopharyngeal tumors) or be conveyed centrally by hematogenous dissemination. Spinal metastases are thought to arise from cells conveyed through the epidural venous plexus of Batson or by direct extension from the vertebrae into the vertebral canal. Tumors of the reticuloendothelial system (such as lymphomas) are presumed to arise intracranially from microglia as there is no cerebral lymphatic system. Spinal lymphomas may arise from paraspinal nodes and extend into the vertebral canal through the intervertebral foramina, or they may arise directly from the vertebral bodies and extend into the extradural space, compressing the adjacent neural structures.

A. General Guidelines

1. Establishment of the Diagnosis

It is essential to establish a definitive diagnosis of the lesion prior to therapy. This should be carried out using those techniques that are associated with the least morbidity and highest potential for providing the information required, so that the therapist can proceed with the most efficacious and rational options (see §7.II).

2. Biopsy

For primary intracranial lesions, a tissue diagnosis is important provided the risks of obtaining tissue do not outweigh the benefits of the interventions. With the advent of CAT scan, stereotactic approaches, and ultrasonic intraoperative localization, even deep lesions can be safely approached from the standpoint of obtaining tissue. A needle biopsy of the lesion has even become an acceptable alternative to surgery in the management of noncurable lesions. There now exists the technological feasibility, using ultrasound transducers in a brain needle, to direct such a needle through a burr hole into the core of a deeply seated neoplasm and sample it at

varying depths; this may be done while actually visualizing the passage of the needle on a screen. With proper medical management of cerebral edema, this procedure carries a low morbidity and a high yield of information. In past years it was customary to follow brain tumor biopsies by an internal decompression procedure to overcome the increased cerebral edema caused by the biopsy; today, using the stereotactic method of needle biopsy done through a burr hole under CAT scan control, this complication is obviated and can be controlled with the administration of corticosteroids.

3. The Curable Lesion

In cases where a complete cure is possible, an all-out effort is made to remove the entire tumor. This directive is modified by judgments that, at times, mandate leaving small fragments of tumor around blood vessels or adhering to the brainstem or spinal cord in order to avoid paralysis or loss of important function. The following are instances in which sacrificing neural function for total tumor removal may be justifiable:

- Facial palsy associated with acoustic neuroma, where removal of the cranial nerve and loss of hearing in the affected ear is acceptable.
- Transecting one optic nerve in instances of optic glioma or where tumor masses are found to be encasing the nerve or severely compressing it.
- One olfactory nerve is routinely sectioned in the subfrontal approaches, and occasionally one needs to section both olfactory nerves.
- An occipital lobectomy may be required, which would result in a contralateral homonymous hemianopsia.

It is usual to try, at all costs, to preserve motor centers, and the brainstem must never be compromised during surgery.

It may be stated, for example, that most meningiomas, with the exception of those located in certain areas such as the clivus ridge, can be totally removed. Every effort should be made to affect such a removal, even if staging the surgery over a period of time proves necessary. In the case of particularly lengthy procedures or whenever difficulties are encountered, staging of the procedure is an acceptable option.

4. The Incurable Lesion

Where a complete cure cannot be effected and palliative therapy is the only alternative, quality of survival should take precedence over simple survival time. This concept is not universally accepted, and some will advocate radical tumor removals for malignant gliomas regardless of the neurological consequences. One may then question whether it is proper to perform a nondominant hemispherectomy with residual hemiplegia if a glioma could presumably be "cured" (i.e., before infiltration has occurred in the corpus callosum); although most surgeons would not embark on this type of resection, some will condone less "radical" removals, even where associated with significant functional losses.

It may be stated that, with the exception of certain cystic lesions with mural nodules, gliomas cannot be totally removed. It would seem, therefore, that to operate with the intention of "cure" and incur additional severe or incapacitating deficit is to defeat the notion of helping a patient live as well as possible through the course of his or her illness.

5. Nonintervention

There are instances where no therapy is warranted. The elderly individual who is obtunded from early cerebral herniation and who has multiple intracranial masses is such an example. To make an attempt to restore such a patient to wakefulness for a few days of life does not seem warranted. Likewise, patients who will clearly not benefit from therapy because of the stage or extent of their disease should be permitted to die in dignity.

6. Rehabilitation

Rehabilitation must be an integral part of the total management of all patients with CNS tumors. The aid of the rehabilitation therapists must be enlisted as early as possible to help the patient during the recovery phase. The need for encouragement is particularly important since certain recuperative periods may be drawn out for a year or more.

B. Common Pitfalls

The following are some of the errors in management that may lead to unnecessarily increased morbidity and that should be recognized and avoided.

1. Lack of Recognition of the Biologic Behavior of the Tumor

The treatment approach must be based on the likely short- and long-term behavior of the lesion.

2. Inadequate Evaluation of the Patient

Insufficient radiodiagnostic assessment of the tumor in preparation for surgery constitutes inadequate evaluation of the patient. Full radiological evaluation is essential even in the most urgent clinical settings. All studies should be reviewed with the neuroradiologist to gain the greatest amount of information. The diagnosis, vascularity, exact localization, and surgical approach must be based on effective x-ray visualization.

3. Unwarranted Delay in Treatment

This is a controversial issue among neurosurgeons and between neurologists and neurosurgeons. There are those who feel that neurosurgery is often more harmful than the underlying disease process; they stress other alternatives to their patients until a desperate situation arises. Such an approach is often detrimental, and if surgery is to be deferred at first, the patient must be maintained under very close observation and referred for surgery at the slightest indication of deterioration. On the other hand, a conservative approach is warranted in the asymptomatic lesions, particularly in the elderly, provided the patient is followed closely. It must be emphasized that one should not rush into a neurosurgical procedure in these cases, but one must keep in mind that it is easier to prevent neurological deficits than to restore them once they have occurred. Just where the balance lies is a matter of refined judgment.

Decompression surgery (drainage or shunt procedure) is indicated in cases of papilledema, hydrocephalus, or a posterior fossa lesion, even though asymptomatic or minimally symptomatic, since sudden death may occur if pressure is not relieved.

Likewise, patients with large supratentorial tumors are at risk of uncal or central herniation. They must be carefully watched and monitored until the intracranial pressure is satisfactorily controlled and then promptly treated.

4. Inadequate Preoperative Preparation

This may take two forms:

- Lack of control of cerebral edema with all its consequences.
- Inadequate anticonvulsant levels pre- and intraoperatively, which may result in postoperative seizures and Todd's phenomenon.

5. Unwarranted Aggressive Treatment

It is most important to keep in mind at all times the quality of survival of the patient when contemplating potentially crippling surgery in diseases that are most often noncurable. There are some situations for example where aggressive therapy is unwarranted:

- Functionally disabling resections.
- Aggressive surgery in the elderly patient.

6. Inadequate Intraoperative Management

This may take several forms:

- Failure properly to position the patient may result in sciatic or ulnar nerve palsy.
- Pressure on the globes of the eyes or carotid bulb, with the risk of cerebral accidents, must be avoided.
- Inadequate maintenance of the blood pressure while bringing the patient to a sitting position may result in increased neurological deficit with a risk of stroke.

7. Inadequate Evaluation of the Available Histological Material

Review of the slides with the pathologist is the obligation of all treating physicians since the histologic findings are often the most important factor in deciding on a therapeutic approach.

8. Failure to Replace Bone Flaps

Occasionally, one may be tempted to leave out the bone flap because of the brain swelling and pressure. This may lead to a fungating mass of tumor and brain when the lesion begins its regrowth, and one must not attempt to achieve decompression by failing to replace a bone flap that was raised for surgical exposure.

C. Selection of Treatment Modality

1. Brain Tumors

Surgery is the main modality of treatment of most primary brain tumors when one is attempting to achieve a cure, provided excision of the tumor-bearing area is technically possible, with reasonable assurances that resulting functional impairment is acceptable. A few tumors, such as ependymomas, medulloblastomas, and malignant lymphomas, prevalent in children, are radiosensitive. The role of surgery in these cases is generally one of biopsy and debulking prior to radiotherapy.

In highly malignant tumors or those affecting areas of the brain that are not resectable, a number of palliative methods are available. Therapeutic goals are to improve the quality of life and prevent urgent life-threatening complications of increased intracranial pressure and/or herniation. These include

- Medical management of cerebral edema, seizures, and/or other symptoms, using corticosteroids, anticonvulsants, etc.
- Palliative radiotherapy or chemotherapy, whenever applicable.

- Ventriculoperitoneal shunt for drainage of the ventricles and relief of hydrocephalus.
- Partial debulking resections.

Whenever surgical exploration is undertaken for benign or low-grade malignant tumors, an attempt at total surgical excision should be carried out. It is often, however, prudent to perform a subtotal excision of the tumor rather than chance crippling functional impairment. This may be followed by radiotherapy and will often achieve the desired effect for several years.

Reoperation for regrowth of a benign tumor is often quite effective and may be repeated as necessary. The question of reoperation on malignant lesions is moot, however, and most surgeons would probably not undertake secondary resections unless significant prolongation of good quality of life could be anticipated. Secondary operations are usually recommended in certain selected lesions, such as lesions of the posterior fossa in children. When there has been an incomplete removal of an astrocytoma or incomplete relief of obstructive hydrocephalus caused by a fourth-ventricle ependymoma or medulloblastoma, a shunt procedure is necessary.

In instances of multiple malignant intracranial lesions, surgical intervention is not felt to be warranted unless it is necessary to distinguish neoplasia from other pathological processes.

Management of tumors in specific locations depends on whether they are benign or malignant and whether they can safely be separated from the surrounding neural tissue. The approach will vary greatly, and some locations require a very specific surgical approach:

- Pituitary lesions can be dealt with in many cases through a transsphenoidal approach; occasionally a subfrontal exposure combined with a transsphenoidal approach will allow removal of lesions that could not be managed entirely by either alone.
- Tentorial lesions may be approached by transsecting the transverse sinus and elevating the occipital lobe.
- Glial lesions in vital centers (such as the brainstem) are known to be reasonably radiosensitive, especially when occurring in children. Radiotherapy is often the modality of choice since surgery is not feasible in certain sites.

Radiotherapy is not advisable as a primary modality in cranial lesions where surgery is being considered, since there are claims that this may be associated with increased surgical morbidity.

2. Tumors of the Spine

- Benign lesions of the spinal cord should be approached with the notion of total excision.

- Intradural extramedullary lesions such as neurofibromas and meningiomas may be completely excised with, if need be, sacrifice of a sensory root (e.g., in the case of neurofibromas).
- Intramedullary lesions can be approached through local and extensive myelotomies with some degree of success. Microscopic visualization has assisted these procedures. Ependymomas may thus be removed prior to radiation, and approximately 20% of astrocytomas may be delineated from the surrounding normal neural tissue and removed.
- In spinal metastases, a single locus of compression may be dealt with either by initial surgical decompression or by radiotherapy. The benefits and hazards are equally shared by both methods, and most practitioners will opt for initial radiotherapy, unless the diagnosis is in question or when there has been no benefit derived from a previous course of radiotherapy. Radiotherapy is indicated for
  - Multiple spinal lesions.
  - Situations where the overall longevity of the patient is limited to months.
  - Where there is severe radicular pain.
  - When the lesion is known to be highly radiosensitive (e.g., myeloma or lymphoma), although even in these cases, a decompressive laminectomy as an adjunctive procedure is sometimes necessary.
- Since most metastatic lesions to the spine arise from local deposits in the epidural space or as a result of direct extension into the vertebral canal from adjacent bone, anterior surgical approaches for excision of the vertebral bodies and decompression are being considered as alternatives to the more traditional laminectomy.
- Steroids, useful in controlling edema, are of questionable usefulness in spinal-compression problems; nevertheless, in an acute situation, 100 mg of dexamethasone given intravenously, followed by 4 mg every 6 hours throughout the periods of surgery and the early phases of radiotherapy, are routinely administered. Steroid doses are traditionally tapered to avoid problems of adrenal insufficiency.

D. Surgical Therapy

Surgical intervention in the management of CNS neoplasms is based on strict criteria. The notion of exploratory surgery does not exist as it does in general surgery. Procedures are precisely calculated so that the craniotomy or laminectomy allows for full exposure of the underlying pathology. The criteria governing the surgery include a complete radiographic investigation as previously described, including CAT scan imaging that provides the surgeon with reasonably precise information on which to base a diagnosis and surgical approach. The surgeon must also be thoroughly acquainted with the natural

history and course of the pathological entity at hand and must be in a position to make an objective assessment of the dynamic mechanical factors involved in the presenting symptoms and the threat they pose to the patient. These elements, along with a sense of the time frame in which the neurological signs are evolving, provide the appropriate setting for judging the need and format for surgical intervention.

1. Goals of Surgical Management

Surgical therapy for CNS tumors has four essential goals:

- Obtaining a tissue diagnosis.
- Relief of mechanical pressure on neural tissues, with its varying neurological deficits, and of pressure or distortion of the cerebral vasculature, with its associated ischemia or edema.
- Relief of increased intracranial pressure, hydrocephalus, or impending herniation.
- Elimination of the tumor, either completely, if possible and safe, or partially to permit more effective use of adjuvant modalities of treatment.

2. Urgent Situations

In the urgent neurological situations resulting from CNS tumors, surgical and medical therapies are primarily designed to relieve the mechanical and distorting effects of the tumor on the blood vessels and the adjacent neural tissues, thereby relieving the surrounding pressure, cerebral edema, and any associated hydrocephalus. The urgency of intervention depends solely on the surgeon's assessment of the clinical profile and the radiographic studies.

The patient with incipient or full-blown cerebral herniation syndrome should be given large doses of dexamethasone and mannitol to buy time, intubated, and given hyperventilation with supplemental oxygen during preparation for surgery.

Seizures should be controlled with appropriate amounts of anticonvulsant medication, preferably phenytoin or carbamazepine, as barbiturates may alter the level of consciousness. If status epilepticus ensues, general anesthesia may be required.

In cranial lesions associated with hydrocephalus, an external ventricular drainage procedure or a ventricular shunt may get the patient through the crisis of increased intracranial pressure so that the tumor may be dealt with on an elective basis. Increased intracranial pressure due to hydrocephalus may produce a frontal lobe syndrome of reluctance to cooperate, mutism, and fluctuating somnolence (in addition to papilledema). This pattern should be recognized, for it is potentially as dangerous as the dilated pupil of an oculomotor nerve palsy associated with uncal herniation. In a similar vein, the tonic extensor movements heralding decerebration, formerly termed "cerebellar fits" by Hughlings Jackson, should not be confused with the tonic clonic movements of epilepsy. They imply a posterior fossa mass effect and tonsillar herniation. These are signs of extreme urgency demanding immediate action.

Spinal lesions must be urgently dealt with when the progression of weakness is rapid and when the myelogram or CAT scan confirms the presence of a compressive lesion or complete blockage to the flow of metrizamide or Pantopaque. Sensory disturbances and pain are not necessarily urgent criteria for surgical intervention; however, Lhermitte's sign and parascapular pain may be indicative of high-cervical spinal cord compression. Bony spinal stenoses producing a complete epidural type of myelographic block are usually stable lesions and need not be addressed as urgently. In situations where one cannot distinguish an epidural tumor from bony stenosis, or where complete evaluation is impossible, one can justify proceeding with a decompression of the bone and, if present, neoplastic elements. If the nature of the lesion is established with some certainty without surgery, high-voltage radiotherapy may, in selected cases of radiosensitive lesions (malignant lymphomas), be the preferred choice of initial management.

3. Surgical Approach

a. Preparation for Surgery

Patients should be placed on prophylactic antibiotics a few hours prior to the surgery. Intraoperative drainage of spinal fluid may be helpful in relieving intracranial tension in some instances and is useful in permitting the brain to retract, thus allowing more room and facilitating operative manipulation. Loupes and the operating microscope are important adjuncts in approaching the lesions and should be available.

b. Incisions and Flaps

For intracranial procedures, various types of incisions may be made, and unilateral bone flaps are raised except in certain cases of subfrontal or parasagittal tumors, where a bilateral bone flap may be required.

c. Method of Dissection

Major dissection is carried out with the use of an electrocautery with bipolar current attached to a bayonet forceps. Additional methods being advised include the use of laser beams and ultrasonic tools such as the Cavitron. Whether they will replace the more traditional tools remains to be seen. The most significant improvements in surgical technology to date have been the bipolar coagulator, the dissecting microscope, and the availability of medical therapies (e.g., dexamethosene, furosemide, mannitol, and urea) to control cerebral edema. The tumor is separated from the surrounding brain, and bridging vessels are cauterized in such a manner as to prevent bleeding that might obscure the field. In benign lesions, the first efforts are directed at curtailing the arterial blood supply to the tumor. Tumor removal is usually piecemeal, with internal decompression followed by separation of the capsule from the surrounding neural tissue. Topical hemostatic agents are used including Avitene, Gelfoam, and Surgicel.

Despite all these newer techniques, three basic questions must always be considered by the surgeon: Can the lesion be removed with relative safety? What is the proper timing for the operation? Should the surgery be staged?

4. Results

The overall results of treatment vary according to the specific lesion. In malignant glioblastomas, for example, the medium survival is between 10 and 15 months with surgical resection followed by radiotherapy. Some reports indicate a significant 3-year survival with aggressive surgery. They fail, however, to stress the quality of life. On the other hand, patients with meningiomas who survive for 1 month postoperatively have a 1-year survival rate of over 90% and a 15-year survival rate of over 60%. In addition, there has been a clear improvement in the surgical mortality, which was staggering in the 1940s but dropped to a reasonable rate (<3%) by the 1960s.

E. Adjuvant Therapy

1. Radiotherapy

Irradiation of the CNS usually raises several questions related to the possibility of radiation damage. In order to dispel these fears, this aspect is discussed in some detail.

a. Tolerance of CNS Tissues to Radiation

The response of the normal nervous system to irradiation has been established from experimental irradiation of animal nervous systems and extrapolation of the results to the human nervous system. Tolerance was also determined by observing the effect of irradiating a part of the nervous system included while treating extranervous tissue. Often, the effect of disease and surgery makes it difficult to evaluate the damage caused by the radiation therapy. The following, however, are recognized changes that result from radiotherapy.

i. Brain.

- Acute changes. Edema of all intracranial structures is thought to be proportional to the daily dose, the volume irradiated, and the fractionation (or number of treatment sessions). These changes may be related to vascular alterations, but with the usual daily therapeutic dose, these acute effects are well tolerated, and symptoms are controlled by the concomitant use of corticosteriods.

- Chronic changes. These take 6–24 months to develop but may occur even later. The latent period depends on the total dose (higher doses are worse), the fractionation, the age of the patient (older patients have a poorer tolerance), and the treatment volume (larger volumes have a more pronounced effect). There are functional and behavioral changes thought to be caused by either vascular occlusion or injury to the glial cells.
- Brain necrosis. This can occur following re-treatment (especially following an intensive course) or after an initial intensive course to a large volume in a short period of time. The mechanism is probably through damage of the supporting vascular structures and takes 8 months to 9 years to occur, with a peak incidence between 1 and 3 years. A period of improvement of the patient's symptoms or even total recovery may occur over a period of 1–5 years, and this is then followed by a sudden or gradual deterioration of brain function without signs of increased intracranial pressure or papilledema. These symptoms have to be differentiated from recurrent tumor, hemorrhage, abscess formation, or other inflammatory processes before incriminating brain necrosis induced by the radiotherapy.

Under ordinary circumstances, brain damage due to irradiation is relatively rare. The range of tolerance varies from the brainstem, which is the most sensitive, through the more resistant motor cortex to the most resistant frontal cortex. This tolerance is volume and fractionation dependent. The normal pituitary gland is extremely radioresistant; doses up to 10,000 rads may, on occasion, fail to cause hypopituitarism.

ii. Spinal Cord.   The functional tolerance of the spinal cord to irradiation is probably 10–15% lower than that of the brain. The dorsal cord is more sensitive than the rest of the spinal cord. Spinal cord damage goes through several stages.

- Early transient myelopathy. Complaints of electric shocks radiating down the back and over the extremities after neck flexion (Lhermitte's sign) may occur 2–4 months after irradiation of the cervical cord and persist for several months. These symptoms are probably due to demyelination within the spinal cord and are self-arresting, wih spontaneous recovery.
- Late irreversible injury. Lhermitte's sign may be the first indication of the onset of a permanent dysfunction, but irreversible changes are preceded by a relatively longer latent period (1–2 years). Symptoms are similar to those of partial or complete cord transection. Radiographs are normal; spinal fluid pressure is normal; the fluid protein is normal; and no obstruction in the canal can be demonstrated. Radiation

myelitis depends on the length of the cord segment irradiated, the dose per fraction, the number of fractions, the interval between fractions, the total dose, and the overall time. Older patients suffering from arteriosclerotic changes may be somewhat more prone. A poorly directed beam, especially in treating adjacent areas with overlapping fields, increases the risk of this complication. Radiation myelitis is a rare complication of curative radiotherapy.

iii. The CNS in Children.   The CNS in children is more sensitive than in adults. The younger the child, the more radiosensitive the brain, and dosages have to be adjusted accordingly. Neuropsychological testing demonstrates gross intellectual function to be satisfactory in most patients, but some children show a shortened attention span, poor short-term memory, and specific learning disabilities. Controlled studies, however, are necessary to define the role of cranial irradiation in children since medical and social factors may have a role in the poor performance of a child treated for a malignant disease. Prophylactic cranial irradiation in acute leukemia in children may alter the blood–brain barrier, and patients receiving high doses of intrathecal methotrexate after radiotherapy have an increased risk of developing leukoencephalopathy.

b. Indications for Radiation Therapy

The response of various primary intracranial tumors to radiation therapy differs. Medulloblastomas are the most radiosensitive, whereas glioblastomas are the least. When radiation therapy is used for glial tumors, it is usually instituted as a postoperative modality. Radiation may be used as the sole modality in lesions inoperable by virtue of the site or extent of the tumor. The following are the usual indications for radiotherapy in CNS tumors.

i. Tumors of Limited Radiosensitivity.   These are the glial tumors. Radiotherapy is applicable for

- Patients who have undergone incomplete resection of their tumor.
- Tumors located in a critical area such as the midbrain, the pons, or the motor area of the cerebral cortex. Surgery here carries high risks and is usually limited to obtaining a biopsy for definitive histological diagnosis.
- Patients presenting with definitive clinical evidence but without histological proof of a tumor situated in the pons or brainstem.
- Recurrence after surgical removal, unless further surgery is indicated (as in cystic tumors or in some meningiomas).
- Medical problems that preclude surgery.

Glial tumors usually need high-dose radiation, on the order of 6000–6500 rads.

ii. Tumors of Moderate Radiosensitivity. Craniopharyngioma and pituitary tumors fall into this group. These lesions usually respond well to moderate doses of about 5000 rads.

iii. Radiosensitive Tumors. Medulloblastoma and, to a lesser degree, ependymomas fall into this group. They usually respond to doses on the order of 3000 rads. Malignant lymphomas are also in this category.

c. Contraindications to Radiation Therapy

- Inadequate diagnosis, where a serious doubt exists as to the nature of a space-occupying lesion (e.g., brain abscess versus neoplasm).
- Previous intensive irradiation of an intracranial tumor.
- Inadequate facilities for radiation therapy.

Radiation therapy should be delivered with high-energy machines using complex and sophisticated treatment plans. These are necessary to deliver optimum doses to the tumor while sparing normal tissues. The specific application of radiotherapy to the various CNS tumors will be presented with the discussion of therapy for the individual tumors.

2. Chemotherapy

The role of chemotherapy in tumors of the CNS is decidedly limited. Clearly, local therapy, i.e., surgery and/or radiotherapy, is the primary mode of therapy in these disorders, chemotherapy being added as an adjuvant in the hope of achieving additional benefit. An important factor limiting the efficacy of chemotherapy is the blood–brain barrier, which may prevent penetration of the drug into tumor deposits within the CNS. Consequently, lipid-soluble drugs, such as the nitrosoureas or procarbazine, have proven to be the most useful agents. However, it is not clearly established that the blood–brain barrier is absolute and that some continuity does not exist with respect to brain tumors. The tumor-enhancing effect of contrast material in brain CAT scanning is an obvious result of blood–brain continuity; it is, therefore, possible that other drugs with clinical efficacy in the treatment of brain tumors may be identified in the future. The cerebral neoplasms that can be treated with chemotherapy include malignant gliomas, meningeal carcinomatosis, and medulloblastomas.

The standard treatment of high-grade astrocytoma consists primarily of surgical resection (if feasible) plus radiotherapy. Any additional benefit contributed by chemotherapy is surely modest. Clinical cooperative group studies have shown that the addition of nitrosourea compounds such as bichloroethyl nitrosourea (BCNU) or chloroethyl chlorohexyl nitrosourea (CCNU) prolongs median patient survival by a few months. More importantly, the proportion of patients who survive 18 months or more has been as high as 20%, as compared with less than 10%

in those patients receiving radiotherapy alone. Treatment with a nitrosourea compound such as BCNU is, therefore, recommended in most cases of high-grade (Grades 3 and 4) astrocytoma. Dexamethasone has no demonstrable antitumor effect but is an additional drug used to treat the serious symptoms caused by increased intracranial pressure; it is known to decrease edema around tumor deposits, resulting in reduction of intracranial pressure.

Oligodendrogliomas are quite rare, accounting for only 1.5% of all brain tumors. When they dedifferentiate into high-grade tumors, they assume the clinical characteristics of other high-grade gliomas and should be similarly treated with appropriate local therapy followed by chemotherapy with a nitrosourea compound.

Meningiomas are usually benign tumors that are treated surgically. Postoperative radiotherapy is recommended if surgical resection is incomplete. Occasionally, these tumors can regrow and undergo sarcomatous degeneration. In such cases, chemotherapy with agents appropriate for sarcomas should be considered. Adriamycin seems to be the agent of choice in these cases.

Medulloblastoma accounts for 25% of all pediatric brain tumors. It commonly spreads intracranially by way of the CSF pathways, as well as along the spinal neuraxis. Appropriate treatment includes surgical resection, if possible, followed by irradiation. Despite the general impression that these tumors are quite chemosensitive, improved survival conferred by chemotherapy has not yet been demonstrated. It is, therefore, recommended that such patients be entered into clinical trials so that the role of chemotherapy can be better defined before a firm recommendation is made.

Leptomeningeal metastatic disease represents a special management problem in the patient with disseminated cancer. This diagnosis is suggested by neurologic findings of widespread symptoms and signs rather than by those of a single focal lesion. Malignant cells are usually found on cytological examination of the CSF, and CSF protein concentration is almost always elevated. Treatment consists of intrathecal methotrexate, cytosine arabinoside, or both, given twice weekly until normalization of the CSF is achieved. The interval between doses is then gradually lengthened until maintenance therapy is given at monthly intervals. Radiotherapy is also delivered concomitantly to the site of major neurological symptoms. Treatment response of leukemia and lymphoma of the CNS is considerably better than that of solid-tumor or leptomeningeal metastases. In responding patients, consideration should be given to insertion of an Ommaya reservoir. This simplifies the technical problems of access to the CSF and avoids frequent, painful lumbar punctures.

Because of the severe toxicity of the various chemotherapeutic agents, their high morbidity in patients who are already seriously impaired, and the marginal and even questionable benefits to be derived from their use, chemotherapy must be used with great discrimination and clinical judgment in patient selection to avoid treating end-stage bedridden patients who are unlikely to benefit from this modality.

V. SPECIFIC NEUROLOGIC TUMORS

A. Astrocytic Tumors

Tumors of the astrocytic series, especially the highly malignant glioblastoma multiforme (astrocytoma, Grade 4), are the most frequently encountered primary brain tumors. In adults, they almost always arise in the supratentorial compartment.

1. Glioblastoma Multiforme

Glioblastoma multiforme is an extremely aggressive, uniformly fatal tumor, presenting most often in the late fifth and sixth decade. Males are affected twice as often as females.

Glioblastoma multiforme (also classified as astrocytoma, Grade 4) is a very anaplastic, highly cellular tumor composed, in any combination, of fusiform cells; small, poorly differentiated round cells; or pleomorphic cells. Other pathological features that characterize this tumor are necrosis, pseudopalisading, fistulous vessels and vascular endothelial proliferation, hemorrhage, and invasive growth. While no further pathological staging of glioblastoma multiforme is possible, it is important to note that any astrocytoma may be characterized by various histologic grades in different portions of the tumor. The tumor is always graded according to its most malignant area.

a. Clinical Presentation

The clinical presentation is generally progressive over a few weeks or months; occasionally the tumor may declare itself acutely, presumably because of hemorrhage within the mass or rapid expansion of a cystic component.

i. Increased Intracranial Pressure. Because the tumor results in extensive cerebral edema, symptoms of increased intracranial pressure often predominate. Headaches are the leading symptom in approximately one-third of patients, and a large majority have this complaint at the time of admission. Not infrequently, the patient shows decreased alertness or even frank impairment in the level of consciousness because of raised intracranial pressure at the time of presentation. Papilledema is often evident on initial examination.

ii. Seizures. Seizures, either generalized or of focal onset, are another frequent presenting feature of glioblastoma multi-

forme and occur in approximately one-third of patients at the time of admission.

iii. Focal Signs. The tumors arise more commonly in frontal and temporal lobes than in parietal lobes and much less commonly in occipital lobes. Symptoms and signs at presentation often reflect these sites of origin. Focal motor weakness is evident in more than one-half of the patients on admission; aphasia may also be noted in those patients with dominant-hemisphere lesions. Because frontal tumors have a particular predilection to involve the corpus callosum and, hence, both cerebral hemispheres (a situation virtually pathognomonic of glioblastoma), rapidly developing confusion or dementia is often seen.

b. Diagnostic Evaluation

The CAT scan of the head may be virtually diagnostic of glioblastoma multiforme. It will generally show an irregular mixed-density lesion, accompanied by a surrounding zone of decreased nonhomogeneous enhancement after the infusion of IV contrast material. Mass effect, manifested by distortion of the lateral ventricles and a shift of midline structures, will usually be apparent. The so-called butterfly pattern of tumor spreading through white matter from one hemisphere to the next seldom represents a lesion other than glioblastoma multiforme. In some cases, particularly those where surgery is not indicated, the CAT scan may be sufficient for diagnostic purposes.

Cerebral arteriography will confirm the presence of the mass, provide supportive evidence of the malignant nature of the tumor, and aid the surgeon in therapeutic planning.

Other investigations such as EEG, brain scan, CSF studies, etc. add little of diagnostic importance.

c. Therapeutic Management

Unfortunately, despite vigorous therapy, glioblastoma multiforme must still be regarded as an invariably fatal disease: survival beyond 18 months is considered very unusual. Nonetheless, in all cases, treatment should be individually tailored to increase the possibility of comfortable, functional survival for as long as possible. To this end, optimal therapy usually begins with surgery designed to remove as much tumor as possible while maintaining neurological function. Radiotherapy is used in inoperable cases or following surgery. Chemotherapy may have some usefulness as an adjunctive measure.

i. Surgery. Prior to surgery, and as an adjunct to all treatment programs, corticosteroids are administered; this often produces a dramatic clinical improvement because of the reduction of cerebral edema. One widely used regimen is dexamethasone, 4 mg orally 4 times a day. Some evidence exists to suggest that much higher doses of dexamethasone (i.e., 100 mgd) may benefit the patient when lower doses do not produce adequate responses. Unfortunately, corticosteroids do not appear to effect any shrinkage of the neoplasm itself. The surgeon should attempt to remove as much of the tumor as possible while preserving essential brain function. At the conclusion of the craniotomy, the dura is closed completely and the bone flap is secured, as the external decompression of the tumor upon its inevitable regrowth is undesirable. Extensive surgery is seldom indicated for tumors that are bilateral or deeply situated within the brain because of the unacceptable neurological deficits that result from the removal. In such cases, stereotactically guided needle biopsy provides an alternative method to establish a tissue diagnosis.

ii. Radiotherapy. After recovery from the craniotomy (usually about 2–3 weeks), whole-brain irradiation with a tumor booster should be administered. The dose is in the range of 5500–6000 rads, delivered over 5 weeks. Radiotherapy is also indicated when the diagnosis is highly likely but surgery is contraindicated. There is convincing evidence that radiotherapy prolongs survival, albeit for only a few months.

iii. Chemotherapy. The role of chemotherapy is less well established in the treatment of glioblastoma. Most currently available chemotherapeutic agents do not cross the blood–brain barrier. The nitrosoureas do, however, and BCNU has proved to be somewhat effective. Although studies have not shown statistically an increased mean survival in patients treated with BCNU in addition to surgery and radiotherapy, there seems to be an increase in the small number of patients with prolonged (18 months) survival. It is recommended, therefore, that current optimal therapy should include:

- Corticosteroids.
- Surgical removal of as much tumor as possible.
- Whole-brain irradiation.
- Chemotherapy with BCNU, alone or in combination, when the patient is in satisfactory clinical condition.

2. Astrocytomas

Astrocytomas are tumors of glial tissue composed predominantly of astrocytes. Histologically as well as clinically, they are less malignant than the glioblastoma multiforme. Pathologically, the tumors are subclassified by the appearance of the predominant cell:

- Fibrillary astrocytomas are composed of astrocytes with many intracytoplasmic fibrils (demonstrable by special stains).

- Protoplasmic astroyctomas consist of cells with few, if any, intracytoplasmic fibrils.
- Gemistocytic astrocytomas consist of large, plump astrocytes with abundant eosinophilic cytoplasm and one or more, usually eccentric, nuclei.

These tumors are usually considered Grade 2, histologically. Occasionally, a Grade 1 tumor consisting of increased nuclei within nearly normal appearing astrocytes that are poorly delineated from surrounding normal brain is encountered.

a. Clinical Presentation

Supratentorial astrocytomas are usually encountered at the convexity of the brain. At times, they present as large fluid-filled cysts with a small mural nodule of tumor and are then characterized by slow growth. Any astrocytoma, however, may dedifferentiate into a more malignant lesion.

The peak incidence of astrocytomas is in the fourth decade, and the most common mode of presentation is with seizures (over 50% in most series), either focal or generalized. The insidious development of other neurological signs or symptoms of increased intracranial pressure are less commonly encountered as initial manifestations.

b. Diagnostic Evaluation

Investigations can provide substantial clues that a relatively low-grade astrocytoma is present, but only histological examination is definitive.

- Plain-skull radiographs show calcification in approximately 12% of cases.
- Results of CAT scans are variable, but decreased-attenuation lesions are often seen, especially with cystic lesions. Less heterogeneity within the mass and less contrast enhancement than is seen with more malignant tumors are typical features. Many of these tumors are invasive and therefore often show little mass effect.
- Angiographically, the larger astrocytomas will be evident only by local vascular displacement. Few will demonstrate any foci of pathological circulation.
- Electroencephalography should be performed in suspected cases of astrocytoma, especially in patients with seizures. Although variable, recordings typically show minor changes compared with the much more severe slowing associated with more rapidly growing malignant tumors.

c. Therapeutic Management

Clear guidelines for the therapeutic management of patients with astrocytomas are not firmly established. Patients with seizures and no progressive neurologic deficit, and without well-defined mass effect, are probably best treated with appropriate anticonvulsant medication and close observation. On the other hand, patients with progressive neurologic signs or increased intracranial pressure, associated with the probability of macrocystic astrocytoma in the cerebral hemisphere should undergo a craniotomy with an attempt at total removal of all gross tumor. Radiotherapy appears to have some effect in prolonging survival, but little definitive information is available on this point. Chemotherapy has no role in the management of the lower-grade astrocytomas.

B. Oligodendrogliomas

Oligodendrogliomas are relatively uncommon tumors composed predominantly of oligodendroglial cells. These are uniform cells with round-to-oval nuclei, clear cytoplasm, and well-defined cell membranes, giving the appearance of halos in a honeycomb pattern. The tumors tend to be very slow growing and may reach enormous sizes. Although they may occur anywhere in the supratentorial compartment (and much more rarely, infratentorially), they are most frequently found in the frontal lobes.

1. Clinical Presentation

The majority of patients present with seizures. The current practice of screening most adult patients with newly developing seizures by CAT scan should result in the detection of these tumors at an earlier stage. Much less frequently, patients present with symptoms of increased intracranial pressure or, even less commonly, with focal neurologic symptoms.

2. Diagnostic Evaluation

The usual investigations for patients with epilepsy or a suspected mass are undertaken, but it must be emphasized that the work-up cannot reliably identify the histologic nature of the mass.

- Plain-skull radiographs should be taken in suspected cases because of the tendency of these tumors to calcify.
- The CAT scan appearance is nonspecific, but again, the presence of calcium density within the tumor suggests the diagnosis.
- Angiography may be valuable for surgical guidance but is unlikely to clarify the diagnosis.

3. Therapeutic Management

Treatment of oligodendroglioma is surgical extirpation to whatever extent is consistent with preservation of function. Surgery should be followed by irradiation, although no con-

clusive studies have been done that demonstrate improved survival rates.

C. CNS Metastases

1. Brain Metastases

The most frequently encountered intracranial tumors today are cerebral metastases. These secondary deposits, which usually result from hematogenous spread of aggressive peripheral tumors, generally arise at the junction of gray and white matter where tumor emboli tend to lodge. The distribution of metastases within the brain approximates the relative blood supply; over 80% of tumors are found in the cerebrum, and approximately 15% are located in the cerebellum. Occasionally, metastases arise in the brainstem. The incidence of brain metastases appears to be rising, probably because of the longer survival of patients with systemic cancer.

While virtually any malignant tumor may metastasize to the brain, melanoma, lung, breast, and renal carcinomas have a particularly strong tendency to do so. As a result of their high frequency of occurrence, as well as their propensity to spread to the brain, lung cancers, followed by breast cancers, are the most common primaries in various series of metastatic brain tumors.

a. Clinical Presentation

The mode of presentation of metastatic brain tumors does not differ significantly from that of primary cerebral malignancies (e.g., glioblastoma multiforme). Symptoms generally arise subacutely over days or weeks, though they may begin suddenly (i.e., with seizures) or develop more insidiously. Patients may present with nonlocalizing symptoms such as headache, confusion, lethargy, or vomiting due to increased intracranial pressure, or hydrocephalus in the case of posterior fossa metastases. Alternatively, focal symptoms and signs, such as hemiparesis, visual-field defects, aphasia, ataxia, or focal seizures may predominate. Generalized convulsions may also be seen.

b. Diagnostic Evaluation

The diagnostic approach to the patient with possible brain metastases varies, depending on whether or not a primary is known to exist. However, CAT is always the cornerstone of the investigation. Asymptomatic patients with known pulmonary carcinoma, especially oat cell carcinomas, should undergo a screening CAT scan of the head to detect early brain metastases. This is not warranted in patients with other primary sites. Neurologically symptomatic patients should have a CAT scan as the initial investigative test. Although brain metastases vary in their density relative to normal brain tissue and will show on a noncontrast scan, nearly all metastases will show enhancement with intravenous contrast, and this should be administered routinely as part of the study. If the CAT scan indicates metastases, treatment should be immediately initiated.

If the clinical onset was gradual and the initial CAT scan is negative, the study should be repeated with overlapping sections. If still negative, the patient should be followed and the CAT scan again repeated after 3–4 weeks. Occasionally a radioactive technetium brain scan will show deposits not demonstrated by a CAT scan. If the patient presents with an acute, strokelike onset and the initial CAT scan is negative, a follow-up scan in 7–10 days may indicate a vascular lesion. At times, angiography may be indicated in addition to the CAT scan.

The approach differs somewhat in the symptomatic patient who may be suffering from brain metastases but in whom no primary cancer has previously been identified. Here, it is important to identify the source of the metastasis, if at all possible. If the CAT scan is positive and suggestive of metastases, the patient should have a thorough, comprehensive history and physical examination, with special attention to the skin (melanomas), and the breasts in women, as well as

- Chest radiography with CAT scan or tomography.
- Cytological examination of the sputum.
- Examination of the stool for occult blood.
- An intravenous urogram.
- Serologic tests for biochemical markers (e.g., chorionic gonadotrophins, carcinoembryonic antigen, etc.) as indicated.

If these investigations prove negative, it is unlikely that any additional study will identify the primary site, and the small yield of positive results from more sophisticated (and costly) studies makes them unwarranted.

c. Therapeutic Management

Although very rare exceptions occur, the patient with metastatic cancer to the brain must be considered incurable, and most patients survive only a few months. Therapy should begin with high-dose corticosteroids (i.e., 16 mg of dexamethasone per day or 120 mg of methylprednisolone per day). Therefore, the choice lies between radiotherapy alone or surgical extirpation followed by radiotherapy.

Surgery is almost always indicated when the diagnosis is uncertain, especially so if an infection is under consideration. It should also be given serious consideration in a patient with evidence of only one cerebral lesion suspected of being metastatic, especially in the case of certain radioresistant primary tumors and when there is no evidence of disseminated cancer elsewhere. A relatively short time interval between the primary diagnosis and the discovery of the metastasis should, however,

dissuade the clinician from surgical treatment. The presence of multiple cerebral metastases, extensive or disseminated extracerebral disease, and stupor or coma are also absolute contraindications to surgery.

Several protocols of whole-brain irradiation have been advocated with somewhat similar results. A typical regimen is one in which 200 rads are administered daily for a total of 4500 rads in about 4 weeks. Sometimes a shorter course of therapy, such as 3000 rads in 2 weeks, is given. Similar regimens have been suggested electively (i.e., without definite evidence of brain metastases) in cases of cancers with a very high incidence of brain involvement (e.g., oat cell carcinoma of the lung).

In making a decision about therapy, the physician must consider many aspects of the patient, including

- Functional status.
- Emotional desires, needs, and perspective.
- Expected duration of survival.
- Probability of recovery from neurologic deficit.
- Time/benefit ratio (e.g., considering that surgery will prolong hospitalization).

2. Meningeal Carcinomatosis

With improved survival from treatment of their primary cancer, more patients are developing symptoms or signs of meningeal carcinomatosis. The physician should be alert to this possibility in patients presenting with headache, changing mental status, or cranial or spinal neuropathies. Cerebrospinal fluid examination should be performed after CAT scan has eliminated the possibility of a focal mass. Cytological examination will provide a definitive diagnosis in many cases, especially if several CSF specimens are examined. Unfortunately, the CSF may be negative for tumor cells and with a profile is otherwise nonspecific. The CSF profile often demonstrates pleocytosis, elevated proteins, and occasionally, a depressed glucose concentration. Rarely, the CSF can even be entirely normal. Opportunistic CNS infection must be excluded, particularly since many of these patients are immunosuppressed.

Optimal management of this condition includes local irradiation to symptomatic areas of the CNS as well as administration of intrathecal or intraventricular methotrexate via an Ommaya reservoir. Despite this therapy, mean survival is only about 7 months.

3. Spinal Epidural Metastases

a. Clinical Presentation

Among the most serious and disabling complications of metastatic cancer is epidural spinal cord compression. The physician caring for a patient with a known primary neoplasm must be especially vigilant in order to recognize this problem early, at a point where a good therapeutic outcome can still be achieved. Although most primary tumors can cause epidural spinal cord compression, carcinomas of the lung, breast, and prostate are most likely to do so. Recently, evidence surfaced to suggest that there has been increased incidence among patients suffering from oat cell carcinoma who were treated successfully by a combination of radiotherapy and chemotherapy for their primary tumor. Lymphomas and myelomas are also overrepresented among such primary neoplasms.

Four principal symptoms characterize the syndome of spinal cord compression:

- Pain. The physician must be particularly attentive to the complaint of pain, which is often the initial symptom and may precede any other neurological symptom by many weeks. Pain may be either local, often accompanied by vertebral tenderness, or radicular.
- Weakness. Weakness of one or, usually, both lower extremities is symptomatic in 75% of patients at the time of diagnosis, but nearly 90% of patients will have demonstrable paresis on neurological examination.
- Sensory deficits. Most patients will also have a sensory deficit at the time of presentation, and the upper limit of the sensory disturbance is usually within two vertebral bodies of the site of the lesion.
- Bladder and bowel dysfunction. At the time of presentation, 50% of patients will have this unfavorable prognostic sign.

b. Diagnostic Evaluation

Although plain spine radiographs are usually helpful in showing probable associated bony lesions, lumbar myelography is the most definitive diagnostic procedure. This should be performed with a small volume of nonreabsorbable contrast material (iophendylate) and will usually show complete or high-grade partial blockage. When a complete obstruction to the flow of contrast material is demonstrated, cisternal myelography, when performed, may identify the upper end of the block. The contrast material should be left in the subarachnoid space for subsequent repeat myelography to evaluate the effectiveness of therapy.

c. Therapeutic Management

Patients suspected of having epidural cord compression should immediately receive very high dose corticosteroid therapy: dexamethasone 100 mg for the first day. This can then be tailored to the patient's progress.

Once the site of pathology has been identified, therapy should be instituted immediately. Some studies have now indicated that radiotherapy alone yields, in most situations, results that are as good or better than decompressive laminectomy

followed by radiotherapy. Radiotherapy must be started within hours of the diagnosis and administered rapidly (i.e., 500 rads daily on 3 consecutive days, followed by more conventional fractionation).

Because the metastatic tumor arises in the vertebral body and its bulk lies anterior to the spinal cord, laminectomy will often not allow complete removal of the tumor. It can, however, rapidly relieve the compression of the spinal cord prior to more definitive treatment with irradiation. Decompressive laminectomy should, therefore, be reserved for the following situations:

- The nature of the tumor is unknown or the diagnosis is uncertain.
- Immediate radiotherapy is not available for a paraparetic patient.
- Relapse has occurred following completion of radiotherapy, and the patient cannot tolerate further irradiation.
- Symptoms continue to progress after several doses of radiation therapy and high doses of steroid therapy have been administered.

Early recognition and prompt institution of therapy for epidural spinal cord compression cannot be overemphasized. Successful outcome of therapy (i.e., the ability of the patient to recover original function) is highly correlated with the degree of weakness present prior to treatment and the duration of deficit. Furthermore, once signs of cord compression are present, the patient's clinical status may deteriorate rapidly and irreversibly because of the superimposition of spinal cord infarction (due to vascular compromise by pressure) to the occurrence of paraplegia or quadriplegia.

D. Meningiomas

1. Clinical Presentation

Meningiomas are largely benign, slow-growing tumors that do not ordinarily infiltrate or metastasize. Symptoms are, therefore, due to compression and are related to the exact location of the lesion. Several distinct types (or sites) of meningiomas can thus be distinguished.

a. Parasaggital and Falx Meningiomas

These constitute 24% of all meningiomas and are usually silent until they reach a significant size. Symptoms will depend on the actual site of the tumor.

- Anterior-third lesions will give rise to
  - Headaches.
  - Frontal lobe syndrome with dementia, incontinence, atax-

ia, and tremor (which may be confused with cerebellar symptoms).
- Grand mal seizures.
- Middle-third lesions will give rise to
  - Headaches.
  - Focal seizures, often affecting the foot before the hand.
- Posterior-third lesions will give rise to visual disturbances in the form of hemianopsia.

b. Meningiomas of the Convexity

These tumors represent 18% of meningiomas and may remain asymptomatic until they reach the size of a walnut or may cause a variety of symptoms:

- Seizures (focal or grand mal).
- Slowly progressing hemiparesis.
- Aphasia (if the dominant side is affected).
- Papilledema and other signs of increased intracranial pressure (in large lesions).

c. Sphenoid Wing Meningiomas

Sphenoid wing meningiomas constitute another 18% of all meningiomas. These lesions, when large enough, will cause orbital and visual disturbances. The following may occur:

- Bony deformation of the orbit, with hyperostosis.
- Optic atrophy with progressive loss of visual acuity. On rare occasion, a Foster Kennedy's syndrome (ipsilateral blindness and contralateral papilledema) may develop.
- Diplopia and paralysis of cranial nerves III, IV, and VI.
- Exophthalmos and proptosis.
- Seizures, hemiparesis, and speech disturbances may be seen when a laterally placed lesion develops a globular growth pattern.

d. Olfactory Groove Meningiomas

Constituting 10% of all meningiomas, olfactory groove meningiomas generally reach large sizes before causing anosmia but can result in progressive blindness, dementia, incontinence, and the witzelsucht syndrome (inappropriate facetiousness and lack of concern for physical disability).

e. Tuberculum and Suprasellar Meningiomas

These lesions represent 10% of all meningiomas and may give use to

- Visual disturbances due to optic nerve compression
  - Bitemporal hemianopsia.
  - Diplopia (due to involvement of oculomotor nerves).
- Hypothalamic manifestations with pituitary endocrine abnormalities.

f. Posterior Fossa Tumors

These tumors comprise 8% of meningiomas.

i. Cerebellopontine Angle.   These lesions need to be distinguished from acoustic neuroma or cysts. Symptoms include

- Hearing loss.
- Ataxia.
- Facial paralysis.
- Trigeminal neuropathy.

ii. Clivus Tumors.   These tumors compress the brain from its ventral surface and should be distinguished from basilar artery aneurysms and chordomas of the area. They produce

- Headaches and ataxia.
- Multiple cranial neuropathy: dysphagia, facial weakness, etc.
- Hemiparesis and paraparesis.
- Papilledema (when there is obstruction to flow of CSF).

iii. Ventral and Dorsal Foramen Magnum Lesions.   These tumors produce occipital and cervical pain occasionally radiating to the C-2 dermatome along the occiput. Brown-Séquard's syndrome progressing to asymmetrical hemiparesis and respiratory disturbances are common.

g. Meckel's Cave and Tentorial Incisura Dumbell Lesions

These lesions (2% of all meningiomas) produce trigeminal neuralgia along with cranial neuropathies and exophthalmos if the cavernous sinus is invaded. Hydrocephalus may occur with secondary ataxia and dementia. Cerebellar signs imply growth into the posterior fossa.

h. Intraventricular Lesions

Another 2% of meningiomas are intraventricular lesions. These tumors are most commonly found in the atrium of the lateral ventricle and occasionally in the third or fourth ventricles. Symptoms are due to obstructive hydrocephalus with dementia and occasionally homonymous hemianopsia.

i. Primary Intraorbital Meningiomas

These tumors constitute only 1% of all meningiomas and are associated with proptosis and decreased visual acuity in the involved eye.

j. Spinal Meningiomas

These lesions comprise approximately 25% of all intraspinal tumors and are about one-tenth as common as intracranial meningiomas. A large majority occur in the thoracic region, where the symptoms include radicular pain and degrees of paresis varying from Brown-Séquard's syndrome to complete paraplegia. The remarkable element in chronic spinal compression from meningioma is that even the deeply paraparetic patients may recover function once decompressive laminectomy and tumor removal have been achieved.

k. Other Meningiomas

Ectopic meningiomas have been reported and are presumably due to nests of arachnoidal cells in epithelial tissues occurring as a developmental abnormality. They have been reported in cutaneous locations on the scalp, in the sinuses, and about the eyes.

Multiple meningiomas (meningiomatosis) have also been reported, and they are usually associated with von Recklinghausen's disease. When meningeal meningiomatosis is seen, it has been regarded as a variant of primary sarcoma of the leptomeninges.

l. Metastatic Spread

Although meningiomas are histologically benign tumors, metastatic spread has been reported on rare occasions and seems to suggest a malignant variant. Invasion of the great sinuses permits spread of the tumor cells to the lungs, liver, and bone. It should be mentioned that in examining the dura under magnification at the time of surgery, one often sees tiny satellite nodules surrounding the major mass. Whether this influences recurrence or not cannot be absolutely stated, but it remains a surgical principle to remove the tumor with a reasonably wide margin of "normal" dura to ensure the removal of all these satellite nodules.

2. Diagnostic Evaluation

The diagnostic evaluation of patients suspected of harboring a meningioma should include

- Plain-skull x-rays or spine radiographs. These may delineate areas of hyperostosis, erosion, or enlargement of the foramina for cranial and spinal nerves or for the middle meningeal artery, which often nourishes these tumors.
- CAT scan of the head. This will usually reveal a lesion of increased attenuation that enhances homogeneously with intravenous contrast. Spinal CAT scanning may be aided by the infusion of metrizamide via lumbar puncture.
- Angiography. Prior to surgical removal, the vascular anatomy must be carefully analyzed by selective arteriography, including, in many cases, direct external carotid artery visualization. Specific attention must be paid to the patency of the venous sinuses when meningiomas are adjacent to them.
- Electroencephalography. This is indicated when seizures are present.

- Electromyography. In the case of suspected spinal meningiomas, electromyography may be useful.
- Routine chest x-rays. These must always be obtained. They may reveal evidence of a dumbbell tumor growing retropleurally, or they may identify a primary pulmonary neoplasm, which might have metastasized to the brain or spinal column, mimicking meningioma.

3. Therapeutic Management

For all practical purposes, surgery is the only treatment for CNS meningiomas. If the lesion can be totally resected, this should be done, provided essential brain function is preserved. Otherwise, debulking procedures are justified, followed by observation.

E. Hemangioblastomas

A true neoplasm of vascular origin, the hemangioblastoma occurs most frequently, though not exclusively, in the cerebellum. It is a histologically benign tumor composed of various sizes of blood vessels separated by stromal cells with clear cytoplasm. Grossly, the tumors may be either solid or cystic, often with a mural nodule, the latter indicating a somewhat better prognosis.

Because of their usual location in the cerebellum, these tumors most often cause symptoms of gait or appendicular ataxia. Alternatively, patients may present with a syndrome of increased intracranial pressure. Polycythemia is present in a small percentage of these patients.

Many patients with this tumor have evidence of the Hippel-Lindau disease complex, which may include angiomatosis of the retina; cysts of the pancreas, kidney, and liver; hepatic angiomas; tumors in the epididymis; hypernephromas; or pheochromocytomas. Thus, patients presenting with such cerebellar tumors should be screened for retinal or visceral involvement. A careful family history should also be taken, for the familial incidence may be as high as 20%.

The CAT scan will generally show a contrast-enhancing posterior fossa mass, with or without associated hydrocephalus. Angiography should be done to further elucidate the vascular pattern and supply of the tumor.

Treatment of these tumors is essentially surgical whenever possible. The role of radiotherapy, though reported in some cases, must be considered minimal, if any.

F. Pituitary Tumors

Pituitary tumors are benign lesions arising within the capsule of the pituitary gland. These sellar tumors and other intra- or parasellar tumors constitute between 6 and 15% of all intracranial neoplasms.

Although pituitary adenomas were formerly classified according to the tinctorial properties of their predominant cells of origin, recent advances have permitted a more useful classification according to the hormones secreted. Because of the peculiar nature of these lesions, a multispeciality approach is needed. It should include a neurologist, an endocrinologist, an ophthalmologist, a neurosurgeon, and often a gynecologist. The radiation oncologist often plays an important role in therapy.

Several unique features of pituitary tumors must be considered in the evaluation of these patients:

- Location. The tumor is strategically located at the base of the brain within the sella turcica, superior to the sphenoid sinus, inferior to the optic chiasm and/or optic nerves, and sandwiched between the paired cavernous sinuses that contain cranial nerves III, IV, and VI as well as the internal carotid artery. It is also adjacent to the temporal lobes and anterior and inferior to the hypothalamus.
- Endocrine properties. A large variety of endocrine syndromes can be observed as a result of hypo- or hypersecretion of the many hormones produced by the pituitary.
- Treatment. The potential for absolute cure with medical and/or surgical intervention is important to bear in mind.

1. Clinical Presentation

Presenting symptoms of pituitary tumors are a result of the location of the tumor and the endocrine properties of the pituitary gland.

a. Compression Symptoms

Headaches, presumably due to stretching of the dura mater, are a common presenting symptom. Other findings are dependent on the local spread of tumor in one or more directions, which gives rise to various symptoms.

- Spread through the floor of the sella turcica into the sphenoid sinus leads to CSF rhinorrhea and potential CNS infection.
- Upward spread toward the optic chiasm leads to the stereotypical bitemporal hemianopsia, usually beginning in the superior temporal fields. Of patients with this direction of spread, 70% complain of blurred vision, and 95% of those will be found to have field defects. Involvement of one optic nerve anterior to the optic chiasm would lead to progressive unilateral blindness with an afferent pupillary defect (so-called Marcus Gunn pupil). The subsequent development of a superior temporal–field cut in the opposite eye would then

represent an early sign of spread to the optic chiasm (by involving "von Willebrand's knee").
- Extension laterally into the cavernous sinus can lead to oculomotor palsies.
- Growth superolaterally into the temporal lobe can cause seizures or focal neurological signs.
- Posteriorly, extension into the hypothalamus may result in disturbances in sleep, eating and drinking habits, or behavior.

b. Endocrine Disturbances

i. Hypersecretion Syndromes.

- Prolactin. This represents the most common form of pituitary adenoma in females. The majority of patients present with the characteristic amenorrhea/galactorrhea syndrome. In males, on the other hand, where tumors tend to be slightly larger at the time of diagnosis, galactorrhea is rarely seen; those patients present with hypogonadism reflected by loss of libido and impotence. Headache and visual disturbance may be seen with or without hypogonadism.
- Growth hormone. In children, excess GH will lead to gigantism, while in adults, it results in acromegaly.
- ACTH. Excess secretion of ACTH will lead to the familiar picture of Cushing's syndrome, with truncal obesity, hypertension, weakness, amenorrhea, hirsutism, abdominal striae, glucosuria, and osteoporosis.
- TSH and gonadotrophins. Hypersecretion of those hormones is exceedingly rare.

ii. Hyposecretion Syndromes. These are usually due to pituitary gland compression from a true nonsecreting tumor and are less common than the hypersecretion syndromes.

- Hypogonadism, the most common clinical manifestation of a nonfunctioning tumor.
- Hypoadrenalism.
- Hypothyroidism.
- Growth failure in childhood (reduced secretion of GH in the adult does not produce clinical signs).

2. Diagnostic Evaluation

Needless to say, a complete neurologic and endocrinologic history must be obtained. This must be supplemented by a thorough medical and neurologic exam. Special attention should be paid to delineating early changes in visual field or acuity, which almost invariably will mandate a more aggressive therapeutic approach. Appropriate neurologic, endocrinologic, and ophthalmologic consultations should, of course, be obtained.

a. Laboratory Investigation

Basal hormonal levels should be evaluated, including

- Prolactin.
- Thyroxine, TSH.
- ACTH, plasma and urinary steroid levels.
- Testosterone.
- FSH, LH.

Various stimulant tests have been employed to better assess pituitary function and reserve.

- Prolactin. Intravenous TRH (thyrotrophin-releasing hormone) is administered. Patients with a prolactinoma often do *not* respond with an appropriate elevation of prolactin. This test is usually performed in the presence of moderately increased serum prolactin and a normal x-ray.
- Growth hormone. Stimulation of secretion can be carried out by insulin-induced hypoglycemia or administration of L-dopa. Although GH deficiency does not cause a clinical syndrome in adults, it is the most common laboratory abnormality in nonfunctioning tumors.
- TSH. Stimulation by administration of TRH. (TSH level should normally double).
- ACTH. Stimulation by administration of metyrapone (which prevents the feedback inhibition of ACTH) and measuring the 24-hour urinary cortisol. In addition, the dexamethasone supression test is useful in diagnosing the nonsuppressibility of the hyper-ACTH–secreting adenoma.
- Gonadotrophins. Stimulation by administration of lutenizing hormone–releasing hormone (LH–RH) (basal LH should normally double).

b. Radiological Investigation

i. CAT Scan. Radiological study of the sella region has advanced dramatically over the past decade as a result of the development of CAT. In most cases, the CAT scan is the definitive radiological test. Earlier, scanners were useful in identifying relatively large sellar and parasellar lesions, especially after contrast injection. The newer machines, however, now provide higher resolution and permit thin slices and coronal or sagittal reconstruction; they can thus confirm the presence of microadenomas. These tumors are less than 10 mm in size, located exclusively within the sella, and often have not resulted in bony changes that can be appreciated on routine skull x-rays or polytomograms. Intrathecal injection of metrizamide will visualize the subarachnoid spaces sufficiently to exclude the "empty-sella syndrome."

ii. Skull X-ray. Lateral view, with cone down, of the sella turcica often demonstrates enlargement of the sella with thinning of the bony walls.

iii. Lateral and Coronal Polytomography. These will reveal asymmetry, erosion, or irregularity in the sella's shape.

iv. Angiography. Angiography is basically employed to exclude a para- or intrasellar carotid aneurysm, which can masquerade as a pituitary tumor. It should also be done prior to definitive surgery.

v. Pneumocephalogram. This is rarely indicated, as it has been replaced by CAT scanning.

3. Therapeutic Management

As a prerequisite, patients must receive endocrine replacement therapy when indicated and must always be given additional corticosteroids prior to treatment. The definitive treatment of some pituitary lesions is still somewhat controversial. As these tumors are being identified at progressively earlier stages, the advocated treatments have varied from close observation to medical therapy to surgical intervention. Implicit in this controversy is the lack of data documenting the natural history of these smaller lesions when untreated. In addition, the availability of transsphenoidal microsurgery has made feasible the selective removal of the tumor with preservation of the normal gland and its function and is as a safe procedure in experienced hands.

a. Medical Treatment

The major controversy surrounds the treatment of microadenomas (most often prolactin-secreting) that are confined within the sella. Some treat these microprolactinomas with the dopamine agonist bromocriptine, which has been shown to suppress prolactin secretion and, in some reported cases, to shrink tumor size as documented by high-resolution CAT scan. The long-term results and possible eventual need for surgery are unknown, and in many centers, transsphenoidal surgery is still advocated as the primary modality.

b. Surgery

Most authorities agree that patients with visual disturbance, acromegaly or Cushing's disease, or those tumors that have a limited extension beyond the confines of the sella should undergo transsphenoidal surgery. If extensive extrasellar growth is present, a craniotomy is then indicated and should probably be followed by radiotherapy.

c. Radiotherapy

Radiotherapy for pituitary tumors is also a controversial issue. Some therapists advocate the use of high-dose irradiation using a proton beam or an interstitial implant directed precisely at the tumor as the definitive therapy for intrasellar adenomas or those with minimal suprasellar extension. Availability of proton beam and interstitial irradiation is, however, limited, and long-term follow-up results are scarce. Standard multiple-field supervoltage radiotherapy is usually employed postoperatively when the tumor has not been completely excised, as documented by the surgeon, endocrinologic markers, or radiological studies. It may also be used for tumor recurrences but is not recommended as the initial treatment unless surgery is not possible (i.e., as in the case of a tumor unresectable because of widespread cerebral invasion) or is otherwise contraindicated.

G. Pineal Region Tumors

Typical and atypical teratoma, pineocytoma, pineoblastoma, glioma, cysts, and chorionepithelioma comprise the most common tumor types involving the pineal region. Classically, the presentation is with Parinaud's syndrome of impaired upward gaze, impaired convergence, decreased pupil reactivity to light combined with headaches, hydrocephalus, and papilledema. If an ectopic pinealoma arises near the hypothalamus, then diabetes insipidus, hypopituitarism, hypersomnia, and visual failure due to invasion of the optic chiasm may ensue. Additionally, precocious puberty may appear in young males. Chorionepitheliomas secrete large amounts of human chorionic gonadotrophin into the CSF and thus may be definitively diagnosed by measuring that hormone.

Therapy consists, first, of management of the hydrocephalus and increased intracranial pressure with a shunt or drainage procedure. Craniotomy by a suboccipital, supracerebellar approach may then be carried out to attempt removal of the lesion. Radiotherapy is usually recommended postoperatively, and intrathecal methotrexate can also be used in chorionepitheliomas. Occasionally it is possible to treat a pinealoma with a radioactive implant (gold-198 or ytrium-90) using steriotactic methods.

H. Craniopharyngiomas

Craniopharyngioma (CPH) is a tumor thought to arise from the congenital remnants of Rathke's pouch. In the majority of cases, it is at least partially cystic and often marked by characteristic calcifications. Because of the tumor's location in the sellar region, it can often be initially mistaken for a pituitary lesion, and its anatomic topography accounts for the variable clinical presentations. The tumor lies in proximity to the pituitary gland, the hypothalamus, the optic nerve or chiasm, the foramen of Monro and third ventricle, and the temporal and frontal lobes. The direction of growth is also totally unpredictable.

1. Clinical Presentation

A common misconception holds that CPHs are restricted to the childhood years. In fact, in some series, as many as one-third of the patients were over 40 years old, and 10% were over age 60. Thus, CPH can be divided for consideration into those presenting, respectively, in children or adults:

a. Childhood Tumors

In children, the presenting symptoms usually include any or a combination of the following, in order of frequency:

- Symptoms related to increased intracranial pressure.
- Visual disturbances due to chiasmatic or optic nerve compression.
- Endocrine deficiencies secondary to pituitary compression, with consequent hypopituitarism.
- Neurological signs resulting from invasion of the frontal or temporal lobes, or extension into the brainstem.

b. Adult Tumors

In adults, the following symptoms may be seen:

- Visual disturbances are the most common presenting symptoms, occurring in more than 75% of patients.
- Mental symptoms include dementia, amnesia, depression, and mild intellectual deterioration.
- Hormonal disturbances, of which the most commonly seen are gonadal dysfunction. Other hormonal changes account for obesity, diabetes insipidus, and hypopituitarism.
- Increased intracranial pressure is commonly related to obstructive hydrocephalus with consequent headaches and papilledema.
- Focal signs as noted for children may also be seen in adults.

2. Diagnostic Evaluation

Because of the complex nature of the evaluation of patients with CPH, a multispeciality approach is advisable. This should include neurology, neurosurgery, endocrinology, and ophthalmology. As with pituitary tumors, a complete neurological history and physical examination is essential. Special attention should be paid to the visual system, and laboratory investigation should include a full battery of endocrine tests, including basal hormone levels and appropriate stimulation tests (see §7.V.F.2.a).

Radiological investigations should include CAT scan of the head and angiography. As with pituitary lesions, the CAT scan is the most important study. It has virtually replaced several other tests such as tomographic skull series, radionuclide scans, electroencephalography, and pneumoencephalography. The variable calcification and cystic components of CPH are easily demonstrated by CAT scan. Angiography is employed in the presurgical evaluation of the tumor.

3. Therapeutic Management

The treatment of CPH is primarily surgical if, based on preoperative studies, the total removal of tumor is thought to be a reasonable goal. If complete removal is not feasible, partial tumor removal with aspiration of the cyst fluid is indicated. This should be followed by a full course of radiotherapy. Radiotherapy is rarely employed as a primary therapeutic modality in CPH but may be employed as a postoperative modality.

Peri- and posttreatment management must include careful monitoring of both anterior and posterior pituitary function. It is uncommon to see diabetes insipidus or relative glucocorticoid deficiency develop at this time. Alterations of pituitary function are corrected by the administration of the appropriate hormone(s).

I. Malignant Lymphomas

Any of the variants that are usually included under the heading of malignant lymphoma can occur as a primary tumor in the CNS. However, the most common type is histiocytic non-Hodgkin lymphoma, or reticulum cell sarcoma.

Reticulum cell sarcomas or microgliomas are rare. The age of presentation is generally between 40 and 60 years, with occasional cases over 70 years of age and rare cases under the age of 20. The incidence of this tumor seems to be greater in patients on immunosuppressive agents and especially in those following renal transplantation.

1. Clinical Presentation

A remarkable feature of this tumor is its rapidly progressive nature. Untreated, most patients die within 9 months. The clinical presentation is variable and depends upon the site of the tumor involvement.

- Headache is the initial symptom in most cases.
- Dizziness, fatigue, and anorexia are often seen.
- Alterations in mental status.
- Meningeal irritation with cranial nerve palsies.
- Seizures are also present in some cases.

2. Diagnostic Evaluation

The work-up begins with the CAT scan with and without contrast. This usually reveals homogeneously enhancing lesions, involving, most commonly, the basal ganglia, the thalamus, the periventricular white matter, or the corpus callosum. Lumbar puncture may reveal an elevated protein with occasional pleocytosis or malignant cells in the CSF.

3. Therapeutic Management

Treatment consists of radiotherapy. The tumor is remarkably radiosensitive, and long-term survivals can be achieved. Surgical extirpation should be reserved for well-localized tumor masses and is rarely indicated except when the diagnosis is in doubt. Systemic and intrathecal chemotherapy should be considered as adjuvants to radiation.

J. Neuromas and Neurofibromas

1. Acoustic Neuromas

These tumors, in most instances, arise from the superior vestibular nerve in the internal acoustic meatus. They account for approximately 8% of all intracranial neoplasms. During the course of their growth, they produce the following sequence of symptoms:

- Hearing loss, usually demonstrable at presentation.
- Tinnitus and intermittent vertigo may be present, but the latter is less prominent than might be expected in view of the tumor's origin from the vestibular portion of the nerve.
- Ataxia and facial numbness (including corneal anesthesia) will appear as the tumor reaches significant size and protrudes in the cerebellopontine angle. Tic douloureux-like pain and paresthesia may also be seen at this point.
- Dysphagia and loss of ipsilateral gag reflex will appear if there is downward extension of the tumor.
- Communicating and noncommunicating hydrocephalus with ataxia, slurred speech, dementia, and papilledema will develop as a result of distortion of the cerebellum and brainstem and impaction into the tentorial notch leading to deviation and compression of the fourth ventricle.

Bilateral acoustic neuromas may occur in the setting of neurofibromatosis. This is more often seen in young individuals.

2. Trigeminal Neuromas

These occur at a frequency of approximately 3–4 for every 100 neuromas of the acoustic nerve. The initial symptoms are sensory disturbances affecting the trigeminal nerve distribution:

- Paresthesias.
- Vague numbness and pain simulating tic douloureux.

• Impaired facial sensation and wasting of the masticatory muscles.

Tumors arising from the ganglion may spread into the middle cranial fossa, producing ophtalmoparesis and proptosis, optic atrophy, and visual-field disturbances. Tumors arising from the roots extend posteriorly and may mimic acoustic neuromas. On occasion, the tumor may have a dumbbell configuration with both middle fossa and posterior fossa components.

3. Spinal Neuromas

These tumors account for 16–30% of all vertebral canal tumors and occur most commonly in the thoracic area. They can be multiple in patients with neurofibromatosis. The cardinal initial symptom is radicular pain, with a significant interval between the onset of pain and the development of any further symptom. At a later date, weakness, atrophy, numbness, and bladder dysfunction may develop. Occasionally, the tumors may grow in an hourglass fashion through the intervertebral foramen and into the paraspinal tissues, causing spinal compression; those lesions require the greatest attention. Treatment is surgical removal.

4. Neuromas of Peripheral Nerves

In this category of tumors, distinction must be made between benign and malignant lesions. The benign tumor usually presents as a swelling accompanied by pain of a neuritic or radicular type. Single neurofibromas and neurilemmomas fall into this category. The neurilemmoma is usually ovoid, eccentrically placed in the nerve, and can be enucleated from its bed in the nerve with the sacrifice of one or at most two fascicles, leaving no residual paresis. Neurofibromas, on the other hand, are soft and centrally placed within the nerve, which, on inspection, has a globular or fusiform shape. These cannot be excised without compromising the nerve.

The malignant lesions—neurosarcoma and sarcoma supervening on the substrate of neurofibromatosis—are potentially lethal lesions. Over 50% of solitary neurosarcomas are fatal, whereas sarcoma occurring in neurofibromatosis has a mortality rate of about 90%. The features suggesting this occurrence are rapid increase in a lesion's size and, to a lesser extent, increase in pain accompanied by a firm, hard, immobile swelling.

The recommended procedure is a block resection of the tumor with wide margins. If the lesion is extensive, or if there is recurrence after bloc resection in an extremity, amputation might be necessary.

5. Neurofibromas

These tumors originate from Schwann cells of cranial, spinal, and peripheral nerves. Their malignant counterparts act as sarcomas and originate virtually exclusively from the peripheral nerves. Neurofibromas can occur independently or in conjunction with full-blown Von Recklinghausen's disease involving multiple nerves.

K. Other Brain Tumors

1. Epidermoid and Dermoid Cysts

These lesions arise from epiblastic cells destined to form skin that have become detached and included in mesenchyme at about the third-to-fifth week of life. Epidermoid cysts contain desquamated keratin and cholesterol crystals. Dermoids have thicker walls and may contain hair, sebaceous glands, or sweat glands, and they may have a narrow epithelium-lined stalk connecting them to the overlying skin.

The epidermoids, or cholesteatomas, can occur extradurally in the skull, producing a radiographic appearance of osteolysis with dense, scalloped margins; in the frontal bone they may produce proptosis; at the apex of the petrous bone they may involve multiple cranial nerves. Intradurally, they may be located in the chiasmal, parasellar, supracallosal, and sylvian areas. The cerebellopontine angle and the ventricles may also harbor these cysts.

Dermoid cysts can be found in the posterior fossa in children, in which case one must examine the scalp closely for a sinus tract. Aseptic meningitis can be seen with intracranial epidermoids after the release of keratin into the spinal fluid; these episodes may be recurrent. Spinal dermoids with sinus tracts have also given rise to episodic meningitis, both aseptic and bacterial. Seizures and cranial nerve signs are frequently presenting symptoms, depending on the location of these cysts. Wherever feasible with respect to location, the treatment is surgical removal.

2. Colloid Cysts

Colloid cysts account for less than 0.5% of all intracranial tumors. They are composed of an external connective tissue coat and an internal epithelial lining with a viscous mucicarminophilic intracystic fluid containing exfoliated epithelial cells, histiocytes, and lymphocytes. The present hypothesis is that this cyst arises from the junction of the choroid plexus of the lateral ventricle and the third ventricle, occurring at the foramen of Monro, where evagination or invagination of the neuroepithelial layers may occur.

Clinically, they may remain small and silent throughout an individual's life. On the other hand, they may be associated with a rapid demise due to a full blown ventricular crisis. The presumed mechanism is an acute obstructive hydrocephalus due to blockage at both foramina of Monro. Headaches often occurring with changes in position, vomiting, and loss of consciousness comprise the acute attacks. More chronic instances present with early-morning headaches, nausea, mental disturbance, and papilledema on examination.

These lesions are amenable to surgical removal and, whenever possible, should be excised via frontal craniotomy and a transventricular approach to the foramen of Monro.

L. Chordomas

Chordomas are tumors arising from remnants of the notochord occurring most frequently along the clivus (60%) and in the sacrococcygeal region (30%). The remainder occur elsewhere along the spine. When they spread along the base of the skull, they may compress the brainstem and emerging cranial nerves in both the middle and posterior fossae. In the spine, they will produce lumbosacral radicular syndromes and cauda equina and/or spinal cord compression. They may undergo malignant degeneration and metastasize as sarcomas to other parts of the body, but their usual course is indolent, though associated with considerable pain. Treatment is surgical, whenever possible.

The place of radiotherapy in the treatment of chordomas is controversial, especially since the tumor is relatively radioresistant. Tumors originating in the base of the skull (the clivus region) may be inoperable or only partially removable by virtue of their site and extent, leaving radiotherapy as the only modality available or as an adjuvant treatment. For radiation to be effective, treatment will have to be carried to high doses, necessitating meticulous planning and a high-quality supervoltage beam (linear accelerator sharp beams are preferred).

M. Intracranial Neoplasms in Children

Brain tumors in children rarely occur before 1 year of age and have their peak incidence in the latter half of the first decade. Frequently, the onset of symptoms is correlated by parents to an episode of an acute nonneoplastic illness. Since the overwhelming majority of brain tumors in infants and children are located in the posterior fossa, the preponderance of symptoms are related to cerebellar disturbances and obstruction of CSF flow, with secondary hydrocephalus and increased intracranial pressure. Symptoms in infancy are often delayed due to the ability of the cranial bones to separate at their suture lines in response to the increased pressure. These symptoms are predominantly headache, unsteady gait, vomiting, and abnormal oculomotor function.

Cerebellar (cystic) astrocytomas, medulloblastomas, fourth-ventricle ependymomas, and pontine gliomas are the most common tumors of the posterior fossa.

Pretreatment evaluation and work-up of brain tumors in children include cranial CAT scan as the single most important neurodiagnostic test. Electroencephalograms usually do not help clarify the diagnosis, as posterior fossa tumors produce nonspecific projected slow dysrhythmias. Selective cerebral angiography is usually indicated to clarify the tumor's blood supply for the neurosurgeon.

1. Cerebellar Astrocytomas

This tumor is the single most common neoplasm in children. It occurs most frequently between 6 and 8 years of age and there is usually a history of symptoms for some months or weeks duration before the diagnosis is established. The tumor is slow growing, usually cystic, and laterally located in the cerebellum.

At present, after the diagnosis is confirmed by CAT scan, the treatment is usually by surgical removal. Unless there are large numbers of mitotic figures present microscopically, irradiation of these tumors is not recommended. Follow up by CAT scan is usual, and should the tumor regrow, it is conceivable to reoperate, debulk the tumor, and then consider radiation therapy. Occasionally radiotherapy is the only alternative, especially when the tumor is located dangerously close to the brainstem.

2. Medulloblastomas

Medulloblastomas occur in younger children including infants; there is usually short interval between clinical symptoms and diagnosis. The prognosis is worse in children younger than 1 year of age. An acute illness is frequently associated with the onset of symptoms. Unlike the relatively benign cerebellar astrocytomas, the medulloblastomas are highly undifferentiated malignant tumors that spread throughout the neuraxis. With operation and exposure to the outside, the tumor may even spread elsewhere.

Medulloblastomas are now being studied and staged by

- Presence of free cells in the CSF, as noted by millipore cytological analysis.
- Myelography, looking for nodular implantation along the spinal roots.
- CAT scan to look for nodular implantation along the ventricular system or cerebral hemispheres.

A debulking operation in which as much tumor is removed as possible and communication between the third and fourth ventricles is reestablished is necessary in most cases. Radiotherapy is also administered to the whole craniospinal axis, with a tumor dose of 3000 rads and with booster doses to areas of known gross disease intracranially or in the spinal cord. The dose is adjusted to age and often reduced to 2500 rads in infants and often given to the cord when there is no evidence of gross involvement. Steroids and chemotherapy are used as adjunctive modalities. With combined surgical removal and radiotherapy, survival rates are approaching 70% at 5 years. Several centers are currently studying the effectiveness of chemotherapy for medulloblastomas, and it is urged that patients be entered into clinical trials whenever possible. Early results are encouraging.

3. Fourth-Ventricle Ependymomas

These tumors are variable in presentation. They may appear quite malignant with a short clinical course and are indeed often found to have spinal implantation manifested by asymmetrical reflexes and painful nerve-root syndromes. Or they may grow very slowly, causing a chronic syndrome of headache and vomiting. The primary therapy is surgical removal and reestablishment of the spinal fluid pathways; cranial irradiation of the entire neuraxis has thus far proved more effective than chemotherapy.

4. Brainstem Gliomas

These tumors frequently have no signs of increased intracranial pressure and usually present as cranial nerve dysfunctions associated with gait disturbance. Examination subsequently tends to demonstrate ipsilateral cranial nerve palsies associated with a contralateral hemiparesis and an ipsilateral cerebellar syndrome.

Surgical removal of brainstem gliomas has been considered unfeasible in the past. More recent microscopic techniques and better localization by CAT scan have made it possible for some brainstem gliomas to be either surgically approached and resected or else debulked prior to radiation therapy. It is recommended, however, that such attempts be made only by neurosurgeons with specialized experience in microsurgery. Chemotherapy has, to date, failed to alter significantly the outcome of this disease.

Radiotherapy is effective in controlling this tumor, especially in children. Steroids are sometimes necessary to permit delivery of full doses properly fractionated (200 rads per fraction). Some authors claim 5-year survival rates that exceed 50%.

VI. POSTOPERATIVE CARE, EVALUATION, AND REHABILITATION

A. Postoperative Care

Ideally, the patient should be managed in a neurosurgical postoperative unit with nurses specially trained as clinical practitioners.

- Regular recording and charting of all parameters is mandatory: vital signs, blood gases, serum electrolytes and blood chemistries, fluid balance, urine output and specific gravity, drainage, etc.
- Corticosteroids must be used, but once the patient is well, they may be tapered after 2–3 days and over a period of 1 week.
- Anticonvulsant medications are usually continued for 6 months to 1 year. A repeat EEG is warranted before stopping the anticonvulsant, and if paroxysmal activity is present, then the medication should be continued.
- Antibiotics are continued as indicated.
- Drainage and suction tubes are removed in 2 days, the dressing and sutures on the seventh postoperative day.
- Tube feedings are instituted in cases of prolonged coma or inability to eat because of neurological disturbance. In this regard, patients with an impaired gag reflex must be carefully observed for aspiration.
- Patients with endocrine disturbances must receive replacement hormones, and patients with diabetes insipidus must be followed closely in order to avoid electrolyte disturbances.

B. Nursing Care and Psychosocial Aspects

Care of the patient with a brain tumor is a challenge to the nurse because of the devastating effects of these tumors. Nursing care in general is based on the signs and symptoms and is directed toward the early recognition, prevention, and treatment of complications. It is most important for the nurse to be aware of the patient's history, objective findings, subjective complaints, suspected and confirmed diagnosis, and proposed treatment in order to plan and administer effective nursing care intelligently.

The following physical observations are made routinely by the nurse:

- State of consciousness.
- Vital signs.
- Presence of absence of pain.
- Seizure activity.
- Ocular Signs.
- Presence or absence of vomiting.
- Motor function.

Problems may result from any one of a number of factors including the altered neurological status, treatment, complications, or the crisis of the situation. The following problems deserve special consideration in the care of the patient and significant other.

1. Changes in Mental Status

Patients with brain tumors frequently demonstrate irritability, mood swings, inappropriate behavior, memory deficits, impaired judgment, disorientation, communication disorders, and/or decreased levels of consciousness. To deal effectively with these problems, the following goals must be met:

- Understanding the reasons for the behavioral changes and explaining them to the family members.
- Ability to cope with the behavior.
- Provisions for safety.
- Maintenance of effective communication.

It is important to involve members of the interdisciplinary health care team (social workers, nurses, clergy, physical and occupational therapists, nutritionists, pharmacists, volunteers). The team approach is important, as it gives its members an opportunity to reinforce the physician's instructions to the patient and his or her family, to help the family to learn ways of coping with behavioral changes, and to eliminate environmental hazards and prepare the family to supervise the patient's care at home.

If the patient becomes aphasic or has difficulty in understanding, it is important for the team to

- Keep conversation short and simple.
- Leave written instructions for the patient and family (preferably using large letters).
- Teach the patient one concept at a time, with a chance for return demonstration if needed.
- Consult with a speech pathologist, if necessary.

2. Changes in Motor and Sensory Function

Patients with tumors of the cerebral hemispheres and the cerebellum may often encounter motor function changes. Symptoms include weakness, paralysis, decreased muscle tone, involuntary movements, and ataxia. These patients frequently sustain injuries due to falls. It is important to teach the patient and significant others methods of proper ambulation and transfer and to encourage the use of aids such as canes, braces, etc. The nurse must also provide nursing care in order to prevent complications of immobility, such as edema, pneumonia, thrombophlebitis and pulmonary embolism, renal calculi, and skin breakdown.

Patients may experience changes in sensory function, such as tactile sensory deficits or disturbances of the special sense organs. Again, it is the responsibility of the nurse to intervene, teach the patient, and provide a safe environment.

3. Changes in Appearance

Patients with brain tumors may often develop change in their appearance that may in turn have an effect on their body image. Facial asymmetry, uncoordinated movements, alopecia, and cushingoid symptoms are examples of such changes. These changes cause anxiety, particularly because our society places such emphasis on physical appearance. The health pro-

fessional must present a caring and accepting attitude in order to encourage the patient to maintain his or her self-concept. Some suggestions for the health professional include

- Demonstrating competence and confidence in caring for the patient.
- Facilitating ventilation of feelings by encouraging the patient to ask questions.
- Preparing and supporting the patient for any changes that might occur.
- Informing the patient and family about the use of cosmetics, wigs, etc.
- Including the family and clergy (if the patient so requests) in the teaching sessions.

It is also important to take the age of the patient into consideration. Teenagers especially may have problems dealing with any change in body image, as peer group pressure is particularly important at this stage of life. Again, honest, caring intervention is required.

4. Changes in Roles

Most victims of chronic illness experience some type of role change, either in the family or the community. Patients may experience feelings of worthlessness, guilt, and anger at these changes. Again, it is important for the health professional to help the patient maintain his or her self-esteem. The patient should be encouraged to verbalize fears and anxieties, and the family should be included in these discussions whenever possible. It may even be necessary at times to explore new roles for the patient. It is often desirable for the health professionals to request the advice of a vocational counselor, if the patient cannot resume his or her roles at work. Resumption of social activities should also be encouraged.

5. Isolation

Patients and families may isolate themselves due to anxieties from altered body image, fear of seizures, and exhaustion. They may also isolate themselves from the health care team and seek out the use of unproven methods for the hope of a promised cure. It is important for the health professional to be honest with the patient and family and provide them with as much information as possible so that they may be able to make an intelligent decision regarding the treatment.

6. Side Effects and Complications of Treatment

Side effects from chemotherapy, radiotherapy, and the use of corticosteroids often pose a problem for the patient and his or her family. It is important to make sure that patient and family are made aware of anticipated effects, including toxic effects.

C. Rehabilitation

Tumors of the central and peripheral nervous system have the potential for causing considerable functional morbidity. Depending on the anatomic localization, the clinical spectrum may include signs and symptoms that range from mild sensory or motor impairment to monoplegia, hemiplegia, paraplegia, or quadriplegia. In addition, a significant degree of disability may result from the neurosurgical intervention, from radiation therapy, or from the side effects of medications. Rehabilitation medicine provides a variety of techniques and well-standardized treatment modalities that can help to restore the patient's level of function (completely or partially), maintain function, or delay functional deterioration. Therapy must be tailored, however, to the patient's individual degree of disability.

The present concern with quality of life has extended the application of rehabilitation programs to patients with shorter life expectancy as well as to the increasing number of those considered cured or controlled. The rehabilitation team (physiatrist, physical therapist, occupational therapist, rehabilitation nurse, speech therapist, social worker, psychologist, and vocational counselor) can prevent, diagnose, and treat a number of physical disabilities. The rehabilitation team–patient interaction adds considerably in alleviating fear and anxiety. The primary barriers to optimal delivery of rehabilitation care are the failure to identify the patient's problems and/or the lack of appropriate referral by physicians who may be unfamiliar with the concepts of rehabilitation.

The mainstays of the physiotherapy rehabilitation programs are

- Therapeutic exercises that are developed in a variety of techniques for each muscle group. These include passive and active range-of-motion exercises aimed at maintaining or improving joint mobility and periarticular joint elasticity. Strengthening of specific muscle groups can be achieved through exercises, including isometrics, isotonics, and isokinetics.
- Training for sitting and standing as prerequisites for ambulation exercises.
- Therapeutic improvement of strength, endurance, and coordination. The latter can be improved by complex sensory motor reeducation exercises using visual and proprioceptive cues.
- Canes, walkers, and braces, which can be individually prescribed, adjusted, and modified to fit the particular needs of the patient.
- A wheelchair, where it is the only means to assure a patient's mobility. Prescribing the proper type of chair and training the patient in its use are essential.
- Physiotherapeutic trials in conjunction with pharmacological agents, for patients with motor disorders such as spasticity and rigidity.

The evaluation for activities of daily living (ADL) is the translation of the neurological and musculoskeletal examination into actual performance in reference to the patient's ability to dress, perform physical hygiene, and groom and feed himself. Training techniques with or without adaptive devices are available to assist the patient to achieve the highest level of ADL, and the patient can achieve considerable levels of independence. Occupational therapists are experts in the ADL evaluation and treatment of functional deficiencies. In real or simulated settings, they attempt to retrain the patient's motor skills. They can select from a vast array of self-helping devices that can enhance functional capabilities and safety and train patients in their use. Bathtub benches, grab bars, special toilet seats, devices that improve prehension and dexterity with minimal effort and maximum efficiency can all be used in selected circumstances. The occupational therapist can also provide splints for support or proper alignment of the various involved segments of the upper extremities and teach specific functional kinetic exercises.

Many of the neurogenic dysfunctions of the bladder and bowel that result from CNS tumors or their treatment are amenable to functional retraining or to other forms of management in a way compatible with social interaction. In many patients, the complications of indwelling catheters can be avoided by using intermittent catheterization or periodic emptying of the bladder by manual pressure. The dynamic study of the voiding mechanism (bladder capacity, intracystic pressure, urethral pressure profile, sphincters' activity, and postvoiding residual) will suggest the most appropriate form of functional rehabilitation. The management will include a combination of pharmacological agents, retraining and time, and when necessary, urologic intervention.

Following neurosurgical interventions, the rehabilitation team should be involved in the process of preventing secondary disabilities, such as

- Weakness from inactivity.
- Contractures.
- Decubiti (use of an air mattress and lamb's wool bedding, frequent change in patient position, intensive local care at pressure points, etc.).
- Thromboembolism secondary to venous stasis (use of elastic stockings, elevation of the legs).
- Complications of indwelling catehters (use of antibiotics).

Pain and suffering can be influenced by the rehabilitation process, and a variety of physical modalities including TENS (transcutaneous electrical nerve stimulation) can diminish the pain experience by the afferent modulation of sensory systems.

Management of disabled patients with stable neurological deficit requires long-range planning that may require the involvement of social services, the family, and specialized agencies.

Table I

Schedule for Follow-Up of CNS Tumor

Management	First year			Second and third years				Thereafter	
	Monthly	6 months	12 months	3 months	6 months	9 months	12 months	6 months	12 months
History									
Neurological, i.e.,									
Headache, pain	X			X	X	X	X	X	X
Nausea, vomiting	X			X	X	X	X	X	X
Seizures	X			X	X	X	X	X	X
State of consciousness	X			X	X	X	X	X	X
Motor or sensory loss	X			X	X	X	X	X	X
Focal signs	X			X	X	X	X	X	X
Cranial nerve deficit	X			X	X	X	X	X	X
Balance and gait	X			X	X	X	X	X	X
Complete review of systems		X	X		X		X		X
Physical									
Complete neurological	X			X	X	X	X	X	X
Fundoscopic exam	X			X	X	X	X	X	X
General physical exam		X	X		X		X		X
Investigation									
CBC, SMA-12			X				X		X
Serumn electrolytes			X				X		X
Chest x-ray			X				X		X
EEG		X	X			X	X		
CAT scan of head		X	X			X			X
Angiography	As indicated by site of tumor or presenting symptoms								
Myelography	As indicated by site of tumor or presenting symptoms								
Spinal tap	As indicated by site of tumor or presenting symptoms								
Visual acuity and fields	As indicated by site of tumor or presenting symptoms								
Endocrine evaluation	As indicated by site of tumor or presenting symptoms								
Other	As indicated by site of tumor or presenting symptoms								

D. Follow-Up Evaluation

Patients who have undergone palliative therapy of any form, surgical or otherwise, will usually remain under the care of their neurologist until their demise. For patients who had a curative procedure and those who had a subtotal excision of a benign or low-grade malignant tumor, a close follow-up system is essential to detect early signs of recurrence and avoid some of the potentially crippling or lethal complications that may result from tumor regrowth. Table I is a suggested schedule for such a follow-up program.

VII. MANAGEMENT ALGORITHM FOR BRAIN TUMORS (see p. 308)

SUGGESTED READINGS

1. Dietz, H. J. Adaptive rehabilitation of the cancer patient. *Curr. Probl. Cancer* **5,** No. 5 (1980).

2. Healey, J. E., and Zislis, J. Cancers. "Handbook of Severe Disability" (W. C. Stolow and M. C. Clowers, eds.), Chapter 28. U.S. Dept. of Education Rehab Services Administration, Washington, D.C., 1981.

3. Lehmann, J. F., Delisa, C. G., Warren, C. G. *et al.* Cancer rehabilitation: Of need, development and evaluation of a model of care. *Arch. Phys. Med. Rehab.* **59,** 410–419 (1978).

4. Northfield, D. W. G. "The Surgery of the Central Nervous System." Blackwell, Oxford, 1973.

5. Post, K. D. *et al.*, eds. "The Pituitary Adenoma." Plenum, New York, 1980.

6. Tindall, G. T., and Collins, W. F., eds. "Clinical Management of Pituitary Disorders." Raven Press, New York, 1979.

7. Vinken, P. J., and Bruyn, G. W., eds. "Handbook of Clinical Neurology," Vol. 16, Part I, Am. Elsevier, New York, 1975.

8. Vinken, P. J., and Bruyn, G. W., eds. "Handbook of Clinical Neurology," Vol. 16, Part II. Am. Elsevier, New York, 1975.

9. Vinken, P. J., and Bruyn, G. W., eds. "Handbook of Clinical Neurology," Vol. 19, Part I. Am. Elsevier, New York, 1975.

10. Vinken, P. J., and Bruyn, G. W., eds. "Handbook of Clinical Neurology," Vol. 20, Part II. Am. Elsevier, New York, 1976.

11. Walker, M. D., Green, S. B., Byai, D. P. *et al.* Randomized comparisons of radiotherapy and nitrosoureas for the treatment of malignant glioma after surgery. *N. Engl. J. Med.* **303,** 1323–1329 (1980).

12. Weiss, L. *et al.* "Brain Metastasis." G. K. Hall, Boston, Massachusetts, 1980.

ALGORITHM FOR TUMORS OF THE CENTRAL NERVOUS SYSTEM

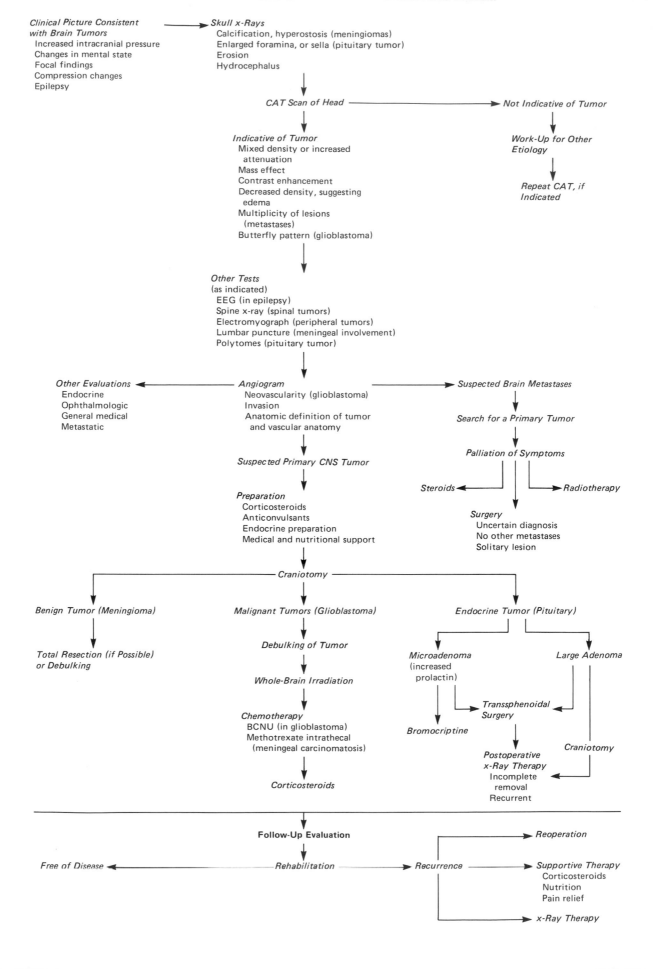

Section 8

Pediatric Tumors

BERTRAM D. COHN AND FELIX FELDMAN

With Contributions By

Susan Goldfine	Radiology
Chanchal Malhotra	Pathology

309

In the United States, cancer is second only to trauma as the leading cause of death in children. There is an annual incidence of 12.5 new cases per 100,000 Caucasians and 9.78 new cases per 100,000 blacks.

The tumors that are most commonly seen in adults are "carcinomas." These are usually of an ectodermal or endodermal origin. These types of tumors are rarely seen in infants and children, whose solid tumors are usually "sarcomas," most often originating from mesodermal tissue. Many of the tumors that are seen almost exclusively in children, such as Wilms's tumor and neuroblastoma, appear to be embryonal in origin.

Leukemia is the single most frequent malignancy of childhood (about 40% of all malignant conditions); its incidence is greatest in children under 5 years of age. It represents 35% of malignancies in the age group between 5 and 10 years; this incidence falls to 22% between 10 and 15 years old. Tumors of the CNS are at their peak (27%) in children 5–10 years old. Neuroblastoma and renal tumors are most frequent in children under 5 years of age. They decrease progressively with age and are rarely seen after age 10.

Section 8. Pediatric Tumors

Part A: Solid Tumors

I. Early Detection and Screening   315
  A. Predisposing Factors
    1. Genetic
    2. Environmental
  B. Early Detection
  C. Education and Screening
II. Pretreatment Evaluation and Work-Up   316
  A. History and Physical Examination
    1. History
    2. Physical Examination
  B. Laboratory Findings
  C. Radiological Evaluation
    1. Plain Abdominal Films
    2. Intravenous Pyelogram
      a. Wilms's Tumor
      b. Neuroblastoma
      c. Soft-Tissue Sarcomas (Rhabdomyosarcomas)
    3. Ultrasound
    4. Computerized Axial Tomography Scan
    5. Inferior Venacavography
    6. Arteriography
  D. Metastatic Evaluation
  E. General Assessment
  F. Multidisciplinary Evaluation
III. Preoperative Preparation   319
IV. Therapeutic Management   319
  A. General Considerations
  B. Biopsy
  C. Staging
  D. Principles of Surgical Management
  E. Adjuvant Therapy
    1. Radiotherapy
    2. Chemotherapy
  F. The Price of Successful Therapy
V. Postoperative Care, Evaluation, and Rehabilitation   320
  A. Postoperative Care
  B. Nursing Care
  C. Follow-Up Evaluation
  D. Rehabilitation
VI. Solid Pediatric Tumors: Type-Specific   322
  A. Wilms's Tumor (Nephroblastoma)
    1. Pathological Considerations
      a. Macroscopic Features
      b. Staging

      c. Microscopic Characteristics
      d. Prognostic Features
    2. Site-Specific Data Form for Wilms's Tumors
    3. Surgical Considerations
    4. Radiotherapy
    5. Chemotherapy
    6. Bilateral Wilms's Tumor
    7. Treatment of Advanced Disease
    8. Management Algorithm for Wilms's Tumors
  B. Neuroblastomas
    1. Pathological Considerations
    2. Staging and Classification
    3. Prognostic Features
      a. Age
      b. Stage
      c. Distant Metastases
      d. Location
      e. Degree of Histologic Differentiation
    4. Therapeutic Management
      a. Surgical Management
      b. Radiotherapy
      c. Chemotherapy
    5. Follow-Up Evaluation
  C. Rhabdomyosarcomas
    1. Pathological Considerations
      a. Embryonal Cell Rhabdomyosarcoma
      b. Alveolar Rhabdomyosarcoma
      c. Pleomorphic Rhabdomyosarcoma
    2. Staging and Classification
    3. Prognostic Features
      a. Age
      b. Site
      c. Histology
      d. Stage
    4. Therapeutic Management
  D. Other Solid Tumors
    1. Liver Tumors
    2. Teratomas
      a. Sacrococcygeal Teratoma
      b. Teratomas of the Neck
      c. Mediastinal Teratomas
      d. Ovarian Teratomas
      e. Retroperitoneal Teratomas

Suggested Readings   338

I, EARLY DETECTION AND SCREENING

A. Predisposing Factors

1. Genetic

Cancer is, in general, uncommon in children. Certain population groups, however, are at increased risk for specific types of malignancies.

Wilms's tumor is associated with various patterns of congenital anomalies and should be suspected in the presence of aniridia (absence or hypoplasia of the iris), hemihypertrophy, and genitourinary anomalies (hypospadias, cryptorchidism, duplication of the collecting system, fusion anomalies). Association of the aniridia–Wilms's tumor syndrome with chromosome 11 deletion is a situation in which a carrier state is detectable; in theory, Wilms's tumor predisposition could even be determined on prenatal analysis.

Retinoblastoma is a rare retinal tumor that occurs in young children and is highly malignant. Of patients with retinoblastoma, 5–10% have a family history of this tumor. It is of interest that when retinoblastoma follows a genetic pattern, it acts as an autosomal dominant with almost complete penetrance. Thus, a parent with bilateral retinoblastoma has a 50% chance of transmitting retinoblastoma to each child. Of individuals with this tumor, 5% have other anomalies associated with a deletion of chromosome 13 (mental retardation, supernumerary digits, imperforate anus, failure to thrive). In this small minority of cases, the relationship between oncogenesis and teratogenesis is manifest. Tumor predisposition may even be determined prenatally. It seems likely that further studies and refinements in chromosome analysis will yield additional correlations and groups of suspect individuals.

Xeroderma pigmentosum is a condition transmitted by autosomal recessive inheritance, associated with an increased incidence of skin malignancies at an early age, as a result of exposure to sunlight. Individuals with this condition have a genetically determined defect in DNA repair, which would otherwise normally follow exposure to ultraviolet light.

There are also those conditions that are associated with nonspecific chromosomal abnormalities, e.g., breaks, gaps, en-doreduplication, etc. They include ataxia, telangiectasia, Fanconi's (constitutional aplastic) anemia, and Bloom's syndrome. All of these are associated with an increased incidence of leukemia, lymphoma, and various solid tumors, which do not necessarily manifest themselves during childhood.

There is also a group of conditions associated with various kinds of immunodeficiency syndromes such as the Wiskott-Aldrich and the Chédiak-Higashi syndromes that are also known to have an increased incidence of malignancy.

2. Environmental

There are numerous environmental factors that appear to predispose to an increased cancer risk. Among these are irradiation and an exposure to a long list of carcinogenic chemical substances. The nonpredictability of clinical manifestations of cancer following contact with such carcinogens has led Knudsen to postulate the "two-hit theory" for emergence of cancer. He proposed that two discrete mutational events must occur to induce carcinogenesis. These insults might be genetically determined or the result of environmental factors such as radiation, chemical carcinogens, etc. The first "hit" would render the cells precancerous; the second "hit" would produce clinical cancer. Those individuals who carry a hereditary cancer mutation would thus already have tissues in a precancerous state and would require only a single additional insult to trigger malignant transformation.

B. Early Detection

Early detection of tumors of the pediatric age group depends on an alert attitude on the part of the primary physician and the willingness of the parent to seek medical help at the time of onset of symptoms that may be subtle. There is no place for so-called cancer-detection examinations as such (except in families with a high genetic risk factor), though the well-informed pediatrician or primary physician must always be on guard for the possible existence of a cancer in each patient seen, whatever the presenting complaint.

Unfortunately, many tumors will present in a detectable form only at a time when advanced spread has already occurred; others, however, can be diagnosed before the onset of metastases and are curable with surgical excision or combined modalities.

The most important sign of malignancy in an infant or child is the presence of a mass. Early detection requires careful, thorough examination of a small patient who may be totally uncooperative; it is through such efforts that an individual is offered the greatest chance of early detection of an asymptomatic cancer. If any possible question exists that a flank mass may be present, it is essential that a screening intravenous pyelogram (IVP) be performed. Similarly, any unusual muscle mass in an extremity must be evaluated with extreme suspicion; rhabdomyosarcoma of the extremities presents as an extremely subtle deep mass producing asymmetry and minimal findings on physical examination. Again, the initial physician must be highly suspicious and consider early surgical exploration and biopsy under these circumstances. General availability of computerized axial tomography (CAT) scanners and sonographic studies has made the early evaluation of these suspicious masses by noninvasive methods more accurate than in the past. The dated and dangerous advice to "wait and see" and return at some unspecified future date cannot be condoned.

Other signs that demand further investigation include

- Hematuria.
- Unexplained anemia.
- Vaginal bleeding or mass.
- Failure to thrive.
- Unexplained increase in abdominal girth.
- Rectal bleeding, intussusception, and bowel obstruction (suggesting intestinal lymphosarcoma).
- Headaches and neurological symptoms.

C. Education and Screening

Every pediatrician and primary care physician must, with neoplasm in mind, screen each child. Parents generally bring their children to a physician periodically for regular check-ups; this, in itself, is a screening opportunity that should be used to advantage by the physician; thus, delay in diagnosis often stems from delay in appropriate medical intervention rather than from patient or parental neglect.

II. PRETREATMENT EVALUATION AND WORK-UP

A. History and Physical Examination

1. History

Most solid pediatric tumors are clinically silent until a mass is identified on physical examination. It is important, however,

to try to elicit the subtle symptoms that might be helpful in the diagnosis:

- Failure to thrive, weight loss, pallor, and anemia.
- Enlargement of abdominal girth (indicative of a mass or ascites).
- Hematuria (indicative of renal tumors).
- Signs of intussusception, rectal bleeding (intestinal tumors).
- Lymphadenopathy, easy bruisability (lymphomas, leukemias).
- Vaginal bleeding (sarcoma botryoides).
- Diplopia and gait disturbances (neuroblastoma of orbit).
- Headache and neurological symptoms (brain tumor).

2. Physical Examination

The most important physical finding is that of a mass. The physician should carefully examine each patient at every visit to detect early signs of a flank mass or a tumor of the extremities. Wilms's tumors or neuroblastomas present with a fullness or mass in the flank; hepatic tumors present with hepatic enlargement, usually of an asymmetrical configuration; rhabdomyosarcomas of the extremities first present as deep soft-tissue masses in the muscle; those that originate in the pelvic area present as lower abdominal masses or, in the botryoid types, as a mass protruding from the vaginal region. Retroperitoneal masses include Wilms's tumors, neuroblastomas, teratomas, sarcomas, and even benign lesions such as hydronephrosis or polycystic kidneys.

B. Laboratory Findings

Routine laboratory investigation will yield little information except in certain specific instances:

- Complete blood count (CBC) (in leukemias or cases associated with insidious bleeding).
- SMA-18.
- Urinalysis [identification of red blood cells (RBCs), suggestive of a renal tumor].
- Chest x-ray (lymphomas, neuroblastomas, or lung metastases).

The measurement of urinary catecholamines and vanillylmandelic acid (VMA) may be useful in identifying neuroblastomas. Likewise, identification of specific markers [e.g., human chorionic gonadotrophins, alpha-fetoproteins (AFP), etc.] is useful in the diagnosis of the various endocrine tumors.

C. Radiological Evaluation

The radiological work-up of the pediatric patient will depend largely on the type of tumor suspected and its site. Discussed in other sections are radiological work-ups for neurological tumors (§7.II.A.2), bone tumors (§5.III.C), lymphomas (§9.II.B), and endocrine tumors (§4, Vol.1). For other solid tumors, the most important evaluation is that of an abdominal or flank mass.

When a clinical diagnosis of a retroperitoneal mass is established or even suspected, immediate films of the chest and abdomen without contrast material are essential. Intravenous pyelography should be done without delay. Additional studies as outlined below (particularly CAT scanning) are then selectively indicated. Arteriography, sonography, and venography of the vena cava may be performed when it is believed that the information to be gained justifies possible delay in definitive treatment; they are particularly useful to the surgeon in planning the surgical approach.

1. Plain Abdominal Films

These will identify the soft-tissue mass and may show

- Bulging of the flank stripe.
- Obliteration of the psoas muscle.
- Displacement of the abdominal viscera.

Calcifications are often noted (15% in Wilms's tumor; 65% in neuroblastoma, where they are usually stippled and punctate).

2. Intravenous Pyelogram

This will often permit a distinction between the various retroperitoneal tumors.

a. Wilms's Tumor

Most importantly, the lesion presents as an intrinsic renal tumor; it disturbs the internal architecture of the collecting system, flattening and causing distortion of the calyces and the renal pelvis.

If it arises at the periphery of the kidney, it can grow in an extrarenal direction with loss of the renal outline but leaving the collecting system intact.

From 10 to 20% of Wilms's tumors present as a nonfunctioning kidney with a renal mass suggesting hydronephrosis. This may be secondary to an extensive tumor that involves the renal pelvis and ureter, often with extension into the renal vein and inferior vena cava.

b. Neuroblastoma

Neuroblastomas of the abdomen are, in reality, extrinsic renal tumors. The IVP will reveal an upward and lateral displacement of the lower pole of the kidney or a downward and lateral displacement of the upper pole. There is usually no distortion of the calyces or renal pelvis. Neuroblastomas can, however, be difficult to differentiate from the "intrinsic" Wilms's tumor.

c. Soft-Tissue Sarcomas (Rhabdomyosarcomas)

The IVP may identify the presence of a retroperitoneal mass or pelvic tumor. The following are classical images suggestive of the diagnosis:

- Pyeloureterectasis secondary to ureteral obstruction from tumor.
- Angulation, or "fish-hooking," of the terminal ureter secondary to outlet obstruction.
- An excretory or retrograde cystogram may show negative lobulated filling defects in the lumen of the bladder.
- Typical "botryoid sarcoma" shows multiple smooth, round shadows filling the lower half of the bladder and posterior urethra.
- Larger lesions can displace the bladder upward. This is usually suggestive of a primary lesion located in the prostate or vagina in cases where there is also an associated stretching of the urethra.

3. Ultrasound

An ultrasound examination will confirm the solid nature of the lesion but is of limited value in determining the local extension of the tumor or its margins.

4. Computerized Axial Tomography Scan

The CAT scan can clearly define the morphology of the lesion and document its extent and any evidence of spread, either by direct extension or by nodal involvement. It is particularly helpful in defining the extent of a pelvic neuroblastoma, and in Wilms's tumor CAT examination is, by and large, the most accurate method of diagnosis. It will identify one or more of the following features:

- The intrarenal origin of the tumor evidenced by distortion and splaying of the remaining renal parenchyma. A peripherally arising mass is the same density as the kidney, but the center of the mass is irregular in shape and has decreased density, especially after enhancement with contrast media.
- Small calcifications not revealed on conventional x-rays can be seen.
- A prominent pseudocapsule is demonstrated.
- The extent of the disease is easily noted.
- When enhancement scanning is done using a bolus of contrast, the inferior vena cava can be seen and traced through its intrahepatic portion and the right atrium, to exclude intra-

venous tumor extension. The renal veins, however, are inconsistently seen because the patients do not have much fat. If a thrombus is identified, it is diagnostic, but if it is not noted, it cannot be excluded.

• Enlarged lymph nodes can be identified.
• Detection of liver metastases. The CAT scan may reveal liver metastases as effectively as the isotopic liver scan and more frequently than ultrasonography.
• Evaluation of the opposite kidney. CAT is excellent for the initial evaluation and follow-up of the contralateral kidney, although this is controversial, and not much has been published on the subject.

CAT scan can thus replace IVP, inferior venacavography (IVC), and isotopic studies, resulting in a more accurate staging of the disease at a lower cost.

In soft-tissue sarcomas the CAT scan is invaluable in defining the exact nature, location, and extent of the disease. It will also identify the presence or absence of involvement of adjacent structures and neurovascular bundles when the lesion is in an extremity, thus allowing for better preoperative planning.

5. Inferior Venacavography

At the time of the IVP, IVC can be done by injecting contrast material into a foot vein, or it can be done by retrograde method at the time of angiography. Its value is to identify the extension of the disease by displacement of the vena cava, involvement of the vein, or intraluminal tumor thrombi.

6. Arteriography

This is a useful modality to establish the diagnosis of malignancy and to define the vascularity and the blood supply of the mass. (The tumor is usually supplied by the renal arteries; it may, however, be supplied by the lumbars, intercostals, or suprarenals). In 90% of cases, neovascularity is demonstrated.

Arteriography may also be particularly useful in the preoperative assessment of sarcomas of the extremities (see §6.II.B.3).

D. Metastatic Evaluation

Most malignant solid tumors in the pediatric age are either sarcomas or embryonal tumors, both of which have a very great propensity for metastatic spread. Neuroblastomas will spread primarily to bone and liver, whereas Wilms's tumors, rhabdomyosarcomas, and bone tumors will usually spread to the lung. A complete metastatic survey is essential prior to embarking on therapy. Treatment will vary if metastases are present, though the prognosis may still be reasonably good despite such spread.

The following evaluation is recommended.

• Chest x-ray with, if indicated, CAT of the chest.
• Bone scan and skeletal survey of any suspicious areas.
• Bone marrow aspiration.
• Liver and spleen scan.
• CAT scan of the abdomen and pelvis.

Bone metastases are usually lytic and destructive, with reactive skull lesions and suture line separation. Liver metastases often present with stippled calcifications.

E. General Assessment

While complete evaluation of each patient is essential, it should be noted that most pediatric patients have one disease process present and do not generally have multisystem disease problems. Blood volume, state of nutrition, electrolytes, etc. must all be evaluated.

F. Multidisciplinary Evaluation

Essential to the care of each patient is the existence of a well-coordinated group involving pediatrician, surgeon, medical oncologist, radiotherapist, nurse, social worker, and psychiatric nursing liaison. Medical specialist coordination is essential for proper therapeutic planning and care; expert support is required from the nursing staff, social worker, and psychiatric nurse. For parents and child suddenly plunged into confronting the elements of cancer treatment, emotional and family support must be furnished along with the other aspects of care. Many of the tumors are rare, the outlook guarded.

Ideally, early, localized tumors can be fully excised with immediate appropriate surgery. However, in most cases, combinations of surgery, chemotherapy, and radiation therapy are required. Radical multimodal therapy and a well-coordinated team approach are essential for the patient's well-being. Based on this concept, and recognizing the need for combined skills, a number of cooperative treatment protocols have been developed. These provide for a uniform standard of care and an exchange of information. As statistical input is also developed within each study group, the protocol can be varied to improve the care of new patients starting treatment. Having the patient entered into one of the national treatment protocols provides a broader base of medical involvement and at the same time reassures the parents that everything currently available is being done.

III. PREOPERATIVE PREPARATION

Attention must be directed to correcting anemia, dehydration, and nutritional depletion if any of these conditions are present. It is unusual that more than 24–48 hours are required to complete the preoperative evaluation and schedule the patient for surgical intervention. Blood typing and cross matching are performed. Venous access is assured by a cut-down or Jelco-type catheter of adequate size; this is best placed in an upper extremity if a retroperitoneal mass is to be approached. The use of prophylactic antibiotics is a matter of individual preference; if used, they should be started intravenously immediately prior to the surgery. Antibiotic bowel preparation may be indicated if a large retroperitoneal mass impinges on the colon so that colon resection may be needed.

IV. THERAPEUTIC MANAGEMENT

A. General Considerations

Probably more than any other group of malignant tumors, cancers of the pediatric age group have gone from diseases with relatively dismal prognoses to cancers that today are curable in a high percentage of cases. This transition has been primarily the result of combining several therapeutic modalities into an integrated treatment program. Improvement in survival with the addition of radiation therapy and/or chemotherapy to surgical resection has further resulted in the promotion of a conservation approach to maximize function and cosmesis. Postoperative radiation therapy effectively extends the "margins" of the surgical resection in the area of the tumor bed, and chemotherapy is meant to affect any potential metastatic disease. Multimodal therapy must always be used with the realization that the undesirable side effects of each treatment and the complications of each modality (e.g., immunosuppression and thrombocytopenia, anorexia, weight loss, altered renal and pulmonary function, etc.) are additive. When cure is achieved, however, the reward is worth the risk.

B. Biopsy

Although a tissue diagnosis is of great value in intelligently planning therapy for pediatric tumors, there are certain circumstances where biopsy of the tumor will decrease the chances of cure.

In early retroperitoneal lesions where surgical cure is the goal there is little place for preliminary biopsy (needle or otherwise) or intraoperative biopsy. Instead, an attempt is made to totally excise the tumor in a one-stage operative procedure. When metastases to lymph nodes are evident, removal of a node is permissible and may be the only surgical procedure necessary before chemotherapy is commenced. Whenever local lymph nodes are available in the operative field, these should be sampled extensively to further provide appropriate staging and prognostic information.

For extremity lesions, limited surgical biopsy (incisional or, for small tumors, excisional) or needle biopsy may be the best initial step before planning a wide local removal of the neoplasm itself.

Biopsies of tumors in other locations will depend greatly on the clinical picture

- Botryoid tumors are easily biopsied.
- Mouth tumors can be punch-biopsied. Other neck tumors may be needle-biopsied.
- Retro-orbital tumors or retinoblastomas are extremely difficult to biopsy.
- Neurological tumors seldom require biopsy prior to therapy (see §7.IV.A.2).

C. Staging

Staging of the various pediatric tumors is entirely different with each tumor and will thus be discussed with the specific lesion. Staging is extremely important in therapeutic planning and frequently requires definition of the surgical findings to complete; thus the staging will often be completed only after surgical therapy.

D. Principles of Surgical Management

These will be defined in greater detail in the discussion of the individual tumors, but several points are common to any surgery for solid tumors in children.

- The first line of treatment, whenever possible, should be total surgical removal of the tumor. Ideally, for example, the early neuroblastoma or Wilms's tumor, localized to one area and not involving adjacent structures, should be excised intact, without preliminary biopsy, thus possibly eradicating the disease with the single surgical procedure alone.
- The enormous tumor that totally envelops the aorta and vena cava and invades the adjacent bowel and lumbar structures, may be left *in situ*. Biopsy in these cases is essential. Reexploration may be possible after chemotherapy and radiation therapy have been administered. Surgical resection can often be completed at this later date.

- Each surgical procedure must be carefully planned, anesthesia properly controlled, blood available for transfusion, and frozen-section pathological studies accessible.
- Generous exposure and meticulous sharp dissection are essential.
- The importance of lymph node sampling cannot be overemphasized.
- Marking of the tumor bed with metal clips for later radiotherapy is extremely important.

Intraoperative chemotherapy and radiation therapy starting immediately after surgery were utilized in the past; there is no evidence, however, that a delay of a few days for chemotherapy or radiotherapy is in any way detrimental.

E. Adjuvant Therapy

Adjuvant therapy in the treatment of solid tumors of the pediatric patient is of the greatest importance. Improvements in cure rates are the direct result of adjuvant therapy, and patients must be treated in a multidisciplinary manner with total treatment planning at the outset.

Radiation therapy and chemotherapy may be used preoperatively to render an inoperable situation resectable or to permit a conservation operation. They may be used postoperatively, electively or for residual disease, and at times, may be recommended for long-term maintenance. The type of radiotherapy administered, the chemotherapeutic agents used, the regimens proposed, and the sequence of treatment will depend entirely on the histologic nature of the tumor, its type, its stage, and its location. These will be individually discussed in the appropriate areas.

The general effects of adjuvant therapy and their complications in this subset of patients are quite unique. The following are some of the risks involved in the use of these modalities in children.

1. Radiotherapy

- Impairment of bone growth and arrest of development of a bone as a result of radiation effects on the epiphysis. Sophisticated dosimetry and three-dimensional treatment planning aided with CAT scanning become critical here.
- Hypothyroidism or Addison's disease may result from irradiation of the thyroid or adrenal areas.
- Renal damage as a result of high-dose irradiation of the kidneys.
- Genetic abnormalities, with risks of congenital anomalies in later generations from effects of the scattered radiation on the development of the gonads. These complications, however, are the result of cummulative exposure and are probably more theoretical than real.
- Risk of oncogenesis.

2. Chemotherapy

The effects of chemotherapy in children are not much different than those in adults:

- Oncogenesis.
- Nephrotoxicity (from actinomycin D).
- Pulmonary fibrosis (from bleomycin).
- Bone marrow suppression, thrombocytopenia, leukopenia, sepsis, hemorrhage, etc.
- GI and other mucosal toxicity.
- Alopecia.

F. The Price of Successful Therapy

Present-day combined therapy has resulted in an expectation of cure rates of 80% in soft-tissue sarcoma and 90% in Wilms's tumors with early, localized disease. The potential life expectancy of these young children requires a careful appraisal of the long-term damaging effects of radiation and chemotherapy. Such damage, resulting from the complications listed above, may manifest itself as impairment of growth of bone and soft tissue, genetic consequences, impaired reproductive potential, and oncogenesis with the possible appearance of second malignancies. (Recovery from childhood malignancy carries a 17% risk of developing a second malignant neoplasm during the subsequent 20 years).

Childhood cancer presents as an immediate and overwhelming threat that appears to require appropriate multimodal therapy to achieve the highest rate of cure. However, with clearer understanding of the natural history of various tumors, when it can be demonstrated that less dangerous combinations are effective, pertinent modifications in approach should be implemented, and therapy should be limited at certain stages of the disease to reduce the risks of toxicity. As an example, based on appropriate statistical evaluation of the National Wilms' Tumor Study (NWTS-1), Group I Wilms's tumors in young patients are no longer given radiation therapy.

Parents must be fully informed regarding the long-term risks and the need for continued observation of the child. The ultimate goal of cure of the disease with minimal risk of side effects is particularly important in the care of the young patient with a life expectancy of many decades.

V. POSTOPERATIVE CARE, EVALUATION, AND REHABILITATION

A. Postoperative Care

Routine postoperative measures include

- Intensive care unit monitoring: vital signs, hemoglobin and hematocrit determinations, central venous pressure (CVP) monitoring, and arterial blood gases.

- Prolonged intubation and respiratory support, as required.
- Monitoring of renal function, particularly after nephrectomy or when surgery is done on a solitary kidney.
- Nasogastric tube drainage is maintained until bowel activity is resumed.
- The relatively large daily fluid turnover makes the young child extremely susceptible to rapid dehydration and electrolyte imbalance. Assessment of the child's fluid status and electrolyte requirement is necessary every few hours in the immediate postoperative period.
- Breathing exercises to prevent atelectasis are essential, and heavy sedation with narcotic medication should be avoided.
- Antibiotics (e.g., aminoglycosides) may be given, but nephrotoxicity must be avoided.
- Sutures must be left in place longer than usual when chemotherapy or radiation is used.
- In children, deep venous thrombosis and pulmonary emboli are extremely rare.

B. Nursing Care

The child or infant with a malignancy presents a large number of problems to the nursing staff, particularly in the area of psychological support of the patient and the family.

Most pediatric or oncology nurses are well prepared for the complexities of nursing assessment and nursing care plans for the patient with a need for radical surgery and subsequent multimodal chemotherapy and radiotherapy. Nutritional support may be required, and central-vein hyperalimentation may be administered through an indwelling catheter. Careful observation for the side effects of chemotherapy and radiotherapy is essential, and isolation techniques may be utilized when indicated.

The greatest burden, however, is often the involvement of the nursing staff with the impact on the family of the cancer diagnosis in a young child or infant. Family members may display reactions varying from total denial to premature grieving in situations where the patient may indeed be fully cured. Maximal support of the family group should be provided. The child, on the other hand, may have needs of expression that require great perspicacity; these may be best managed by a play therapist working with the young child or by a psychiatric nurse clinician and psychiatric social worker working with the older child.

Individual children and individual families vary in their coping abilities and needs. Each situation must be approached with delicacy, infinite care, and deep understanding.

C. Follow-Up Evaluation

Table I is a sample follow-up schedule for Wilms's tumor, presented as a guide to indicate a basic minimum of observations for careful follow-up of this type of patient. More frequent studies should be performed when there is a clinical

Table I

Schedule for Follow-Up of Wilms's Tumor

Management	First and second year					Fourth year		Thereafter, annually
	1–1/2 months	3 months	6 months	9 months	12 months	6 months	12 months	
History								
Pain	X	X	X	X	X	X	X	X
Enlargement of abdomen	X	X	X	X	X	X	X	X
Hematuria	X	X	X	X	X	X	X	X
Pallor	X	X	X	X	X	X	X	X
Other	X	X	X	X	X	X	X	X
Physical								
Mass	X	X	X	X	X	X	X	X
Weight loss	X	X	X	X	X	X	X	X
Other	X	X	X	X	X	X	X	X
Investigation								
CBC	Frequent during chemotherapy (include platelet count)							
Chest x-ray	X	X	X	X	X	X	X	X
SMA-12		X		X	X	X	X	X
Urinalysis	X	X	X	X	X	X	X	X
IVP					X		X	X
CAT	As indicated							
Bone series	As indicated							
Liver scan	As indicated							

suspicion of disease activity or metastatic disease or when a recurrence is under active treatment. Additionally, it should be noted that a bone survey is indicated at the start of therapy when a clear-cell sarcomatous tumor is present, and a brain scan is indicated with the diagnosis of the "rhabdoid" sarcomatous variety of Wilms's tumor. Chest x-rays for Wilms's tumors and bone scans for neuroblastomas must be obtained frequently during follow-up visits to detect metastases in these more common sites.

D. Rehabilitation

The patient who is actively under therapy is under close observation by the physicians involved in his or her treatment. One should not lose site, however, of the intricacy of the factors that impact on the behavior of these patients:

- Psychosocial reaction to the strange environment, loss of the "home sanctuary," contact with strangers, etc.
- Fear, of the illness, its treatment, and of pain.
- Functional disability resulting from the surgery.
- Impact of loss of schooling.

The establishment of good rapport among the child, the family members, the physician, and other hospital personnel is most important. Pain relief and patient comfort are essential. The patience of the staff may be tested by a demand for frequent, repetitive explanations; maintenance of hope and reasonable reassurances are extremely important. Social service, rehabilitation medicine, psychiatric liaison staff, occupational and recreational therapists, and the primary care physician must be involved in the rehabilitation of these children.

Long-term care is usually not necessary in these patients since complete cure is expected after a 2- to 3-year survival. The patients must, however, continue on a follow-up schedule, with particular attention paid to detecting long-term complications of treatment.

The management of the more common solid pediatric malignancies will be individually discussed in the following pages. These are Wilms's tumor, neuroblastoma, rhabdomyosarcoma, hepatic tumors, and teratomas. Leukemias and lymphomas are presented separately in Part B of this section, and other tumors of the pediatric age group are discussed in various other sections:

- Neurological tumors, §7.
- Ewing's sarcoma and other bone tumors, §5.
- Testicular tumors, §13.
- Endocrine tumors, §4.

VI. SOLID PEDIATRIC TUMORS: TYPE-SPECIFIC

A. Wilms's Tumors (Nephroblastomas)

1. Pathological Considerations

Wilms's tumor is an embryonal cancer of the kidney. The classic type is a mixed renal tumor of metanephric blastema and its recognized stromal and epithelial derivatives are at variable stages of differentiation. Some tumors are predominantly or exclusively composed of one histological pattern.

The tumor usually arises between 1 and 4 years of age; however, some cases of Wilms's tumor have been reported in adults. On occasion, extrarenal Wilms's tumors in ectopic nephrogenic rests are found in the retroperitoneal space, the mediastinum, the inguinal canal, and sacrococcygeal teratomas. Involvement of both kidneys has been reported in 3–13% of cases.

a. Macroscopic Features

The typical Wilms's tumor is a large, soft mass in the kidney surrounded by a pseudocapsule composed of fibrous tissue and compressed kidney parenchyma. The cut surface is grayish-pink, slightly mucoid-to-slimy, and bulges out. Some tumors show areas of hemorrhage and necrosis with cystic degeneration. Invasion of the renal vein may occur and is not necessarily related to the size of the tumor.

b. Staging

The NWTS Pathology Center has proposed the following clinical and pathological grouping of patients with Wilms's tumors based upon the degree of gross extension of the disease.

i. Group I. Tumor limited to the kidney and completely excised. The surface of the renal capsule is intact; the tumor was not biopsied or ruptured during surgery. No apparent residual tumor.

ii. Group II. Tumor extending beyond the kidney but completely excised. Includes cases with involvement of the perirenal soft tissues, periaortic lymph nodes, or renal vein.

iii. Group III. Residual nonhematogenous tumor confined to the abdomen with

- Hilar or periaortic lymph node involvement beyond the area of resection.

- Diffuse peritoneal involvement by spillage or tumor growth that has penetrated the peritoneal surfaces.
- Microscopic or gross extension of the tumor beyond the surgical margins.
- Inability to excise the tumor completely due to involvement of vital structures.

iv. Group IV.   Hematogenous metastasis to liver, lung, bone, or brain.

v. Group V.   Bilateral renal involvement at the time of diagnosis or subsequently.

c. Microscopic Characteristics

The classic Wilms's tumor of favorable histology consists of mixed epithelial components with a variable degree of tubular and glomeruloid differentiation with stromal and renal blastema elements, although any one of these may be prominent. Cytopathological evaluation of specimens reviewed by the NWTS Pathology Center have led to the identification of microscopic features that help to predict the clinical course of the disease (excluding mesoblastic nephroma). An 89% survival rate has been recorded for children with so-called favorable histology (FH), while only 39% survival was found for those with "unfavorable histology" (UH).

The unfavorable histology (UH) includes cases with four subtypes of the disease:

- Wilms's tumor with focal anaplastic changes.
- Wilms's tumor with diffuse anaplastic changes.
- "Rhabdoid" sarcoma.
- Clear-cell sarcoma.

The rhabdoid and clear-cell neoplasms have certain clinical features that are unlike those of the usual Wilms's tumor. The rhabdoid tumor tends to be associated with intracerebral disease, either as metastatic deposits or as second, independent small-cell tumors. The clear-cell sarcoma tends to metastasize to bone. The implications of these histological types, therefore, mandate, as part of the evaluation of the patient, a brain scan for the former and a bone scan for the latter.

d. Prognostic Features

According to NWTS, the five most important criteria for prediction of the outcome of treatment in Wilms's tumors are

- Histology (FH or UH).
- Lymph node involvement (gross or microscopic).
- Chemotherapy (early use yields favorable results).
- Age (children 2 years old or over have a less favorable

outcome, while children under 2 years of age have a better prognosis).

The effect of capsular penetration on relapse, while significant, is not as important as other criteria (e.g., lymph node involvement or specimen weight) in the final outcome.

2. Site-Specific Data Form for Wilms's Tumors (see pp. 325–328)

3. Surgical Considerations

Surgery still remains an integral part of the treatment of the patient with Wilms's tumor in spite of the fact that most advances and improved survivals have resulted from improvements in the adjuvant treatment of the disease by radiotherapy and chemotherapy.

The goal of surgery is complete removal of the tumor in a carefully planned and meticulously executed procedure. With care and patience, even large, bulky tumors can often be removed with an intact capsule, avoiding the obvious risk of tumor spillage. Because 5% of these tumors are bilateral, careful palpation and inspection of the contralateral kidney is essential. A generous transverse abdominal incision is ideal to allow for proper exposure and careful dissection. An oblique flank incision has no place in the surgical approach to Wilms's tumor; it does not provide adequate exposure; does not allow careful, sharp dissection; and precludes inspection of the opposite kidney. Much emphasis has been placed on early ligation of the vessels of the renal pedicle; while this is desirable, it is no longer considered essential and should never be attempted if the attempt risks capsular rupture. In large, bulky tumors it is often safer to gradually encircle the tumor to mobilize it and approach the vessels at a later stage in the procedure, when ligation can be achieved with greater ease. If tumor extension precludes excision, one may mark the extent of the lesion with metal clips and consider reexploration after a course of radiation therapy has been given to shrink the tumor. The importance of lymph node sampling should be emphasized. Careful labeling of each specimen, as well as, mapping during the procedure, is necessary.

Outlined below are the basic features of the surgical procedure in a stepwise manner.

- i. Transverse abdominal incision, generous.
- ii. Complete abdominal exploration.
  - a. Contralateral kidney.
  - b. Lymph node involvement.
  - c. Contiguous-organ involvement.
  - d. Plan extended excision, if required.
- iii. Avoid biopsy of the tumor unless it is not resectable.
- iv. Collect peritoneal fluid for cell block.

   v. Total excision with no spillage or capsular damage is the goal.

   vi. Meticulous dissection with adequate exposure.

   vii. Early vessel ligation, if possible (flush to the vena cava).

   viii. Bulky tumors distort the anatomy and may have anomalous blood supply. They may require a "circling technique" prior to vessel ligation.

   ix. Ureterectomy.

   x. Adrenalectomy (usually necessary).

   xi. Handling of lymph nodes.

      a. Mapping in detail.

      b. Excise if suspicious.

      c. Extensive sampling if not suspicious (hilar, para-aortic, etc.).

   xii. Palpate the renal vein and the vena cava for tumor extension; remove them as necessary.

   xiii. Use of metal clips to mark the limits and areas of invasion.

A large measure of success in the management of most cancers is the result of multi-institutional clinical trials that evaluate various therapeutic approaches in a randomized prospective manner. Most of the progress achieved in the treatment of Wilms's tumor has been the result of such clinical trials organized by the NWTS. The NWTS is currently accumulating cases treated throughout the country according to one or another of their protocols and will advise any physician or surgeon wishing to participate as to the nature of these protocols and the procedure to be followed to include his or her patient in their protocol if these are still open for case accumulation. The various protocols will be discussed in §8A.VI.A.5. The accompanying forms (see pp. 327–328) are illustrations of checklists with mapping instructions that must be completed to properly enter a patient in a NWTS study.

4. Radiotherapy

There is still considerable controversy regarding the role of radiotherapy in treating Wilms's tumor, given that there are few reports of the actual rate of local failure following surgery alone. Some reports, however, do indicate a local recurrence rate ranging between 22% (for Stage I) and 100% (for Stage IV) following surgery alone. Recent NWTS protocols have attempted to identify the role of postoperative radiotherapy in Wilms's tumor. Although their studies seem to indicate no advantage to radiotherapy in Stage I or II patients, several other large series seem to indicate that local recurrences can be totally eliminated by the use of proper radiotherapy and chemotherapy postoperatively; chemotherapy alone does not seem to be sufficient to achieve such results. It has been demonstrated that local recurrences carry a grim prognosis indeed (less than 20% salvage).

The following categories of patients must be considered valid candidates for postoperative radiotherapy:

- Patients with gross or microscopic residual disease.
- Patients where biopsy was performed or surgical spillage has occurred.
- Large tumors (over 250 g or T2).
- Capsular penetration or adjacent-organ involvement.
- Unfavorable histology.
- Positive nodes.

It seems reasonable to withhold radiotherapy from all patients with T1, N0 (Stage I) lesions and from patients under 24 months of age with favorable histology.

The technique of radiation is of great importance. Therapy should be started within 1 week of surgery because results indicate that early treatment is more favorable. Appropriate portals must be designed. Generally, treatment is limited to the tumor site in Group II but includes all of the abdomen when spillage occurs or with more advanced disease. A dose of 2500 rads in 3 weeks is given to the tumor bed in 150- to 200-rad increments daily. This may be boosted to 3000 rads for patients with gross disease to particular sites.

5. Chemotherapy

The impact of modern therapy on the outcome in patients with Wilms's tumor represents one of the real successes in cancer treatment. The 2-year survival has risen from 20% 30 years ago to better than 80% during the past decade. This success has been the result of prompt surgery, postoperative radiation therapy when indicated, and the proper use of anticancer chemotherapeutic drugs. A large measure of this successful collaboration must be attributed to the protocols devised by the NWTS. These have been developed in three phases:

- NWTS 1. The results of the first therapeutic trial showed that double-agent chemotherapy using actinomycin D and vincristine was superior to either agent alone.
- NWTS 2. The second NWTS trial established that the addition of Adriamycin in a three-drug regimen along with actinomycin D and vincristine provided significantly better results for children with Group II and III disease. Patients with Group IV disease or those with UH did not do as well. The results of the NWTS 2 protocols C, D, E, and. F are summarized in Table II.

Two-year relapse-free survivals, without reference to treatment or other factors were 88, 78, 70, and 40% for groups I, II, III, and IV, respectively. Patients with unfavorable histology had an overall much worse survival rate (54%) as compared to those with favorable histology (90%), and those pa-

SITE SPECIFIC DATA FORM—WILMS'S TUMOR

HISTORY

Age:_____ Sex:_____

Symptoms
_____ Pain
_____ Enlargement of abdomen
_____ Hematuria
_____ Failure to thrive
Other_____
Duration:_____

Social history
    Race:____White____Black____Oriental____Other
    Marital status:____ Single ____ Married ____ Other
    Occupation:_____
Family history of carcinoma:____ No____Yes
    Relation _____ Site:_____
Previous history of carcinoma:____ No____Yes
    Site _____
    Rx: _____

Previous treatment (describe):
(Surgery, radiation, chemotherapy, tracheostomy, etc.)
_____
_____
_____

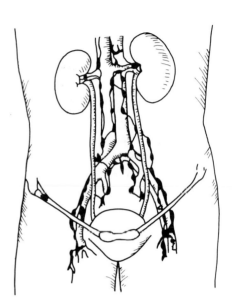

PHYSICAL EXAMINATION AND SURGICAL FINDINGS

Mass: _____ Right _____ Left

Extension to	Yes	No
Contralateral kidney	____	____
Perirenal fat	____	____
Spleen	____	____
Colon	____	____
Peritoneum	____	____
Psoas muscle	____	____
Renal vein	____	____
Vena cava	____	____
Adrenal	____	____
Liver	____	____

Nodes	Yes	No
Hilar	____	____
Periaortic	____	____
Pelvic	____	____
Contralateral	____	____
Other:	____	____

Tumor biopsy:____Yes ____ No
    Type: _____
    When: _____
Tumor spillage or rupture:
    ____Yes ____No

PRETREATMENT EVALUATION

	Pos.	Neg.	Suspicious
CBC	____	____	____
Urinalysis	____	____	____
SMA-12	____	____	____
Chest x-ray	____	____	____
IVP	____	____	____
Sonogram	____	____	____
CAT scan	____	____	____
Arteriogram	____	____	____

	Pos.	Neg.	Suspicious
Liver scan	____	____	____
Bone scan	____	____	____
Brain scan	____	____	____
CAT of chest	____	____	____
Bone marrow aspiration	____	____	____

Classification
  Histology:_____
  _____ T____ N____ M Stage:_____
National Wilms's Tumor Study
    Group (NWTS)_____

Signature:_____
Countersignature:_____
Date:_____

Clinical TNM Classification

Local disease

TX	Inadequate information on the primary tumor
T0	The primary is undetectable by palpation or radiographic procedure
T1	Not crossing midline by palpation and/or IVP area of renal shadow on IVP <80 cm²
T2	Crossing midline by palpation and/or IVP area of renal shadow >80 cm²
*T3	No T3 in Wilms's tumor
T5	Bilateral primary tumors occurring simultaneously

Nodal involvement

NX	Inadequate information (no lymphangiogram)
N0	Para-aortic lymph nodes considered normal on lymphangiogram
N1	Lymph nodes considered to contain tumor

Distant metastases

MX	Not assessed
M0	No (known) distant metastasis
M1	Distant metastasis present (specify)

Postsurgical Treatment—Pathologic TNM

This indicates the local extent of the tumor and lymph nodes and whether complete removal was done and is derived from the first surgical attempt at removal (and from histopathology).

Primary tumor

PT1	Intrarenal tumor (completely encapsulated), excision complete, and margins histologically free
PT2	Tumor extending beyond the capsule or renal parenchyma, excision complete
PT3	Excision incomplete
A	Microscopic residual tumor confined to the tumor bed. To include histologically positive adhesions, previous biopsy or localized operative rupture, if assumed not to have involved the peritoneal cavity
B	Macroscopic residual or widespread contamination of normal tissues during surgery, or evidence of preoperative rupture
C	Cases where attempted nephrectomy proved impossible
PT5	Bilateral disease histologically confirmed

Nodes

PNX	No surgical excision of regional lymph nodes performed, or there is inadequate information on the pathologic findings
PN0	Sampled lymph nodes histologically negative
PN1	Sampled lymph nodes histologically positive, all tumorous regional lymph nodes are considered resected
PN2	Sampled lymph nodes histologically positive, tumorous nodes not considered totally resected (including surgically ruptured nodes)

Metastases

PM0	No distant metastases found at surgery
PM1	Distant metastases confirmed at surgery

NWTS Grouping

Clinical staging

Stage I/II	T1 or T2, N0, M0
Stage III	T1, N1, M0 or T2, any N, M0
Stage IV	Any T or N with M1
Stage V	Bilateral at presentation

Postsurgical treatment—Pathologic staging

Stage I	pT1, pNX or pN0 (Group I)
Stage II	pT2 or pN1 or both (Group II)
Stage III	(Group III)
IIIA	Microscopic residual tumor confined to the tumor or bed, meeting criteria for pT3a, pN0 or pN1
IIIB	pT3b or pN2 or both
IIIC	(Group IV)
Stage IV	(Group IV) — Distant metastasis present beyond the regional lymph nodes (including clinical metastasis)
Stage V	(Group V) — Bilateral tumor at presentation

National Wilms's Tumor Study—3
Surgical Checklist
(To be filled out by operating surgeon)

Identification

Patient's name: _____ NWTS—3 Study # _____

Institution: _____ Clinical stage _____

Surgeon _____

Preoperative blood pressure: _____ / _____

Hematuria: Gross: _____ No _____ Yes

Micro: _____ No _____ Yes

Date of operation: _____ / _____ / _____
                 month day   year

The impression of the operating surgeon may be of as much importance as the pathologist's opinion. We are interested in your operative findings, whether you suspect tumor in lymph nodes or in adherent organs.

1. Tumor site: _____ Right _____ Left _____ Bilateral

2. Was all gross tumor removed? _____ No _____ Yes

SEE EXHIBIT IV FOR GUIDANCE IN COMPLETING ITEMS 3 AND 4

3. In your opinion, was the tumor cut across during operation? _____ No _____ Yes

If yes, please complete table, indicating where the tumor was transected and the extent of peritoneal soilage by appropriate check marks.

	Peritoneal soilage	
	Local	Diffuse †
Renal vein or IVC		
Adjacent structure		
Microscopically verified? _____ No _____ Yes		
Lymph nodes		
Ureter		
Other		

4. In your opinion, was the capsule intact? _____ No* _____ Yes

If no, complete the table following the Exhibit IV guidelines.

	Peritoneal soilage	
	Local	Diffuse †
Penetrated grossly with tumor		
Preoperative rupture		
Biopsy		
Incisional		
Other		
Spillage during surgery		

5. In your opinion was there local extension and/or local nontumor adherence (adhesion)? _____ No _____ Yes

_____ Extension _____ Adhesion

If yes, indicate involved areas:

EXTENSION
- _____ Contralateral kidney
- _____ Peritoneal implant
- _____ Perirenal fat
- _____ Renal vein
- _____ Lumen
- _____ Wall
- _____ Liver
- _____ Spleen
- _____ Adrenal
- _____ Colon
- _____ Psoas muscle
- _____ IVC
- _____ Other_____
- _____

ADHESION
- _____ Contralateral kidney
- _____ Peritoneum
- _____ Wall of renal vein
- _____ Liver
- _____ Spleen
- _____ Adrenal
- _____ Colon
- _____ Psoas muscle
- _____ IVC
- _____ Other_____
- _____

---

* Explain fully in operative note.

† Diffuse soilage implies all peritoneal surfaces are at risk, the patient is stage III, and the radiation field must include the peritoneal parietes and the true pelvis.

6. In your opinion, were the lymph nodes involved? _____ No _____ Yes
   If yes, indicate involved sites below and in the diagram.
   _____ Hilar nodes involved
   _____ Periaortic nodes involved
   _____ Ipsilateral
   _____ Contralateral

7. Were lymph nodes removed?
   Hilar: _____ No _____ Yes
   Periaortic: _____ No _____ Yes

8. Were additional biopsies done? _____ No _____ Yes
   Site: _____

9. Renal vessels ligated before tumor mobilized? _____ No _____ Yes

10. Was cystoscopy performed? _____ No _____ Yes
    Positive findings? _____ No _____ Yes

    Describe: _____
    _____

11. Were there immediate operative or postoperative complications?
    _____ No _____ Yes. If yes, indicate:
    _____ Anesthesia
    _____ Extensive hemorrhage
    _____ Wound. Describe: _____
    _____ Other. Describe: _____

Please draw on figure below the size and position of tumor and any tissue removed

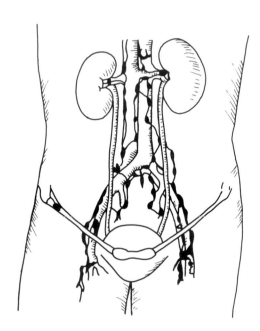

12. Was opposite kidney explored? _____ No _____ Yes
    Was Gerota's fascia opened? _____ No _____ Yes
    Was kidney mobilized? _____ No _____ Yes
    Was posterior surface visualized? _____ No _____ Yes

Signed: _____   Date: _____

Mail together with operative note to:

   National Wilms's Tumor Study Data and Statistical Center
   Fred Hutchinson Cancer Research Center
   1124 Columbia Street
   Seattle, Washington 98104

Table II

Summary of Statistical Analysis for NWTS-2 (May, 1981): Randomized Patients by Regimen

Patient groups	Regimen[a]	Number of patients	Relapse-free survival at 2 years (%)
Group I, FH and UH	E (6 months AMD)	88	88
	F (15 months AMD)	91	
Groups II and III, FH	C (AMD + VCR)	121	74
	D (AMD + VCR + ADR)	111	89
Groups II and II, UH	C	16	35
	D	19	44
Group IV, FH and UH	C	22	43
	D	27	59

[a] C, D, E, and F stand for NWTS-2 protocols. AMD, actinomycin D; VCR, vincristine; ADR, Adriamycin.

tients without nodes also had a higher survival (82%) compared to those with nodal involvement (54%).

- NWTS 3. The present NWTS 3 trial hopes to refine the method of treatment according to staging (or grouping), to identify high-risk patients and families, and to study late consequences treatment of Wilms's tumor.

As far as present-day chemotherapy is concerned, the agents used include actinomycin D (AMD) and vincristine (VCR), which are given to all patients. Adriamcyin (ADR) is still being evaluated in Group II and III disease with favorable histology. All patients with Group IV disease, however, and patients with unfavorable histology should receive all three drugs. The three-drug regimen is at present being compared with a four-drug program that adds cyclophosphamide (CPM) to the other three agents. The drug dosages used are as follows:

- Actinomycin D, 15 μ/kg/day, IV (×5 per course).
- Vincristine, 1.5 mg/m²/week.
- Adriamycin, 20 mg/m²/day IV (×3 per course).
- Cyclophosphamide, 10 mg/kg/day IV (×3 per course).

Table III summarizes the randomized clinical studies currently being conducted by the NWTS group and the present-day recommended approaches to the patient with Wilms's tumor.

Patients with mesoblastic nephromas should receive no treatment other than surgery, and there seems to be a trend to decrease the duration of chemotherapy in those patients with the more favorable histologic type of tumors.

6. Bilateral Wilms's Tumor

Bilateral Wilms's tumors occur in about 5% of cases (33 of 606 in NWTS 1). The histology is generally favorable, and a

Table III

Summary of Current Clinical Studies of NWTS and Recommended Approaches for Patients with Wilms's Tumor

Stage of patient	Recommended therapy			
	Surgery recommended	Radiation	NWTS 2 protocol codes	Chemotherapy
Favorable histology (FH)				
Stage I (any age)	Surgery	No radiotherapy	L	AMD + VCR for 10 weeks
			EE	AMD + VCR for 6 months
Stage II (any age)	Surgery	No radiotherapy 2000 Rads	DD	AMD + VCR + ADR for 15 months
		No radiotherapy 2000 Rads	K	Intensive AMD + VCR for 15 months
Stage III (any age)	Surgery	1000 Rads 2000 Rads	DD	AMD + VCR + ADR for 15 months
		1000 Rads 2000 Rads	K	Intensive AMD + VCR for 15 months
Unfavorable histology (UH) and all stage IV	Surgery	Radiotherapy[a]	DD	AMD + VCR + ADR for 15 months
			J	AMD + VCR + ADR + CPM for 15 months

[a] All FH Stage IV receive 2000-rad flank irradiation and irradiation to other sites as in NWTS 2 (permissible flank dose variations). All UH, all stages, receive age-adjusted flank irradiation and irradiation to other sites as NWTS 2.

survival rate of 87% at 2 years has followed various treatment approaches. Preservation of renal function in this circumstance is given high priority, and a carefully planned approach should be exercised. The following guidelines are recommended:

- Excise all tumor at the first operation if adequate renal function can be preserved.
- If it is not possible to do so because of the extent of the disease, bilateral biopsies should be performed, followed by chemotherapy and subsequent radiotherapy if indicated. Laparotomy at 3–6 months should then be undertaken, with partial nephrectomy for removal of the tumor from the less involved kidney. If this leaves adequate renal function, total removal of the other kidney is then performed if it is extensively involved. If there is hope for some preservation of function of the other kidney, then the extent of the tumor is marked with metal clips. Additional chemotherapy and radiotherapy are given, and a repeat laparotomy is done to evaluate the possibility of preservation of some additional renal function.

7. Treatment of Advanced Disease

Disseminated disease from Wilms's tumor requires aggressive multimodal therapy despite the poor outlook (e.g., cases of unfavorable histology). Within this group, certain features must be noted; rhabdoid tumors are associated with metastases to the brain, and CAT studies of the head should be performed as indicated. Clear-cell tumors are associated with bone metastases, and bone surveys and radioisotope studies are indicated.

In addition to chemotherapy and radiotherapy, surgery must be considered in certain situations of metastatic Wilms's tumor:

- Hepatic metastases amenable to resection should be approached surgically.
- Solitary or limited multiple pulmonary metastases that persist and are resectable should be resected.

Despite the grim prognosis, such an approach is justified by the occasional long-term survival or cure in this group of patients.

8. Management Algorithm for Wilms's Tumors (see p. 331)

B. Neuroblastomas

Neuroblastoma is one of the most common extracranial solid tumors of early childhood. It has its highest incidence during the first 2 years of life, and numerous cases of congenital neuroblastoma have been reported. With this tumor, 80% of cases are seen by 5 years of age, and it is almost never seen after the age of 10.

1. Pathological Considerations

Neuroblastoma is the most common and malignant neoplasm in childhood. It is a congenital tumor that arises in cells of the sympathetic nervous system (sympathetic neuroblasts) derived from the embryonic neural crest. It may be associated with other congenital anomalies or may at times be seen in patients with neurofibromatosis. The tumor is almost always unilateral and occurs at sites within a region extending from the posterior cranial fossa to the coccyx. The most common intra-abdominal sites are within the adrenal gland or in the retroperitoneal area, this location accounts for two-thirds of the cases. The next-most-common site is the posterior mediastinum. Other areas from which the tumor can arise include the head and neck, chest, abdomen, and pelvis.

The tumor is relatively well circumscribed, large, soft, friable, and gray, with areas of hemorrhage, necrosis, and calcification. In 50% of the cases, there is radiographic evidence of calcification. The tumor is composed of masses of small, regular cells with tiny, deeply staining nuclei slightly larger than lymphocytes and scant cytoplasm with poorly defined cell borders. Homer Wright rosettes (collections of tumor cells arranged around central pale eosinophilic areas) are seen in one-third of the cases. Necrosis is usually present, leaving viable tumor around the vessels. Variable degrees of differentiation to mature ganglion cells may be seen in some tumors. Microscopically, this tumor may resemble Ewing's bone tumor, embryonal cell rhabdomyosarcoma, or anaplastic embryonal tumors.

The tumor spreads by local invasion, blood vessels, and lymphatics. The most common sites of metastases include the liver, bone, and lymph nodes. The location of metastases varies with the age of the patient. In the neonate, liver metastases and subcutaneous lesions are common, while bony lesions are rare; in fact, subcutaneous spread seems to be unique to the young infant. The incidence of bony metastases increases with age and may be seen in as many as two-thirds of children over 2 years of age.

2. Staging and Classification

Staging work-up should include chest x-rays, bone survey, bone scan, IVP, and bone marrow aspiration. The Evans classification is the most commonly used method of staging neuroblastomas.

Stage I: Tumor confined to the organ or structure of origin.

ALGORITHM FOR WILMS'S TUMOR

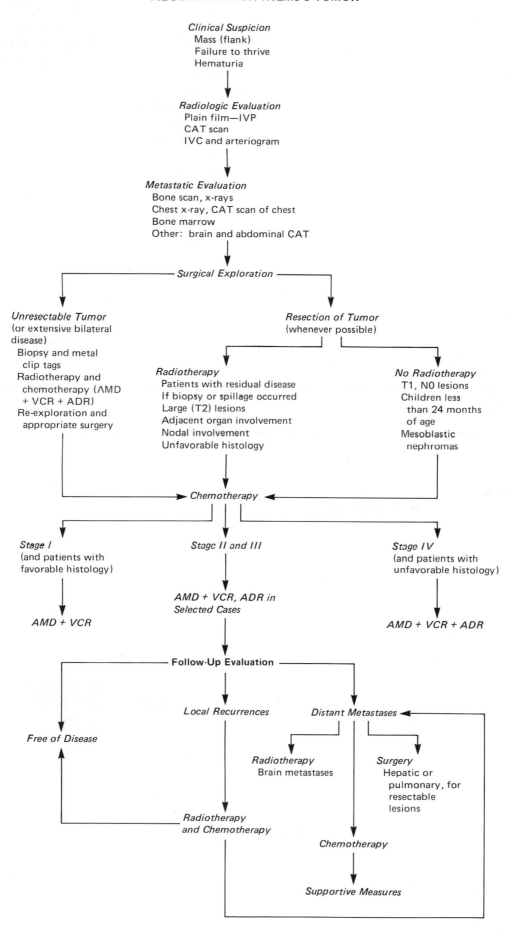

Clinical Suspicion
Mass (flank)
Failure to thrive
Hematuria

Radiologic Evaluation
Plain film—IVP
CAT scan
IVC and arteriogram

Metastatic Evaluation
Bone scan, x-rays
Chest x-ray, CAT scan of chest
Bone marrow
Other: brain and abdominal CAT

Surgical Exploration

Unresectable Tumor
(or extensive bilateral disease)
Biopsy and metal clip tags
Radiotherapy and chemotherapy (AMD + VCR + ADR)
Re-exploration and appropriate surgery

Resection of Tumor
(whenever possible)

Radiotherapy
Patients with residual disease
If biopsy or spillage occurred
Large (T2) lesions
Adjacent organ involvement
Nodal involvement
Unfavorable histology

No Radiotherapy
T1, N0 lesions
Children less than 24 months of age
Mesoblastic nephromas

Chemotherapy

Stage I
(and patients with favorable histology)

Stage II and III

Stage IV
(and patients with unfavorable histology)

AMD + VCR

AMD + VCR, ADR in Selected Cases

AMD + VCR + ADR

Follow-Up Evaluation

Free of Disease

Local Recurrences

Distant Metastases

Radiotherapy
Brain metastases

Surgery
Hepatic or pulmonary, for resectable lesions

Radiotherapy and Chemotherapy

Chemotherapy

Supportive Measures

Stage II: Tumor extending in continuity beyond the organ of origin but not crossing the midline. Regional lymph nodes on the ipsilateral side may be involved.

Stage III: Tumor extending in continuity beyond the midline. Regional lymph nodes may be involved bilaterally.

Stage IV: Remote disease involving skeleton, other organs, soft tissues, or distant lymph nodes.

Stage IVS: Patients under 1 year of age who would otherwise be in Stage I or II but who have remote disease confined to one or more of the following sites: liver, skin, or bone marrow (without evidence of bone metastases on complete radiographic skeletal survey).

3. Prognostic Features

Neuroblastoma is a tumor with a rather grim outlook. There are a number of prognostic indicators of importance in this disease.

a. Age

Infants under 1 year of age have a distinctly better chance of long-term survival; their survival rate may be as high as 60–80%. In children between 1 and 2 years of age, the rate is 20–30%, and in patients over 2 years old, only 10–15% survive.

b. Stage

Patients with Stage I disease have the best prognosis, and those with Stage IV, the worst, except for young infants with Stage IVS disease. The latter category is confined to infants under 1 year of age and demonstrates a spectrum of metastatic lesions that include the liver, subcutaneous tissues, and bone marrow but not cortical bone involvement.

c. Distant Metastases

Metastatic spread at the time of diagnosis is a frequent finding in neuroblastoma. Except in some children under 1 year of age, metastatic spread is an extremely poor prognostic sign. There is also a difference in young infants between bone marrow infiltration such as is seen in children with Stage IVS disease and cortical bone involvement, the former being much less serious. Skeletal lesions apparent on x-ray examinations are a bad prognostic sign at any age. On rare occasions, complete disappearance of bony metastases has been reported following radiation therapy, and there have also been infrequent reports of maturation of bony metastases to ganglioneuroma.

Despite the poor prognosis in children with widespread neuroblastoma, infants with Stage IVS disease have a high rate of survival. The explanation for this improved prognosis is ob-

scure and does not appear to be related to the therapeutic regimen employed. It has been suggested that these lesions may represent multifocal sites of primary tumor rather than metastatic disease, though this does not explain why these tumors should regress spontaneously. An as yet unexplained immunologic rejection phenomenon has also been postulated, and more recently, Knudsen, the proponent of the two-hit theory of malignancy, suggested that children with Stage IVS neuroblastomas might be victims of a single mutational event rather than the two that are necessary to produce true malignancy.

d. Location

The primary site of neuroblastoma is also of great prognostic importance. Tumors of extra-adrenal, extra-abdominal origin and, in particular, mediastinal tumors seem to be associated with a significantly higher rate of survival. This may be a result of earlier diagnosis of the nonabdominal tumor, before metastatic spread has occurred.

e. Degree of Histologic Differentiation

This also has a distinct effect upon ultimate outcome. In this regard, primary tumors of the adrenal are usually poorly differentiated, and that may account, in part, for the poor prognosis in patients with adrenal neuroblastoma. There is also an association between survival and lymphocytic infiltration of the tumor, implying that an immune mechanism with greater lymphocytic infiltration may favorably influence the prognosis.

The chances of long-term survival in patients with neuroblastoma range from over 90% in patients under 1 year of age with Stage I disease to less than 15% in patients with Stage III disease at 5 years of age (see table below):

Percentage Survival of Patients with Neuroblastomas

	Stage		
Age	I	II	III
0–1	90	70	50
1–2	80	50	35
2–5	60	30	15

4. Therapeutic Management

The treatment of neuroblastoma must be tailored to the age of the child and the stage of the disease. Surgery, radiotherapy, and chemotherapy are all useful modalities. Wide surgical excision, even if it is incomplete, is associated with improved survival. Some patients, especially those with Stage III disease, seem to benefit from postoperative radiation, and neuroblastomas seem to be quite responsive, at least initially, to a number of chemotherapeutic agents including CPM, VCR, and the anthracyclines.

a. Surgical Management

Surgery is the mainstay of therapy in Stage I and II disease. The surgeon must attempt to remove the entire tumor with any involved adjacent organ (kidney, pancreas, etc.).

Abdominal primary tumors are approached through a generous transverse incision. While total removal of the lesion is the goal, it may at times be necessary to leave some tumor behind when contiguous organs are involved, such that resection would result in a prohibitive surgical morbidity or in situations where hemostasis would be impossible with such wide resection. The aortic blood supply to the tumor should preferably be controlled as the initial step; this may be facilitated by the use of hemoclips when the exposure is limited. Most neuroblastomas that arise in the adrenal gland involve the adjacent kidney and require a nephrectomy in continuity. However, in tumors that do not involve the kidney, there is no absolute requirement that the kidney be removed.

Thoracic tumors are approached through a standard thoracotomy, preferably with resection of the rib adjacent to the tumor mass.

Epidural extensions must be identified preoperatively and should be treated by laminectomy before removal of the primary abdominal or thoracic tumor is undertaken.

When laparotomy or thoracotomy have apparently allowed total removal of the tumor, it is important to sample and map the lymph nodes in the surgical area to provide an accurate assessment of the extent of the lesion. If residual tumor is left behind, metal clips are used to mark these areas.

When it is clinically apparent that the liver is massively involved, preoperative confirmation by CAT scan followed by precutaneous needle biopsy may obviate the need for surgery.

b. Radiotherapy

Neuroblastomas are ordinarily radiosensitive, and 2-year survivals following biopsy and irradiation have been reported in about 38% of cases. Traditionally, however, radiotherapy is reserved for use in Stage I and II disease as a postoperative modality if there is a suspicion of residual disease. In addition, it may be of use for palliation of symptoms in patients with Stage IV disease (bone, or even liver, metastases) or in the unresectable Stage III lesion in an attempt to render an unresectable tumor operable. Patients less than 18 months of age can tolerate 1800–2400 rads; those over 30 months can be given as much as 3000–4000 rads.

c. Chemotherapy

Various chemotherapeutic agents have, to date, failed to improve survival significantly in patients with neuroblastoma.

This being so, it is important not to injure with chemotherapy those patients who have an intrinsically good prognosis, namely, patients with Stage I, II, or IVS disease. Most oncologists treat such patients with minimal or no chemotherapy and confine their treatment entirely to surgical resection plus postoperative radiation therapy. Single-drug therapy has not been shown to be effective in Stage I and II disease.

Chemotherapy for neuroblastoma is ordinarily confined to oral or IV CPM (10 mg per kilogram) either alone every 4 weeks or alternating with VCR (1.5 mg per square meter, weekly ×4) every 12 weeks. The patients are carefully hydrated to avoid the potentially dangerous complications of chemical cystitis that may occur with the use of CPM. The anthracyclines, a group of drugs that have potentially serious side effects including myelosuppression, skin ulceration, and cardiotoxicity are recommended only for patients with Stage IV disease. The total dose should be restricted to a maximum of 450 mg per square meter to avoid cardiotoxicity.

More recent reports seem to indicate a slightly better response with more aggressive combination protocols such as

- DTIC (dacarbazine), 250 mg/m^2, IV daily for 5 days.
- Cyclophosphamide, 750 mg/m^2 on day 1.
- Vincristine, 1.5 mg/m^2 on day 5.

This regimen can be repeated every 21 days. Some investigators have even added Adriamycin, 40 mg per square meter on day 3, and lowered the dose of DTIC to 200 mg per square meter. Responses with these aggressive regimens have been reported in about 80% of cases, with 35 to 40% complete responses. The median overall survival, however, was only around 12 months, with only 18% surviving 2 years disease free. Such regimens are extremely toxic and must only be considered for patients with Stage III or IV disease.

5. Follow-Up Evaluation

Following treatment, patients should be monitored periodically both clinically and with bone and liver radionuclide scans and urinary catecholamine determinations. Most children who are free of tumor for 2 years after completion of therapy remain tumor free. However, the term *cure* must be used with caution in this disease, since on very rare occasions, there are late recurrences. The table of follow-up evaluation suggested for Wilms's tumor (Table I) can also be used in neuroblastoma with some modification.

C. Rhabdomyosarcomas

Soft-tissue sarcomas are a group of tumors that arise from the fibrous and adipose tissue, blood vessels and lymphatics, smooth and striated muscle, fascia and synovial tissue, all derived from the primitive mesenchyme. They represent 6–7% of all malignant disease of infancy and childhood.

Rhabdomyosarcoma is the most common of this group of malignancies and represents about 12% of malignant pediatric tumors. It arises from the embryonal mesenchyme, which produces striated skeletal muscle, and it represents well over half the soft-tissue sarcomas. Four morphological varieties have been described: embryonal, alveolar, pleomorphic, and mixed. The first two resemble normal fetal skeletal muscle at various stages of development.

Rhabdomyosarcoma may occur at anytime during childhood, with a peak incidence in the 1- to 5-year age group. It can arise from a primary site almost anywhere in the body, but the most common sites include the ear, the orbit, the genitourinary tract, the chest wall, the pelvis, and the extremities. Clinical manifestations will depend on the site of origin. It spreads locally and metastasizes via the lymphatic or venous system. The most frequent sites of metastatic involvement include regional lymph nodes, lung, liver, bone, bone marrow, and brain.

1. Pathological Considerations

Rhabdomyosarcoma is a malignant tumor arising from rhabdomyoblasts. Three distinct histological types are seen in childhood: embryonal cell, alveolar, and pleomorphic. The first two types account for 90% of rhabdomyosarcomas. It is not uncommon to see mixed histological patterns, particularly in the embryonal group.

a. Embryonal Cell Rhabdomyosarcoma

This is the least differentiated type, while often cellular. The botryoid type (sarcoma botryoides) is common in the urogenital tract, nasopharynx, oropharynx, ear canal, and rarely, in the gallbladder. Grossly, sarcoma botryoides appear as large, polypoid, myxomatous and edematous grapelike masses growing in a body cavity and projecting from the mucosal surface of that cavity.

Embryonal rhabdomyosarcoma consists essentially of primitive mesenchymal blastema with some rhabdomyoblastic differentiation and a myxomatous matrix. Short or long fusiform cells with abundant eosinophilic cytoplasm may be arranged parallel or in interlacing bands. The diagnostic feature is the presence of longitudinal or transverse striations in eosinophilic cytoplasm.

The prognosis in embryonal cell rhabdomyosarcoma is extremely poor. It infiltrates aggressively locally and disseminates with ease through blood vessels and lymphatics.

b. Alveolar Rhabdomyosarcoma

This type arises mainly in the extremities and less commonly in the trunk, perineum, orbit, occipital area, and tunica vaginalis. Grossly, it is a grayish-white, moist, firm, relatively encapsulated mass with areas of necrosis and cystic degeneration.

Microscopically, it consists of round-to-oval cells with prominent eosinophilic cytoplasm around nuclei arranged in groups separated by thin, fibrous strands. When central cells drop out, the alveolar pattern becomes more prominent. Invariably, strap cells with cross striations can be demonstrated.

Alveolar rhabdomyosarcoma is an extremely rapidly growing tumor with grave prognosis. It spreads via blood vessels and lymphatics.

c. Pleomorphic Rhabdomyosarcoma

This is the rarest variety occurring in childhood, and almost all these tumors arise in skeletal muscle. It is characterized by extreme pleomorphism of the nuclei and abundant cytoplasm with prominent cross striations. The cells are usually arranged irregularly but may be aligned in parallel groups.

2. Staging and Classification

Several staging systems are commonly utilized. The standard TNM classification (see.§6.II.F) takes into account the size (T1 < 5 cm, T2 > 5 cm) and local infiltration (T3), the status of the regional lymph nodes, and the presence or absence of distant metastases. Tumor grading is also commonly used for staging.

The Intergroup Rhabdomyosarcoma Study has suggested classifying these lesions in children according to the completeness of the resection:

Group I:	Localized disease completely resected with margins free of tumor.
Group Ia:	Confined to one organ or muscle group.
Group Ib:	Infiltrating but with no lymph node involvement.
Group II:	Regional disease, grossly resected.
Group IIa:	Microscopic disease at the margin of resection.
Group IIb:	Regional nodes involved but all disease removed.
Group IIc:	Regional nodes and microscopically involved margins.
Group III:	Incomplete resection with gross residual disease.
Group IV:	Distant metastases.

In pediatric tumors, a postsurgical histopathological classification has further been recommended with

- PT-1 corresponding to Group Ia.
- PT-2 corresponding to Group Ib.
- PT-3 corresponding to Group IIa or III.

- PN-1 corresponding to Group IIb.
- PN-2 corresponding to Group IIc.
- PM-1 corresponding to Group III.

3. Prognostic Features

The prognosis of rhabdomyosarcoma is influenced by several factors.

a. Age

Children between 1 and 7 years of age have the best record of survival. Unlike some of the other solid tumors of childhood, infants under 1 year of age have a particularly poor prognosis.

b. Site

The site of origin of the tumor also has prognostic significance since it can influence the onset of symptoms and the pattern of metastases. A tumor appearing in a confined, obvious area like the orbit is likely to be diagnosed promptly. In addition, the orbit does not have many lymphatics so that spread via that route tends to be minimal. Orbit lesions, therefore, are likely to have a relatively good prognosis. By contrast, lesions of the nasopharynx and adjacent areas have no anatomic barriers and may grow undetected for a considerable period of time. They frequently show evidence of lymphatic spread at the time of diagnosis. Tumors of the pelvis have an intermediate prognosis, but even there, variations occur: Rhabdomyosarcomas of the prostate have a particularly poor prognosis because they tend to spread both locally and to distant sites in a large percentage of cases. Bladder tumors, on the other hand, remain superficial, and metastases tend to be a late occurrence; therefore, they tend to have a relatively good prognosis. Extremity lesions also have an intermediate prognosis, though patients who require amputations do particularly poorly.

c. Histology

The histologic type seems to influence the prognosis to some extent. Embryonal rhabdomyosarcoma, especially sarcoma botryoides, for example, has better survival statistics than the alveolar type, which has the poorest prognosis of the entire group.

d. Stage

The stage of the disease is most important. Stage I and II disease is frequently curable, although multidisciplinary treatment has recently resulted in long-term survivals even in Stage III and occasionally in Stage IV disease. The presence of metastases is, of course, associated with the poorest outcome.

4. Therapeutic Management

Modern treatment stresses a multidisciplinary approach. When complete surgical resection is not immediately feasible, initial use of radiation and multiple chemotherapeutic agents may permit complete surgical removal of the tumor at a later date; it has certainly been established that it is possible to eradicate local residual disease with both radiation and chemotherapy. Chemotherapy and radiation may also be useful in eradicating distant metastases. While complete surgical resection is probably still the most effective therapeutic modality for the treatment of localized rhabdomyosarcoma, the current tendency is to avoid overly radical surgical procedures like amputations or exenteration whenever possible. With the use of combination chemotherapy and radiation, less extensive surgical procedures may be sufficient to achieve long-term survival. In the past, when surgery was used as the sole modality, less than 20% of patients operated upon (or less than 10% of all patients) remained free of disease following surgery, except in such favorable lesions as orbital or bladder tumors.

a. Surgical Therapy

It is important to stress several important points that today govern surgery for rhabdomyosarcoma:

- Biopsy, with surgery postponed until a definitive diagnosis, accurate staging, and multidisciplinary opinions are obtained, is strongly recommended.
- Preoperative radiotherapy, chemotherapy, or both, with split therapy and interdigitating courses, may prove extremely useful.
- Liberal use of node sampling, mapping, and marking with metal clips after completion of the resection is encouraged to facilitate postoperative therapy.
- Maximal conservation of normal anatomy and function should be considered. Preservation of bladder and sexual function in genitourinary tumors; vision in orbital tumors; voice, deglutition, and cosmetic appearance in head and neck tumors; etc.; must be seriously considered.
- Total removal of all disease should be attempted. When this is impossible, debulking with maximal tumor excision consistent with reasonable conservation principles should be carried out.
- Elective prophylactic node resections are not usually recommended since adjunctive modalities can control subclinical disease in local and regional sites.

Within that context, a slightly different approach must be considered in rhabdomyosarcomas of various specific sites.

i. Extremities. Tumors of the extremities are associated with a high incidence of lymphatic and vascular spread and have a poor prognosis. Clinically, they present as soft-tissue masses, often relatively small and subtle in nature. Lymphangiograms, arteriograms, and CAT scans can be very useful in evaluating the extent of the lesion.

The initial surgical procedure usually consists of a biopsy of the lesion with minimal dissection and avoidance of mobilization of tissue planes; this allows for a better planned total excision after the histologic diagnosis is established. There is no place for a procedure based on a quick section reading by the pathologist (fasciitis, a benign condition, is occasionally difficult to differentiate from sarcoma), and careful, leisurely examination of the tissue is essential. Amputation offers no advantage over wide local removal; the ultimate goal is total removal of the tumor with preservation of limb function and appearance, to the greatest extent possible. When the extent of the tumor precludes this goal, biopsy followed by appropriate radiation and chemotherapy may allow later surgical excision of the neoplasm with the possibility of cure and preservation of the limb.

ii. Pelvis. Pelvic tumors should be totally excised whenever possible but not with sacrifice of the anorectum, bladder, or female genital tract. The current approach entails biopsy alone for the more extensive lesions, followed by chemotherapy and radiation therapy. Further surgery of a mutilating type should only be considered if the tumor continues to grow and destroy the local structures.

Tumors of the bladder are ordinarily of the botryoid type. They are usually only superficially invasive, and radical procedures should be avoided. Combination radiotherapy and chemotherapy have permitted limited endoscopic procedures used as the sole surgical modality to be carried out with great success.

Tumors of the prostate often spread to the retroperitoneal nodes. Suspicious nodes should be biopsied, but lymphadenectomy should be avoided in order to preserve sexual function. Treatment of positive nodal disease should, rather, be with radiotherapy and chemotherapy.

Vaginal rhabdomyosarcoma (sarcoma botryoides) must also be approached with conservation in mind. Primary chemotherapy with limited surgery (hysterovaginectomy) or interstitial implantation of radioactive seeds has lessened the indications for the exenterative procedures. Small lesions might even be treated exclusively by these methods, avoiding resection, altogether.

Paratesticular tumors require more aggressive surgery because of their intense tendency for lymphatic spread. Radical orchiectomy with unilateral or even bilateral aortoiliac node dissection is recommended.

iii. Head and Neck. The overly aggressive radical resections have given way to more conservative resections with either preoperative or postoperative adjuvant radiotherapy and chemotherapy. Total surgical excision of the tumor still re-

mains the primary objective of the surgeon. The timing and extent of surgery, however, will depend on the exact site and extent of the tumor, and cosmetic and functional conservation have become major considerations.

b. Radiotherapy

Radiotherapy has been adequately demonstrated as extremely effective in controlling locoregional residual disease following surgery. Proper evaluation and planning is essential since the disease tends to spread widely along fascial planes. Plain x-rays, CAT scans, and angiography may be used to properly define the volume to be treated, and wide margins must be allowed to include all surgical and biopsy sites, all involved compartments, total muscle bundles, and lymphatic reservoirs.

Dosages must reach 5500–6000 rads in 5–6 weeks for gross disease (or 5000 rads for microscopic disease). Younger children may be treated with reduced dosages (4000–4500 rads in 4 weeks). Megavoltage units should be employed with multiple fields. Isocentric techniques and shrinking fields should be used to avoid complications, and interstitial irradiation can also be used as booster treatment or for the treatment of recurrences or metastases.

c. Chemotherapy

Effective drugs for the treatment of rhabdomyosarcoma include

- Vincristine.
- Actinomycin D.
- Cyclophosphamide.
- Adriamycin.
- DTIC.

The Intergroup Rhabdomyosarcoma Study suggest the use of a modified "Pulse" VAC (vincristine, 2 mg per square meter, IV on day 0 and day 4; actinomycin D, 0–015 mg per kilo, IV on days 0, 1, 2, 3, and 4; cyclophosphamide, 10 mg per kilo, on days 0, 1, and 2), alternating every 4 weeks with V-Adr-C for 1 year; then repetitive Pulse VAC is continued for 1 year. This regimen has resulted in long-term survivals even in Stage III and Stage IV disease. It may also make possible secondary definitive surgical procedures in cases that were originally inoperable.

Aggressive multimodality therapy may be expected to cure 75% of all patients with rhabdomyosarcomas.

D. Other Solid Tumors

1. Liver Tumors

Hepatic tumors of children are usually asymptomatic until they attain a large size. They are generally not curable unless they can be completely resected. Malignancies predominate with a ratio of 2 : 1.

Of malignant tumors, hepatoblastoma occurs in the infant under 3 years of age; hepatocellular carcinoma (histologically identical to hepatoma in adults) is seen in older children, usually over 5 years of age. The most common benign tumors are vascular in nature, either hemangioendothelioma or cavernous hemangioma. Hamartomas are next in frequency.

Abdominal enlargement is the usual presenting complaint, though the vascular lesions may present with cardiac failure as a result of arteriovenous shunting or with thrombocytopenia. Radiologic studies are diagnostic and helpful in assessing resectability; IVP, CAT scan, sonography, isotope scan, and selective celiac angiography should be performed as indicated.

Alpha-fetoprotein levels are elevated in two-thirds of children with malignant hepatic epithelial neoplasms. This is a useful diagnostic marker and may be helpful in postoperative follow-up.

Surgical resection of the tumor offers the only hope of cure, and exploration is indicated in all cases, except in the face of extensive metastatic disease. In those cases with massive local disease, preoperative chemotherapy and radiotherapy may convert an inoperable tumor to one that may be resectable. The timing of postoperative adjuvant therapy must be carefully considered with regard to anticipated hepatic regeneration. Following radical resection, hepatic regeneration is rapid and is complete in about 3 months; serial isotope scans are useful to document progress of repair before adjuvant therapy is started.

The prognosis in cases of hepatic malignancy in children is determined by the extent of the tumor. When complete resection is achieved, a 50% cure rate is possible. When recurrent disease occurs, however, death usually occurs within 1 year. Diffuse hepatic involvement or pulmonary spread preclude resection, though recently anecedotal reports of total hepatectomy with liver transplantation with apparent success have been appearing. This is strictly an experimental procedure, and not enough time has elapsed to fully assess its validity.

2. Teratomas

a. Sacrococcygeal Teratoma

Teratomas may present in many locations and are usually benign. The most common site is in the sacrococcygeal region (sacrococcygeal teratomas occur once in 30,000–40,000 live births; 75% of them are in females; and 80% overall are benign). The age at the time of diagnosis is related to the incidence of malignancy; the diagnosis is made at birth in 50% of cases; in those cases where the diagnosis is made between the time of birth and the age of 2 months, the tumor is associated with a 10% rate of malignancy. If the diagnosis is made after age 2 months, there is a 90% rate of malignancy.

The preoperative evaluation should include an IVP, a CAT scan, and myelography whenever intraspinal extension is suspected. Immediate surgical excision through a posterior sacrococcygeal approach is performed with removal of the coccyx. A V-shaped "chevron" incision provides excellent exposure. Larger tumors press against the rectum, and care must be taken to protect this structure during the resection; occasionally an additional abdominal incision may be required. The identification of malignant tissue at the margins of resection calls for postoperative chemotherapy. Before initiation of subsequent radiotherapy, a second-look procedure is recommended whereby, after 3–6 months, the residual site of disease, is reassessed and localized, using metal clips to facilitate the administration of radiotherapy, should that be necessary.

b. Teratomas of the Neck

Cervical teratomas are rare lesions in the newborn. They may be alarmingly large in size but are usually benign and technically resectable in most cases.

c. Mediastinal Teratomas

Mediastinal teratomas are usually anterior in location and may reach large sizes. Surgical removal is indicated (see §10).

d. Ovarian Teratomas

Ovarian teratomas are usually benign and may reach massive size. Bilateral lesions are present in 15–20% of cases and pose a surgical challenge to the gynecologist who wishes to preserve ovarian function. When malignancy is present, complete removal is indicated, in which case no radiotherapy is needed. Likewise, radiotherapy is not indicated if a low-grade malignancy is noted. After an interval of 3–6 months, a second-look procedure may be indicated to evaluate the need for postoperative radiotherapy. Serial sonography and CAT scans are also useful in the postoperative follow-up of these patients. In the postoperative evaluation of the benign group where metachronous contralateral teratomas often occur, frequent examination with sonography and CAT scans must be carried out to identify contralateral tumors early enough to perserve function of the remaining ovary at the time of resection.

e. Retroperitoneal Teratomas

Retroperitoneal teratomas are rarely malignant (5–10%). The malignant type usually presents as an embryonal carcinoma and may require aggressive postoperative chemotherapy and radiotherapy. Alpha-fetoprotein levels may be elevated in the presence of embryonal carcinoma and may serve as a valuable postoperative marker in the follow-up of these patients.

Generally speaking, the true malignant teratoma acts as a highly malignant embryonal carcinoma with a poor prognosis. Aggressive postoperative chemotherapy and radiotherapy are indicated, and second-look operations are recommended. One must exercise caution in those tumors that show cellular pleomorphism and disorganization of cellular pattern but that are not characteristic of embryonal carcinoma. In these cases, there is no invasion of the capsule or of adjacent tissues. The pathology report may read "malignant," but one must be careful in recommending the use of postoperative adjunctive therapy.

SUGGESTED READINGS

Solid Tumors of Childhood

1. D'Angio, G. J., Evans, A., Breslow, N., Beckwith, B., Bishop, H., Farewell, V., Goodwin, W., Leope, L., Palmer, N., Sinks, L., Sutow, W., Tefft, M., and Wolfe, J. The treatment of Wilm's tumor: Results of the Second National Wilm's Tumor Study. *Cancer* **47,** 2302–2310 (1981).
2. Beckwith, J. B., and Palmer, N. F. Histopathology and prognosis of Wilms' tumor. *Cancer* **41,** 1987–1948 (1978).
3. Belasco, J., and D'Angio, G. J. Wilms' tumor. *Ca—Cancer J. Clin* **31,** No. 5, 258–270 (1981).
4. Bishop, H. C. Survival in bilateral Wilms' tumor. *J. Pediatr. Surg.* **12,** 631 (1977).
5. Cline, M. J., and Golde, D. W. A review and reevaluation of the histiocytic disorder *Am. J. Med.* **55,** 49 (1973).
6. D'Angio, G. J., Beckwith, J. B., Breslow, N. E. *et al.* Wilms tumor: An update. *Cancer* **45,** 1791 (1980).
7. Evans, A. Staging and treatment of neuroblastoma. *Cancer* **45,** 1799 (1980).
8. Exelby, P. R. Retroperitoneal malignant tumors: Wilms' tumor and neuroblastoma. *Surg. Clin. North Am.* **61,** 1219 (1980).
9. Exelby, P. R. *et al.* Liver tumors in children. *J. Pediatr. Surg.* **10,** 329 (1975).
10. Filler, R. M. *et al.* Liver tumors. *Surg. Clin. North Am.* **61,** 1209 (1981).
11. Gehan, E. *et al.* Prognostic factors in children with rhabdomyosarcoma. *Natl. Cancer Inst. Monogr.* **56,** 83–92 (1981).
12. Gerson, J. M., and Koop, C. E. Neuroblastoma. *Semin. Oncol.* **1,** 35 (1974).
13. Hays, D. M. Pelvic rhabdomyosarcomas in childhood. Diagnosis and concept of management reviewed. *Cancer (Philadelphia)* **45,** 1810 (1980).
14. Jaffe, N. Late side effects of treatment. *Pediatr. Clin. North Am.* **23,** 233 (1976).
15. Maurer, H. The intergroup rhabdomyosarcoma study, update. *Natl. Cancer Inst. Monogr.* **46,** 61–68 (1981).
16. "National Wilm's Tumor Study—3 Protocol." Children's Cancer Research Center, Philadelphia, Pennsylvania.
17. Raney, R. B., Schnaufer, L., and Donaldson, M. H. Soft tissue sarcoma in childhood. *Semin. Oncol.* **1,** 57 (1974).
18. Sieber, W. K., Dibbins, A. W., and Wiener, E. S. "Pediatric Surgery," 3rd ed., Chapter 99, p. 1082. Yearbook Publ., Chicago, Illinois, 1979.
19. Sutow, W. W., Lurdberg, R. D., Sehan, S. A. *et al.* Three year relapse-free survival rates in childhood rhabdomyosarcoma of the head and neck. Report from the intergroup rhabdomyosarcoma study. *Cancer (Philadelphia)* **49,** 2217 (1982).

Section 8. Pediatric Tumors

Part B: Leukemias and Lymphomas

I. Leukemias of Childhood 341
  A. Introduction and Classification
  B. Acute Lymphoblastic Leukemias
    1. Typing of Acute Lymphoblastic Leukemia
      a. Morphological Classification
      b. Surface Markers
      c. Monoclonal Antibodies
    2. Clinical Characteristics
      a. CNS Involvement
      b. Testis
      c. Skeleton
    3. Prognostic Factors
      a. Age
      b. White Blood Count
      c. Race
      d. Morphology
      e. Cell Surface Markers
      f. Cytogenetics
      g. Summary
    4. Therapeutic Management
      a. Remission Induction Phase
      b. Consolidation Phase
      c. Maintenance Phase
      d. Treatment of High-Risk Patients
      e. Relapse

  C. Acute Myeloblastic Leukemia
    1. Classification
    2. Therapeutic Management
  D. Acute Undifferentiated Leukemia
  E. Chronic Myelocytic Leukemia
    1. Adult Type
    2. Juvenile Type
II. Lymphomas in Childhood 345
  A. Hodgkin's Disease
    1. Pretreatment Evaluation
    2. Therapeutic Management
  B. Non-Hodgkin's Lymphoma
    1. Clinical Characteristics
    2. Pathological Considerations
      a. Histologic Type
      b. Staging
    3. Therapeutic Management
  C. Histiocytoses
    1. Histiocytosis X
      a. Clinical Characteristics
      b. Prognostic Factors
      c. Therapeutic Management
    2. Familial Hemophagocytic Lymphohistiocytosis

Suggested Readings 349

CURRENT GUIDELINES
FOR THE MANAGEMENT OF CANCER

I. LEUKEMIAS OF CHILDHOOD

A. Introduction and Classification

The leukemias of childhood are a group of malignant conditions usually involving segments of the white blood cell population, although erythrocyte precursors are also involved in erythroleukemia. Leukemias can be classified in a variety of ways.

The classification as "acute" or "chronic" originally referred to the behavior of the disease before the availability of modern chemotherapy. The acute leukemias then tended to be fulminating and rapidly fatal, whereas the chronic leukemias were more indolent, permitting a prolonged survival often measured in years.

Today, the acute leukemias refer to conditions with a predominance of undifferentiated blast cells, while the chronic leukemias are characterized by a proliferation of more mature lymphoid or myeloid elements. The terms *acute* and *chronic* no longer reflect the anticipated length of survival.

The morphological classification of the leukemias begins with the identification of the type of cell involved. Acute leukemias of childhood are about 80% lymphoblastic, 15% myeloblastic, and 5% undifferentiated. Blast cells, which are the hallmark of the acute leukemias, are undifferentiated cells; distinguishing among the various types of leukemic blasts may be difficult using ordinary light microscopy and the usual Wright Giemsa staining. It is of more than academic interest to identify the type of blast cell present, since different types of acute leukemia require different therapeutic approaches and have different prognostic implications. Accordingly, a variety of methods have been developed for the identification of the various types of blasts, including cytological criteria, special stains, enzymatic determinations, and immunologic determinants including surface markers and reactions with monoclonal antibodies.

Currently, the most widely accepted theory of the leukemic process involves the emergence of a single abnormal precursor cell that gives rise to a self-perpetuating, poorly differentiated cell line. The clonal origin of the leukemic cells can often be demonstrated by the presence of an abnormal chromosome pattern confined to the abnormal cells. For example, 90% of patients with adult-type chronic myelocytic leukemia (CML) show the Philadelphia chromosome (9:22 translocation); a 15:17 translocation is present in the malignant cells of patients with acute promyelocytic leukemia; and the 8:14 translocations have been reported in patients with Burkitt's lymphoma. With improved banding techniques, a much higher percentage of nonrandom chromosomal abnormalities have been identified among the various types of leukemia. These cytogenetic abnormalities tend to disappear during remission and reappear during relapse.

B. Acute Lymphoblastic Leukemias

1. Typing of Acute Lymphoblastic Leukemia

Acute lymphoblastic leukemia (ALL) is a heterogeneous condition that is classified in numerous ways. Classification is crucial in order to establish the best plan of treatment and to predict the outcome.

a. Morphological Classification

A "morphological classification" (Table I) has recently been established by the French American British (FAB) Cooperative Group. The following cytological criteria have been suggested for separating ALL into three types. L1 is the usual type of ALL seen in children. L2 is the type more commonly seen in adults. There were no consistent differences reported in surface markers between L1 and L2 ALL; however, cases classified as L3 were shown to have B-cell markers and are indistinguishable from the leukemic cells seen in Burkitt's lymphoma.

b. Surface Markers

Classification by surface markers also separates ALL into three groups:

- B-cell leukemias, which are rare in infants and children, have blasts with immunoglobulins on their surfaces.
- T-cell leukemia, which represents about 15% of childhood ALL. The cells in T-cell ALL were originally identified by

Table I

Morphological Classification of Acute Lymphoblastic Leukemia

	Classification		
Characteristic	L1	L2	L3
Cell size	Small cells predominate; occasionally mixed pattern	Large cells predominate; occasionally mixed pattern	Large cells
Nuclear chromatin	Fine or clumped, usually homogeneous	Fine, usuallly homogeneous	Fine, homogeneous
Nuclear shape	Regular, with clefts or convolutions	Regular, oval-to-round, occasionally with clefts	Regular, oval-to-round
Nucleoli	Indistinct or not prominent	Large, prominent, one or more per cell	Prominent, one or more per cell
Cytoplasm	Scanty	Moderately abundant	Moderately abundant
Basophilia	Slight	Slight	Deep
Vacuolization	Variable	Variable	Prominent

rosetting of sheep erythrocytes. They are now identified serologically as well.

- Non–B-, non–T-cell ALL. The bulk of children with ALL have neither mature B-cell nor T-cell markers on their surface membranes. Molecular hybridization studies of the cellular DNA of most of these have recently been reported to show rearrangements of the genes controlling immunoglobulin synthesis, indicating that these cells belong to the B cell lineage at an early stage of differentiation.

Cells in all these groups are positive for terminal deoxynucleotidyl transferase, an enzyme usually found in normal T-cells.

c. Monoclonal Antibodies

The recent development of a group of monoclonal antibodies that react with specific cell-surface antigens has added a new dimension to the classification of ALL. CALLA, the common acute lymphoblastic leukemia antigen, is found on the blasts of most children with non-B, non-T ALL. This antibody does not react with normal cells; it does, however, react with certain other malignant cells including (TDT)-positive lymphoblasts seen in some patients with CML in blast crisis.

Other monoclonal antibodies have been prepared that react with other surface antigens on ALL blasts. The T-cell leuke-

mias, for example, are themselves a heterogeneous group of leukemias that can be sorted out by the use of monoclonal antibodies, e.g., the human thymic leukemia (HTL) antigen, the TH2+ and TH2− surface markers or the OKT system of surface markers.

The non-B, non-T CALLA-positive ALL makes up about 80–85% of the leukemias of childhood. T-cell leukemia tends to occur in older children and affects males significantly more frequently than females. Generally, they have higher WBC counts at the time of diagnosis (often in excess of 100,000 per cubic millimeter); many have anterior mediastinal masses, and some have normal or even elevated hematocrits at the time of diagnosis. The rate of induction of initial remission is similar to non-B, non-T ALL, but many of these patients relapse in less than 2 years.

2. Clinical Characteristics

The presenting findings in ALL at the time of diagnosis typically include fever, pallor, and ecchymosis; hepatosplenomegaly and joint pains may also be present, and most children have some degree of anemia. The WBC count may vary from less than 1000 per cubic millimeter to greater than 100,000 per cubic millimeter, and in most cases, blasts are found in the peripheral blood. Bone marrow aspirates show the classical monotonous picture; the usual pleomorphic marrow with mature lymphocytes and myeloid and erythroid precursors in various stages of development is replaced, almost entirely, by lymphoblasts.

Despite the fact that ALL involves primarily the bone marrow, extramedullary leukemic infiltration can occur anywhere in the body.

a. CNS Involvement

Among the more common sites of extramedullary involvement is the CNS. Signs and symptoms referable to the CNS such as headache, vomiting, nuchal rigidity, sixth cranial nerve palsy, etc. are an indication for lumbar puncture and appropriate treatment with intrathecal methotrexate if leukemic cells are found in the cerebrospinal fluid. The differential diagnosis includes hemorrhage, infection, aseptic or septic meningitis, and neurotoxicity from chemotherapeutic agents such as vincristine.

Prior to the availability of modern chemotherapy, CNS leukemia was rarely seen, probably because the patients failed to survive long enough for this complication to become manifest. As better treatment methods evolved and survival was prolonged, more and more CNS leukemia was seen. This was particularly true in infants under 2 years of age and in patients with T-cell leukemia. CNS involvement in all types of ALL is recognized as such a threat that measures for its prevention with intrathecal medication or cranial irradiation are routinely included in all the therapeutic regimens for ALL.

b. Testis

The testis is another relatively common site for leukemic infiltration. Like the CNS, it is considered to be a "sanctuary area" because chemotherapeutic agents reach the testis in less than maximal amounts. Testicular involvement manifests itself as a painless enlargement. It is sometimes discovered as part of the routine evaluation done when a patient has been in remission for several years and therapy is about to be discontinued.

c. Skeleton

Bone and joint involvement is not an infrequent occurrence. In fact, many leukemic children present with painful bone and joint manifestations or with bony radiological changes. X-ray findings include subperiosteal new-bone formation, osteolytic lesions, diffuse demineralization, and growth-arrest lines. The pain and swelling of the joints, which is sometimes migratory, can be confused with juvenile rheumatoid arthritis or rheumatic fever.

3. Prognostic Factors

a. Age

Children between 2 and 10 years of age have the best prognosis. Children between 1 and 2 years of age or between 10 and 15 years have an intermediate prognosis. Patients over 15 years of age have a more dire prognosis.

b. White Blood Count

Patients with white blood counts (WBC) less than 20,000 per cubic millimeter at the time of diagnosis tend to be good-risk patients. Patients with higher WBC counts, especially with hepatosplenomegaly and/or lymphadenopathy, presumably have a higher body burden of leukemic cells and have a poorer prognosis.

c. Race

Black children have a poorer prognosis than Caucasians in the same risk category. This may be related to a higher incidence of the B-cell and T-cell ALL in black children.

d. Morphology

Patients with L1 morphology appear to have the best prognosis. L3 morphology is associated with Burkitt's type leukemia with B-cell markers, and these patients tend to do poorly. Patients with L2 morphology have an intermediate prognosis.

e. Cell Surface Markers

Patients with TDT-positive, non-B, non-T cells appear to have a better prognosis. The recent availability of monoclonal antibodies has added a new dimension to the immunologic classification of ALL, and patients whose blasts are CALLA positive also seem to have a better outlook. Absence of glucocorticoid receptors on the surface of leukemic blasts appears to be associated with a poorer prognosis; where these receptors are absent, cells tend not to be responsive to corticosterid therapy.

f. Cytogenetics

Patients with ALL are often found to have chromosomal abnormalities. Patients with hypodiploidy tend to have a poor prognosis; those with hyperdiploidy tend to have a better one. Patients with chromosomal structure changes (i.e., 8q−14q+) seen in Burkitt's lymphoma, or with the Philadelphia chromosome (22Q− 9q+), tend to do poorly.

g. Summary

The patient with ALL with the best prognosis is thus the one between 2 and 10 years of age whose initial WBC count is less than 20,000 per cubic millimeter; whose blast morphology is L1 cells; whose surface markers are non-B, non-T, TDT, CALLA, and Ia positive; who has no extramedullary involvement; and whose cytogenetic studies show a normal pattern or hyperdiploidy.

4. Therapeutic Management

Treatment is aimed at the total eradication of all leukemic cells. To some extent, the therapeutic plan is influenced by the prognostic factors previously mentioned; obviously, in patients who have a poor prognosis, more intensive treatment plans must be devised. Primary therapy is divided into three phases: remission induction, consolidation, and maintenance.

a. Remission Induction Phase

The remission induction phase is the first phase of therapy; during this phase, the total number of leukemic cells is reduced dramatically. A patient with overt manifestations of acute leukemia is converted to one who is in clinical remission with no clinically detectable signs of leukemia. By using combination therapy with prednisone, VCR and L-asparaginase, clinical remission can be achieved in over 90% of good-risk patients.

Central nervous system prophylaxis has become an important part of the treatment regimen. A number of different CNS prophylaxis schedules have been tried: intrathecal methotrexate (MTX), cranial irradiation, and combinations of the two. More recently, long-term effects of cranial irradiation were found to include loss of IQ, learning disabilities, and atrophic defects demonstrable on CAT scan. Its use has, on a trial basis, been largely replaced in the "standard-risk" ALL by intrathecal MTX either alone or in concert with intermediate-dose MTX given parenterally with citrovorum rescue. The treatment in the unfavorable group continues, however, to be a combination of intrathecal MTX and cranial irradiation. Currently, the use of drugs to enhance movement of therapeutic agents across the blood–brain barrier is also under investigation to obviate the problems of "sanctuary" areas.

b. Consolidation Phase

This phase is begun within a few days after clinical remission is achieved. It may consist of the use of intermediate-dose MTX, either alone or with additional intrathecal MTX. The purpose is to further reduce the total-body leukemic burden and bring therapeutic levels of MTX to "sanctuary areas" like the CNS and testis. Patients who have received this type of therapy have a significantly lower incidence of delayed testicular involvement. Other consolidation regimens are under study.

c. Maintenance Phase

Maintenance therapy consists of the use of mercaptopurine given daily and MTX given weekly. In addition, periodic pulses of VCR and prednisone are given, initially every 4 weeks, later every 12 weeks. In most studies, maintenance is discontinued after 3 years. It has been demonstrated that once therapy is discontinued, the relapse rate is about 25%, mostly occurring within the first year.

d. Treatment of the High-Risk Patient

Patients in high-risk categories because of elevated white blood cell counts in excess of $50,000/mm^3$ at the time of diagnosis, or because their disease has lymphomatous characteristics (T-cell markers, mediastinal widening, etc.) are achieving better results with more intensive treatment. For example the West German (BMF) protocol calls for a multiple drug regimen including remission induction with vincristine, prednisone, daunomycin, and L asparginase plus intrathecal cytosine arabinoside and intrathecal methotrexate. If there is a good bone marrow response, this is followed by a consolidation phase using cyclophosphamide, 6 mercaptopurine, and cytosine arabinoside. Additional intrathecal methotrexate and cranial irradiation are also given during this time. There is then a 3-week period of interim maintainance using 6 mercaptopurine and methotrexate. This is followed by a period of delayed intensification using dexamethasone, vincristine, adriamycin, L asparginase, cyclophosphamide, 6 thioguanine, cytosine arabinoside, and intrathecal methotrexate. Finally the patient is maintained on daily 6 mercaptopurine, weekly methotrexate, and monthly vincristine and prednisone, with periodic intrathecal doses of methotrexate.

Using intensive treatment programs like this or the Memorial LSA_2-L_2 protocol much better long term results have been achieved in children with ALL who are at high risk.

e. Relapse

Patients who have a bone marrow relapse while on therapy have, to date, no chance for long-term survival with standard chemotherapy. A large percentage of them can be reinduced into further clinical remissions, particularly if anthracyclines are added to the induction regimen with vincristine and prednisone. VM-26 (epipodophyllotoxin analogue) and cytosine arabinoside have also reportedly prolonged the remission in these patients, but virtually none have survived past 27 months from the date of relapse, except for patients undergoing successful bone marrow transplants.

Bone marrow transplantation (BMT) has become a more accepted therapeutic modality in various types of leukemia. Currently, it is a viable alternative that is available to children with ALL who relapse while on therapy, since there is no chemotherapy regimen that has consistently produced prolonged survival in this group of patients. The technique of BMT is complex and is associated with a large number of problems in the transplanted patient, especially problems related to infection and to graft-versus-host reactions, which remain formidable. The major problem with BMT to date, however, remains donor availability; only about one third of patients will have a histocompatible family donor. The use of autologous bone marrow of treated patients, which is harvested during clinical remission and treated with monoclonal antibodies to remove leukemic cells, is now under intensive investigation and may prove to be an answer to the donor problem.

Patients who relapse after completion of therapy have a somewhat better prognosis. Most relapses occur within the first year after treatment, and they are extremely rare after 4 years. Most of these delayed relapses are bone marrow relapses, and long-term survival occurs in about 30% of these patients.

C. Acute Myeloblastic Leukemia

1. Classification

Acute myeloblastic leukemia (AML) can be classified morphologically and enzymatically. The FAB morphological classification ranges from M1 through M6:

- M1 myeloblasts may closely resemble L2 lymphoblasts; they are large cells with relatively abundant cytoplasm with one or more prominent nucleoli and minimal evidence of differentiation and maturation. However, myeloblasts, unlike lymphoblasts, are peroxidase positive, and they react poorly or not at all with *p*-aminosalicylic acid (PAS).

- M2 cells show evidence of differentiation to the promyelocyte and the myelocyte stage; most cells have numerous granules or, more rarely, Auer rods.
- M3 (promyelocytic leukemia) cells have very abundant azurophilic granules. A specific chromosomal translocation (15 : 17) is present in most cases. An occasional patient will have the microgranular variant with inapparent granules on routine light microscopy but abundant granules and the typical karyotypic abnormality on electron microscopy. DIC is very common and can result in severe bleeding once treatment is initiated.
- The M4 type has characteristics of both myeloid and monocytoid elements and is often called "acute myelomonocytic leukemia."
- The M5 form is called "acute monocytic leukemia" and has both poorly and well-differentiated monocytic elements. Monocytoid cells can be distinguished from myeloid elements by the presence of nonspecific esterase activity in the cytoplasm. These patients often have gum hypertrophy and skin infiltration.
- The M6 form is called "erythroleukemia" (Di Guglielmo's syndrome). Erythroblastosis in the marrow and peripheral blood, dyserythropoiesis and megaloblastic erythroid hyperplasia in addition to myeloblasts are noted in the M6 type of AML.

2. Therapeutic Management

Children with AML do not do as well as those with ALL. Remission can be induced in about 75% of patients with the use of cytosine arabinoside, 6-thioguanine, and the anthracyclines; some pediatric hematolgists feel that there is also a place for the addition of VCR and prednisone in the remission-induction regimen. The three main drugs are potent agents, and considerable support of the patient is needed during the prolonged periods of myelosuppression associated with their use. Prevention and treatment of sepsis is regularly required during the remission-induction phase. Maintenance therapy requires the continued intermittent use of this same group of agents, but only 30–40% of patients with AML who achieve clinical remission can be expected to have prolonged leukemia-free survival.

Better results appear to be achievable with BMT; the major problem is still donor availability, but about 60% of children with AML in clinical remission who are treated with BMT reportedly have prolonged survivals and may be cured. Many investigators feel that children with AML who have a histocompatible family donor should be given a transplant whenever a first clinical remission is achieved; this view, however, is still controversial.

D. Acute Undifferentiated Leukemia

The undifferentiated types of acute leukemia make up 5% of all cases. Little can be said about their behavior. They are unclassified though in many respects they resemble the non–B-, non–T-cell ALL of the L1 type. Therapeutic approaches are the same as for ALL.

E. Chronic Myelocytic Leukemia

Two types of CML are seen in childhood, the adult and the juvenile type.

1. Adult Type

The adult type is characterized by a very high WBC count, frequently in excess of 200,000 per cubic millimeter. All myeloid elements are well represented in great profusion in both the peripheral blood and the bone marrow, but there are comparatively few blast forms seen. These patients are rarely thrombocytopenic and are more likely to be thrombocythemic with platelet counts in excess of 500,000 per cubic millimeter. Proliferating cells in the peripheral blood and bone marrow show the characteristic cytogenetic abnormality: the Philadelphia chromosome (22q− 9q+). They do not produce erythrocytes, which contain an unusually large amount of fetal hemoglobin.

The leukemic cells are sensitive to busulfan, and the disease tends to run an indolent course with a mean survival of 5–7 years. Although the adult type of CML responds well to busulfan and hydroxyurea, neither of these agents have altered the ultimate fatal outcome of this disease.

At present, the only way to achieve a cure in children with adult-type CML is with early BMT. The timing of the transplantation, even when a histocompatible family donor is available, remains controversial. Once blastic transformation has occurred, successful BMT is not likely to be achieved. Unfortunately, there are no reliable indicators of when blastic transformation will occur, although changes in the cytogenetic patterns may suggest an imminent transformation. Many investigators therefore feel that, in the presence of a histocompatible family donor, early transplantation should at least be offered.

2. Juvenile Type

The juvenile type of CML usually presents with a lower WBC count (usually below 100,000 per cubic millimeter. While there is a profusion of myeloid elements, there tends to be a substantial percentage of myeloblasts, and the patients are frequently thrombocytopenic. The Philadelphia chromosome is absent, and levels of fetal hemoglobin are characteristically elevated (levels in the 30% range are not unusual). The "i" antigen is also present on the reds cells, another indication of fetal erythrocytosis.

The leukemic cells of juvenile-type CML are not responsive to busulfan. In fact, there is no chemotherapeutic regimen that will produce a prolonged remission, and the disease tends to run a fulminating course with virtually no chance of prolonged survival except with BMT, which should be offered whenever a suitable donor is available.

II. LYMPHOMAS IN CHILDHOOD

Lymphomas may be seen in infants and children and require a somewhat different perspective than when found in adults. In recent years, it has been demonstrated that both Hodgkin's disease and non-Hodgkin's lymphomas are often curable using available chemotherapeutic programs and/or radiation therapy. It must be recognized, however, that these therapeutic modalities when used in children can produce severe problems in growth and development. Furthermore, there are major differences in the classification as well as in the management of non-Hodgkin's lymphoma in infants and children as compared with adults.

A. Hodgkin's Disease

1. Pretreatment Evaluation

Hodgkin's disease presents in a manner similar to the disease in adults. Cervical lymphadenopathy is most common, whereas systemic manifestations (i.e., fever, night sweats, weight loss, and pruritis) are rare. All of the histologic types reported in adults (i.e., lymphocyte predominant, nodular sclerosis, mixed cellularity and lymphocyte depletion) are seen in childhood.

Staging procedures include:

- Careful history and physical examination.
- Lymph node biopsy.
- Chest x-ray.
- Staging laparotomy, including splenectomy.
- Bone marrow biopsy.
- Lymphangiography.
- Abdominal CAT scan.

All these methods are potentially useful and selectively indicated in infants and children, as well as in adults. Splenectomy in children is hazardous, mainly because of the increased risk of serious subsequent infection. If splenectomy is done, prophylactic amoxicyllin should be given; pneumococcal vaccine may also be useful in preventing pneumococcal infection in these children, and should be given prior to the splenectomy. However, most patients with Hodgkin's disease are immunosuppressed and do not produce adequate titers of antipneumococcal antibodies.

2. Therapeutic Management

Treatment often includes radiation therapy. It must be recognized, however, that wide-field and mantle radiation can have serious undesirable side effects in the growing child, including shortening and incomplete bony development. Radiotherapy, when used, should be confined to local and limited-field radiation.

A number of chemotherapeutic regimens involving the use of multiple agents have been recommended. These include

- MOPP (nitrogen mustard, VCR, procarbazine, and prednisone).
- MVPP (vinblastine, instead of the VCR).
- ABVD (ADR, bleomycin, vinblastine, and DTIC).
- CVPP (chlorambucil, vinblastine, procarbazine, and prednisolone).

All of these combinations have been used with very satisfactory results.

Children with bulky mediastinal involvement, often with nodular sclerosis histology, are particularly likely to relapse and require more intensive therapy by combined modalities.

B. Non-Hodgkin's Lymphoma

1. Clinical Characteristics

Unlike Hodgkin's disease, the pattern of presentation of non-Hodgkin's lymphoma in children is quite different from that seen in adults. Many children present with disease at extranodal sites, most commonly abdominal, mediastinal, and nasopharyngeal. Intra-abdominal involvement is likely to affect the small bowel in children, rather than the stomach, which is more commonly affected in adults.

Non-Hodgkin's lymphoma in children is frequently associated with a leukemialike picture, a mediastinal mass, spread to the bone marrow and peripheral blood, and perhaps meningeal and gonadal involvement as well. Except for the Burkitt's type, abdominal lymphomas do not tend to spread to the bone marrow. The non-African Burkitt's lymphoma often involves both intra-abdominal sites and bone marrow; the cells in the marrow are L3-type blasts with dark-blue cytoplasm and prominent vacuolization; marked hyperuricemia can occur with, at times, uric acid nephropathy. Meningeal involvement also occurs frequently in Burkitt's lymphoma.

2. Pathological Considerations

a. Histologic Type

Histologically, the non-Hodgkin's lymphomas in children are distinctly different from the adult forms. Follicular patterns, which are so common in adults, are extremely rare in the pediatric age group. Instead, lymphomas of childhood have diffuse histology and highly malignant courses. According to Murphy (5a), they may be categorized in one of three groups:

- Lymphoblastic, with convoluted or nonconvoluted muclei.
- Undifferentiated, either Burkitt's or non-Burkitt's.
- Histiocytic, consisting of large lymphoid cells.

Lymphoblastic lymphomas frequently present with mediastinal masses, and the cells are often identifiable as one of the several T-cell types. The undifferentiated B-cell type tends to present with abdominal involvement. The presence of B- or T-cell markers on the cells is a poor prognostic sign in lymphoma of childhood.

b. Staging

The purpose of staging is to define the extent of the disease, to help gauge the prognosis, and to aid in the process of selecting the most appropriate therapy. Since laparotomy is usually not done as part of the staging procedure in children with non-Hodgkin's lymphoma, the Ann Arbor classification (see §9A.II.C.1.a), which is so useful in Hodgkin's disease, has serious limitations. Other more appropriate staging classifications have been described, notably by the groups from St. Jude's Children's Research Hospital and Memorial Sloan-Kettering Cancer Center. Staging evaluation must include

- A complete history.
- A thorough physical examination.
- CBC.
- X-ray of the chest.
- Bone marrow aspiration and biopsy.
- Examination of spinal fluid.
- Uric acid, blood urea nitrogen (BUN), creatinine, and liver function tests.
- Review of the histology of all biopsy material.

If indicated, further studies might include

- Radionuclide bone scan.
- Gastrointestinal series.
- IVP.
- Ultrasonography.
- Abdominal CAT scan.
- Laparotomy to biopsy an intra-abdominal tumor.

Since all of the suggested staging systems have limitations, some groups use no specific staging system but instead have a

Table II
Two Systems of Staging of Non-Hodgkin's Lymphoma in Children

	St. Jude's Children's[a] Research Hospital	Memorial Sloan-Kettering[b] Cancer Center
Stage I	A single tumor (extranodal) or single anatomic area (nodal) excluding the mediastinum or abdomen.	One single site.
Stage II	A single tumor (extranodal) with regional node involvement. Two or more nodal areas on the same side of the diaphragm. Two single (extranodal) tumors with or without regional node involvement on the same side of diaphragm. A primary gastointestinal tract tumor usually in the ileocecal area, with or without mesenteric node involvement, grossly (>90%) resected.	Two or more sites above or below the diaphragm.
Stage III	Two single tumors (extra-nodal) on opposite sides of the diaphragm. All primary intrathoracic tumors (mediastinal, pleural, or thymic). All extensive primary intra-abdominal disease. All paraspinal or epidural tumors regardless of other tumor sites.	Two or more sites above and below the diaphragm. Extensive intrathoracic disease. Extensive intra-abdominal disease.
Stage IV	Any of the above with initial CNS and/or bone marrow involvement.	One of the above with bone marrow and/or CNS involvement.

[a]Murphy, S. B. Prognostic factors and obstacles to care of children non-Hodgkin's lymphoma. *Semin. Oncol.* **4**, 265, (1977).
[b]Wollner, N. Non-Hodgkin's lymphoma in children. *Pediatr. Clin. North Am.* **23**, 371, (1976).

uniform treatment approach. Table II is a comparative description of two of the most commonly used staging systems.

3. Therapeutic Management

Treatment regimens commonly recommended in children are based on the use of multiple drugs including VCR, prednisone, CPM, anthracyclines, MTX, and others; in addition, involved-field irradiation is often indicated. Intrathecal MTX with or without cranial irradiation is also frequently used for CNS prophylaxis. Treatment is continued for much longer than in adults, most often for 2 to 3 years. Unlike adults, where the disease has a prolonged natural history with late patterns of relapse, relapse in childhood occurs most frequently during the first 12 months of illness and hardly ever after 2 years. Furthermore, a substantial number of children are curable. Some recently reported series, including children of all ages and diseases of various stages and histological patterns, reported an overall 2-year survival of 60–75%.

With increasing success in managing lymphomas of childhood with modalities that include radiation therapy and polydrug chemotherapy that may themselves be potential carcinogens, there is clearly a risk that second independent tumors may develop in the future. Investigative studies are assessing a number of problems including appropriate limitations of therapy in children with good prognoses, the role of combined therapy (radiation therapy and multiple chemotherapeutic regimens), and possible alternatives to the use of prophylactic cranial irradiation.

C. Histiocytoses

This is a group of diseases characterized by the proliferation of tissue macrophages.

1. Histiocytosis X

Eosinophilic granuloma, Hand-Schüller-Christian disease, and Letterer-Siwe disease have been considered as varying manifestations of a single entity and have been lumped together under the designation "histiocytosis X." The condition runs the gamut from a localized benign lesion to a disseminated and often fatal systemic disorder.

The diagnosis depends upon histological appearance of biopsy material from the involved areas, which may include skin, lymph nodes, or bone. Histologically, there is a proliferation of well-differentiated histiocytes. In eosinophilic granulomas there are, in addition, a large number of eosinophils present. In Letterer-Siwe disease, there is little phagocytosis by the histiocytes. In Hand-Schüller-Christian disease, there is prominent lipid phagocytosis with foamy histiocytes.

a. Clinical Characteristics

Typically, eosinophilic granuloma is a single, benign, localized lytic lesion of bone without any systemic manifestations. Hand-Schüller-Christian disease, on the other hand, is a chronic progressive and multifocal disease; skeletal and mucocutaneous lesions often occur, but the classical triad of lytic bone lesions in the skull, exophthalmos, and diabetes insipidus is seen only rarely. Letterer-Siwe disease is an acute, systemic, nonlipid histiocytosis that is often fatal; it affects mainly infants and is characterized by fever, lymphadenopathy, hepatosplenomegaly, skin rash, and draining otitis media that is resistant to therapy. Overlapping manifestations are sufficiently common in the three conditions that the disease complex has been appropriately designated histiocytosis X.

The following features are commonly encountered in patients with histiocytosis X:

- Bony lesions are common, and their clinical manifestations will depend upon which bony structures are involved, e.g., chronic otitis, exophthalmos, etc.
- Cutaneous involvement is also common. The rash is reddish-brown and maculopapular; often involves the scalp, neck, and diaper area; and may often be mistaken for the seborrheic dermatitis of diaper rash.
- The liver, spleen, and lymph nodes are frequently involved in the diffuse, systemic form of the disease.
- The blood and bone marrow are usually normal, although there may be an increase in histiocytes in the bone marrow.
- Pituitary function is often compromised in the chronic form of the disease, with diabetes insipidus and short stature as the major manifestations.

b. Prognostic Factors

The prognosis in this disease depends upon a number of factors.

i. Age. In general, the younger the patient, the poorer the prognosis. The great majority of patients who expire are under 3 years of age. In patients under 6 months, the mortality is reported at approximately 80%.

ii. Extent of Disease. It has been noted that the more extensive the disease, the poorer the prognosis. Lahey outlined a scoring system based on the number of organ systems involved: prognosis was best in the patients with scores of 1 or 2 and became progressively poorer as the scores rose. It has also been reported that presence or absence of dysfunction in the liver, lung, or hematopoietic system have prognostic significance. Patients who have no involvement of any of those three systems responded well to therapy, and most of those patients survived; patients with evidence of dysfunction in any of those three systems responded poorly to treatment, and many of them died.

iii. Histological Criteria. A system has been devised for classifying patients into two groups based on the presence or absence of three histological characteristics:

- The formation of sheets by the histiocytes, giving a syncytial appearance.
- Prominent fibrosis and focal necrosis.
- Multinucleated giant cells.

The prognosis was more favorable when those three characteristics were present.

c. Therapeutic Management

Chemotherapy with vinblastine and prednisone or 6-mercaptopurine and prednisone has succeeded in lowering the mortality of histiocytosis X. Response to treatment may be slow with, at times, periods of increased disease activity; this does not necessarily indicate therapeutic failure. Therapy should be continued for 6–12 months after all disease activity has ceased. Radiotherapy is effective in the control of individual lesions and may be used to relieve local symptoms or to help achieve complete regression.

2. Familial Hemophagocytic Lymphohistiocytosis

This is a rare autosomally recessive disorder characterized by the infantile onset of progressive hepatosplenomegaly, fever, pancytopenia, bleeding, and irritability; most cases have been rapidly fatal. It is distinguishable from Letterer-Siwe disease by the finding of prominent erythrocyte phagocytosis, lymphohistiocytic meningoencephalitis, and the absence of skin involvement. At times, abnormal cells are found in the CSF after cytocentrifugation. Hypofibrinogenemia has been documented in a number of these patients studied. There is only one report of a favorable outcome, following the use of vinblastine.

SUGGESTED READINGS

1. Chaganti, R. K. Significance of chromosome changes to hematopoietic neoplasms. *Blood* **62,** 515 (1983).
2. Lampkin, B. C., Woods, W., Strauss, R. *et al.* Current status of the biology and treatment of acute non-lymphocytic leukemia in children. *Blood* **61,** 215 (1983).
3. Miller, D. R. Acute lymphoblastic leukemia. *Pediatr. Clin. North Am.* **27,** 269 (1980).
4. Molpas, J. S. Lymphomas in children. *Semin. Hematol.* **19,** 301 (1982).
5. Moretta, L., Mingari, M. C., Moretta, A., and Fanco, S. Human lymphocyte surface markers. *Semin. Hematol.* **19,** 273 (1982).
6. Murphy, S. B., Frizzerag, G., Evans, A. E. A study of childhood non-Hodgkin's lymphoma. *Cancer* **36,** 2121–2131 (1975).
7. Roper, M., Crist, W. M., Metzgar, R. *et al.* Monoclonal antibody characterization of surface antigens in childhood T-cell lymphoid malignancies. *Blood* **61,** 83 (1983).
8. Weinstein, H. J., and Link, M. P. Non-Hodgkin's lymphomas in childhood. *Clin. Haematol.* **8,** 699 (1979).

Section 9

Neoplastic Disorders of the Blood, Bone Marrow, and Lymphatic System

NICHOLAS LEONE and SAMUEL KOPEL

With Contributions By

Ismat Nawabi	Hematology-Oncology
Sameer Rafla	Radiotherapy
Aurelia Cacatian	Medical Oncology
Adolfo Elizalde	Hematology
Karl Jindrak	Pathology
Irene Sweeney	Radiology
Margaret Amato	Nursing Oncology
Randi Moskowitz	Nursing Oncology

351

Section 9. Neoplastic Disorders of the Blood, Bone Marrow, and Lymphatic System

Part A: Hodgkin's Disease and Non-Hodgkin's Lymphomas and Related Disorders

I. Early Detection and Screening   355
  A. Signs and Symptoms
  B. Patient Education
II. Pretreatment Evaluation and Work-Up   356
  A. Establishment of the Diagnosis
  B. Staging Work-Up
    1. Complete Physical Examination
    2. Chest X-ray and/or Chest Computerized Axial Tomography (CAT) Scan
    3. Intravenous Urogram
    4. Abdominal CAT Scan
    5. Lymphangiogram
    6. Bone Marrow Aspiration or Biopsy
    7. Closed Liver Biopsy
    8. Staging Laparotomy
    9. Liver and Spleen Scan
    10. Gallium Scan
  C. Staging and Classification
    1. Hodgkin's Disease
      a. Clinical Anatomic Staging (Ann Arbor System)
      b. Symptoms Substaging
      c. Histopathology and Typing of Hodgkin's Disease
    2. Non-Hodgkin's Lymphomas
  D. Pretreatment Preparation
  E. Multidisciplinary Evaluation
  F. Site-Specific Data Form for Lymphomas
III. Therapeutic Management of Hodgkin's Disease   362
  A. Basic Principles
  B. Treatment Modalities
    1. Radiotherapy
      a. Treatment of Early Stages Hodgkin's Disease
      b. Potential Complications of Radiotherapy
      c. Special Circumstances
    2. Chemotherapy
      a. General Concepts
      b. Drugs Active in Hodgkin's Disease
      c. Various Drug Combinations
      d. Maintenance Chemotherapy
      e. Late Effects of Treatment
  C. Specific Management Guidelines
    1. Stages I and IIA
    2. Stage IIB
    3. Stage IIIA

    4. Stages IIIB and IV
    5. Treatment of Recurrent Disease
    6. Treatment Controversy
IV. Therapeutic Management of Non-Hodgkin's Lymphoma   369
  A. Criteria for Therapy
  B. General Recommendations
    1. Nodular Lymphomas
    2. Diffuse Lymphomas
  C. Specific Management Guidelines
    1. Stages I and II
    2. Stages III and IV
      a. Aggressive Types (Unfavorable Histology)
      b. Nonaggressive Types (Favorable Histology)
  D. Potential Curability
  E. Radiotherapy
    1. Stages I and II
    2. Stages III and IV
    3. Treatment of Extranodal Sites (Stages IE and IIE)
      a. Gastrointestinal tract
      b. Waldeyer's Ring
      c. Bone
      d. Central Nervous System
      e. Orbit
      f. Skin
      g. Testes
  F. Other Therapeutic Considerations
    1. Involvement of the CNS
    2. Hyperuricemia
V. Other Specific Types of Lymphoma and Related Disorders   376
  A. Burkitt's Lymphoma
    1. General Considerations
    2. Clinical Characteristics
    3. Pathological Features
    4. Therapeutic Management
  B. Immunoblastic Lymphadenopathy
  C. Sézary Syndrome
  D. Mycosis Fungoides
  E. Histiocytic Medullary Reticulosis (Malignant Histiocytosis)
  F. Waldenström's Microglobulinemia
VI. Follow-Up Evaluation and Rehabilitation of the Patient with Lymphoma   378
  A. Psychological Support

B. Complications of the Disease and Its Treatment
C. Rehabilitation
   1. Decreased Energy Level Due to Anemia
   2. Susceptibility to Infection Due to Leukopenia
   3. Risk of Bleeding Due to Thrombocytopenia
   4. Exacerbation of the Disease

   5. Need for Blood Component
D. Follow-Up Evaluation

VII. Management Algorithm for Lymphomas   379

Suggested Readings   379

I. EARLY DETECTION AND SCREENING

There is, to date, no known specific screening procedure that will facilitate the early detection of Hodgkin's disease or other lymphomas. Education of the patient and the general public, however, is of prime importance, and health professionals must assume the responsibility of informing the public about cancer warning signs, the necessity of early reporting of any such signs, and the importance of routine periodic medical check-ups.

A. Signs and Symptoms

The typical presentation of Hodgkin's disease or non-Hodgkin's lymphoma is characterized by painless lymph node enlargement. Cervical lymph nodes are most commonly (60–80% of cases) enlarged at the onset of the disease. Mediastinal, axillary, and inguinal nodes are less commonly (6–20% of cases) enlarged at presentation. In a small minority of cases, involvement of the liver, spleen, lungs, or bone marrow is the presenting syndrome. Rarely, lymphoma may present primarily in an extralymphatic site such as bone, soft tissue, breast, gastrointestinal tract, endocrine gland, or salivary gland.

Other symptoms suggestive of lymphoma include:

- Unexplained chronic low-grade fever.
- Drenching night sweats.
- Generalized malaise with weight loss and anemia.
- Pruritus.
- Intolerance to alcohol, which evokes mediastinal or vague chest pains.

In addition, some symptoms unusual for Hodgkin's disease may be seen in non-Hodgkin's lymphoma:

- Gastrointestinal symptoms: bleeding, obstruction, masses, etc.
- Bone pain.
- Peripheral edema, ascites, or pleural effusion (mainly due to lymphatic obstruction).
- Skin manifestations: rashes, tumors, etc.

None of these early symptoms, however, is distinctively specific for lymphoma. If any are present, it is important for the patient to be examined by a knowledgeable physician, and additional work-up should be instituted to elucidate the diagnosis.

When lymphomas become progressive or refractory to treatment, late symptoms will appear that will depend on the organ systems most heavily involved.

- Liver infiltration with jaundice and eventually hepatic failure may occur.
- Pulmonary involvement may result in respiratory failure.
- Neurologic signs and symptoms can develop.
- Repeated infections with a variety of organisms is a common problem in advanced, uncontrolled Hodgkin's disease and non-Hodgkin's lymphoma, especially after heavy previous chemotherapy.
- Pancytopenia, developing as a result of progressive bone marrow involvement and/or previous therapy, and immunologic defects account for a notable propensity toward infection in patients with advanced lymphoma.
- Ureteral obstruction or compression may result in decreased renal function; renal involvement itself is a rare cause of renal failure.

Occasionally, lymphoma may manifest as an oncologic emergency in the form of a life-threatening situation:

- Superior vena cava syndrome.
- Spinal cord compression.
- Hypercalcemia (infrequent).

B. Patient Education

This must be promoted through the various channels available (hospitals, clinics, community groups, employment or industrial complexes, etc.). The public must be informed of the importance of the above signs and symptoms, particularly as regards the presence of a "lump," and stress must be laid on regular yearly physical examinations, especially in high-risk population groups (age, prior immosuppressive treatment, etc.).

II. PRETREATMENT EVALUATION AND WORK-UP

A. Establishment of the Diagnosis

Prior to lymph node biopsy, the following diagnostic tests are recommended for all patients who present with any of the previously mentioned symptoms:

- Complete blood count (CBC), including examination of the peripheral blood smear.
- Biochemical profile (SMA-18, including liver function tests, renal profile, uric acid, serum calcium, serum electrolytes, etc).
- Chest ex-ray.
- PPD.
- Serum electrophoresis and urine protein electrophoresis.
- Serologic tests to rule out certain viral infections (e.g., infectious mononucleosis or cytomegalic viral infection) and toxoplasmosis, especially if a "viral syndrome" is present.

Lymph node biopsy is the next step in establishing the diagnosis. Once a diagnosis of lymphoma is established, the histologic type and grade of the tumor needs to be ascertained.

Careful histological examination of the biopsied tissue, using different staining techniques, even including monoclonal antibody–based tests, is essential. Various technical problems may add to the already substantial difficulty of establishing a histologic diagnosis. These include

- Lack of adequate or accurate clinical information about the patient.
- Improperly chosen site of biopsy (e.g., a small, nonrepresentative node).
- Insufficient biopsy (needle biopsy is not an effective means of obtaining tissue for accurate diagnosis and typing in the case of lymphomas).
- Damage to the specimen during surgery.
- Improper fixation; mercury-based fixatives (e.g., B3) are recommended.

The following general criteria should be adhered to when considering the question of nodal biopsy:

- In cases of generalized lymphadenopathy, the inguinal and upper cervical lymph nodes should be avoided because of the frequent chronic inflammatory changes in these sites that may modify the features of the node and lead to misinterpretation. Furthermore, the likelihood of removing a nonrepresentative node is high in the case of inguinal nodes.
- From a group of enlarged lymph nodes, the largest one should be taken, since the smaller nodes may show only reactive changes.

- Crushing of the specimen by forceps or traction may render the diagnosis impossible and must be carefully avoided.
- Needle biopsy has no place in the diagnosis of malignant lymphomas.
- Fixation should be started immediately unless the node can be immediately delivered fresh to the pathology department for processing.
- Since microbiologic examination may be important in a large hospital setting, the lymph node should be sent immediately by a special messenger to the pathology laboratory along with adequate clinical information so that cultures and imprints can be made and the lymph node sliced for thorough fixation.
- A practitioner removing a lymph node in the office should immerse it immediately in a large volume of fixative, preferably a 3% solution of neutral, buffered formalin. For a lymph node 1 cm in diameter, about 30 ml of fixative should be adequate. After an hour of fixation of the capsule, the lymph node should be sliced in 4- to 5-mm-thick slices. Certain specific tests, however require special processing of the fresh tissues, and it is therefore preferable, whenever possible, to deliver the fresh specimen immediately to the pathologist.
- Frozen-section diagnosis has no place in the diagnosis of lymphoma or various other lymphadenopathies. Large pieces of valuable tissue can be lost by this method. It should be used only if a possible lymphoma has to be differentiated from metastatic carcinoma, which needs to be recognized at the time of operation.

B. Staging Work-Up

There is still some controversy concerning the types of diagnostic procedures needed to complete the staging process in patients with lymphoma. However, staging is mandatory prior to instituting therapy.

It must be made perfectly clear that the recommendations cited here are merely guidelines. Patients with Hodgkin's disease or other lymphomas must be evaluated and treated by a qualified oncologist with input from a multidisciplinary team that must include a medical and radiation oncologist. This is all the more important in view of the fact that many of these diseases are potentially curable when properly treated.

1. Complete Physical Examination

All lymph node chains must be carefully examined: cervical, supraclavicular, axillary, epitrochlear, inguinal, femoral, etc.

A full examination of the head and neck region must not be overlooked, and disease in Waldeyer's ring (tonsil, nasopharynx, etc.) must be noted.

Abdominal examination is also most important. Enlargement of the liver or spleen must be identified and other masses noted.

2. Chest X-ray and/or Chest Computerized Axial Tomography (CAT) Scan

The latter must be done if routine chest x-ray is positive or suspicious.

3. Intravenous Urogram

In view of other examination currently available (CAT scan in particular), an IVU may not be necessary for staging unless radiotherapy is contemplated (see §9A.III.B.1.a).

4. Abdominal CAT Scan

This will provide information about the liver and spleen as well as the status of the kidneys and the pelvic and aortic lymph nodes. It may also identify pelvic disease that may have escaped routine clinical examination.

A normal abdominal CAT examination does not rule out pathological involvement of unenlarged or minimally enlarged (<2 cm) nodes. A markedly positive CAT scan, however, can obviate other invasive staging procedures.

5. Lymphangiogram

The indications for this test are rather controversial in view of its invasive nature and the technical expertise that is required. It is felt that it is most productive after a CAT scan suggests the presence of intra-abdominal disease. It is urged that the physician ordering a lymphangiogram first consult with the radiologist as to the necessity of the test. It is more commonly employed in the staging of Hodgkin's disease (localized to nodes in a large proportion of cases) than in the non-Hodgkin's lymphomas (disseminated to extranodal sites in a substantial number of cases). In expert hands, the procedure carries minimal risk and provides important information necessary for staging and radiation treatment planning. Follow-up is possible with plain films of the abdomen.

6. Bone Marrow Aspiration or Biopsy

It is widely accepted, though not uniformly, that bone marrow aspiration or biopsy should be performed in all patients. The importance of medical oncological consultation is stressed, and such decisions must be left in the hands of a trained oncologist. A bone marrow study is strongly recommended in the following situations:

- Patients exhibiting B symptoms (low-grade fever, weight loss, night sweats).
- Patients with unexplained anemia, leukopenia, or thrombocytopenia.
- Patients with an unexplained elevated alkaline phosphatase.
- Patients with generalized disease (Stage III or IV—see §9A.II.C.1.a).

In experienced hands, bone marrow studies carry very little morbidity and should be considered necessary in the proper staging of all lymphoma cases.

7. Closed Liver Biopsy

If the patient is suspected of having Stage IV Hodgkin's disease and no exploratory laparotomy is being done, one should undertake a closed liver biopsy. This biopsy is also recommended in patients with B symptoms (see §9A.II.C.1.b) or when the spleen and para-aortic nodes are positive on the abdominal scan. The procedure is not usually done on children or if the abdominal CAT scan shows a normal liver and spleen. In the absence of liver biopsy and for purposes of clinical staging, an abnormal liver scan and altered liver function tests may be accepted as evidence of liver involvement.

8. Staging Laparotomy

Controversy persists as to the need for laparotomy as a mechanism for staging patients with lymphoma. It is uncommonly used in non-Hodgkin's lymphomas since a substantial number of patients already have obviously disseminated disease at the time of presentation. Laparotomy would only serve a purpose if the findings (positive or negative) would result in a major change in therapeutic approach. For example, clinical Stage I or II Hodgkin's lymphoma is generally treated with radiotherapy alone; if unsuspected lower abdominal disease or liver involvement is found at laparotomy, the patient would then receive additional therapy. Likewise, at least 20% of enlarged spleens (clinical Stage III) are found *not* to be involved with Hodgkin's disease at laparotomy, and that would result in a change in therapy. If such circumstances are considered likely and cannot be satisfactorily assessed by CAT scan or lymphangiogram, then laparotomy is indicated. On the other hand, if it has already been decided, based on initial evaluation, that systemic chemotherapy is indicated (primarily in Stages IIIB or IV), laparotomy would serve no great purpose.

The procedure is a major undertaking and includes detailed inspection of the abdomen, splenectomy, wedge and core biopsies of both lobes of the liver and any abnormal tissue, and right and left para-aortic node inspection and sampling even if entirely normal in appearance; the same holds true for iliac and pelvic nodes, splenic hilar nodes, and hepatic hilar nodes. Females should undergo oophoropexy, a procedure that entails relocating the ovaries to a region easy to protect during subsequent radiotherapy, in order to prevent sterility. The surgeon should remove any identifiable abnormal node seen on lymphangiogram, and this may require intraoperative radiography. Surgical clips should be placed in involved (or biopsied) areas to help delineate future radiation portals. The surgical mortality is less than 1%, but morbidity may be in excess of 10%, even in experienced hands. The procedure should be considered with great reserve in patients with large mediastinal masses (high anesthesia risk) and in children where there is a high incidence of postsplenectomy infection. All patients should receive pneumococcal vaccine although its efficacy remains unproven in lymphoma.

The most common area of unsuspected involvement is the spleen. About 25% of patients with clinically normal spleens are found to have involvement, whereas a significant fraction of patients with enlarged spleens will be found not to be involved. Para-aortic, spenic hilar, iliac, and portahepatic lymph nodes are sometimes found to be involved despite negative lymphangiograms and CAT scans.

If a laparotomy is not done, treatment must be so tailored as to include potential areas of involvement. For example, patients with clinical Stage II disease (i.e., neck and mediastinum involved, negative lymphangiogram, CAT scan, etc.) might be cured by radiation directed only at the mantle portal; but because the status of the spleen and the upper para-aortic areas remain in doubt, the radiotherapy fields are generally extended to encompass these areas. The decision as to whether to recommend staging laparotomy is a complex one and requires multidisciplinary consultation.

9. Liver and Spleen Scan

This scan is not necessary as a routine in early cases since there are many false negative results. The test gives accurate description of the *size* of the organs, but even extensive involvement may be missed. Abdominal CAT examination has largely supplanted this procedure.

10. Gallium Scan

A gallium scan is not necessary. It is held by some to be more accurate in histiocytic than lymphocytic lymphoma, but false positives abound.

C. Staging and Classification

Hodgkin's disease and non-Hodgkin's lymphomas share certain features and thus have been discussed together in the pre-

ceding sections. However, the two groups are so dissimilar with regard to pathological classification, modes of spread, staging, clinical behavior, and treatment as to warrant separate discussion.

1. Hodgkin's Disease

In staging of Hodgkin's disease, one must differentiate between clinical stage (CS) and pathologic stage (PS). Clinical stage is based on physical examination, laboratory tests, and radiographic interpretation. As stated above, as many as one-quarter to one-third of patients will be under or overstaged if one relies on CS alone: 20% of enlarged spleens turn out to be negative on pathological examination, and 10%–20% of negative lymphangiograms and abdominal CAT scan examinations are false negatives. Pathological staging includes laparotomy; splenectomy and sampling of nodes from the para-aortic, splenic hilar, iliac, pelvic, and portahepatic areas; wedge and core liver biopsies; wedge biopsy of the iliac crest; and thorough abdominal exploration. Thus, in a significant proportion of patients, staging laparotomy adds important information that may lead to a change in the actual stage of the disease and in the treatment protocol.

a. Clinical Anatomic Staging (Ann Arbor System)

A generally accepted clinical classification of Hodgkin's disease according to the anatomic sites involved is important to facilitate meaningful communication and to aid in planning therapy. In 1971 the Ann Arbor Symposium on Staging of Hodgkin's Disease recommended the following system, utilizing CS and PS, the latter being based on the surgical sampling of tissues during staging laparotomy. Literature published prior to 1970 should be interpreted carefully because of the varying definitions of stages. The following is the currently accepted anatomic classification of Hodgkin's disease.

Stage I: Involvement of a single lymph node region (I) or a single extralymphatic organ or site (I_E).

Stage II: Involvement of two or more lymph node regions on the same side of the diaphragm (II), or localized contiguous involvement of an extra-lymphatic organ or site and of one or more lymph node regions on the same side of the diaphragm (II_E). An optional recommendation is that the number of nodal regions involved be indicated by a subscript (i.e., II_3).

Stage III: Involvement of lymph node regions on both sides of the diaphragm. These cases may be divided into III_1, involvement of upper abdominal and para-aortic nodes, and III_2, involvement of nodes of the lower abdomen and pelvic nodes. Stage III may also be accompanied by localized involvement of the extralymphatic organs or sites (III$_E$) or by involvement of the spleen (III$_S$) or both (III$_{SE}$).

Stage IV: Diffuse or disseminated involvement of one or more extralymphatic organs or tissues, with or without associated lymph node enlargement. The involved extralymphatic site should be identified by symbols used for pathological staging.

b. Symptoms Substaging

Each stage defined above is further subdivided into A or B categories, B for those with certain general symptoms and A for those without symptoms. B symptoms include

- Unexplained weight loss of more than 10% of body weight in the 6 months preceding diagnosis.
- Unexplained fever with temperature above 38°C.
- Drenching night sweats.

c. Histopathology and Typing of Hodgkin's Disease

Hodgkin's disease is classified histologically into four major subtypes depending upon the histologic appearance of the disease in the involved lymph nodes. These subtypes are

- *Nodular sclerosis (NS):* This constitutes 30–75% of the cases in most series and is more common in females than in males. Annular bands of collagen are prominent. Reed-Sternberg cells are typically seen in free spaces (lacunar cells). Nodular sclerosis has a strong propensity to involve mediastinal nodes and is often seen in the young. The prognosis is generally good.
- *Mixed cellularity (MC):* This is the next-most-common histological type. Moderate numbers of Reed-Sternberg cells are found associated with eosinophils, plasma cells, and benign histiocytes. Males predominate in this group, and systemic symptoms are common. The prognosis is intermediate.
- *Lymphocyte predominant (LP):* This is an uncommon type of disease, often localized, and consisting of many mature lymphocytes with very few Reed-Sternberg cells. Prognosis is excellent.
- *Lymphocyte depletion (LD):* This is also a relatively uncommon type that occurs predominantly in older patients and is often associated with systemic symptoms and widespread tissue involvement. Prognosis is relatively poor.

The prognosis of Hodgkin's disease depends on both the stage and the histologic type of the disease, as well as on a few other less important factors such as the presence of bulky dis-

ease or mediastinal masses. Although histologic types are sometimes considered exclusively, there is good correlation between the favorable or unfavorable histologic subtypes and the stage of the disease. Thus, it is uncommon to find stage IA LD-type Hodgkin's disease and rare to identify an LP Hodgkin's lymphoma in a patient with advanced-stage disease. It has been suggested that Hodgkin's disease tends to propagate itself from one lymph node–bearing area to contiguous areas through normal lymphatic channels in an orderly fashion (at least in its early development). There is also some evidence to suggest that as the disease progresses, its histology may evolve from LP to MC to LD. Such a progression from early to late stage and from favorable to unfavorable histology may account for the correlation between histology and stage of disease. Those patients who present with an advanced stage and poor histology may have had rapid progression of the disease during the preclinical (prediagnostic) phase, whereas the patient who presents with Stage IA LP disease comes to our attention early because of very slow evolution. It is important to keep in mind that the pleomorphic infiltrate of normal lymphocytes, polymorphs, eosinophils, plasma cells, etc. is probably a host reaction to the malignant Reed-Sternberg cell. Thus, the predominant component in early-stage Hodgkin's disease of the LP type is normal reactive tissue. As the disease evolves (or the histological subtypes evolve), the normal reactive component diminishes while the number of Reed-Sternberg cells increases. Whether the pleomorphic infiltrate plays a role in keeping the disease in check early on is still a matter of conjecture.

2. Non-Hodgkin's Lymphomas

Though the Ann Arbor System may be used for staging non-Hodgkin's lymphomas (NHLs), there exists no generally acceptable, practical system of classification. Different groups of physicians use different terminology and classifications, frequently to the detriment of common understanding. The number and complexity of the more recent classifications is exasperating, and novel terms expressing novel concepts and interpretations of the identity of the cells forming the lymphoma only add to the confusion. The clinical usefulness of any classification is limited by the fact that lymphomas classified pathologically as the same type may vary in response to treatment, and occasionally the type itself may transform during the course of the illness, generally to a more aggressive variety. The general physician responsible for the treatment of the patient is usually concerned about two basic questions: whether the patient has a malignant lymphoma or not and how likely it is to respond to treatment.

Currently, there are several classifications of NHL in use that have scientific merit:

- Henry Rappaport's (Washington, Armed Forces Institute of Pathology) classification, probably the most widely used.
- Dorfman classification, mostly morphological.
- Lukes and Collins classification, scientifically more accurate but so far only reluctantly accepted because of its novel terminology.
- Lennert *et al.* (Kiel) classification, used mainly in Europe.

The latter two systems relate to the functional characteristics of the cells within the tumor. Modern immunohistochemical methods allow the differentiation of the cells, in histological sections, into B, T, and undifferentiated (U) lymphocytes. The results of these studies on lymphomas have not been sufficiently sorted so far as to yield a unifying, clinically useful, relevant, and reproducible classification. Furthermore, the progress in this field of research is hampered by the fact that, much as a loss of differentiation in a carcinoma may result in loss or appearance of specific new features, so the various B- or T-cell markers may be lost or possibly appear in a lymphocytic neoplasia.

Recently, an attempt aimed at creating an internationally accepted histological classification was sponsored by the National Cancer Institute (NCI), but the outcome, known as the "International Formulation," is still under debate, and its relevance is yet to be proven. In order to retain relevance and usefulness, any pathologic classification must be reproducible and should predict prognosis.

Recent progress in this field has resulted in a deeper understanding of the function and structure of the lymphocyte and its relation to the immune system; this will ultimately permit a more "biologic" classification. In the meantime, we still rely in most cases on the morphologic appearance of cells in stained sections and on the overall architecture of the involvement. These criteria are often difficult to quantify, resulting in a fair amount of disagreement, even when trained observers review the same slides. Not every community hospital will have a fully equipped immunologic surface-marker laboratory in the forseeable future, and it is therefore important to understand the current classifications, whatever their faults.

Rappaport's classification has the benefit of being relatively easy to remember; furthermore, it has the important qualification of accurately predicting the prognosis. Its major failing resides in the concept that there are two distinct types of cells: lymphocytes and histiocytes. "Histiocytes" are large cells that are generally agreed to be of monocyte/reticular cell lineage; it has been demonstrated, however, that a "histiocyte," in histiocytic lymphoma is, in the overwhelming majority of cases, a transformed lymphocyte of the T or B (usually B) types and not really a monocyte. Thus, "histiocytic lymphoma" in the Rappaport scheme is, in reality, a form of lymphocytic lymphoma. In most other respects, the Rappaport classification remains acceptable and is still in use in most clinical trials.

The Rappaport scheme divides lymphomas into two main groups: those with a nodular (follicular) pattern and those in which no nodularity is observed—a diffuse pattern. The histology in *nodular lymphomas* is marked by nodules (follicles) that are visible on gross examination or low-power magnification. In contrast to normal germinal centers, the growth of malignant nodules is chaotic; it is found in all areas of the node (rather than being concentrated in the cortical areas) and shows malignant lymphocytes both within the nodule and in the surrounding areas. There may be residual normal lymph node tissue between the nodules, in which case, differentiation between lymphoma and hyperplasia may be difficult; in the former, however, the nodules tend to be homogeneous and abnormal cells tend to be found outside the nodules. All nodular lymphomas are of B-cell origin. Depending on the predominant cell type, nodular lymphomas are subclassified as

- *Poorly differentiated lymphocytic,* where the malignant lymphocytes are small with indented ("cleaved") nuclei, inapparent nucleoli, and few large cells.
- *Nodular histiocytic,* where the cells are larger, frequently with a prominent nucleolus and a vesiculated nucleus. Small lymphocytes are few in number.
- *Nodular mixed lymphoma,* in which both poorly differentiated lymphocytes and large "histiocytes" are seen in fairly equal proportions.

In Diffuse Lymphomas, on low-power magnification there is no evidence of a nodular pattern. The architecture of the node is effaced by sheets of malignant tissue. Depending on cell type, diffuse lymphomas are subdivided into

- *Well-differentiated lymphocytic lymphoma:* The solid counterpart of chronic lymphocytic leukemia. This type is usually a B-cell disorder but of a different stage of development than the nodular poorly differentiated lymphocytic lymphoma, which is still associated with follicles. Patients with this subtype tend to have early bone marrow and vascular invasion; their cases comprise less than 5% of NHLs.
- *Diffuse poorly differentiated lymphocytic lymphoma:* The cells are similar to those of nodular poorly differentiated lymphoma, cleaved and small. Most adult cases are of B-cell type and is of intermediate prognosis. In adolescents and young adults, a T-cell type of diffuse poorly differentiated lymphocytic lymphoma is seen. This type is frequently accompanied by mediastinal masses, rapidly progressive disease, and early transformation into a leukemic phase. The prognosis is very poor.
- *Diffuse lymphocytic-histiocytic malignant lymphoma:* Cell types are similar to the cells of nodular mixed lymphoma and may represent an evolution of nodular mixed lymphomas. Most cases are B-cell type ("histiocytic," or transformed B-lymphocyte).

- *Diffuse histiocytic lymphomas:* Large cells, vesiculated nuclei, and prominent nucleoli are features of the predominant cell type. They may be of B, T, or unknown subtypes. In some patients, cells of different sizes are present with basophilic nucleoli, lobulated nuclei, and frequent mitotic figures. This type has been referred to as pleomorphic. Diffuse histiocytic lymphoma comprises a number of subtypes categorized separately in other classifications schemes (see Table I).
- *Undifferentiated lymphomas:* Burkitt's type, a B cell with round or oval nucleis, strikingly uniform in size and in "starry-sky" appearance on low-power magnification. The starry-sky effect is due to less densely staining macrophages in a dark carpet of malignant cells.

The Lukes and Collins as well as the Kiel classifications are based on functional characteristics and require the backup of an immunology laboratory in order to take full advantage of the proposed changes. There is general agreement that these classifications are based on more scientific data and concepts than the Rappaport scheme, which is based on morphology alone. On the other hand, many pathologists and hematologists are comfortable with the latter and have been somewhat reluctant to adopt the new terminology associated with the former two systems.

Table I is a comparative tabulation of the three more commonly used classifications for NHL.

A collaborative effort to bridge the differences between the competing classifications was issued in the recent publication of a new "International Working Formulation of Non-Hodgkin's Lymphoma," which incorporates some of the better features of the existing systems and attempts to reduce esoteric terminology to a minimum by grouping the various subtypes by prognostic implication (see Table II).

It is necessary to stress that accurate subtyping of NHL is rather difficult. However, with good material and careful sectioning and staining, excellent concordance can be achieved, especially as regards differentiation of Hodgkin's disease from NHL, diffuse from nodular varieties, and "good prognosis" from "poor prognosis" cases.

D. Pretreatment Preparation

Most patients with early Hodgkin's disease will require little or no preparation since they are often in apparent good health. Patients with advanced disease and Stage B symptoms must be treated without delay. Any needed symptomatic and/or sup-

Table I

A Comparison of Classification of Non-Hodgkin's Lymphomas[a]

Popular terminology	Rappaport (1966)	"Kiel classification" (1974)	Lukes and Collins (1974)
Giant follicle lymphoma	Nodular lymphomas (b-F) Lymphocytic, poorly differentiated (c-F) Mixed lymphocytic-histiocytic (e-F) Histiocytic	Low-grade malignancy (a) Lymphocytic (a) Lymphoplasmacytoid (b) Centrocytic	Undefined cell type T-cell types (b) Convoluted lymphocytic (e) Immunoblastic sarcoma (T-cell)
Lymphosarcoma	Diffuse lymphomas (a) Lymphocytic, well-differentiated (b) Lymphocytic, poorly differentiated (c) Mixed lymphocytic-histiocytic	(c) Centroblastic-centrocytic follicular (b-,c-,e-,F), follicular and diffuse, diffuse High-grade malignancy (e) Centroblastic	B-cell types (a) Small lymphocytic (a) Plasmacytoid lymphocytic Follicular center cell (follicular, follicular and diffuse, diffuse, sclerotic):
Reticulum cell sarcoma	(d) Histiocytic, well-differentiated (e) Histiocytic, poorly differentiated (f) Undifferentiated, pleomorphic	Lymphoblastic (q) Burkitt's type (b) Convoluted cell type (e) Immunoblastic	(b) Small cleaved (e) Large cleaved
Burkitt's tumor	(g) Undifferentiated, Burkitt's type		(q) Small noncleaved (e) Large noncleaved (e) Immunoblastic sarcoma (B-cell) Histiocytic (d) Unclassifiable

[a] Note: letters in parentheses allow comparison of entries in recently proposed systems to those in the modified Rappaport system.

Table II

International Working Formulation of Non-Hodgkin's Lymphoma

Working formulation	Rappaport terminology
Low Grade	

A. Malignant lymphocytic
    Small lymphocytic consistent with
    chronic lymphocytic leukemia
    plasmacytoid
	Diffuse well-differentiated
	lymphocytic

B. Malignant lymphoma, follicular
    Predominantly small cleaved-cell
    diffuse areas; sclerosis
	Nodular poorly differenti-
	ated lymphocytic

C. Malignant lymphoma, follicular
    Mixed, small cleaved- and large-cell
    diffuse areas; sclerosis
	Nodular mixed lympho-
	cytic-histiocytic

Intermediate grade	

D. Malignant lymphoma, follicular
    Predominantly large-cell diffuse
    areas; sclerosis
	Nodular histiocytic

E. Malignant lymphoma, diffuse Small cleaved-cell	Diffuse poorly differenti- ated lymphocytic

F. Malignant lymphoma, diffuse
    Mixed, small- and large-cell scle-
    rosis; epitheloid cell component
	Diffuse mixed lympho-
	cytic-histiocytic

G. Malignant lymphoma, diffuse
    Large-cell, cleaved-cell, non-
    cleaved-cell; sclerosis
	Diffuse histiocytic

High grade	

H. Malignant lymphoma
    Large-cell, immunoblastic, plas-
    macytoid, clear-cell, poly-
    morphous; epitheloid cell
    component
	Diffuse histiocytic

I. Malignant lymphoma
    Lymphoblastic, convoluted-cell,
    nonconvoluted cell
	Diffuse lymphoblastic

J. Malignant lymphoma
    Small noncleaved cell, Burkitt's fol-
    licular areas
	Diffuse undifferentiated

portive therapy may be instituted immediately and simultaneously but should not delay therapy.

Likewise, most patients with NHL will require no preparation prior to treatment. An exception is the patient with a rapidly growing tumor of poor histology—most commonly Burkitt's lymphoma—in whom massive lysis of tumor is anticipated once chemotherapy is initiated. In order to prevent or ameliorate the serious metabolic consequences resulting from the "tumor lysis syndrome," patients should be kept very well hydrated, should be started on massive (600–900 mg) doses of allopurinol, and should be monitored very frequently during the first few days of treatment.

E. Multidisciplinary Evaluation

The importance of a multidisciplinary approach for consultation, evaluation and treatment of the patient with Hodgkin's disease or NHL must be stressed. Besides the traditional areas of medical oncology, radiotherapy, and general surgery, other specialties can offer the patient additional desirable expertise. Pediatrics, nursing oncology, social services, rehabilitation, psychology, radiology, pathology, psychiatry, and immunology are of importance.

It is most desirable to introduce this concept of multidisciplinary consultation to those health professionals involved in the diagnosis and care of the patient with lymphoma.

F. Site-Specific Data Form for Lymphomas
(see pp. 363–364)

A site-specific data sheet should include all pertinent information relating to the disease, histology, physical findings, laboratory data, and classification. This sheet should be completed prior to therapy for all patients with lymphoma; it must also include staging parameters and mapping of the disease.

III. THERAPEUTIC MANAGEMENT OF HODGKIN'S DISEASE

The treatment of Hodgkin's disease has improved dramatically in the past 20 years, illustrating the value of coordinated multidisciplinary approaches consisting of meticulous pathological classification, careful clinical staging, a team approach to therapy, and the clinical trial method. Prior to the development of modern radiotherapy and chemotherapy, the median survival of patients with Hodgkin's disease was about 2 years. At present, most patients with localized disease are cured with radiation therapy, and a majority of those with disseminated disease are apparently cured with combination chemotherapy.

Nevertheless, the optimum treatment of Hodgkin's disease in any stage is complicated and is still in a state of transition. Current investigational efforts are directed toward finding treatment programs that maximize remission rates and durations while, at the same time, minimizing immediate and long-term complications.

A. Basic Principles

- In many cases, the disease appears to spread in an orderly fashion from one group of nodes to the next contiguous group.

SITE-SPECIFIC DATA FORM—HODGKIN'S DISEASE AND NON-HODGKINS LYMPHOMA

HISTORY

Age: _____

Symptoms
- _____ Fever
- _____ Weight loss _____ lbs.
- _____ Night sweats
- _____ Pain
- _____ Pruritis
- _____ General malaise
- _____ GI symptoms
- _____ Skin manifestations
- _____ Other

Social history
  Occupation: _____
  Race: _____ White _____ Black _____ Oriental _____ Other
  Marital status: _____ Single _____ Married _____ Other
Family history of carcinoma
  Relation: _____ Site: _____
Previous history of carcinoma:
  _____ No _____ Yes   Site: _____
Previous treatment (describe): _____
_____
_____
_____

PHYSICAL EXAMINATION

Weight: _____
Palpable adenopathy: _____ No _____ Yes

Area	R	L	Size (cm)
Preauricular	_____	_____	_____
Occipital	_____	_____	_____
Upper cervical	_____	_____	_____
Lower cervical	_____	_____	_____
Submental	_____	_____	_____
Supraclavicular	_____	_____	_____
Infraclavicular	_____	_____	_____
Axillary	_____	_____	_____
Epitrochlear	_____	_____	_____
Para-aortic	_____	_____	_____
Hilar	_____	_____	_____

Area	R	L	Size (cm)
External iliac	_____	_____	_____
Inguinal	_____	_____	_____
Femoral	_____	_____	_____
Waldeyer's ring	_____	_____	_____
Lung parenchyma	_____	_____	_____
Splenomegaly	_____	_____	_____
Bone marrow involvement:	_____ No	_____ Yes	
Other: _____			

Distant metastasis: _____ No _____ Yes
Histologic Diagnosis: _____

PREOPERATIVE WORK-UP (Check, if done)

Investigation	Neg.	Pos.	Suspicious
CBC, differential	_____	_____	_____
Chemistry profile	_____	_____	_____
PPD	_____	_____	_____
Chest x-ray	_____	_____	_____
Chest tomogram	_____	_____	_____
Chest CAT scan	_____	_____	_____
IVP	_____	_____	_____

Investigation	Neg.	Pos.	Suspicious
Adb/pelvic CAT scan	_____	_____	_____
Lymphangiogram	_____	_____	_____
Liver scan	_____	_____	_____
Total body bone scan	_____	_____	_____
Bone marrow biopsy	_____	_____	_____
Bone marrow aspirate	_____	_____	_____
Staging laparotomy	_____	_____	_____
Staging: _____ No _____ Yes			

Classification
  Hodgkin's stage (Ann Arbor): _____
  Symptom classification: _____ A _____ B
  Non-Hodgkin's histologic classification
    _____ Nodular _____ Diffuse
    Cell type (Rappaport): _____
    Other classification: _____
Signature: _____
Countersignature: _____
Date: _____

Staging Classification of Lymphomas

<u>Hodgkin's Disease</u>

Staging—Ann Arbor classification

Stage I: Involvement of a single lymph node region or a single extralymphatic organ or site (IE)
Stage II: Involvement of two or more lymph node regions (number to be stated) on the same side of the diaphragm
            or localized involvement of extralymphatic organ or site and one or more lymph node regions on the same
            side of the diaphragm (IIE)
Stage III: Involvement of the lymph node regions on both sides of the diaphragm, which may also be accompanied
            by localized involvement of extralymphatic organ or site or by involvement of the spleen or both.
            Subclassification into 1 and 2 indicates lower or upper abdominal nodes involved
Stage IV: Diffuse or disseminated involvement of one or more extralymphatic organs or tissues with or without
            associated lymph node enlargement. The reason for classifying the patient as stage IV is identified
            further by defining sites: pulmonary (PUL), brain (BRA), pleura (PLE), osseous (OSS), skin (SKI),
            hepatic (HEP), lymph nodes (LYM), eye (EYE), bone marrow (MAR), other (OTH)

Systemic Symptoms

Each stage is subdivided into A and B categories, B for those with defined general symptoms and A for those without.
The B classification will be given to those patients with unexplained weight loss of more than 10% of the body weight
in the 6 months before admission, or unexplained fever with temperatures above 38°C, night sweats, or any combination
of those. Note: pruritis alone does not qualify for B classification. Also, a short febrile illness associated with infection
will not qualify for B classification.

Pathologic Staging (PS)

Involvement found at laparotomy or by any further removal of tissue for histologic examination other than that
taken for the original diagnosis.

N+ or N−   Lymph node positive (+) or negative (−) for disease by biopsy
H+ or H−   Liver positive or negative by liver biopsy
S+ or S−   For spleen, positive or negative after splenectomy
L+ or L−   For lung, positive or negative by biopsy
M+ or M−   For marrow, positive or negative by biopsy or smear
P+ or P−   For pleura, involved or negative by biopsy or cytologic examination
O+ or O−   For osseous involvement or its absence by biopsy
D+ or D−   For skin involvement or its absence by biopsy

Examples

CSIAPSI   Clinical stage I without symptoms, and pathologic stage I with negative spleen after
S−H−N−M−   splenectomy, liver biopsy negative, additional lymph node biopsy negative, and
               marrow biopsy negative

CSIIA₃PSIIIA   Clinical stage IIA with three lymph node regions involved, pathological stage III
S+N+H−M−   with spleen positive, abdominal lymph node positive, liver biopsy
               negative, bone marrow biopsy negative

Histologic Types

1. Lymphocyte predominant (LP)
2. Nodular sclerosis   (NS)
3. Mixed cellularity   (MC)
4. Lymphocyte depleted   (LD)

<u>Non-Hodgkin's lymphoma</u>

Although lymphomas are staged as described above, non-Hodgkin's lymphomas are usually classified according
to Rappaport's schema into the following:

1. Nodular lymphoma
2. Diffuse lymphoma

Futher subclassifications will depend on the predominant cell type:

Nodular lymphoma   Diffuse lymphoma
Poorly differentiated lymphocytic   Well-differentiated lymphocytic
Nodular histiocytic   Poorly differentiated lymphocytic
Nodular mixed   Diffuse lymphocytic histiocytic
                                      Diffuse histiocytic
                                      Undifferentiated lymphoma (Burkitt's)

- Radiotherapy in sufficient doses can sterilize a given mass of Hodgkin's disease; in other words, a tumoricidal dose of radiation exists.
- Combined chemotherapy is capable of curing patients with disseminated disease.

B. Treatment Modalities

1. Radiotherapy

a. Treatment of Early Stages of Hodgkin's Disease

With few exceptions, irradiation is the primary form of treatment for all localized stages of Hodgkin's disease (Stages I, II, and III1A). Several forms of the disease exist, however, where, even in early-stage presentation, radiotherapy needs to be supplemented or modified, for example, cases with large mediastinal masses or those where the condition of the spleen is uncertain. Whether patients with limited extranodal disease (e.g., bone or pulmonary lymphoma) should be treated by radiation alone or by a combination of radiation and chemotherapy is still controversial. It is strongly recommended that all the investigational steps previously described be taken prior to undertaking therapy. Furthermore, an IVU and lymphangiogram are necessary for treatment planning and shielding of important structures (e.g., kidneys).

The *technique* of radiotherapy is extremely important, and several authors have demonstrated conclusively that cure rates are affected substantially by changes in technique. To wit, the introduction of accelerator beam therapy; the use of a large-field, high-dose approach; and the inclusion of several neighboring nodal regions that are apparently uninvolved have been credited with the highly satisfactory outcome (80% to over 90% cure rates) often reported in early-stage disease.

It is because of the complexities of the technique, the need for careful protection of neighboring sensitive organs (lung, kidney, etc.), and the potential for permanent radiation damage to those organs that treatment of Hodgkin's disease should be carried out by qualified radiation therapists equipped with state-of-the-art tools of treatment planning, beam-directing devices, and an array of different types of radiation beams, preferably photons originating from an accelerator or a highly collimated γ beam. The main advantage of these modalities is essentially in the sharp demarcation (or small penumbra) that enables careful and accurate beam volume delineation and limitation of the irradiation to areas of interest. This, coupled with the use of lead blocks to protect vital structures, assures safe delivery of high-dose radiation to the needed volumes.

The *volume* that is treated usually includes several adjoining areas in addition to the site primarily involved. Whether all the nodal sites should be treated (total nodal irradiation) or only

nodes of the upper trunk (mantle field) or of the lower trunk (inverted Y field encompassing the para-aortic and pelvic nodes) is still unsettled and generally depends on the stage of the disease. However, most authors agree that total nodal irradiation should only be used in Stage IIIA disease and should include the splenic pedicle (if the spleen was removed) or a complete splenic portal (if the spleen is present) in addition to a porta hepatis portal. Mantle or inverted-Y irradiation seems to be adequate in Stage II disease; however, the addition of a field to treat the upper para-aortic nodes is essential in the case of mediastinal Stage II disease (especially if the lower mediastinal nodes are involved. The choice of treatment volume in Stage I Hodgkin's disease is debatable. There is evidence to suggest that the use of "extended-field" irradiation, which includes several neighboring sites in addition to the presenting site, is followed by a higher incidence of cure and disease-free survival than is seen after the use of "involved-field" irradiation (field encompassing only the site of the presenting disease) only. However, survival rates are not statistically different, indicating that patients whose disease recurs after the use of involved-field irradiation are salvaged (or cured) by further therapy (radiation or chemotherapy).

The *doses* of radiation given to these volumes are rather critical if one is to avoid substantial myelosuppression and achieve the highest level of cure rates. Many factors are taken into consideration. Generally, a dose of 4000–4500 rads (40–45 grays) is essential for sterilization of gross disease, but smaller doses on the order of 3500 rads are adquate for control of microscopic disease.

b. Potential Complications of Radiotherapy

A large number of complications and late effects of radiotherapy have been reported; these include

- Radiation effect on bone growth in childhood.
- Sterility in young patients.
- Leukemia, particularly when radiotherapy is used in conjunction with chemotherapy.
- Chronic myelosuppression, in patients treated by total nodal radiotherapy.
- Renal impairment, if the spleen is irradiated.
- Lung fibrosis and perimyocarditis, if the chest and mediastinum are treated.
- Hypothyroidism.
- Transverse myelitis.

These are rarely seen when radiation planning is carefully carried out and when the proper precautions are taken.

c. Special Circumstances

i. Cases with Large Mediastinal Masses. It is now recognized that the presence of a large mediastinal mass (especially when it exceeds one-third of the diameter of a chest x-ray) at the level of T5 is accompanied with a high incidence of failure if treatment is limited to a routine mantle portal. Therapy must consist either of a combined chemotherapy/radiotherapy approach or of the extension of the radiation fields to include both lungs, which must receive low-dose radiation (2000 rads in 4 weeks). While both approaches seem to yield comparable cure rates (or disease-free survivals), treatment complications and organs at risk are somewhat different. The choice of treatment in any particular case needs the input of an expert multidisciplinary team and must be carried out in all cases by a proficient therapist.

ii. Hodgkin's Disease in the Young. While the prospects for cure in young patients are particularly good, even in advanced stages, complications of treatment can be severe, and in some cases, the long-term effects can be most undesirable. Of these, the most important is the effect on the bone growth centers, leading to possible stunted growth when treating the very young (<10 years of age). However, recent studies have demonstrated that sitting height (or torso length) is the only parameter affected, and a compensatory mechanism in lower limb growth centers alleviates that effect, with the resultant average standing height being normal (or even higher).

Gonadal effects with possible sterilization is another undesirable long-term effect. This is particularly dreaded in patients receiving a full inverted-Y irradiation for pelvic or inguinal nodal disease. Such sterility is preventable in the female by relocation of the ovaries but only partially preventable in the male, even with heavy scrotal shielding. However, in most cases, testicular function does eventually recover adequately after 1–2 years, if the scrotum has been fully shielded during treatment. The use of semen banks is an effective method of bridging this gap of 1–2 years and would also insure the complete absence of potential genetic radiation-induced teratogenetic effects.

The incidence of leukemia or second malignancies (especially nonlymphocytic leukemias) that was noted in patients undergoing combined therapy (chemotherapy and radiation) for Hodgkin's disease is now accepted to be a hazard attached to the chemotherapy, particularly after the prolonged use of alkylating agents.

iii. Extranodal Presentation. Many notable authors argue that extranodal localized disease presentations (i.e., E stage) do not affect the results of treatment. Nevertheless, the presence of such a presentation may necessitate large-volume treatment carried to high doses to a sensitive organ such as the lungs or spine, an approach accompanied by a high risk of serious complications. The treatment of these patients by radiation must be planned very carefully and is better left in the hands of therapists accustomed to managing such complex problems.

iv. Consolidation Radiotherapy. This term is applied to the use of radiation in conjunction with chemotherapeutic agents, usually in the treatment of advanced stages (Stage IV or IIIB) and generally in patients presenting with bulky disease. The use of radiation in these situations is planned jointly with the medical oncologist; timing is of the utmost importance (for example, whether treatment is started after three courses or six courses of chemotherapy), and the particular drugs used will have a considerable impact (for example, when Adriamycin is used in patients with mediastinal disease). Rest periods after chemotherapy and the patient's tolerance must also be taken into account. Generally, radiation is only applied to limited volumes (essentially, to regions of presenting bulky disease), and doses are limited to about 2000–2500 rads).

2. Chemotherapy

Over 15 years of experience with the four-drug regimen nitrogen mustard, oncovin, procarbazine, and prednisone (MOPP), which was developed by DeVita and his associates at NCI, has demonstrated the attainment of complete remissions in 80% of patients with advanced disease and an apparent cure in more than half. The success of this regimen illustrates the basic concepts underlying modern combination chemotherapy.

a. General Concepts

- A combination of active single agents is used, resulting in added therapeutic benefit without entirely additive toxicity.
- Drugs are given intermittently, permitting bone marrow, gastrointestinal tract, and other tissues to repair damage during a 2- to 4-week drug-free period of each cycle.
- Complete remissions occur much more frequently in response to combinations than to single agents.

b. Drugs Active in Hodgkin's Disease

Alkylating agents	Antibiotics
nitrogen mustard	Adriamycin
cyclophosphamide	bleomycin
chlorambucil	
nitrosoureas (BCNU, CCNU)	
dacarbazine (DTIC)	
	Corticosteroids
Vinca alkaloids	Miscellaneous
vincristine	VM-26 (epipodophyllotoxin
vinblastine	analogue) procarbazine

c. Various Drug Combinations

Tables III and IV may help to summarize existing information about the type of drugs used for treatment of these patients.

It must be stressed that the above are merely guidelines and that any patient with this disease should be evaluated and treated by a qualified medical oncologist and/or radiation oncologist.

In general, treatment with combination chemotherapy must be continued for at least 6 months, though some programs require a year of treatment. Most chemotherapists will give at least two full courses of treatment after demonstrable complete remission is achieved. If complete remission is *not* attained after six courses of chemotherapy, it is advised that treatment be switched to a non–cross-resistant regimen, for example, ABVD (Adriamycin, bleomycin, vinblastine, and dacarbazine) after MOPP.

Ascertaining the adequacy of clinical complete remission is most important. It is necessary to evaluate all the areas known to be involved before therapy was instituted to assure that disease control has been attained in all areas. This generally requires repetition of all initial staging procedures that were positive, though a laparotomy is generally not repeated. Careful attention must be paid to any previously involved site that is not easily accessible for restaging after treatment. Most relapses occur in

Table III

Drug Combinations in Hodgkin's Disease[a]

Regimen[b]	Dose
MOPP	
Nitrogen mustard	6 mg/m^2, IV on days 1 and 8
Vincristine	1.4 mg/m^2, IV on days 1 and 8, maximum 2 mg per dose
Procarbazine	100 mg/m^2, PO on days 1–14
Prednisone (cycles 1 and 4)	40 mg/m^2, PO on days 1–14
MVPP	
Nitrogen mustard	6 mg/m^2, IV on days 1 and 8
Vinblastine	6 mg/m^2, IV on days 1 and 8
Procarbazine	100 mg/m^2, PO on days 1–15
Prednisone (each cycle)	40 mg/m^2, PO on days 1–15
BCVPP	
BCNU	100 mg/m^2, IV q. 28 days
Vinblastine	5 mg/m^2, IV q. 28 days
Cyclophosphamide	600 mg/m^2, IV q. 28 days
Procarbazine	100 mg/m^2, PO on days 1–10
Prednisone (each cycle)	60 mg/m^2, PO on days 1–10

[a] Modified from Rosenthal and Bennett (14).
[b] Repeat every 28 days; minimum of six cycles.

Table IV

Drug Combinations in MOPP-Resistant Hodgkin's Disease[a]

Regimen	Dose
ABVD (repeat every 28 days)	
Adriamycin	25 mg/m^2, IV on days 1 and 15
Bleomycin	10 mg/m^2, IV on days 1 and 15
Vinblastine	6 mg/m^2, IV on days 1 and 15
Dacarbazine	375 mg/m^2, IV on days 1 and 15
CVB (repeat every 28 days)	
CCNU	100 mg/m^2, PO on day 1
Vinblastine	6 mg/m^2, IV on days 1 and 8
Bleomycin	15 mg, IM on days 1 and 8
B-DOPA (repeat every 21–28 days)	
Bleomycin	4 mg/m^2, IV on days 2 and 5
Dacarbazine	150 mg/m^2, IV on days 1–5
Vincristine	1.5 mg/m^2, IV on day 1
Prednisone	40 mg/m^2, PO on days 1–6
Adriamycin	60 mg/m^2, IV on day 1
BVAS (repeat every 28 days for 12 cycles)	
Bleomycin	5 mg/m^2, IV on days 1 and 15
Vinblastine	6 mg/m^2, IV on days 1 and 15
Adriamycin	30 mg/m^2, IV on day 1
Streptozotocin	1500 mg/m^2, on days 1 and 15
B-CAVe (repeat every 42 days to total Adriamycin dose of 450 mg/m^2)	
Bleomycin	2.5 mg/m^2, IV on days 1, 28, and 35
CCNU	100 mg/m^2, PO on day 1
Adriamycin	60 mg/m^2, IV on day 1
Vinblastine	5 mg/m^2, IV on day 1

[a] Modified from Rosenthal and Bennett (14).

previously involved sites, especially if "bulky" disease was present.

d. Maintenance Chemotherapy

There is currently no conclusive evidence that maintenance therapy is of any benefit in Hodgkin's disease patients after a complete remission has been induced by intensive chemotherapy. Studies done at NCI show no difference in survival between patients in complete remission receiving no maintenance therapy and those placed on long-term BCNU or additional MOPP. Most patients who relapse after 1 year of apparent remission will respond again to one or another of the combinations described previously. This "salvage chemotherapy" approach is preferred to "maintenance therapy," since the latter is often associated with increased bone marrow suppression, infectious complications, and an increased risk of acute leukemia.

e. Late Effects of Treatment

i. Leukemia. A disturbingly high incidence of late-onset acute leukemia has been reported in patients treated for Hodgkin's disease. While the incidence of the dread complication is not significant in patients treated with radiation alone, it is seen more commonly in patients receiving chemotherapy, and its incidence rises markedly in patients who receive combined-modality treatment (radiotherapy and chemotherapy). This knowledge has fostered considerable debate on what constitutes the optimum current treatment of advanced Hodgkin's disease. In most studies comparing combined-modality treatment with chemotherapy alone, the complete remission rate is higher for the combined-modality group. Thus, one segment of opinion maintains that the optimum treatment is that which yields the highest complete remission rate, i.e., combined modality. The opposing view is that the higher initial complete remission rate does not necessarily imply higher ultimate survival rates. This view maintains that, given the effectiveness of subsequent salvage regimens, a policy of applying combined-modality treatment exclusively in cases of disease recurrence can confine the increased leukemia risk to this subgroup of patients only rather than the whole population. At present, the issue remains unresolved.

ii. Sterility. This is a likely consequence of any standard combination chemotherapy program. Several recent papers, however, indicate that fertility may still be possible (with the issue of normal offspring) if the patients are treated in their teenage years or their early 20s.

Women undergoing staging laparotomy should have an oophoropexy performed in case abdominopelvic radiation becomes necessary at a later date. Males should be offered the opportunity to store sperm before chemotherapy is started.

C. Specific Management Guidelines

1. Stages IA and IIA

All patients in Stages IA and IIA, except those with lymphocyte-depleted histology, should be treated with radiotherapy. The fields used will be the standard mantle or inverted Y field for Stage IA or extended mantle for Stage IIA. Patients with lymphocyte depletion histology (rare) should be treated more aggressively (total modal radiotherapy or chemotherapy), especially if not staged by laparotomy.

2. Stage IIB

Patients with IIB disease should be treated by subtotal or total nodal irradiation. If a large mediastinal mass is present, combined-modality therapy should be considered.

3. Stage IIIA

Those patients with PSIIIA$_1$ disease (upper para-aortic nodes only) should be treated with total nodal irradiation. The same holds true for patients with IIIA$_s$ (where only the *removed* spleen was involved). In patients with PSIIIA$_2$ disease, some recommend total nodal irradition, with chemotherapy reserved for patients who fail radiation. Others feel these patients are best treated with chemotherapy.

4. Stages IIIB and IV

Hodgkin's disease at these stages is treated by chemotherapy. Radiation is reserved for areas of massive involvement.

5. Treatment of Recurrent Disease

a. Chemotherapy for MOPP-Resistant Hodgkin's Disease

The need for regimens effective in MOPP-resistant cases is evident from the observation that about 20% of the patients with advanced Hodgkin's disease do not enter complete remission with MOPP, and another 30% will fail sometime after apparent complete remission.

A widely used combination, after MOPP failure, is the ABVD regimen (see Table IV) studied by Bonnadonna and his associates (9). Other combinations include CVB, B-DOPA, and BVAS (see Table IV also). However, the response to combination chemotherapy of patients suffering recurrent disease after prior intensive chemotherapy is far from satisfactory. This is particularly noticeable in whose who failed after only a short initial remission (<1 year) and if they are older than 60 years of age.

b. Recurrent Nodal Disease

All patients deserve periodic evaluation for retroperitoneal disease if that area was not electively treated. All radiation failures in nodal sites (e.g., para-aortic extensions or marginal recurrences) must always be treated by intensive chemotherapy in addition to moderate-dose radiation therapy to the involved site of relapse if this is outside of the previously irradiated field. Chemotherapy will salvage approximately 50% of radiation failures, and more when nodal sites are the first site of relapse.

6. Treatment Controversy

A number of controversies still exist and have been alluded to above. These have to do with philosophical approach as much as scientific information. Some prefer to give maximum therapy initially (both radiotherapy and chemotherapy) in hopes of achieving higher complete remission rates and, it is hoped, a higher percentage of cures. Others point out that combined-modality therapy carries unacceptable risks of late complications and that it is preferable to treat Stage IIIA and IIB patients with radiation initially (because of low risk of late complications), accept a relatively high risk of relapse (as high as 50%), and then treat all failing patients with chemotherapy, "rescuing" a significant proportion and not exposing all patients who do *not* relapse to chemotherapy. Such a strategy may lead to a similar percentage of cures and lower the risk of late complications, such as acute leukemia and sterility. At present, neither strategy has been shown to be superior to the other. In general, combined-modality studies show higher *complete remission* rates than radiotherapy alone, but overall survival has not yet been shown to be improved, largely owing to the effectiveness of "rescue" chemotherapy.

IV. THERAPEUTIC MANAGEMENT OF NON-HODGKIN'S LYMPHOMA

A. Criteria for Therapy

Non-Hodgkin's lymphoma is, in the great majority of cases, disseminated at the time the patient is first seen. For all practical purposes, it must be considered incurable, except for the diffuse histiocytic type. The object of treatment is therefore dual: an attempt at cure for those patients falling in a favorable group (Stage I or II without bulky disease) and prolonged complete remission in the unfavorable group (Stages III and IV, especially in the elderly and those with bulky disease). Approximately 10% of patients with NHL, especially those with lymphocytic disease, have a slow-growing, indolent disease with a history of lymphadenopathy being present for months or years; in this group of patients, observation without treatment has been recommended by some, especially when cure is not anticipated.

Several factors need to be ascertained in order intelligently to institute treatment best suited to the disease at hand:

- Are the anticipated benefits from treatment expected to be palliative or curative?
- Is the disease symptomatic, and do the complications at hand require rapid relief (e.g., ureteral obstruction, GI bleeding, effusions, hypersplenism, bone pain, exophthalmous, etc.)?
- Is there an impending disaster requiring emergency action (e.g., superior vena cava compression or spinal cord compression)?
- What is the likely biologic behavior of the disease (i.e., indolent, progressive, recurrent, etc.)?

- Is the disease nodular or diffuse, and is there evidence of systemic disease?
- What is the patient's age and general health?

B. General Recommendations

In spite of the absence of a uniform classification of lymphomas and the resultant lack of comparability in the various reported publications, Rappaport's classification is the one on which most of the long-term studies are based; until a new classification is adopted as final, it will continue to be the reference pathological classification for malignant NHL.

1. Nodular Lymphomas

The nodular lymphomas, except for the histiocytic and possibly mixed histiocytic–lymphocytic types, have a better prognosis. They respond to both chemotherapy and radiotherapy, though they are generally not curable with present regimens. Nodular poorly differentiated lymphocytic (NPDL) lymphoma forms the majority of these, whereas the well-differentiated (NWDL) type is very uncommon. For early-stage disease (Stages I and II), especially when it is not considered bulky, the results of wide-field high-dose radiation therapy (4500 rads) are satisfactory, with a 5-year disease-free survival of over 40%; results are usually better in younger patients with 5-year survivals rising as high as 70%. However, over 80% of these lymphomas present with Stage III or Stage IV disease, and there is no concensus on how they should be treated. Available policies include

- Initial observation.
- Single chemotherapeutic agents such as cyclophosphamide or chlorambucil.
- Combination chemotherapy with these agents plus prednisone and vincristine.
- More aggressive combinations such as MOPP, C-MOPP (cyclophosphamide, nitrogen mustard, vincristine, procarbazine, and prednisone), CHOP (cyclophosphamide, doxorubicin, vincristine, bleomycin, and prednisone), or CHOP with bleomycin.
- Local radiotherapy (to clinically important masses) or total-body irradiation.

Each of these policies is valid under certain circumstances. Although the results of C-MOPP, especially in nodular mixed lymphoma, have been encouraging, there is no general agreement that this more aggressive chemotherapy is necessarily any better than more limited therapy. These various regimens are still under study, and proposals are being made for multimodality treatment in the hope of achieving higher cure rates.

The choice of whether to treat or not to treat is not at all easy.

Certainly, for elderly patients with indolent, widespread disease, a policy of observation seems reasonable, and many such patients will not require treatment for months or years. The decision to withhold treatment is buttressed by the fact that no curative treatment exists. Essentially, all patients will respond to any of the above-mentioned modalities, and apparent complete remissions will regularly be achieved. However, long-term follow-up shows a constant progressive relapse rate over time.

Although a substantial fraction of patients are elibible for a no-treatment policy, most patients either present with symptoms, or presently develop symptoms, that require intervention. This is not necessarily a reflection of the initial stage of the disease, and it is quite possible that patients with advanced Stage IV disease can be observed initially, especially if they are in Stage IV by virtue of bone marrow involvement, whereas the development of massive, unsightly adenopathy in the neck or axilla, of fever and night sweats or weight loss, of abdominal masses that threaten to obstruct a viscus or a ureter will require therapeutic intervention regardless of the stage of the disease.

For an isolated mass lesion, a local course of radiation seems reasonable. For disseminated disease, one or another chemotherapy program can be tried; it is not known how long such therapy should be continued after a remission has been induced, but most treatment programs last 18–36 months.

As a result of natural evolution or because of treatment-induced reaction, the disease may, in some patients, take on a more aggressive course. This is generally accompanied by a change in the histology of the tumor, most often to a *diffuse* large-cell (histiocytic) or immunoblastic type. Such patients should be treated with intensive chemotherapy programs designed for poor-histology lymphomas, and some long-term remissions may thus be produced. Unfortunately, if the patient has received extensive chemotherapy during the "indolent" phase, the chances of a meaningful remission once the histology has converted are correspondingly diminished.

2. Diffuse Lymphomas

The diffuse lymphomas are more aggressive tumors; that is, they have a much more aggressive *natural history* than their nodular counterparts, but there has been some success in their treatment with a variety of combination chemotherapy programs, such as BACOP (bleomycin, Adriamycin, Cytoxan, vincristine, and prednisone), CHOP bleomycin, and C-MOPP, and a variety of newer, even more aggressive regimens. This is especially the case in diffuse histiocytic lymphoma, less so in the other subgroups. Thus, for a majority of patients with advanced disease, a fatal outcome is anticipated. Better treatment regimens, combinations as well as multimodality approaches, must be explored until at least a rate of cure approaching that of Hodgkin's disease is reached.

The most aggressive forms of malignant lymphoma such as undifferentiated, lymphoblastic, immunoblastic, Burkitt's, and non-Burkitt's malignant lymphomas are the most rapidly progressive generalized diseases, with systemic and metabolic manifestations that require immediate attention upon diagnosis. The remission rate in these types varies from 20 to 70%, but early relapses are the rule.

In summary, when faced with malignant lymphoma, cases with bulky but localized disease can often be controlled with radiotherapy. The more advanced and aggressive tumors require one or another form of chemotherapy. If the institution is participating in a national or regional protocol designed to explore better classification and treatment, all eligible patients should be encouraged to enter such protocols. If protocols are not locally available, or if the patient cannot be entered in a study protocol, our current recommendations are presented in the following paragraphs.

C. Specific Management Guidelines

1. Stages I and II

Radiotherapy may be the best form of treatment in these localized forms of lymphoma (i.e., those with involvement of a single lymph node region, or two or more regions on the same side of the diaphragm). The 5-year survival rate is reported as high as 70%, though some histologic types do better than others. When cure is the goal, the extent of the disease should be clearly delineated. If radiation is to be the chosen modality, an occasional patient with Stage IA clinical presentation may even be a candidate for staging laparotomy when other procedures (i.e., lymphangiogram or CAT scan) suggest, but do not prove, intra-abdominal disease. If the latter is confirmed, treatment would have to include chemotherapy.

In those selected few cases (patients in poor general condition or those with other debilitating disease, etc.) where the goal is palliative, one needs to determine whether it is necessary to initiate the treatment altogether. The symptoms that need to be palliated—frequency of recurrence, size and bulkiness of disease, gradual or rapid progression, etc.—will dictate the therapy. Radiotherapy is the choice of treatment of local bulky disease. Single-agent chemotherapy may also be suitable when the desired response can be gradual.

Combination chemotherapy has been recommended for Stage I and II diffuse histiocytic lymphomas; complete remission rates of >90% have been reported in this subgroup of patients. It is too early, as yet to judge the likelihood of cure in such remissions, but chemotherapy is obviously more toxic than radiotherapy for Stage I and II diffuse lymphoma. No published studies are available comparing radiotherapy to chemotherapy in a prospectively controlled clinical trial.

2. Stages III and IV

Treatment of patients with advanced stages of lymphoma (i.e., with involvement on both sides of the diaphragm with or without extralymphatic involvement or diffuse disseminated disease), both nodular and diffuse, will depend on the histological type of the tumor.

a. Aggressive Types (Unfavorable Histology)

- Nodular histiocytic lymphoma (NodHL).
- Diffuse histiocytic lymphoma (DHL).
- Diffuse mixed lymphoma (DML).
- Undifferentiated lymphoma (UL).
- Diffuse poorly differentiated lymphoma (DPDL).
- Lymphoblastic lymphoma.
- Burkitt's and non-Burkitt's lymphoma.

The preceding categories of lymphoma require aggressive combination chemotherapy (see Table V). Newer regimens using up to 10 drugs in very intensive schedules are currently being studied.

Table V

Combination Chemotherapy Regimens for Non-Hodgkin's Lymphoma

Regimen	Drug	Dose	Day	Cycle length
CVP	Cyclophosphamide	400 mg/m², PO	1 to 5	21 days
	Vincristine[a]	1.4 mg/m², IV	1	
	Prednisone	100 mg/m², PO	1 to 5	
COPP (C-MOPP)	Cyclophosphamide	650 mg/m², IV	1 and 8	28 days
	Vincristine[a]	1.4 mg/m², IV	1 and 8	
	Procarbazine	100 mg/m², PO	1 to 14	
	Prednisone	40 mg/m², PO	1 to 14 (cycles 1, 4 and so forth)	
CHOP	Cyclophosphamide (Cytoxan)	650 mg/m², IV	1 and 8	28 days
	Doxorubicin (Adriamycin)	25 mg/m², IV	1 and 8	
	Vincristine[a]	1.4 mg/m², IV	1 and 8	
	Bleomycin	5 mg/m², IV	15 and 21	
	Prednisone	69 mg/m², PO	15 to 28	

[a] Maximum total single dose of vincristine < 2.0 mg.

b. Nonaggressive Types (Favorable Histology)

In nonaggressive Stage III or IV malignant lymphomas, which include most of the nodular lymphomas but only the well-differentiated type of diffuse lymphomas (DWDL), initial observation may be sufficient depending on the patient's condition and disease status. This may be followed, when indicated, by one of the following types of chemotherapy:

- Single-agent.
- Single-agent in combination with prednisone.
- Multiple-drug chemotherapy.

The following types of lymphomas may be considered nonaggressive:

- NPDL.
- DWDL.
- Nodular mixed lymphoma. (NML)

The recommended chemotherapeutic agents are

- Cytoxan alone or with prednisone, particularly in the older patient with relatively indolent disease.
- Chlorambucil alone or with prednisone.
- CVP (Cytoxan, vincristine, and prednisone).
- CHOP or CHOP with bleomycin. ⎫
- BACOP. ⎬ rarely
- C-MOPP. ⎭

Dosages, schedules, and length of therapy will depend on the individual tumor and require an experienced medical oncologist to achieve the best possible results with the minimum of morbidity.

Table VI is for quick reference on the most commonly employed chemotherapeutic agents. It details their toxicity, modes of administration, and special considerations required in their use.

D. Potential Curability

It is something of a paradox that lymphomas with better prognosis, i.e., nodular and lymphocytic subtypes, are precisely those for which a modern chemotherapy treatment program has not as yet made a significant contribution in improving cure rates in the advanced stages (III and IV); whereas these lymphomas almost always respond to whatever treatment modality is applied, long-term follow-up shows a steady, progressive relapse rate, so that it is premature to talk of a "cured" subgroup. On the other hand, among the poor-prognosis lymphomas, there apparently exists a subgroup, within the broad category of DHL, that is subject to durable, complete remission with intensive combination chemotherapy. Com-

Table VI

Antineoplastic Agents: Toxic Reactions and Special Considerations

Drug name	Myelosuppression	Stomatitis	Nausea, vomiting, diarrhea	Alopecia	Side effects and other toxicities	Routes of administration	Special considerations
Actinomycin D (Dactinomycin, Cosmegen)	$+^a$ +++	+ +	+ +++	+ +	Skin necrosis	IV through the side-arm of a freely running line Avoid extravasation	Use of water containing a perservative to reconstitute results in the formation of a precipitate
5-Azacytidine	+++	+	++	0	Hepatotoxic	IV or subcutaneous.	
Bleomycin	0	+	0	+	Pulmonary fibrosis, skin rash, anaphylaxis, fever	IV (administer slowly over a period of 10 mins), IM, subcutaneous, or intra-cavitary	
Busulfan (Myleran)	++	0	0	0	Pulmonary fibrosis	Oral.	
Chlorambucil	++	0	0	0	—	Oral.	Toxicity may be increased in a setting of prior barbiturate use
Chlorozotocin (DCNU)	+	0	++	0	Nephrotoxic	IV	
Cisplatin	+	0	++++	+	Nephrotoxic, peripheral neurophathy, anaphylaxis, ototoxic	IV infusion with mannitol. (Do not use needles or IV sets containing aluminum; a precipitate may form)	Insure adequate hydration
Cyclophosphamide (Cytoxan)	+++	+	‖	+	Sterile hemorrhagic cystitis	IV or orally. Intraperitoneal and intrapleural routes have been used but are not recommended	Keep patient well hydrated for at least 24 hours following administration to minimize cystitis Cytoxan for injection contains no antimicrobial agents; care must be taken to insure the sterility of prepared solutions
Cytosine arabinoside (Ara-C)	+++	+	++	+	—	IV, subcutaneous, IM, or intrathecally	Discard any solution in which even a slight haze appears
Dacarbazine	+	0	+++	0	Hypotension, skin necrosis, flulike syndrome	*See* actinomycin D	

(continued)

Table VI (*Continued*)

Drug name	Myelosuppression	Stomatitis	Nausea, vomiting, diarrhea	Alopecia	Side effects and other toxicities	Routes of administration	Special considerations
Daunorubicin (Daunomycin, Rubidomycin)	+++	++	+++	+++	Cardiotoxic skin necrosis	*See* actinomycin D	Impaired excretion with hepatic dysfunction
Doxorubicin (Adriamycin)	+++	++	+++	+++	Cardiotoxic	*See* actinomycin D	See daunorubicin
5-Fluorouricil (5-FU)	++	++	+	+	—	IV	Incompatible with Cytosar, methothrexate, Adriamycin, and Valium. Do not mix with IV additives.
Hexamethylmelamine	0	0	+++	+	Peripheral neuropathy	Oral	Due to GI toxicity, drug is often given in 4 divided doses (after meals and h.s.)
Hydroxyurea (Hydrea)	++	+	+	0	—	Oral	Unusually high incidence of neurotoxicity when used with 5-FU
L-Asparaginase	0	0	++	0	Major organ failure, anaphylaxis, clotting disorders, pancreatitis	IV (infuse over a period of not less than 30 mins); IM (if a volume 2 ml is to be administered, use 2 sites)	
Melphalan (Alkeran)	+	0	rare	0	—	Oral	Long-term continuous dosing may cause acute leukemia
Mercaptopurine (6-MP)	++	+	+	0	—	Oral	Reduce dose to ⅓–¼ usual dose if concurrent allopurinol is given
Methotrexate	++	+++	+	+	Nephrotoxic, hepatoxic, Lung toxicity	Oral, IV, IM, intrathecal, and intra-arterial	Use preservative-free diluent for CNS
Mitomycin C	+++	+	++	+	Nephrotoxic, skin necrosis	*See* actinomycin D	Myelosuppression may be cumulative with successive doses. Long term delayed myelosuppression
Nitrogen mustard (Mustargen, mechlorethamine)	+++	++	+++	++	Skin necrosis	*See* actinomycin D	Avoid contact with skin and eyes. Antidote: sodium thiosulfate

(continued)

Table VI (*Continued*)

Drug name	Myelosuppression	Stomatitis	Nausea, vomiting, diarrhea	Alopecia	Side effects and other toxicities	Routes of administration	Special considerations
Procarbazine	minimal	0	+	0	—	Oral	Concurrent use with: ethanol sympathomimetics, antidepressants, tyramine-rich foods (cheese, wine, banana), or CNS depressants is not recommended
Rubidazone	+++	++	+++	+++	GI bleeding, renal failure, anaphylaxic, skin necrosis, fever, chills and hives; nephrotoxic; skin necrosis	IV; avoid extravasation	Total cumulative dose of 3500 mg/m^2 in patients not previously treated with anthracyclines
Streptozotocin	+	0	+++	+	—		
6-Thioguanine	++	+	+	0	—	Oral (between meals or in one dose)	Doses do not generally need to be reduced with concurrent allopurinorl administration
Vinblastine (Velban)	++	+	+	+	Neurotoxic; skin necrosis. muscle aches	*See* actinomycin D	Dose-limiting myelosuppression
Vincristine (Oncovin)	0	0	0	+	Neurotoxic; skin necrosis	*See* actinomycin D	Neurotoxicity is dose limiting
Vindesine	+	+	+	+	Neurotoxic	IV	*See* vincristine
VM-26	+	+	+	+	Acute cardiovascular collapse, anaphylaxis	IV	Severe hypotension can occur. Administer over a period of 45 min
VP-16 (Etoposide)	+	0	+	+	Anaphylaxis, severe hypotension	IV infusion; avoid extravasation	
BCNU (Carmustine)	+	0	+	+	Hepatotoxic; rare lung toxicity	IV drip over 1–2 hours to avoid pain over injection site	Causes delayed myelosuppression. Vials contain no preservatives, should not be used for multiple dosing
Lomustine (CCNU)	+	+	+	+	Hepatotoxic	Orally, on an empty stomach	Causes delayed bone marrow toxicity

[a] Relative levels of toxicity: from least toxic (+) to most toxic (+++).

[b] 0, none or no effect.

plete remission rates of 40–70% are commonly reported, and a large proportion of these patients stay in remission for extended periods. Given the rapidly progressive nature of uncontrolled disease in this histologic category, failure of the disease to recur in the first 3–4 years after treatment suggests that cure may be possible. Thus, all chemotherapy programs for DHL are given with curative intent. There is substantial agreement that the dose–response curve is relatively steep, implying that high doses, at the very edge of serious toxicity, are necessary to achieve the best results. This contrasts with the situation that prevails in the nodular lymphomas, in which low-dose single-agent therapy is as effective as more intensive therapies.

The aforementioned multiagent programs require that treatment be carried out only under the supervision of trained oncology practitioners. Serious toxicity is commonplace, and one must be prepared to deal with leukopenia-related sepsis and able to provide, at a moments notice, whatever support might be required.

E. Radiotherapy

The curative role of radiation therapy in the treatment of NHL is quite different from that in Hodgkin's disease. While NHL is quite responsive to radiation, only a small proportion of patients present with early disease (Stages I and II) or with small enough bulk to render them amenable to cure with local or regional radiation.

1. Stages I and II

The technique of radiation therapy is different from that used with Hodgkin's disease. Wide-field irradiation, rather than mantle or inverted-Y, is usually necessary since most relapses will occur distally rather than contiguous to the involved areas.

For extranodal sites, the regional lymphatics are usually included in the treatment volume. Involved-field treatment for extranodal or nodal Stages I and II lymphoma (localized) in the abdomen is most often done by total abdominal irradiation.

2. Stages III and IV

Patients with symptomatic progressive nodular disease or those with massive disease who are in good general condition should be treated. Treatment may consist of radiation therapy, chemotherapy, or both modalities combined. Radiation therapy for Stage III malignant lymphoma can be delivered in one of two strategies: total, comprehensive lymphatic irradiation (CLI) or total-body irradiation.

a. Comprehensive Lymphatic Irradiation

This strategy, which covers mantle, total abdomen, Waldeyer's ring, and epitrochlear nodes, starts with the area of gross involvement and is pursued for several weeks. A rest period consistent with changes in white blood cell (WBC) and platelet counts is inserted after treatment of each region. Early liver involvement is not an absolute contraindication for CLI since the entire liver can be irradiated to a low dose. However, this must be handled carefully and within the context of a comprehensive plan. Recovery of the bone marrow takes 4–8 weeks after completion of the treatment; full recovery of marrow can be expected in most patients since the total dose of irradiation is rather low.

b. Total-Body Irradiation

This is an effective palliative treatment for those patients who are in an advanced age group and have medical problems. The patient receives 10–15 rads to the total body twice weekly, up to a total dose of 150 rads. This procedure is still experimental, and it carries a substantial morbidity, with bone marrow depression, severe bowel reaction, sensitive organ damage (e.g., to lungs, eyes), etc. and results in questionable long-term effect.

3. Treatment of Extranodal Sites (Stages IE and IIE)

a. Gastrointestinal Tract

Although resection of the the stomach or segments of the bowel is usually carried out for malignant lymphoma, it is not always necessary since local cure can be effectively achieved with radiation, especially when the disease is not bulky. In cases where the disease is limited to the stomach, radiation therapy is delivered to the stomach and the regional lymph nodes. If the regional nodes are involved, whole abdominal irradiation is indicated, and the patient may benefit from adjuvant chemotherapy. In cases of intestinal involvement, surgery may be performed, followed by whole abdominal irradiation. The prognosis in these patients is worse than that of lymphoma of the stomach.

b. Waldeyer's Ring

Waldeyer's ring includes the nasopharynx, the tonsil, and base of the tongue. The treatment is by radiotherapy and should encompass all areas in Waldeyer's ring as well as the neck nodes bilaterally.

c. Bone

Lymphoma of bones is almost always a DHL. It spreads by distant bone-borne metastases, although some patients may develop regional node involvement. The entire bone should be treated.

d. Central Nervous System

Primary intracranial lymphoma is uncommon. The entire brain and the spinal axis should be irradiated for primary CNS lesions, especially if there is evidence of meningeal involvement.

e. Orbit

The entire orbit and lids are irradiated for localized eye presentations. Patients with bilateral presentation seem to do as well as those with unilateral disease.

f. Skin

The lesions are present either as small nodules clustered together or as a single tumor mass. Solitary tumors are occasionally seen in the head and neck area or in the skin of the posterior chest wall; the prognosis in these cases is exceptionally good if the lesions are isolated. Likewise, lesions localized in the scalp have a good prognosis; the entire scalp should be treated.

g. Testes

The prognosis is poor since the disease shows widespread dissemination at an early stage.

F. Other Therapeutic Considerations

1. Involvement of the CNS

This serious complication is very rare in the good-prognosis (mainly nodular) lymphomas but is seen in high-grade lymphomas, particularly in lymphoblastic lymphomas and in large-cell lymphomas with bone marrow involvement. It is routine, nowadays, to include *prophylactic* therapy to the CNS in childhood (and adolescent) lymphoblastic lymphomas and in the Burkitt's type of malignant lymphomas. Similarly, treatment with intrathecal chemotherapy has been advocated, as a prophylactic measure, to adult patients with DHL (or one of its variants), especially if the bone marrow is involved. Another potential approach is the use of high-dose methotrexate (3 g) with citrovorum rescue in combination with standard CHOP-like regimens. High-dose IV methotrexate is capable of achieving therapeutic levels in the cerebrospinal fluid and may be useful as prophylaxis to the CNS, as well as systemic antilymphoma therapy. The long-term benefits of these approaches are yet to be proven.

The treatment of established CNS involvement includes intrathecal therapy with methotrexate and cytosine arabinoside as well as radiation therapy. The prognosis, however, tends to be dismal.

2. Hyperuricemia

Patients with NHL generally have a large tumor load. Chemotherapy may cause rapid cell destruction, resulting in a marked release of uric acid, leading to uric acid nephropathy and acute renal failure. To avoid such disastrous consequences, these patients must be adequately hydrated and given allopurinol (300–900 mg per day) several days before induction of chemotherapy.

V. OTHER SPECIFIC TYPES OF LYMPHOMA AND RELATED DISORDERS

A. Burkitt's Lymphoma

1. General Considerations

African Burkitt's lymphoma is generally classified as a UL and has been known for many decades to occur in children in Uganda, Nigeria, and West Africa. It is endemic in the so-called "lymphoma belt" of Africa south of the Sahara and in Papua, New Guinea. Sporadic cases, though, do occur throughout the world. There is a distinct relationship to climatic conditions and a coincidence with endemic malaria.

The peak occurrence of "Western" adult Burkitt's lymphoma is between the fourth and eighth years of life. Individuals with sickle cell trait have half the chance of developing the tumor as those with AA hemoglobin.

The Epstein-Barr virus operating with a climate-dependent cofactor, possibly another infection appears implicated in the pathogenesis of the disease. The patient usually has a high titer of circulating antibodies against this virus, much higher than is seen in patients with infectious mononucleosis.

2. Clinical Characteristics

The lesions of the "African" Burkitt's lymphoma are most frequent in the jaws (55%), the ovaries (38%), the testes, the thyroid, the adrenals, and the breasts. This distribution is quite distinct from that of other lymphomas. In autopsied cases, the CNS is frequently involved.

Clinically, the presentation will depend on the site of the disease:

- Mandibular or maxillary tumors.
- Facial distortion.
- Exophthalmos and ophthalmoplegia resulting from spread into the retro-orbital space.
- Ascites, retroperitoneal tumors, mesenteric mass, etc.

- Paraplegias (in 15% of cases), sphincteric dysfunction, cranial neuropathies (more rare).

3. Pathological Features

Histologically, the most striking characteristic is the "starry-sky" appearance of the tumorous infiltrates; this is due to regular scattering of single, pale macrophages throughout an infiltration of densely packed, dark tumor cells with very scanty cytoplasm and nuclei with granular chromatin and two to five small nucleoli. It is to be noted that a well-differentiated lymphocytic lymphoma may simulate this histological appearance.

Clinical Staging is important.

Stage A: Single, extra-abdominal site.
Stage B: Multiple, extra-abdominal site.
Stage C: Intra-abdominal tumor.
Stage D: Intra-abdominal tumor with one or more extra-abdominal involvements.

Patients diagnosed as having Burkitt's lymphoma must be thoroughly investigated to establish the actual extent of the disease. Such investigation should include the following:

- CBC, chest x-ray, SMA-12.
- Skeletal survey, or bone scan.
- Intravenous pyelogram, or CAT scan of the abdomen.
- Bone marrow aspiration.
- Spinal tap and fluid for cytology.

In the United States, Burkitt's lymphoma typically presents with abdominal disease with involvement of the terminal ileum and abdominal masses. The process tends to generalize quickly, and CNS involvement is common.

4. Therapeutic Management

This is a highly responsive neoplasm. It can be cured with modern, very intensive chemotherapy programs including agents such as cyclophosphamide or vincristine, methotrexate, and cytosine arabinoside. Patients should be referred to centers where such treatment is available. Adults with this neoplasm fare very poorly, however.

B. Immunoblastic Lymphadenopathy

Immunoblastic lymphadenopathy occurs predominantly in the sixth and seventh decade of life. It develops as febrile lymphadenopathy with skin rashes and hepatosplenomegaly. Hemolytic anemia, as well as polyclonal hypergammaglobulinemia, are often present.

The prognosis is dismal, and about 80% of patients will die within a period of 1 month to several years after the onset of the disease, death usually resulting from infection facilitated by immunodeficiency. Exceptionally, a true lymphoma may develop, and, at times, spontaneous remissions have been reported to have occurred.

The disease is believed to be a nonneoplastic proliferation of B lymphocytes that become massively transformed into immunoblasts. In some cases, the onset of the disease follows medication with agents such as penicillin, oral antidiabetics, hydantoin, cyclophosphamide, sulphonamides, thiazides, and others. A history of a "viral syndrome" is sometimes elicited.

Histologically, the disease is marked by complete obliteration of the normal architecture of the lymph nodes by pleomorphic cellular infiltrates with large quantities of immunoblasts. The infiltrate involves the capsule, thus giving the impression of a lymphoma. Plasma cells, lymphocytes, eosinophils, and neutrophils are also abundant. Other characteristic features are abnormal proliferation of numerous branching blood vessels and deposits of amorphous eosinophilic, PAS (P-aminosalicylic (p-aminosalicyclic acid)-positive material. Similar changes can be found in the spleen, liver, bone marrow, and other lymphoid tissues. If an erroneous diagnosis of lymphoma is made, treated subsequently by radiation or chemotherapy, disastrous consequences may ensue. Prednisone has been advocated to control symptoms and is certainly useful to control hemolytic anemia when present. Infections should be treated vigorously.

C. Sézary Syndrome

This is a rare, chronic, infiltrative proliferative neoplastic disorder characterized by large, atypical lymphocytes of T-cell origin infiltrating the upper dermal layer and giving rise to a diffuse progressive pruritic erythroderma with exfoliative lesions and lymphadenopathy (see §3.V.B, Vol. 1). It is the visceral and leukemic counterpart of mycosis fungoides.

D. Mycosis Fungoides

This type of cutaneous lymphoma is a progressive neoplastic proliferation of histiocytes that begin in the skin and remain there for many years. As the disease progresses, destructive lesions, fungating tumors, and nodules develop in the skin. Eventually, lymph nodes, bone marrow, and visceral involvement (lungs, liver, etc.) occurs. These lesions are also dealt with in §3.V.B, Vol. 1.

E. Histiocytic Medullary Reticulosis (Malignant Histiocytosis)

This is a disorder of acute onset and short course caused by a neoplastic proliferation of sinusoidal histiocytes that retain their phagocytic functional capacity. Marked marrow infiltration and erythrophagocytosis will result in anemia, granulocytopenia, and thrombocytopenia. Infiltration of the skin will also give a skin rash, and at times, atypical histiocytes may be identified in the peripheral blood. This is the true histiocytic neoplasm and thus technically not a lymphoma. The course is usually relentlessly downhill.

Some cases resembling histiocytic medullary reticulosis have been reported with infections caused by tuberculosis or a number of viruses. In these instances, however, the treatment of the underlying disease resulted in cure. Histiocytic medullary reticulosis accounts for less than 1% of all lymphomas.

F. Waldenström's Macroglobulinemia

This disease is the result of proliferation of lymphocytoid plasma cells. The abnormal cell is a B lymphocyte that overproduces a monoclonal immunoglobulin (IgM, macroglobulin). The bone marrow and other organs are infiltrated, causing hepatosplenomegaly and lymphadenopathy. The IgM protein, because of its large size, accumulates almost entirely in the intravascular compartment, causing an increase in blood volume and plasma viscosity. Hyperviscosity syndromes will ensue, with peripheral neuropathy, congestive heart failure, retinal hemorrhages, mucosal bleeding, and anemia. Bence Jones proteins are found in about 10% of cases.

Treatment is essentially by chemotherapy: cyclophosphamide, melphalan, and chlorambucil are the drugs of choice. The hyperviscosity syndrome and complications may respond to plasmapheresis. The average survival after onset of the disease is 4–6 years, with several reported survivals beyond 10 years.

VI. FOLLOW-UP EVALUATION AND REHABILITATION OF THE PATIENT WITH LYMPHOMA

A. Psychological Support

Even though there are high cure rates for early stages of the disease, particularly in Hodgkin's lymphoma, it is imperative that the physician, nurse, and other health professionals involved in the patient's care recognize the fact that the patient and family will be affected by the diagnosis of cancer.

Patients should be made aware of the fact that various health professionals are available to assist them and their families to cope with the diagnosis, prognosis, and any degree of altered body image or life cycle.

Support groups such as Make Today Count or Living with

Cancer may assist the patient to work out feelings of hopelessness and despair. Patients that have been successfully treated for Hodgkin's disease may also be called on to offer support to acutely ill patients through the aforementioned groups.

B. Complications of the Disease and Its Treatment

Many patients under therapy for Hodgkin's disease will have various deficiencies, symptoms, and complications that require correction. Some of the required interventions include

- Nutritional support, oral or parenteral as need be.
- Symptomatic relief of fever, pain, nausea, vomiting, etc.
- Blood transfusions as required.
- Treatment of intercurrent infections with judicious antibiotic usage.

The usual complications proper to the various chemotherapeutic agents are outlined in Table VI; these must be detected, recognized, and promptly treated. Prevention of the complications of radiotherapy has been previously discussed.

An increased incidence of second malignancies in patients with lymphoma has been recognized in recent years. Wtih combined-modality therapy, the risk of developing acute leukemia increases with time; furthermore, these leukemias are extremely refractory to therapy, and survival is rarely more than a few months following diagnosis. The use of combined radiotherapy and chemotherapy, therefore, should be extremely selective.

Although complications of treatment are significant and unfortunate, a large proportion of patients with advanced Hodgkin's disease and some with NHL will be cured by therapy; carefully monitored intensive chemotherapy and/or radiotherapy should therefore be made available to virtually all patients. As previously mentioned, the optimal planning of such therapy is best assured by employing a multidisciplinary approach involving the medical oncologist, hematologist, radiation oncologist, diagnostic radiologist, surgeon, nurse, social worker, physical therapist, occupational therapist, nutritionist, pharmacist, psychologist, vocational counselor, etc.

C. Rehabilitation

The following problems, goals, and interventions need to be addressed in the rehabilitation of the patient with lymphomas.

1. Decreased Energy Level Due to Anemia

- Goal: Conservation of energy.
- Intervention

- Assess the degree of limitation; explain the reasons for decreased energy level; encourage activity within limits.
- Include adequate rest periods in daily schedule.
- Identify and change architectural barriers that may contribute to decreased energy requirements.
- Assess nutritional status and refer to dietician.
- Explain the need for consultation with the physician, if the patient becomes weaker.

2. Susceptibility to Infection Due to Leukopenia

- Goal: Prevention of infection.
- Intervention:
  - Monitor WBC; explain the reasons for the increased risk of infection.
  - Assess the lifestyle patterns regarding hygiene and work.
  - Instruct the patient regarding dental propylaxis; need for daily inspection of mouth and skin; scrupulous personal hygiene; avoidance of crowds and people with upper respiratory infections; care of cuts and wounds; need to report symptoms of infection to the physician promptly.
  - Use of strict aseptic technique when performing any procedure.

3. Risk of Bleeding Due to Thrombocytopenia

- Goal: Prevention of bleeding.
- Intervention:
  - Monitor the platelet count and coagulation profiles; explain the reason for increased risk of bleeding.
  - Instruct the patient regarding avoidance of aspirin-containing products (except as instructed by the physician); use of an electric razor; possibility of menstrual irregularities; need to inspect mouth, skin, stool, and urine for signs of bleeding; use of a stool softener recommended by the physician.
  - Assist the patient to modify and plan his or her activities.
  - If the patient bleeds, instruct him or her not to remove the clots that have formed.

4. Exacerbation of the Disease

- Goal: Provision of support to the patient and significant others.
- Intervention:
  - Reinforce the physician's instructions.
  - Anticipate the patient's needs, and involve the family in his or her care.
  - Interact with the family members to answer questions, clarify any misconceptions, and allay their fears.
  - Involve a spiritual counselor if the patient desires such services.

5. Need for Blood Components

- Goal: Understanding of the purpose of the transfusion; reduction of anxiety.
- Intervention:
  - Reinforce the explanations given to the patient.
  - Involve the social worker or financial counselor to counsel on available medical insurance coverage.

D. Follow-Up Evaluation of the Patient with Lymphoma

It must be emphasized that any guidelines for follow-up of the patient with Hodgkin's disease or NHL must be very individualized and will depend upon the stage of the disease, the histological classification, and how well the patient responds to the treatment.

The patient should be informed that any new symptoms or deviations from normal should be reported to the physician promptly, regardless of how insignificant they may seem or of previously recommended follow-up time intervals. At that time, decisions about more sophisticated tests may be made and should be based on sound clinical judgment.

Table VII presents a follow-up schedule for lymphoma patients.

VII. MANAGEMENT ALGORITHM FOR LYMPHOMAS (see p. 381)

SUGGESTED READINGS

Hodgkin's Disease

Pathology

1. Lukes, R. J., Butler, J. J., and Hicks, E. D. Natural history of Hodgkin's disease as related to its pathologic picture. *Cancer (Philadelphia)* **19,** 317–344 (1966).

Staging

2. Brogadir, S., Fialk, M. A., Coleman, M., Vinciguerra, V. P., Degnan, T., Pasmantier, M., and Silver, R. T. Morbidity of staging laparotomy in Hodgkin's disease. *Am. J. Med.* **64**(3), 429–433 (1978).
3. Carbone, P. P., Kaplan, H. S., Musshoff, K. *et al.* Report of the committee on Hodgkin's disease staging. *Cancer Res.* **31,** 1860–1861 (1971).
4. Johnson, R. E. Is taging laparotomy routinely indicated in Hodgkin's disease? *Ann. Intern. Med.* **75,** 459 (1971).
5. Stein, R. S., Golomb, H. M., Diggs, C. H. *et al.* Anatomic substages of Stage III-A Hodgkin's disease. *Ann. Intern. Med.* **92,** 159–165 (1980).

Table VII

Schedule for Follow-Up of Lymphoma

Management	First 3 months: monthly	First and second year				Third-to-fifth year		Thereafter, annually
		3 months	6 months	9 months	12 months	Semiannually	Annually	
History								
Complete	X	X			X		X	X
Fever	X	X	X	X	X	X	X	X
Weight loss or gain	X	X	X	X	X	X	X	X
Night sweats	X	X	X	X	X	X	X	X
Pruritis	X	X	X	X	X	X	X	X
Lymphadenopathy	X	X	X	X	X	X	X	X
Pain	X	X	X	X	X	X	X	X
Cough	X	X	X	X	X	X	X	X
Abdominal distention	X	X	X	X	X			
Physical								
Complete					X		X	X
Peripheral lymph nodes	X	X	X	X	X	X	X	X
Lungs	X	X	X	X	X	X	X	X
Abdomen	X	X	X	X	X	X	X	X
Skin	X	X	X	X	X	X	X	X
Oropharynx	X	X	X	X	X	X	X	X
Investigation								
Chest x-ray		X			X		X	X
Urine	X	X	X	X	X	X	X	X
CBC, platelets	X	X	X	X	X	X	X	X
SMA-12		X			X	X	X	X
Other tests or procedures				A S I N D I C A T E D				

Radiotherapy

6. Kaplan, H. S. Role of intensive radiotherapy in the management of Hodgkin's disease. *Cancer (Philadelphia)* **19,** 356–367 (1966).
7. Peters, M. V. A study of survival in Hodgkin's disease treated radiologically. *Am. J. Roentgeonol. Radium Ther.* **63,** 299–311 (1950).
8. Rosenberg, S. A., and Kaplan, H. S. Evidence for an orderly progression in the spread of Hodgkin's disease. *Cancer Res.* **26,** 1225–1231 (1966).

Chemotherapy

9. Bonadonna, G., Zucali, R., Monfardini, S. *et al.* Combination chemotherapy of Hodgkin's disease with adriamycin, bleomycin, vinblastine, and imidazolc carboximidc versus MOPP. *Cancer (Philadelphia)* **36,** 252–259 (1975).
10. Coleman, C. N., Williams, C. J., Flint, A. *et al.* Hematological neoplasia in patients treated for Hodgkin's disease. *N. Engl. J. Med.* **300,** 452–458 (1979).
11. DeVita, V. T., Serpick, A. A., and Carbone, P. P. Combination of chemotherapy in the treatment of advanced Hodgkin's disease. *Ann. Intern. Med.* **73,** 891–895 (1970).
12. DeVita, V. T., Jr., Lewis, B. J., Rozencweig, M. *et al.* The chemotherapy of Hodgkin's disease: Past experiences and future directions. *Cancer (Phildadelphia)* **42**(2), 979–990 (1978).
13. Rosenberg, S. A., Kaplan, H. S., Portlock, C. S. *et al.* Combined modality therapy of Hodgkin's disease: A report on the Stanford trials. *Cancer (Philadelphia)* **42**(Suppl. 2), 991–1000 (1978).
14. Rosenthal, S. N., and Bennett, J. M. "Practical Cancer, Chemotherapy." Medical Examination Publication Co., Inc., 1981.

Non-Hodgkin's Lymphoma

Pathology

15. Lennert, K., Stein, H., and Kaiserling, E. Cytological and functional criteria for the classification of malignant lymphomata. *Br. J. Cancer* **31**(II), 29 (1975).
16. Lukcs, R. J., and Collin, R. D. Immunologic characterization of human malignant lymphomas. *Cancer (Philadelphia)* **34,** 1488 (1974).
17. National Cancer Institute. The non-Hodgkin's lymphoma pathologic classification group: NCI sponsored study of classifications of non-Hodgkin's lymphomas: Summary and description of a working formulation for clinical usage. *Cancer (Philadelphia)* **49,** 2112 (1982).
18. Rappaport, H. Tumors of the hematopoietic system. *In* "Atlas of Tumor Pathology" (M. 0. Dayhoff, ed.), Sect. III, Fasc. I. Armed Forces Inst. Pathol., Washington, D.C., 1966.

Staging

19. Chabner, B. A., Johnson, R. E., Young, R. C. *et al.* Sequential nonsurgical and surgical staging of non-Hodgkin's lymphoma. *Ann. Intern. Med.* **85**(2), 149–154 (1976).
20. Herman, T. S., and Jones, S. E. Systematic re-staging in the management of non-Hodgkin's lymphoma. *Cancer Treat. Rep.* **61,** 1009–1015 (1977).
21. Jones, R., Hubbard, S. M., Osborne, C. *et al.* Histologic conversions in non-Hodgkin's lymphoma: Evolution of nodular lymphomas to diffuse lymphomas. *Clin. Res.* **26,** 437 (1978).
22. Jones, S. E., Fuks, Z., Bull, M., Kadin, M. E., Dorfman, R. F., Kaplan,

ALGORITHM FOR HODGKIN'S DISEASE AND NON-HODGKIN'S LYMPHOMAS

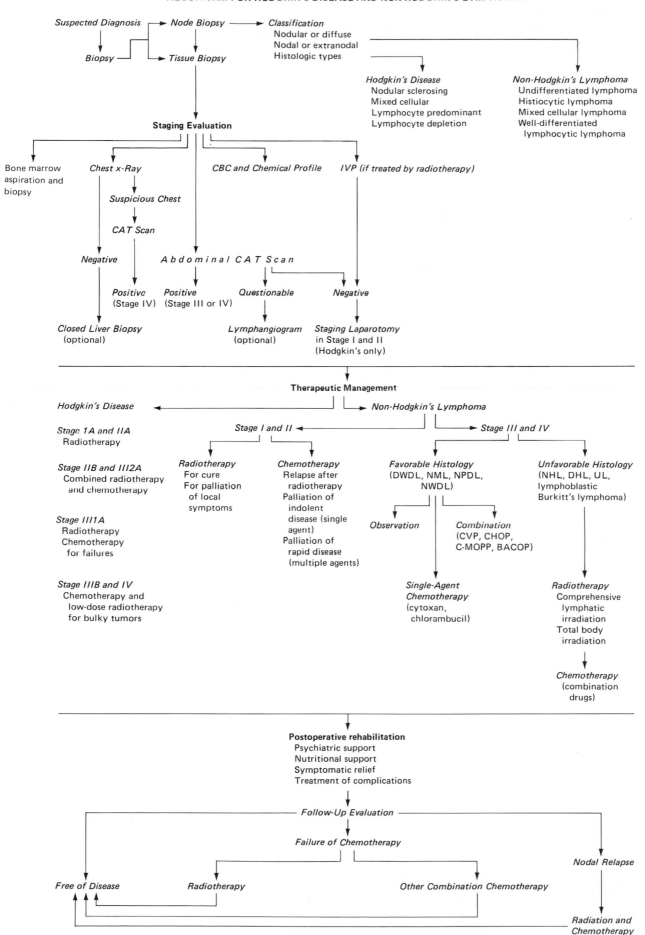

H. S., Rosenberg, S. A., and Kim, H. Non-Hodgkin's lymphomas. IV. Clinicopathologic correlation in 405 cases. *Cancer (Philadelphia)* **31,** 806–823 (1973).

23. Veronesi, U., Musumeci, R., Pizzetti, F. *et al.* The value of staging laparotomy in non-Hodgkin's lymphomas (with emphasis on the histiocytic type). *Cancer (Philadelphia)* **33,** 446–469 (1974).

Therapy

24. Bagley, C. M., DeVita, V. T., Berard, C. W. *et al.* Advanced lymphosarcoma: Intensive cyclical combination chemotherapy with cyclophosphamide, vincristine and prednisone. *Ann. Intern. Med.* **76**(2), 227–234 (1972).
25. DeVita, V. T., Canellos, G. P., Chabner, B. *et al.* Advanced diffuse histiocytic lymphoma, a potentially curable disease. Results with combination chemotherapy. *Lancet* **1,** 248–250 (1975).
26. Portlock, C. S., and Rosenberg, S. A. No initial therapy for stage III and IV non-Hodgkin's lymphomas of favorable histologic types. *Ann. Intern. Med.* **90,** 10–13 (1979).
27. Schein, P. S., DeVita, V. T., Hubbard, S. *et al.* Bleomycin, adriamycin, cyclophosphamide, vincristine and prednisone (BACOP): Combination chemotherapy in the treatment of advanced diffuse histiocytic lymphoma. *Ann. Intern. Med.* **85**(4), 417–422 (1976).

28. Sweet, D. L., Golomb, H. M., Ultmann, J. E. *et al.* Cyclophosphamide, vincristine, methotrexate with leucovorin rescue and cytosine arabinoside (COMLA) combination sequential chemotherapy in the treatment of advanced diffuse histiocytic lymphoma. *Ann. Intern. Med.* **92,** 985–790 (1980).

Radiotherapy

29. Carabell, S. C., Chaffey, J. T., Rosenthal, D. S. *et al.* Results of total body irradiation in the treatment of advanced non-Hodgkin's lymphomas. *Cancer (Philadelphia)* **43,** 994–1000 (1979).
30. Johnson, R. E., O'Conor, G. T., and Levin, E. Primary management of advanced lymphosarcoma with radiotherapy. *Cancer (Philadelphia)* **25,** 787–791 (1970).
31. Peters, M. V., Bush, R. S., Brown, T. C. *et al.* The place of radiotherapy in the control of non-Hodgkin's lymphoma. *Br. J. Cancer* **31,** Suppl. II, 386–401 (1975).

Section 9. Neoplastic Disorders of the Blood, Bone Marrow, and Lymphatic System

Part B: Leukemias

I. Acute Leukemias 385
  A. Early Detection and Screening
    1. Clinical Presentation
    2. Screening
  B. Pretreatment Evaluation and Work-Up
    1. Baseline Investigation
    2. Additional Studies
    3. Bone Marrow Studies
    4. Special Investigation
    5. Prognostic Factors
      a. Unfavorable Factors
      b. Favorable Factors
  C. Pretreatment Preparation
  D. Therapeutic Management: General Considerations
    1. Acute Myelogenous Leukemia
    2. Acute Adult Lymphoblastic Leukemia
  E. Therapeutic Guidelines: Special Considerations
    1. Central Nervous System Leukemia
    2. Smoldering Leukemia
    3. Bone Marrow Transplantation
    4. Treatment of Relapsed Acute Leukemia
  F. Radiotherapy
    1. Adjuvant Radiotherapy
    2. Salvage Radiotherapy
II. Chronic Myelocytic Leukemia 391
  A. Clinical Considerations
    1. Presenting Symptoms
    2. Hematologic Manifestations
    3. Evolution of the Disease
  B. Initial Work-Up
  C. Therapeutic Management
    1. Chronic Phase
      a. Busulfan
      b. Hydroxyurea
      c. Combination Chemotherapy

    d. Splenectomy
    e. Leukophoresis
    f. Bone Marrow Transplantation
    2. Accelerated Phase
      a. Drug Therapy
      b. Bone Marrow Transplantation
      c. Cryopreservation of the Patient's Own
        Harvested Bone Marrow
IV. Chronic Lymphocytic Leukemia 394
  A. Clinical Considerations
  B. Natural History
  C. Pretreatment Evaluation and Work-Up
    1. Initial Work-Up
    2. Classification
    3. Staging
      a. Early CLL
      b. Advanced CLL
  D. Therapeutic Management
    1. Initiation of Treatment
    2. Chemotherapy
    3. Radiotherapy
      a. Palliative Radiotherapy
      b. Total-Body Irradiation and Splenic Radiation
    4. Therapy Complications
      a. Autoimmune Disorders
      b. Hypersplenism
      c. Pleural Effusion
      d. Masses
      e. Infectious Complications
      f. Other Complications
IV. Hairy Cell Leukemia 398
  A. Clinical Considerations
  B. Therapeutic Management

Suggested Readings 399

Leukemias constitute a large, varied group of diseases characterized by the neoplastic proliferation of one or several of the cellular elements of the blood or bone marrow. In general terms, leukemias are divided into the acute or chronic types, though the word *chronic* may be misleading given that some chronic leukemias may be lethal in a short period of time. Some types of leukemia affect children predominantly, and these are discussed also in §8.B. The reader is referred to that section for the management of childhood leukemias.

I. ACUTE LEUKEMIAS

Acute leukemias constitute a group of diseases that result from extensive replacement of the bone marrow by the neoplastic proliferation of undifferentiated or precursor hematopoietic stem cells over a short period of time. This accumulation of stem cells that have lost their capacity to mature into normal blood cells results in a relentless overgrowth of cells that, in failing to follow the normal path to maturation and destruction, thus crowds the bone marrow and suppresses the growth of normal blood cells.

Several classifications have been suggested for acute leukemias. These are mostly based on the morphology of the leukemic cell, or on the predominant cell line in the bone marrow, since mixed forms are not uncommon. The following classification is recommended by Bennett *et al.* (1).

- Acute myelogenous leukemia (AML—constituting 75% of cases in the adult).
  - M1   Myeloblastic.
  - M2   Myeloblastic with differentiation.
  - M3   Promyelocytic.
  - M4   Myelomonocytic.
  - M5   Monocytic, monoblastic.
  - M6   Erythroleukemic.
- Acute lymphoblastic leukemia (ALL—constituting 10–15% of cases and sometimes called acute nonmyeloblastic leukemia, or ANL).
  - L1   Lymphoblastic, small and homogeneous (childhood ALL).

- L2   Lymphoblastic, small and heterogeneous (adult ALL).
- L3   Burkitt's.
- Acute undifferentiated leukemia (AUL—5–10% of cases).

A. Early Detection and Screening

1. Clinical Presentation

Since the disease results in the crowding and elimination of the normal cellular elements of the blood, anemia, thrombocytopenia, and granulocytopenia constitute the basis of the clinical picture of acute leukemia. The early signs to look for are thus

- Pallor from the anemia.
- Fever, with or without documented infections, resulting from neutropenia. Typical signs and symptoms of infection may be scarce as a result of the paucity of inflammatory cells.
- Abnormal bleeding or bruising, from the thrombocytopenia or consumption coagulopathy.
- Enlargement of lymph nodes, spleen, or liver.
- Pains, due to bone marrow expansion.

Later symptoms are the results of organ failures due to leukemic infiltration:

- Organomegaly.
- Hyperuricemia and renal failure due to kidney infiltration.
- Neurological symptoms from intracerebral leukostasis or leukemic growth in the arteriolar walls, with subsequent rupture and cerebral hemorrhage.
- Hypocalcemia with elevated serum potassium and serum phosphate.

The diagnosis is usually easily established by examination of the peripheral blood smear and bone marrow.

2. Screening

Early detection is based primarily on a high degree of awareness and quick evaluation of patients with persistent symptoms, particularly in the pediatric age group. No specific screening for leukemia is recommended beyond what is included in a routine check-up as suggested both in the pediatric age group and in the older population. This usually will include a CBC, usually the first test in which aberrations suggesting leukemia can be detected.

B. Pretreatment Evaluation and Work-Up

1. Baseline Investigation

Initial studies, beyond a comprehensive history and physical examination, include

- CBC and morphology (review of the peripheral blood smear).
- WBC differential count and platelet count.
- Coagulation profile.
- Serum electrolytes, blood urea nitrogen, and uric acid.
- Chest x-ray.
- Serum and urine electrophoresis with immunoelectrophoresis, if necessary.
- Urinalysis.

2. Additional Studies

Certain specific tests must be obtained, based on the clinical presentation of the patient at the time of diagnosis:

- Blood grouping and typing.
- Spinal tap.
- Cultures (blood, urine, sputum, perineum, throat, etc.) and renal function tests.
- Other x-rays or scans, as indicated.

3. Bone Marrow Studies

The most indispensable part of the evaluation of the leukemic patient is the study of the bone marrow by both aspiration and biopsy. Biopsies of other organs are usually contraindicated in patients suspected of having acute leukemia. For more accurate typing and classification of the leukemia, multiple staining procedures have been suggested. These include

- Cytochemical stains
  - Peroxidase or Sudan black.
  - PAS (p-aminosalicylic acid).
  - Leukocyte alkaline phosphatase (LAP) and acid phosphatase.
  - Chloracetate and alpha naphthyl acetate esterase, with or without fluoride inhibition.
- Serum and urine muramidase.

- Lymphocyte suface markers for ALL; other surface markers for myeloid leukemias are under development.
- Determination of terminal deoxynucleotidyltransferase (TDT), positive in most cases of ALL but negative in AML.
- Karyotyping.

Table I describes the differential findings identified by the most commonly performed typing procedures.

4. Special Investigation

Additional investigations, carried out in specialized centers and research laboratories, have proven very useful in identifying certain subtypes of leukemia and certain prognostic features (e.g., insufficient patterns, etc.). These investigative approaches include

- Cytogenetic analysis, with more sophisticated banding and synchronization techniques.
- Immunologic markers and labeling indices.
- Electron microscopy.
- Cell cultures and patterns of growth, in semisolid growth media.

5. Prognostic Factors

The likelihood of response to therapy in a patient with adult acute leukemia depends on several factors:

a. Unfavorable Factors

- Elderly, febrile, debiliatated patients.
- Major bleeding episodes.
- Organomegaly or renal insufficiency.
- Prolonged phase of "smoldering leukemia" prior to diagnosis.
- Lack of normal metaphase.
- Immunoincompetence.
- High blast cell count.
- Secondary (therapy related) leukemia.

b. Favorable Factors

- Females.
- Young patients.
- High labeling index (>9%).

C. Pretreatment Preparation

The role of the internist or pediatrician in the management of the patient with acute leukemia is primarily to control the infections; correct the fluid, electrolyte, and acid-base defects; monitor vital functions, including the CNS, cardiopulmonary

Table I

Cytochemical Typing of Various Leukemias

Cytochemical reaction	Discrimination	Interpretation	Acute myelocytic leukemia	Acute myelomono-leukemia	Acute monocytic leukemia	Acute lymphocytic leukemia
Peroxidase and sudan black	Lymphoid versus myeloid	Positive = dark granular cytoplasmic reaction = nonlymphoid process (granulocytic-monocytic)	Positive	Positive	Usually positive	Negative
Specific esterase (Chloracetate esterase)	Granulocytes versus monocytes	Positive = pink cytoplasmic reaction = granulocytic differentiation	Usually positive	Usually positive	Negative	Negative
Nonspecific esterase (a-naphtylbutyrate)	Granulocytes versus monocytes	Positive = brown cytoplasmic reaction = monocytic-histiocytic differentiation Exceptions: May see weak rxns in Megs, plasma cells, etc. Also "Block" positivity in T lymphs	Negative	By FAB criteria 30% of leukemia cells positive.	Positive (inhibited by fluoride).	Negative
PAS (with and without diastase)	In some cases, may discriminate lymphoid versus non-lymphoid; usually not of value	Block positivity = diastase digestible, i.e., glycogen = lymphoid process				
		Other rxns = granular positivity and diastase-resistant products are nonspecific	May see granular positivity	May see granular positivity	Often see granular positivity	Ideally see block positive
Acid phosphatase	May be of value in discriminating T- from null-all, otherwise non-discriminatory	Block positivity = T-cell process. Tartrate-resistant granular positivity found in hairy cell leukemia	Often granular positivity	Often granular positivity	Often strong granular positivity	T-cell ALL block positives; other ALL may show granular positives

function, kidneys, etc.; and attend to the patient's general care. The chemotherapy of acute leukemia is too complicated to be carried out in places other than those medical centers prepared to deal with the serious complications of the disease and its therapy—centers that have the resources to provide intensive hematologic support and personnel specially trained and experienced in the treatment of leukemia. It is required that one become familiar with the disease, the drug regimens, and the psychological strain that it creates for the patient and the patient's family. A physician not trained to handle all of these aspects adequately should not attempt to manage these patients.

The diagnosis of acute leukemias mandates quick action and meticulous attention to details, both in terms of nonspecific and specific therapy. A WBC of over 100,000 or severe thrombocytopenia constitutes an emergency because of the risks of impending serious complications. The following modalities must be utilized without delay in the appropriate cases:

- Empirical bacteriocidal antibiotics must be started immediately in febrile neutropenic leukemia patients, once appropriate cultures are taken. Carbenicillin plus an aminoglycoside with or without a cephalosporin are the best current choice since the most common offending organisms are pseudomonas, *Klebsiella, Escherichia coli,* and to a lesser degree, *Staphylococcus aureus.*
- Prophylactic platelet transfusions are indicated in thrombocytopenic patients (those with 20,000 or fewer platelets per cubic millimeter).
- Prophylactic heparinization should be considered in selected cases where there is a high risk of consumption coagulopathy due to the release of thromboplastic materials from dying cells (e.g., acute promyelocytic leukemia and some AML).
- Hydration, alkalinization of the urine, and allopurinol must be started in all patients with or without hyperuricemia.
- Renal dialysis in cases of renal failure.
- Prophylactic isoniazid in PPD-positive patients should be considered, since reactivation of tuberculosis is a potential hazard after chemotherapy.

D. Therapeutic Management: General Considerations

With present-day chemotherapy, remissions in acute leukemia are not uncommon, and it is projected that 25% of patients who achieve a complete remission will be alive and still in remission at 2 years, with an excellent chance of prolonged survival.

1. Acute Myelogenous Leukemia

The major advances in the treatment of AML in adults have been attributed to the use of cytosine arabinoside (ARA-C), the anthracycline antibiotics daunorubicin—(DNR), and Adriamycin (ADR), all of which, when used as single agents, will yield a 20–30% rate of remission. Combinations with thioguanine (TG) have increased the response rate to 80% in expert hands.

The following combinations have been reported to yield high response rates by various cooperative groups:

- DNR, 45 mg/m², daily for 3 days.
  ARA-C, 100 mg/m², daily for 7 days, by continuous infusion.
- The addition of TG to the above regimen (100–200 mgm/M², PO daily for 5–7 days) resulted in an 82% complete response rate in 28 patients in one reported series.
- ADR (usual dose, 30–60 mg/m², for 2–3 days).
  ARA-C (usual dose, 100–200 mg/m², IV every 8–12 hours).
  Vincristine (usual dose, 1.4 mg/m², on day 1 of each cycle).
  Prednisone.

The treatment objective is to induce severe bone marrow aplasia, thus reducing the body burden of leukemic infiltrates by at least 99 or 99.9% (by a factor of 100–100). It is assumed that a normal population of stem cells continues to exist and that it can repopulate the bone marrow with normal cells once the leukemic population has been largely eliminated. That this occurs can be demonstrated by the reversal (normalization) of karyotypic abnormalities once a remission is established and by its reappearance when the leukemia relapses. If the bone marrow continues to show leukemic infiltrates on two consecutive aspirations, another course of chemotherapy is given, recognizing that chances of success are less bright.

The severe marrow aplasia consistently induced by modern chemotherapy programs virtually always results in a period of profound pancytopenia. The latter is relieved only with repopulation of the marrow by normal elements. The period of aplasia generally starts within a week to 10 days after therapy is initiated and lasts between 1 and 3 weeks. It is during this period that the patients experience the most dangerous complications of treatment:

- Serious bleeding complications. These have been reduced by prophylactic platelet transfusions. Patients should be given platelet concentrates when the platelet count reaches $20,000/\mu^3$ or less and should be treated even with higher platelet counts in the event of serious bleeding. Patients receiving antibiotics may become vitamin K deficient. If coagulation tests suggest vitamin K deficiency, it should be given parenterally (IV).
- Infection. Neutropenic patients developing fever, with or without laboratory or clinical evidence of infection, must be started on a program of broad-spectrum antibiotics. Antibiotics must be continued until such time as the peripheral blood shows evidence of regenerating marrow (>500 granulocytes per cubic millimeter). If there is *no* response to broad-spectrum antibiotics and if the site of infection is unknown or if no organism is identified on multiple cultures, some recommended that granulocyte transfusions be given.

Single-donor, HLA-matched granulocytes are ideal but generally unavailable. Single-donor granulocytes are preferable to pooled multiunit granulocytes obtained from regional blood centers.

- If there is no response to the combination of antibiotics and granulocytes and the patient continues to be profoundly granulocytopenic, a trial of amphotericin B is probably indicated in addition to the antibiotic because of a high incidence of intercurrent fungal infections. Antibiotics are discontinued when there is evidence of marrow recovery (>500 granulocytes) and when the patient's fever resolves.

Other precautions are necessary when caring for a patient treated for leukemia:

- Attention must be paid to transfusion of packed red blood cells.
- Fluid and electrolyte balance must be carefully maintained (e.g., replacing potassium for patients receiving carbenicillin or ticarcillin).
- Coagulation tests must be carried out, and defects other than platelets deficiency (e.g., vitamin K deficiency in patients on prolonged antibiotic therapy) must be identified.
- All manipulations, especially all venipunctures, must be done with sterile technique. Manipulation of the perianal area must be prohibited (no rectal temperatures, endoscopies. etc.).

Reverse isolation procedures, as practiced in most general hospitals, are unnecessary and serve mainly to increase the patient's anxiety and sense of isolation. Physical isolation provisions, such as laminar flow rooms, do reduce the incidence of infection when combined with a program of gut sterilization but are very expensive and cumbersome. They have not been shown to increase the complete remission rate; some have recommended the prophylactic use of trimethoprim/sulfamethoxazole to reduce the number of infections, and this remains under study.

Bone marrow examination should be performed frequently after the remission-induction chemotherapy is completed. The marrow is usually found to be severely hypoplastic for 1–2 weeks (sometimes longer) and then gradually shows signs of recovery. This is generally heralded by improvement in the peripheral blood and manifested by the appearance of granulocytes and by a reduction in transfusion requirement. Remission is defined as complete when the peripheral blood is free of leukemic cells, has at least 11–12 gram % Hb, at least 3000 WBC with 2000 granulocytes, and over 100,000 platelets. The bone marrow must be cellular, pleomorphic, show evidence of normal maturation, and have fewer than 5% blast cells. The remission is defined as partial if any of the above criteria, especially the percentage of blast cells, is not met. Patients achieving only a partial remission are retreated in order to establish complete remission (CR). Only a CR offers a chance at prolonged survival.

The search for more effective treatments of AML continues. Whenever possible, newly diagnosed patients with acute leukemia should be referred to centers where newer treatment programs are under active investigation, keeping in mind that all the major strides made in the last 20 years are directly attributable to the clinical trial methods employed. Further research efforts will continue to lead to improvement in the percentage of long-term survivors. For example, new drugs are now being incorporated into primary induction therapy schemes, and early and late intensification programs are also being tested.

2. Acute Adult Lymphoblastic Leukemia

The management of patients with ALL varies slightly from that of AML: patients are younger, and the immediate prognosis is better. Vincristine (VCR), corticosteroids, methotrexate (MTX), and L-asparaginase (L-ASP) are all individually active in ALL, with response rates around 30%. Various combinations and the addition of ADR have increased the response rates significantly.

- VCR-P (prednisone) alone, response rate around 50%.
- MP(mercaptopurine)-VCR-MTX-P, response rate around 60%.
- DNR-VCR-P, response rate around 80%.
- ADR–VCR–P–L-ASP, response rate around 70%.

The most common regimen is to employ intravenous VCR (1.4 mg per square meter, maximum 2 mg) once a week for 3–4 weeks. Prednisone is started on day 1 at 40 or more mg per square meter and continued for 3–4 weeks before being tapered off. It has been suggested that the addition of an anthracycline early in the induction period will increase the complete remission rates from 50–60 to 70–80%. Treatment with VCR and prednisone tends to be very well tolerated, and patients tend to require little hematologic support. Some attain remission without a discernible episode of marrow aplasia or severe pancytopenia. The addition of an anthracycline virtually guarantees marrow aplasia, and the induction course will then resemble more closely an AML induction with the attendant need for intensive hematologic support.

Once remission is established, most protocols call for a course of treatment with L-ASP and CNS prophylaxis as outlined below.

Maintenance therapy generally consists of courses of 6-MP and MTX with reinforcement courses of VCR and prednisone every 3–4 months. Under study at the present time are a variety of consolidation studies using ARA-C and DNR shortly after remission has been induced. Maintenance therapy is usually continued for 2 years. If the patient is in complete remission at the end of the second year, all therapy is discontinued.

E. Therapeutic Guidelines: Special Considerations

1. Central Nervous System Leukemia

Central nervous system prophylaxis and treatment is of great importance in the management of the patient with acute leukemia. A spinal tap at the time of complete remission will identify some, but not all, patients with CNS disease. Over 25% of patients with ALL will have CNS leukemia, as compared to 10% of patients with AML. It has been suggested that patients with AML be treated with one dose of ARA-C, 100 mg intrathecally, after one has performed a diagnostic tap and that one observe them for CNS disease. Patients with ALL or ANL, on the other hand, must be treated more aggressively, even in the absence of a positive spinal tap. Intensive intrathecal therapy using MTX (12 mg per square meter, maximum dose 15 mg) delivered by serial lumbar punctures or an Ommaya reservoir is the standard method, and prophylactic cranial irradiation (2400 rads) has been recommended.

Treatment of the patient with confirmed CNS disease must be prolonged. Intermittent intrathecal chemotherapy is given every 3 days until the cerebrospinal fluid is clear of leukemic cells, then weekly for 1 month, biweekly for 2 months, and monthly for 1 year. Cranial irradiation is also recommended.

2. Smoldering Leukemia

This "preleukemic" phase of the disease, often seen in the elderly patient, presents with anemia, pancytopenia, and hypercellularity of the bone marrow with a mild increase in blasts and promyelocytes. It augurs a poor prognosis, and 50–70% of patients will progress to frank AML within 6–12 months. During the smoldering chemotherapy phase is ineffective and contraindicated; therapy with hematinics, though generally ineffective, may be occasionally beneficial. Several recent reports suggest that treatment with low-dose ARA-C (20–30 mg per day) for 14 days may cause the bone marrow to differentiate, resulting in relief of pancytopenia. These reports need to be confirmed by more observations.

3. Bone Marrow Transplantation

Experimental clinical trials with allogenic transplantation of bone marrow in patients with leukemia are being undertaken in several centers. The patient is pretreated with intensive chemotherapy and/or radiotherapy in an attempt to eliminate the entire leukemic cell population; this is then followed by an infusion of bone marrow cells closely matched at HLA-A, B, C, and D loci from selected donors, usually siblings. The results are promising, particularly if the donor is an identical twin.

The centers practicing bone marrow transplantation (BMT) claim that 30–50% of patients so treated will have prolonged remissions, free of any maintenance chemotherapy. This contrasts with the 20% long-term remission rates usually obtained with the chemotherapy described above. On the other hand, BMT results in an immediate 20–30% mortality from the rigors of the conditioning regimen ("lethal" doses of chemotherapy plus radiation), from acute complications such as infections (bacterial, fungal, and especially viral), from idiopathic interstitial pneumonitis, and from graft versus host (GVH) disease. Furthermore, only those patients who have an HLA-identical (or compatible) donor are eligible for the procedure. Finally, the procedure is generally available only for patients less than 40 years of age, and the best results are obtained in patients less than 20 years old.

BMT has *not* been effective therapy for patients in relapse. Thus, a difficult decision faces the patient and the treating physician who has a young patient with AML in remission and with a potential bone marrow donor. Continuing maintenance on chemotherapy will result in a *median* remission duration of 14–20 months and a 20% chance of prolonged survival. Referral for BMT will result in an immediate mortality of 20–30%, yet successful, complication-free engraftment of the donor marrow may double the chances for ultimate cure.

Major efforts are underway to improve the methodology and technology of BMT and to increase the safety of the modality. One distressing problem is that efforts to reduce GVH disease may result in an increase of leukemic relapse: it appears that those donor cells responsible for GVH disease also exert an antileukemia effect. Nonetheless, if BMT can be accomplished with less morbidity and mortality in future studies, it will prove to be a major contribution in the treatment of acute leukemia.

Bone marrow harvesting from leukemic patients in a chemotherapy-induced complete remission, for later reinfusion following intensive cytotoxic chemotherapy for relapse, is also actively being investigated and offers the distinct advantage of minimizing the "graft" rejections often seen with allogenic transplantation.

4. Treatment of Relapsed Acute Leukemia

If the relapse occurs after a relatively durable remission, one usually attempts to induce a second remission with the same (or similar) agents as those that produced the initial response. This is particularly effective in the case of patients who have been off maintenance chemotherapy or whenever the maintenance schedule did not include the same agents as initially employed to induce the remission. If, on the other hand, the patient recently received a maintenance course including ARA-C and an anthracycline in moderate doses, and a frank relapse supervenes in short order, it is rather unlikely that the use of the same agents, even in higher doses, will result in a remission. In such cases, a therapeutic trial of different agents is reasonable; this generally involves the use of those new investigational agents that have shown antileukemic activity in preclinical screening and in early testing in human subjects (Phase I and II clinical trials).

When the leukemia becomes refractory, it becomes pointless to subject the patient to further chemotherapy procedures. At such times, a judicious program of transfusions and other measures to assure patient comfort, is recommended. Whether or not to employ aggressive (and necessarily toxic) treatments— as opposed to the more gentle approaches, which offer no, or little, hope of a second complete remission—is not always easy. The patient and his, or her, family should be participants in any such deliberations.

F. Radiotherapy

The role of radiotherapy in the management of acute leukemia is essentially one of adjuvant therapy. It is also indicated for salvage after failure of chemotherapy to extinguish aggregates of leukemia cells in sites such as the brain or testicles, where a so-called barrier exists that prevents the free diffusion of effective cytotoxic agents. This barrier may be overcome by using increasing doses of the cytotoxic agent or by adding ionizing radiation. In children, the use of high-dose chemotherapy is often preferred to radiotherapy; external irradiation to the brain, with its potential risks of late neuropsychiatric deficiencies (memory defects, slow mentation, and stunted intellectual growth), may thus be avoided. However, high-dose chemotherapy is frequently associated with severe, acute, and sometimes fatal toxicity, and control of the disease is not assured. Even in adults, high-dose chemotherapy is less desirable, since the effects of low-dose radiation on the adult brain are minimal, whereas tolerance to high-dose chemotherapy is even less than that of children.

1. Adjuvant Radiotherapy

Adjuvant radiotherapy in the treatment of leukemia is primarily used in the management of potential disease within the CNS. This is particularly true for the intracranial component of the CNS (the brain), since the spinal axis seems to be accessible to intrathecal MTX therapy. The application of radiation to the whole cerebrospinal axis (brain and spinal cord) is still in use in certain centers. The doses aimed at are usually low, in the range of 24 grays (2400 rads) given in 2.5 weeks. These

doses are reduced in very young children to 1800 rads in order to minimize long-term side effects.

2. Salvage Radiotherapy

Since leukemic cell aggregates are highly sensitive to low-dose radiation, the use of radiation to control local aggregates that fail to respond to systemic therapy is highly effective. However, the ultimate cure of the patient will depend on the control of the systemic disease by chemotherapy.

The two most common sites of failure after systemic chemotherapy are the cerebrospinal meninges and the testes. Both sites are easily accessible to external irradiation, with good results achieved with rather limited doses; 24 grays (2400 rads) in 2.5 weeks.

Generally, cranial irradiation is combined with intrathecal MTX, a combination that is preferred to irradiation of the entire cerebrospinal axis; the latter entails the irradiation of a large volume of bone marrow, with the danger of subsequent prolonged periods of marrow depression. It must be emphasized that cranial irradiation must include treatment of the posterior orbital compartment, including the retina and optic nerves, as well as the upper two segments of the spinal cord, since these regions are all at high risk.

Irradiation of both testes for control of leukemic aggregates is rather simple and effective, with the delivery of the same low dosages. The long-term side effect of sterility is almost theoretical since long-term survival after such a clinical presentation, is rare.

II. CHRONIC MYELOCYTIC LEUKEMIA

The word *chronic* in leukemias should be carefully interpreted. The median life span of a patient with chronic myelocytic leukemia (CML) is about 3 years, and it affects a younger age group. Though "chronic" may be comforting to the patient at the time of diagnosis, the physician must be aware that the disease is lethal in a relatively short period of time.

Chronic myelocytic leukemia is a disease of the hemopoietic stem cell; the latter is a self-renewing population of cells that are also capable of producing other stem cells committed to differentiate into the various hematic cell lines: erythroid, granulocytic, macrophagic, lymphoid, and megakaryocytic.

Chronic myelocytic leukemia is characterized, in about 90% of cases, by the presence of the Philadelphia chromosome (Ph′, a translocation of the short arm of chromosome 22 to chromosome 9) in bone marrow and blood cells but not in other somatic cells. That the lesion of CML resides in the stem cell is attested to by the fact that all the hematic cells are involved in the leukemic process, even though the myeloid (granulocytic) component tends to dominate the clinical picture.

A. Clinical Considerations

a. Presenting Symptoms

The disease may be discovered incidentally during a patient's periodic health examination or during the course of another illness. The presenting clinical symptoms are frequently due to an enlarged spleen, which can cause one of several complaints:

* Upper abdominal fullness.
* A pulling sensation in the left upper quadrant.
* Pain over the splenic area.
* A mass felt by the patient.
* Early satiety due to pressure on the stomach.

Pain over the splenic area is usually due to stretching of the splenic capsule; however, splenic infarction can also cause pain. Splenic rupture is unusual. The physical examination is generally remarkable for the absence of enlarged lymph nodes.

Other symptoms include:

* Night sweats.
* Weight loss.
* Skeletal pain.
* Easy fatigability.

b. Hematologic Manifestations

The stem cell origin of the disease accounts for the hematologic manifestations. Most patients have a leukocytosis, which, on occasion, may be severe (several hundred thousand). The peripheral smear will show the entire spectrum of granulocytic maturation (from myeloblast to polymorphonuclear granulocyte); an increased relative and absolute number of eosinophils and basophils is almost always present. Hemoglobin levels are generally normal or slightly lower at presentation; the platelet count may be normal, high, or low; and megathrombocytes may be seen. The red blood cell morphology may be normal but may show teardrop poikilocytes.

Serum chemistries usually show an increased uric acid and lactate dehydrogenase (LDH), as evidence of the massive cell turnover in the bone marrow.

The bone marrow aspirate is uniformly hypercellular with massive expansion of the granulocytic line. Erythroid activity is less pronounced. Megakaryocytes are increased, as are basophils (mast cells) and eosinophils.

c. Evolution of the Disease

The disease usually passes through two phases: a chronic, relatively indolent phase that may last several months or years and an accelerated, fulminant phase indistinguishable from acute leukemia in its late stages and characterized by a rising WBC, a decreasing hemoglobin and platelet count, and an increased blast percentage (>30%). If a patient presents primarily in "blastic crisis," it may be erroneously labeled acute myelogenous leukemia. The presence of an enlarged spleen or hepatosplenomegaly and lymphadenopathy, associated with symptoms of fatigue or weight loss of some months duration, should alert the physician to the possibility of a CML in blastic crisis. An increased number of basophils and eosinophils, thrombocytosis, and changes in red cell morphology are also clues to a preexisting CML. The diagnosis can be confirmed by the presence of the Philadelphia chromosome.

Most patients with CML are initially diagnosed in the "chronic" phase of the illness. Patients will present as outlined above and tend to be easily treated into a "remission," i.e., symptoms are promptly relieved, and the blood counts can be brought back close to normal ranges. However, remissions are practically never of importance to the ultimate survival chances. The Philadelphia chromosome is essentially always demonstrable in the bone marrow, indicating that the abnormal clone has not been eliminated but simply controlled. There is no evidence whatsoever that chemotherapy during the chronic phase is able to delay or prevent the most dreaded evolution of this disease, the transformation into an acute blastic leukemia. At present, the recommended treatment during the chronic phase remains the use of single agents (most commonly busulfan and/or hydroxyurea). At some point in the course of an otherwise well-controlled chronic phase, one notes that the blood counts are more difficult to manage, that the spleen enlarges, that symptoms recur, that the platelet count drops, and most obviously, that the percentage of blast cells increases. Such changes may progress over several months to a picture of an acute blastic leukemia, which is generally refractory to regimens otherwise effective in *de novo* acute leukemia.

It is impossible to predict whether a particular patient will have a short or prolonged chronic phase. About 25% of a particular population of patients will convert into the blastic phase in each successive year of observation. Thus, there is a steady attrition, apparently uninfluenced by therapy, with some patients surviving less than 1 year, while others remain in the chronic phase for a decade or more.

During the transformation into the acute phase, additional chromosomal abnormalities are frequently noted. Most commonly these consist of extra Philadelphia chromosomes, changes in the number of chromosomes, etc. It has been suggested that treatment for the acute phase ought to be instituted as soon as such new karyotypic abnormalities are noted, though prospective studies on this question are still lacking.

Most patients will manifest a conversion into an acute myeloid-type leukemia. A minority (20–30%) will convert into an acute lymphoid leukemia, emphasizing again the pluripotential nature of the underlying affected cell. Morphological evaluation alone is inadequate to distinguish one type of conversion from another (i.e., many cases of lymphoid conversion will look like myeloblastic), though such distinction is important in planning subsequent therapy. Determining TDT activity has been useful in this regard—the enzyme is detectable in almost all cases of ALL but tends to be absent (or low) in AML. Surface marker analysis may also be useful. If the diagnosis of lymphoid conversion is confirmed, treatment with vincristine and prednisone, as in ALL, is more likely to induce a remission with substantially less toxicity than the standard treatments for myeloid leukemia. Unfortunately, remission, even with lymphoid-type transformation, tends to be relatively short lived.

About 10% of patients are Philadelphia chromosome negative. Their prognosis appears to be worse than Ph' + patients.

B. Initial Work-Up

- CBC and peripheral smear.
- Serum chemistries.
- LAP (very low or absent in CML; tends to be normal or elevated in other myeloproliferative diseases).
- Serum B_{12} and B_{12} binding capacity (elevated in CML).
- Bone marrow aspiration for microscopy and for karyotyping.
- Bone marrow biopsy: histology and check for fibrosis.

C. Therapeutic Management

1. Chronic Phase

A. Busulfan

Busulfan is the classic agent for the treatment of CML. Remissions tend to be relatively smooth and side effects very few, and many patients can be managed with several tablets per week. It is particularly effective for controlling thrombocytosis but can cause chronic, sometimes severe, myelosuppression, which sometimes persists for weeks or months following cessation of therapy. A small minority of patients develop progressive, severe interstitial lung fibrosis.

b. Hydroxyurea

This agent is preferred by some because it may do less damage to the bone marrow. Its effects are short lived and are readily reversible. It has no proven advantage over busulfan, however, and is more difficult to control. Some physicians prefer to combine both agents.

c. Combination Chemotherapy

Many agents and combinations of cytotoxic drugs have been employed in the treatment of CML, but there has been no clear advantage over the use of single agents. Several group have employed very intensive chemotherapy during the chronic phase in hopes of eradicating the Philadelphia chromosome. Others have cryopreserved the chronic-phase marrow for reinfusion after ablative therapies for the blastic phase, and most intensive programs have also employed splenectomy. The ultimate value of these intensive treatments, however, is not yet established.

d. Splenectomy

The enlarged spleen seem initially in patients with CML generally shrinks readily with the initial treatment for the chronic phase. During the blastic transformation, however, it tends to enlarge again, sometimes to enormous size, causing severe symptoms. These may be due to mechanical obstruction and pressure, to hypersplenism with resultant anemia and thrombocytopenia, or may be related to severe pain secondary to stretching of the capsule or to splenic infarcts. Some hematologists favor early splenectomy, as the operation is well tolerated in this generally young group of patients. If one waits until the spleen is very large and cytopenias are well established, the risk of splenectomy increases markedly. An alternative approach to splenectomy is irradiation to the spleen.

e. Leukopheresis

Mechanical removal of white blood cells is indicated as the initial treatment for any patient with very high WBC counts ($>300,000/mm^3$) or for patients exibiting signs of leukostasis in the pulmonary or cerebral circulations. The early use of hydroxyurea has also been recommended in such cases to control the leukocytosis rapidly.

f. Bone Marrow Transplantation

The application of BMT in the chronic phase of CML is an approach that holds out the promise of permanent eradication of the Philadelphia-positive clone. The same arguments discussed in §9A.I.E.3 are relevant here; furthermore, it should be kept in mind that the chronic phase will occasionally last for many years, and the decision to carry out a BMT, even when a match donor is available, is not a clear-cut or easy choice.

2. Accelerated Phase

a. Drug Therapy

Therapeutic management of the CML patient in an accelerated phase will require more aggressive therapy, which will vary depending on the type of conversion. For patients with lymphoid conversion, treatment with vincristine and prednisone is indicated. Some hematologists will add MTX, 6-MP, and generally L-ASP (see §9A.I.D.2). Remission can be achieved but generally tends to last less than 12 months. For patients with myeloid conversion, on the other hand, treatment with standard AML regimens has yielded less than a 20% complete remission rate. Newer agents are under constant scrutiny for effectiveness in this situation.

b. Bone Marrow Transplantation

Bone marrow transplantation is generally unsuccessful when carried out in the full-blown blastic phase because of the inability to eradicate the transformed clones. More recently, however, the transplant group at the University of Minnesota has reported a series of successful BMTs in patients in the "early accelerated" phase. Since most such patients in blastic crisis survive less than 1 year, the decision in favor of BMT is certainly more appropriate and easily made than for a patient in the pure chronic phase. If the early reports of success (elimination of the Ph'+ clone) meet the test of time, BMT will be strongly recommended for early transformation of CML.

c. Cryopreservation of the Patient's Own Harvested Bone Marrow

Cryopreservation of the chronic-phase marrow for reinfusion after vigorous ablative therapy during the accelerated phase is an intriguing and promising approach. Unfortunately, relapse of the acute blastic leukemia almost inevitably occurs after a very brief restoration of the chronic phase. It appears that whatever stimulus was responsible for inducing the acute transformation still persists and remains capable of transforming the cryopreserved chronic-phase stem cell.

In point of fact, the only approach that has shown any promise over single-agent chemotherapy is BMT. The great majority of patients with early-phase CML will respond dramatically to chemotherapy, and remissions may be prolonged. Progression into an accelerated phase, however, is an ominous sign with complete responses ranging between 5 and 20% and lasting no more than 6–10 months.

There is great need for research to improve treatment of CML. So far the various treatments have done little to prolong the chronic phase or prevent acute blastic transformation.

III. CHRONIC LYMPHOCYTIC LEUKEMIA

Chronic lymphatic leukemia (CLL) is a term applied to a heterogeneous group of proliferative disorders of well-differentiated lymphocytes. It is characterized by lymphocytosis and progressive, diffuse infiltration of the bone marrow and lymphoid organs and is frequently associated with disturbance of the immune system.

A. Clinical Considerations

The disease is frequently discovered fortuitously during a routine physical examination or when the blood is examined for an unrelated illness. Chronic lymphatic leukemia may also present with

- Enlargement of the lymph nodes, spleen, and liver.
- Anemia, hemolytic or myelophthisic.
- Thrombocytopenia, autoimmune or myelophthisic.
- Pyogenic infection (pneumonia being the most common) as a result of granulocytopenia and hypogammaglobulinemia.
- Constitutional symptoms: night sweats, fevers, weight loss, etc.

B. Natural History

Chronic lymphocytic leukemia is an accumulative disease of long-lived lymphocytes—B cells in over 98% of cases—with slowly progressive infiltration of the bone marrow, the lymphatic tissues, and eventually, all other organs, with the notable exception of the CNS. The proposed and most widely accepted disease classification reflects the accumulative nature of the disorder. Thus Stages I and II indicate involvement of the bone marrow but no significant suppression of function, whereas the later stages are reserved for situations in which further infiltration results in relentless organ failure unless effective therapy is applied.

Early-stage CLL is associated with a prolonged survival (>10 years), whereas patients presenting with Stage IV disease typically survive for less than 2 years, emphasizing the heterogeneous nature of this rather common disease. Many elderly patients present with asymptomatic lymphocytosis and encounter few, if any, clinical problems attributable to the CLL. In contrast, young patients tend to present with more aggressive symptomatic disease requiring treatment at once.

The vast majority of CLLs arise from B cells (see Table II). The lymphocytes express monoclonal immunoglobulin on the

Table II

Differential Diagnosis of Chronic Lymphocytic Leukemia[a]

	B cell "common type"	B cell prolymphocytic	"Lymphosarcoma" cell leukemia	T Cell "knobby" Japanese type	T Cell cytoplasmic	Hairy cell leukemia
Clinical						
Age	40+	50+	50+	50 (34–68)	54 (19–80)	40–60
M : F	2 : 1	>5 : 1	1 : 1	?	1 : 1	4 : 1
Spleen	Stage II–>	Prominent	30%	80%	80%	80%
Nodes	Stage I–>	Slight	90%	80%–90%	10%	<10%
Skin	Rare	Rare	Rare	Common	Common	Rare
Laboratory lymphocyte count	>10,000	>100,000	Below normal to >100,000	80,000 (11,000–700,000)	12,000 (3,000–300,000)	Below normal to >40,000
Markers						
SIg	IgM,IgD	IgM,IgD	IgM,IgD	0	0	IgG
EAC rosettes	1+	4+	2+	—	—	0
E rosettes	0	0	0	4+	4+	0
Others		Nucleolus prominent	Nucleolus prominent		Azurophilic granules	Tartrate-resistant acid phosphatase
Survival	2–20 years	3–42 months	2–5 years	1 year	>25 years	5–7 years or better

[a] Adapted from R. G. Gale *et al.*: Chronic leukemias. *In* Hematology 1981, Education Program, American Society of Hematology, pp. 22–27.

cell surface, but the number of molecules per cell is reduced. A fraction of patients will have a monoclonal paraprotein in the serum, corresponding in class and light-chain type to the immunoglobulin on the cell surface. With progressive replacement of the bone marrow and normal lymphoid tissue, the immunologic deficiencies come, in time, to dominate the clinical picture. Granulocytopenia and deficiency of normal immunoglobulins contribute susceptibility to a variety of infections: pyogenic, viral (e.g., herpes zoster, cytomegalovirus [CMV]), and those resulting from a variety of opportunistic agents. Severe infection is probably the most common cause of death in CLL.

The problems of anemia and thrombocytopenia are the result of two distinct mechanisms. Autoimmune thrombocytopenia and hemolytic anemia are fairly common and are indistinguishable in immune pathogenesis from their idiopathic counterparts, idiopathic thrombocytopenic purpura and acquired idiopathic hemolytic anemia. Perhaps more ominous are the cytopenias resulting from progressive marrow infiltration; whereas autoimmune thrombocytopenia and anemia respond quite readily to treatment, the cytopenias produced by progressive infiltration are generally a consequence of late-stage relentlessly advancing disease and are more resistant to treatment.

Only 1 or 2% of patients with CLL have T-cell CLL. These cells are E rosette positive and surface Ig negative (see Table II). Several clinical features serve to distinguish this group of patients from the common B-cell type:

- Adenopathy is less prominent in T-cell-type CLL.
- Splenomegaly is more prominent in T-cell-type CLL.
- Infiltration of the skin is often present in T-cell-type CLL.

A particular type of T-CLL is seen more commonly in Japan. Prolymphocytic leukemia is another rare variant of CLL. The cells are larger, tend to have prominent nucleoli and heavy Ig staining on the cell surface, and almost always presents with very high WBC counts. The patients generally have markedly enlarged spleens and surprisingly inconsequential peripheral lymph node enlargement. The diagnosis is confirmed by surface-marker analysis, and the prognosis is substantially worse than that for CLL in general (see Table II).

C. Pretreatment Evaluation and Work-Up

1. Initial Work-Up

- History and complete physical examination. Fever, night sweats, weight loss, weakness, jaundice, etc. should be noted. The examination should record the location and size of lymph nodes, liver, and spleen.
- CBC, differential WBC, platelets, and careful study of lymphocyte morphology. The lymphocytes in CLL are mature-appearing, small lymphocytes for the most part, though larger and atypical lymphocytes are frequently seen. The absolute number of granulocytes should be noted. Red blood

cell morphology should be scrutinized for the presence of microspherocytes and polychromasia, which indicate a possibility of hemolysis. Rouleaux formation may indicate the presence of a paraprotein.

- Urinalysis.
- Chemistries and SMA-18.
- Chest x-ray, anterior/posterior and lateral.
- Bone marrow aspiration and, if needed, bone marrow biopsy.
- Serum and urine protein electropheresis and immunoglobulin quantification. The serum and urine protein examinations are necessary to determine the presence and degree of hypogammaglobulinemia, to determine the presence of monoclonal paraproteins, and to recognize Waldenström's macroglobulinemia or heavy chain disease, either of which may present like CLL.
- Immunoelectrophoresis if a paraprotein is identified (both serum and urine).
- Coombs's test and serum haptoglobin.
- Determination of subsets of lymphocytes (T or B cells) and surface markers, if available.

Biopsy of nodes, liver, lung, or kidneys are to be avoided, and lymphangiograms or scans are usually not necessary. Biopsy of nodes, however, may be useful in patients with progressive disease that is not responding to therapy; the biopsy may indicate a change from CLL to an undifferentiated or histiocytic lymphoma (Richter's syndrome), and a change in the therapeutic regimen would then be indicated.

2. Classification

The subtyping of CLL is particularly useful to predict the prognosis. Table II identifies the features of the various types of CLL.

3. Staging

a. Early CLL

Stage 0:   Pheripheral blood lymphocytosis and infiltration of the bone marrow.
Stage I: Lymphadenopathy in addition to the above.

b. Advanced CLL

Stage II: Hepatosplenomegaly.
Stage III: Thrombocytopenia.
Stage IV: Anemias with any of the above.

D. Therapeutic Management

There is some controversy regarding treatment of early CLL. Most hematologists are reluctant to initiate therapy at that stage, and there is no real evidence that treatment actually changes the course of the disease or the length of survival.

1. Initiation of Treatment

Although most authorities recommend withholding therapy until the disease is active and using "gentle" therapy to avoid aggravating the abnormal immune state that is usually present, complete remissions are rarely observed once the disease reaches a late resistant phase. Recently, some oncologists have recommended a more aggressive approach in the early stages of the disease, using single agents or combinations with minimal hematologic toxicity to achieve a higher rate of complete remission with the hope of improving the long-term survival. The ultimate goal of therapy would be to reverse all abnormal functions, and a "complete remission" must include

- Disappearance of all constitutional symptoms (fever, malaise, sweats, etc.).
- Regression of all nodes and liver and spleen enlargement; return to normal of peripheral blood count and bone marrow.
- Restoration of immune function to normal and reversal of autoimmune complications.

Regardless of one's approach to the treatment of patients with early-stage CLL, or even of those patients with Stage II disease who are asymptomatic, therapy should be initiated as soon as the patient shows evidence of thrombocytopenia or anemia, whether these are the result of progressive disease or of an autoimmune process. Treatment must be directed at correcting the disease and the abnormal immune mechanism. In addition, pressure symptoms from enlarged nodes or splenomegaly and hypersplenism are indications for active treatment. The lymphocyte count itself, even if greater than 100,000 per cubic millimeter does not have the same grave connotation as it would have in acute leukemia or in CML; it does, however, have an unsettling effect on both the patient and the physician and may lead to earlier initiation of therapy.

2. Chemotherapy

To date, the treatment that best maintains the patient's health and probably modestly prolongs the patient's life is the administration of single cytotoxic agents alone or in combination with corticosteroids. Chlorambucil (Leukeran) is the drug of choice and is given either as a continuous daily dose or in large single doses at monthly intervals, along with 5- to 7-day courses of prednisone. Chlorambucil is administered orally in doses of 0.1–0.2 mg per kilogram per day with a downward adjustment of dose as the disease responds. Myelotoxicity is significant, however, and represents the major drawback to the drug. Cyclophosphamide has been used in cases of chlorambucil resistance, particularly in combination regimens.

The use of corticosteroids is limited by their toxicity over prolonged periods of time. They are rarely used alone and are preferably administered intermittently or on alternating days in decreasing quantities.

Combinations of multiple cytotoxic agents in CLL have not shown significant advantages, although cyclophosphamide, vincristine, and prednisone (CVP) as brief courses of "pulsed therapy" are frequently used in refractory CLL and have been reported to yield significant rates of complete remissions in previously untreated patients.

3. Radiotherapy

a. Palliative Radiotherapy

The role of radiation in chronic leukemia is essentially palliative and is aimed at the relief of symptoms and the improvement of the quality of life. To that effect, radiotherapy is indicated in a variety of circumstances:

- Large nodes or masses causing symptoms, functional disability, or cosmetic deformity.
- Pressure symptoms.
- Organomegaly, large spleen, mediastinal masses, etc.
- Total or impending obstruction.

Leukemic infiltrates are highly radiosensitive, with responses occurring at very low dose levels, on the order of a few hundred rads. Treatment is usually suspended when the WBC is maximally around 20,000 because of the lag factor in radiation effect (more effect appearing after the end of radiation). A more important indicator is the rate of reduction of the abnormal WBC after each dose increment. Because of the large variation of the dose/response curve, it is recommended that treatment be carried out only by experienced personnel in centers equipped with good support services.

b. Total-Body Irradiation and Splenic Irradiation

Several authors have reported trials at disease control utilizing total-body irradiation that resulted in claims of increasing rates of patient survival and of disease control akin to that achieved by multiple-drug chemotherapy. The radiotherapy is given in 10- to 15-rad increments, one to three times a week for 1 year (total dose not to exceed 200 rads), or once a month with intermittent chlorambucil and prednisone. The gains reported so far are still far from satisfactory. Moreover, complications such as radiation pneumonitis and dysfunction of sensitive organs (e.g., the bowel) are not insignificant. Such an approach, with or without the addition of systemic chemo-

therapy, must be considered experimental and is better left in specialized hands.

Occasionally disease control can be achieved by irradiating the spleen with small doses (1000–2000 rads) at intervals when the disease is considered active. This approach is successful only when the spleen is enlarged with an excessive WBC and is self-limiting since the spleen will eventually become fibrotic, making further irradiation futile. The simplicity of this approach, however, and its relative safety and effectiveness, especially in cases resistant to chemotherapy, should persuade the treating oncologists to consider it as a useful alternative.

4. Therapy Complications

a. Autoimmune Disorders

Autoimmune hemolytic anemia or thrombocytopenia may complicate the course of CLL and require prompt administration of corticosteroids in large doses (60 mg of prednisone or more daily) for 1–2 months. Splenectomy may be necessary if a response is not achieved with steroids, particularly if significant splenic sequestration is demonstrated by a radioactive Cr-tagged RBC survival study. Radiotherapy to the spleen may also be tried in these cases.

Sjögren's disease, cryoglobulinemia, and rheumatoid arthritis are also treated with steroids in conjunction with an aggressive combination chemotherapy regimen to achieve a remission.

b. Hypersplenism

Hypersplenism is identified by splenomegaly and cytopenia in the blood, in the face of adequate hematopoietic cell lines in the bone marrow; a tagged RBC survival study may be necessary to clarify the diagnosis. Treatment of the condition is primarily through effective chemotherapy, sometimes for as long as 6 months or a year, during which time transfusions are administered as necessary. Some patients will, however, require splenectomy. Splenic irradiation may also be considered.

c. Pleural Effusion

Infiltration of the pleural surfaces with leukemic infiltrates will result in pleural effusions that must be distinguished from those resulting from other causes. Treatment, if no response is seen with chemotherapy, is by radiotherapy. Low doses in the range of 1000 rads may be given to the pleural surfaces or to the mediastinum if mediastinal nodes are enlarged. Intrapleural instillation of cytotoxic agents (nitrogen mustard or chloroquine) and, at times, even surgical pleural stripping may be necessary to control the effusion.

d. Masses

Large symptomatic masses (nodes, spleen, liver, etc.) causing pain or pressure symptoms (e.g., nerve pressure, spinal compression, superior vena caval syndrome, obstructive symptoms, etc.) require prompt radiotherapy.

e. Infectious Complications

These can be of serious consequence in the CLL patient with an impaired immune system. Such patients must be appropriately treated with antibiotics promptly and aggressively. Patients with repeated pyogenic and viral infections may benefit from the administration of gamma globulin in high doses, both during the acute infection and as maintenance on a chronic basis. Newer IV preparations of gamma globulin are more convenient to administer than the older IM preparations. One must also remain alert to the possibility of tuberculosis.

f. Other Complications

Most patients with CLL are of middle age or older, and most will have a relatively protracted course. Diseases affecting this age group are seen regularly, and the clinician must not fall into the trap of attributing newly developing problems to progression of the leukemia. For example, the appearance of anemia in an otherwise well-controlled patient with CLL is not necessarily a consequence of hemolysis or marrow infiltration. Careful review of the peripheral smear may disclose hypochromia, and repeat examination of the bone marrow may disclose absent iron stores, thus initiating an investigation that could result in the discovery of an unsuspected carcinoma of the cecum. Second malignancies are perhaps more commonly seen in the course of CLL than any other neoplasm. Skin cancers are particularly frequent and tend to recur repeatedly.

IV. HAIRY CELL LEUKEMIA

Hairy cell leukemia (HCL) is an entity characterized by circulating mononuclear cells with serrated cytoplasm ("hairy cells"). Clinically, the patient presents with splenomegaly and pancytopenia without significant lymphadenopathy.

The hairy cells, which infiltrate the bone marrow and the spleen, stain positively for tartrate-resistant acid phosphatase. Most available evidence suggests that they are of a B-lymphocyte lineage; some authors have described features distinctive of monocytes. Typically, bone marrow aspiration yields poor material, in most cases due both to marrow infiltration by hairy cells and secondary myelofibrosis. The disease is more frequent in males than females (3 : 1), and its peak incidence is between 40 and 60 years of age.

A. Clinical Considerations

The most common problems that bring the patient to the attention of the physician are

- Easy bruising or bleeding tendencies (30%).
- Infective processes (35%).
- Abdominal discomfort secondary to splenomegaly (25%).

The diagnosis is made by recognizing the hairy cells in the blood smear, where they are present in variable numbers. In doubtful cases, bone marrow aspiration and biopsy will confirm the diagnosis.

The normal counterpart of the "hairy cell" is not yet identified, but most agree that it is of B-cell origin, as are most cases of CLL. Likewise, as in CLL, the disease manifestations appear to be due to the slow accumulation of long-lived malignant cells, and HCL causes cytopenias of normal elements, mainly by the effects of marrow replacement and hypersplenism. In contrast to CLL, however, HCL is not associated with autoimmune thrombocytopenia or hemolysis, and it tends not to present with high WBC counts. Most patients have very slowly progressive disease, even after presenting with pancytopenia. Infections are the most common serious complication and should be treated vigorously.

B. Therapeutic Management

In general, chemotherapy should be avoided in the treatment of this dease, at least as first-line therapy. The reason for initiating therapy in most instances is the desire to correct severe pancytopenia, which is present in about 60% of the cases and which is exacerbated, at least in part, by hypersplenism. Splenectomy is, therefore, the initial mode of therapy. Prednisone in large doses (60–80 mg per day) may induce transient improvement of the marrow reserve, and some practitioners use it as a preparative measure for splenectomy. Others, however, have found no response to corticosteroids. Splenectomy will, in most cases, improve the blood picture. Many patients, however, will show later recrudescence of their cytopenias, requiring further therapy.

Due to both leukemic infiltration and secondary myelofibrosis, the marrow reserve in patients with HCL is poor, and cytotoxic chemotherapy, which might further depress the marrow, is thus generally undesirable. Low-dose chlorambucil therapy (4 mg per day), however, has recently been shown useful in some cases following relapse after splenectomy.

Reports in the medical literature indicate occasional cases successfully treated using aggressive chemotherapy. That modality should probably be reserved for desperate situations. In addition, there is at least one report of successful BMT in HCL. Several reports concerning substantial efficacy of α interferon in HCL have recently appeared and the drug is undergoing intensive study in HCL and related diseases (CLL, myeloma) as of this writing.

The duration of the disease is variable, but four recent reviews demonstrated that about half the patients are alive after 4 years. The most common causes of death are infective processes due to neutropenia, monocytopenia, and T-cell dysfunction.

SUGGESTED READINGS

Acute Leukemia

1. Bennett, J. M., Catovsky, D., Daniel, M. T. *et al.* Proposals for the classification of the acute leukemias. *Br. J. Haematol.* **33**, 451.
2. Bernard, J., Weill, M., Boiron, M. *et al.* Acute promyelocytic leukemia: Results of treatment by Daunorubicin. *Blood* **41**, 389 (1973).
3. Gale, R. P., and Cline, M. J. High remission-induction rate in acute myeloid leukemia. *Lancet* **1**, 497 (1977).
4. Gralnick, H. K., Bagley, J., and Abrel, E. Heparin treatment for the hemorrhagic diathesis of acute promyelocytic leukemia. *Am. J. Med.* **52**, 167 (1972).
5. Henderson, E., Williams, *et al.* "Hematology," pp. 221–253. McGraw-Hill, New York.
6. Reiner, R. R., Hoover, R., Fraumeni, J. F., Jr. *et al.* Acute leukemia after alkylating agent therapy of ovarian cancer. *N. Engl. J. Med.* **297**, 17 (1977).
7. Schimpff, S. C., Landesman, S., *et al.* Ticarcillin in combination with Cephalothin or Gentamicin as empiric antibiotic therapy in granulocytopenic cancer patients. *Antimicrob. Agents Chemother.* **10**, 837 (1976).
8. Thomas, E. D., Buckner, C. D., Clift, R. A. *et al.* Marrow transplantation for acute nonlymphoblastic leukemia in first remission. *N. Engl. J. Med.* **301**, 597 (1979).
9. Wiernik, P. H. *In* "Cancer, Principles and Practice of Oncology" (V. T. DeVita, Jr., S. Hellman, and S. A. Rosenberg, eds.), pp. 1402–1426. Lippincott, Philadelphia, Pennsylvania, 1982.

Chronic Myelocytic Leukemia

10. Bloomfield, C. D., Peterson, L. C., Ynis, J. J. *et al.* The Philadelphia chromosome (Phl) in adults presenting with acute leukemia: A comparison of Phl and Phl-patients. *Br. J. Haematol.* **36**, 347–358 (1977).
11. Canellos, G. P. The treatment of chronic granulocytic leukemia. *Clin. Haematol.* **6**, 113–128 (1977).
12. Canellos, G. P., Whang-Peng, J., and DeVita, V. T. Chronic gran-
ulocytic leukemia without the Philadelphia chromosone. *Am. J. Clin. Pathol.* **65**, 467–470 (1976).
13. Fefer, A., Cheever, M. A., Thomas, E. D. *et al.* Disappearance of Phl positive cells in four patients with chronic granulocytic leukemia after chemotherapy, irradiation and marrow transplantation from an identical twin. *N. Engl. J. Med.* **300**, 333–337 (1979).
14. Fialkow, P. J., Jacobson, R. J., and Papayannopoulou, T. Chronic myelocytic leukemia: Clonal origin in a stem cell common to the granulocyte, erythrocyte, platelet and monocyte/macrophage. *Am. J. Med.* **63**, 125–130 (1977).
15. Marks, S. M., Baltimore, D., and McCaffrey, R. Terminal transferase as a predictor of initial responsiveness to Vincristine and Prednisone in blastic chronic myelogenous leukemia. *N. Eng. J. Med.* **298**, 812–814 (1980).
16. Monfardini, S., Gee, T., Fried, J. *et al.* Survival in chronic myelogenous leukemia: Influence of treatment and extent of disease at diagnosis. *Cancer (Philadelphia)* **31**, 492–501 (1973).
17. Spiers, A. S. D. Annotation, Metamorphosis of chronic granulocytic leukemia: Diagnosis; classification of management. *Br. J. Haematol.* **41**, 1–7 (1979).

Chronic Lymphocytic Leukemia

18. Galton, D. A. G., Goldman, J. M., Wiltshaw, E. *et al.* Prolymphocytic leukemia. *Br. J. Haematol.* **27**, 7–23 (1973).
19. Peterson, L. C., Bloomfield, C. D., and Brunning, R. D. Relationship of clinical staging and lymphocyte morphology to survival in chronic lymphocytic leukemia. *Br. J. Haematol.* **45**, 563–567 (1980).
20. Phillips, E. A., Kempin, S., Passe, *et al.* Prognostic factors in chronic lymphocytic leukemia and their implications for therapy." *Clin. Haematol.* **6**, 303–222 (1977).
21. Preud'home, J. L., and Seligmann, M. Surface bound immunoglobulins as a cell marker in human lymphoproliferative diseases. *Blood* **40**, 777–794 (1972).
22. Rai, K. R., Sawitsky, A., Cronkite, E. P. *et al.* Clinical staging of chronic lymphocytic leukemia. *Blood* **46**, 219–234 (1975).
23. Sawitsky, A., Rai, D. R., Glidewell, O. *et al.* Comparison of daily versus intermittent Chlorambucil and Prednisone therapy in the treatment of patients with chronic lymphocytic leukemia. *Blood* **50**, 1049–1059 (1977).

Hairy Cell Leukemia

24. Golomb, M. H., and Hintz, U. Treatment of hairy cell leukemia (leukemic reticloendotheliosis). II. Chlorambucil therapy in postsplenectomy patients with progressive disease. *Blood* **54**, 305–309 (1979).
25. Yam, L. T., Li Cy, and Lam, K. W. Tartrate-resistant acid phosphatase isoenzyme in the reticulum cells of leukemic reticuloendotheliosis. *N. Engl. J. Med.* **284**, 357 (1971).

Section 9. Neoplastic Disorders of the Blood, Bone Marrow, and Lymphatic System

Part C. Multiple Myeloma

I. Definition and Clinical Considerations 403
II. Pretreatment Evaluation and Work-Up 403
  A. Basic Evaluation
  B. Diagnostic Criteria
  C. Staging
III. Therapeutic Management 404
  A. Induction Chemotherapy
  B. Maintenance Therapy
  C. Treatment of Relapse Phase
  D. Other Modalities

    1. Radiotherapy
    2. Surgery
  E. Management of Complications
    1. Orthopedic Complications
    2. Anemia
    3. Hypercalcemia
    4. Renal Insufficiency
    5. Amyloidosis
    6. Cryoglobulinemia
    7. Hyperviscosity

I. DEFINITION AND CLINICAL CONSIDERATIONS

Multiple myeloma is the result of malignant proliferations of plasma cells in the bone marrow; these are usually widely disseminated at the time of diagnosis and are accompanied by serum and/or urine monoclonal hypergammaglobulinemia and lytic bone lesions due to the destruction of structural bone.

The signs and symptoms of multiple myeloma and their order of frequency at presentation are

- Monoclonal immunoglobulin paraprotein with low levels of normal gamma globulin.
- Bone pain or pathological fracture (68%).
- Anemia (62%).
- Renal failure (55%).
- Hypercalcemia (30%).
- Infection (12%).

It is rare for a patient with multiple myeloma to present with leukopenia, thrombocytopenia, fever (due to myeloma per se), weight loss, neuropathy (other than due to compression by myeloma tumor), soft-tissue tumor, hepatosplenomegaly, or lymphadenopathy.

II. PRETREATMENT EVALUATION AND WORK-UP

A. Basic Evaluation

All patients suspected of having multiple myeloma or plasmacytoma require the following laboratory and radiological tests to define the nature and extent of the disease process:

- CBC (including platelet count and review of the peripheral smear).
- Urinalysis.
- Chemistry profile (SMA-18).
- Serum protein electrophoresis.

- Urine protein electrophoresis (and 24 hours urine collection for total urinary proteins).
- Immunoelectrophoresis of serum and urine.
- Chest x-ray.
- Skeletal survey (*not* bone scan, since myeloma bone lesions do not display increased activity.)
- Bone marrow aspiration.
- Biopsy of bone or tumor if a localized plasmacytoma is suspected.

B. Diagnostic Criteria

The diagnosis of multiple myeloma is based on several criteria. These diagnostic criteria have been classified by the Southwestern Oncology Group into three major and four minor criteria:

The major criteria are

- I   Plasmacytosis on biopsy.
- II   Bone marrow aspiration shows >30% of plasma cells.
- III   Monoclonal immunoglobulin of >3.5 gram % for IgG peak on serum electrophoresis and >2 gram % for IgA peak on serum electrophoresis. Unequivocal evidence of kappa or lambda light-chain excretion on urine protein electrophoresis.

The minor criteria are

- a   Bone marrow plasma cells, 10–30%.
- b   Lower *monoclonal* immunoglobulin levels than those listed above but exceeding normal levels.
- c   Lytic bone lesions.
- d   Suppression of normal immunoglobulins below normal levels: (IgM <50 milligram%, IgA <100 milligram%, IgG <600 milligram %).

Diagnosis is confirmed by any of the following combinations:

- I   + (b, c, or d).
- II   + (b, c, or d).
- III   (alone).

- a + b + c,
- a + b + d

C. Staging

The prognosis of myeloma is, in effect, dependent on the actual tumor burden. Thus, it has been possible to divide myeloma patients into three categories by their hematologic findings and the M-component production rate. These clinical criteria correlate well with the measured plasma cell mass (Table I).

The prognosis of the disease is directly related to the level of the tumor burden, with median survivals reported at around 30 months, 55 months, or 75 months, respectively, for patients with high, intermediate, or low tumor burden. A clinical staging system has thus been recommended, taking into account all the factors listed in Table I.

A futher subclassification into A and B has been added:

- A   Normal renal function, creatinine level <2.0 milligram %.
- B   Abnormal renal function, creatinine level >2.0 milligram %.

In addition, this classification may be supplemented by the actual calculation of the cell mass by the exact multivariate regression equations available for this purpose. The initial cell mass can be calculated, and quantitative responses to therapy may be measured.

Immunoelectrophoresis will identify immunologic variants (IgG, IgA, IgM, IdD, and IgE, etc.) as well as light-chain myeloma and heavy-chain disease.

III. THERAPEUTIC MANAGEMENT

Management of the patient with myeloma, although standard in many respects, is riddled with unanswered questions. There are a large number of multi-institutional cooperative studies trying to clarify the situation; interpretation of their results, however, is difficult since their methodology, definitions, and qualification of responses vary from one group to another.

The alkylating agent melphalan is still the backbone of therapy for disseminated myeloma. There remain, however, many unanswered questions pertaining to the best method of using the drug:

- Is a loading initial dose necessary?
- Should treatment be continuous, or is "pulse therapy" preferable?
- Are the results improved with the addition of prednisone?
- Are multidrug regimens superior to melphalan alone?
- Is maintenance after complete response desirable? And if so, for how long?
- Is melphalan the drug of choice for relapses?

A. Induction Chemotherapy

A standard regimen yielding a respectable response rate and survival utilizes melphalan in a loading dose of 6–10 mg per day for 8–10 days, followed by a maintenance dose of 2 mg per day together with prednisone (0.8 mg per kilogram per day, halved, every 2 weeks for 6 weeks). Other regimens use pulse therapy with melphalan 0.1–0.15 mg per kilogram per day for 7 days, combined with 15 mg of prednisone q.i.d.,

Table I

Comparison of Myeloma Patients in Relation to Tumor Burden

Tumor burden[a]	Measured myeloma cell mass (plasma cells/m² × 10⁻¹²)	Hemaglobin (g)	Serum Ca (mg %)	Bone survey	M-Component production rates (g %)		Urine light-chain component (g/24 hour by electrophoresis)
					IgG	IgA	
High (1.2 × 10¹² cells/m²)	>1.2	<8.5	>12	Advanced lytic bone lesions >3	>7	>5	>12
Low (0.6 × 10¹² cells/m²)	<0.6	>10.0	Normal	Normal or solitary lesion	<5	<3	<4
Intermediate (0.6–1.2 × 10¹² cells/m²)	0.6–1.2	8.5–10.0	<12	Between high and low categories	5–7	3–5	4–12

[a] Low tumor burden, meets all criteria; high tumor burden, meets one or more criteria category; intermediate tumor burden, fits neither high nor low category.

repeated every 6 weeks for three courses; or Melphalan 0.25 mg per kilogram per day for 4 days, with 40 mg per square meter of prednisone, repeated every 28–42 days.

A program of combination chemotherapy has been recommended by the Memorial Sloan-Kettering Cancer Center as follows:

- Melphalan, 0.25 mg/kg/day, PO for 4 days.
- Prednisone, 1 mg/kg/day, PO for 7 days, then tapered down.
- Vincristine, 0.03 mg/kg, IV on day 1.
- BCNU, 0.5 mg/kg, IV on day 1.

This is repeated every 5 weeks until relapse occurs.

Several other multidrug combinations, including within them vincristine, BCNU, Adriamycin, and cyclophosphamide, have been tried with varying results, some with apparent improvement over melphalan alone and with response yields as high as 70% with a median survival of 36 months. It needs to be kept in mind that absorption of melphalan from the human gastrointestinal tract (bioavailability) varies widely from patient to patient, some absorbing very little (<10%) of an administered dose, others absorbing more than 50%. Thus, some patients never develop leukopenia or thrombocytopenia while on the drug and, presumably, cannot be expected to respond favorably. It is possible that at least part of the apparent improvement noted with multidrug regimens is due to the fact that some of the drugs are given intravenously. When treating a patient with myeloma with melphalan, the physician should use such doses as are necessary to poduce mild-to-moderate myelosuppression (WBC 2500–3500, platelets in the low-normal range). If no myelosuppression is induced and no tumor response is evident, it is recommended that treatment be changed to another alkylating agent, usually cyclophosphamide.

In general terms, the following guidelines seem appropriate when approaching the patient with multiple myeloma:

- Chemotherapy is contraindicated in patients with benign, asymptomatic gammopathy.
- Chemotherapy should be initiated as soon as possible in the patient with progressive disease indicative of active myeloma.
- Melphalan plus prednisone is the standard drug combination for initiation. Cyclophosphamide and prednisone seem to be equally effective.
- Multiple agents in various combinations may yield a better response rate with a higher median survival. They should be considered in patients with high cell mass (Stage III).
- The best treatment schedule is yet to be determined.
- No one has reported cure of the disease with any regimen, with or without maintenance.

- Factors that adversely affect the prognosis include
  - Advanced stage of disease, particularly in the B subgroup (although the SWOG could not correlate stage with rate or duration of response).
  - High and rising M-component protein, especially of the non-IgG type.
  - Anemia, hypercalcemia, and azotemia.
  - CNS involvement.
  - Elevated plasma cell labeling index.
  - Major associated syndromes (e.g., hyperviscosity, amyloidosis).
- Patients with predominately extramedullary disease have a better prognosis and are much more chemosensitive and radiosensitive.

Patients with malignant myeloma should be treated only by experienced hematologists or oncologists and preferably entered into one of the available chemotherapy trial protocols. The physician and his or her institution should be able to manage the acute complications that occur during the course of malignant myeloma such as sepsis, pneumonia, hypercalcemia, hyperviscosity syndrome, cord compression secondary to vertebral collapse or outgrowth of tumor, hip fractures, acute renal failure, acquired Fanconi's syndrome (renal tubular acidosis), aminoaciduria, hypokalemia, and hyperphosphatemia.

B. Maintenance Therapy

With effective induction, tumor regression will usually occur rapidly at first, then slow down and reach a plateau. If the response is good, symptomatic relief will be achieved, though bones rarely recalcify. The plateau phase is stable in less than half of the patients; others may fluctuate or continue in a slow regression phase. The measurement of the M-component, tumor cell mass, and plasma cell labeling index is an accurate method of identifying the actual response of the disease; patients with a stable plateau, disappearance of the M-component, and a labeling index of less than 1% may have their therapy stopped.

In patients with a lesser response, maintenance therapy should be considered. Although the SWOG trials of maintenance therapy for 1 year showed no improved survival, the Memorial Sloan-Kettering Cancer Center M2 protocol suggested early relapse when therapy is interrupted. Some have recommended continuing maintenance therapy until relapse. Others have stopped it 18–24 months after stabilization of the disease.

In patients where the plateau is unstable and the course of the disease fluctuates during induction therapy, shorter intervals must be considered, and the addition of cycle-active drugs (e.g., vincristine) may be considered.

C. Treatment of the Relapse Phase

A relapse will almost always supervene in patients with myeloma, regardless of the maintenance therapy; this may be an indication of resistance to the specific alkylating agent. Patients with initial responses to melphalan and prednisone may respond again to the same agents at increased dosages; repeating Melphalan is particularly indicated if the relapse occurs off therapy. Failure will then necessitate changing to other chemotherapeutic regimens:

- Cyclophosphamide, 1 gm/m², every 3 weeks.
- BCNU (carmustine) and Adriamycin, 30 mg/m² each, every 3 weeks.
- VBAP.
  - Vincristine, 1 mg on day 1.
  - BCNU, 30 mg/m² on day 1.
  - Adriamycin, 30 mg/m² on day 1.
  - Prednisone, 100 mg/day for 4 days.

Responses up to 35% have been observed with these agents. *Cis*-platinum, bleomycin, hexamethylmelamine, and procarbazine have also been used in resistant cases with occasional responses.

In institutions where this is possible, *in vitro* cultures of myeloma stem cell colonies, with cloning assay for kinetic and drug sensitivity information, may give valuable information in the treatment of the refractory patient.

D. Other Modalities

1. Radiotherapy

Localized plasmacytoma is best treated by radiation therapy, which gives excellent results. Solitary lesions are extremely radiosensitive and locally radiocurable; in most cases, however, secondary tumors will appear. Patients presenting with truly solitary plasmacytoma, primarily in the head and neck region, have been claimed to show the best response, with a 5-year survival of about 40%.

Total bone marrow irradiation is in a trial stage. It requires megavoltage equipment with electron beam units for the skull and rib cage, and results are not yet established. It might be considered in totally refractory cases.

Radiotherapy is also indicated for palliation in the following circumstances:

- Severe pain, particularly when the pain is of bony origin.
- Impending fracture (to be used along with orthopedic measures such as fixation and pinning).
- Vertebral disease with risk of compression or intramedullary deposits.

2. Surgery

Surgery may be required in the patient with symptoms of spine compression. It may also be useful in the patient with a solitary plasmacytoma. Of these patients 75%, however, will progress to disseminated disease.

E. Management of Complications

1. Orthopedic Complications

Patients with skeletal lesions do not respond to any supportive measures such as androgens, calcium salts, fluorides, etc. Patients with orthopedic complications must be treated promptly with present-day supportive measures, chemotherapy, and palliative radiotherapy. Patients can tolerate orthopedic procedures very well; if the patient is to be kept ambulatory, it is important to correct any orthopedic complications without delay.

2. Anemia

Transfusion of packed red cells should be given in all cases with a hemoglobin level low enough to cause fatigue or anytime angina or cerebrovascular insufficiency is noted.

3. Hypercalcemia

Simple measures such as hydration, diuresis (with furosemide), and prednisone are usually sufficient to correct the hypercalcemia. Inorganic phosphate may be required, and mithramycin (25 μg per kilogram, IV) can be administered in resistant cases. Hypercalcemia can be reduced in incidence if patients are kept ambulatory.

4. Renal Insufficiency

The goal of therapy should be the control of the myeloma by chemotherapy since this would result in reversing the renal failure. Chemotherapy doses must, however, be adjusted and some agents (e.g., BCNU) deleted. Allopurinol should be given for hyperuricemia, and sodium bicarbonate or Diamox can be used to alkalinize the urine. Renal dialysis should be considered if these measures fail or if the renal damage is irreversible.

5. Amyloidosis

This is a frequent complication in patients with light-chain disease. There is no specific therapy, but amyloidosis may resolve with treatment of the myeloma.

6. Cryoglobulinemia

This complication occurs in 5% of cases, and patients with clinical symptoms must be protected from cold until they respond to their chemotherapy.

7. Hyperviscosity

This is seen in IgA- and rarely in IgG-type myeloma and may simulate macroglobulinemia. The treatment of choice is plasmapheresis, either by multiple phlebotomies with return of the red blood cells to the patient or by using blood cell separators. Plasmapheresis is essential in the symptomatic patient with oozing from minor cuts, blurring of vision, central-vein thrombosis, depletion of plasma-clotting factors, or neurological symptoms.

Section 9. Neoplastic Disorders of the Blood, Bone Marrow, and Lymphatic System

Part D. Other Neoplastic Disorders of the Blood

I. Polycythemia Vera 411
  A. Pretreatment Evaluation
    1. Clinical Considerations
    2. Laboratory Findings
    3. Differential Diagnosis
  B. Therapeutic Management
II. Melofibrosis and Myeloid Metaplasia 413
  A. Pretreatment Evaluation
    1. Clinical Considerations

    2. Laboratory Findings
  B. Treatment
    1. Androgens and Corticosteroids
    2. Splenectomy
    3. Radiotherapy
    4. Chemotherapy
III. Acute Myelofibrosis 415
IV. Essential Thrombocythemia 415

I. POLYCYTHEMIA VERA

Polycythemia vera is included in this manual because of recent evidence pointing to a monoclonal origin for this disease. Thus, strictly speaking, polycythemia vera is a neoplastic process involving the pluripotential hematopoietic stem cell. The evidence resides in several characteristics of the disease and particularly in the fact that there is involvement of all three cell lines: the erythrocytic, granulocytic, and platelet lines. In some patients, the bone marrow ultimately becomes involved by a fibrotic process, but the fibroblasts responsible for the fibrosis are not derived from the same clone of cells as the hematopoietic elements. Hematopoietic cells, including red cell precursors, white cell precursors, and platelets, have only one type of G6PD isozyme, indicating that the disease is indeed monoclonal, i.e., presumably originated from one cell or one clone of cells, whereas fibroblasts and other somatic cells show both isozymes in female heterozygotes.

The pathogenesis of the increased blood formation is as of yet, not well understood. Studies with colony-forming units of the erythroid series (CFU-E) done in semisolid culture media disclosed that, unlike normal stem cells, those of patients with polycythemia vera seem to be relatively independent of the action of erythropoietin. Erythropoietin is absolutely necessary to obtain growth of normal colonies. Under suitable culture conditions, it is possible to show that normal stem cells persist in the marrow but are apparently suppressed by the polycythemia vera clone.

A. Pretreatment Evaluation

1. Clinical Considerations

Polycythemia vera tends to have an insidious onset and is frequently discovered in a routine complete blood count. This will almost always show an increase in the hematocrit and will generally also show an increase in white cell and platelet counts. Patients are sometimes diagnosed after an acute thrombotic or hemorrhagic event. Individuals affected by polycythemia are more likely than the general population to suffer from thrombovascular disorders such as strokes, myocardial infarctions, thromboembolic disease, mesenteric thrombosis, or the Budd-Chiari syndrome.

The history will often identify complaints of headaches, dizziness, vertigo, and/or tinnitus. A fraction of patients will complain of blurred vision. Others will have histories of angina or intermittent claudication. It is said that there is a high incidence of peptic ulcer disease in patients with polycythemia vera, and some patients will have abdominal symptoms ascribable to an enlarged spleen, including early satiety, a dragging feeling in the left upper quadrant, etc. Another prominent symptom is pruritus. This is particularly troublesome in hot weather and after a bath.

The physical examination will disclose facial plethora in almost all individuals. This is due to engorged capillaries and venules by the markedly increased red cell mass. Many patients will show ruddy cyanosis. Fundoscopic examination discloses engorged veins and a hyperemic retina. The most important physical finding is splenomegaly, the presence of which serves to differentiate polycythemia vera from secondary polycythemia (see below). The splenomegaly is not massive, is present in about 60–75% of the patients at presentation, and becomes palpable in almost all patients at some point during the illness. Mild-to-moderate hepatomegaly is generally also present.

It must be remembered that elective surgery must be avoided if at all possible in any patient with uncontrolled polycythemia vera. There is a 50–75% risk of serious, even fatal, complications if the hematocrit is not brought down to normal levels.

2. Laboratory Findings

The *sine qua non* of laboratory investigations for the diagnosis of polycythemia is the finding of an increased RBC mass. The test is done with radioactively labeled red cell methods and not deduced from simple measurements of the hematocrit. The peripheral smear will generally show normal red cell morphology, though in some patients it may disclose hypochromic microcytic red cells indicating iron deficiency, presumably from utilization of iron stores to produce the excessive amounts of blood, or from blood loss secondary to peptic ulcer disease.

Some 60% of patients will have increased WBC counts,

generally in the 10,000–30,000 per cubic millimeter range, and most patients will have an increase in the absolute and relative basophil count in the blood. It is thought by some that the basophilia is associated with the pruritus.

An increase in the platelet count is found in about 50% of patients. In general, the platelets appear normal morphologically. Platelet aggregation studies show, in a large fraction of the patients, the so-called storage pool defect: aggregation with low-dose Adenosine diphosphate (ADP), epinephrine, and collagen is impaired. The bleeding time is usually within normal limits, and coagulation tests tend to be normal.

The bone marrow aspirate is hypercellular and shows hyperplasia of all three cell lines. In contrast to patients with secondary polycythemia, patients with polycythemia vera have much more cellular marrows because of hyperplasia of the granulocytic line in addition to the erythrocytic line. Iron stores tend to be normal or decreased. A fraction of the patients will have some fibrosis in the bone marrow biopsy.

Serum chemistries display an increase in the uric acid. Arterial oxygen saturation is normal.

Specialized laboratories capable of measuring erythropoietin have generally found very low to absent levels of the hormone in patient's blood or urine. It is to be remembered that erythropoietin is increased in essentially all patients with secondary polycythemia. Unfortunately, reliable tests for erythropoietin levels are not widely available.

Leukocyte alkaline phosphatase is generally within normal limits or maybe slightly elevated. Its main value lies in differentiating polycythemia vera from early-stage chronic myelogenous leukemia, in which very low levels of LAP are found. Most patients will have moderately increased levels of vitamin B_{12} and vitamin B_{12}–binding capacity; the latter is due to an increase in transcobalamin III.

3. Differential Diagnosis

Once a diagnosis of polycythemia is established by the finding of an increased RBC mass, it is necessary to distinguish polycythemia vera from secondary polycythemia.

The Polycythemia Vera Study Group has published diagnostic criteria; these include

A1   Increased RBC mass.
A2   Normal arterial oxygen saturation.
A3   Splenomegaly.
B1   Increased platelet count above 400,000.
B2   Increased WBC count above 12,000.
B3   Increased LAP.
B4   Increased vitamin B_{12}.

Polycythemia is diagnosed if all three criteria of Category A are met or if the increased RBC mass and one other criterion from Category A is found along with any two criteria from Category B.

Most patients referred to hematologists for evaluation of increased hematocrits will turn out not to have polycythemia at all. On evaluation, these patients will be found to have a normal RBC mass with diminished plasma volume (Gaisböck's syndrome, stress polycythemia, or spurious polycythemia) resulting in a high hematocrit. This is not considered to be a disease, nor is it understood how such patients develop a decreased plasma volume. Many of these patients will have been treated with diuretics for hypertension, but even after discontinuing the diuretics, their hematocrits tend to remain elevated. Most individuals with this syndrome are middle aged, stressed, and male; many of them have arterial hypertension, and most are smokers.

If the criteria for polycythemia vera are not met in a patient with a documented increased RBC mass, it is necessary to consider the various causes of secondary polycythemia. Most commonly, secondary polycythemia is seen in patients with the following conditions:

- Severe chronic obstructive pulmonary disease.
- Individuals living at high elevations.
- Patients with cyanotic heart disease.
- Patients with erythropoietin-producing tumors.

In most instances, the history and physical examination will be sufficient to elucidate the nature of the problem. However, when the initial evaluation fails to produce an explanation of the polycythemia, it is reasonable to undertake a series of investigations:

- Intravenous pyelogram.
- Liver scan.
- Measurement of the P50 (in order to rule out abnormal hemoglobins with increased oxygen affinity).
- Test for carboxyhemoglobin.

In difficult or doubtful cases, it is reasonable to perform marrow culture studies and to check the level of erythropoeitin.

B. Therapeutic Management

The course and prognosis of polycythemia vera is such that most patients will require a variety of treatments over a relatively long duration of time. Polycythemia is a disease of middle-aged and elderly persons and has a marked propensity for cardiovascular and thromboembolic complications; this has to be taken into account in choosing among the available treatment modalities; namely phlebotomy or myelosuppressive agents such as alkylating agents or radioactive phosphorus.

In newly diagnosed patients with uncontrolled polycythemia vera and very high hematocrits and especially in those patients who show evidence of cerebral or cardiovascular compromise, a rapid program of phlebotomy is indicated: 500 ml of blood can be removed every other day with relative safety until a hematocrit of less than 50% is reached. Because each phlebotomy removes several hundred miligrams of iron, an iron deficiency state is eventually induced, and an occasional patient will have symptoms of iron deficiency, such as glossitis, dysphagia, abdominal pain, etc. Replacement of iron will quickly improve the symptoms but will also result in an increased phlebotomy requirement. It is generally agreed that it is best to keep the hematocrit in the low-to-mid 40s whenever possible, as it is thought that this will reduce the risk of vascular accidents. Some authors have claimed that a therapeutic program of phlebotomy alone will increase the risk of thrombotic complications. This may be due in part to the fact that despite normal hematocrits, these patients have a very much increased number of red blood cells (6–8 million per cubic millimeter), mainly severely microcytic, hypochromic cells. Controlled studies have shown that patients treated by phlebotomy alone do have a somewhat increased risk of thrombotic events during the course of the disease. Unfortunately, the other alternative, myelosuppressive treatment with either radioactive phosphorus or alkylating agents, results in an increased incidence of late onset acute leukemia, although it correspondingly seems to offer protection from thrombovascular complications. Thus, the best single treatment for polycythemia vera is not established at present, and treatment has to be tailored for individual patients.

An elderly patient with a high platelet count and a history of angina or cerebrovascular disease is probably best treated, after initial phlebotomy has controlled the hematocrit, by a myelosuppressive regimen consisting of either radioactive phosphorus, alkylating agents or hydroxyurea. On the other hand, a young patient, for whom the risk of late leukemia is relatively more important, ought to be treated with phlebotomy alone, possibly with iron supplementation to prevent severe microcytosis. It has been known for a long time that among chemotherapy agents, the alkylating agents are the most leukemogenic. Some recent studies have employed hydroxyurea instead of the alkylating agents (chlorambucil or busulfan). At the present, no conclusions are warranted as to the potential leukemogenic effects of hydroxyurea. It should be kept in mind that at least 10–20 years of follow-up are necessary in this chronic illness before firm conclusions can be drawn.

A significant proportion of patients will have a high platelet count. Such patients are somewhat paradoxically prone to suffer from serious hemorrhage in addition to thrombotic events. Busulfan is a particularly valuable agent for thrombocytosis. There are as yet no data to suggest that "prophylactic" use of antiplatelet agents such as aspirin or Dipyridamole will result in a reduction of thrombotic complications; randomized studies in that direction are in progress.

Most patients who have had polycythemia vera for more than 5 years will be noted to have a slowly progressive transformation of the illness into a syndrome indistinguishable from myelofibrosis and myeloid metaplasia. The spleen increases in size; progressive anemia may develop; the WBC count tends to increase; and the platelet count will frequently decrease as the spleen enlarges. Myeloid metaplasia will be found in its usual sites in the spleen, liver, etc. The treatment of this phase of the illness is particularly difficult, as one has to contend with progressively increasing white counts at the same time that the patients tend to become anemic and thrombocytopenic. The average survival during this phase is on the order of 2–3 years.

About 15% of patients will ultimately suffer a conversion of the illness into an apparent acute leukemia. Such a "secondary" leukemia tends to be particularly resistant to therapy.

II. MYELOFIBROSIS AND MYELOID METAPLASIA

This syndrome, related to polycythemia vera and chronic myelogenous leukemia and included in the "myeloproliferative syndromes," is discussed here because, like polycythemia vera, it too is a monoclonal disease. Although the clinical picture is dominated by progressive bone marrow fibrosis, it is agreed that the fibrosis is a secondary phenonomon, probably relating to growth factors elaborated by an increased pool of megakaryocytes. Such platelet-derived growth factors are known to be able to stimulate fibroblasts *in vitro,* and as in polycythemia vera, fibroblasts from patients who are heterozygous for the glucose 6-phosphate dehydrogenase enzymes are found to contain both isozymes A and B, whereas the hematopoietic cells contain either A or B enzymes.

A. Pretreatment Evaluation

1. Clinical Considerations

This is also a disease of middle-aged and elderly individuals and is slightly more predominant in males. About one-third of patients are asymptomatic at diagnosis and present with the finding of an enlarged spleen. Most of the remainder of the patients come to clinical attention because of the markedly enlarged spleen, which produces left upper quadrant symptoms such as a dragging feeling, pressure on the stomach, and occasionally, an acute pain due to splenic infarction. Most patients will also have moderate hepatomegaly.

About two-thirds of patients are anemic at presentation. A small fraction of patients will present because of purpura due to diminished platelet counts.

2. Laboratory Findings

As mentioned above, most patients have mild-to-moderate anemia. Review of the peripheral smear will disclose the typical teardrop cells characteristic of this disease. In addition, there will be an increase in the WBC count, generally higher than those observed in polycythemia vera, and a leukoerythroblastic blood smear. In an occasional patient, the anemia is due to a hemolytic process that tends to be Coombs's negative.

About one-third of patients have a decreased platelet count, and about one-third of patients have an increased platelet count. Studies of platelet aggregation will generally show abnormalities with ADP, collagen, and epinephrine similar to those observed in other myeloproliferative diseases. The bleeding time tends to be normal but may be prolonged, especially if there is thrombocytopenia. This needs to be kept in mind in case surgery is indicated. The bleeding time may be prolonged even in the face of very high platelet counts. It is paradoxic, therefore, that the patients may require transfusion of platelets although they have platelet counts in excess of a million per cubic millimeter.

Coagulation tests will frequently show an increased prothrombin time, and some patients will have laboratory evidence of disseminated intravascular coagulation.

The LAP and the uric acid tend to be elevated. A fraction of patients will have a monoclonal immunoglobulin paraprotein.

Typically, the bone marrow is inaspirable as a result of the relatively dense fibrosis seen in most areas. On occasion, however, very cellular marrow aspirates are obtained, and these will show hyperplasia of all three cell lines, with areas of dense fibrosis and islands of bone marrow. When chromosomal studies are feasible on marrow aspirates, they will be Philadelphia-chromosome negative. The latter test is the most important one in the differentiation of myeloid metaplasia from chronic myelogenous leukemia, the disease with which it is most often confused. Another aid in the differential diagnosis is the very low LAP seen in chronic myelogenous leukemia.

B. Treatment

If the patient is asymptomatic, it is reasonable simply to observe the course of the disease. Many patients will not require any therapeutic interventions for 5 years or more.

1. Androgens and Corticosteroids

Androgens are useful for patients whose sole clinical problem is anemia. Corticosteroids are of benefit if there is evidence of a hemolytic process. In our experience, the combination of nandrolone decanoate and prednisone has yielded remissions of anemia in a significant fraction of patients who were resistant to either medication alone. Many of these patients were transfusion dependent but managed to do without transfusions after therapy.

2. Splenectomy

In most patients, the spleen, which is frequently very large at the outset of the illness and which enlarges progressively during its course, will require some attention. Cytopenias, especially anemia and thrombocytopenia, ultimately develop and are caused at least in part by hypersplenism; the clinician is frequently faced with the question of the need for splenectomy. It needs to be kept in mind that splenectomy is a formidable procedure in this population of patients, most of whom are middle aged and elderly, many of whom have hemorrhagic and thrombotic diathesis, and many of whom have had previous chemotherapy. The indications for splenectomy include

- Severe abdominal pain and pressure symptoms causing malnutrition.
- Refractory hemolytic anemia.
- Refractory thrombocytopenia.
- Severe portal hypertension.

Prior to splenectomy, the patient must have a complete hemostatic evaluation, including coagulation studies to rule out disseminated intravascular coagulopathy, and platelet function studies. Transfusion of platelets and plasma may well be life saving.

3. Radiotherapy

Patients who develop acute left upper quadrant pain secondary to splenic infarcts are easily treated with a short course of several hundred rads of radiation to the area in question. Other indications for radiotherapy include the development of ascites when it can be demonstrated that the ascitic fluid contains megakaryocytes, indicating that the ascites is due to areas of myeloid metaplasia within the peritoneal surfaces.

4. Chemotherapy

The use of chemotherapy in this disease remains a controversial issue. Many will agree that it is indicated for the "hypermetabolic symptoms" including fever, night sweats, weight loss, etc. In addition, it occasionally has a salutory effect on the size of the spleen. It is certainly indicated for the control of markedly increased platelet counts (above a million).

The chronic management of myelofibrosis and myeloid metaplasia taxes the skill and judgment of the hematologist to the utmost. Correction of one problem frequently results in exacerbation of others: chemotherapy employed for extreme leukocytosis or thrombocytosis will aggravate the anemia; splenectomy may correct the anemia but may also produce extreme leuko- or thrombocytosis, making chemotherapy necessary, etc.

The most common complications of myelofibrosis and my-

eloid metaplasia are similar to those mentioned for polycythemia vera and include cardiovascular, thrombotic, and
hemorrhagic phenomona. Acute leukemia supervenes in about
25% of patients, fatal infectious complications in about 15%.

III. ACUTE MYELOFIBROSIS

This is a syndrome characterized by pancytopenia, a rapidly
progressive course, and absence of plenomegaly in most patients. The bone marrow biopsy shows markedly increased
proliferation of megakaryocytes and fibrosis. The peripheral
blood will frequently show some young myeloid cells, including myeloblasts. The disease generally evolves into an acute
leukemia in short order (6–18 months) and tends to be quite
refractory to treatment. Many feel that the acute leukemia that
supervenes is a megakaryoblastic leukemia.

IV. ESSENTIAL THROMBOCYTHEMIA

This is another entity in the spectrum of the myeloproliferative diseases and shares many features of the preceding syndromes. Essentially, the clinical picture is dominated by
markedly increased platelet counts (more than 1 million, frequently more than 2 or 3 million). The white cells and the
platelets are affected much less severely and generally do not
constitute problems by themselves.

The clinical features are caused by the markedly increased
platelet mass. Platelet clumps are seen on the peripheral smear,
and presumably, aggregates of platelets are responsible, by
occluding distal arterioles, for the blue toe and blue finger
syndrome seen so commonly in this entity. Despite the markedly increased platelet counts, these patients are also prone to a
serious risk of bleeding because of the severe platelet function
defect many of them display. The bleeding time is frequently
elevated, and platelet aggregation studies show abnormalities
similar to those described for polycythemia and myeloid
metaplasia.

The differential diagnosis is between reactive thrombocytosis and essential thrombocytopenia. Reactive thrombocytosis
is seen in patients with a number of chronic illnesses, including
cancers of all kinds, chronic infections, etc. In most instances
of reactive thrombocytosis, the platelet counts do not exceed 1
million; the platelet morphology is entirely normal on the
blood smear; and one tends not to see platelet aggregates. In
essential thrombocythemia, the platelet count is generally well
in excess of 1 million; the peripheral smear discloses a variety
of morphological abnormalities; and frequent platelet clumps
are seen in blood smears. The bone marrow aspirate will generally show a marked increase in megakaryocytes and in
platelet aggregates. The bone marrow biopsy will confirm the
marked increase in megakaryocytes and will show a variable
amount of fibrosis.

The course of the illness tends to be relatively indolent.
Many patients will live for a decade with minimal treatment.

The treatment requires a lowering of the platelet count to
relatively normal values. Busulfan is an excellent choice, as it
generally results in a smooth reduction in the platelet count and
tends to be sparing of the white cell and red cell series.

The usefulness of antiplatelet agents in this disease has not as
yet been established.

Section 10

Chest Tumors

MICHAEL GOLDING

With Contributions By

John Addrizzo	Chest Disease and Rehabilitation
Samuel Kopel	Hematology-Oncology
Ezzat Youssef	Radiotherapy
Sameer Rafla	Radiotherapy
Bernard Gussof	Hematology-Oncology
Karl Jindrak	Pathology
Linda Rogando	Nursing Oncology

Section 10. Chest Tumors

Part A: Cancer of the Lung

I. Early Detection and Screening   421
  A. Predisposing Factors and Prevention
    1. Smoking
    2. Industrial Hazards
  B. Detection
    1. Routine History and Physical Examination
    2. Chest X-Rays
    3. Cytology
  C. Screening
  D. Patient Education
II. Pretreatment Evaluation and Work-Up   422
  A. Radiological Evaluation of the Pulmonary Lesions
    1. Pulmonary Infiltrates
    2. Pulmonary Masses
  B. Preoperative Establishment of the Diagnosis
    1. Bronchoscopy
      a. Open-Tube Bronchoscopy
      b. Flexible Fiberoptic Bronchoscopy
    2. Biopsy
      a. Brush Biopsy
      b. Transbronchial Biopsy
      c. Transcutaneous Needle Biopsy
      d. Bone Marrow Biopsy in Bronchogenic Cancer
      e. Thoracoscopy
      f. Limited Open Thoracotomy or Minithoracotomy
  C. Metastatic Evaluation of the Patient
  D. Evaluation of Operability
    1. Mediastinal Evaluation
      a. Special Radiological Procedures
      b. Transcervical Mediastinoscopy
      c. Anterior Thoracic Mediastinal Exploration
    2. Scalene Node Biopsy
    3. Celiotomy or Laparoscopy
    4. Venography
  E. Histological Evaluation of the Tumor
    1. Epithelial Tumors
      a. Squamous Cell Carcinoma
      b. Small-Cell Carcinoma
      c. Adenocarcinoma
      d. Large-Cell Carcinoma
      e. Adenosquamous Carcinoma
      f. Carcinoid Tumors
      g. Bronchial Gland Carcinoma
    2. Soft-Tissue Tumors
    3. Miscellaneous Tumors
    4. Tumorlike Lesions
  F. Classification and Staging

  G. Cardiopulmonary Evaluation
    1. Pulmonary Functions
    2. Cardiac Status
  H. Multidisciplinary Evaluation
  I. Site-Specific Data Form for Lung Cancer
III. Preoperative Preparation   431
  A. Nutritional Assessment
  B. Pulmonary Physiotherapy
  C. Antibiotics
  D. Correction of General Medical Disabilities
IV. Therapeutic Management   431
  A. Surgical Therapy
    1. Evaluation for Surgery
      a. Absolute Contraindications for Surgery
      b. Relative Contraindications for Surgery
      c. Indications for Surgery
    2. Type of Surgery
      a. Palliative Surgery
      b. Curative Surgical Resection
  B. Radiotherapy
    1. Indications for Radiotherapy
      a. Radiation Therapy for Cure
      b. Adjunctive Radiation Therapy
      c. Palliative Radiation Therapy
    2. Dose and Technique
    3. Small-Cell Carcinoma
  C. Chemotherapy
    1. Chemotherapeutic Agents Used
    2. Prognostic Factors
    3. Guidelines for Chemotherapy of Non–Oat Cell Carcinoma
    4. Treatment of Small-Cell Anaplastic Carcinoma of the Lung
      a. Localized Disease
      b. Extensive Disease
      c. Superior Vena Cava Syndrome
  D. Management of Metastatic Lung Cancer
    1. Selection of Patients for Surgery
    2. Preoperative Evaluation
    3. Surgical Treatment
      a. Operative Approach
      b. Technique
      c. Operative Risk
V. Postoperative Care, Evaluation, and Rehabilitation   437
  A. Postoperative Care
  B. Rehabilitation
    1. Psychosocial Support
    2. Physical Rehabilitation
  C. Follow-Up Evaluation
VI. Management Algorithm for Chest Tumors   439

Cancer of the lung is the most common visceral malignancy in men. There is an increase in incidence of this disease worldwide, as well as an increasing incidence among women, with statistics suggesting that since the year 1984, lung cancer in women causes more deaths per year than breast cancer. Furthermore, cure rates in lung cancer are rather poor, and it is estimated that less than 1 in every 10 patients with an established diagnosis of cancer of the lung will be alive 5 years later. Recent epidemiologic studies suggest that the incidence of pulmonary tumors is higher in southwest Brooklyn than in any other part of New York City.

In the past 25 years, some advances have been made in the establishment of an early diagnosis, in the preoperative assessment and preparation of the patient, and in the postoperative management. The dismal 5-year survival rates, however, make it obvious that most patients are still diagnosed at a stage of the disease that is already beyond any hope of cure with current forms of therapy.

For the physician involved in the management of this disease, a number of important objectives can be identified that might improve the end results in the management of lung cancer:

- Early detection.
- Improvement in the selection of patients for surgical treatment, thus diminishing the morbidity and mortality associated with fruitless operations and avoiding unnecessary surgery in patients that are beyond surgical cure.
- Determination of the cell type, stage, and extent of the tumor prior to instituting any therapy and precise staging of the disease at the time of surgery by both surgeon and pathologist. This is of great importance in selecting subsequent adjunctive therapy.
- Learning more about the natural history of cancer of the lung in order to make logical decisions for appropriate treatment at various stages of the disease.

I. EARLY DETECTION AND SCREENING

A. Predisposing Factors and Prevention

Carcinoma of the lung, which is among the most common visceral cancers and one of the most lethal, is eminently preventable in a large majority of the population.

1. Smoking

It has been estimated that 25% of all deaths from cancer are related to cigarette smoking. It is well recognized that, with relatively few exceptions, lung cancer is seen all but exclusively in heavy smokers and that the risk of lung cancer is directly related to the amount and duration of smoking. Massive campaigns by health-related groups and social organizations are underway to try and curb the use of cigarettes. Although these have been somewhat effective in decreasing the number of male adults who smoke, there appears to be a distressing increase in young smokers, particularly among females. There is a great need for strong education campaigns to discourage patients from smoking and possibly even for legislative action to curb the use of tobacco.

2. Industrial Hazards

Some industries are recognized as being associated with a definite increase in incidence of lung cancer. Exposure to nickel, uranium, and asbestos has resulted in a high risk of lung cancer. Regular screening of all individuals working in these environments and strict adherence to safety precautions are mandatory.

B. Detection

Aside from prevention, only early diagnosis is likely to modify the present mortality rates; early detection and screening are thus of the greatest importance.

1. Routine History and Physical Examination

These are of primary importance in the detection of lung cancer and must be carried out diligently with a high degree of awareness and suspicion. It is recommended that all adults over the age of 40 be examined yearly by a competent internist.

Questions about occupational history; family history; smoking and drinking habits; coughing (its pattern and duration); the character of sputum; hemoptysis; dyspnea; fever; chest pains (dull, pleuritic, or radiating), and unexplained general malaise, anorexia, weight loss are all of importance and may identify an early lung cancer. A thorough physical examination with particular attention to the chest, neck, lymphatics, and skeletal system may uncover signs suggestive of lung cancer. The following are red alert signs:

- Subtle findings at percussion and auscultation of the chest.
- Signs of superior vena cava obstruction.
- Clubbing.
- Hypertrophic osteoarthropathy.
- Lympadenopathy of the neck or axillae.
- Organomegaly, masses, etc.

These are, however, late findings, and patients identified as having lung cancer by the above signs are rarely subjects for surgical cure.

2. Chest X-Rays

The use of multiple chest x-ray examinations, even in high-risk populations, has generally been disappointing. A significant percentage of cases are incurable when the neoplasm is first identified on chest x-ray, and the value of routine yearly chest x-ray for screening is now being seriously questioned. It must, however, be obtained at the slightest suggestion during the yearly physical examination.

3. Cytology

Sputum cytology has improved the diagnosis of radiologically occult carcinoma of the lung. Tumors such as squamous cell carcinomas arising from the epithelial surface of a bronchus are those most likely to yield a positive diagnosis on cytology. In adenocarcinomas or large-cell cancers, sputum cytology is of little use in making the diagnosis.

Induced cytology has improved the diagnosis of radiologically occult carcinoma of the lung. Specimen collections should follow an early-morning heated-aerosol inhalation mixture of NaCl/15% propylene glycol solution for a required period (approximately 15 min) to induce a deep, productive cough. Alternatively, the use of ultrasonic nebulization of normal saline can be used in mass-screening series. Whenever indicated, chest percussion with increased numbers of sputum samples and postural drainage of specific areas will induce a higher yield of positive cytology. Three to six specimens are needed for thorough cytological evaluation.

C. Screening

High-risk patients such as heavy smokers and those with a strong family history or industrial exposure to nickel, uranium, or asbestos should be evaluated frequently and subjected to routine screening with early-morning deep-cough cytology and repetitive chest x-ray as well as to careful examination including flexible fiberoptic bronchoscopy under fluoroscopic control.

Routine screening of large segments of the population that are not at high risk has not proven very effective. Chest x-rays are still done on a large scale, but the yield has been small; yearly physical examinations are also widely recommended, yet early detection of lung cancer has so far eluded the physician.

D. Patient Education

As with most other cancers, an intensive program of patient education in all of the above aspects of lung cancer would be of great value in achieving the earliest possible diagnosis for the greatest number of patients.

II. PRETREATMENT EVALUATION AND WORK-UP

If bronchogenic cancer is suspected on the basis of chest x-ray findings, clinical symptoms, or both, treatment should not be started without histological confirmation of the diagnosis and a thorough systemic evaluation of the patient. The diagnostic work-up should proceed in an orderly fashion in an attempt to obtain tissue diagnosis, establish the stage of the disease, and determine the appropriate mode of therapy. A deep-cough early-morning specimen for sputum cytology may provide diagnosis of malignant cells and may even identify the cell type, but it will lack accuracy of histological diagnosis and localization of the neoplasm.

A. Radiological Evaluation of the Pulmonary Lesions

The diagnosis of pulmonary tumors is primarily radiological, and therefore, a logical stepwise plan of evaluation is mandatory.

1. Pulmonary Infiltrates

Lesions with an infiltrative appearance are usually treated with antibiotics for at least 6 weeks before further studies are undertaken, unless there is strong evidence of neoplasms such as bronchioloalveolar cell carcinoma or lymphoma or of postobstructive pneumonia. In patients with an endobronchial disease causing obstruction, sputum cytology may prove to be positive; otherwise, chest x-rays at 2-week intervals are suggested until complete resolution of the infiltrate occurs. Lack of complete clearance or recurrent infiltrate in the same area suggest a possible endobronchial lesion and tomography (or a computerized axial tomography [CAT] scan of the chest) and bronchoscopy are then indicated.

2. Pulmonary Masses

Comparison with prior chest x-rays is critical before calling any coin lesion cancer, and every effort to obtain previous chest x-rays must be made. Radiographic stability of a pulmonary lesion for more than 18 months is a reliable indication that the lesion is benign. If no previous chest x-rays are available, or if a change is noted, expeditious work-up should be undertaken to rule out a pulmonary neoplasm.

After the initial discovery of a coin lesion on chest x-ray, a low-kV (about 70 kV) chest film is required. Homogeneous or central calcification discovered at this time suggests a benign lesion. If this film is not diagnostic, tomography should be carried out. This should be performed as whole-chest tomography, with a mediastinal trough, using a linear (20°) mode at 1-cm intervals from the posterior rib to the anterior rib. The rationale is a search for other lesions and an evaluation of the hilum and mediastinum. The lesions of interest, once localized, should have cone pluridirectional tomography at 2- to 3-mm intervals with low kV. Tomography of the hilum at 55° posterior oblique projections is advised for evaluation of hilar adenopathy. Nowadays CAT has superseded these tests.

If a question of mediastinal adenopathy exists, a CAT scan of the mediastinum is most useful. Open-field CAT scan of the lungs can also better delineate small nodules and define the shape and relationships of the pulmonary mass. It is now preferred by many to standard tomography and has widely replaced it in most medical centers.

Some lesions of the mediastinum can be visualized on barium esophagography, and this should be required for any patient with suggestive symptoms.

Angiography, venography and isotopic or contrast studies are reserved for patients with symptoms suggesting vascular involvement, e.g., superior vena cava syndrome, pulmonary thromboembolism, oligemic-appearing lung, or a mass located in the proximity of the great vessels.

B. Preoperative Establishment
of the Diagnosis

It is very important to establish a tissue diagnosis prior to any therapy. Attempts should be made to visualize the tumor through a rigid or flexible bronchoscope. Bronchoscopic aspiration and washings for cytology, bronchial biopsy, brushing,

transbronchial biopsy (under fluoroscopic control), and transcutaneous aspiration biopsy with a fine needle are all techniques that may be used to obtain a preoperative histological diagnosis. On occasion, the results of these procedures may establish a sufficient diagnosis and determine the stage of the disease, thus avoiding an unnecessary thoracotomy.

1. Bronchoscopy

An experienced endoscopist should achieve a 70–80% diagnostic accuracy when assessing primary bronchogenic cancer.

a. Open-Tube Bronchoscopy

Open-tube bronchoscopy can often be done under topical anesthesia using a 5–10% cocaine solution. If a general anesthesia is required, side-arm-ventilation bronchoscopes provide adequate tidal volumes and should be used.

Open-tube bronchoscopy has the advantage of permitting identification of a tumor in a central location and of providing sufficient biopsy material for accurate diagnosis. There is better control of the airway, and viscid secretions or massive hemoptysis can be better managed. The main indications for open-tube bronchoscopy are

- Removal of a foreign body.
- Dilatation of tracheal and bronchial stenosis.
- Hemoptysis.
- Need for more adequate biopsy material.
- Evaluating the "feel" of the carina.

The disadvantages of this technique are the patient's discomfort, if general anesthesia is not used, and the limitation of the diagnostic evaluation to the large central bronchi. The rigid scope is not good for visualization of subsegmental bronchi. Telescopes or angled scopes are not as useful or versatile as the current generation of flexible fiberoptic bronchoscopes; therefore, satisfactory diagnostic accuracy cannot always be obtained with the rigid scope.

b. Flexible Fiberoptic Bronchoscopy

This is usually done under local anesthesia, but it is preferable to have the patient well premedicated; atropine, 0.6–0.8 mg; Demerol, 50–100 mg; Vistaril, 25–50 mg; and diazepam, 10 mg, may be given 30 min prior to the procedure. Topical 0.5% tetracaine can then be used for anesthesia. General anesthesia is only necessary when a prolonged search for an *in-situ* cancer is required.

Insertion of the bronchoscope can be either oral, through a preloaded uncuffed endotracheal tube (the endotracheal tube providing airway control for supplemental ventilation and suctioning, as needed), or nasopharyngeal, which has the advantage of permitting better visualization of the epiglottis and larynx as well as the tracheobronchial tree.

Fiberoptic flexible scopes are not good for infants because of their small airway. Sutures cannot be removed, nor can strictures be dilated, through them. In the presence of significant hemoptysis or viscid secretions, control of the airway is not possible, and an inferior examination results.

The complications of fiberoptic bronchoscopy include

- Laryngospasm.
- Cardiac arrhythmias.
- Bronchospasm.
- Bleeding.
- Pneumothorax (with transbronchial biopsy only).

2. Biopsy

a. Brush Biopsy

Brush biopsies require at least four separate vigorous and accurate brushings. The brush is passed over the area of suspected malignancy several times and then immediately rubbed on a slide, which is dropped into an alcohol solution. Separate brushes are used for each brushing.

b. Transbronchial Biopsy

Under fluoroscopic control, transbronchial biopsies using the fiberoptic scope may be taken. This is more applicable to diffuse infiltrates than to isolated masses. Multiple small bronchial biopsies are taken to diminish the chance of a false negative biopsy. There is a 5% incidence of pneumothorax associated with this biopsy technique.

c. Transcutaneous Needle Biopsy

There are two situations where precutaneous biopsy of a pulmonary lesion is of established value: when significant pleural effusion is associated with an underlying neoplasm and in tumors close to the chest wall that can be aspirated with little risk of bleeding or pneumothorax. Needle aspiration in these circumstances may help in identifying the cell type and making a decision regarding operative therapy.

Complications of transcutaneous needle biopsy of the lung are often minor but can delay or complicate definitive therapy.

- Pneumothorax is a common complication of needle aspiration biopsy, particularly in deep-seated tumors. Some air may enter the pleural cavity through the open needle, but the more likely cause is puncture of the lung with the needle and continued air leak into the pleural cavity.
- Hemorrhage is rare; however, significant hemorrhaging may result from the needle causing injury to an intercostal vessel, biopsy of a vascular tumor, and/or inadvertent penetration of the diaphragm.
- Pleural shock. True pleural shock is very rare and may result from the aspirating needle penetrating simultaneously the

lung and a branch of the pulmonary vein, thus allowing air to leak into the pulmonary veins, producing a left-sided air embolism.
- Inadequate tissue for diagnosis via the needle.
- Pleural seeding with possible infection or malignant cell implantation prior to definitive treatment.

d. Bone Marrow Biopsy in Bronchogenic Carcinoma

Iliac crest bone marrow aspiration and biopsy should be considered as a primary tool in the tissue diagnosis and overall hematologic evaluation of the patient with bronchogenic carcinoma. This is especially important in small-cell and anaplastic carcinoma, where the frequency of involvement ranges from 10 to 50%.

Bone marrow examination combined with flexible fiberoptic bronchoscopy has a positive yield of 92%.

e. Thoracoscopy

This is useful for Stage III (see § 10A.II.F) unclassified tumors and may be carried out with a flexible fiberoptic bronchoscope (7.5 mm) inserted into the thorax under local anesthesia for inspection and biopsy. Biopsy of pleural or peripheral masses is thus possible for diagnosis.

f. Limited Open Thoracotomy or Minithoracotomy

Failure to establish a diagnosis with any of the above procedures might result in the need for a diagnostic thoracotomy and open biopsy of the lung. This is particularly true in cases with diffuse lesions, lymphagitic disease, or small tumors. In the latter case, a minimal incision can be made over the lesion for biopsy, and it can then be extended if resection is indicated.

C. Metastatic Evaluation of the Patient

Recent literature suggests limited value for routine liver–spleen, brain, and bone radionuclide scans in the absence of organ-specific symptoms, physical findings, or biochemical abnormalities. It has been our policy to eliminate routine liver scans from the work-up of the patient in the absence of abnormal liver function tests. Bone scan (with coned down skeletal views of any abnormality identified on the bone scan) and cranial CAT scan are essential components of the evaluation of any patient with carcinoma of the lung prior to surgery because of the relatively frequent occurrence of occult metastases to bone and brain. Computerized axial tomography scans are positive in 5–10% of lung cancer patients who are asymptomatic.

Beyond the above mentioned tests, patients considered for

curative surgery should then undergo CAT scans of the chest, mediastinum, and upper abdomen (including the adrenal glands), which may be the site of hidden metastases.

D. Evaluation of Operability

1. Mediastinal Evaluation

a. Special Radiological Procedures

Prior to the widespread use of mediastinoscopy, approximately 50% of the patients selected for thoracotomy for cure were found to be unresectable due to unsuspected tumor in the mediastinum. The outlook for those patients was dismal, and 90% were dead within a year. A tumor spreads through the ascending chain of parabronchial, subcarinal, and paratracheal lymphatics. These are the main routes of spread that preclude curative resection of a bronchogenic carcinoma. Invasion of the capsule of the lymph nodes results in secondary fixation and deposits of tumor in the mediastinum and limits any possibility of a surgical cure.

Oblique views of the hilum and CAT scan of the mediastinum are most helpful in identifying mediastinal node involvement. In those patients with demonstrable mediastinal node involvement, a tissue diagnosis and staging can then be accomplished by means of a limited mediastinal procedure.

With the advent of mediastinoscopy, now augmented by tomography and CAT scan, it has been possible, with a few exceptions, to avoid thoracotomy in patients with involved mediastinal nodes especially when extensive.

b. Transcervical Mediastinoscopy

Transcervical mediastinoscopy (TCM) provides direct access to the paratracheal and occasionally the subcarinal lymph node areas. The plane of dissection of the scope on the anterior surface of the trachea in the middle mediastinum is also the pathway for lymphatic drainage of the tumor as far down as the proximal 3 cm of each main-stem bronchus. This proximal portion of the main-stem bronchi can thus be readily examined during mediastinoscopy.

The anterior mediastinum, on the other hand, cannot be safely reached in many instances because the aorta and great vessels intervene between the sternum and the paratracheal plane, where the mediastinoscope is passed. It has, therefore, been suggested that to establish the diagnosis and operability of left-sided tumors, an anterior thoracic mediastinal exploration be used rather than a TCM.

Transcervical mediastinoscopy is performed under general endotracheal anesthesia after complete prep and drape to allow for a sternum-splitting incision should emergency exploration become necessary for control of hemorrhage. Transcervical mediastinoscopy is usually a safe and well-tolerated procedure with a mortality of less than 0.1% and few serious complications. The following are the complications that can be avoided with proper care and technique:

- Hemorrhage. Minor-vessel bleeding in the neck can be controlled by ligation and electrocautery. Major-vessel bleeding in the mediastinum can be avoided by careful palpation and needle aspiration prior to biopsy. Failure to establish the correct plane of cleavage can result in increased bleeding and poor visibility, resulting in serious risks of complication. The proper plane of dissection on the anterior tracheal surface allows for a clean, safe procedure.
- Pneumothorax.
- Esophageal injury, which is not common but may occur from failure to enter the proper pretracheal plane and inadvertently swaying from the midline.

The following are the situations in which TCM is primarily indicated:

- A centrally located mass lesion more than 3.0 cm in diameter.
- Evidence of mediastinal or hilar adenopathy on oblique views of the hilum, or positive CAT or gallium scan of the mediastinum. If the above studies are not remarkable, we do not feel that TCM is necessary.

We do not recommend the procedure for patients with peripheral nodules or patients with a normal hilum and mediastinal studies. The yield is far too low to justify the small, but definite, mortality and morbidity of the procedure. Transcervical mediastinoscopy is definitely contraindicated in any patient with previous neck surgery, such as thyroidectomy.

c. Anterior Thoracic Mediastinal Exploration

It has been claimed that anterior thoracic mediastinal exploration (ATME) gives an increased accuracy of predicting operability for left-sided lesions. This procedure is performed under general endotracheal anesthesia by way of a small anterior thoracotomy; the mediastinoscope is then inserted through a parasternal extrapleural incision.

There is a greater morbidity and increased pain and disability associated with ATME. It is, however, indicated for the following conditions:

- Left-sided lesions. The claim that there is increased accuracy for predicting operability of left-sided lesions by ATME is, however, somewhat exaggerated. Experience revealed an equal percentage of positive biopsies doing TCM in both left- and right-sided lesions. Moreover, patients with a negative TCM were rarely found to be unresectable at thoracotomy because of tumor invasion of the anterior mediastinum.

- When transcervical mediastinoscopy is contraindicated because of previous surgery in the neck.

The procedure is done through an incision made over the third costal cartilage on the appropriate side. A segment of cartilage is resected, and the extrapleural plane of dissection is developed toward the hilum. Biopsy may then be taken through the scope.

The complications of ATME include

- Hemorrhage. Hemorrhage from the internal mammary, intercostal or great vessels can occur if care is not taken to identify and avoid these structures.
- Pneumothorax.
- Esophageal injury.
- Wound infection.

There remains some controversy concerning the results of resection in patients with involved mediastinal lymph nodes. Most of the reports describing results of resection do not identify the precise location or extent of such involvement but generally report a dismal outcome. There may be a place for surgery in selected patients with ipsilateral superior mediastinal lymph node involvement. For resection to be considered, the mediastinal involvement must be ipsilateral, completely resectable, and not extending above the midtracheal level, and this only in non–oat cell carcinoma.

2. Scalene Node Biopsy

The removal of the lymph nodes from the prescalene fat pad for biopsy purposes is based on the concept that lymphatic drainage of lung cancer is to the mediastinal and scalene nodes. The yield of positive results is very low in the absence of readily palpable nodes, but the procedure can be easily and safely performed under local anesthesia, and a positive biopsy will provide the histological diagnosis and establish the stage of the disease, precluding unnecessary surgery. Scalene node biopsies should be done on the right side for all lung cancers, except those in the left upper lobe.

Complications of scalene node biopsy are rare but may be quite formidable and include

- Hemorrhage.
- Lymph or chylous fistula.
- Brachial plexus injury.
- Phrenic nerve injury.
- Pneumothorax.

3. Celiotomy or Laparoscopy

If a patient has a pulmonary tumor with or without a histological diagnosis and is found to have abnormal liver function tests, a liver scan is indicated. If the scan is positive, a diag-

nostic minilaparotomy can be done for tissue diagnosis. This procedure can be done under local anesthesia with minimal risk and a very low morbidity and mortality. Its indications and utilization are limited and rare.

4. Venography

Superior venacavograms and azygosvenograms may be of value in studying upper lobe tumors. They are particularly useful in patients with superior vena cava obstruction and can often differentiate between extrinsic pressure from a tumor mass and tumor thrombosis. Superior venacavography using radioactive material is rapidly replacing the routine venogram because of its simplicity and the additional information generated by subsequent lung scan.

E. Histological Evaluation of the Tumor

1. Epithelial Tumors

Benign pulmonary tumors include

- Papillomas, squamous cell or transitional. The latter type has a tendency to be multiple and recur after resection. Dysplasia can at times be seen, and maligant degeneration may occur.
- Adenomas. These tumors arise from the mucous glands of the tracheobronchial tree and, as in salivary gland tumors, they can present as monomorphic adenomas or pleomorphic adenomas.

Dysplasias and epithelial abnormalities similar to those seen in the cervix or larynx can also be seen in the tracheobronchial tree. They may occur in the normal bronchial mucosa, in mucous glands, or within papillary growths. Carcinomas *in situ* can also be identified.

The malignant epithelial tumors are of several varieties.

a. Squamous Cell Carcinoma

This malignant epithelial tumor, which shows keratinization and/or intercellular bridges, was, until recently, the most common of all lung cancers. It may be well differentiated, moderately differentiated, or poorly differentiated and generally arises from the large bronchi. It is usually centrally located and can often be seen on bronchoscopy and easily sampled cytologically. Squamous cell carcinomas frequently develop extensive central necrosis and can cause substantial hemorrhage; they can also produce a parathyroidlike hormone and result in hypercalcemia. The tumor metastasizes primarily to regional lymph nodes.

A variant of the squamous cell carcinoma of the lung is the "spindle cell carcinoma" with a spindle cell component suggestive of a sarcoma. This tumor often shows pleomorphism and abnormal mitoses but carries a somewhat better prognosis than the usual squamous cell cancer. It can, at times, form polypoid projections in the large bronchi.

b. Small-Cell Carcinoma

- Oat cell carcinomas composed of small, uniform lymphocytoid cells with minimal cytoplasm are the most aggressive lung tumors. They metastasize early and widely (to brain and bone marrow as well as regional lymph nodes). Their cytoplasm can contain dense (neurosecretory) granules, and they frequently produce various biologically active substances (e.g., ACTH, serotonin, antidiuretic hormone, calcitonin, melanocyte-stimulating hormone, etc.) In some ways, this tumor may be related to apudomas.
- Intermediate-cell carcinoma composed of polygonal, irregular cells with more cytoplasm than the oat cell carcinoma.
- Combined oat cell carcinoma with squamous or glandular components.

c. Adenocarcinoma

These can show tubular, acinar, or papillary features with mucin production and frequent psammoma bodies. They may simulate a metastasis from a variety of sites: pancreas, stomach, ovary, breast, etc. These tumors are usually more peripheral in the lungs, metastasize early and widely, and are most often associated with migratory thrombophlebitis and hypertrophic osteoarthropathy. They can be divided into

- Acinar adenocarcinoma.
- Papillary adenocarcinoma.
- Bronchioalveolar adenocarcinoma with cylindrical mucous-secreting cells lining the walls of the alveoli (a rapidly spreading tumor).
- Solid adenocarcinoma, a poorly differentiated tumor with mucin-containing vacuoles and a compact growth pattern.

d. Large-Cell Carcinoma

This group of tumors includes other malignant epithelial tumors that do not fall in the previous three categories. They have large, nucleated cells with abundant cytoplasm. Several variants are recognized: giant cell carcinoma with multinucleated pleomorphic cells and clear cell carcinoma.

e. Adenosquamous Carcinoma

These show features of both squamous and adenomatous carcinomas but behave as adenocarcinomas.

f. Carcinoid Tumors

This very specific tumor can be seen in the lung and is usually centrally located. It may show considerable metaplasia (osteoid or amyloid), is often multiple, frequently affects younger patients, rarely metastasizes, and is considered of low grade. A carcinoid tumor of the lung does not usually result in a carcinoid syndrome unless it has metastasized.

g. Bronchial Gland Carcinoma

These are similar to salivary gland carcinomas and include adenoid cystic carcinoma and mucoepidermoid carcinoma. They are characterized by slow growth.

2. Soft-Tissue Tumors

Soft-tissue tumors are less common than the epithelial tumors but can assume any of the reported histological types of sarcomas.

3. Miscellaneous Tumors

- Benign clear-cell tumors, rich in glycogen.
- Paragangliomas, solitary or multiple and located in the interstitium of the lung.
- Teratomas.
- Carcinosarcomas.
- Pulmonary blastomas, which resemble mesenchymomas, occur in the periphery of the lung and show various degrees of malignancy.
- Malignant melanomas.
- Lymphomas.
- Unclassified tumors.
- Metastatic carcinomas.

4. Tumorlike Lesions

- Hamartomas, either chrondromatous or leiomyomatous. They consist of cartilagenous or leiomyomatous nodules associated with fibrous, adipose, or bronchial epithelium. They clinically present as coin lesions and constitute a major differential diagnosis with carcinomas.
- Lymphoproliferative disease or lymphomatoid granulomatosis.
- Eosinophilic granulomas, often part of a systemic disease (histiocytosis X).
- Sclerosing hemangioma.
- Inflammatory pseudotumors, plasma cell granulomas, or fibroxanthomas.

F. Classification and Staging

The classification (see the Site-Specific Data Form, § 10A.II.I) should be based on the extent of the primary tumor (T), the nodal status (N), and the metastatic sites (M). Not only is clinical staging important for prognosis, data collection, postsurgical treatment, and retreatment therapeutic management, but it is also useful to better understand the nature of carcinoma of the lung and apply the optimum treatment.

Stage I disease is a discrete peripheral tumor, squamous or adenocarcinoma in cell type, with no mediastinal lymphadenopathy, no segmental or lobar atelectasis, and no pleural effusion. These lesions are usually resectable with a 35–50% 5-year survival (staging of lung cancer, 1979 manual of the American Joint Committee on Cancer Staging and End-Results Reporting Task Force on lung).

Stage II disease is possibly resectable, and a 20–25% 5-year survival may be expected. For a tumor to be classified as Stage II, there can be no pleural effusion or proven mediastinal metastases, no sternal or vertebral involvement, no total lung atelectasis; a bilateral iliac crest biopsy for bone marrow aspiration to detect bone marrow spread must also be negative. The tumor can be >3 cm with ipsilateral hilar nodes.

Stage III disease is unresectable, and a 0–10% 5-year survival may be expected. This stage is characterized by T3 lesions with any N, N2 lesions with any T, and any T or N with distant metastases. Criteria for this stage include any of the following:

- A histological diagnosis of oat cell carcinoma established preoperatively.
- A tumor that has spread to any intrathoracic structure that would preclude resection.
- Contralateral disease.
- Involvement of the bronchus in its proximal 2 cm from the carina on bronchoscopic examination.
- Pleural effusion, which may be negative for malignant cells.
- Recurrent laryngeal or phrenic nerve paralysis.
- Microscopic metastases in mediastinal nodes.
- Tumor involvement of the superior sulcus, apex of the chest, or spine.
- Atelectasis or pneumonitis of an entire lung.
- Distant metastases.

Stage III disease also includes patients who have totally unresectable tumors. There is a 0% 5-year survival if there are proven extrathoracic metastases, contralateral metastases, pulmonary artery obstruction adjacent to the main pulmonary artery, gross tumor in the mediastinal nodes, and aortic or esophageal involvement.

G. Cardiopulmonary Evaluation

Cardiopulmonary evaluation of the candidate for surgical therapy of cancer of the lung is required prior to any plan of definitive therapy.

1. Pulmonary Functions

The initial pulmonary evaluation prior to resectional surgery should include

- Routine pulmonary volumes.
- Ventilatory studies including response to bronchodilators.
- Resting arterial blood gases on room air.
- Exercise stress testing (Bruce protocol with 80% maximum heart rate).

The usual criteria for nonresectability due to poor pulmonary reserve are those where one can identify severe and nonreversible destructive patterns of pulmonary functions:

- Forced vital capacity of <40% predicted.
- Forced expiratory volume at 1 sec of <50% predicted.

In borderline cases, ^{133}xenon ventilation perfusion scan can be utilized by subtraction techniques to estimate residual functional status.

2. Cardiac Status

The cardiac status is determined by a good history and physical examination, a resting EKG, and exercise stress testing for ischemia and arrhythmia. Nuclear studies with thallium testing will be the basis for estimating cardiac reserve and left ventricular functions. Criteria for nonresectability due to cardiac status are intractable chronic congestive failure or uncontrolled atrial/ventricular arrhythmias.

Massive obesity is not necessarily a contraindication to surgery and can be managed with proper anesthesia and vigorous postoperative care.

H. Multidisciplinary Evaluation

Prior to mapping out a course of therapy, a multidisciplinary evaluation of the patient is mandatory in order to determine the most effective coherent approach. A radiation oncologist and medical oncologist should plan the treatment strategy together with the primary physician and the responsible surgeon. A nurse oncologist, social worker, and rehabilitation therapist can also be of great help in identifying and meeting certain special needs that the patient might have, thus permitting the patient to make the optimum recovery.

I. Site-Specific Data Form
for Lung Cancer (see pp. 429–430)

SITE SPECIFIC DATA FORM—LUNG CANCER

HISTORY

Age: _____

Symptoms
- _____ Cough
- _____ Sputum
- _____ Hemoptysis
- _____ Dyspnea
- _____ Fever
- _____ Chest pains
- _____ Wheezing
- _____ Clubbing
- _____ Lymphadenopathy
- _____ Weight loss
- _____ Arthropathy
- _____ Other

Duration _____

Social history
Occupation: _____
Race: ____White ____Black ____Oriental ____Other
Marital status: ____Single ____Married ____Other
Smoking habits: ____Nonsmoker ____Exsmoker
Present smoker ____ Packs/day ____
Duration (in years): _____

Family history of carcinoma
Relation: _____ Site: _____

Previous history of carcinoma
_____No _____Yes Site: _____

Rx: _____

Previous treatment (describe):
(Surgery, radiotherapy, chemotherapy, etc.)
_____
_____
_____

PHYSICAL EXAMINATION

General condition: _____

Chest examination (describe findings)
- _____ Auscultation
- _____ Percussion

Other findings: _____
_____

Tumor size: _____Occult _____<3 cm _____>3 cm _____Massive

Actual size _____

Tumor location:	Right	Left
Upper lobe	_____	_____
Middle lobe	_____	_____
Lower lobe	_____	_____

Tumor extension:	Right	Left
Visceral pleura	_____	_____
Pleural effusion	_____	_____
Parietal pleura	_____	_____
Chest wall	_____	_____
Main bronchus within 2 cm from carina	_____	_____
Mediastinum	_____	_____
Atelectasis or pneumonitis	_____	_____
Localized	_____	_____
Whole lung	_____	_____

Nodal involvement
- _____ Peribronchial
- _____ Hilar
- _____ Subcarinal
- _____ Paratracheal
- _____ Paraesophageal
- _____ Aortic

Distant metastases
- _____ No _____ Yes _____ Brain _____ Bone _____ Liver _____ Other

PREOPERATIVE WORK-UP (Check, if done)

	Neg.	Pos.	Suspicious		Neg.	Pos.	Suspicious
Skin tests							
Coccidiomycosis	_____	_____	_____	Candida	_____	_____	_____
Histoplasmosis	_____	_____	_____	Mumps	_____	_____	_____
Tuberculosis	_____	_____	_____	Trich	_____	_____	_____
CBC	_____	_____	_____	Sputum C and S	_____	_____	_____
Biochemical profile	_____	_____	_____	Pulmonary function study	_____	_____	_____
Chest x-ray	_____	_____	_____				
Electrocardiogram	_____	_____	_____	Lung CAT scan	_____	_____	_____
Sputum cytology	_____	_____	_____	Lung tomogram	_____	_____	_____
Brain scan	_____	_____	_____	Bone scan	_____	_____	_____
Liver scan	_____	_____	_____	Mediastinoscopy	_____	_____	_____
CEA	_____	_____	_____	Bronchoscopy	_____	_____	_____
Bone marrow aspiration	_____	_____	_____	Type _____			
				Biopsy	_____	_____	_____
Blood gases	_____	_____	_____	Type _____			
Mediastinal CAT	_____	_____	_____	Other _____			

Classification
_____ T _____ N _____ M

Stage: _____

Histologic diagnosis: _____

Signature: _____

Countersignature: _____

Date: _____

Classification and Staging of Lung Cancer

Classification

Primary tumor (T)

T0   No evidence of primary tumor
TIS Carcinoma *in situ*
TX   Tumor proven by presence of malignant cells in the bronchopulmonary secretion
       but not seen on chest x-ray or bronchoscopy
T1   A tumor is 3.0 cm or less in greatest diameter, surrounded by lung or visceral pleura,
       and without evidence of invasion proximal to a lobar bronchus at bronchoscopy
T2   A tumor that is greater than 3.0 cm in greatest diameter with the following provisions:
       at least 2.0 cm distal to the carina
       any associated atelectasis or obstructive pneumonitis must involve less than an entire lung
       no pleural effusion present
T3   A tumor of any size with the following:
       direct extension into adjacent structures such as chest wall, diaphragm, or mediastinum
       a tumor whose proximal end is less than 2.0 cm distal to the carina
       a tumor with associated atelectasis or obstructive pneumonitis of an entire lung
       the presence of pleural effusion

Regional lymph node involvement (N)

N0   No demonstrable metastases to regional nodes
N1   Metastases to lymph nodes in the ipsilateral hilar nodes; no direct extension to the tumor
N2   Metastases to lymph nodes in the mediastinum

Distant metastases (M)

  For example, scalene node, cervical and contralateral hilar lymph nodes, as well as brain, bone, liver,
or adrenal metastases.

Staging Groupings of Lung Cancers

Stage I (probably resectable, expected 30–35% 5–year survival)
  TX, N0, M0   An occult cancer with malignant cells in the bronchopulmonary secretions, but with
                   no evidence of metastases to the regional lymph nodes or distant metastases
  T1, N0, M0   Tumor that is 3.0 cm or less
  T2, N0, M0
  T1, N1, M0

Stage II
  T2, N1, M0   Tumor classified as T2 with metastases to the ipsilateral hilar region only or in the
                   peribronchial lymph nodes

Stage III
  T3 with any N
  Any T with N2
  Any T or N with M+ or contralateral disease or scalene node positive

III. PREOPERATIVE PREPARATION

Patients with Stage I and II lung cancer, who have resectable tumors, are usually in good general and nutritional state and require little preoperative preparation. Patients with advanced lung cancer are most often debilitated and require more supportive care during their palliative therapy.

A. Nutritional Assessment

Nutritional assessment is necessary, and hyperalimentation is sometimes advisable to correct a negative nitrogen balance prior to surgery, especially in patients with a history of malnutrition, heavy drinking, and smoking.

B. Pulmonary Physiotherapy

Following the pulmonary function tests, respiratory therapy to attain optimum pulmonary function is desirable, and patients must be taught to use the various respirators that they might require postoperatively.

- Bronchial toilet, coughing, and suctioning is essential.
- Bronchodilators may be used as indicated.
- Use of various incentive respirators and nebulizers may be initiated preoperatively.
- Instruction in function and use of various respirators is best given preoperatively.
- Helping the patient to stop smoking before and after surgery. Because most patients with lung cancer are heavy smokers, this type of preoperative respiratory therapy is of great importance.

C. Antibiotics

Preoperative antibiotics are often indicated in the management of lung cancer to resolve pulmonary processes that may have resulted from bronchial obstruction.

D. Correction of General Medical Disabilities

- Cardiac arrhythmias and myocardial insufficiency must be corrected and compensated.
- Any liver damage from drinking must be assessed and corrected, as indicated.
- Hematologic evaluation must be carried out to identify any blood volume deficits, leukopenias, or coagulopathies, and these must be corrected prior to surgery.

IV. THERAPEUTIC MANAGEMENT

A. Surgical Therapy

1. Indication for Surgery

a. Absolute Contraindications for Surgery

A tumor is not curable surgically if it has spread beyond the confines of the lung and, as such, is inoperable. The criteria of inoperability basically include Stage III disease:

- Known oat cell carcinoma preoperatively.
- Pleural effusion.
- Evidence of distant metastases.
- Positive scalene nodes.
- Evidence of intrathoracic spread that would preclude resection: superior vena cava obstruction, phrenic nerve palsy, recurrent laryngeal nerve palsy, myocardial involvement, aortic or esophageal invasion, and tracheal spread.

b. Relative Contraindications for Surgery

The various criteria of an advanced Stage II disease constitute relative contraindications:

- Mediastinal node involvement, especially in patients with adenocarcinoma. Epidermoid carcinomas with mediastinal node involvement may be considered resectable under special circumstances if the extent of involvement is limited, though survival figures are extremely low.
- Involvement of main-stem bronchi within 1 cm of the carina.
- Chest-wall invasion. In a superior sulcus tumor, combined radical resection following preoperative x-ray treatment may be considered. Such an approach might be indicated in other lung tumors that have invaded the chest wall but that have no other signs of inoperability or distant metastases. There seems to be some suggestion that survival depends more on mediastinal invasion and other criterias of incurability than on chest-wall invasion per se.

c. Indications for Surgery

Surgery is primarily indicated in Stage I cancer of the lung.

2. Type of Surgery

a. Palliative Surgery

With very few exceptions, resection is indicated only when it can be presumed to be complete and potentially curative. The indications for palliative surgery are only for unrelieved symptoms from the secondary effects of the tumor, where less invasive methods (i.e., radiotherapy or chemotherapy) have failed and only in patients where there is a likelihood of the patient surviving the procedure. The following complications are the usual indications for palliative resection:

- Distal bronchial obstruction with sepsis.
- Massive hemoptysis.
- Refractory hypercalcemia.
- Disabling pulmonary osteoarthropathy.

b. Curative Surgical Resection

Several types of resections are possible in lung cancer. The most desirable one is lobectomy, whenever possible. If this is technically not possible, or if the margins of resection are positive on frozen section, a pneumonectomy must be carried out.

Lesser resections with frozen section control of the margins, the nodes, and pulmonary veins are of definite value in the treatment of early lung cancer. These include sleeve resection, segmentectomy, and open-wedge resection. Initially, these procedures were proposed as a compromise in patients with poor cadiopulmonary reserve, but there are increasing numbers of reports suggesting that there may be a definite role for these procedures as the surgical treatment of choice in well-selected cases.

Extended resection is only rarely indicated and then only for cure in young patients where a direct extension of the primary tumor necessitates removal en bloc of the lung and adjacent tissues (e.g., with pericardial involvement, Pancoast tumors, chest-wall resections, etc.). It should never be carried out for local or regional spread.

A posterolateral thoracotomy incision and exposure is advisable for all resections except those that require bilateral exploration. If bilateral exploration is necessary, a full-length median sternotomy is the incision of choice for the simultaneous exposure of both the right and left lungs.

Since most operations are for cure, it is important to assess the status of the regional nodes and resection margins during the procedure; frozen section of the bronchial stump, regional nodes, and pulmonary vein is often indicated. These biopsies are particularly important if conservative lung-sparing resections are being contemplated. The more limited resections, such as lobectomy, sleeve resection, and segmentectomy will have resection margins that lie closer to the tumor and will require more frozen sections.

B. Radiotherapy

1. Indications for Radiotherapy

The long experience of treating lung cancers with radiotherapy has been both rewarding and frustrating. The rewards are seen early in the form of substantial tumor regression or complete disappearance; relief of symptoms such as hemoptysis, pain, shortness of breath (when caused by obstructive lesions); and general improvement in the patient's health, appetite, and weight. The frustrations, however, follow after a short interval in time in the form of disease spread primarily to areas outside the thorax such as brain, liver, bones, and other organs. Local intrathoracic recurrences do also contribute to this dismal picture, especially when the dose originally given was limited. For cure, epithelial tumors (squamous cell and adenocarcinoma) need a radical dose of about 6500 rads in 6.5 weeks. Small-cell (or oat cell) lesions are controlled by slightly smaller doses. The application of radical radiotherapy is hampered when the tumor is of a large size or when mediastinal structures are substantially involved, since the midline dose has to be curtailed due to the presence of the spinal cord. The tolerance of the cord is limited to about 4500 rads (given in about 4 weeks) and appropriate steps, for its protection should be taken to avoid radiation myelopathy when such doses are reached. Other side effects of radiotherapy are rather limited, and although heavily irradiated pulmonary tissue will fibrose and shrink, the subsequent compensatory reaction, along with the normal pulmonary reserve, will minimize the clinical impact of such changes on the patient.

a. Radiation Therapy for Cure

Radiation therapy is the treatment of choice in the following circumstances:

- Locally advanced disease.
- Ipsilateral supraclavicular node involvement.
- Inoperable patients due to medical complications.
- Patient's refusal of surgery.

Radiation therapy is delivered to the site of the primary, the mediastinum, and the supraclavicular area in upper lobe lesions or in cases of involvement of the supraclavicular nodes. This is usually followed by a coned down beam to the site of the primary in order to spare the spinal cord from excessive irradiation.

Interstitial implants using ^{222}radon or ^{125}iodine are utilized in some centers, particularly for apical tumors. They have the advantage of delivering high doses of radiation to relatively localized areas, sparing the surrounding tissues. They have been advocated for small and moderate-sized lesions and in postirradiation recurrences.

b. Adjunctive Radiation Therapy

Postoperative radiation therapy appears to be indicated in the following circumstances:

- Patients with hilar or mediastinal node involvement.
- Gross residual disease.
- Microscopic involvement of the bronchial stump.

Oat cell carcinomas are treated with a combination of radiation therapy and chemotherapy. Prophylactic elective brain irradiation in these patients is also indicated and decreases the incidence of brain metastases. Brain irradiation may also be given electively in cases of adenocarcinoma of the lung as an adjunctive modality.

c. Palliative Radiation Therapy

The superior vena cava syndrome occurs with mediastinal involvement in right upper lobe lesions. Radiation therapy alone is usually quite effective, and there is often no need for diuretics, steroids, or nitrogen mustard injections. About 70% of the patients are well palliated by radiation therapy.

Hemoptysis, chest pain, dyspnea, and cough respond well to the same treatment, if the symptoms are directly related to the tumor. Dyspnea will be relieved if it is the result of an obstructive bronchial tumor (intraluminal obstruction or external pressure), and cough relief will occur if the cough is directly related to the presence of the tumor.

Symptoms due to distant metastases (e.g., bone metastases, brain metastases, spinal cord compression due to extradural metastases, soft-tissue metastases, and jaundice due to porta hepatis metastases) are all relieved by radiation therapy in a high percentage of patients. Spinal cord compression is an urgent indication for palliative radiation therapy, sometimes in combination with surgical decompression.

2. Dose and Technique

The dose and technique depend on the site of involvement and the intent of therapy. Adjuvant and palliative treatments do not require a very high dose, and simple parallel opposed portals can be used. For curative therapy, higher doses, in the range of 6500 rads, must be given. For central tumors or when there is gross mediastinal adenopathy, where the volume to be treated lies near such sensitive structures as the spinal cord, elegant techniques, often aided by computer planning and dosimetry, are used to achieve maximum tumor control with minimal complications. For upper lobe lesions, the entire mediastinum and the supraclavicular fossa are treated to a dose of 4500 rads followed by a booster dose to areas of gross disease, using such spinal cord–sparing techniques as two posterior oblique fields.

3. Small-Cell Carcinoma

This lesion has long been known to be very radiosensitive, necessitating only modest doses to achieve complete regression in a large number of cases. However, the high incidence of widespread disease has prompted several national protocols to determine the best treatment, and several points seem clear.

- Combination therapy with chemotherapy and radiotherapy is most effective.
- In those regimens where chemotherapy alone has been used with apparent complete regression, very often the primary tumor site is the first area of relapse. This occurs much less often when radiotherapy is integrated into the original treatment plan and when the dose is carried to an adequate level.
- Many studies have shown that prophylactic cranial irradiation reduces the incidence of clinically undetected brain metastases, although any impact on survival is yet to be seen.

The exact sequence and optimum timing of combination therapy in this histological subtype of lung cancer is still under investigation, but a combined approach of radiotherapy and chemotherapy should be routinely considered.

C. Chemotherapy

Chemotherapy of lung cancer is based on the cell type of the tumor and the stage of the disease. Curative surgery is usually the most desirable treatment whenever possible, and with the exception of small-cell cancers, it should be used for all Stage I and II lung cancer unless there are specific contraindications. Radiation therapy is also useful in non–small-cell carcinomas for the palliation of symptoms: pain, obstruction, atelectasis with pneumonitis, hemoptysis secondary to local erosive or infiltative disease, superior vena cava syndrome, brachial plexus symptoms, osseous or brain metastases. Radiotherapy is also effective in small-cell carcinoma in controlling local and regional disease and, when used in combination with multiagent chemotherapy, may accomplish long-term survivals in limited-stage small-cell carcinoma. As a result of the generally poor outcome of curative therapy of lung cancer, however, chemotherapy is often utilized.

With the exception of small-cell cancer of the lung, the results obtained to date with combined chemotherapy in lung cancer remain disappointing. Unlike the case of small-cell lung carcinoma, in which there is a definite improvement in the median survival, including a small fraction of patients with long-term remission (possibly even cures, as a result of treatment with chemotherapy), similar results have not been forthcoming in the treatment of non–small-cell carcinoma. In fact, the biology and natural history of these diseases are quite separate. For this reason, it has been the convention to group epidermoid, adenocarcinoma, and large-cell undifferentiated carcinoma together and to separate these histologies from small-cell anaplastic carcinoma (oat cell carcinoma).

1. Chemotherapeutic Agents Used

In recent years, multiple combination chemotherapy regimens have been studied for the treatment of non–small-cell lung carcinoma. Active agents include Adriamycin, bleomycin, cyclophosphamide, methotrexate, nitrosoureas, vinca alkaloids, hexamethylmelamine, procarbazine, *cis*-platinum, 5-fluorouracil (5-FU), and etoposide (VP-16). Most combinations have included two to five of the above agents, the intention being, whenever possible, to follow the general guidelines of combination chemotherapy: that is, to combine agents with convergent toxic effects on the tumor but divergent toxic effects on the host. Many of the agents listed above, when studied as single agents, have activities in the neighborhood of 10–20%. Unfortunately, a combination of two, three, or four agents, each with a relative response rate of 20%, has, to date, done little to further enhance the response rate. Furthermore, these agents have considerable toxicity.

The following combinations are some of the commonly used regimens:

MACC—methotrexate, Adriamycin, lomustine (CCNU), and cyclophosphamide

Methotrexate	30 mg/m^2, IV
Adriamycin	30 mg/m^2, IV
Cyclophosphamide	400 mg/m^2, IV
CCNU	30 mg/m^2, PO

All agents are administered together, one dose of each every 3–4 weeks.

FAM—5-FU, Adriamycin, and mitomycin-C

5-FU	600 mg/m^2, IV on days 1, 8, 29, and 36
Adriamycin	30 mg/m^2, IV on days 1 and 29
Mitomycin C	10 mg/m^2, IV on day 1 *only*

This cycle is repeated every 56 days.

Other combination programs in use include CAP (cyclophosphamide, Adriamycin, *cis*-platinum [DDP]) and CAMP (cyclophosphamide, Adriamycin, methotrexate, and procarbazine).

Chemotherapy for lung cancer, using single agents or combinations of drugs, may be continued until evidence of disease progression is objectively demonstrated. Patients may then be placed on alternate agents, or therapy may be discontinued.

2. Prognostic Factors

Nearly all human malignancies have prognostic factors that are useful to predict the clinical behavior of the disease. These include the performance status of the patient, the extent of the disease, the sites of involvement, the histology, the age of the patient, and the presence or absence of weight loss. Although many of these factors are interrelated, any analysis of treatment results and ultimate survival must include information pertaining to these prognostic factors. In patients with lung cancer, it has been shown that some prognostic factors are, by themselves, more important variables in the ultimate determination of the duration of survival than is any particular treatment applied to this disease.

a. Performance Status

The performance status is a measure of the patient's ability to ambulate and to care for him or herself. Numerous studies have amply documented the fact that patients whose performance status is normal, or close to normal, have a total survival of at least twice that of patient's who spend 50% of their day in bed. Consequently, any chemotherapy program applied to the former group is more likely to result in longer survival than any chemotherapy, efficacious or not, applied to the latter group.

b. Weight Loss

Closely allied to the performance status is the presence or absence of significant weight loss, i.e., weight loss greater than 10% of body weight. Patients who have no weight loss fare better than those who have minimal weight loss, and these fare better than those who have lost more than 10% of their body weight.

c. Extent of Disease

The conventional TNM classification system is not entirely satisfactory when analyzing patients with advanced disease. For instance, patients whose disease is limited to one hemithorax but is unresectable have Stage III disease; so do patients who have multiple metastases in visceral organs. The latter group of patients has a worse survival than the former group. It is, therefore, important, when judging any chemotherapy program, to have information as to the true extent of the disease.

d. Histology

Although claims have been made that one chemotherapy program or another is more active for a particular histological subtype within the general group of non–small-cell lung cancers, such differences have, to date, not been very relevant.

e. Combination of Prognostic Factors

Using a variety of models, it has been estimated that the median survival may vary between 6 and 70 weeks when three prognostic factors are considered together. For example, a group of patients with an initial performance status of 100, with no evidence of weight loss, and with disease limited to one hemithorax has a median survival in excess of 70 weeks. On the other hand, patients with a performance status of less than 50, more than 10% body weight loss, and extensive metastatic disease have a mediam survival of only 6 weeks.

3. Guidelines for Chemotherapy of Non–Oat Cell Cancer

It appears clear that major improvements in the treatment of lung cancer are not likely to be forthcoming unless new and effective agents are developed for the treatment of this disease. Research is hampered in trying to find novel combinations of agents because prior treatment with any chemotherapy will preclude the possibility of determining the efficacy of a new agent. As a result, many centers have adopted a policy of treating newly diagnosed Stage III patients with non–small-cell lung cancer with new agents as a first line of treatment; such an approach is justified when one considers that a drug such as *cis*-platinum was considgred to be inactive when it was tested in Phase II trials in previously treated patients but has been found to be an active agent in previously untreated patients. The same may be said for VP-16. Consequently, it is suggested that, whenever feasible, patients be entered on investigative protocol studies, whether these be in the nature of Phase II trials or Phase III combination chemotherapy regimens. The poor outlook for patients with advanced non–small-cell lung cancer makes an investigative approach ethically and therapeutically justified.

At present, due to the fact that no agent or combination of agents has been demonstrated to produce significant response rates, there is no clear indication for the use of chemotherapy as an adjuvant following the completion of definitive local therapy such as surgery or radiotherapy. If a new agent, or combination of agents, can be shown to have definite activity in prolonging the median survival of patients, when prognostic factors are taken into account, then it might be reasonable to consider such a combination of agents for use in an adjuvant setting. A controlled trial comparing local treatments against local treatments and chemotherapy would then have to be considered.

4. Treatment of Small-Cell Anaplastic Carcinoma of the Lung

In contrast to the lack of progress achieved in the treatment of non–small-cell carcinoma, the situation in small-cell carcinoma shows grounds for optimism. This disease, with less than a 2% 5-year survival rate and a mediam survival of less than 6 months in the prechemotherapy era, is now one in which significant palliation is currently achievable for the majority of patients and a long-term survival, possibly including occasional cure, is a real possibility for a minority of patients.

The list of active agents in this disease parallels the one given above for non–small-cell lung cancer. The response rates, however, in small-cell lung cancer tend to be double those of non–small-cell lung cancer. In addition, additive and possibly even synergistic effects are achievable with various combinations of agents. Most active regimens have combined an alkylating agent, usually cyclophosphamide, with Adriamycin and a vinca alkaloid. More recent combinations have, in addition, included agents such as *cis*-platinum, VP-16, mitomycin, hexamethylmelamine, methotrexate, and nitrosoureas. Most recent studies of active combinations show a response rate

between 60 and 90% and a complete response rate of between 15 and 30%.

In this disease, as in any other, the role of prognostic factors must be borne in mind. It has been conventional to divide small-cell lung cancer for the purposes of chemotherapy studies into "localized" versus "extensive" disease. Although it is assumed that virtually all patients have early dissemination of their disease, the outlook for patients with *apparently* localized disease appears to be better than that for patients with obvious extensive disease.

a. Localized Disease

In general, the treatment of "localized" oat-cell carcinoma (Stages I and II) has employed combination chemotherapy with radiotherapy. Most studies today employ combination chemotherapy as first-line treatment in order to establish a rapid tumor reduction and control micrometastases; following several courses of chemotherapy, most patients are referred for radiation therapy to the primary site and, prophylactically, to the brain. Upon completion of radiation therapy and depending on the tolerance of the host, chemotherapy is resumed. If remission is achieved, particularly if complete remission ensues, therapy is continued for anywhere from 1 to 2 years after such remission. In general, complete and partial response rates utilizing such an approach may be expected to reach as high as 80% of patients so treated; between 15 and 35% of these patients will still be alive at the end of a year, and many of them will have a prolonged disease-free survival. It is an interesting and as yet an unexplained observation that women have a higher likelihood of entering a complete remission than men.

Among the problems still to be elucidated are the following:

- The optimum chemotherapy regimen(s).
- The best mode of interdigitation of chemotherapy with radiation therapy. In fact, although many patients will achieve an apparent complete remission, a significant fraction of these will have their first recurrence in the primary site; such an event is taken as a justification for the early use of radiation therapy to the primary site. However, in order to achieve adequate doses of radiotherapy in the tumor bed, a significant hiatus must be taken from the chemotherapy program; such an approach may allow the disseminated metastases to reactivate. In addition, the enhanced toxicity of combining radiation therapy and chemotherapy is rather significant. Several modern studies are attempting to give radiation therapy and chemotherapy simultaneously; although it may eventually be shown that such an approach improves the remission rate, it certainly augments the toxicities, and it remains to be seen if it is justifiable.
- The length of chemotherapy. At present, it is not known how long one should give chemotherapy for those patients who achieve complete remission.

Thus, many unresolved questions remain, and it is clear that further studies of this disease are absolutely essential. The recommendations contained in these guidelines are such that, if a properly controlled clinical protocol study of oat-cell carcinoma is available in the institution, physicians are urged to consider their patients for entry into such protocols.

b. Extensive Disease

Extensive disease is defined as those patients who have demonstrable metastases outside of one hemithorax. The outlook for complete remission in this group of patients is not as good as in the group with localized disease; nevertheless, the principles of chemotherapy treatment are similar, and significant palliation is achievable, even in patients with far-advanced disease. Complete remission may be seen in 10% of patients. A number of questions remain as yet unresolved in this category and include the following:

- Optimum chemotherapy regimens and optimum treatment time. It is recommended that a minimum of six cycles of combination chemotherapy be used before abandoning treatment, and if a response is noted, treatment should be continued for at least 1 year.
- The use of combination chemotherapy and radiation therapy. Because these patients have widely disseminated disease and because they are more likely to succumb to these metastases than to central nervous system metastases, prophylactic radiation therapy to the whole brain is not warranted. However, for patients who achieve a remission, it is entirely reasonable to consider prophylactic whole-brain irradiation, as a significant number of them will relapse primarily in the CNS.
- At present, there is no resolution regarding the advisability of radiation therapy to the primary site and, if it is indicated, when such therapy should be given. Because these patients tend to relapse in multiple metastatic sites, control of the primary is of subsidiary importance. However, as for CNS radiation therapy, similar arguments apply with respect to patients who achieve complete remission. They may well be candidates for "adjuvant" radiation therapy to the primary site.

c. Superior Vena Cava Syndrome

Radiation therapy has traditionally been the first line of therapy in patients with superior vena cava (SVC) syndrome. However, because of the high response rate seen in oat cell carcinoma of the lung treated by chemotherapy and the consistency with which responses are seen, the presence of SVC syndrome is not a contraindication to combination chemotherapy. In fact, most patients with SVC syndrome caused by oat cell carcinomas—in contrast to that seen in patients with non–oat cell carcinoma—are manageable with prompt institution of combination chemotherapy. Because a large fraction of such patients have widely disseminated metastatic disease, it is rea-

sonable to consider combination chemotherapy instead of radiation therapy for this group of patients.

D. Management of Metastatic Lung Cancer

Primary malignant tumors originating in any organ in the body are capable of causing metastatic spread to the lung. Those lesions most often responsible for pulmonary metastases are

- Breast carcinoma.
- Soft-tissue and osteogenic sarcomas.
- Renal cell carcinoma.
- Colon carcinoma.
- Uterine carcinoma.
- Testicular or extratesticular gonadal carcinomas.

Traditionally, the presence of pulmonary metastases precludes any attempt at curative therapy. Radiotherapy may be used if the primary tumor is radiosensitive and if the area of lung involved is small enough, but is only rarely beneficial. Metastases from primaries of epithelial origin (squamous cell carcinoma or adenocarcinoma) and those from the more sensitive lesions (e.g., seminomas) respond well to adequate doses (6000 rads). Pulmonary fibrosis will almost always develop in the area irradiated, which, therefore, must be kept to a small size. Chemotherapy is advisable if the patient is in a reasonable general state of health and particularly if the primary tumor is responsive to chemotherapy (e.g., gonadal tumors, breast cancer).

More recently, an aggressive surgical approach has evolved in the treatment of the patient with pulmonary metastases, and preliminary reports tend to indicate an increased salvage rate in highly selected cases of certain types of primary tumors. The results of surgery in the treatment of pulmonary metastases as reported in the literature are significant when the case selection is highly discriminating.

1. Selection of Patients for Surgery

The following criteria are mandatory in order to consider a patient a reasonable candidate for resection of a metastatic tumor in the lung:

- Long disease-free interval between the treatment of the primary and the development of the metastases.
- Solitary metastasis or multiple adjacent lesions limited to one lung. In the case of a solitary lesion, it is often not possible to rule out a second primary in the lung, and surgery, therefore, becomes almost mandatory.
- Disease at the primary site must be controlled.

- No other distant metastases are identified.
- Satisfactory general condition and good surgical risk.

2. Preoperative Evaluation

- A complete physical evaluation, cardiopulmonary, nutritional, hematologic, etc. must be done.
- Metastatic work-up including liver and bone scans.
- Evaluation of the lung
  - Chest x-ray. The least sensitive of all tests but carries a low false positive index (10%).
  - Tomograms. Significantly more accurate in identifying multiple lesions. False positive findings, however, are significant.
  - CAT scan of the lungs. The most sensitive of all the studies, identifying over half of the total number of nodules found at surgery. The false positive rate, however, is high.

3. Surgical Treatment

a. Operative Approach

A median sternotomy is indicated in most cases to examine both lungs thoroughly. A posterolateral thoracotomy should only be done if there is absolutely no question as to the unilaterality of the pulmonary metastases.

b. Technique

The most desirable procedure is a lung-sparing operation, if possible, wedge resection or segmental resection. A lobectomy may be done if necessary but only when the patient is in condition to tolerate the procedure; the patient should be otherwise free of disease and maintaining a stable weight. Subsequent rehabilitation in terms of the quality of life is necessary. Pneumonectomy is rarely, if ever, indicated for pulmonary metastatic disease.

c. Operative Risk

An overall mortality rate of 1% or slightly over may be anticipated, with a morbidity in the range of 10% in terms of the usual complications.

V. POSTOPERATIVE CARE, EVALUATION, AND REHABILITATION

A. Postoperative Care

A postoperative chest x-ray before leaving the operating room is recommended to determine whether the position of the chest tube is adequate and to confirm full reexpansion of the remaining lung tissue as well as the status of the contralateral lung. These x-rays are repeated daily until all chest drains have been removed.

Until consciousness is regained, the primary consideration is the maintenance of an adequate airway, and vital signs must be carefully monitored. The pleurovacs, if employed, should stay well below the level of the chest. The patient should be maintained flat with the head slightly raised and turned frequently: side–back–side. Intravenous fluids and transfusions should be administered as needed to avoid overhydration and pulmonary edema.

The respiratory status of the patient should be frequently assessed. The rate of respiration, tidal volume, and gas exchange must be recorded, and arterial blood gas determinations must be carried out as often as necessary. The patient should be encouraged to cough and practice deep breathing; thoracic incisions are painful, and frequently patients will splint and not allow for full inspiratory excursion of the affected side. This leads to atelectasis and retained secretions; vigorous suctioning and adequate analgesia help prevent these problems. It is also useful, at times, to block the intercostal nerves with long-acting local anesthetics at the end of the surgical procedure. If these measures fail to expand the lung fully, bedside bronchoscopy can be extremely helpful in resolving atelectatic changes postoperatively and establishing full expansion of the lungs.

The patient should be mobilized and out of bed the day following surgery. This helps clearing of bronchial secretions and aids in the stabilization of the altered pulmonary circulation, thus avoiding hypostatic pneumonia and thromboembolism.

If there is an indwelling chest tube for postoperative drainage, the quantity and quality of the drainage should be determined hourly. Hemorrhage is a complication that may occur after thoracic surgical procedures, it should be identified early and dealt with aggressively; drainage of more than 100 cc per hour of blood via the chest tube for several hours is considered a hemorrhage and requires reexploration of the patient and ligation of the source of bleeding. The intercostal arteries are often identified as the source of such postthoracotomy bleeding. The chest tube is removed when it stops tidaling, drainage is less than 50–75 cc per 24 hours, and the lung is reexpanded without fluid collections. It is desirable to clamp the last tube for 24 hours prior to removing it in order to make sure that there is no air leak and that the lung remains expanded.

In the case of a pneumonectomy, usually no chest tube is used; the empty hemithorax fills with blood and serous fluid. This will eventually organize and fibrose, which is the desired outcome since it stabilizes the chest and prevents mediastinal shift on hyperinflation of the remaining lung. There is, however, a definite danger of mediastinal shift or even herniation toward the resected side in the immediate postoperative period. Frequent physical examination, chest x-rays, and close follow-up are necessary to prevent these potentially fatal complications.

Wound infections and infections of the pleural space are serious complications of chest surgery, and every effort should be made to prevent them. The use of a broad-spectrum antibiotic postoperatively is desirable. If wound infection does occur, it should be laid open and treated vigorously with local irrigation and frequent dressing changes. Acute empyema should be aspirated after localization by fluoroscopy, and open drainage with rib resection is only instituted after the presence of frank pus has been established and more conservative forms of therapy have failed.

Sound wound healing must be achieved before permitting the use of adjunctive postoperative radiotherapy or chemotherapy; this will usually require about 2 weeks.

B. Rehabilitation

Rehabilitation of the patient after resection of a malignant pulmonary tumor has two objectives:

- A concerted effort by the physician and the family has to be made to help the patient accept the diagnosis of a malignancy and its threat to long-term survival.
- The patient should be kept in the best possible physical condition for as long as possible to enjoy a reasonable quality of life.

1. Psychosocial Support

It must be stressed that the management of psychosocial issues in relation to carcinoma of the lung demands coordination of an interdisciplinary team. Many patients and their families still associate cancer with disfigurement, pain, suffering, hopelessness, and death. These attitudes must be taken into consideration before intervention takes place. Other threats include expenses, loss of work and family roles, changes in bodily functions or appearances, and prolonged disability.

A major factor in the etiology of lung cancer (in 80% of cases) is cigarette smoking. The risk is more pronounced for persons who begin smoking in their teens, who inhale deeply, and who smoke half a pack or more a day. It is essential that the health professional caring for the patient be aware of the potential for feelings of guilt. The patient may feel that he or she has played a major role in the development of the cancer and that if he or she had never started smoking, or had quit sooner, the disease would not have occurred. The patient should be encouraged to stop smoking, but a nonjudgmental attitude should be maintained by the caring professional. The importance of cessation of smoking is supported by the high

incidence of second primaries in other sites of the aerodigestive tract that are noted in long-term survivors from the first pulmonary tumor (15%). It would also be helpful both physically and psychologically if the immediate cohabitants of the patients were also to stop smoking.

2. Physical Rehabilitation

The following problems should be addressed in the care of the patient with lung cancer:

a. Decreased Activity Tolerance

This is due to the limited lung reserve that results from the surgery or the disease process. The goal of rehabilitation here would be the resumption of activities within the patient's physical limitations. The patient should be encouraged to conserve energy whenever possible and to increase activity gradually, as tolerated. One must evaluate the need for oxygen and refer the patient to a chest physical therapist and/or occupational therapist, if needed.

b. Shoulder Dysfunction Due to Surgery

The maximum range of motion and function should be restored, and preoperative posture should be encouraged. The surgeon must provide referral to the physical therapist and reinforce the information given about range-of-motion exercises.

c. Atelectasis Due to Disease Process

Maximum ventilation of the remaining lung tissue must be achieved. Prevention and treatment of this condition is of great importance to obtain optimum rehabilitation. The patient should be encouraged to report untoward signs and symptoms promptly to his or her physician. Referral for chest physical therapy should be made early, and a structured program of appropriate exercises to support the patient should be instituted.

d. Decreased Cardiopulmonary Reserve

A carefully designed program of active cardiopulmonary rehabilitation to increase the patient's functional capacity should be instituted whenever possible. This program should include general exercises, to improve muscular tone and an overall sense of fitness, as well as pulmonary physiotherapy; it should be regulated by a trained physiotherapist.

e. Failure of Nutritional State

A diet rich in protein and caloric content helps the patient withstand the rigors of adjuvant therapy and keeps him or her

Table I

Long-Term Follow-Up Schedule for Lung Cancer

Management	First three months			First and second year				Third year and thereafter	
	1 month	2 months	3 months	3 months	6 months	9 months	12 months	6 months	12 months
History									
Cough and sputum	X	X	X	X	X	X	X	X	X
Weight loss	X	X	X	X	X	X	X	X	X
Hemoptysis	X	X	X	X	X	X	X	X	X
Pain	X	X	X	X	X	X	X	X	X
Dyspnea	X	X	X	X	X	X	X	X	X
Temperature	X	X	X	X	X	X	X	X	X
Other (update on general history)					X		X	X	X
Physical									
Complete physical examination			X		X		X		X
Examination of head and neck			X	X	X	X	X	X	X
Chest exam	X	X	X	X	X	X	X	X	X
Investigation									
CBC, SMA-12			X		X		X		X
Chest x-ray			X		X		X	X	X
Tomograms or CAT of chest					As indicated				
Liver scan					As indicated				
Bone scan					As indicated				
Brain scan					As indicated				
Bronchoscopy					As indicated				

in a positive nitrogen balance; this should be developed early with the help of a dietician.

f. Infection Due to the Treatment or Disease Process

Prevention and control of infection is extremely important. The patient should be encouraged to report signs and symptoms of upper respiratory infections and to continue chest physical therapy.

g. Smoking

An attempt to discourage smoking must be pursued.

C. Follow-Up Evaluation

Table I is the recommended schedule for follow-up evaluation necessary to care for the patient properly following therapy for lung cancer.

VI. MANAGEMENT ALGORITHM FOR CHEST TUMORS (see p. 440)

ALGORITHM FOR CHEST TUMORS

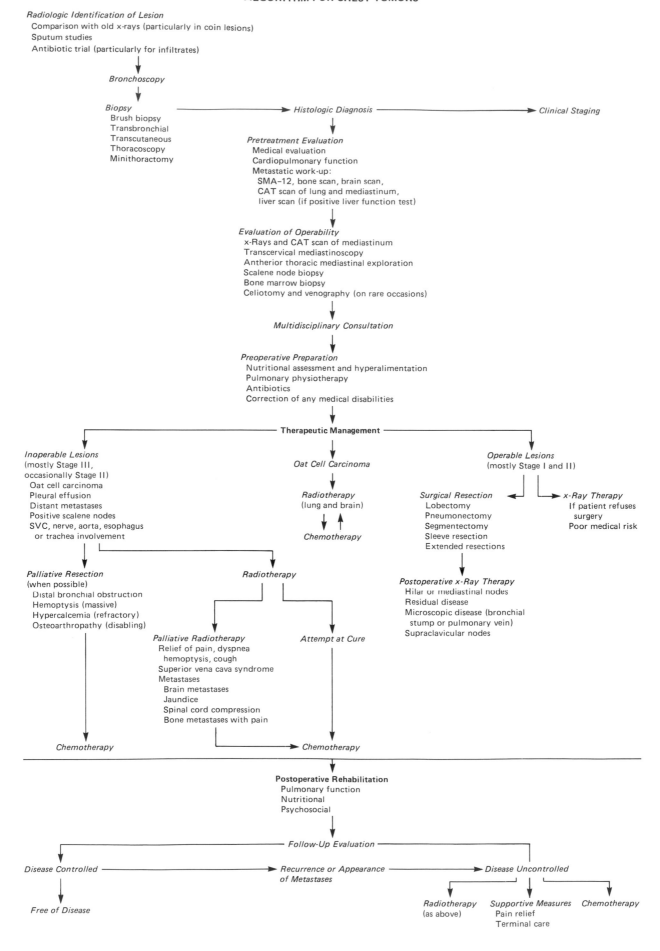

Radiologic Identification of Lesion
Comparison with old x-rays (particularly in coin lesions)
Sputum studies
Antibiotic trial (particularly for infiltrates)

Bronchoscopy

Biopsy
Brush biopsy
Transbronchial
Transcutaneous
Thoracoscopy
Minithoractomy

Histologic Diagnosis

Clinical Staging

Pretreatment Evaluation
Medical evaluation
Cardiopulmonary function
Metastatic work-up:
SMA–12, bone scan, brain scan,
CAT scan of lung and mediastinum,
liver scan (if positive liver function test)

Evaluation of Operability
x-Rays and CAT scan of mediastinum
Transcervical mediastinoscopy
Antherior thoracic mediastinal exploration
Scalene node biopsy
Bone marrow biopsy
Celiotomy and venography (on rare occasions)

Multidisciplinary Consultation

Preoperative Preparation
Nutritional assessment and hyperalimentation
Pulmonary physiotherapy
Antibiotics
Correction of any medical disabilities

Therapeutic Management

Inoperable Lesions
(mostly Stage III,
occasionally Stage II)
Oat cell carcinoma
Pleural effusion
Distant metastases
Positive scalene nodes
SVC, nerve, aorta, esophagus
or trachea involvement

Oat Cell Carcinoma

Radiotherapy
(lung and brain)

Chemotherapy

Operable Lesions
(mostly Stage I and II)

Surgical Resection
Lobectomy
Pneumonectomy
Segmentectomy
Sleeve resection
Extended resections

x-Ray Therapy
If patient refuses
surgery
Poor medical risk

Palliative Resection
(when possible)
Distal bronchial obstruction
Hemoptysis (massive)
Hypercalcemia (refractory)
Osteoarthropathy (disabling)

Radiotherapy

Postoperative x-Ray Therapy
Hilar or mediastinal nodes
Residual disease
Microscopic disease (bronchial
stump or pulmonary vein)
Supraclavicular nodes

Palliative Radiotherapy
Relief of pain, dyspnea
hemoptysis, cough
Superior vena cava syndrome
Metastases
Brain metastases
Jaundice
Spinal cord compression
Bone metastases with pain

Attempt at Cure

Chemotherapy

Chemotherapy

Postoperative Rehabilitation
Pulmonary function
Nutritional
Psychosocial

Follow-Up Evaluation

Disease Controlled

*Recurrence or Appearance
of Metastases*

Disease Uncontrolled

Free of Disease

Radiotherapy
(as above)

Supportive Measures
Pain relief
Terminal care

Chemotherapy

Section 10. Chest Tumors
Part B: Tumors of the Mediastinum

I. General Considerations 443
  A. Epidemiology
  B. Pathological Considerations
    1. Neurogenic Tumors
    2. Teratodermoids
    3. Thymomas
    4. Lymphomas
    5. Mediastinal Cysts
      a. Pericardial Cysts
      b. Bronchogenic Cysts
      c. Enteric Cysts
    6. Mesenchymal Tumors
    7. Carcinoma
    8. Miscellaneous Tumors
      a. Thyroid Lesions
      b Parathyroid Adenomas
      c. Germ Cell Tumors
      d. Other Rare Mediastinal Tumors
II. Early Detection and Screening 445
III. Pretreatment Evaluation and Work-Up 446
  A. Radiological Evaluation
    1. Routine Studies
    2. Barium Swallow
    3. Ultrasound
    4. Computerized Axial Tomography
    5. Radioisotope Scans
    6. Special Procedures
      a. Pneumomediastinum
      b. Angiocardiography
  B. Laboratory Findings
  C. Biopsy
  D. General Evaluation of the Patient
IV. Therapeutic Management 447
  A. Surgery
  B. Radiotherapy
    1. Thymomas
    2. Germ Cell Tumors
    3. Neuroblastomas
    4. Lymphomas
  C. Chemotherapy
    1. Thymomas
    2. Germ Cell Tumors
      a. Nonseminomatous Germ Cell Tumors
      b. Mediastinal Seminomas
  D. Management of SVC Syndrome
    1. Cause of SVC Syndrome
    2. Evaluation of the Patient
    3. Management

I. GENERAL CONSIDERATIONS

A. Epidemiology

The mediastinum, defined as the space between both lungs in the thoracic cavity, contains a large number of anatomic structures and organs. A variety of neoplasms occur within the mediastinum and are being recognized with increasing frequency. There are several tumorlike lesions that simulate neoplasia (e.g., cysts) and a large number of benign and primary malignant tumors. In addition, metastases from malignant tumors in other areas of the body may also present in the mediastinum and in the mediastinal nodes. An orderly evaluation is thus essential to try and establish a reasonable differential diagnosis of a mass lesion within the mediastinum. Many mediastinal tumors are highly curable in their early stages, and it is, therefore, imperative to establish an early diagnosis as often as possible and institute appropriate therapeutic measures to achieve the highest cure rates.

The incidence, as well as the location, of the more common primary mediastinal tumors are listed in Table I. Metastatic tumors, however, are considerably more common in the mediastinum than are primary tumors.

Other tumors, which occur less frequently, include thyroid or parathyroid masses in the superior mediastinum. Hiatus hernias at the esophageal hiatus in the posterior mediastinum or, more rarely, in the subcostosternal or retrosternal space, when they are congenital in nature, may simulate a mediastinal tumor. Likewise, eventration of the diaphragm, traumatic perforation, and tumors of the diaphragm may present as mediastinal tumors; these are easy to differentiate and will not be considered in this section.

B. Pathological Considerations

1. Neurogenic Tumors

Neurogenic tumors constitute the most common mediastinal tumor. They occur at any age but are more likely to be malignant in children. Classically, they are found in the posterior mediastinum along the paravertebral gutter, and they usually arise either from the intercostal nerves or the dorsal sympathetic chain.

Most neurogenic tumors produce no symptoms. When symptomatic, the clinical picture will be related to either pressure by the tumor or humoral factors. For example, ganglioneuromas and neuroblastomas may give rise to a picture of abdominal distention and diarrhea or to one of hypertension, troublesome sweating and flushing, and an elevation of the urinary vanillylmandelic acid (VMA).

The majority of neurogenic tumors are benign; only the neuroblastomas and the rarer sarcomatous variant of the usually benign neurogenic tumors are truly malignant. The following are the primary neurogenic tumors presenting in the mediastinum:

- *Neurofibromas.* Arising from the nerve sheaths and fibers, these lesions may be solitary or present as part of generalized von Recklinghausen's disease.
- *Neurilemmomas.* Arising from the Schwann cells of the nerve sheath, these are usually benign lesions that rarely change into neurosarcomas, the malignant counterpart of neurilemmomas.
- *Ganglioneuromas.* Constituting the most frequent neurogenic tumors in children, these arise from the sympathetic chain and are invariably found in the posterior mediastinum. These lesions are usually benign, though a rare case of ganglioneurosarcoma can be seen.
- *Neuroblastomas.* A common tumor in children, these are more often found in the retroperitoneal area than in the

Table I

Incidence and Location of Common Primary Mediastinal Tumors

Tumor	Incidence (%)	Location
Neurogenic tumors	25	Posterior mediastinum
Cysts (enteric, pericardial, bronchogenic)	20	Middle mediastinum
Teratomas or dermoids	17	Anterior mediastinum
Lymphomas	13	Anterior mediastinum
Thymomas	12	Superior mediastinum

mediastinum. This tumor is extremely aggressive and may occur at any level of the sympathetic nervous system (see § 8A.VI.B, Vol. 2).

- *Paragangliomas and Pheochromocytomas.* Tumors that originate from the sympathetic nervous system and may occur in the mediastinum, many of them are chromaffin positive and can secrete epinephrine and/or norepinephrine.
- *Meningoceles.* Saccular protrusions of the dural sac through a normal or enlarged intervertebral foramen, projecting as a paravertebral mass into the thoracic cavity, these lesions are usually asymptomatic, only identified by serendipity during a chest x-ray, and are extremely rare.
- *Chemodectomas.* Tumors of the chemoreceptor organs found in the vicinity of the aortic arch, similar to the carotid body tumors in the neck, they are composed of neuroepithelium, which probably arises from vagus nerve fibers. Though usually asymptomatic, their location in the superior mediastinum poses a threat if they achieve a large size, resulting in a SVC syndrome. Resection of these lesions is extremely difficult because of their extremely vascular nature and their proximity to the great vessels.

A diagnosis of neurogenic tumor of the mediastinum is often simple; the precise histological nature of the tumor, however, can only be determined at surgery and often requires study of its standard and ultrastructural morphology.

2. Teratodermoids

A *teratoma* is a tumor composed of multiple histological tissue types foreign to the area in which the tumor is found. The tumor is usually located in the anterior mediastinum, though it has been described on rare occasions in the posterior mediastinum; it may be solid or cystic and ordinarily contains microscopic evidence of endoderm, mesoderm, and ectoderm in varying amounts. It is not unusual to identify hair or teeth within the tumor. Teratomas in the mediastinum are usually benign, though malignant aggressive variants are seen, where one element of the teratoma acquires invasive characteristics.

Teratomas may, with catastrophic results, rupture into the pericardial sac, the pleural cavity, and/or one of the major vessels.

3. Thymomas

Thymoma, a common mediastinal tumor, usually presents in adults and is located in the anterior superior mediastinum, though on occasion it has been reported in the posterior mediastinum. The relationship of this tumor to myasthenia gravis and other autoimmune diseases is well known:

- Patients with thymomas have a 10–15% incidence of having myasthenia gravis.

- Patients with myasthenia have an 8–15% incidence of thymomas, and the incidence of thymomas in myasthenics undergoing thymectomy is in excess of 20% (in comparison to an incidence of 1 in 2000 in the population at large).

Tumors of the thymus may be cystic, benign, or malignant thymomas. Histologically, it is almost impossible to distinguish the benign from the malignant thymoma; the distinction must be made at the time of surgery and is based on the gross characteristics of the tumor and its local invasiveness as demonstrated by infiltration of the adjacent tissues: lung, pericardium, blood vessels, etc. Distant metastases are rare.

4. Lymphomas

Lymphoma may present as a primary lesion in the mediastinum without evidence of its presence in any other part of the body, or as part of a disseminated lymphoma. Histologically, the disease may assume the form of any one of the Hodgkin's (the most common type) or non-Hodgkin's lymphomas. These tumors are characteristically found in the anterior mediastinum but may involve lymph nodes elsewhere, especially around the bronchi.

5. Mediastinal Cysts

These cysts represent a significant percentage of mediastinal masses and must be considered in any differential diagnosis. Cysts may arise from the pericardium, bronchial epithelium, trachea, esophagus, and/or thymus.

a. Pericardial Cysts

These cysts are common mediastinal lesions that occur in the cardiophrenic angles, especially on the right side. They usually have a characteristic x-ray appearance and are ordinarily benign, rarely causing symptoms.

b. Bronchogenic Cysts

These cysts are lined by respiratory epithelium and rarely communicate with the bronchial lumen. They usually arise in close proximity to the main-stem bronchi, most commonly posterior to the carina. They are benign but often symptomatic; dough, dyspnea, and respiratory stridor are common.

c. Enteric Cysts

These cysts originate from the dorsal division of the foregut and arise along the course of the esophagus. They are lined with gastric or intestinal mucosa and tend to be attached to the wall of the esophagus; sometimes, they are completely embedded within the muscular layer of the esophagus.

Enteric cysts may present with pressure symptoms on the

esophagus; in addition, since they are lined by gastric mucosa, acid secretion and peptic ulceration is a common complication, with perforation and/or bleeding within the cyst. Enteric cysts are occasionally associated with vertebral anomalies, with occasional attachment of the cyst to the meninges or spinal cord by a tract containing neural elements. A myelogram may show this tract to be patent and communicate with the spinal cord. Dumbbell enteric cysts may also occur in the posterior mediastinum and extend below the diaphragm to involve both the thoracic and abdominal cavities.

6. Mesenchymal Tumors

These tumors account for about 5% of mediastinal tumors. They affect both sexes equally and involve virtually all age groups. Over 50% of these tumors found at surgery are malignant, and there is a higher incidence of malignancy in children under 15 years of age. Tumor size varies widely, though size does not correlate with malignancy. The presence of symptoms due to pressure, on the other hand, usually indicates a malignant mesenchymal tumor (liposarcomas, fibrosarcomas, etc.), which is almost universally fatal.

7. Carcinoma

Carcinoma arising within the mediastinum with the absence of any other primary source has been reported to account for 3–11% of primary mediastinal tumors. The origin of these carcinomas is unclear, although they seem to occur more frequently in male smokers and are squamous cell carcinomas; the primary point of origin may, therefore, be within the lung. It is also possible that these carcinomas may arise in preexisting benign epithelial cysts. The prognosis of epidermoid carcinoma of the mediastinum is very poor, and the disease progresses very rapidly.

8. Miscellaneous Tumors

a. Thyroid Lesions

Substernal goiters are quite common and usually are quite apparent on physical examination of the neck where an enlarged palpable thyroid can often be identified. Occasionally, there is no enlargement of the gland in the neck, and a substernal thyroid is found entirely within the superior mediastinum. The diagnosis, however, is easy to make by routine chest x-ray and thyroid scan. Rarely, an abberrant thyroid has been reported as a solitary mass in the posterior mediastinum; these lesions are more difficult to diagnose.

b. Parathyroid Adenomas

Parathyroid adenomas are usually found in the anterior and superior mediastinum, where they are frequently embedded within the thymus. These adenomas are usually benign and have hormonal activity resulting in hyperparathyroidism. Very rarely have there been reports of a functioning parathyroid cyst or a carcinoma of the parathyroid gland in the mediastinum.

c. Germ Cell Tumors

Primary mediastinal tumors of germ cell origin are not uncommon, particularly in the young adult; they are usually found in the anterior mediastinum. They may be seminomatous, nonseminomatous (embryonal or choriocarcinomic), or mixed tumors, and they have all the characteristics of their testicular counterpart, though they seem to be more aggressive in their behavior. Germ cell tumors are notable by their production of specific marker proteins: alphafetoproteins (AFPs) in the case of embryonal carcinomas and human chorionic gonadotrophin (HCG) in the case of the choriocarcinomas. These serum markers are easily identifiable and can be of great help in establishig the diagnosis preoperatively, in assessing the effect of therapy, and in evaluating the patient after treatment to identify early recurrences of the disease.

d. Other Rare Mediastinal Tumors

A variety of rare neoplasms are found in the mediastinum; they include lipomas, xanthomas, and mesotheliomas. These diagnoses are usually established after exploratory surgery or postmortem examination.

II. EARLY DETECTION AND SCREENING

Screening for mediastinal tumors is neither practical nor possible because of the relative rarity of these lesions and the wide variation of pathology, none with identifiable high-risk populations, predisposing factors, or any common denominator besides the presence of a mass.

Routine chest x-rays obtained on a yearly basis as discussed in § 10A.I.B.2, are the only possible means of identifying an asymptomatic mediastinal mass. The majority of mediastinal tumors, however, present in the younger population, a group not ordinarily subjected to routine chest roentgenograms.

The alertness of the physician in recognizing the early signs and symptoms of a mediastinal mass and the education of the primary care physician and the population at large are the only avenues available to achieve early detection in this group of tumors.

The symptoms and signs of mediastinal masses vary widely from no signs at all to very ominous presentations that have been recognized as specific syndromes associated with mediastinal tumors (e.g., SVC syndrome). Less than one-third of all patients with a mediastinal mass will be totally asymptomatic, and the mass will be found on a routine chest x-ray; more than two-thirds of patients will have some symptoms. The most common early symptoms are

- Chest pain.
- Nonspecific malaise, weight loss, fatigue.
- Fever or night sweats.
- Cough.
- Dyspnea.

These symptoms are often associated with malignant tumors, yet they are often ignored for long periods of time because of their apparent insignificance. More severe symptoms are caused by nerve invasion, compression, or evidence of major vena cava pressure and obstruction. These symptoms might include

- Back pain.
- Hoarseness or Horner's syndrome.
- Superior vena cava obstruction syndromes.
- Spinal cord compression with various neurological symptoms.
- Chylothorax or pleural effusion.

These findings are usually indicative of aggressive malignant tumors and are usually evidence of advanced disease.

Mediastinal tumors are, in addition, often associated with various specific syndromes that must alert the physician to the presence of a tumor:

- Intermittent fever (Pel-Ebstein fever), characteristic of Hodgkin's disease.
- Hypertrophic osteoarthropathy, commonly seen in association with neurogenic tumors and lung cancer.
- Hypertension and diarrhea or flushing and intensive sweating may occur with mediastinal pheochromocytomas or ganglioneuromas.
- Myasthenia gravis, hypogammaglobulinemia, Cushing's disease, Whipple's disease, and red blood cell aplasias have all been reported to be associated with thymomas.
- Von Recklinghausen's disease may be associated with mediastinal neurofibromas.
- Enteric cysts are often found in association with vertebral anomalies.

Screening of selected groups of patients with some of the above syndromes is desirable, specifically in cases of myasthenia gravis, hypertension, or carcinoid syndrome patients.

III. PRETREATMENT EVALUATION AND WORK-UP

Though most mediastinal tumors will require surgical exploration at some point, almost all are definable preoperatively, and most may be diagnosed with accuracy prior to surgery. A good history might reveal one or more of the symptoms described in the preceding sections; the physical examination rarely offers any significant information; and the main evaluation is actually radiological.

A. Radiological Evaluation

1. Routine Studies

A good-quality anteroposterior, lateral, and oblique view of the chest will show the shape, size, and density of the lesion as well as its relationship to the adjacent structures. The location of the lesion will already direct the physician toward the most likely diagnosis:

- Posterior masses → neurogenic tumors.
- Anterior masses → teratomas, lymphomas, or dysgerminomas.
- Middle mediastinal masses → cysts.
- Superior mediastinal mass → goiters or thymomas.

Tomography and fluoroscopy might further aid in identifying the location and relationship of the tumor.

2. Barium Swallow

This is sometimes useful in supplementing the information obtained from the chest roentgenograms.

3. Ultrasound

Sonography is an extremely useful diagnostic modality for mediastinal tumors, particularly in the differentiation of cystic versus solid tumors. It has recently been largely supplanted by the CAT scan.

4. Computerized Axial Tomography

The CAT scan, used with or without contrast enhancement techniques, has today replaced most other diagnostic imaging procedures for mediastinal lesions. It can give an excellent anatomic definition of the tumor, its location, size, density, infiltration, and involvement of adjacent structures. The CAT scan will also identify metastatic nodes and/or pulmonary metastases.

5. Radioisotope Scans

These may be useful to identify substernal thyroid glands (^{131}I), thymomas (radioactive selenium), and rarely, parathyroid tumors (radioactive selenium). They can also identify the presence of a SVC obstruction (SVC scan).

6. Special Procedures

a. Pneumomediastinum

This procedure is only of historical interest. It has been completely replaced by the CAT scan.

b. Angiocardiography

This is useful in the diagnosis of aneurysms or vascular malformations.

B. Laboratory Findings

In certain selected cases, specific laboratory tests may confirm a suspected diagnosis. This is particularly true in patients with endocrine-producing tumors or those that produce specific markers:

- Thyroid profile studies or serum calcitonin in suspected substernal thyroid masses.
- Serum calcium and phosphorus and parathyroid hormone assays (sometimes with selective venous catheterization) in parathyroid tumors.
- Urinary catecholamines and VMA for suspected pheochromocytoma.
- Alpha-fetoproteins for embryonal carcinomas or human chorionic gonadotrophins for choriocarcinoma.
- Myasthenia gravis studies in case of suspected thymomas.

C. Biopsy

A definitive tissue diagnosis is not always available prior to thoracotomy, but it is extremely desirable in order better to plan and coordinate a multidisciplinary attack on the disease from the outset. Several procedures are available to obtain tissue specimens. These have been described at length in § 10A.II.B.2 and include the following:

- Transcutaneous fluoroscopically guided needle aspiration biopsy or needle biopsy with CAT scan control.
- Mediastinoscopy (transcervical, or TCM).
- Anterior exploration of the mediastinum (ATME).
- Exploratory thoracotomy or minithoracotomy.

It must be pointed out that bleeding is a dreaded complication of mediastinal biopsies, particularly when they are closed biopsies (e.g., needle biopsy); aneurysms must be ruled out first, and care must be taken not to enter the major vessels. The surgeon must be prepared to operate following the biopsy.

D. General Evaluation of the Patient

Evaluation here is identical to that of patients with pulmonary tumors. The general medical status must be assessed, and pulmonary function tests, measurement of blood gases at rest and following exercises, evaluation of coagulation factors, nutritional assessment, and metastatic work-up must all be carried out. Any deficiency must then be corrected preoperatively. In addition, patients must be evaluated from a neurological and endocrinologic standpoint when there is the possibility of the presence of an endocrine or neurological tumor.

IV. THERAPEUTIC MANAGEMENT

A. Surgery

Surgery is the primary treatment of all primary mediastinal tumors, with the exception of lymphomas and germ cell tumors, once the diagnosis is established. In most instances, a precise histological diagnosis is not established before surgery, although a reasonably accurate impression may exist as to the nature of the tumor, its exact location, and its extent. Thoracotomy is thus usually indicated for both diagnosis and definitive management.

Exposure is gained by one of several approaches, depending on the location of the tumor. The incision should be planned after careful review of the chest x-ray, CAT scan, or angiogram: for anterior and middle mediastinal tumors, sternotomy or lateral thoracotomy if the tumor projects to one side or the other; for posterior mediastinal tumors, appropriate posterolateral thoracotomy. An attempt should be made to resect all tumors, benign or malignant, with the exception of lymphomas. It is important to emphasize the need to resect all benign tumors since some may ultimately become malignant and others will enlarge progressively, causing pressure symptoms, hemorrhage, chronic infections, or serious rupture. In some cases of malignant tumors, it may, at times, be impossible to carry out a total resection. An attempt should be made to remove the tumor even if that means resecting pericardium, lung, or nodes; the benefits of such extended radical surgery must, however, be balanced against its morbidity and long-term results. If total resection is not possible, debulking is justified in most cases, particularly in those with demonstrable sensitivity to adjuvant therapy (e.g., germ cell tumors or thymomas) or those slow-growing tumors that may be causing pressure (e.g., chemodectomas) and where incomplete resection is compatible with long-term survival.

In some instances where the tumor is totally unresectable, the undertaking of heroic surgery may be necessary to palliate urgent complications (for example, severe SVC obstruction has been treated by a Teflon bypass shunt from the right innominate vein to the right atrial appendage for palliation). Such procedures must, however, be tempered by their high morbidity and mortality in a subset of patients with dismal ultimate outcome, and other forms of palliation should be considered first.

Postoperative care and rehabilitation is much the same as that for patients with lung cancer, and follow-up evaluation of these patients may be patterned after that of lung cancer, with the addition of measurement of tumor markers where appropriate.

B. Radiotherapy

Many of the most common mediastinal tumors are radiosensitive, some of them exquisitely so (for example, thymomas, seminomatous germ cell tumors, neuroblastomas, and lymphomas). Radiotherapy in most of these cases, however, must be considered as part of a multidisciplinary approach in order to achieve the highest success rate.

1. Thymomas

Thymomas are highly radiosensitive, especially when the lymphoid component predominates. Relatively high doses are necessary, however, to achieve a reasonable control rate. The radiotherapy approach to the management of each individual patient will thus depend primarily on the clinical stage of the disease as well as on its expected biologic behavior. The indications for radiotherapy in thymomas are

- The inability to complete the surgical resection.
- Evidence of invasion and aggressive behavior (i.e., lymph node metastases or invasion of the pericardium or large vessels).
- The associated presence of myasthenia gravis.

Generally, radiation is advised when any of the above factors is present. At times, radiation therapy to the mediastinum may even be recommended in cases of refractory myasthenia gravis, in the absence of thymoma, though the benefits of such therapy are not always consistent. While the dose of radiation recommended for malignant thymic tumors is about 5000 rads in 5 weeks, higher doses have been recently recommended since this dose has been demonstrated to be inadequate for the elimination of the epithelial component of the tumor.

2. Germ Cell Tumors

Among the germ cell tumors, seminomas in males and dysgerminomas in females are those lesions most sensitive to radiation therapy. Complete responses are easily achieved following a very modest dose (3000 rads). Embryonal carcinomas also respond to irradiation; the necessary dose, however, is higher (4500 rads), and the recent success obtained by the use of chemotherapeutic agents justifies their use as the definitive therapeutic modality either in conjunction with, or instead of, radiotherapy. It is important to establish the extent of disease spread prior to the institution of therapy; this is especially true in the seminomatous type of germ cell tumors, since the volume to be irradiated primarily depends on the stage of the disease.

3. Neuroblastomas

These are lesions that are highly radiosensitive as well as chemosensitive. The combined treatment of this tumor by surgical extirpation, radiotherapy, and chemotherapy has led to markedly improved results, especially in children. Radiotherapy is indicated when the lesion is extensive, not fully excised, or involves both the posterior mediastinum and the abdominal cavity. The dose is rather substantial (about 5000 rads) but is generally modified in children.

4. Lymphomas

In malignant lymphomas, whether of the Hodgkin or non-Hodgkin's variety, the role of radiotherapy is dependent on the extent of disease as well as on the tumor type. For Hodgkin's lymphoma, particularly in the advanced stages or unfavorable cell types (lymphocyte depletion and mixed cellularity), the treatment is generally by a combination of radiotherapy and chemotherapy. Radiation is the only treatment necessary when the disease is early (Stage I or II) and is limited in size without hilar or parenchymatous involvement. In early non-Hodgkin's lymphoma, radiotherapy is also the primary modality, except that here chemotherapy is used in combination with radiotherapy in Stage II disease. The dose of radiotherapy is about 4000 rads, though this must be modified if chemotherapy (especially Adriamycin or bleomycin) is given simultaneously or soon thereafter.

The technique for treating mediastinal lesions is rather simple, entailing the use of direct anterior and posterior portals, which is extended in lymphomas to treat the supraclavicular and neck nodes as well as the mediastinum in one setup (mantle field). The mantle portal is usually custom planned with special lead shields to protect the adjoining lung, and care must be exercised not to exceed a dose of 4000 rads to the spinal cord, in order to avoid radiation myelopathy (see §§ 9A.III.B.1 and 9A.IV.E., Vol. 2).

C. Chemotherapy

The great majority of mediastinal tumors are benign (cysts, neurogenic tumors, chemodectomas, thyroid lesions, etc.). Furthermore, the largest number of malignant tumors of the mediastinum are lymphomas that are dealt with at length in §

9A.III.B.2 . Thymomas and germ cell tumors are, thus, the only two other categories of mediastinal tumors that will be considered here. The reader is referred to §§ 8B.II, 9A.III, and 9A.IV, for chemotherapy of lymphomas and § 8A.VI.B.4 for neuroblastomas.

1. Thymomas

The great majority of thymic tumors are benign lesions in which a cure might be anticipated from surgical extirpation; furthermore, in those patients with associated syndromes (in particular, myasthenia gravis), one might expect a significant rate of remission of the syndrome following surgery. In the case of myasthenia gravis, it has been even demonstrated that thymectomy in the absence of a thymoma will result in a significant rate of improvement in the disease. This improvement is more consistent in patients where the gland is found to be hyperplastic.

Surgery is, therefore, always the primary therapeutic modality in all cases of thymomas. In those cases where the tumor appears encapsulated (and is therefore considered to be benign), the prognosis with surgery alone should be excellent. Even in cases where the tumor is invasive but can be completely resected, surgical cure can usually be achieved. In patients where the lesion is unresectable or in those who develop local recurrences following surgery, multimodality therapy is definitely indicated. Debulking or an attempt at resection should be the first step, followed by radiotherapy if it has not been previously employed. The value of chemotherapy is as yet not totally established, and it is only indicated in recurrent or residual malignant thymomas following surgery and radiotherapy. There is no indication for the use of adjuvant chemotherapy at the present time.

Reports relative to chemotherapy of thymoma are, by the very nature of the rarity of the disease, extremely fragmentary. The series reported in the literature contain only a handful of patients, such that systematic evaluation of the various chemotherapeutic agents is not available. Nevertheless, it appears that both Adriamycin and cyclophosphamide have yielded some responses, and more recently, *cis*-platinum has been reported to be an active agent. It is noteworthy that multiple studies related to other cancers have suggested synergism between *cis*-platinum and Adriamycin or *cis*-platinum and cyclophosphamide; whether such synergism would prevail in metastatic or recurrent malignant thymoma is as yet undetermined.

2. Germ Cell Tumors

With the exception of the difference in location, germ cell tumors arising in the mediastinum (or in other extragonadal sites) behave and appear to respond in the same manner as germ cell tumors arising in the testicle. Many of the chemotherapy guidelines as outlined in this section are also applicable to metastatic carcinoma arising from the testicle. The reader is also referred to that section for a more detailed discussion of the chemotherapy of germ cell tumors (Section 8).

Previous literature had seemed to indicate a worse prognosis for extragonadal germ cell tumors, particularly for embryonal cell carcinomas; this impression was most likely a result of the fact that these latter tumors were discovered at a more advanced stage than their testicular-origin counterparts. With the advent of effective combination chemotherapy in the mid 1970s, it has been reported that mediastinal germ cell tumors have a prognosis similar to that of their ordinary testicular counterpart.

Because most of these patients require thoracotomy for diagnosis (bronchoscopic or mediastinoscopic biopsies generally yield insufficient tissue for diagnosis and could be dangerous because of the vascularity of the tissue), it has been our conviction that the tumor should be removed, or at the very least maximally debulked, whenever in the opinion of the operating surgeon this can be accomplished with reasonable safety. It has already been noted that frequently these lesions manifest different histologies in different areas, sometimes showing teratoma mixed with embryonal carcinoma and/or choriocarcinoma elements. Since the cytotoxic agents used may vary with the cell type, it is preferable to await final pathology reports before starting therapy. In addition, any patient presenting with a large anterior mediastinal mass without significant lymphadenopathy (which would suggest a diagnosis of lymphoma), should have serum markers (HCG and AFP) determined as a preoperative baseline.

A thorough staging work-up is necessary in all cases to rule out the possibility that the disease began as a testicular primary. In patients who have a negative clinical examination of the testes and scrotum and a negative examination of the retroperitoneum by CAT scan and/or lymphangiography, one may be reasonably confident that one is not dealing with metastatic disease from the testicle but with a mediastinal primary. If the disease is confined to the mediastinum, it may be difficult (if not impossible) to have objective tumor-size measurements accurate enough to assess the response to chemotherapy and to ascertain the completeness of remission. One would have to rely on serum markers to judge the latter.

a. Nonseminomatous Germ Cell Tumors

Spectacular strides have been made within the last decade in the chemotherapeutic management of this disease. The progress has been particularly noteworthy in the embryonal cell variant of germ cell tumors in young men. This has been directly related to the introduction of *cis*-platinum into clinical practice. A number of recent reports further indicate that combination chemotherapy can, in this disease, achieve complete remission in as many as 70–80% of patients, the vast majority of these remaining in complete remission for several years, thus suggesting a conceivable clinical cure.

The most effective combination appears to be that of the *cis*-platinum, bleomycin, and vinblastine, a regimen popularized by the investigators from the University of Indiana. *Cis*-platinum is given at 20 mg per square meter of body surface area daily for 5 consecutive days. Bleomycin is given at a dose of 30 units IV once a week for 12 weeks. Vinblastine is given at a dose of 0.15 mg per kilogram, IV on the first and second day of the *cis*-platinum infusions. Patients must be kept in the hospital for intensive hydration to prevent renal damage consequent to *cis*-platinum infusions. The toxicity of this regimen (in terms of myelosuppression, nausea, vomiting, and weight loss) is formidable, but the results have been worthwhile. The courses of chemotherapy are repeated every 3 weeks if the myelosuppression has been tolerable, and a total of four courses are given. If there is clinical and pathological evidence of complete remission (x-rays, markers, etc.), no further therapy is necessary. The overall results of such treatment are that about 60–70% of patients achieve complete remission with the chemotherapy alone and that another 10–20% of the patients achieve complete remission following the subsequent surgical removal of any residual tumor mass(es). Some of these are found to contain viable tumor, but many of the masses are found to have matured either into teratomas or simply fibrous tissue. A small percentage of patients who achieve complete remission are destined to recur; it has been observed that almost all of the recurrences will have occurred within the first 18–24 months.

Other chemotherapy programs with results similar to the Indiana experience include the VAB protocols developed at the Memorial Sloan-Kettering Cancer Institute. In addition to high-dose *cis*-platinum, these regimens include dactinomycin, bleomycin, Adriamycin, and vinblastine in a complex schedule; the results obtained are similar to those of the University of Indiana. Several other major centers have reported chemotherapy regimens based on this same group of agents with similar results.

Although germ cell tumors of the mediastinum, as well as primary tumors of the testicles, are relatively rare, the patient population is predominantly made up of young men whose entire lives and careers are still to come. Complete remission in such cases is obviously of great sociologic, emotional, and economic importance. In addition, because of the substantial likelihood that intensive chemotherapy programs such as the one outlined above will result in azospermia, which may or may not be reversible, it has been the practice that young men be given an opportunity to bank several specimens of sperm for future use. It should be mentioned, however, that many times the sperm counts in such specimens are deficient even before chemotherapy is begun.

b. Mediastinal Seminomas

This tumor is discussed separately from the other germ cell tumors because the management principles differ significantly. Most patients with seminoma of the mediastinum have extensive local invasion such that complete surgical removal is generally not feasible. Radiation therapy remains the treatment of choice, as this tumor is one of the most radiosensitive neoplasms known. Cure rates between 50 and 80% are achievable with the use of limited surgery and radiation alone. As a result, very few cases are available for evaluation of chemotherapy in this disease. Some investigators claim that seminomas are also responsive to chemotherapy and that the use of this modality should be considered early on in cases of extensive disease with poor prognosis. Certainly, the use of chemotherapy is indicated in any patient who has metastases in sites difficult to irradiate or whose disease recurs after radiation.

D. Management of SVC Syndrome

1. Cause of SVC Syndrome

Superior vena cava syndrome may present as an acute emergency or as a subacute progressive swelling of the neck, face, and upper trunk often associated with dyspnea and hoarsness. The SVC is contained in a relatively restricted and tight compartment of the right anterior mediastinum. The most common cause of SVC syndrome is malignant disease that metastasizes to the lymph node chains surrounding the vena cava and can easily lead to compression and eventually complete obstruction of the vessel. In some cases, the syndrome results from intravascular coagulation or tumor thrombus within the SVC. In the past, nonmalignant diseases such as syphilitic aortitis with aneurysm and sclerosing mediastinitis secondary to tuberculosis were significant etiologic factors. With better antibiotic control of both of these infectious diseases, 97% of cases of SVC syndrome are now related to malignant disease. On rare occasions, benign mediastinal masses (thyroid, thymus, etc.) may result in an SVC syndrome. By far the most common neoplasm resulting in the SVC syndrome is lung cancer, and of the various histological subtypes of lung cancer, oat cell carcinoma is the most common variety, followed by epidermoid carcinoma. Other entities that may give rise to the SVC syndrome are the various mediastinal tumors including lymphomas, teratomas, thymomas, etc. It is rare for metastatic disease in the mediastinum to cause an SVC syndrome.

2. Evaluation of the Patient

The clinical onset of symptoms may either be acute or subacute. In patients who present with severe shortness of breath, hypoxia, cyanosis, and evidence of thrombosis in the upper venous circulation, it may not be possible to pursue a complex range of diagnostic procedures. Noninvasive studies such as chest x-ray and CAT scan should be obtained and will help establish a reasonable working clinical diagnosis as to the probable nature of the underlying tumor, and therapy should be started immediately. This will most often consist of radiation, although in some cases, especially if oat cell cancer is thought to be the underlying disease, combination chemotherapy may also be considered. If the clinical situation is emergent enough to preclude attempts at establishing a pathological diagnosis prior to treatment, one should still endeavor to get histological confirmation after treatment has started and the patient's symptoms have subsided somewhat. It is unlikely that the histological nature of the underlying neoplasm will change markedly after limited radiation or chemotherapy.

Most cases of the SVC syndrome do not present with a clinical syndrome as abrupt as that described above. One, therefore, has a chance to pursue a systematic work-up and attempt to obtain an accurate histological diagnosis on which rational therapy is based. The chest x-rays will show a mass, most commonly in the right upper mediastinum. In about half of the patients, this will be associated with an obvious primary tumor in the adjacent lung field. About 20–25% of the patients will have an associated pleural effusion. Sonography and CAT scans will compliment the findings of the chest x-ray. In cases of doubt, a superior venacavogram and/or a nuclear flow study will readily establish the presence of obstruction.

It must be recognized that the increased venous pressure in the thoracic circulation makes certain biopsy procedures more hazardous; for instance, mediastinoscopy in a patient with dilated thoracic veins may well be fraught with great danger.

3. Management

The definitive treatment of the SVC syndrome will naturally depend on the underlying primary tumor type, and the reader is referred to the sections regarding each of those neoplasms for the appropriate management guidelines. The overall prognosis depends largely on the underlying disease; the prognosis for lymphomas, for example, is obviously better than that for most lung cancers.

Although radiotherapy is usually the first line of treatment, in selected cases, chemotherapy may be the initial treatment of choice (for example, in patients presenting with a highly responsive neoplasm such as lymphoma or small-cell carcinoma of the lung). In addition, in patients who present with very large mediastinal masses, there may be some benefit to using chemotherapy first in order to allow for smaller radiation portals to be employed, thus sparing some normal lung tissues. A caveat should be introduced regarding the injection of chemotherapy into centrally obstructed veins. It is generally best to avoid injections in the right arm or in any of the circulation system that is obviously completely obstructed. If the drugs remain in the local circulation, substantial local toxicity may ensue, including phlebitis and necrosis of the soft tissue. In such cases, it is sometimes advisable to make use of the veins in the lower extremities.

Patients who present with a SVC syndrome associated with back pain should have a careful neurological examination, including myelography, if necessary, to rule out spinal cord pathology. In a small percentage of cases there is an association of spinal cord compression (usually high thoracic or low cervical).

Other general measures that have sometimes been advocated include

- Anticoagulation, especially in the rapidly progressive cases, and fibrinolytic agents have been suggested. The rationale behind these suggestions is that the obstruction of the vena cava is not simply the result of pressure due to the underlying tumor but is also the result of a thrombotic occlusion of the vessel.
- Diuretics may be judiciously used to reduce severe facial edema and are sometimes temporarily effective.
- Corticosteroids have been suggested early on in the course of treatment. These may well be indicated in patients having respiratory distress since many patients are seen with acute bronchospasms as the initial manifestation; a trial of steroids with bronchodilators would certainly seem reasonable.

Section 10. Chest Tumors

Part C: Pleural Tumors (Mesotheliomas)

I. General Considerations   455
   A. Epidemiology
   B. Clinical Considerations
   C. Pathological Considerations
II. Pretreatment Evaluation and Work-Up   455
   A. Physical Evaluation
      1. History
      2. Physical Examination
   B. Radiological Tests
   C. Thoracentesis
   D. Biopsy

E. Bronchoscopy
F. Sputum Cytology
G. Thoracoscopy and Open Thoracotomy
III. Therapeutic Management   456
   A. Surgery
   B. Radiotherapy
      1. External Radiotherapy
      2. Intracavitary Radiotherapy
      3. Interstitial Implants
   C. Chemotherapy
   D. Combined Treatments

I. GENERAL CONSIDERATIONS

A. Epidemiology

There is now a substantial rise in the incidence of mesothelioma of the pleura, which was once thought to be an unusual disease. There appears to be a definite increase in incidence associated with exposure to asbestos. This is of particular importance in southwestern Brooklyn, where many people have been employed in situations where there existed direct exposure to asbestos: construction industry, shipyards, and the U.S. Navy Yard, where asbestos was commonly used. A substantial risk for asbestos exposure has been documented. Although lung cancer does not seem increased in asbestos workers who are nonsmokers, asbestos workers who do smoke have a very high incidence of lung cancer (60–100 times higher than nonsmokers). Mesotheliomas, on the other hand, are definitely increased in asbestos workers even if they are nonsmokers.

B. Clinical Considerations

Thoracic mesotheliomas spread quickly around the chest wall but do not as readily metastasize to other areas of the body. They primarily involve the pleura but can also affect the pericardium, lung, and diaphragm by direct extension onto their serous surfaces. On occasion, they can involve the mediastinum and cause pericardial tamponade.

This insidious disease, which has a slow growth rate and a long latency period, may initially present as a localized pleural mass and/or mild chest pain of a pleuritic nature. As the mass increases in size, it may result in effusion and cause dyspnea. With advancing disease, there can be spread through the diaphragm to involve the abdomen, spread to the pericardium, or even to the contralateral lung. As the disease progresses, dyspnea may increase because of shunting of inadequately oxygenated blood. If the pericardium becomes involved, congestive heart failure, pericardial effusion, atrial arrhythmias, and on rare occasions, cardiac tamponade may occur. The cause of death in pleural mesothelioma is usually a direct result of the growth of tumor and fluid effusions.

C. Pathological Considerations

Mesotheliomas arise from the surface lining cells, or mesothelium. Histological identification can be difficult, however, because of their diverse microscopic appearance. They may be classified as purely sarcomatous in about one-fifth of the cases, as epithelial or tubulopapillary in one-half of the cases, and as mixed in the remainder. Some specimens display an epithelial configuration and may even resemble metastatic carcinoma; the diagnosis may then require a careful search for other potential primary tumor sites. The use of special stains, electron microscopy, and immunoperoxidase changes may help establish an accurate pathological diagnosis.

Mesotheliomas are divided into two categories: localized solitary tumors and diffuse malignant tumors. While localized lesions may extend to involve the entire pleura, their identification and early management are most rewarding in this otherwise highly fatal disease.

II. PRETREATMENT EVALUATION AND WORK-UP

A. Physical Evaluation

This should include a comprehensive history taking and physical examination.

1. History

The history should include a social and occupational history to identify occupational exposure or "bystander" contact with asbestos. In addition, the following symptoms may be identified:

- Chest pain (nonpleuritic and of an aching nature). The pain is frequently referred to the shoulder or upper abdomen.
- Cough and dyspnea.
- Fatigue and weight loss.
- Osteoarthropathy or clubbing of the fingers (may occasionally be present).

- Symptoms of congestive heart failure, arrythmias, and pericardial effusion.
- Intermittent hypoglycemia (associated with the benign form of this disease).

2. Physical Examination

A physical examination should be complete to evaluate the patient's general condition as well as to assess the chest findings accurately:

- Identification of a mass by percussion and auscultation.
- Changes in breath sounds.
- Detection of pleural effusion.
- Cardiac evaluation and detection of effusion.

B. Radiological Tests

These will include a chest x-ray and a thoracoabdominal CAT scan for identification of the extent of disease. It is preferable to perform these tests after aspiration of as much pleural fluid as possible.

C. Thoracentesis

Mesothelioma frequently presents with a pleural effusion as a primary finding. Control of this effusion is important lest the patient develop a tension effusion, trapped lung, or nonfunctioning lung. The pleural effusion caused by a mesothelioma does not respond to closed thoracotomy drainage because of the presence of adhesions and compartmentalization. A thoracentesis is immediately indicated in all patients, and the following evaluation is carried out:

- Nature of the fluid (often hemorrhagic).
- Hyaluronic acid, which is often increased in the pleural fluid of patients with mesothelioma.
- Cytological examination of the fluid is not as helpful in mesothelioma as it is in metastatic carcinoma and is often negative for identifiable malignant cells. Normal pleural fluid contains mesothelial cells, and both false positive and false negative pleural cytology are possible.
- Needle aspiration biopsy of the pleura. This technique is simple but not without complications (hemorrhage, infection, pneumothorax). It is highly successful in experienced hands but will not always yield a diagnosis.

D. Biopsy

A good pleural biopsy is necessary to prove the diagnosis of mesothelioma. Biopsy of the identifiable mass is best done with fluoroscopic control and requires cooperation between the thoracic surgeon, the radiologist, and the pathologist to achieve the highest rate of accuracy in the diagnosis.

E. Bronchoscopy

This is necessary to rule out a radiologically occult bronchogenic carcinoma. Flexible fiberoptic bronchoscopy is the choice procedure in these cases.

F. Sputum Cytology

Examination of the sputum cytology may also identify a bronchogenic carcinoma.

G. Thoracoscopy and Open Thoracotomy

If the above less invasive measures fail to establish the diagnosis of malignant mesothelioma, invasive procedures such as thoracoscopy or even open thoracotomy and biopsy may be required. The tendency of mesothelioma to infiltrate needle tracts, thoracotomy sites, and thoracotomy scars appears to be overrated and should not discourage attempts to obtain a definitive diagnosis or symptomatic relief in patients with recurrent pleural effusions.

III. THERAPEUTIC MANAGEMENT

A. Surgery

It is generally agreed that there is often a need to carry out an open thoracotomy for adequate biopsy of pleural mesotheliomas; the real value of attempting a total tumor excision, however, remains in dispute. The morbidity and mortality from very extensive procedures tend to negate any potential benefit that might accrue. Surgical procedures for mesotheliomas might include any one of the following procedures:

- Open thoracotomy and biopsy.
- Partial resection of pleural malignant mesotheliomas. This approach has led to an apparent increase in survival, though it is not universally accepted.
- Radical extrapleural pneumonectomy and pleurectomy, followed by radiotherapy and chemotherapy. This has been advocated, and a small number of 5-year survivals have been reported by some.

B. Radiotherapy

1. External Radiotherapy

There is some evidence that the median survival is increased and palliation of pain may be achieved following radiotherapy (4500–5000 rads) delivered to the involved hemithorax. A report by Schlienger noted that the study group survived a median of 13 months as compared with the historical 9.8 months. Nonrandomized studies seem to suggest a slightly longer median survival with the use of megavoltage radiation than with conventional radiation therapy. The overall consensus, however, is that external radiotherapy alone is useful for palliation but ineffective in significantly prolonging survival. External radiotherapy used as an adjuvant following surgical resection has been recommended; though it appears to be effective in preventing local recurrences, its use is not without risk to the underlying lung since the doses required are substantial (5000 rads). Special techniques and electron beams are essential to avoid serious damage.

2. Intracavitary Radiotherapy

Since malignant mesothelioma arises from the mesothelial lining of the pleura, instillation of radioactive colloidal gold (^{198}Au) into the pleural space has been attempted; colloidal gold has an affinity for the serosal lining cells, making this a theoretically ideal method. The instillation of radioactive colloidal gold (^{198}Au) requires an intact pleura with residual fluid to be successful. It can, therefore, only be expected to succeed in early cases. In late cases, the tumor enlarges and obliterates the pleural space, prohibiting the low-energy irradiation from ^{198}Au to penetrate through the thick plaque of tumor and be therapeutically effective.

3. Interstitial Implants

Radioactive iodine grains or after-loading catheter techniques are particularly useful for some localized unresectable tumors.

C. Chemotherapy

Because most published series on mesotheliomas involve a relatively small number of cases, it is difficult to assess accurately the effectiveness of various agents or combinations of agents. Response rates approaching 30–40% have been obtained with combination regimens incorporating Adriamycin, achieving palliation and a longer median survival for the responding patients. Adriamycin (doxorubicin) and alkylating agents, notably cyclophosphamide, are probably the most active single agents against mesotheliomas. Azacytidine and 5-fluorouracil have also been reported to be somewhat effective. The potential efficacy of other standard chemotherapeutic agents has not been established in the management of malignant mesotheliomas. Several encouraging case reports of responses to standard and investigational agents suggest that mesotheliomas, unlike other related sarcomas, may be somewhat sensitive to a range of chemotherapeutic agents; *cis*-platinum is currently undergoing Phase II efficacy trials in this disease. The use of chemotherapy in malignant mesothelioma must still be considered experimental.

D. Combined Treatments

Surgery and intracavitary radiotherapy has resulted in a few 5-year disease-free survivals. Patients treated with surgery, cyclophosphamide, and radiotherapy appear to survive longer than those treated with only one or two of those methods. Since Adriamycin appears to be more effective than cyclophosphamide, its use in place of cyclophosphamide may increase the number of long-term disease-free survivors.

The following stepwise guidelines can therefore be recommended in the treatment of pleural tumors:

1. Control the effusion and establish a definitive diagnosis, without prolonged chest tube drainage. A thoracentesis to clear the chest, followed by pleural biopsy for diagnosis is thus the first step.

2. If all other less invasive diagnostic techniques fail, early open thoracotomy to establish a definitive diagnosis is indicated.

3. If a localized fibrosarcomatous lesion is identified, radical surgical excision is the procedure of choice.

4. If a diffuse malignant mesothelioma is present, a parietal pleurectomy removing as much tumor as possible and reestablishing an expanded lung should be the first order of therapy.

5. Following pleurectomy, radiotherapy by one modality or another should be utilized.

- Implant techniques using iodine seeds (useful for unresectable cases).
- After-load catheters inserted during pleurectomy are especially useful over the diaphragm, where the pleura could not be completely removed. These catheters provide a route of insertion of intense local treatment with radioactive seeds to areas not surgically resectable or otherwise accessible.

- External radiotherapy preferably with particle beam machines to extend just past the pleura, in order to preserve lung function as much as possible, may be useful.
- Intracavitary radiation (in early cases with an open pleura).

6. Chemotherapy, preferably in combination, administered following surgery and/or radiotherapy, should be used in all instances, whether the disease is advanced or not, since neither surgery nor radiotherapy has been able to cure more than a small fraction of patients with diffuse mesothelioma.

The results of treatment depend to a great extent on the nature of the disease. Patients with localized mesothelioma (either fibrosarcomatous or epithelial) do reasonably well, with some being long-term survivors, whereas patients with diffuse mesothelioma have a much more serious prognosis, with the majority surviving less than 12 months.

Section 10. Chest Tumors
Part D: Cancer of the Esophagus

I. Epidemiology   461
II. Pathological Considerations   461
III. Pretreatment Evaluation and Work-Up   462
   A. Signs and Symptoms
   B. X-ray
   C. Esophagoscopy
   D. Biopsy
   E. Bronchoscopy
IV. Preoperative Preparation   462
   A. Nutritional Status
   B. Hematologic Status
   C. Cardiopulmonary Status
   D. Status of the Gastrointestinal Tract
   E. General Considerations
   F. Metastatic Evaluation
   G. Site-Specific Data Form for Cancer of the Esophagus
V. Therapeutic Management   463
   A. Surgery
      1. Cervical Esophagus
         a. Curative Surgery

         b. Palliative Operations
      2. Thoracic Esophagus
      3. Lower Esophagus and Esophagogastric Junction
   B. Radiotherapy
      1. Radiation for Cure
      2. Adjuvant Radiotherapy
         a. Preoperative Radiotherapy
         b. Postoperative Irradiation
   C. Chemotherapy
VI. Postoperative Care and Evaluation   467
   A. Immediate Postoperative Care
   B. Late Postoperative Care
   C. Follow-Up Evaluation
VII. Management Algorithm for Cancer
     of the Esophagus   468

I. EPIDEMIOLOGY

Carcinoma of the esophagus is predominately a disease of men 50–70 years of age. The incidence of the disease in the United States is 10 per 100,000 population; in Japan, however, the disease rate is 46 per 100,000. It is also more prevalent in China, Scotland, the U.S.S.R., Scandinavia, and among the native Bantu of South Africa. The factors for this increased incidence are not clear, though it has been suggested that dietary influences are important.

Risk factors that have been identified with cancer of the esophagus include

- Smoking and alcohol consumption.
- High intake of nitrosamines, which have been shown to be highly carcinogenic for the esophagus. This compound is found predominantly in preserved meats (e.g., bacon) and smoked fish.

There is also an increased incidence of carcinoma of the esophagus in patients with the following conditions:

- Paterson-Kelly syndrome.
- Tylosis.
- Esophageal achalasia.
- Corrosive lye strictures.
- Columnar epithelial–lined lower esophagus.
- Other epithelial carcinomas of the upper aerodigestive tract.

A high degree of suspicion should be aroused when evaluating any patient with the above predisposing factors. Although no mass screening is available or recommended, evaluation of patients in the above categories should be carried out at the slightest suggestion.

Public awareness and education should be encouraged to increase the number of cases detected early that might be amenable to cure. Symptoms include

- Dysphagia. Any dysphagia in a male over 45 years of age is almost synonymous with cancer of the esophagus and requires immediate work-up.
- Regurgitation.
- Weight loss.
- Blood or blood streaks *per os*.

II. PATHOLOGICAL CONSIDERATIONS

Carcinoma of the esophagus presents in the lower third of the esophagus in over 50% of the cases. About 40% will present in the middle third, whereas only 8–10% are found in the cervical esophagus.

The tumors are usually ulcerated and exophytic, rapidly growing circumferentially to encircle the esophagus and result in obstruction. Submucosal growth to involve large segments of the esophagus is not uncommon. The great majority of carcinomas of the esophagus are squamous cell carcinomas. Primary adenocarcinomas are rare, usually arising from a columnar epithelial–lined lower esophagus; more often, adenocarcinomas in the lower esophagus arise from cells of gastric origin situated about the esophagogastric junction that spread proximally by direct extension.

Polypoid lesions of the esophagus are rare and could represent one of the following conditions:

- Carcinosarcoma (which has a more favorable prognosis).
- Pseudosarcoma.
- Leiomyosarcoma.
- Melanoma.

The primary routes of spread of esophageal carcinoma are by direct extension, lymphatic permeation, and hematogenous spread. Direct extension and lymphatic spread are most important in determining the therapy and ultimate outcome.

It is well recognized that direct extension of esophageal carcinoma may result in long segments of apparently normal esophagus being microscopically involved by tumor; skip areas are not unusual, and frozen sections must be resorted to at the time of resection to assure that the margins of resection are free of tumor.

Lymphatic spread is predictable and often early.

- Cervical esophageal carcinomas spread to the cervical nodes, including the anterior jugular and supraclavicular nodes. Upper mediastinal nodes are also at risk.
- Thoracic esophageal carcinoma spreads to local and mediastinal nodes early in the course of the disease, usually before hematogenous spread or direct extension that would

preclude resection. Later, there may be wider spread to su-praclavicular and/or subdiaphragmatic nodes, making the disease unresectable for cure.
- Carcinoma arising at the esophagogastric junction may involve local and mediastinal nodes as well as subdiaphrag-matic nodes, celiac nodes, and nodes at the hilus of the spleen.

Hematogenous spread may produce lung, liver, and bone metastases.

III. PRETREATMENT EVALUATION AND WORK-UP

A. Signs and Symptoms

Early symptoms are quite characteristic and include dys-phagia, weakness, and weight loss, though patients presenting with symptoms of short duration do not always have early lesions.

Late symptoms and signs will depend on the location of the tumor and the extent of involvement of adjacent structures. Evaluation should seek to identify the following:

- Aspiration pneumonia; cough, fever, dyspnea, etc.
- Recurrent laryngeal nerve palsy; hoarseness.
- Pulmonary symptoms resulting from compression or inva-sion of the trachea or bronchi (tracheoesophageal fistula, atelectasis), etc.
- Symptoms of pericardial involvement (rare).

B. X-ray

A barium esophagogram will usually provide the diagnosis. An annular luminal constriction with an irregular ragged mucosal pattern is seen. Proximal dilation is usually not striking.

Chest x-rays, tomograms, and CAT scans of the chest are useful in identifying the extent of local spread and the status of adjacent structures.

C. Esophagoscopy

Esophagoscopy (either rigid or flexible fiberoptic) is essen-tial to identify the tumor, establish the histological diagnosis, and determine the anatomic limits of the lesion. There have been fewer complications with the newer flexible fiberoptic endoscopes then with the rigid esophagoscope.

D. Biopsy

Cytology taken during endoscopy is occasionally helpful to establish a tissue diagnosis, especially if a gross tumor cannot be identified or when obstruction is such that it will not allow passage of the scope.

Punch biopsy of a lesion during endoscopy is the best meth-od of obtaining a tissue diagnosis. Multiple biopsies might be indicated to identify the extent of local spread or the nature of secondary lesions.

E. Bronchoscopy

This might be useful to identify the spread of the tumor and the presence of a fistula.

IV. PREOPERATIVE PREPARATION

A. Nutritional Status

Preoperative assessment of the state of nutrition is most important, as dysphagia usually results in severe nutritional depletions. The following parameters are indications of nutri-tional deficit that should preferably be corrected preoperatively.

- Weight loss of over 5 kg.
- Skin test for anergy. A simple skin test with a universal antigen to establish immunocompetence may be used; if the patient is found to be anergic, nutritional status should be corrected preoperatively by either feeding tube or intra-venous hyperalimentation.

B. Hematologic Status

Blood volume determination and appropriate preoperative transfusion of packed red blood cells and blood products as indicated must be arried out. Coagulation screening should be done to detect any hidden coagulopathy that might complicate the surgery or postoperative recovery.

C. Cardiopulmonary Status

An EKG and Holter monitor should be used as indicated. If these identify any abnormality, or if there is a history of car-diac disease, appropriate studies should be undertaken. Ar-rythmias, congestive failure, or other cardiac decompensation must be corrected prior to surgery.

Pulmonary function studies and testing is necessary preoperatively, and an attempt should be made to improve pulmonary function as much as possible. Preparation of the patient should include the following:

- Discontinuation of smoking.
- Clearing of bronchial secretions and elimination of infection with antibiotics.
- Bronchodilators and mucolytic agents, as necessary, in cases of chronic bronchitis or pulmonary emphysema.
- Pulmonary physiotherapy and instruction in the use of various respirators.

D. Status of the Gastrointestinal Tract

If there is any history of gastrointestinal disease, a barium enema, as well as an upper GI series, should be done to establish the presence of a normal GI tract. This is particularly important should it be necessary to carry out an interposition of colon or stomach and also to restore postesophagectomy continuity of the GI tract.

E. General Considerations

General considerations in preoperative preparation include dental consultation to find and eliminate any sites of oral sepsis and ear, nose, and throat (ENT) consultation and examination of the oro- and hypopharynx to exclude the presence of coexisting oropharyngeal cancers.

F. Metastatic Evaluation

Computerized axial tomography scan of the thorax and upper abdomen is most important in the identification of local disease extension (particularly spread to the celiac axis nodes) and pulmonary metastases. These would be contraindications for an attempt at curative resection.

Preoperative staging of carcinoma of the esophagus has been improved with the use of isotopic scanning of the liver and spleen. Liver scans are rarely positive, however, unless a blood chemistry profile (SMA-12 or SMA-18) identifies abnormalities of the liver function tests.

Bone and head CAT scans are only indicated if symptoms seem to suggest such metastases.

G. Site-Specific Data Form for Cancer of the Esophagus (see pp. 464–465)

V. THERAPEUTIC MANAGEMENT

There is some controversy concerning the proper role of surgery, radiotherapy, and chemotherapy in the management of carcinoma of the esophagus. Several factors are important in determining the appropriate modality of sequence of modalities to be used:

- The level of the lesion (i.e., cervical, upper thoracic, midthoracic, or esophagogastric junction).
- Whether therapy is intended to be curative or palliative.
- The nutritional condition and cardiopulmonary status of the patient.
- The local extent of the lesion and symptoms present.

A. Surgery

Surgery remains the mainstay of curative therapy for esophageal carcinoma, either alone or in combination with radiotherapy or rarely chemotherapy.

1. Cervical Esophagus

a. Curative Surgery

Curative surgery entails resection of the cervical esophagus with adequate margins often extending from the pharynx to below the thoracic inlet. The larynx is almost always simultaneously resected, and a radical neck dissection (unilateral or modified bilateral) might also have to be performed. Restoration of continuity of the upper GI tract may be achieved by one of many methods:

- Local or regional flaps: tubed deltopectoral flap or myocutaneous flaps (pectoralis or trapezius). These can only be done if the resection does not extend below the thoracic inlet, and they are indicated particularly following laryngopharyngoesophagectomy. Temporary ostomies might be necessary with staged reconstruction, and failure of primary healing is a significant problem.
- Pull-up procedures with esophagogastrostomy. The stomach may be pulled up into the neck, either subcutaneously, transpleurally, or retrosternally. Some have recommended constructing a tube out of the greater curvature of the stomach to bring up to the neck and anastomose to the pharynx.
- Intestinal interposition operations of left colon (which has a more constant and adequate blood supply and a more even lumen) or transverse colon (isoperistaltic), pedicled on the left colic artery.
- Free small intestinal graft with microvascular anastomosis.

It must be recognized that any one of these procedures constitutes surgery of the greatest magnitude, with significant

SITE-SPECIFIC DATA FORM FOR CANCER OF THE ESOPHAGUS

HISTORY

Age:

Symptoms
_____ Dysphagia
_____ Pain
_____ Weight loss
_____ Weakness
_____ Aspiration
_____ Hoarseness
_____ Hematomesis
Duration _____

Associated conditions
_____ Tylosis
_____ Lye stricture
_____ Achalasia
_____ Paterson–Kelly
       syndrome

Social history
  Occupation:
  Race: ____ White ____ Black ____ Oriental ____ Other
  Exposure to sun _____
  Allergies: ____ Arsenic ingestion: _____
Family history of carcinoma
  Relation: _____ Site: _____
Previous history of carcinoma
  _____ No _____ Yes Site: _____
  Rx: _____
Previous treatment (describe):
(Surgery, radiotherapy, chemotherapy,
PUVA, phototherapy, etc.)
_____
_____

PHYSICAL EXAMINATION

Positive clinical findings: _____
  Pulmonary status: _____
  Cardiac status: _____
  Head and neck status: _____
  Esophagoscopy status: _____
Location of tumor (distance from incisors): _____
Character: ____ Ulcerated ____ Constricting ____ Exophytic
Size: _____
Biopsy: ____ Yes ____ No

	Yes	No
Extension to:		
Nodes	____	____
Pericardium	____	____
Lung	____	____
Stomach	____	____

RETREATMENT EVALUATION

	Pos.	Neg.	Suspicious		Pos.	Neg.	Suspicious
CBC	__	__	__	Bronchoscopy	__	__	__
SMA-12	__	__	__	Chest and abdominal			
Chest x-ray	__	__	__	CAT scan	__	__	__
Barium swallow	__	__	__	Pulmonary function			
EKG and holter				tests	__	__	__
monitor	__	__	__	Liver scan	__	__	__
Esophagoscopy	__	__	__	Bone scan	__	__	__
				Head scan	__	__	__

Classification: ____ T ___ N ___ M
  Histologic diagnosis: _____
  Stage: _____

Signature: _____
Countersignature: _____
Date: _____

TNM Classification

Primary tumor (T)

TO   No demonstrable tumor in the esophagus
T1S   Carcinoma *in situ*
T1   A tumor 5 cm or less in esophageal length with no obstruction,*
        no circumferential involvement, and no extraesophageal spread†
T2   A tumor more than 5 cm in esophageal length with no extraesophageal spread† or a tumor of any size
        which obstructs* or has circumferential involvement with no extraesophageal spread
T3   Any tumor with extraesophageal spread†

Nodal involvement (N)

Cervical esophagus: The regional lymph nodes in the cervical esophagus are the cervical and
supraclavicular nodes.

N0   No clinically palpable nodes
N1   Movable, unilateral, palpable nodes
N2   Movable, bilateral, palpable nodes
N3   Fixed nodes

Thoracic esophagus

NX   (Clinical evaluation.) Regional lymph nodes for the upper, midthoracic and lower thoracic
        esophagus that are not ordinarily accessible for clinical evaluation
N0   (Surgical evaluation.) No positive nodes
N1   (Surgical evaluation.) Positive nodes

Distant metastases (M)

MX   Not assessed
M0   No (known) distant metastasis‡
M1   Distant metastasis present (specify).

Histopathology

Squamous cell carcinoma, adenocarcinoma. Rarely do sarcomas and melanomas occur.

Grade

Well-differentiated, moderately well differentiated, poorly differentiated, or very poorly differentiated
(grade numbers 1, 2, 3, or 4, respectively)

Stage grouping

Stage I   T1S N0 M0   Carcinoma *in situ*
             T1   N0 M0   Tumor in any region of the esophagus that involves 5 cm or less of esophageal
             T1   NX M0   length, produces no obstruction, has no extraesophageal spread, does not
                            involve the entire circumference, and shows no regional lymph node
                            metastases or remote metastases
Stage II   A tumor of any size with no extraesophageal spread and with no distant metastases.
                            Cervical esophagus:
                            T1   N1 M0
                            T1   N2 M0
                            T2   N1 M0, T2, N2, M0
                            T2   N0 M0
                            Thoracic esophagus:
                            T2   NX M0
                            T2   N0 M0
Stage III   Any esophageal cancer at any level with:
                            Any T3
                              Extraesophageal spread
                            Any N3 (cervical)
                            Any N1 (thoracic)
                              Any intrathoracic esophageal carcinoma including either upper and midthoracic
                              region or lower thoracic region with any positive findings in regional lymph nodes
                            Fixed lymph node metastases
                            Any M

---

*Roentgenographic evidence of significant impediment to the passage of liquid contrast material past the tumor
or endoscopic evidence of esophageal obstruction.
†Extension of cancer outside the esophagus is seen by clinical, roentgenographic, or endoscopic evidence of
(1) recurrent laryngeal, phrenic, or sympathetic nerve involvement; (2) fistula formation; (3) involvement of
the tracheal or bronchial tree; (4) vena cava or azygos vein obstruction; and (5) malignant effusion. Mediastinal
widening itself is not evidence of extraesophageal spread.
‡For the cervical esophagus, any lymph node involvement other than that of cervical or supraclavicular
lymph nodes is considered distant metastasis. For the thoracic esophagus, any cervical, supraclavicular, scalene,
or abdominal lymph node is considered distant metastasis.

morbidity and mortality and a relatively low yield in terms of long-term cure. Selection of patients is therefore critical, and the procedure should only be done after very careful consideration.

b. Palliative Operations

- Esophagogastrostomy without resection, for bypass of obstruction. This should be done only if no other palliation (i.e., radiotherapy) is possible, if the tumor is unequivocally unresectable, and if the patient is otherwise in satisfactory general condition.
- Diversion without resection, which involves cervical esophagostomy to facilitate management of oropharyngeal secretions, and also a feeding gastrostomy. This should only be done in extreme cases, very poor risk patients, and when no other method is available.

2. Thoracic Esophagus

The procedures available for treatment of the patient with cancer of the thoracic esophagus are many:

- Palliative resection.
- Palliative bypass operations.
- Insertion of a Celestin tube.
- Total thoracic esophagectomy for cure with esophagogastrostomy or colon interposition (left, transverse, or right).
- Cervical esophagogastrectomy.

The choice of procedure is dependent on the local factors found at the time of surgery. The patient is first explored through a right posterolateral thoracotomy through the bed of the resected fifth rib. Resectability is assessed, and if the tumor is resectable, the esophagus is mobilized. The abdomen is then explored via a midline incision; the absence of celiac or splenic nodes, as well as the absence of metastses to the liver, must be established. Biopsies and frozen sections for staging of the cancer are often useful at this point. The stomach and the colon are then examined to determine the length and suitability for mobilization as an esophageal replacement. Only then can one make a final decision as to the type of surgery to be carried out.

If the tumor is not resectable for cure as a result of unresectable local extension or extensive celiac or liver metastases, a decision must be made whether to proceed with a palliative resection, a bypass operation, or insertion of a Celestin tube as a palliative procedure. The extent of metastatic disease identified, the overall condition of the patient, and the availability of other palliative modalities will together determine if the patient ought to be subjected to a palliative resection. Otherwise, an esophagogastrostomy to relieve the patient of the disabling dysphagia and the difficulty in handling saliva, which invariably complicates the terminal days of the patient with cancer of

the esophagus, is a superior way of achieving palliation, provided it can be tolerated and the patient has enough time to live, to leave the hospital, and to enjoy the palliation that is offered. In all other cases, the simplest method of palliation is the insertion of a Celestin tube under direct vision during the exploration and fastening it securely in place.

If the tumor is resectable, a total esophagectomy performed through the pleural cavity should be carried out. The margins of the resected specimen should be examined histologically by frozen section. Reconstruction can be carried out by one of the many methods above. In order to offset the effect of truncal vagotomy, which by necessity accompanies any esophagectomy, the pylorus should be rendered patulous either by a simple manual transmural dilation or by an extramucosal pyloromyotomy or Heineke-Mikulicz pyloroplasty.

3. Lower Esophagus and Esophagogastric Junction

Wide resection of the tumor and reanastomosis with esophagogastrostomy is the treatment of choice of lower esophageal and gastroesophageal junction lesions, whether it be for cure or for palliation. The patient is explored through the left chest and through the bed of the resected seventh rib. Intrathoracic resectability for cure is assessed by direct palpation. The diaphragm is then divided radically from the hiatus, and the abdomen is thoroughly examined for metastases. If metastases are present, and the patient's condition warrants it, a modest palliative resection should be carried out (i.e., esophagogastrectomy with esophagagogastrostomy). If there are no metastases in the liver, celiac axis or spleen, a radical esophagogastrectomy including the removal of all node-bearing tissue in the periaortic area and gastric ligament, as well as splenectomy, is indicated. A separate, additional midline abdominal incision is sometimes necessary for adequate exposure of the upper abdomen in cases of radical esophagogastrectomy. Intraoperative frozen section studies and pyloromyotomy are indicated just as in resections of the thoracic esophagus.

B. Radiotherapy

1. Radiation for Cure

Radiation therapy has been widely utilized in the treatment of carcinoma of the esophagus, most often for palliation or as an adjunctive modality, though the use of radiotherapy as the sole and definitive modality of treatment has been substantiated by several reports (e.g., Pearson, 1971, in *Br. J. Surg.* **58,** 794) that suggest that there might be as much as 20% 5-year survival with radiotherapy alone. The selection of cases, however, is extremely important in order to achieve the best results. Ideal cases are those limited lesions of the cervical esophagus without involvement of the postcricoid area.

Doses of curative radiotherapy have to be high (in the range of 6000 rads), and treatment planning must avoid exposure of the spinal cord. The tumor is radiosensitive, as attested by postmortem examinations that fail to identify residual cancer following radiation; the healing process, however, results in marked fibrosis and frequent strictures that require repeated dilatation. Other complications of radiotherapy such as hemorrhage and perforation are rare. The role of radiotherapy for palliation is much clearer. Dysphagia, hemoptysis, and pain are easily relieved by modest doses (4000–5000 rads), and careful attention to nutrition and supportive care will ensure acceptable recovery and quality of life.

2. Adjuvant Radiotherapy

a. Preoperative Radiotherapy

The combination of surgery and radiation therapy for carcinoma of the esophagus has been found to be preferable to either modality alone. Several regimens have been recommended:

- A 3-day course of irradiation to a dose of 2400 rads, followed 7 days later by resection (Nakayama *et al.*, 1967, in *Cancer* **20,** 778).
- A dose of 4000–7000 rads over a period of four to seven weeks, followed by resection 4 weeks later (Parker *et al.*, 1976, in *JAMA* **235,** 1018).

Both approaches necessitate careful tretment planning and tumor localization in order to achieve optimum results.

b. Postoperative Irradiation

There is an opportunity to increase the 5-year survival of patients with carcinoma of the esophagus by the administration of postoperative megavoltage radiation therapy. This should be particularly urged when patients are found to have residual tumor after resection or when the margins of resection are found to be microscopically involved by tumor. This modality may be used even in cases where preoperative irradiation has been administered, provided the approach is carefully pre-planned and integrated.

C. Chemotherapy

There have been some recent enthusiastic reports of remissions obtained with various combinations used in other squamous cell carcinomas of the aerodigestive tract (see § 1). Methotrexate, bleomycin, and *cis*-platinum have been used and may be administered on an outpatient basis under close observation.

Combination chemotherapy and megavoltage radiation therapy has also been investigated. One regimen combines therapy as follows:

- Mitomycin C, 10 mg, IV on day 1 of radiation.
- 5-Fluorouracil, 1000 mg/m², on days 1, 2, 3, and 4 of radiation.
- 3000 rads are then administered over 3 weeks.

If the patient becomes operable, resection is then advised after recovery from bone marrow depression. Otherwise, a second course of therapy with the same agents and an additional 2000 rads of megavoltage radiation therapy is administered after a rest period of 3 weeks.

Several cancer centers have reported encouraging results with anterior chemotherapy, i.e., patients receive chemotherapy before radiation or surgery, the advantage being that the primary lesions are more susceptible to chemotherapeutic attack before radiation and there is the possibility of controlling micrometastases already established outside the surgical or radiation fields. It is generally conceded that chemotherapy is quite ineffective in previously irradiated patients. The treatment plan employs intensive chemotherapy with a combination generally including bleomycin, *cis*-platinum, methotrexate and/or a vinca alkaloid. Responding patients are treated for 2–3 courses before being subjected to definitive local procedures: surgery, radiation, or both. Multimodal therapy, as outlined above, involves formidable toxicity, and one must be prepared to support these patients intensively with hyperalimentation, blood products, etc. before embarking on such an aggressive approach. Whether these intensive regimens will result in a higher fraction of cured patients is not yet known.

VI. POSTOPERATIVE CARE AND EVALUATION

A. Immediate Postoperative Care

- A nasogastric tube is passed through the anastomosis and kept on low suction for the first 2–3 days. The tube can be removed after restoration of peristaltic activity of the GI tract. The patient, however, should be maintained NPO until one is certain that healing has occurred.
- Chest tubes must be put in place (right pleural cavity for thoracic esophagus resections, left pleural cavity for thoracoabdominal resections) for drainage of air and blood. The tubes can be removed as soon as drainage ceases.
- Antibiotics should be administered by IV until the last IV line is removed (usually on postoperative day 4).
- A direct arterial line and a Swan-Ganz catheter are necessary for monitoring and can be removed as soon as the patient's

hemodynamic and pulmonary status are stable. The usual supportive measures for any major thoracic operation are given: fluids, blood transfusions, pulmonary toilet, physiotherapy, etc.

- Prior to ingestion of any food by mouth, a Gastrografin esophagogram must be done to establish the patency of the anastomosis and to rule out any anastomotic leak. Only then can feeding be started and progressively increased to a 6-feeding ulcer diet with additional high-protein supplements and vitamins.

B. Late Postoperative Care

- The nutritional status of the patient is closely monitored by a carefully recorded daily weight and diet diary.
- Exercise is encouraged, particularly walking, stretching, in addition to arm and girdle exercises.
- The patient usually may return to work on or about the eighth postoperative week. The patient must be cautioned to avoid smoking, drinking, or binge eating.

C. Follow-Up Evaluation

- The patient should be thoroughly examined every 3 months the first 2 years, every 6 months until 5 years, and yearly thereafter. Any other test required according to the patient's symptoms should be done.
- If the patient remains asymptomatic, an upper GI series is repeated every 12 months, and any positive findings are followed up.
- A careful ENT examination, as is done preoperatively, should be repeated at 1- to 2-year interval, looking for an occult carcinoma of the oropharynx or hypopharynx.

VII. MANAGEMENT ALGORITHM FOR CANCER OF THE ESOPHAGUS
(see p. 469)

ALGORITHM FOR CANCER OF THE ESOPHAGUS

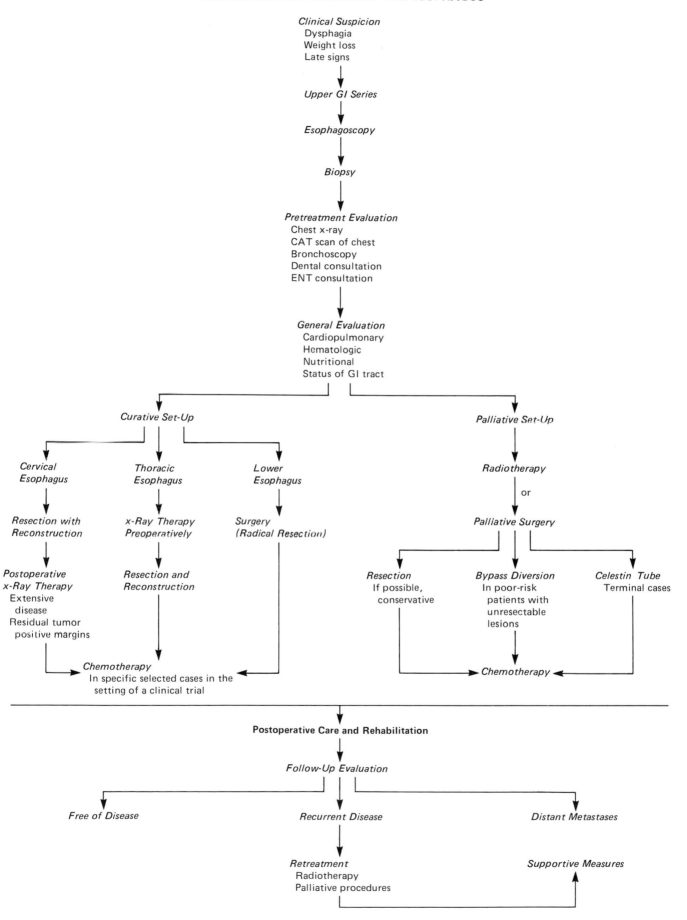

Section 11

Carcinomas of the Alimentary Tract

IRVING ENQUIST

With Contributions By

Felix Siegman	Surgery
Rene A. Khafif	Surgical Oncology
Joseph Giovaniello	Radiology
Karl Jindrak	Surgical Pathology
Baroukh Kodsi	Gastroenterology
Samuel Kopel	Hematology-Oncology
Hosny Selim	Radiotherapy
Thomas Reynolds	Oncology
Marilyn Draxton	Nursing Oncology

Section 11. Carcinomas of the Alimentary Tract

Part A: Carcinoma of the Stomach

I. Early Detection and Screening   475
   A. Epidemiology and Predisposing Factors
      1. Diet
      2. Genetic Factors
      3. Polyps and Pernicious Anemia
      4. Atrophic Gastritis, Metaplasia, and Dysplasia
      5. History of Gastric Ulcer
   B. Early Signs and Symptoms
   C. Screening
II. Pretreatment Evaluation, Work-Up, and Preparation   476
   A. Evaluation and Work-Up
      1. History and Physical Evaluation
      2. Identification of the Lesion
         a. Gastrointestinal X-Rays
         b. Fiberoptic Endoscopy
      3. General Medical and Metastatic Evaluation
   B. Preoperative Preparation
   C. Multidisciplinary Evaluation
   D. Site-Specific Data Form for Carcinoma
      of the Stomach
III. Therapeutic Management   478
   A. Pathological Considerations
      1. Histological Types of Gastric Carcinoma
         (according to the World Health Organization)

      2. Biological Behavior of Gastric Cancer
         a. Early Gastric Carcinoma
         b. Lymphatic and Vascular Spread
         c. Prognosis
   B. Surgery
      1. Goals of Surgery
         a. Curative Resection
         b. Palliation
      2. Extent of Surgical Procedure
      3. Surgical Reconstruction
      4. Complications of Surgery
   C. Radiotherapy
   D. Chemotherapy
IV. Postoperative Care, Evaluation, and Rehabilitation   483
   A. Immediate Postoperative Period
   B. Evaluation of the Patient
V. Management Algorithm for Cancer of the Stomach   484

Suggested Readings   484

I. EARLY DETECTION
AND SCREENING

A. Epidemiology and Predisposing Factors

Although incidence of carcinoma of the stomach has been decreasing over the past three to four decades in this country, it is still a relatively common visceral cancer and leads to approximately 14,000 deaths per year. It affects men more commonly than women and is seen more often in the elderly. There is considerable variation in the frequency of gastric cancer among various countries. During the last 30 years, its incidence rate has been steadily declining in the United States, while in some other regions (e.g., Eastern Europe or Japan) it is still the leading cause of cancer deaths. In the United States, gastric cancer is most frequently encountered among recent immigrants from those countries; the incidence among white American males is 12.7/100,000 population per year, rising to 47.3/100,000 among Hawaiians of Japanese extraction.

Several predisposing factors seem to influence the risk of genetic carcinoma:

1. Diet

The major factor influencing the incidence of gastric cancer is diet. Daily intake of milk, meat, and green and yellow vegetables seems to lower the risk of stomach cancer, while consumption of smoked, salted, and pickled foods seem to increase the risk. The one main carcinogenic group of chemicals recognized as significant in gastric cancer is nitrosamines, which are commonly found in unrefrigerated foods in which sodium nitrite is often used as preservative.

2. Genetic Factors

Genetics also seem to play a role in the incidence of gastric cancer, although a less important one. Persons of blood group A appear to be at a higher risk for some types of gastric carcinoma (the diffuse type).

3. Polyps and Pernicious Anemia

Among various types of gastric polyps, only adenomas are considered premalignant, and these are exceedingly rare; they occur more frequently in patients with pernicious anemia, a disease that may represent a predisposing factor for gastric carcinoma, particularly for tumors that present in the body and fundus of the stomach.

4. Atrophic Gastritis, Metaplasia, and Dysplasia

A significant association of gastric carcinoma with atrophic gastritis does exist: the latter is frequently associated with intestinal metaplasia of the gastric mucosa. Although dysplastic changes can occur in normal gastric mucosa, they more frequently develop from metaplastic epithelium. In the process of carcinogenesis, dysplasia can increase in severity until it reaches the stage of "carcinoma *in situ*." Invasion of malignant cells into the lamina propria takes place rather quickly, so that "*in-situ* carcinoma" is a rather ephemeral phase in the progress of the disease, and this term should not be used in the classification of early gastric carcinoma.

5. History of Previous Gastric Ulcer

A history of gastric ulcers contributes little to the incidence of stomach cancer; less than 1% of all gastric ulcer become malignant.

B. Early Signs and Symptoms

The importance of early diagnosis in the management of gastric cancer cannot be overemphasized. Long-term survival of patients with gastric cancer is dismal, and the majority of patients are not curable when first seen; less than one-fourth of those that are resectable will survive 5 years. The Japanese have been reporting significantly better results, a finding that may be ascribed to early detection. The use of the gastrocamera, fiberoptic endoscopy, and double-contrast gastrointestinal x-rays, for example, were promoted by them and have resulted in achieving detection of 36% of cases at Stage I and another 36% at Stage II; their overall cure rates in 1971 were thus reported at 65%.

Early cancers of the stomach are usually asymptomatic so that the prognosis for those with symptoms is not good. The most common symptoms of gastric cancer are vague and nonspecific: anorexia and weakness; bloating and feeling of fullness; dull epigastric pains. Other symptoms are usually indications of late complications such as pyloric obstruction or bleeding (hematemesis, melena, or anemia).

Because the symptoms are often nonspecific and resemble those caused by other common abdominal conditions—peptic ulcer, cholecystitis, functional bowel disease, etc.—it is important that all patients with abdominal symptoms be studied by barium swallow or gastroscopy early in their investigations. Increased public and physician education is necessary to raise the index of suspicion and promote the early evaluation of the upper gastrointestinal tract.

C. Screening

There is no systematic screening program for gastric cancer in the United States. The screening that is performed in cancer screening centers or among hospitalized patients is limited to a history and physical examination, augmented by examination of the stool for occult blood. A positive screen would then lead to further investigations that may uncover a gastric cancer.

All patients with pernicious anemia, others with achlorhydria, and those with a strong family history of gastric cancer should be screened biennially with barium studies or fiberoptic gastroscopy.

II. PRETREATMENT EVALUATION, WORK-UP, AND PREPARATION

A. Evaluation and Work-Up

1. History and Physical Evaluation

As indicated in the early signs of gastric cancer, the history offers few clues of a specific nature unless bleeding or pain can be elicited. The physical examination is usually negative, except in the most advanced disease, where one or several of the following findings may be observed:

- Abdominal mass.
- Enlarged liver with nodularity.
- Umbilical mass.

- Left supraclavicular nodes.
- Blumer's shelf identified on rectal examination.

2. Identification of the Lesion

a. Gastrointestinal X-Rays

Radiological barium studies of the stomach still constitute the initial diagnostic procedure in the detection of gastric tumors. A 20–40% false negative has been reported, but this should be significantly reduced by double-contrast studies. False positives are in the range of 5–15%.

i. Methodology. For many years, the traditional method of examination of the stomach has consisted of a combination of fluoroscopy and radiography following the administration of a barium meal. During the past 10–15 years, the emphasis previously placed on fluoroscopy has been reduced, and more emphasis is now placed on the study of high-quality radiographs obtained with the double-contrast technique. Though certain information, such as peristaltic activity and flexibility of the gastric walls, is best seen under fluoroscopy, the most important use of fluoroscopy is to permit the radiologist to obtain films in optimal position and to obtain spot films with compression.

The double-contrast barium-air examination of the stomach has been developed by Japanese workers, and this technique has recently gained acceptance in the United States. The principal requirements for a good-quality double-contrast examination of the stomach are an adequate volume of barium and air and frequent positional changes of the patient. The air for the barium-air double contrast study may be introduced in one of several ways: it could be the air that the patient has normally swallowed with the barium; it could be aspirated by placing a pinhole in the straw through which the patient drinks the barium suspension; it may be introduced through a nasogastric tube or by the ingestion of gas-producing tablets or powder (which will produce the required amount of 300–400 ml of CO_2). The amount of barium suspension required for this type of study is approximately 200–300 ml. Frequent positional changes should be made in order to wash away adherent mucus from the mucosal surface of the stomach and allow mixing of the barium suspension with the gastric juices. An antispasmodic agent (Glucagon, 1 mg, IM) is usually administered approximately 5 min before the examination. Multiple films are taken with the patient in different positions (upright, supine, prone, oblique); and then under fluoroscopy, several compression films are also taken (especially of the gastric antrum).

The double-contrast technique is particularly valuable for the demonstration of infiltrating lesions and of tumors of the proximal portion of the stomach; these are lesions that require particularly accurate radiological diagnosis since they frequently yield negative endoscopic biopsies and cytological results. The double-contrast study is also helpful in the differential diagnosis of benign and malignant gastric ulcers.

ii. Radiological Diagnostic Features

- Changes in the caliber of the stomach may be manifested by either narrowing or dilatation. Narrowing of the distal third is more frequently encountered. Gastric malignancies rarely cause obstruction, unless they are located in the distal third of the stomach.
- Intraluminal radiolucencies may be identified. They vary in size from the very small and barely visible defect to the very large and almost obstructing one. They may be caused by a variety of benign or malignant tumor masses and may be single or multiple, sessile or pedunculated.
- Intrinsic lesions of the stomach may produce changes in the marginal contour, resulting in out-pouching of barium (where there are ulcerations) or encroachment of the lumen (where there is a mass). These may vary greatly in size, and their configuration may be smooth or irregular.
- The normal mucosal pattern of the stomach has a wide variation in width and redundancy, especially along the greater curvature of the upper half of the stomach. If the folds are unusually prominent or nodular and this appearance persists despite overdistention or the application of compression, malignant involvement of the mucosa or of the submucosa should be suspected (e.g., lymphoma).
- Usually peristalsis begins in the middle third of the body of the stomach. A deeply infiltrating lesion may interrupt peristalsis.
- Benign or malignant tumors of the stomach may displace the stomach if there is a large extragastric component. This is likely to occur with a leiomyosarcoma. Enlargement of adjacent organs (especially pancreas) may also cause displacement of the stomach.
- The sites of predilection of gastric cancer are the pyloric and the prepyloric region of the stomach.

The radiological appearances of gastric carcinoma are summarized as follows:

- A mass projecting into the gas bubble of the fundus of the stomach in the erect position.
- Ulceration of the stomach with irregular, rolled edges.
- Marked irregularity or nodular margination of the stomach.
- Ulcer crater within a mass not extending outside the confines of the stomach.
- Shallow crater that does not hold fluid in the erect position.
- Rigidity of the area of the stomach involved.
- Ulcer within a rigid area of the stomach.
- Ulcer crater with interruption of gastric folds toward the crater.

- Evidence of perigastric mass indenting the stomach.
- "Leather-bottle" type stomach suggesting scirrhous carcinoma.
- Lymphoma of the stomach presents as a diffuse or infiltrating variety but occasionally may be nodular, polypoid, or pedunculated. Radiologically there may be a "fingerprint impression" pattern due to diffuse intramural invasion, or there may be broad ulcerations and moderate rigidity with loss of peristaltic activity.

b. Fiberoptic Endoscopy

This diagnostic modality, which has supplanted the gastric lavage and cytology procedures, allows for direct visualization of the stomach and permits tissue sampling under vision, with either brushing or forceps biopsy of any suspicious lesion. The yield of accuracy is in the 90–95% range, with a slightly lower yield in ulcerated and infiltrating tumors (as compared with exophytic ones) and in lesions of the cardia.

3. General Medical and Metastatic Evaluation

Most patients with gastric cancer are malnourished, anemic, and frequently have extensive disease beyond the ability of cure. They therefore require a thorough preoperative assessment:

- Cardiopulmonary status, EKG, pulmonary function tests, blood gases, and chest x-ray.
- Nutritional assessment.
- Complete blood count (CBC), hematocrit, and blood volume determinations.
- Serum electrolytes and blood chemistries.
- Coagulation profile.

Extensive metastatic evaluations are of little value since most patients are locally incurable. Bone scans, gallium scans, liver scans, etc. are therefore not routinely indicated. Abdominal computerized axial tomography (CAT) scans may, however, be useful in identifying the local spread of the disease.

If possible, every patient with gastric cancer should have an exploratory laparotomy with resection carried out for cure or palliation. The degree and location of any spread or metastases can then be determined at that time.

B. Preoperative Preparation

This must take into account the various parameters that need to be corrected:

- Because gastric cancer seriously affects the caloric intake of most patients, intensive study of the patient's nutritional status must be made before exploratory laparotomy. If the patient is malnourished, a period of 2–3 weeks of vigorous nutritional support, enteral or parenteral, may be required before any operative intervention.

- Anemia must be corrected with appropriate blood transfusions.
- Respiratory therapy is given, as needed.
- Correction of any intercurrent illness must be initiated immediately.
- Coagulopathies must be corrected.
- Antibiotics are not usually indicated.

C. Multidisciplinary Evaluation

Though the treatment of gastric cancer is primarily surgical, a multidisciplinary approach is most important in the evaluation of the patient as well as in the later phases of the disease. The radiologist, gastroenterologist, surgeon, chemotherapist, radiotherapist, nurse oncologist, social worker, nutritionist, and psychiatric liasion nurse all have significant resources to offer the patient and must be properly consulted and appropriately utilized.

D. Site-Specific Data Form for Carcinoma of the Stomach (see pp. 479–480)

III. THERAPEUTIC MANAGEMENT

A. Pathological Considerations

Within the stomach, carcinoma occurs most frequently in the antrum and pylorus (47%), then with decreasing frequency in the body and cardia, and finally least frequently in the fundus (2%). Diffuse involvement of the linitis plastica type is found in 7% of cases.

The gross appearance of the carcinoma may be nodular (44%), ulcerated (40%), fungating (7%), linitis plastica (7%), or superficially spreading (2%). The tumor may extend into both the esophagus and the duodenum.

1. Histological Types of Gastric Carcinoma (according to the World Health Organization)

- Adenocarcinoma.
  - Papillary.
  - Tubular.
  - Mucinous.
  - Signet-ring cell.

- Adenosquamous carcinoma.
- Squamous cell carcinoma (which has to be differentiated from carcinoma extending from the esophagus).
- Undifferentiated carcinoma.
- Unclassified carcinoma.

Other tumors of the stomach are

- Carcinoid. This tumor, most frequently found in the antrum, usually behaves in a malignant fashion. It may be combined with adenocarcinoma.
- Leiomyosarcoma. This is a nonephithelial malignant tumor, which may become ulcerated and cystic due to central necrosis.
- Malignant Schwannoma.
- Choriocarcinoma.
- Melanoma (extremely rare).
- Lymphoma. Among the primary lymphomas of the stomach, the non-Hodgkin's type predominates over Hodgkin's disease.

It is important to be aware of benign lesions that may be clinically misinterpreted as carcinoma. They include hyperplastic polyps, inflammatory fibroid polyps ("eosinophilic granuloma"); lymphoid hyperplasia ("pseudolymphoma"); various heterotopies: pancreas, Brunner's glands, and submucosal gastric glands; and hamartomas: Peutz-Jeghers polyps, juvenile polyps, giant rugal hypertrophy (Ménétrièr's disease), parasitic granuloma, and Cronkhite-Canada syndrome.

2. Biological Behavior of Gastric Cancer

a. Early Gastric Carcinoma

This is defined as a carcinoma confined to the mucosa or mucosa and submucosa, regardless of the presence of lymph node metastases. Microscopically, it can be subdivided into intramucosal and submucosal carcinoma. The term *carcinoma in situ* cannot be used with confidence since invasion of the lamina propria by tumor cells had been found after many serial sections from the specimen were examined in cases presumably diagnosed as carcinoma *in situ*.

The macroscopic types of early gastric carcinoma that are important for the endoscopist and radiologist are

- Type I: polypoid.
- Type II: elevated, flat, depressed.
- Type III: excavated.

The majority of these early tumors are 2.0 cm or less in diameter, yet in about 10% of gastrectomies for early gastric carcinoma, there will be multiple focal lesions present.

b. Lymphatic and Vascular Spread

The lymph nodes of the lesser curvature are those most frequently involved, followed by those of the greater curvature,

SITE-SPECIFIC DATA FORM—STOMACH

HISTORY

Age: _____

Symptoms
- _____ Weight loss _____ lbs.
- _____ Pain
- _____ Nausea
- _____ Vomiting
- _____ Anorexia
- _____ Bloating
- _____ Hematemesis
- _____ Eructation

Duration _____

Past history
- _____ Pernicious anemia
- _____ Gastric ulcer
- _____ Gastric polyps

Social history
Occupation: _____
Race: ____ White ____ Black ____ Oriental ____ Other
Smoker: ____ No ____ Yes How much? _____
Drinker: ____ No ____ Yes How often? _____
Family history of carcinoma
Relation: _____ Site: _____
Previous history of carcinoma
_____ No ____ Yes Site: _____
Rx: _____
Previous treatment (describe):
(Surgery, radiotherapy, chemotherapy, etc.)
_____
_____

PHYSICAL EXAMINATION

General condition: _____
Abdomen
- _____ Tenderness
- _____ Distension
- _____ Mass
- _____ Hepatomegaly
- _____ Umbilical mass

Rectal exam: _____ Negative _____ Positive
Neck nodes: _____ Negative _____ Positive

PREOPERATIVE WORK-UP (Check, if done)

	Neg.	Pos.	Suspicious		Neg.	Pos.	Suspicious
UGI	_____	_____	_____	SMA–12	_____	_____	_____
Gastroscopy	_____	_____	_____	Liver scan	_____	_____	_____
Biopsy	_____	_____	_____	Chest x-ray			
Laparotomy	_____	_____	_____	or CAT	_____	_____	_____
CAT of abdomen	_____	_____	_____	Bone scan	_____	_____	_____
Ultrasound	_____	_____	_____	Other	_____	_____	_____

OPERATIVE FINDINGS

Tumor
Site: _____
Size (in cm): _____
Depth of penetration: _____

	Yes	No
Limited to mucosa and submucosa	_____	_____
Extends to or into serosa	_____	_____
Penetrates through serosa	_____	_____
Invades contiguous structures	_____	_____

Specify _____
_____

Lymph nodes:	Yes	No
None involved	_____	_____
Perigastric (within 3 cm of the stomach)	_____	_____
Lesser curvature	_____	_____
Greater curvature	_____	_____
Regional (more than 3 cm from tumor)	_____	_____
Left gastric	_____	_____
Splenic	_____	_____
Celiac	_____	_____
Common hepatic	_____	_____
Intra-abdominal (not removed)	_____	_____
Para-aortic	_____	_____
Hepatoduodenal	_____	_____
Retropancreatic	_____	_____
Mesenteric	_____	_____

Distant metastasis. _____ Liver _____ Peritoneum _____ Omentum _____ Lungs _____ Pancreas _____ Adrenals _____ Spleen
Histologic diagnosis: _____

Classification: ____ T ____ N ____ M
Stage: _____

Signature: _____
Countersignature: _____
Date: _____

Classification of Stomach Cancer

TNM Classification

Primary tumor (T)

T0	No evidence of primary tumor
T1	Tumor limited to mucosa and submucosa, regardless of its extent or location
T2	Tumor involves the mucosa and the submucosa (including the muscularis propria) and extends to or into the serosa but does not penetrate through the serosa
T3	Tumor penetrates through the serosa without invading contiguous structures
T4	Tumor penetrates through the serosa and invades the contiguous structures

Nodal involvement (N)

NX	Metastases to intra-abdominal lymph nodes not determined (e.g., laparotomy not done)
N0	No metastases to regional lymph nodes
N1	Involvement of perigastric lymph nodes within 3 cm of the primary tumor along the lesser or greater curvature
N2	Involvement of the regional lymph nodes more than 3 cm from the primary tumor that are removed or removable at operation, including those located along the left gastric, splenic, celiac, and common hepatic arteries
N3	Involvement of other intra-abdominal lymph nodes that are not removable at operation, such as the para-aortic, hepatoduodenal, retropancreatic, and mesenteric nodes

Distant metastasis (M)

MX	Not assessed
M0	No (known) distant metastasis
M1	Distant metastasis present (specify)

Grade

Well-differentiated, moderately well differentiated, poorly differentiated, or very poorly diferentiated (grade numbers 1, 2, 3, or 4)

	Stage Grouping	
Stage	Clinical–diagnostic staging	Postsurgical treatment pathologic staging
I	T1, N0, M0	pT1, N0, M0
II	T2, N0, M0 T3, N0, M0	pT2, N0, M0 pT3, N0, M0
III	N1–3, M0 Any T with any N	pT1–3, N1, M0 pT1–3, N2, M0 pT1–3, N3, M0 (resected for cure)
IV	T4, M0 (probably not resectable) Any T or N, M1	pT1–3, N3, M0 pT4, N0–3, M0 (not resectable) pT1–4 or pTX or N0–3 or NX, M1

porta hepatis, and celiac axis. In surgical specimens, lymph nodes have been found to be involved in 3% of cases of intramucosal cancers, 12% of submucosal cancers, and 60–70% of advanced gastric cancers.

Bloodstream metastases are found most frequently in the liver, lung, skin, and ovaries. The latter can also be involved by transperitoneal spread (Krukenberg tumor).

c. Prognosis

The prognosis depends mainly on lymph node involvement, the 5-year survival rate in early gastric carcinoma being about 93%, while in advanced carcinoma with lymph node involvement, it is only about 12%. Tumors measuring less than 2 cm have a better prognosis than larger ones, but there is no relationship between survival and macroscopic appearance of the tumor, its location, or the duration of symptoms prior to surgery. Histological patterns have little prognostic value, though the diffuse types have a worse prognosis. On the other hand, the stromal reaction of the host to the presence of the tumor cells, both in the form of lymphoplasmocytic infiltrates and the formation of young, fibroblastic tissue around invasive parts of the tumor is a favorable sign.

B. Surgery

Surgery is the mainstay of treatment of gastric cancer. It may be palliative or curative, with the potential for cure being directly related to the extent of the disease. Approximately 80% of patients diagnosed with gastric cancer are operable; only 50% are found to be resectable at the time of operation; and only 60% of these are considered curative resections. In other words, less than 25% of all gastric cancers are resected for cure. The only real cures of gastric cancer ever achieved have been by resection of all or part of the stomach with the tumor.

1. Goals of Surgery

a. Curative Resection

The type of gastric resection performed will depend on the actual site of the tumor:

- Subtotal gastectomy (Billroth II type), for lesions of the antrum and pylorus.
- Proximal subtotal gastrectomy, rarely performed for cancer.
- Total gastrectomy or esophagogastrectomy, indicated for lesions of the cardia or fundus of the stomach.

Mortality for these procedures is significant (5% in subtotal gastrectomy and as much as 15–25% in total gastrectomy), and 75–80% of all patients will recur within 5 years. Super-

ficial gastric cancer (T1), which represents less than 10% of all cases, is curable in 85–90% of cases; thus any series with a higher number of T1 or T2 lesions will have a significantly better overall cure rate (e.g., in Japan). The following factors seem to affect the end result of curative surgery:

- Location of the tumor and macroscopic appearance (antral or polypoid being more favorable).
- Type of operation.
- Nodal involvement (50% overall cure rate in the absence of nodal involvement).
- Degree of penetration of the tumor in the gastric wall.
- Size of the tumor.

b. Palliation

One third of patients undergoing surgery will end up with palliation only. Surgical palliation may be of two types:

i. Palliative Resection. This procedure is preferred any time the tumor can be completely removed, even though peritoneal seeding. liver involvement, or node metastases are present. Median survival ranges between 4 and 9 months.

ii. Bypass Procedures. Gastrojejunostomy to bypass obstruction and gastrostomy or jejunostomy for drainage or feeding have all been tried in unresectable patients. Results are disappointing, and these procedures offer little in the way of relief of symptoms.

2. Extent of Surgical Procedure

There is little to substantiate claims of improved results from more radical operations:

- Total gastrectomy is only indicated in proximal stomach tumors.
- Resection of the lesser and greater omentum is routinely performed for gastric cancer, though its value is debatable.
- Systematic removal of nodal reservoirs is not ordinarily performed in this country, though in Japan lymph node dissections are clearly defined in the "Rules of Gastric Cancer Surgery." The Japanese report a 5-year survival rate of 33% in patients with positive nodes who have had radical en-bloc resections. The concept of a "radical" subtotal gastrectomy should, therefore, not be discounted.
- Splenectomy is only indicated in proximal stomach cancer.
- Distal esophageal resection. This is most important in tumors of the cardia and gastroesophageal junction. Submucosal spread is common in these tumors, and a long segment of disease-free esophagus should be resected and verified with frozen-section control of the margins.

3. Surgical Reconstruction

Reconstruction following subtotal or total resections is ordinarily accomplished using the jejunum. If a total resection is done, creation of some type of pouch from the jejunum (Roux-en-Y anastomosis or jejunal loop with jejunojejunostomy) may help the patient ingest and digest more food postoperatively and prevent regurgitation of the bile into the esophagus.

4. Complications of Surgery

With the loss of much of the stomach and continuous suction from the GI tract, fluid and electrolyte problems may easily develop and must be attended to.

Leakage from an anastomosis (gastrojejunostomy or esophagojejunostomy) is a very serious complication, which again must be recognized early and treated vigorously. Treatment may include laparotomy, placement of drainage tubes, and/or hyperalimentation.

Other possible complications are those associated with any major laparotomy: subphrenic abscess, atelectasis, intestinal obstruction, etc.

Because of the loss of storage volume following gastric resection, patients may have trouble with fullness after eating and difficulty in consuming sufficient food, resulting in an inability to gain or maintain weight. In some, the symptoms of a dumping syndrome may present. The patient will then require considerable psychosocial support and guidance from the physician and operating surgeon, including intensive counseling and advice about diet and eating habits.

C. Radiotherapy

Radiotherapy of the GI tract is restricted by the poor tolerance of gastric and intestinal mucous membranes to the high doses that are necessary to achieve an adequate response. As such, radiotherapy is relatively ineffective as a curative modality for stomach cancer and is therefore not recommended as primary treatment. It has been sporadically recommended, however, for the palliation of selected patients: for treatment of the unresectable primary tumor for the relief of pain or bleeding, which may be helped by modest doses (obstruction, on the other hand, is a difficult symptom to palliate with radiotherapy) and for treatment of symptomatic metastatic disease (e.g., painful bone or subcutaneous lesions).

Palliative radiotherapy for the elective treatment of unresectable disease has not been encouraging, though recent studies combining radiotherapy with 5-fluorouracil (3500–400 rads and 45 mg per kilogram of 5-FU given in 3 days) suggest an advantage in terms of median survival and have claimed a 56% response rate.

Some newer methods of radiation therapy might open up new horizons: fast neutron beams, combination neutron and gamma beams, intraoperative radiotherapy, addition of radiation sensitizers, etc. Preliminary data, however, are still very sketchy.

D. Chemotherapy

It is very difficult to determine the response of patients with adenocarcinoma of the stomach to nonsurgical therapy. Physical examination is often unrevealing because these tumors are deep seated in the midabdomen and are usually partially resected by the surgeon. Liver metastases must be larger than 2 cm in diameter before they can be seen on nuclear or CAT scans. Most patients with easily measurable disease have far advanced cancer with poor performance status, anorexia, and weight loss; such patients are the least likely to respond well to chemotherapy. Even so, objective response rates to combination chemotherapy have been in the range of 20–40%, making stomach cancers one of the most sensitive tumors of the GI tract to this kind of therapy. The three most active drugs are 5-FU, Adriamycin, and mitomycin-C. Until recently, most physicians treated advanced disease with single drugs only; duration of response, however, was only 3–6 months, and there were very few long-term survivors.

In 1980 Georgetown University reported significantly better results using the above three drugs in combination in patients with advanced measurable disease. The objective response rate was 42%, with a median duration of response of 9 months; the median survival of responders was 12.5 months as compared with 3.5 months for nonresponders. These results have been confirmed in studies from other institutions, and some long-term survivors have been reported. Therefore, combination chemotherapy with FAM (5-FU, Adriamycin, and mitomycin-C) is now being studied in patients with residual disease after surgical resection of a bulky cancer. Preliminary reports show significant prolongation of the symptom-free interval, as compared with simultaneous control groups treated without FAM, though definitive results are not yet available, and it is unknown whether there will be any cures rather than just a prolongation of the disease-free period before the appearance of recurrent symptomatic cancer.

Another promising approach in clinical research is chemotherapy combined with radiation therapy. Early studies from the Mayo Clinic compared radiation therapy alone to radiation plus 5-FU in patients with inoperable cancer. Their median survival for combined therapy was 12 months, versus 6 months after radiation therapy alone. In addition, 3 of 25 patients with radiation therapy and 5-FU were alive 5 years later, while none of the 23 with radiation alone survived. A major problem with combined therapy, especially when the modalities are used simultaneously, is the marked increase in acute toxicity and treatment-related death. Nevertheless, current improvements in irradiation techniques and in chemotherapy delivery and monitoring have allowed the initiation of new studies using two and three drugs along with radiation therapy. These studies are still ongoing, and combined therapy with FAM and radiation must still be considered experimental.

Another experimental area is the use of adjuvant chemotherapy in patients with fully resected stomach cancer who are at high risk of recurrence because of microscopic metastases to perigastric lymph nodes or direct extension to the serosal surface of the stomach. Early reports from a study by the Gastrointestinal Tumor Study Group (Ref. 4), comparing observation alone to 5-FU plus methyl lomustine (CCNU), show a projected 4-year survival of 36% for the control group and 55% for the chemotherapy-treated group. More definitive results must be awaited before a recommendation can be made.

The impact of chemotherapy on patients with metastatic disease from gastric cancer is not yet clear. Though most of the reported series are incomplete, it appears that combination chemotherapy has a growing role in the treatment of adenocarcinoma of the stomach. It appears to be most effective in intraabdominal metastatic disease (liver) and subcutaneous areas. Lung metastases respond but to a lesser degree, whereas bone metastases are relatively resistant. Of all patients so treated, 40–50% show response, sometimes with dramatic palliation of several months duration and increased survival.

IV. POSTOPERATIVE CARE, EVALUATION, AND REHABILITATION

A. Immediate Postoperative Period

Resections for gastric carcinoma are very major operative procedures and are attended by major organic and metabolic changes. Highly professional and attentive care must be given by the medical and nursing staff during the early postoperative period. Close observation in an intensive care unit is essential:

- Vital sign monitoring, hemoglobin and hematocrit determinations, serum electrolytes, blood gases, and serum chemistries must all be obtained at frequent intervals.
- Blood transfusions, fluids, and electrolytes are administered as needed.
- Pulmonary ventilation and inhalation therapy is used as needed.
- Antibiotics may be prescribed prophylactically.
- Renal function and urinary output is carefully monitored.
- Surgical wounds, drains, and abdomen are checked regularly.
- Early ambulation and activity is encouraged.

When normal GI activity is resumed and the patient is allowed nutrition by mouth, fluids in moderation are given first, followed by soft food and ultimately by a regular diet. Because of the markedly limited capacity of the stomach after subtotal or total resections, the patients must be instructed as to the need to eat and drink frequently, but in small amounts.

B. Evaluation of the Patient

Patients who are treated for palliation require long-term supportive care until their demise. Several parameters need to be attended to:

- Nutritional support. This might require IV hyperalimentation or jejunostomy feedings in extreme cases. Vitamin and enzyme supplements are also essential.
- Relief of pain.
- Psychosocial support.

In the later stages, the assistance of social service for home health care, custodial care, and hospice placement is invaluable, and the clergy is most helpful in the terminal stage of the disease. The assistance of a well-planned supportive care team as illustrated in §1.VIII.D.4, Vol. 1 can go a long way toward making the few months of life available to these patients a tolerable interlude.

Table I

Long-Term Follow-Up Schedule for Cancer of the Stomach

Management	First year			Second and third year		Thereafter, annually
	Every 6 weeks	Every 3 months	Annually	Every 6 months	Annually	
History						
Complete	X			X		X
Anorexia	X			X		X
Weight loss	X			X		X
Vomiting	X			X		X
Diarrhea	X			X		X
Bleeding	X			X		X
Pain	X			X		X
Physical						
Abdomen	X			X		X
Neck	X			X		X
Rectal	X			X		X
General		X			X	X
Investigation						
Stool guaiac	X			X		X
CBC	X			X		X
SMA-18		X		X		X
Chest x-ray			X		X	X
GI series			X		X	X
Gastroscopy			X		X	X

When curative surgery has been carried out and the patient is discharged, a systematic plan of regular evaluation must be established to detect and correct any complication of the surgery (e.g., dumping, anemia, bile reflux, esophagitis, etc.) and to identify recurrences of distant metastases. Table I suggests such a schedule of follow-up evaluation.

V. MANAGEMENT ALGORITHM FOR CANCER OF THE STOMACH

(see p. 485)

SUGGESTED READINGS

1. Aird, I., Benthall, H. H., and Roberts, J. A. H. A relationship between cancer of the stomach and the ABO blood groups. *Br. Med. J.* **1,** 799–801 (1953).

2. Desmond, A. M. Radical surgery in the treatment of carcinoma of the stomach. *Proc. R. Soc. Med.* **69,** 867 (1976).
3. Devesa, S. S., and Silerman, D. T. Cancer incidence and mortality trends in the United States 1935–74. *J. Natl. Cancer Inst. (U.S.)* **60,** 545 (1978).
4. Douglas, H. O., Stablein, D. M. *et al.* Randomized controlled trial by the G.I. Tumor Study Group of adjuvant chemotherapy in gastric cancer. *Proc. Am. Soc. Clin. Oncol.* **22,** 430 (1981).
5. Dupont, J. B., Jr., and Cohn, I., Jr. Gastric adenocarcinoma. *Curr. Probl. Cancer* **4,** 25 (1980).
6. Hitchcock, C. R., and Scheiner, S. L. Early diagnosis of gastric cancer. *Surg., Gynecol. Obstet.* **113,** 665, (1961).
7. Moertel, C. G. Chemotherapy of gastrointestinal cancer. *Clin. Gastroenterol.* **5,** 777 (1976).
8. Shahon, D. B., Horowitz, S., and Kelly, W. D. Cancer of the stomach: An analysis of 1152 cases. *Surgery (St. Louis)* **39,** 204 (1956).

ALGORITHM FOR CANCER OF THE STOMACH

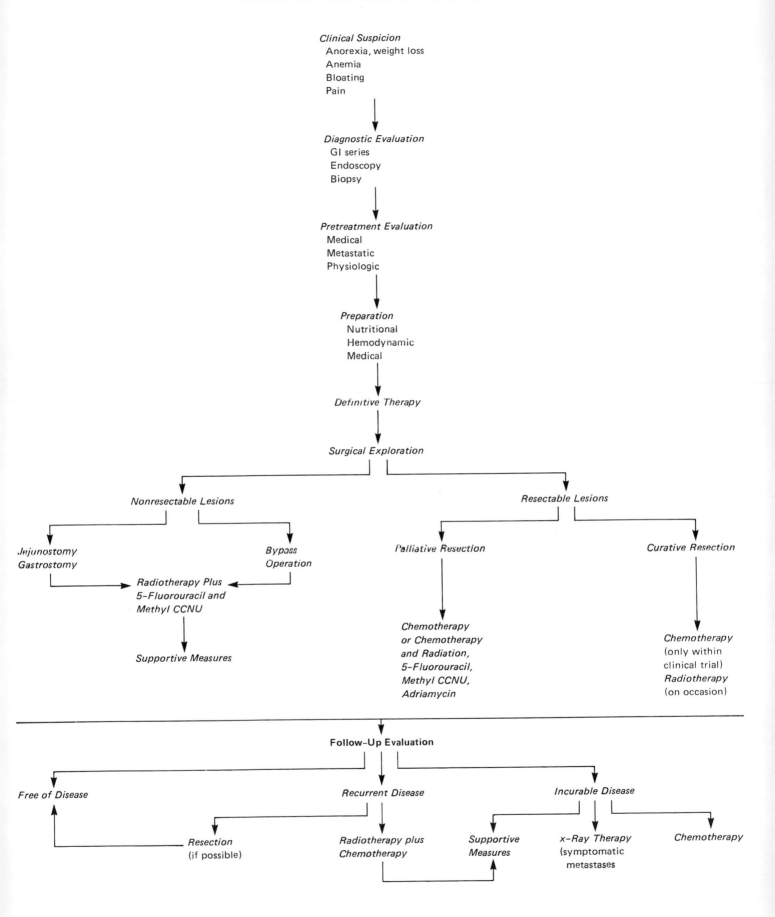

Clinical Suspicion
  Anorexia, weight loss
  Anemia
  Bloating
  Pain

Diagnostic Evaluation
  GI series
  Endoscopy
  Biopsy

Pretreatment Evaluation
  Medical
  Metastatic
  Physiologic

Preparation
  Nutritional
  Hemodynamic
  Medical

Definitive Therapy

Surgical Exploration

Nonresectable Lesions

Jejunostomy
Gastrostomy

Bypass Operation

Radiotherapy Plus 5-Fluorouracil and Methyl CCNU

Supportive Measures

Resectable Lesions

Palliative Resection

Curative Resection

Chemotherapy or Chemotherapy and Radiation, 5-Fluorouracil, Methyl CCNU, Adriamycin

Chemotherapy (only within clinical trial) *Radiotherapy* (on occasion)

Follow-Up Evaluation

Free of Disease

Recurrent Disease

Incurable Disease

Resection (if possible)

Radiotherapy plus Chemotherapy

Supportive Measures

x-Ray Therapy (symptomatic metastases)

Chemotherapy

Section 11. Carcinomas of the Alimentary Tract

Part B: Colorectal Cancer and Tumors of the Anus and Small Intestine

I. Early Detection and Screening of Colorectal Cancer   489
  A. Early Signs of Colorectal Cancer
  B. Screening
    1. Examination of the Stool for Occult Blood
    2. Proctosigmoidoscopy
  C. High-Risk Patients
II. Preoperative Evaluation, Work-Up, and Preparation of Patients with Colorectal Cancer   490
  A. Pretreatment Evaluation
    1. History and Physical Examination
    2. Laboratory Findings
    3. Carcinoembryonic Antigen
    4. Proctosigmoidoscopy
    5. Radiological Studies
      a. Barium Enema with Air Studies
      b. Intravenous Pyelography with Retrograde Studies
      c. Abdominal CAT Scan
      d. Lymphangiogram
    6. Metastatic Evaluation
    7. Staging
  B. Pretreatment Preparation
    1. General Preparation and Systemic Support
    2. Local Bowel Preparation
    3. Ureteral Catheterization
    4. Psychological Preparation
    5. Preparation of the Obstructed Patient
    6. Antibiotics
  C. Multidisciplinary Evaluation and Consultation
  D. Site-Specific Data Form for Colorectal Carcinoma
III. Pathological Considerations of Colorectal Carcinoma   492
  A. Gross Characteristics of the Tumor
  B. Microscopic Features
  C. Dukes's Classification
  D. Prognosis in Carcinoma of the Large Bowel
  E. Polyps of the Large Intestine
    1. Adenomatous Polyps
    2. Familial Polyposis
    3. Gardner's Syndrome
    4. Turcot Syndrome
    5. Villous Adenomas
IV. Therapeutic Management of Colorectal Carcinoma   496
  A. Surgery for Colorectal Carcinoma
  B. Radiotherapy in Colorectal Carcinoma
    1. Rationale

    2. Methodology
    3. Special Modalities and Newer Approaches
      a. Interstitial Therapy
      b. Intracavitary Irradiation
      c. Radiation Sensitizers
      d. Sandwich Techniques
      e. Intraoperative Irradiation
    4. Surgical Considerations Pertaining to Radiotherapy
  C. Chemotherapy for Colorectal Carcinoma
    1. Adjuvant Chemotherapy
    2. Treatment of Advanced Carcinoma
V. Postoperative Care, Psychological Support, Rehabilitation, and Evaluation of Patients with Colorectal Carcinoma   499
  A. Postoperative Care
    1. Immediate Postoperative Care
    2. Complications
    3. Wound and Skin Care
  B. Psychosocial Support
  C. Rehabilitation
    1. Skin Excoriation
    2. Odor and Gas
    3. Purchase of Supplies
    4. Irrigation of Colostomy
    5. Altered Body Image
  D. Follow-Up Evaluation
  E. Management Algorithm for Colorectal Carcinoma
VI. Carcinoma of the Anus   501
  A. General Considerations
  B. Therapeutic Management
    1. Surgery
      a. Excision of the Primary
      b. Groin Dissection
    2. Radiotherapy
    3. Chemotherapy
  C. Prognosis
VII. Neoplasms of the Small Intestine   504
  A. General Considerations
    1. Pathology
    2. Clinical Features
    3. Pretreatment Evaluation
  B. Therapeutic Management

Suggested Readings   504

I. EARLY DETECTION
AND SCREENING
OF COLORECTAL CANCER

Carcinoma of the large intestine in the United States is by and large the most common and most curable tumor of the GI tract, although only one-third of patients with these cancers are cured by present therapy. We must, therefore, actively explore various screening methods of detecting cancers earlier and thereby improving results.

A. Early Signs of Colorectal Cancer

The most common symptoms of colorectal cancer are

- Rectal bleeding.
- Constipation.
- Diarrhea or mucoid stools.
- Abdominal pain.
- Anemia.
- Anorexia and weight loss.
- Late onset of hernia in the elderly.

Intensive educational campaigns should be mounted to make *all* physicians and nurses well acquainted with these early signs so that they will constantly be alert to recognize them. Education of the public by groups such as the American Cancer Society should also be vigorously and widely pursued.

The establishment of the diagnosis of colorectal cancers is relatively easy; the standard diagnostic modalities are

- Digital rectal examination.
- Sigmoidoscopy.
- Fiberoptic colonoscopy.
- Barium enema examination.

B. Screening

To uncover patients with asymptomatic colorectal neoplasms, screening programs can and should be carried out in high-risk populations. Since these cancers are relatively rare in patients under age 40, most screening is done on people 40 years of age and older.

1. Examination of Stool for Occult Blood

The simplest technique for screening is the examination of the stool for the presence of occult blood, using one of several chemical methods (usually the guaiac agent). If the test is positive, the patients should then undergo sigmoidoscopy with barium enema, or total fiberoptic colonoscopy, to try and identify the source of bleeding. Most often, screening for colorectal cancer by fecal occult blood testing is done as part of an annual cancer detection screening examination or during routine annual physical examinations. To achieve the highest possible yield, particularly when the test is done for cancer detection in a high-risk patient, it should be repeated six times over 3 days, with the patient on a high-fiber, meat-free diet.

2. Proctosigmoidoscopy

There are differences of opinion whether all patients (outpatients and inpatients) 50 years of age or older should have a proctosigmoidoscopy examination performed annually as well as the testing for fecal occult blood. At present, it is recommended every 3–5 years or whenever indicated by any suggestive symptoms. Screening evaluations need to be intensified in certain selected groups of patients who are recognized as high-risk patients for colorectal cancer.

C. High-Risk Patients

The percentage of patients in the general population who are at high risk for colorectal cancer is at present unknown. There are, however, several clinical situations where the risk of colorectal cancer is greatly increased. These include

- *Chronic ulcerative colitis.* Patients with chronic ulcerative colitis are well recognized as high-risk patients for colorectal cancer. The process often starts as dysplasia frequently associated with an adenomatous growth pattern. It has been well documented that the chances of carcinoma in those patients increases with the duration of the illness and becomes very real after several years duration.

- *Colonic polyps and adenomas.* There appears to be a real continuum of neoplastic alterations from adenomas of the colon to invasive carcinoma. The "hyperplastic polyps" must be distinguished from the true "adenomatous polyps" in this respect, since they have no real precancerous potential. True adenomas of the colon have a 20–50% chance of being multiple and a 5% chance of having areas of carcinoma within them. The risk of cancer is greater in the larger (>2 cm) adenomas and in patients with multiple adenomas.
- *Multiple familial polyposis.* Gardner's syndrome, Peutz-Jeghers syndrome, Turcot syndrome, or juvenile polyposis have all been associated with a marked increase in incidence of colorectal cancer.
- *Patients with a prior history of colon cancer.*
- *Various pathological lesions of the anal areas.* Carcinoma of the anus proper is often associated with anal fissures, fistulas, condylomats, etc., especially when these are chronic in nature.

The high-risk patient must be approached differently from the general population:

- The patient with chronic ulcerative colitis of more than 7 year's duration should have total colonoscopy and multiple biopsies every year.
- Patients with prior history of adenoma should have total colonoscopy either every year or every other year. Those with prior history of colon cancer should have colonoscopy every year.
- Patients with familial polyposis must be approached even more aggressively. Because the cancer risks are so high, all of these patients should be seriously considered for a total colectomy to be performed before the cancer can develop. The exact timing of the operation will depend on individual circumstances, but until the colon is removed, the physician must be exceedingly vigilant in studying the colon at regular intervals by fiberoptic colonoscopy and/or barium enema, to uncover any developing carcinoma at an early stage.

In addition, there have been many attempts to correlate the incidence of colorectal cancer to dietary habits. There seems to be an increased risk among individuals falling in the following categories: high consumption of red meats (e.g., beef), high cholesterol diet, and obesity. Diets rich in fiber seem to protect against colorectal cancer, and increased selenium in the soil of some geographic farm areas (for example, in the western United States) seem to be associated with a lower incidence of colorectal cancer.

II. PREOPERATIVE EVALUATION AND PREPARATION OF PATIENTS WITH COLORECTAL CANCER

A. Pretreatment Evaluation

Naturally, every patient should have a complete history and physical examination as well as routine blood work profiles. In addition, several studies are required for every patient diagnosed with carcinoma of the colon or rectum:

1. History and Physical Examination

- Anorexia, weight loss.
- Anemia, pallor.
- Constipation.
- Recent onset of a hernia.
- Diarrhea, mucoid stool.
- Rectal bleeding.
- Tenesmus and pain.

These are all symptoms that need to be identified. In addition, a complete physical examination might uncover

- An abdominal mass or an enlarged, nodular liver.
- Ascites.
- A palpable rectal mass on digital examination.

Most patients with colorectal cancer are elderly and often seriously debilitated by their illness or other intercurrent conditions. Their evaluation must, therefore, also include a complete cardiopulmonary assessment and a search for other medical illnesses.

2. Laboratory Findings

A CBC, hematocrit, and blood volume determination must be carried out since many of these patients will have bled significantly. Serum electrolytes and a complete chemical blood profile (SMA-12 or SMA-20) should be obtained. Renal and hepatic function tests should be carefully screened.

3. Carcinoembryonic Antigen

The only tumor-associated antigen that was noted to be of any value as a marker in colorectal cancer is the carcinoembryonic antigen (CEA). The preoperative CEA level in itself is of little value but serves as a baseline for regular comparison with postoperative sequential determinations. These constitute, today, the best noninvasive method of assessing the completeness of the surgical resection, of evaluating the effectiveness of adjunctive chemotherapy or radiotherapy, and of detecting disseminated recurrences of the tumor. If the CEA level drops to a normal range postoperatively and then rises subsequently, a recurrence of the disease must be strongly suspected, and appropriate examinations are indicated to identify the disease.

4. Proctosigmoidoscopy

Sigmoidoscopy, or preferably, fiberoptic colonoscopy, is an integral part of the evaluation of the patient with colorectal cancer. Whenever a lesion, polyp, or cancer is discovered during proctoscopy, it should be biopsied and the histology of the tumor identified before definitive therapy is started. However, since the gross and x-ray appearance of colonic tumors are classic, laparotomy and resection of the tumor of the colon may be carried out in those cases where the diagnosis is established by x-ray, without biopsy if not feasible.

5. Radiological Studies

a. Barium Enema with Air Studies

This is still the pedestal of the work up of patients with colorectal cancer.

b. Intravenous Pyelography with Retrograde Studies

These are useful in identifying the local extent of the disease and any potential involvement or distortion of the urinary passages (particularly the bladder and ureters).

c. Abdominal CAT Scan

This is particularly useful for identifying any hepatic metastases or large, retroperitoneal masses or nodes.

d. Lymphangiogram

Lymphangiography may be indicated in cases of carcinoma of the anus because of the propensity of these tumors to spread to inguinal and iliac lymph nodes.

6. Metastatic Evaluation

The usual work-up for metastases must routinely be done:

- Chest x-ray.
- SMA-12.
- Liver scan (or CAT scan), if the liver function tests or clinical examination suggest any metastases.
- Bone scan, whenever bone metastases are suspected.

7. Staging

On the basis of these studies, a clinical stage can be established that will determine those patients who are amenable to "curative" operations and those who are not. Final staging, however, will only be made at the time of laparotomy, and completion of pathological staging must await the pathology report (see §11B.III. below and the Site-Specific Data Form, §11B.II.D).

B. Pretreatment Preparation

The general health of the patient should be restored to as close to normal as possible prior to therapy. This is particularly essential in patients who will be subjected to laparotomy, but is just as important in those patients treated by chemotherapy or radiation therapy.

1. General Preparation and Systemic Support

This may include blood transfusions, infusions of blood volume expanders (albumin or starch), high doses of vitamins by the oral or parenteral route, and in the occasional patient, a 1- or 2-week course of hyperalimentation. Compensation and correction of any preexisting medical illness should also be carried out (respiratory therapy, cardiac compensation, etc.). Correction of coagulation defects is imperative, and fluid and electrolyte balance must be restored (e.g., in cases of large, villous adenomas or partial obstruction).

2. Local Bowel Preparation

In patients undergoing operations on the colon or rectum, the preparation must include proper cleansing of the bowel for manipulation and possible division and anastomosis. This consists of vigorous mechanical cleansing (cathartics, fluid diet, and enemas) and chemical sterilization (antibiotics).

The regimens for antibiotic sterilization are now rather standardized. Two widely used, totally acceptable, and well-proven schedules are

- Neomycin-erythromycin. The patient is given 1 g of neomycin and 1 g of erythromycin base orally at 1 P.M., 2 P.M., and 11 P.M. on the day prior to the scheduled elective operation.
- Parenteral cefoxitin. The patient is given 2 g of cefoxitin intravenously preoperatively (on call to the operating room), 0.5 g during the operation, and four separate 1-g doses on the first postoperative day.

3. Ureteral Catheterization

If a preoperative intravenous pyelogram (IVP) has shown either displacement or obstruction of a ureter, it is wise to have ureteral catheters inserted prior to the laparotomy.

4. Psychological Preparation

One must not ignore the profound psychological impact that the presence of a colostomy will have on most patients; it is therefore mandatory in cases where a colostomy might be required, whether this be temporary or permanent, that someone, preferably the surgeon, discuss this possibility preoperatively and go over the many aspects of colostomy care with the patient. In addition, males who undergo abdominoperineal resection of the rectum very often suffer from impotence following the operation; this possibility should be presented and discussed with the patient prior to the surgery.

5. Preparation of the Obstructed Patient

Many patients with colorectal cancer first present with partial or complete large-bowel obstruction. If the obstruction is partial, the colon can often be sufficiently decompressed preoperatively to permit an elective operation. However, if the obstruction is nearly complete or complete, an emergency intervention to decompress the bowel must be done without any delay, ignoring any anemia, hypoproteinemia, and malnutrition. These will be corrected in the postoperative period while the patient is prepared for his or her definitive surgery. The decompression could be partial (i.e., cecostomy) or completely diverting (i.e., colostomy) and, at times, may be combined with resection of the tumor itself if the patient's condition allows.

6. Antibiotics

Systemic antibiotics should be used. They must be initiated a few hours preoperatively (or longer, when used for bowel preparation) and continued for 48 hours postoperatively. Antibiotics selected must be those effective against the gram negative organisms found in the lower GI tract.

C. Multidisciplinary Evaluation and Consultation

The importance of a multidisciplinary approach for consultation, evaluation, and treatment of the patient with colorectal carcinoma must be stressed.

Over the years, it has been felt that there has been a lack of cooperation between certain medical specialties when dealing with cancer of the colon. Besides the traditional areas of general surgery, radiotherapy, and medical oncology, other specialties can offer the patient an expertise that is most useful to total patient care. Nursing oncology, social services, gastroenterology, rehabilitation, psychiatry, radiology, and pathology are of prime importance.

The importance of the multidisciplinary approach is underscored by the general acceptance that colon cancer is responsive to radiation and that radiotherapy has an important role to play. The role of adjuvant or palliative chemotherapy is also gaining better precision and wider understanding.

D. Site-Specific Data Form for Colorectal Carcinoma (see pp. 493–494)

III. PATHOLOGICAL CONSIDERATIONS OF COLORECTAL CARCINOMA

A. Gross Characteristics of the Tumor

The usual adenocarcinoma of the large bowel is a bulky tumor with well-defined, rolled margins about an area of central ulceration. There is a sharp dividing line between the carcinoma and the normal bowel wall. The pathologist should determine whether the tumor is confined to the wall or whether it has extended to the pericolic tissues; large veins should be examined for gross invasion. If the tumor secretes a large amount of mucin, it has a mucoid, glairy appearance, and lakes of mucin may separate the layers of bowel wall. The nodes draining the tumor-bearing area are obviously important; if those distal to the tumor are found to be involved, it indicates retrograde involvement as a result of blockage of lymphatics at and above the level of the tumor. The lymph nodes at the highest point of the dissection, where the vessels are ligated, are also examined separately; the presence of tumor in these nodes indicates a great likelihood of spread of the disease beyond the resection.

Carcinoma of the anus may present as a localized ulceration; a small, raised tumor; or in the late stages, a larger exophytic ulcerated tumor with indurated edges.

B. Microscopic Features

The usual carcinoma of the large bowel is a well-differentiated adenocarcinoma secreting variable amounts of mucin. A

SITE-SPECIFIC DATA SHEET—COLORECTAL CARCINOMA

HISTORY

e: _____

mptoms
_____ Rectal pain
_____ Rectal bleeding
_____ Abdominal pain
_____ Weight loss _____ lbs.
_____ Anemia
_____ Diarrhea _____ Frequency _____ Duration
_____ Constipation _____ Frequency _____ Duration
_____ Obstruction
_____ Other
Duration _____
cial history
Occupation: _____
Race: ____ White ____ Black ____ Oriental ____ Other
Marital status: ____ Single ____ Married ____ Other

Family history of carcinoma
  Relation: _____ Site: _____
  _____ Polyps
  Relation: _____
  _____ Polyposis of colon
  Relation: _____
  _____ Chronic ulcerative colitis
  Relation: _____
Previous history of carcinoma
  _____ No _____ Yes Site: _____
  Rx: _____
Previous treatment (describe)
  (Surgery, radiation, chemotherapy, trachea)
  _____
  _____

PHYSICAL EXAMINATION

eneral condition: _____
_____

ectal examination: ____ Yes ____ No
Ray findings
  ize: _____
  olypoid: _____
  Japkin ring: _____
  Obstructing: _____

Abdomen
  Tenderness: _____
  Ascites: _____
  Distention: _____
  Mass: _____

PREOPERATIVE WORK-UP (Check, if done)

	Neg.	Pos.	Suspicious
emoccult	_____	_____	_____
octosigmoidoscopy	_____	_____	_____
rium enema	_____	_____	_____
olonoscopy	_____	_____	_____
EA	_____	_____	_____
AT scan	_____	_____	_____

	Neg.	Pos.	Suspicious
Liver chemistries	_____	_____	_____
Chest x-ray	_____	_____	_____
Bone scan	_____	_____	_____
IVP	_____	_____	_____
Cystoscopy	_____	_____	_____
Liver/spleen scan	_____	_____	_____

OPERATIVE STAGING

ze: _____ Gross character: _____
te: _____
esentery involvement ____ Yes ____ No
djacent involvement ____ Yes ____ No
Describe: _____

Nodal involvement ____ Yes ____ No
Liver involvement ____ Yes ____ No
Ascites ____ Yes ____ No

Fallopian tube
Ovary
Uterus
Bladder
Rectum

assification: ____ Dukes A ____ B1 ____ B2 ____ C ____ D
gnature: _____
ountersignature: _____
ate: _____

Rectum
Bladder
Prostate

Dukes' classification is the most commonly employed staging system for colon cancer and depends on depth of anatomic spread and presence or absence of nodal metastases. Broder's classification depends on the degree of anaplasia microscopically. Either classification may offer a rough guide to prognosis, but both are limited by variations in both depth and anaplasia within a given tumor. There is a new AJCCS classification which is based on surgical-pathologic evaluation.

Dukes' Classification

A. Invasion into submucosa or muscle. No nodal or distant metastases
B. Invasion into serosa. No nodal or distant metastases
C. Invasion through serosa and involvement of regional nodes
D. Distant metastases

TNM Classification

Primary tumor (T)

TX Depth of penetration not specified
T0 No clinically demonstrable tumor
TIS Carcinoma *in situ*
T1 Clinically benign lesion or lesion confined to the mucosa or submucosa
T2 Involvement of muscular wall, or serosa, no extension beyond
T3 Involvement of all layers of colon or rectum with extension to immediate adjacent structures or organs or both, with no fistula present
T4 Fistula present along with any of the above degrees of tumor penetration
T5 Tumor has spread by direct extension beyond the immediately adjacent organ or tissues

Nodal involvement (N)

NX Nodes not assessed or involvement not recorded
N0 Nodes not believed to be involved
N1 Regional nodes involved (distal to inferior mesenteric artery)

Distant metastasis (M)

MX Not assessed
M0 No (known) distant metastasis
M1 Distant metastasis present (specify)

Grade

Well-differentiated, moderately well differentiated, poorly differentiated, or very poorly differentiated (grade numbers 1, 2, 3, or 4, respectively)

Stage grouping

Stage 0   (TIS, N0, M0)
           Carcinoma *in situ* as demonstrated by histologic exam of tissue (biopsy or other)
Stage I   (Stage 1A)
           (T1, N0, M0 or T1, NX, M0)
           Tumor confined to mucosa or submucosa with no demonstrable metastasis, regional lymph nodes and no evidence of distant metastasis
Stage IB   (T2, N0, M0 or T2, NX, M0)
           Tumor involves muscularis but has not extended beyond serosa, with no demonstrable metastasis to regional lymph nodes, and no evidence of metastasis (Dukes' A)
Stage II   (T3-T5, N0, M0 or T3-T5, NX, M0)
           Tumor that has extended beyond the bowel wall or serosa, with no demonstrable metastasis to regional lymph nodes, and no evidence of distant metastasis (Dukes' B)
Stage III (Any T, N1, M0)
           Any degree of penetration of bowel or rectal wall by tumor, with metastasis to regional lymph nodes, but no evidence of distant metastasis (Dukes' C)
Stage IV   Any T, Any N, M1)
           Any degree of penetration of bowel or rectal wall by tumor, with or without metastasis to regional lymph nodes, with evidence of distant metastasis (Dukes' D)

desmoplastic reaction is consistently seen at the edge of the invasive tumor. In a few instances, there may be extremely large lakes of mucin with scattered collections of tumor cells. These mucinous carcinomas comprise 15% of colorectal carcinomas and occur most commonly in the rectum. Their prognosis is worse than for the common variety of adenocarcinoma.

In a few instances of large-bowel carcinoma, areas of squamous differentiation may be present. They can form the entirety of the tumor (epidermoid or squamous cell carcinoma) or be mixed with glandular focuses (adenosquamous carcinoma). In those cases that are located in the low rectum, the possibility of an upward extension or submucosal metastasis from a carcinoma of the anal canal should be considered.

Carcinomas arising in the anal region are epidermoid in nature, in contradistinction to the classical adenocarcinoma arising in the rectum.

There exists in the colon a rare type of carcinoma that is similar to the linitis plastica variant observed in the stomach; it affects younger patients and carries a very poor prognosis. This lesion exhibits poorly defined margins and a pebblelike mucosal surface.

C. Dukes's Classification

Dukes's staging system for rectal carcinomas can also be applied to cancers of the colon:

- Stage A tumors involve the wall of the bowel only.
- Stage B tumors extend through the wall. B1 denotes extension to the serosa only; B2 indicates involvement of the pericolic fat.
- Stage C tumors have lymph node metastases.

The 5-year survival rates average around 90%, 65%, and 20%, respectively in Dukes's A, B, and C carcinomas of the colon.

D. Prognosis in Carcinoma of the Large Bowel

The following is a guideline to the outlook for various colon carcinomas according to their histological nature.

Excellent prognosis	Carcinoma in a polyp without invasion of the stalk. Carcinoma in a villous adenoma limited to the mucosa and submucosa. Carcinoma limited to the mucosa and submucosa.

Only under exceptional circumstances do metastases develop in any of the foregoing groups.

Good prognosis	Carcinoma limited to the wall of the bowel without lymph node metastases (Dukes's A).
Fair prognosis	Carcinoma with lymph node metastases limited to the immediate area of the tumor.
Poor-to-hopeless prognosis	Signet-ring mucin-secreting carcinoma. Extensive lymph node metastases. Gross or microscopic evidence of vein invasion. Microscopic evidence of perineural invasion. Retrograde lymph node metastases. Any evidence of metastatic spread (e.g., liver, mesentery, etc.).

E. Polyps of the Large Intestine

Although the specific relationship is not known, epithelial polyps of the colon are in some way related to the development of cancer of the colon. Because of this fact, it is generally accepted that all polyps in the colon should be removed or destroyed, if the patient's condition permits.

1. Adenomatous Polyps

Adenomatous polyps (tubular adenomas) may be distributed throughout the large intestine. They may be multiple or single, and focal areas of villous configuration are not infrequent in these adenomatous polyps. The incidence of carcinoma appears to be related to the size of the polyp, reaching 75% in lesions larger than 1 cm in diameter. It is further believed that these polyps, even when totally benign, will undergo malignant degeneration.

2. Familial Polyposis

Familial polyposis of the large bowel must be segregated from other polyps. This defect is inherited as an autosomal Mendelian dominant trait with a high degree of penetrance. Carcinomatous change in this lesion occurs early, resulting in carcinomas some 20 years earlier than in the ordinary cases of bowel cancer (usually in the early 30s). A minimum of 100 polyps needs to be present before such a diagnosis can be justified on morphological grounds.

3. Gardner's Syndrome

In rare instances, familial polyposis may involve the entire GI tract. Gardner's syndrome is a familial condition in which adenomatous polyps of the large bowel are seen associated with multiple osteomas of the skull and mandible, multiple keratinous cysts of the skin, and soft-tissue neoplasms, especially fibromatosis. Adenomatous polyps may also be present in the small bowel. The potential for development of large-bowel cancer appears to be as high as in familial polyposis. In addition, patients with this syndrome can develop carcinomas of the small bowel, particularly in the periampullar area.

4. Turcot Syndrome

Turcot syndrome is a combination of colonic adenomatous polyps and brain tumors. The pattern of inheritance is autosomal recessive.

5. Villous Adenomas

Villous adenomas (villous papilloma) is a distinctive, relatively infrequent type of polyp that usually presents as a single lesion and occurs in the rectum or rectosigmoid of older patients. It eventually forms a large, superficial neoplasm that may encircle the bowel. It has papillary villous projections and is usually attached by a wide base. The recorded incidence of carcinoma in villous adenomas has ranged from 29 to 70%.

IV. THERAPEUTIC MANAGEMENT OF COLORECTAL CARCINOMA

A. Surgery for Colorectal Cancer

The backbone of treatment for colorectal carcinoma is surgery. When first diagnosed, nearly all patients will require either resection of a section of colon or rectum, whether curative or palliative, or a colostomy. Upon entering the abdomen, the surgeon must first carry out a careful exploration of the entire abdomen as part of a staging procedure. A careful determination of the size and character of the tumor and any attachments or fistulization should be made; identification of any evidence of clinical spread to lymph nodes or other adjacent organs (ovary, bladder, pancreas, etc.) and a search for any evidence of metastases (especially to the liver) or peritoneal seeding must also be carried out.

A properly executed radical operation for cancer will include resection of a long segment of colon with its mesentery, which includes the regional lymph node draining areas. It is impossible to remove a sufficient number of draining lymph nodes unless a long enough segment of bowel is resected. The extent of resection, however, will depend on the site of the tumor as well as on other pertinent circumstances. Resections are then followed in most instances by end-to-end anastomoses of the intestine. End-to-side anastomoses (Baker's) or side-to-end anastomoses (in low anterior sigmoid resections) are also acceptable. In many palliative resections, the proximal end is brought out as a colostomy; the distal end is closed over and permitted to retract in the abdomen or is brought out as a mucous fistula. Other organs or adjacent tissues that are attached to the cancer should be removed with the colon if there appears to be a chance of removing all the disease; this should be carried out as an en-bloc resection whenever possible.

Patients with colonic obstruction are often operated upon as emergencies. If the lesion is on the right side, an emergency right hemicolectomy can be done with a primary end-to-end ileo transverse colon anastomosis. More often, the obstruction is secondary to a left colon lesion, in which case the best treatment is an emergency transverse colostomy. The cancer operation can then be done electively 2–3 weeks later, and the colostomy can be closed a few weeks after that. It is possible at times to convert this three-stage procedure to a two-stage procedure either by resecting the tumor at the first stage and doing a proximal colostomy to be closed later or by resecting the distal colostomy end during the second stage at the time of the resection of the tumor and using the proximal colostomy end for the permanent anastomosis.

Carcinomas of the rectum require a slightly different surgical approach in that a distal stump is often not available for primary anastomosis; a permanent colostomy thus becomes necessary in many cases. Depending on the level of the tumor and its extent, one of the following procedures can be done:

- Anterior resection with low anastomosis (for lesions above 15 cm from the anocutaneous line, or even lower than that, depending on the habitat of the patient and the surgeon's skills).
- Anterior abdominal resection with pull-through and perineal anastomosis (for intermediate lesions between 8 and 15 cm from the anal verge).
- Sacral exposure with resection and low anastomosis.
- Abdominoperineal resection with permanent colostomy (for all lesions below 8–10 cm from the anal line).

The use of sphincter-saving operations has been demonstrated as being quite effective; cure rates are not likely to be significantly compromised, and functional results are quite satisfactory. It has been suggested that preservation of the lower third of the rectum is necessary for effective control of defecation; much lesser amounts have been spared in pull-through procedures, and control seems eventually to return (within 3–6 months) in most of these patients.

Fulguration of low-lying rectal lesions with or without radiotherapy is also an acceptable procedure in elderly or ill patients and may result in significant symptom-free survival.

Carcinomas arising in patients with multiple polyposis or ulcerative colitis require total colectomy with either low anastomosis or permanent ileostomy.

Although no consensus exists regarding the use of postoperative adjuvant chemotherapy or radiotherapy following "curative" resections of the colorectum, the benefits of postoperative radiotherapy in Stage IIB and Stage IIC carcinomas of the rectosigmoid are now well documented. A multidisciplinary panel, which is consulted either preoperatively or after the resection is completed, is undoubtedly the best way to plan total therapy for any individual case. This committee, however, strongly recommends that—following "curative" resections for Dukes B2 or Dukes C lesions in the sigmoid, rectosigmoid, or rectum—an appropriate course of radiotherapy be given (see §11B.IV.B.3.d).

For patients with lesions that are not amenable to "curative" resections, any combination of palliative surgical procedures may be considered in an effort to remove or destroy the tumor. These might include resection and anastomosis, exteriorization resection, Hartman operation with proximal colostomy and distal blind pouch, pull through or abdominoperitoneal resection, transanal resection and fulguration, etc. Failing this, a colostomy may go a long way to achieve relief of symptoms.

The following general guidelines may be suggested in the surgical treatment of colorectal cancer:

- Generous incision for effective exposure and ease of manipulation (e.g., xyphoid process to pubis incision).
- Thorough abdominal exploration.
- Gentle manipulation and ligation of the bowel above and below the tumor to minimize intraluminal tumor spillage.
- Early control of the venous return and arterial supply of the segment to be resected is desirable whenever possible.
- Wide segments of bowel resected according to the site of the lesion, resection of mesentry and lymphatic drainage sites.
- Bloc resection of all resectable adjacent organs involved (including even liver segments or abdominal wall).
- Placement of metal clips in areas suspected of having residual disease, to guide the radiotherapist.
- Placement of a hepatic artery catheter for postoperative chemotherapy in cases of multiple liver metastases (or ligation of the hepatic artery) should be considered where such clinical trials are available to evaluate intra-arterial chemotherapy.
- Generous use of proximal decompression in tenuous anastomoses.
- Secure abdominal closure.

B. Radiotherapy in Colorectal Carcinoma

1. Rationale

Failures of radical operative procedures appear to be the result of subclinical microscopic disease that is left behind.

Neither the use of radical surgery nor extensive lymph node dissections have significantly improved the survival rates of colorectal carcinoma. Once local recurrence has occurred, the chances of controlling the disease by radiotherapy are almost nil; doses in the amount of 6000–6500 rads are needed to achieve pain palliation and result in complete disappearance of the recurrent masses in only 15% of cases.

Since local-regional failures constitute the major problem with colorectal carcinoma, radiation appears to be the logical adjuvant therapy to "curative surgery." Local failure and/or regional lymph node spread occur as the only failure in 40–50% of cases and in combination with distant metastases in an additional 40%. Once the lesion has extended through the entire bowel wall, infiltration into surrounding tissues or structures occurs readily, and the exact extent of the disease is difficult to diagnose or remove surgically. Likewise, as the number and size of involved lymph nodes increases, tumor extension through the nodal capsule into the adjacent tissues becomes more likely, and complete operative removal also becomes less likely.

There are specific pathological subgroups of colorectal carcinoma that have excellent survival rates and a low incidence of local-regional failure with surgery alone and therefore receive little or no benefit from local-regional adjuvant modalities such as radiotherapy. Many series have shown that this is the case for patients in whom the primary lesion is confined to the bowel wall and nodes are not involved (Dukes's A). Survival rates decrease, however, and local-regional failures increase, when lesions extend completely through the bowel wall, whether nodes are involved or not (Dukes's B; Astler-Coller B2). Radiotherapy, therefore, appears to be indicated as an adjuvant to surgery in all patients, with Dukes's B2 or C tumors, particularly in the rectum.

2. Methodology

Patterns of local-regional failure fall within a distribution suitable for inclusion within an extended radiation field. A field covering the perineum inferiorly and extending upward to the level of LIII–LIV covers most of the sites of the local-regional failures of colorectal cancer.

Data on time and site of failures indicate that any postoperative adjuvant should be started as soon as possible, preferably within 2–6 weeks of surgery. With longer delays, tumor growth could increase to the extent that tolerable moderate doses of radiation therapy would then be inadequate to sterilize residual disease. Several authors have presented data showing that the required curative dose for radiation is dependent on the initial bulk of disease. Subclinical or minimal residual disease can be controlled with doses of only 4500–5000 rads in 4.5–5.0 weeks.

There is a difference of opinion regarding the preferred sequence of surgery and radiation for colorectal carcinoma. Postoperative radiotherapy would have certain major advantages over preoperative irradiation:

- Accurate staging of the disease.
- The total extent of the tumor with regard to the local lesion, lymph nodes, and distant metastases would be known and could be tagged during the surgery.
- Smaller volume of tumor to be treated.
- Those patients who are identified not to be at risk for local-regional failure (15–30% of patients with Dukes's A or B1 lesions).
- Postoperative radiation would not interfere with the operative approach and would permit the removal of all known carcinoma and the placement of clips around any potential residual disease for radiation purposes.
- The postoperative approach could be utilized in patients with very low anterior resections as well as in those with abdominoperineal resections and, therefore, would potentially benefit a larger number of patients. If preoperative radiotherapy is used, even in moderate (4000–5000 rads) doses, abdominoperineal resection seems to be advisable in all cases because of the increased risk of anastomatic leaks with low anterior resections after radiotherapy.

Preoperative radiotherapy is indicated in those patients with bulky, unresectable tumors and may have the advantages of treating virgin well-oxygenated cells and reducing the viability of cells that may be spilled during surgery.

3. Special Modalities and Newer Approaches

a. Interstitial Therapy

Interstitial therapy is useful in the management of low-lying rectal cancers in conjunction with external irradiation to the perineum. Radium, iridium seeds, or occasionally tantalum wires were utilized.

b. Intracavitary Irradiation

This method, introduced in France in 1952, has been reported to yield excellent results in well-selected cases:

- Well-differentiated tumors.
- Tumors less than 5 cm in diameter.
- Tumors no more than 10 cm from the anal verge.
- Only Dukes's A tumors.

Therapy is administered through a 3-cm proctoscope using low-voltage machines. A high dose can thus be delivered to a small volume.

Complications are few when the treatment is carefully applied; mild mucous discharge, local discomfort, and a minimal proctitis may occur. Results with radiation are good and may avoid the colostomy that is usually necessary with surgery for

these lesions. Local control is quite high (>90%), and failures may still be treated surgically.

c. Radiation Sensitizers

5-Fluorouracil, mitomycin, and metronidazole have been used as radiation sensitizers with some promise. Their application is, however, still experimental.

d. Sandwich Techniques

Several trials are presently underway combining the advantage of pre- and postoperative radiotherapy, using a single preoperative dose of 500 rads within 24 hours of the anticipated surgery. This is then followed by 4500 rads in 5 weeks postoperatively for those patients found to have Dukes's B2 or C tumors. Early results in small numbers of patients are extremely promising.

e. Intraoperative Irradiation

There is a good deal of interest being presently expressed in the use of a single large dose of intraoperative irradiation as a boost for the treatment of advanced or recurrent rectal cancer by external irradiation. Electron beam irradiation to a dose of 1500 rads can be delivered to a limited area with effective protection of adjacent organs. The method is cumbersome, however, difficult to institute, and must still be considered experimental.

f. Adjuvant Studies

There are several multi-institutional randomized prospective studies in progress both in Europe and in the United States to evaluate the value of adjuvant radiotherapy and/or chemotherapy in the treatment of colorectal cancer. Results are so far inconclusive, at times conflicting, and require more time for accurate evaluation. The G.I. Tumor Study Group has reported a reduced incidence of local failures in rectal cancer patients randomized to receive postoperative radiotherapy as compared with patients treated by surgery alone.

4. Surgical Considerations Pertaining to Radiotherapy

Postoperative radiation could be utilized following either anterior or abdominoperineal resections but would be less satisfactory following a pull-through procedure. Since a moderate number of patients with pelvic radiation may develop radiation-induced diarrhea during treatment, a patient with a pull-through procedure and initial lack of decent sphincter control is therefore not a good candidate for radiotherapy. The choice of operative procedure should not, however, be dictated by the possibility of adjuvant therapy. Anterior resections are, whenever feasible, preferable to abdominoperineal resections for the following reasons:

- Less disruption of pelvic anatomy with decrease in postoperative scarring, less disruption of the vascular bed, and less of a problem with small bowel dropping within the pelvis;
- Faster rate of healing (unless the perineum was closed primarily at the time of abdominoperineal resection), which allows the institution of radiotherapy at an earlier phase.

C. Chemotherapy for Colorectal Carcinoma

Whereas surgical treatment and radiotherapy have been shown to be very effective in colorectal cancer, the role of chemotherapy is not well established.

1. Adjuvant Chemotherapy

A number of drugs have been evaluated as adjuvant agents in the past, but the results have shown little or no improvement in survival. At the present time, national cooperative groups are studying two different treatment regimens:

- 5-FU plus methyl CCNU. Several studies are already underway. Early reports indicate no benefit resulting from its use.
- A combination of 5-FU plus methyl CCNU plus vincristine. This large study is now well underway, but the code has not been broken and results are therefore not known.

2. Treatment of Advanced Carcinoma

The same drugs, namely, a combination of 5-FU and methyl CCNU, have resulted in approximately 20% objective response in several studies. However, the response is short lived, and the long-term yield is disappointingly poor.

For the treatment of hepatic metastases specifically, perfusion of the hepatic artery with floxuridine (FUDR) (with or without low-dose radiotherapy) has been used with some reported salutory results.

V. POSTOPERATIVE CARE, PSYCHOSOCIAL SUPPORT, REHABILITATION, AND EVALUATION OF PATIENTS WITH COLORECTAL CARCINOMA

A. Postoperative Care

1. Immediate Postoperative Care

The three basic issues that must be addressed during this period are physical needs, metabolic needs, and psychosocial support. Vital signs, urine output, electrolytes, and blood chemistries must be monitored frequently during the initial postoperative phase.

Colostomies that have not been opened during the surgical procedure are usually opened during the second or third day postoperatively. Liquid stool is not usually seen until the fifth day, as mucus and fluid are usually present prior to that time. Fluid loss may be greater from the perineal wound than from the stoma, and this may persist for weeks after the procedure has been carried out.

Nutritional factors should not be overlooked; it is imperative that adequate weight and caloric intake be maintained. Clear liquids are started after the nasogastric tube is removed, and the diet is gradually advanced as tolerated. Instructions about foods to be avoided should be provided to the patient and family. If oral intake is not possible, intravenous hyperalimentation should be considered. Every effort should be made to contact the dietician and include the family members in any teaching sessions.

2. Complications

It is best to attempt to avoid protracted complications through early recognition of signs and symptoms and prompt action. The most common complications seen include

- Damage to ureters and/or bladder (hematuria may be a presenting sign).
- Neurogenic bladder and retention.
- Thrombus formation.
- Electrolyte imbalance.
- Bowel obstruction.
- Wound infection.
- Pulmonary complications.
- Ileus.
- Stoma complications: discoloration; skin excoriation; stoma prolapse, retraction, or separation; necrosis, etc.

3. Wound and Skin Care

After opening of the ostomy, the stoma should be covered to prevent contamination of the operative site (a temporary appliance should be considered). Sterile technique should be maintained during care of the operative site but does not need to be observed for care of the stoma.

If a perineal incision is present, sitting may cause discomfort. Sitz baths should be recommended later on, as they will help the healing process.

If the wound is closed, a drain may be left in place, to be removed by the tenth postoperative day.

Frequent observation, gentleness, and optimum skin care must be provided for these patients. If available, an enterostomal therapist should be consulted to provide skin care, psychosocial support, and adequate information to the patient and family. If appliances do not fit properly, skin integrity cannot be maintained. As mentioned previously, temporary appliances are used in the immediate postoperative period until shrinkage of the stoma is complete. The type of appliance ordered will depend upon the patient's needs. If the patient has a permanent sigmoid colostomy, he or she may be taught to control bowel movements by diet and irrigations and thus perhaps function without the use of an ostomy bag.

B. Psychosocial Support

If the patient is to return to his or her optimum level of health in relation to his or her roles in the community and with family, it is imperative for the hospital staff to consider adequate patient teaching methods and tools during the preoperative period. This important aspect of patient care can relieve anxiety and allay fears. Teaching methods must be geared to the patient's needs, since the patient who is not ready to learn or discuss his or her problems will not benefit from these interventions. The reactions of the patient and family regarding the diagnosis and treatment must be considered.

Privacy should be encouraged, and those health professionals trained in the care of patients with ostomies should be consulted on a regular basis. Nurses, enterostomal therapists, psychologists, social workers, clergy members, and even rehabilitated ostomates should become a part of the health care team.

One area of great importance and one that is very often skipped over by health professionals is the topic of sexuality and body image. Accurate information must be provided in order to decrease beliefs in myths. Health professionals should be aware of resources available for assistance, especially if the subject is a difficult one to approach.

C. Rehabilitation

The following problems and solutions need to be addressed in the rehabilitation of the patient with colorectal cancer:

1. Skin Excoriation

This may occur due to irritation from leakage of feces.
Intervention:

- Consult an enterostomal therapist to check proper fit of appliance.
- Provide diet instruction, and include family and dietician in sessions.
- Keep area surrounding stoma clean and dry.
- Secure appliance to prevent leakage.

2. Odor and Gas

Intervention:

- Instruct patient to chew food slowly with mouth closed to reduce air intake and gas formation.
- Provide patient with information about gas-forming foods to avoid.
- Use appliance anti-odor properties.
- Consider use of external deodorants.
- Instruct patient to use an aspirin or charcoal tablet in the ostomy bag.
- Teach patient to cover stoma with finger when expelling flatus to avoid noise.

3. Purchase of Supplies

Intervention:

- Provide patient and family with telephone numbers of agencies (American Cancer Society), supply companies, ostomy clubs.
- Refer patient to a social worker (the patient may need assistance with financial problems).

4. Irrigation of Colostomy

Intervention:

- Teach the patient to observe the amount, color, and odor of fecal drainage.
- Encourage slow rate of water flow during irrigation, especially if cramping persists.
- Try to determine the reasons for poor returns if that problem presents itself.
- If diarrhea exists, stop irrigations, provide adequate skin care, and encourage patient to use antidiarrheal medications (under the advice of the physician).

5. Altered Body Image

It is important for patients to understand and accept changes in lifestyle, body image, sexual adjustment, and independence.
Intervention:

- Demonstrate confidence and a hopeful attitude.
- Encourage the patient to verbalize his or her feelings, taking cues from the patient's behavior.
- Assist the patient to look at the stoma for the first time.
- Encourage self-care with support and teaching methods.
- Encourage visits from a rehabilitated ostomate.
- Refer the patient to a psychologist, clergy member, nurse oncologist, and/or social worker for counseling, if needed.

Table I

Long-Term Follow-Up Schedule for Colorectal Carcinoma

Management	First two years			Third to fifth years		Thereafter, annually
	Every 3 months	Every 6 months	Annually	Every 6 months	Annually	
History						
Complete		X		X	X	X
Appetite and digestion	X			X		X
Condition of stool	X			X		X
Abdominal pain	X			X		X
Weight loss	X			X		X
Performance	X			X		X
Other						
Physical						
Complete			X		X	X
Abdomen and liver	X			X		X
Rectal or stoma	X			X		X
Andenopathy	X			X		X
Female-breast			X		X	X
Female-pelvic			X		X	X
Female pap smear			X		X	
Sigmoidoscopy or colonoscopy		X			X	X
Investigation						
CBC-urine		X			X	X
Stool for blood	X			X		X
Chest x-ray, barium enema			X		X	
CEA			A s i n d i c a t e d			
SMA 12		X			X	X
Liver scan		Monthly for the first 2 years; every 3 months for the next 3 years; then annually				
CAT scan		Monthly for the first 2 years; every 3 months for the next 3 years; then annually				

D. Follow-Up Evaluation

See Table I for the recommended follow-up schedule.

E. Management Algorithm for Colorectal Cancer (see p. 502)

VI. CARCINOMA OF THE ANUS

A. General Considerations

Carcinomas arising in the anal area are predominantly epidermoid (squamous cell) in type in contradistinction to the adenocarcinomas that arise in the rectum. They are seen more commonly in men and are very often associated with other pathological lesions in the anal area, such as fistulas, fissures, condylomas, etc. The lesions may present as a localized ulceration; as a small, raised firm or soft tumor; or in the late stages, as a large, ulcerated tumor with indurated edges. Because of the lymphatic drainage of the region, the inguinal lymph nodes on one or both sides are often enlarged; the adenopathy may be the result either of a benign inflammatory swelling as a result of drainage from an ulcerated lesion or of involvement by metastatic carcinoma.

Other malignant neoplasms of the anus and perianal skin area are less common but worthy of mention:

- Bowen's disease (intraepithelial squamous cell cancer).
- Basal cell cancer, usually locally invasive.
- Paget's disease, which represents the skin manifestation of an underlying glandular carcinoma of skin appendages or of the rectum itself.
- Malignant melanoma, usually noted for its aggressive behavior and poor prognosis, especially when it presents with palpable nodes in the groin.
- Malignant lymphoma.
- Giant malignant condyloma.

There are no characteristic symptoms of anal carcinoma. Most patients present with symptoms that mimic those of hemorrhoids, fissures, fistulas, hypertrophied papillae, etc. Delay in diagnosis is very common, either because the patient has

ALGORITHM FOR CANCER OF THE COLORECTUM

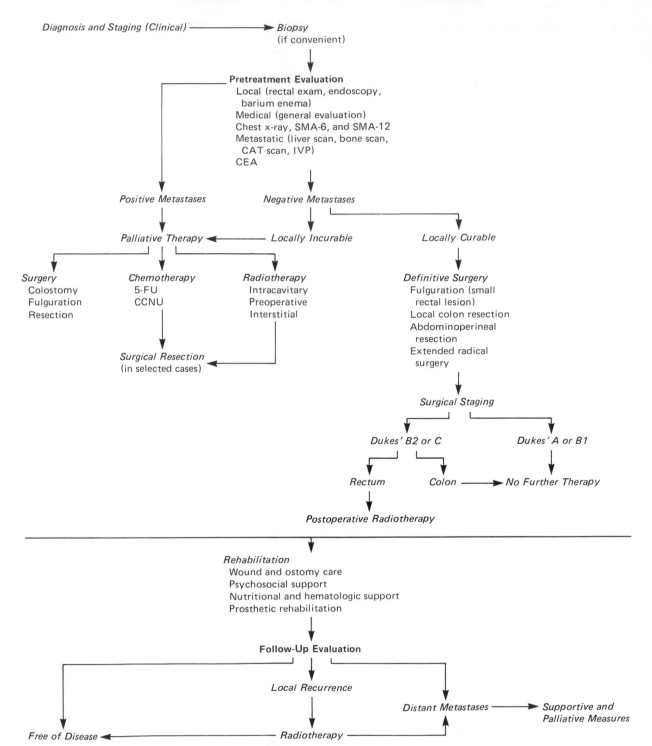

attributed the symptoms to "hemorrhoids" or because the clinician, even after examination, believes that a benign pathological condition exists. The large, indurated lesions that are seen late in the course of the disease will raise strong suspicion.

Early detection can only be encouraged by public education and by a high degree of alertness on the part of the primary care physician. All patients with anorectal complaints must be carefully examined to rule out the presence of cancer and, at the slightest suspicion, a biopsy should be carried out without delay.

The pretreatment evaluation of the patient must include

- Biopsy of the tumor (punch biopsy or incisional biopsy) to confirm the diagnosis.
- Proctosigmoidoscopy to assess the extent of the disease.
- Inguinal and abdominal examination to identify any groin or intra-abdominal masses (iliac nodes, enlarged liver, etc.).
- Total physical examination.
- Routine blood work (CBC, SMA-12 and liver profile, renal function tests, etc.).

Once the diagnosis is made, the usual screening for metastases similar to that obtained for other colorectal tumors is carried out prior to therapy. In addition, because the lymphatic drainage from the anal area is to the inguinal nodes, as well as upward along the rectum, a bipedal lymphangiogram of the inguinal and iliac nodes may be helpful in determining the extent of spread and the type and magnitude of surgical therapy.

Blood, vitamin, and protein stores are replenished preoperatively and, because in most instances a rather major operation on the rectum will be carried out, careful preparation of the colon by mechanical cleansing and preoperative sterilization will be indicated.

B. Therapeutic Management

1. Surgery

a. Excision of the Primary

For many years the accepted treatment for anal carcinoma has been wide surgical excision; the extent will depend on the location and stage of the disease. For lesions extending above the pectinate line, standard abdominoperineal resection of the rectum is necessary because these tumors can and do spread to the lymph nodes in the mesosigmoid as well as to lymph nodes along the internal and common iliac vessels. For tumors confined to the anus or perianal region, a wide local excision is usually adequate, although on occasion an abdominoperineal resection might be needed. These tumors rarely metastasize to the internal pelvic structures.

b. Groin Dissection

The frequency with which the inguinal nodes are involved in carcinoma of the anus dictates a therapeutic approach that selectively includes these nodes in most patients. Because the morbidity of bloc dissections in the groin is so high (i.e., because of poor healing, infection, lymphedema of the extremity, etc.), it is unwise to perform routine inguinal node dissections. The present-day approach includes dissection of these nodes in selected patients:

- If the nodes are obviously involved on clinical examination, a bloc dissection in one or both groins is done after the patient has recovered from the original operation.
- If the nodes are not clinically involved, no prophylactic bloc dissection is done.
- If, in the course of follow-up, the nodes become enlarged, the bloc dissection is done at that time.

The use of adjuvant radiotherapy to the groin is under trial in cases where there is no palpable disease and might obviate the need for inguinal lymphadenectomy.

2. Radiotherapy

Patients with anal carcinoma have been treated by radiotherapy for various forms in a large number of centers throughout the world. The results, however, are insufficient for conclusive recommendations, and surgical therapy continues to be the standard approach. Squamous cell cancers, however, respond well to radiotherapy, and adequate control may be expected in early cases. Combined approaches using preoperative radiotherapy followed by surgery have been embarked upon in more advanced cases, but results from such studies have not as yet been reported in significant numbers.

For large or extending tumors that cannot be removed by surgery, radiation therapy should be the primary approach. Palliation is often the only accomplishment in such cases since the delivery of radical or curative irradiation is rarely possible. Supportive therapy, particularly drugs to relieve pain, is also necessary, and if pain, odor, or drainage are serious problems, a sigmoid colostomy to redirect the fecal stream is often very helpful for the relief of symptoms.

3. Chemotherapy

There is a paucity of data regarding chemotherapy in carcinoma of the anus. Scattered case reports indicate activity for several agents, including 5-FU, Adriamycin, bleomycin, etc., a list of agents similar to those employed in epidermoid cancers of the head and neck. The use of induction preoperative chemotherapy, with or without postoperative radiotherapy, is presently under clinical trial investigation.

C. Prognosis

If patients are seen early enough so that "curative" surgical resection can be done, 5-year cure rates of 50–55% can be realized. Results with radiotherapy in limited lesions are also very similar.

VII. NEOPLASMS
OF THE SMALL INTESTINE

A. General Considerations

1. Pathology

Neoplasms of the small bowel are rare if one compares their incidence with that of the stomach, colon, rectum, and pancreas. They do, however, present a fascinating array of tumors representing all the cell types seen in the intestine. About half the primary tumors are benign; these include adenomatous polyps, fibromas, hemangiomas, lymphangiomas, leiomyomas, neurofibromas, and neurilemmomas and lipomas. The polypoid tumors found in the Peutz-Jeghers syndrome are not true tumors but constitute hamartomas. The malignant counterpart of these benign tumors can also be seen, and in addition, there are primary lymphomas of the small intestine and carcinoid tumors arising from the Kulchitsky cells. All malignant tumors can spread through the lymphatics to the nodes in the mesentery and via the bloodstream to the liver and distant tissues. Metastases to the small intestine are quite rare but have been seen with melanoma and breast cancer.

2. Clinical Features

Many benign neoplasms are asymptomatic and are only discovered by serendipity or at autopsy. The most common symptoms of small-bowel tumors are

- Pain, resulting from obstruction or intussusception.
- Gastrointestinal bleeding resulting from ulceration. This is often manifested by anemia and gross or microscopic evidence of rectal bleeding.
- Small-bowel obstruction, distention, nausea, vomiting, etc.
- Periorbital pigmentation may be noted in association with Peutz-Jeghers syndrome.
- Diarrhea can be seen in functioning carcinoid tumors that produce serotonin. If there are widespread metastases from carcinoid tumors, the "carcinoid syndrome" (i.e., diarrhea, flushing, vasomotor instability, asthma, and cardiac lesions) can result.
- Obstructive jaundice. Because the majority of malignant ad-

enocarcinomas of the small intestine arise in the duodenum, they can lead to obstruction of the common bile duct, resulting in jaundice. These tumors can only be differentiated from other lesions causing jaundice by extensive work-up, by fiberoptic endoscopy, or at the operating table. These periampullary lesions are described in §11C.V.A.3.

3. Pretreatment Evaluation

Most diagnoses of small-bowel tumors are made at the operating table or in the autopsy room. In the patient with vague, nonspecific abdominal pain due to small-bowel tumor, a barium study of the intestine will occasionally uncover the lesion, and elective surgery can then be undertaken; sometimes the study will uncover multiple tumors. It is, however, nearly impossible to determine if a tumor is benign or malignant by x-ray or any other studies.

If a carcinoid tumor is suspected preoperatively, quantitative measurement of the urinary 5-hydroxyindoleacetic acid (5-HIAA) is required. If enough serotonin is being elaborated, anesthesia may accentuate any vasomotor instability, and it is wise in these patients to plan proper drug management pre- and perioperatively (see §§4G.V.A and 4G.V.C.3).

B. Therapeutic Management

Surgical exploration with removal of all neoplastic tissue is the only curative therapy of small-bowel tumors, except in lymphomas, where chemotherapy and/or radiotherapy have been shown to be extremely effective.

- Local enucleation of small benign tumors may be all that is necessary.
- Large benign and all-malignant tumors will require resection of an appropriate segment of intestine with all of its attached mesentery.
- Patients with the carcinoid syndrome may respond to serotonin antagonists or antitumor chemotherapy (see §§4G.V.A. and 4G.V.C.3).

There is no evidence of any role for radiotherapy or chemotherapy in the treatment of epithelial tumors of the small bowel. In the case of lymphoma, the primary treatment is surgical resection followed by postoperative radiotherapy of the field, or chemotherapy in the more extensive disease.

SUGGESTED READINGS

Colorectal Cancer

1. Beahrs, O. H. Low anterior resection for rectal carcinoma. *Surg., Gynecol. Obstet.* **23**, 593 (1966).

2. Dennis, C., and Karlson, K. E. Cancer risk in ulcerative colitis: Formidability per patient-year of late disease. *Surgery (St. Louis)* **50,** 568 (1961).

3. Dukes, C. E. Cancer of the rectum. An analysis of 1000 cases. *J. Pathol. Bacteriol.* **50,** 527 (1940).

4. Gilbertson, V. Colon cancer screening: The Minnesota experience. *Gastrointest. Endoscopy* **26,** 315 (1980).

5. Gilbertson, V. A., and Nelms, J. M. The prevention of invasive cancer of the rectum. *Cancer* **41,** 1137 (1978).

6. Goligher, J. C. "Surgery of the Anus, Rectum and Colon." Thomas, (Springfield, Illinois, 1975.

7. Greegor, D. H. Occult blood testing for detection of a symptomatic colon cancer. *Cancer* **28,** 131 (1971).

8. Grinnell, R. S., and Lane, N. Benign and malignant adenomatous polyps and papillary adenomas of the colon and rectum. An analysis of 1856 tumors in 1335 patients. *Int. Obstet. Surg.* **106,** 519 (1958).

9. Higgins, G. A., Conn, J. H., Jordan, P. H. *et al.* Preoperative radiotherapy for colorectal cancer. *Ann. Surg.* **181,** 624 (1975).

10. Lawrence, W., Jr., Terz, J. J., and Horsley, S. Chemotherapy as an adjuvant to surgery for colorectal cancer. *Ann. Surg.* **181,** 616 (1975).

11. Madden, J. L., and Kandalaft, S. I. Electrocoagulation as a primary curative method in the treatment of carcinoma of the rectum. *Surg., Gynecol. Obstet.* **157,** 164 (1983).

12. Moertel, C. G. Chemotherapy of gastrointestinal cancer. *N. Engl. J. Med.* **299,** 1049 (1978).

13. Spratt, J. S., Ackerman, L. V., and Mozer, C. A. Relationship of polyps of the colon to colonic cancer. *Ann. Surg.* **148,** 682 (1958).

14. Stearns, M. W., and Deddish, M. Five-year results of abdominopelvic lymph node dissection for carcinoma of the rectum. *Dis. Colon Rectum* **2,** 169 (1959).

15. Wynder, E. L., and Shigematsu, T. Environmental factors in cancer of colon and rectum. *Cancer* **20,** 1520 (1967).

Cancer of the Anus

1. Stearns, M. W., Urmacher, C. *et al.* Cancer of the anal canal. *Curr. Probl. Cancer* **4,** 4 (1980).

Cancer of the Small Intestine

1. Herbsman, H., Wetstein, L., Rosen, Y. *et al.* Tumors of the small intestine. *Curr. Probl. Surg.* **17,** 121 (1980).

2. Mittal, V. K., and Bodzin, J. H. Primary malignant tumors of the small intestine. *Am. J. Surg.* **140,** 396 (1980).

Section 11. Carcinomas of the Alimentary Tract

Part C: Carcinoma of the Pancreas (Eccrine Gland) and the Biliary Tree

I. Early Detection and Screening
   for Pancreatic Carcinoma   509
   A. Epidemiology
   B. Early Signs and Symptoms
II. Pretreatment Evaluation and Work-Up for Patients
   with Pancreatic Carcinoma   510
   A. Physical Evaluation
   B. Laboratory Findings
      1. CBC and Stool Examination for Occult Blood
      2. SMA-12
      3. Pancreatic Enzymes and Pancreatic
         Function Tests
      4. Serodiagnosis
   C. Radiological Diagnosis
      1. Ultrasound
      2. Computerized Axial Tomography
      3. Radionuclide Scintiscanning
      4. Gastrointestinal Studies
      5. Angiography
      6. Percutaneous Transhepatic Cholangiography
   D. Endoscopy
   E. Cytological Diagnosis
   F. Overview of the Diagnostic Approach
   G. Metastatic Evaluation
   H. Site-Specific Data Form for Pancreatic Carcinoma
III. Preoperative Preparation with Pancreatic Carcinoma   515
   A. Nutritional and Hemodynamic Status
   B. Intercurrent Illness
   C. Correction of Coagulation Defects
   D. Diabetes
   E. Biliary Decompression
   F. Antibiotics
   G. Immediate Preoperative Preparation
IV. Therapeutic Management of Carcinoma of the Pancreas
   and Periampullary Region   516
   A. Pathological Considerations
      1. Duct Cell Carcinomas
      2. Carcinomas of Acinar Cell Origin
      3. Cancers of Uncertain Origin

      4. Sarcomas
      5. Metastatic Malignant Tumors
   B. Prognostic Implications
   C. Pitfalls in Therapy
   D. Goals of Surgery
      1. Palliation
      2. Attempt at Cure
   E. Types of Surgical Resection of the Pancreas
      1. Whipple's Operation
      2. Total Pancreatoduodenectomy
      3. Extended Regional Pancreatectomy
      4. Pylorus-Preserving Operations
      5. Reconstruction
   F. Other Therapeutic Modalities
      1. Radiotherapy
      2. Chemotherapy
V. Postoperative Care and Evaluation of Patients
   with Pancreatic Carcinoma   520
   A. Immediate Postoperative Care
   B. Supportive Care
   C. Postoperative Evaluation
VI. Management Algorithm for Pancreatic Carcinoma   520
VII. Therapeutic Management of Carcinoma of the Gallbladder
   and Extrahepatic Biliary Tree   522
   A. Pathological Considerations
      1. Benign Tumors and Tumorlike Lesions
      2. Carcinoma of the Gallbladder
      3. Extrahepatic Biliary Tree Carcinoma
   B. Evaluation of the Patient with Carcinoma
      of the Biliary Tree
   C. Therapeutic Considerations
      1. Preoperative Preparation
      2. The Role of Radiologist in the Care
         of the Patient with Obstructive Jaundice
      3. Surgical Treatment
      4. Radiotherapy
      5. Chemotherapy

Suggested Readings   525

I. EARLY DETECTION AND SCREENING FOR PANCREATIC CARCINOMA

A. Epidemiology

Pancreatic cancer has in the past 15 years climbed to fourth place as a cause of death from cancer in the United States and accounts for over 20,000 deaths per year. The incidence of the disease has continued to climb over the past decade but at a much slower pace than in earlier years. Available incidence rates in black populations show a significantly higher incidence than for whites, and rates for males in each race are higher than those for females. Socioeconomic factors have little influence on the incidence of the disease, and the rates are not significantly different in urban areas as compared with rural areas.

Pancreatic cancer is a disease of the elderly and is quite rare in individuals under the age of 40. The incidence ranges from 2 cases per 100,000 population between the ages of 40 and 44, to over 100 cases per 100,000 population between the ages of 80 and 84. There does not appear to be a genetic background or a strong family predisposition to the disease.

Factors that have been identified as being possibly significant in influencing the incidence of pancreatic cancer include

- Diabetes, though diabetes is more likely to be a result of cancer of the pancreas than a causal factor.
- Diet. Diets rich in meat seem to be more frequently associated with this disease.
- Tobacco appears to be the most clearly established risk factor; with heavy smoking more than doubling the risk of pancreatic cancer. Although the relationship between smoking and pancreatic cancer is weaker than that seen in lung or larynx cancer, it is significant nonetheless.
- Caffeine. Heavy consumption of coffee was reported to be associated with a significantly higher risk (a threefold increase) of pancreatic cancer.

The use of alcohol was not found to be associated with an increased incidence, and no occupational or environmental factors have so far been identified as pertinent to pancreatic cancer.

Although new techniques in diagnosis have emerged in the past decade, early detection remains elusive. Furthermore, advances in surgical technique, chemotherapeutic agents, and radiotherapy have, to date, made no great dent in the dismal outcome of the disease.

B. Early Signs and Symptoms

The earliest manifestations of carcinoma of the pancreas are actually nonspecific for the disease. These may be in the form of diminished appetite, indigestion, and minor weight loss (less than 10%). The sudden onset of diabetes mellitus in the absence of a family history in a patient above the age of 50 should attract one's attention to the disease. In addition, thrombophlebitis is rather common and may precede any other manifestations of the disease.

More specific symptoms of pancreatic cancer include

- Unexplained upper abdominal and/or midback pain; these are present in roughly half of the patients seeking medical attention.
- Obstructive jaundice, pruritis, dark urine, and clay-colored stools are the presenting manifestations in about 50% of patients with carcinoma of the head of the pancreas.
- Unexplained steatorrhea and weight loss of over 10% should be considered as warning signs suspicious for carcinoma of the pancreas, and the patient must be thoroughly investigated.
- A mass in the upper abdomen (epigastric region) or right upper quadrant (liver mass) is rarely an early finding in the course of the disease but must arouse suspicion.

It is extremely rare that carcinoma of the pancreas is detected at an early stage of the disease, and this, undoubtedly, is the main reason for the dismal results of treatment. No prevention or screening is available, and early detection is all but impossible because of the nonspecific nature of the symptoms. Less than 15% of patients consult a physician within one month of onset of symptoms, and the duration of symptoms prior to diagnosis ranges from 2 to 18 months, indicating "physician delay" in addition to "patient delay." A strong program of public and physician education is essential to overcome the problem in the hope of improving end results.

II. PRETREATMENT EVALUATION AND WORK-UP FOR PATIENTS WITH PANCREATIC CARCINOMA

A. Physical Evaluation

A thorough history and physical examination may be helpful in identifying a carcinoma of the pancreas if it is suspected because of

- General GI malaise, anorexia, weight loss, and diarrhea.
- Pain, particularly epigastric or midback, sometimes extremely severe in nature and penetrating.
- Jaundice, obstructive in character.
- Abdominal mass.

The character of the pain, mass, and jaundice may even identify the location of the tumor within one area of the pancreas.

Patients with pancreatic cancer are ordinarily elderly and debilitated individuals. Intercurrent disease is common, and a complete physical evaluation is essential to assess their general status as well as their ability to tolerate any major surgical procedure. One must evaluate the following parameters:

- State of nutrition, weight, and nitrogen balance.
- Fluid and electrolyte balance, blood volume, and hematocrit.
- Cardiopulmonary status, state of cardiac reserve, pulmonary function, blood gases, etc.
- Liver function and coagulation profile.
- Renal diseases, etc.

B. Laboratory Findings

1. CBC and Stool Examination for Occult Blood

Anemia and positive stool guaiac are rarely present in early cases. In advanced cases, about 40% have a positive stool guaiac and/or anemia, which is usually mild. This is quite significant and might indicate the presence of a lesion detectable on endoscopy.

2. SMA-12

The earliest abnormality in liver function tests is the elevation of the alkaline phosphatasc; this may precede bilirubin

elevation by 1–2 months. When the bilirubin is elevated, the alkaline phosphatase is always elevated. Aspartate aminotransferase (SGOT) and alanine aminotranfertase (SGPT) are usually mildly elevated, unless cholangitis supervenes.

3. Pancreatic Enzymes and Pancreatic Function Tests

The serum lipase and serum amylase are elevated in a minority of cases (less than 10%). On occasion (approximately 2% of cases), an attack of mild pancreatitis is the presenting manifestation of carcinoma of the pancreas and that can be associated with an elevated serum amylase.

Pancreatic function tests may be carried out with duodenal intubation and stimulation of pancreatic secretion by intravenous secretin or cholecystokinin or by a test meal (the Lundt test). Duodenal contents can then be analyzed for volume, pH, and bicarbonate and enzyme concentrations to assess pancreatic function. Although various modifications of the test seem to have a 90% accuracy in identifying various pancreatic diseases, it is of little value in the diagnosis of pancreatic cancer, since only patients with obstruction of more than 60% of the length of their main pancreatic duct can be so detected. Pathological study of the material obtained in an attempt to identify malignant cells is probably the most valuable part of this examination.

4. Serodiagnosis

The measurement of the serum level of various tumor markers in the systemic or portal circulation has been studied. These include

- Carcinoembryonic antigen.
- Alpha fetoprotein (AFP).
- Pancreatic oncofetal antigen (POA).

None of these markers is sufficiently sensitive and specific to be of use in the diagnosis or screening of pancreatic cancer, although POA has been reported by some investigators to rise with the occurrence of recurrent or metastatic disease and may thus be of some value in monitoring the effectiveness of surgical therapy and in predicting recurrences.

C. Radiological Diagnosis

Until recent years, the radiological demonstration of the pancreas has been difficult, and the early diagnosis of carcinoma of the pancreas has continued to represent a challenge, not only to the clinician, but also to the radiologist. In recent years, a variety of highly accurate imaging procedures have been developed in an attempt to reach an earlier diagnosis and obtain improved survival rates. These include

- Sonography.
- CAT scan.
- Pancreatic scanning.
- Hypotonic duodenography.
- Angiography.
- Percutaneous transhepatic cholangiography (PTC).
- Endoscopic retrograde cholangiopancreatography (ERCP).

1. Ultrasound

Ultrasound is a totally noninvasive diagnostic procedure that may be performed as a static laminographic study with images in transverse and saggital planes at 1-cm intervals or as "real-time" sonography that relies on identification of the vascular anatomy. Sonography will reveal changes in size, shape, and echo texture of the gland as well as dilatation of the pancreatic duct proximal to the carcinoma.

Ultrasound is particularly useful for carcinomas of the head of the pancreas and can detect lesions as small as 2 cm that have not distorted the contour of the pancreas as yet and that would thus escape detection by CAT scanning. Ultrasonography is preferable to CAT scanning in the following circumstances:

- Smaller tumors.
- Tumors of the head of the pancreas.
- Emaciated patients who have no fat around the pancreas, making CAT visualization difficult.
- Immobile or uncooperative patients.
- Patients who have had previous surgery or have metal clips in an old operative site.

Sonography is technically unsuccessful in 15% of cases. Successful sonograms have a positive predictive value of around 80% and a negative predictive value of over 90%. In the elderly, a successful ultrasound procedure allows reliable exclusion of the disease in a noninvasive way. Added advantages of sonography are that it permits the simultaneous identification of other abdominal structures (liver, kidney, adrenals, nodes, etc.) and also the assessment of the biliary ductal system in patients with jaundice.

2. Computerized Axial Tomography

The most reliable single test for carcinoma of the pancreas is the CAT scan. The CAT diagnosis of pancreatic cancer relies entirely on alterations of pancreatic contour caused by the tumor. It is often the initial procedure of choice for evaluation of patients with known or suspected pancreatic carcinoma. CAT is approximately 90% accurate in detecting a mass in patients with carcinoma of the pancreas; it will reveal deformity of the size and shape of the pancreas secondary to the focal mass, dilatation of the pancreatic duct proximal to the carcinoma, evidence of metastatic spread into the retropancreatic fat

planes, involvement of the peripancreatic lymph nodes, and metastatic deposits within the liver.

Computerized axial tomography is better suited in the following circumstances:

- Lesions of the tail and body of the pancreas.
- Obese patients.
- Presence of ascites or excessive bowel gas.

The use of contrast, both oral and intravenous, enhances the value of CAT scans immensely and helps define the adjacent vessels and structures, thus offering valuable information regarding operability.

3. Radionuclide Scintiscanning

The standard selenomethionine scan of the pancreas is today totally defunct. ^{11}C-tryptophan scanning as an enhancement in conjunction with CAT or ultrasound is still being evaluated.

4. Gastrointestinal Studies

The upper GI series (including hypotonic duodenography) may be helpful in ruling peptic ulcer disease in or out and in identifying a mass effect or a mucosal deformity of the duodenum or posterior gastric wall. Its value, however, is limited to large tumors or those affecting the duodenal mucosa, and it has been largely replaced by CAT scanning and sonography.

5. Angiography

Celiac and superior mesenteric arteriography using selective catheterization of the pancreatic vessels, is an extremely accurate diagnostic modality, particularly when combined with image magnification and digital subtraction. The complexity of the procedure and of the necessary equipment make it inaccessible to the majority of the patients, however; its main value remains as a tool to predict unresectability in patients who have otherwise been selected for laparotomy and to help in the planning of the surgical procedure.

6. Percutaneous Transhepatic Cholangiography

This procedure, widely used prior to the advent of the CAT scan, is presently advocated primarily for the differential diagnosis of obstructive jaundice and offers little information about the pancreas itself. It is only indicated if sonography identifies large, dilated intrahepatic ducts and when ERCP is not feasible.

The advent of interventional radiology in conjunction with PTC, however, has opened up new horizons in its use for therapeutic noninvasive biliary decompression; this may be desirable as a preliminary preparatory step prior to surgery in patients with serum bilirubins over 20 mg/100 cc, in those who need further preoperative preparation, or as a definitive palliative procedure in the nonresectable patient.

D. Endoscopy

Gastroduodenoscopy is becoming more and more popular in the diagnostic evaluation of patients with pancreatic disease, especially with the more recent advances made in fiberoptic instrumentation and techniques that have permitted actual cannulation, radiographic studies, and even biopsies within the pancreatic duct itself. Endoscopic retrograde cannulation of the pancreas should only be instituted after the less invasive studies have been perfomed because it carries a significant morbidity, particularly in the presence of pancreatitis or cholangitis. X-rays of the pancreatic duct by retrograde cannulation will identify stenosis or obstruction, but cytological confirmation of the diagnosis is the most important potential benefit of the procedure; this can be achieved by cytological sampling of the tumors of the ampulla or pancreatic duct.

ERCP is a complex procedure with a high (15%) failure rate even in experienced hands. It should be performed only by experienced operators with the proper radiological and backup facilities and only when specifically indicated.

E. Cytological Diagnosis

Establishing a tissue diagnosis in carcinoma of the pancreas is of the utmost importance, since palliation is often the best that can be achieved. This is particularly true in carcinomas of the body and tail, where curative resection is of very little avail. Tissue from the pancreas may be obtained in one of several ways:

- Duodenal drainage studies with secretin stimulation and cytological examination of the pancreatic juices. The procedure has a yield of 71% in tumors of the had of the pancreas but only 33% in tumors of the body or tail.
- Material collected from the pancreatic duct during ERCP has a slightly higher yield (47–84%) and should be examined whenever ERCP is done. Direct biopsy of an intraductal tumor identified on endoscopy is another method of tissue diagnosis during ERCP.
- Fine percutaneous needle biopsy with sonographic or CAT guidance. This procedure is particularly useful in tumors of the body and tail of the pancreas, particularly in the frail elderly patient and when a mass is palpable. It should be performed in the young, fit patient where surgical resection will be attempted or in those patients who would require surgery for palliation regardless.
- Laparoscopy with direct needle aspiration biopsy. This procedure has the advantage of permitting visualization of the whole peritoneal cavity in an attempt to assess operability.

The value of achieving a tissue diagnosis must be tempered with good judgment. It must not be a substitute for surgical exploration if there is any chance of helping the patient surgically by attempting a curative resection or by carrying out a palliative procedure. Some tumors of the pancreas (e.g., islet cell tumors, lymphomas) have a better prognosis than the usual adenocarcinoma if properly treated; an inaccurate needle biopsy might miss such lesions and deny the patient proper management.

F. Overview of the Diagnostic Approach

The choice and sequence of examinations are actually determined in part by the availability of equipment and expertise in individual institutions. The complete clinical picture and whether surgery is feasible or not are also important factors.

In a patient who presents with jaundice and is in good medical condition, an ultrasound followed by thin-needle biopsy may be all that is necessary to document the diagnosis before the patient is operated upon. A similar approach may be undertaken in a very elderly individual in poor medical condition in whom surgery is not feasible.

The radiologist should be able to suggest an approximate sequence of examinations that will permit a rapid, accurate diagnosis with the least number of tests and with minimum expense and discomfort to the patient. The following algorithm has been recommended.

- In a patient with a history and physical examination suggestive of a pancreatic carcinoma, the first imaging study should be sonography or CAT. If these are negative, hypotonic duodenography and a GI series may be performed followed by ERCP.
- If the sonography or the CAT reveals a pancreatic mass, an ERCP may be performed. Percutaneous transhepatic cholangiography may also be indicated in a jaundiced patient if the intrahepatic ducts are dilated.
- Duodenal cytology, preferably during endoscopy, might confirm the diagnosis; otherwise, a needle biopsy may be performed and might obviate the need for ERCP.
- If the ERCP or the needle biopsy identify a pancreatic carcinoma, pancreatic angiography should be performed to assess resectability of the tumor. If the ERCP is technically unsatisfactory, the angiogram is still done to establish the diagnosis as well as the operability.
- If pancreatic angiography shows the tumor to be resectable, the patient should undergo surgery. If pancreatic angiography shows the tumor to be unresectable, a percutaneous fine-needle biopsy must then be performed to establish the histological diagnosis before the patient is treated for palliation.

G. Metastatic Evaluation

The majority of patients with carcinoma of the pancreas are not candidates for curative therapeutic modalities, and in most cases this is the result of local extension of the disease to adjacent structures, regional node involvement, or liver metastases. These areas are usually thoroughly assessed during evaluation of the pancreatic lesion itself (CAT scan, sonograms, laparoscopy, etc.), and little additional metastatic survey is actually indicated:

- Chest x-ray and CAT scan of the chest.
- SMA-12.
- Bone scan and skeletal surgery, if indicated by routine studies or clinical suggestion of bone metastases.

Furthermore, the identification of distant metastases in the evaluation of the patient with pancreatic cancer is often not a contraindication for surgery since most surgical procedures are performed for palliation rather than for cure.

H. Site-Specific Data Form for Pancreatic Carcinoma (see pp. 515–516)

III. PREOPERATIVE PREPARATION OF PATIENTS WITH PANCREATIC CARCINOMA

Most patients with pancreatic cancer are elderly, debilitated individuals with advanced disease and multiple intercurrent illnesses. They are, therefore, likely to require significant preparation prior to definitive therapy.

The preparation of the patient with cancer of the pancreas for surgery varies with the anticipated scope of the surgery. Most patients are not candidates for resection, either because of the advanced stage of the disease or because of their inability to tolerate a major procedure. In this group, where only palliation is sought, the preoperative preparation is straightforward: in addition to the routine baseline chemistries, EKG, chest x-ray, and SMA-12, a coagulation profile and correction of vitamin K deficiency are indicated. Preparation of the patient in these cases is primarily supportive. If the patient is deemed a candidate for surgical resection, the preoperative preparation must then be much more rigorous.

A. Nutritional and Hemodynamic Status

Preoperative hyperalimentation is often necessary for several days prior to surgery. This may be carried out orally with the use of enzyme supplements or intravensouly, either peripherally or centrally.

Anemia and hypovolemia should be corrected by blood transfusions, bringing the hemoglobin level to a minimum of 12 gram %.

B. Intercurrent Illness

The patient needs to be brought back to as normal a state of health as possible. Cardiopulmonary therapy must be initiated preoperatively, and any decompensation must be corrected; pulmonary toilet and physiotherapy are better instituted before therapy. Other problems must also be corrected as they are encountered.

C. Correction of Coagulation Defects

This is particularly important in the jaundiced patient and in those with hepatic insufficiency. Most often, the parenteral administration of vitamin K is all that is necessary; if this fails to correct the coagulopathy, severe liver damage may be present, and that might militate against any major surgery. A complete coagulation profile then becomes necessary, with replacement of any deficient factor or transfusion of fresh-frozen plasma.

D. Diabetes

Diabetes is often present in patients with pancreatic carcinoma. Monitoring of blood sugars pre- and postoperatively is essential, and insulin is used for correction as needed.

E. Biliary Decompression

Surgery in the presence of hyperbilirubinemia in excess of 20 mg % carries significant risks. Any patient with these levels should have an attempt at decompressing the biliary tree by percutaneous transhepatic cannulation of the intrahepatic dilated ducts under x-ray control. If the decompression is to be temporary, the catheter may be left in place and permitted to drain externally until the bilirubin drifts to an acceptable level. Internal drainage has, of late, been developed by the intervention radiologist for use in cases where decompression might be required as a prolonged or definitive palliative procedure, especially in those patients where surgical decompression is contraindicated. In such cases, the catheter is introduced through PTC and advanced all the way down to the ampulla of Vater and into the duodenum, thus bypassing the obstruction and permitting the bile to drain into the gut.

F. Antibiotics

Prophylactic antibiotics are indicated since the procedures are usually quite lengthy and entail several bowel anastomoses. They should be started prior to surgery and continued for 48 hours postoperatively, or longer if the operative findings so indicate.

G. Immediate Preoperative Preparation

Intraoperative leg compression with elastic supports or pneumatic compression is desirable. Miniheparin used prophylactically to prevent thromboembolic disease should be considered. The patient should be instructed in deep breathing and leg exercises. Central venous pressure (CVP) and arterial lines should be in place, and Swan-Ganz catheter introduction may be considered.

IV. THERAPEUTIC MANAGEMENT OF CARCINOMA OF THE PANCREAS AND PERIAMPULLARY REGION

A. Pathological Considerations

Tumors of the pancreas can arise from the duct cells, acinar cells, islet cells, or stroma. Over 90% of pancreatic tumors are of epithelial origin. Tumors of the islet cells are fully discussed in §4A, Vol. 1 and will not be included in this presentation.

1. Duct Cell Carcinomas

About 90% of all pancreatic carcinomas are of duct cell origin. This type of carcinoma is histolgically divided into several subtypes:

• Ductal adenocarcinoma.
• Giant-cell carcinoma.
• Adenosquamous carcinoma.
• Microadenocarcinoma.
• Mucinous (''colloid'') carcinoma.
• Cystadenocarcinoma (mucinous).

The majority of cases are represented by the first type. Giant-cell carcinoma, adenosquamous carcinoma, and micro-adenocarcinoma represent about 3–5% of cases each. Other types are even more rare. The 1-year survival rate is highest for the mucinous cystadenocarcinoma, which occurs predominantly in women. ''Colloid'' adenocarcinoma has also a rela-

tively good 1-year survival rate (around 33%). The overall survival for carcinoma of the pancreas is otherwise dismal.

2. Carcinomas of Acinar Cell Origin

Acinar cell carcinoma comprises about 1% of cancers of the pancreas. The 1-year survival rate is 14%. This tumor occurs in two subtypes: acinar cell carcinoma and cystadenocarcinoma (acinar cells).

3. Cancers of Uncertain Origin

These tumors comprise about 9% of the total. Most of them belong to the group of unclassified carcinomas and may be large-cell, small-cell, or celar-cell type of anaplastic carcinomas.

4. Sarcomas

Sarcomas comprise about 1% of pancreatic cancers.

5. Metastatic Malignant Tumors

Approximately two-thirds of all malignant tumors found in the pancreas at autopsy are metastatic in nature.

B. Prognostic Implications

Carcinoma of the head of the pancreas constitutes about 79% of all pancreatic cancers and carries a significantly better prognosis than that of the body or tail of the gland. This may be the result of the earlier identification of the tumors in the head of the pancreas as a result of obstructive jaundice. The generally dismal prognosis of pancreatic cancer is to a great extent related to the rich lymphatic drainage of the gland, which empties directly into the large collecting channels (cysterna chyli and thoracic duct) and to the early vascular spread to the liver via the portal vein, which is found within the substance of the pancreatic gland. Death is often the result of liver failure from either biliary obstruction or metastatic disease. The median survival of patients treated by palliative measures alone is 3.5 months, with only 8% being still alive at 1-year.

It is most important to distinguish carcinoma of the head of the pancreas from carcinoma of the ampulla of Vater, intrahepatic bile ducts, or duodenal mucosa. The latter lesions (periampullary tumors) are frequently resectable, with a reasonable chance of cure, whereas carcinomas of the head of the pancreas are rarely cured, and surgical resection is considered futile by many surgeons.

Carcinoma of the body and tail of the pancreas is practically never curable by present day modalities, whether surgical or otherwise.

SITE–SPECIFIC DATA FORM—PANCREAS

HISTORY

Age:_____

Symptoms

_____ Jaundice

_____ Pain

_____ Mass

_____ Anorexia

_____ Weight loss _____ lbs.

_____ Diarrhea, steatorrhea

_____ Thrombophlebitis

_____ Diabetes

_____ Other

Duration:_____

Social history

   Occupation:_____

   Race:____ White____ Black____ Oriental____ Other

   Smoker:____ No____ Yes How much?_____

   Drinker:____ No____ Yes How often?_____

   Coffee drinker:____ No____ Yes How often?____

Family history of carcinoma

   Relation: _____ Site: _____

Previous history of carcinoma

   _____ No____ Yes Site:_____

Rx:_____

Previous treatment (describe)

   (Surgery, radiotherapy, chemotherapy, etc.)

_____

_____

_____

PHYSICAL EXAMINATION

General condition:_____

Mass:_____ Yes_____ No

Site:_____

Size:_____

Palpable liver_____ Yes_____ No

Ascites:_____ Yes_____ No

Common duct

Pancreatic duct

RADIOLOGIC STUDIES

	Location	Extension
Mass		
Head	_____	_____
Body	_____	_____
Tail	_____	_____

Characteristics

_____ Soft_____ Multiple

_____ Hard_____ Soft _____ Cystic

_____ Fixed _____ Mobile

	Yes	No	Description
Involvement of			
Adjacent organs	_____	_____	_____
Adjacent vessels	_____	_____	_____
Lymph nodes	_____	_____	_____

PREOPERATIVE WORK-UP (Check, if done)

	Neg.	Pos.	Suspicious		Neg.	Pos.	Suspicious
CBC	___	___	___	Endoscopy	___	___	___
SMA 12	___	___	___	ERCP	___	___	___
Pancreatic				PTC			
function tests	___	___	___	Biopsy	___	___	___
CAT scan	___	___	___	Type:	___	___	___
Sonogram	___	___	___	Laparoscopy	___	___	___
GI series	___	___	___	Laparotomy	___	___	___
Angiogram	___	___	___				

Classification:_____ T ___ N ___ M

Stage: _____

Histology:_____

Grade: _____

Signature:_____

Countersignature: _____

Date:_____

Classification of Pancreatic Cancer

TNM Classification

Primary tumor (T)

TX   Minimum requirements not met
T1   Tumor measuring 2 cm or less, limited to the pancreas
T2   Tumor measuring 2–6 cm in diameter
T3   Tumor measuring greater than 6 cm
T4   Extrapancreatic extension

Nodal involvement (N)

N0   No nodal involvement
N1   One regional group involved at laparotomy
N2   Two or more regional groups involved at laparotomy
N3   Clinical evidence of node metastases
N4   Juxtaregional nodes

Distant metastasis (M)

MX   Not assessed
M0   No (known) distant metastasis
M1   Distant metastasis present (specify site)

Grade

I   Well differentiated
II   Moderately well differentiated
III   Poorly differentiated
IV   Undifferentiated

Stage

I   Local disease only
II   Invasion to surrounding tissue
III   Metastases to regional nodes
IV   Generalized carcinoma, liver metastases, peritoneal implants, etc.

C. Pitfalls in Therapy

Since therapeutic attempts for pancreatic carcinoma are rarely curative, the motto Primum non nocere is of greatest importance. Palliation and quality of life become the main concerns, and relief of symptoms, the goal of treatment.

Pancreatic resections should not be undertaken in the following circumstances:

- Clinical, laparoscopic, or operative evidence of metastatic disease.
- Patients over 70 years of age.
- Frail and otherwise seriously ill patients.
- Life expectancy estimated at less than 2 years.

Nevertheless, major surgery for palliation is often indicated, and keen judgment is required in these cases to weigh the risks of such surgery against the benefits that might ensue.

The need for operative biopsy is an issue of great controversy. If the diagnosis is not established preoperatively, the surgeon must decide at the time of surgery whether to biopsy and rely on the frozen-section study of the tissues or to make a decision on the basis of the gross findings. The problem is particularly acute in deep-seated masses of the head of the pancreas, where differentiation between pancreatitis and carcinoma may be extremely difficult. One or two needle biopsies may be attempted, but a negative result may not be representative of the true nature of the pathology because of the difficulty in sampling. An open biopsy is traumatic and time consuming and often a final decision still needs to be made on clinical grounds. Thus, a decision to resect in the absence of a tissue diagnosis may be necessary in small, favorable pancreatic tumors in order not to miss the opportunity of curing an early cancer. Each surgeon, based on personal experience and philosophy, must be permitted to make this decision in selected clinical situations.

D. Goals of Surgery

1. Palliation

a. Biliary Decompression

The symptoms of biliary obstruction—jaundice, pruritis, and cholangitis—are most stressful and need to be corrected. In the severely ill or debilitated patient, decompression by percutaneous transhepatic needle access, with external or internal drainage, might suffice; in all other cases, surgical decompression is essential in cases of biliary obstruction. This can be done in one of several ways:

- Cholecystojejunostomy, using a jejunal loop with jejunojejunostomy or a Roux-en-Y procedure, is the procedure of

choice if there is an intact gallbladder and a patent cystic duct.
- Cholecystectomy and choledocojejunostomy is necessary if there is no adequate communication between the gallbladder and the common bile duct.

b. Gastrointestinal Bypass

Identifiable or impending duodenal obstruction recognized at laparotomy must be corrected. Approximately 30% of patients with carcinoma of the head of the pancreas require some bypass procedure, and some would even advise performing a gastrojejunostomy electively on all patients who are operated upon. This seems desirable in young patients with a reasonable projected survival, even when no immediate obstruction is noted.

c. Palliative Resection

Surgical treatment for carcinoma of the body and tail of the pancreas is, for all practical purposes, always palliative. By the time the patient presents with clinical symptoms, the disease is invariably at a late stage. The purpose of surgery, therefore, is twofold: to establish a tissue diagnosis and to achieve relief of pain. If the tumor can be mobilized from the parietes, a palliative pancreatectomy and splenectomy is the procedure of choice for palliation. The surgical margins must be outlined with metal clips for postoperative radiation. If the tumor is too extensive to permit resection, adequate tissue should be obtained for diagnosis, and no further surgery should be carried out.

2. Attempt at Cure

Because of the extremely low cure rates and short survival, it has been suggested that curative resection for pancreatic cancer is seldom indicated. Most surgeons, however, feel that resections for carcinoma of the head of the pancreas should be undertaken whenever possible; it appears unequivocal that the only appreciable survival has been in patients where some form of resection was undertaken.

E. Types of Surgical Resection of the Pancreas

Four basic operations have been recommended in the treatment of carcinomas of the pancreas and periampullary areas: pancreatoduodenectomy (Whipple's operation), total pancreatectomy, regional extended pancreatectomy, and pylorus-preserving operations.

1. Whipple's Operation

This procedure entails an en-bloc resection of the head and neck of the pancreas with the gastric antrum, duodenum, gallbladder, distal bile ducts, and upper jejunum, together with the regional lymphatic nodal basin. The procedure is ideally suited for ampullary or periampullary carcinomas; whether it is adequate for carcinomas of the head of the pancreas is questionable, and many have even argued the advisability of resection altogether in cancers of the head of the pancreas.

2. Total Pancreatoduodenectomy

This procedure is an extension of Whipple's operation to include resection of the entire pancreas, spleen, and regional nodes. The arguments given for its use include

- Frequent identification of tumor at the cut end of the specimen in Whipple's operation.
- Multicentricity of the tumor (in 30% of cases).
- Seeding and local recurrences from viable cancer cells present in the obstructed pancreatic duct.
- A better regional node dissection.
- Avoiding the anastomosis of the pancreatic remnant, with its potential complications.

There seems to be little difference in 5-year survival rates between Whipple's operation and the more aggressive total pancreatectomy for carcinoma of the head of the pancreas (6.5 and 8.2% respectively), but the operative mortality of the total pancreatectomy (15%) far exceeds that of the pancreatoduodenectomy. In addition, in patients free of diabetes preoperatively, a total pancreatectomy would result in the occurrence of diabetes. Total pancreatectomy is therefore not generally accepted as the procedure of choice for carcinomas of the head of the pancreas.

3. Extended Regional Pancreatectomy

a. Type I Operation

This includes resection of the retropancreatic portion of the portal vein.

b. Type II Operation

This operation involves resection of segments of the celiac axis, mesenteric artery, or hepatic artery. Such heroic surgery has been reported in selected cases of advanced pancreatic cancer; one must await objective data to support its use, particularly in view of its extreme risks in patients who are rarely curable.

4. Pylorus-Preserving Operations

This operation, which saves the entire stomach, the pylorus, and the first portion of the duodenum, is only possible in the smallest, most localized tumors of the periampullary area. Anytime less than 60% of the stomach is resected, a bilateral truncal vagotomy must be performed.

5. Reconstruction

Reestablishment of the continuity of the GI, biliary, and pancreatic tracts requires reconstruction regardless of which type of resection has been performed. There are innumerable variants to this reconstruction, and the choice is often a preference of the surgeon:

- The pancreatic remnant in a pancreatoduodenectomy must be reanastomosed to the jejunum. This may be done either by plugging the pancreatic end into the jejunal lumen as an end-to-end pancreatojejunostomy, holding it together with sutures in the capsule and serosa only, or by performing an end-to-side pancreatojejunostomy with suturing of the intestinal mucosa to the duct and splinting of the anastomosis with a small Silastic tube.
- The common duct is anastomosed to the jejunum in an end-to-side fashion.
- Gastrojejunostomy must also be performed in one of the standard methods.

F. Other Therapeutic Modalities

Although surgery to date is the mainstay of therapy for carcinoma of the pancreas, the dismal results reported have encouraged numerous attempts at evaluating the efficacy of radiotherapy and chemotherapy as substitutes or adjuvant modalities.

1. Radiotherapy

Until recently, the role of radiation therapy in the treatment of carcinoma of the pancreas has been largely palliative. The reasons for this include the relative radioresistance of pancreatic carcinomas, necessitating high doses for control of the tumor, and the deep-seated location of the organ and its close proximity to vital radiosensitive structures such as the bowel, spinal cord, liver, and kidneys. Until the advent of megavoltage radiotherapy, these factors limited the amount of external beam radiation that could effectively be delivered to the pancreas, and conventional doses (3000–4000 rads) have had no effect on the course of the disease.

High-dose, small-volume radiation therapy with high-energy

beams can improve the survival of patients with localized or regional pancreatic cancer. The 1-year survival statistics are comparable to those for patients with resectable disease treated surgically, who usually have more limited disease and a more favorable prognosis. Haslam, from Duke University, in a series of 23 patients, reported a 12-month survival rate of 34% and a median survival period of 7.5 months after 6000 rads in 10 weeks by a split course. Dobelbower, from Thomas Jefferson University, reported a 12-month survival rate of 59% and a median survival of 11.8 months for a group of 18 patients.

For patients to be considered for radical treatment, the disease must be fairly localized with no extension to the liver. Radiopaque clips should be placed around the tumor during laparotomy to outline the tumor volume for radiotherapy, and CAT scanning of the upper abdomen is a must for accurate treatment planning. Multiple high-energy megavoltage fields are used to encompass the tumor volume and avoid other sensitive structures (spinal cord, kidneys, liver, and bowel). A minimum tumor dose of 6000–6500 rads in 6–7 weeks should be delivered.

Interstitial implantation of radioactive seeds (iodine-125 and gold-198) directly into the locally unresectable tumor mass has the theoretical advantage of delivering a very high dose to the tumor-bearing area with little radiation exposure to the surrounding vital structures. This approach may be of value to irradiate the tumor bed following surgical resection and could be of value for boosting the dose to residual tumor areas after or before external beam therapy.

Newer radiotherapeutic techniques using fast neutron beam therapy are currently under study and hold some promises. Likewise, several studies for the evaluation of two new radiosensitizers (metronidazole and Roche compound R0-07-0582) might open up new horizons.

Intraoperative radiotherapy is also currently under investigation in several centers. This has the advantage of delivering a very high single dose of radiation to the tumor volume (using an electron beam) with practically no radiation exposure to other sensitive organs that can be moved outside the radiation field during surgery. This is usually followed by a course of external irradiation.

Patients with more extensive disease or with liver involvement and patients with distant metastases can still get pain relief by shorter courses of local radiotherapy to areas of involvement. In addition, limited recurrent disease following surgery can be treated with radical radiotherapy as described above.

2. Chemotherapy

Adenocarcinoma of the pancreas is the least curable neoplasm of the GI tract, with less than 3% of patients alive 2 years after diagnosis. Until very recently, chemotherapy has had a very small role in the treatment of this disease, as a result of the paucity of active agents and the great difficulties in measuring objective responses in patients with a retroperitoneal tumor. Only three drugs—5-Fluorouracil, mitomycin C, and Streptozotocin—have demonstrated an objective response rate greater than 20% when used as single agents. Such responses rarely last more than 2 or 3 months, and there has been no effect on median survival when compared with untreated control groups, despite clinically objective tumor shrinkage. Current clinical research, therefore, has focused on three areas:

- Experimental Phase II drugs as initial chemotherapy.
- Combination chemotherapy.
- Simultaneous chemotherapy and radiation therapy.

Several Phase II trials have been reported, and only Adriamycin was found to have some activity, with 2 out of 15 patients responding.

The two currently used combination chemotherapy regimens are FAM and SMF (Streptozotocin, mitomycin C, 5-FU). Two separate reports of FAM gave a response rate of 40% with a median survival in responders of 12 months, compared with 3.5 months in nonresponders. The SMF regimen caused objective response in 43% of 23 patients treated, but there were similar survivals for responders and nonresponders. These reports await confirmation from ongoing large, multi-institutional prospective randomized trials using treatment and control groups.

The last area of investigation is the combination of radiation therapy plus chemotherapy. A Mayo Clinic report compared irradiation with irradiation and 5-FU. The mean survival after radiation therapy alone was 25 weeks as compared with 42 weeks when radiation and 5-FU were combined. Another study of the same drug, with a different radiation schedule, gave similar results, with prolongation of life measured only in weeks. Clearly, new drugs or new ways of irradiation are essential if there is to be any hope for long-term survival and possible cure.

The following guideline is suggested as a reasonable approach to carcinoma of the pancreas according to stage:

Stage I   Pancreatoduodenectomy (or total pancreatectomy in selected cases), ideally suited for ampullary or periampullary carcinomas.

Stage II   Total pancreatectomy, with consideration given to regional extended procedures in selected cases. Postoperative or combined intraoperative and postoperative radiotherapy may be desirable at this stage.

Stage III   Total pancreatectomy, or preferably regional pancreatectomy, would be the required surgical procedure if one is inclined to carry out surgery for cure. This must be followed by adjuvant radiotherapy, chemotherapy, or both, and high-dose combined radiation methods must be considered. These patients are best treated in specialized centers within the scope of randomized clinical trials when available.

Stage IV Combination chemotherapy, radiotherapy for palliation of pain, palliative surgical or nonsurgical procedures, and supportive measures.

It must be made perfectly clear that surgical resection for cure in carcinoma of the pancreas (with the exception of ampullary and periampullary tumors) is considered inappropriate by a large number of surgeons who treat the disease. This is particularly true for Stages II and III, where cure rates are almost nil and surgical mortality and morbidity extremely high. It is often felt that effective palliation can often be achieved by a lesser procedure, with a minimum of morbidity and a significant improvement in the quality of life and that there is very little to be gained by adopting a more radical approach.

V. POSTOPERATIVE CARE AND EVALUATION OF PATIENTS WITH PANCREATIC CARCINOMA

A. Immediate Postoperative Care

The usual postoperative care pertinent to any major intraabdominal and gastrointestinal operation applies to these patients as well:

- Careful monitoring of all physiological parameters: cardiac, pulmonary, blood gas determinations, fluid loss, urinary output, blood chemistries and serum electrolytes, CBC, etc. Fluid and electrolyte balance must be maintained. Blood volume should be replaced as needed, and respiratory assistance should be utilized as indicated.
- Prevention of thromboembolic disease, elastic support stockings, elevation, early ambulation, and miniheparin should be utilized.
- Local wound and drain care.
- Oral alimentation is withheld until normal bowel function is resumed.

In addition, the bilirubin level should be monitored until its return to normal, and the patient must be closely observed for anastomotic leaks. The fluid draining from the operative site may be tested for bile and amylase. If a leak is suspected, it must be confirmed with contrast studies of the sinus or the GI

tract. Hyperalimentation must be continued postoperatively until the patient is in a positive nitrogen balance, and supportive measures of longer term value must be instituted as early as possible.

Postoperative diabetes must be identified and treated by the appropriate use of insulin and diet.

B. Supportive Care

The patient with pancreatic cancer is the prototype of the patient who will require intensive supportive care for a variety of reasons:

- The disease is usually not curable.
- Patients are elderly and emaciated.
- The pain is often excruciating.
- A downhill course, with all its psychological impact, is obvious to the patient and the family.

The assistance of a support care team is invaluable in such cases (see §1.VII.D.4, Vol. 1). The nurse oncologist, social worker, nutritionist, psychiatric liasion, and clergy member may all be needed at one time or another during the patient's illness.

Relief of pain is of the greatest importance, and any one of several modalities may be used:

- Oral or parenteral analgesics.
- Narcotics.
- Analagesic cocktails that include narcotics (methadone), sedatives, mood elevators (tricyclics), phenothiazine, and caffeine have been used in any one of several combinations, with effective results.
- Intravenous morphine in small doses.
- Intrathecal morphine. This has even been described with the use of an indwelling catheter for repeated injections 2–3 times daily or as a totally implantable continuous-pump infusion system.
- Phenol or alcohol injection around the celiac plexus.

C. Postoperative Evaluation

Most patients following treatment of pancreatic carcinoma remain under the continuous care of their primary physician, as well as their surgeon, throughout their demise. For those fortunate few who have had curative resection, a system of close follow-up is essential to detect any early recurrence or delayed postoperative complications (e.g., diabetes, ulcer, pancreatic pseudocyst, pancreatitis, dumping syndrome etc.). Table I is a recommended schedule follow-up.

VI. MANAGEMENT ALGORITHM FOR PANCREATIC CARCINOMA

(see p. 521)

MANAGEMENT ALGORITHM FOR PANCREATIC CANCER

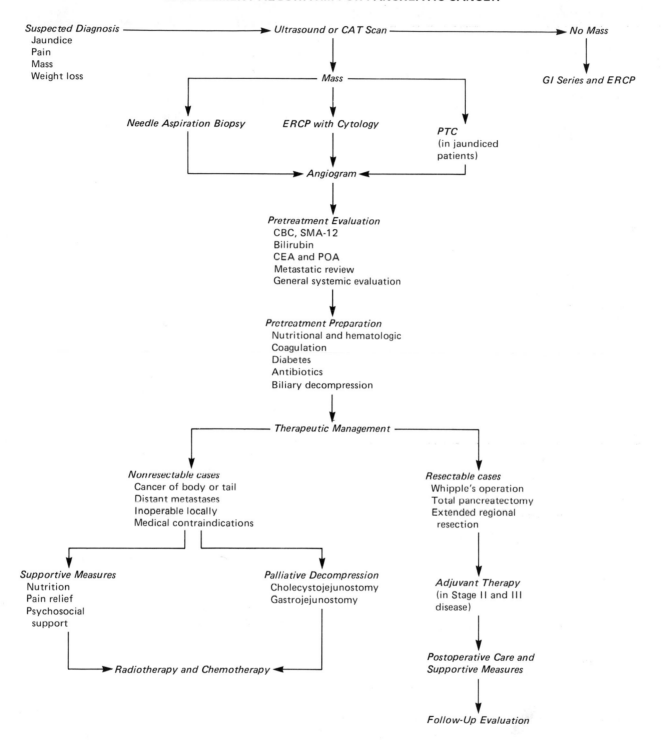

Table I

Long-Term Follow Up Schedule for Pancreatic Cancer

Management	First six months		Six Months to two years		Thereafter	
	Monthly	Every 3 months	Every 3 months	Every 6 months	Every 6 months	Annually
History						
Complete		X		X	X	X
Pain	X		X		X	
Pruritis	X		X		X	
Weight loss	X		X		X	
Diarrhea	X		X		X	
Other	X		X		X	
Physical						
Complete		X		X		X
Abdomen	X		X		X	
Liver	X		X		X	
Jaundice	X		X		X	
Nutritional assessment	X		X		X	
Investigation						
CBC	X		X		X	
SMA-12	X		X		X	
Fasting blood sugar and serum					X	
					X	
bilirubin	X		X		X	
Chest x-ray		X		X		X
CAT scan	As indicated					
Liver scan	As indicated					
PTC, ERCP	As indicated					
Endoscopy	As indicated					
Needle biopsy	As indicated					

VII. THERAPEUTIC MANAGEMENT OF CARCINOMA OF THE GALLBLADDER AND EXTRAHEPATIC BILIARY TREE

A. Pathological Considerations

1. Benign Tumors and Tumorlike Lesions

- Adenoma or papillary adenoma, sometimes pedunculated. These are very rare.
- Polyps, frequently associated with cholecystolithiasis; they may be of cholesterol type, fibrous type, inflammatory, or xanthogranulomatous.
- Local thickening of the gallbladder wall, which may be due to adenomatous or adenomyomatous hyperplasia and is usually seen in the fundus.

2. Carcinoma of the Gallbladder

Carcinoma of the gallbladder constitutes less than 4% of all carcinomas, resulting in 6500 deaths per year in the United States. It is unusual for it to appear before the age of 50, and it is about three times more frequent in women than in men. Approximately 90% of cases are associated with cholecystolithiasis, and the presence of gallstones has been considered a precursor of gallbladder cancer, resulting in the frequent recommendation of routine prophylactic cholecystectomy in all young and middle-aged patients with gallstones.

Grossly, the tumor may present as a polypoid mass protruding into the lumen, or as an infiltrative growth causing focal or diffuse thickening of the gallbladder wall. It often invades the adjacent structures very early, frequently penetrating into the liver. It also frequently extends along the viscus to the cystic duct and toward the extrahepatic bile ducts.

Histologically, the tumor is usually a moderately well-differentiated adenocarcinoma or a papillary adenocarcinoma. Mucinous metaplasia occurs in about 10% of cases, and some tumors are completely undifferentiated and may even mimic a sarcoma. True carcinosarcoma can occur but is extremely rare. Metastases tend to appear first in the lymph nodes of the cystic duct and porta hepatis, and the tumor also tends to extend along the nerves. The only malignancy of the gallbladder with a favorable prognosis is carcinoma *in situ;* it is usually diagnosed incidentally to cholecystectomy performed for cholelithiasis, and the cholecystectomy is usually curative treatment if the malignant change did not extend to the margins of resection. In those patients where the diagnosis is established pre- or perioperatively during laparotomy, the tumor is usually advanced, often inoperable, and usually has a poor prognosis.

3. Extrahepatic Biliary Tree Carcinoma

These tumors are about one-quarter as common as carcinoma of the gallbladder. They do not show any significant sex predilection, and lithiasis does not appear to be of significance. A number of investigators have reported a frequent association of ulcerative colitis and biliary tree cancer; it is interesting to note that ulcerative colitis is also frequently associated with sclerosing cholangitis. The most frequent sites are

- The junction of the cystic and common hepatic ducts.
- The ampulla of Vater.
- The retropancreatic portion of the common bile duct.

As with tumors of the gallbladder, there are virtually no benign tumors of the extrahepatic bile ducts, and only one type of malignant tumor—adenocarcinoma—usually of scirrhous character, prevails. For the purpose of organization and management, we tend to consider all tumors of the right and left hepatic ducts and most of the common bile duct as one group and the tumors of the distal 2 cm of the duct as another. The latter tumors are managed as tumors of the ampulla, duodenum, and head of the pancreas—the so-called periampullary tumors.

The tumors at the ampulla of Vater are papillary, projecting into the duodenum as soft masses. Besides producing obstructive jaundice, they can also obstruct the pancreatic duct, with subsequent atrophy of the eccrine pancreas. Other parts of the extrahepatic ducts are usually involved by tumors that present as sclerotic thickening of the duct wall, sometimes involving long segments of the ducts, at times even extending into the liver. They spread intramurally, mimicking sclerosing cholangittis. Histologically, they are scirrhous adenocarcinomas, but even in biopsy specimens it is extremely difficult to differentiate this type of tumor from inflammatory fibrosis.

A very rare but interesting tumor found in the extrahepatic bile ducts is the embryonal rhabdomyosarcoma, counterpart of a similar more-frequent tumor of the vagina of young girls (botryoid sarcoma). The tumor forms polypoid masses and at the same time infiltrates the wall. Most of the cases occur in infancy and carry a very poor prognosis.

B. Evaluation of the Patient with Carcinoma of the Biliary Tree

Most patients with carcinoma of the gallbladder are detected incidentally during laparotomy, and the evaluation usually ensues the treatment. When work-up for vague symptoms of cholecystitis reveals a tumor on oral cholecystogram, additional investigation should include sonography and CAT scanning of the upper abdomen as well as intravenous cholangiography in order to identify the extent of the disease.

In the case of carcinoma of the extrahepatic biliary tree that presents with jaundice, the work-up should proceed in the same fashion as that of patients with carcinoma of the pancreas or periampullary region. Sonography, CAT scan, PTC, and ERCP are all valuable in selected situations (see §11C.II).

Surgery (i.e., exploratory laparotomy) is often the only finite method of determining the exact nature and extent of the tumor. It should always be carried out, unless there are severe medical contraindications; surgery is the only possible hope for cure and is often necessary even if palliation alone is achievable.

C. Therapeutic Considerations

1. Preoperative Preparation

Preparation is rarely possible in patients with carcinoma of the gallbladder that is detected at surgery. The indications for surgery, in these cases, are those of cholecystitis and cholelithiasis. Patients with ductal carcinomas, particularly when there is associated jaundice, require the same preparation as that described for pancreatic cancers.

2. The Role of the Radiologist in the Care of the Patient with Obstructive Jaundice

The radiological diagnostic approach to the patient with jaundice has been significantly altered by the introduction of several accurate noninvasive screening procedures, in particular ultrasound and computerized axial tomography, which are now used prior to the more invasive direct forms of cholangiography. The role of the radiologist in the care of these patients has recently been expanded to include a large variety of interventional procedures including drainage, biopsy, stricture dilatation, and stone extraction. The most important role of the radiologist as a therapist is in the palliative treatment of the patient with jaundice due to obstruction of the bile ducts.

Biliary obstruction can be present without ductal dilatation, such as in patients with sclerosing cholangitis or intermittent obstruction due to a stone; in such cases there is no place for interventional radiology. A variety of neoplasms, however, will produce biliary obstruction with proximal dilation of the ducts. These include primary ductal tumors (cholangiocarcinoma); neoplasms that involve the duct by direct extension, such as gallbladder or pancreatic carcinoma; and neoplasms that metastasize to periductal lymph nodes, producing ductal obstruction.

In patients with jaundice due to biliary obstruction, percutaneous biliary decompression (PBD) during PTC can provide access to the bile ducts for a number of therapeutic procedures:

- Preoperative biliary drainage.
- Palliation of obstructive jaundice.
- Biopsy of ductal lesions.
- Intraductal radiotherapy.

The commonest use of PBD is in the palliation of obstructive jaundice due to unresectable carcinoma; PBD can be a substitute or a valuable adjunct to surgery in the management of such patients with obstructive jaundice. A preliminary PTC is performed to identify the site of obstruction and to allow selection of a favorably located duct for PBD. Under fluoroscopic control, a guidewire is inserted into a biliary duct and advanced past the site of the obstruction. A drainage catheter is then inserted over the guidewire and, if possible, introduced all the way to place its tip into the duodenum. The catheter has multiple side holes located above and below the obstruction, and internal biliary drainage is thus accomplished. If the guidewire cannot pass the obstruction, a catheter is introduced up to that point and secured in place for external drainage. Patients with external drainage must collect, strain, and ingest their bile, and the catheters used for internal and external drainage should be irrigated daily with saline; they are replaced when they occlude or deteriorate, which usually occurs in 6 months to 1 year.

3. Surgical Treatment

a. Carcinoma of the Gallbladder

Surgical treatment offers the only hope for cure, although the prognosis is grim and the reported 5-year survival rates rarely exceed 5–7% overall. When the malignancy is identified by surprise in patients undergoing cholecystectomy for stones, the reported survival rates are in the range of 25–35%, whereas they are less than 1–2% when the diagnosis is recognized clinically. Median survival in those patients that are resectable is in the range of 20 months, compared with 2–3 months for those with unresectable disease.

When the diagnosis is available, the recommended procedure is a cholecystectomy with partial (or total right lobe) hepatectomy and en-bloc resection of the regional nodes. If the liver is grossly involved, it becomes highly questionable whether radical surgery is of any value, and its mortality and morbidity are extremely high.

In those cases where no curative resection is possible, palliation for jaundice should be considered, and one of the following biliary bypass or drainage procedures should be attempted:

- T-tube or straight-tube drainage of a dilated proximal duct.
- Choledocojejunostomy.
- Hepaticojejunostomy.

b. Carcinoma of the Bile Ducts

Carcinomas of the distal part of the common bile ducts are treated much the same as pancreatic and periampullary carcinomas. Radical pancreaticoduodenectomy has been reported to yield as 25–30% 5-year survival rate in selected series. The prognosis is better in well-differentiated papillary tumors and when regional nodes are not involved.

Carcinomas of the upper two-thirds of the biliary tree have a much worse prognosis, which is a reflection of the usually advanced stage of disease at the time of diagnosis. The 5-year survival is less than 5%, and most survive little after diagnosis. Cure can only be achieved surgically, although rarely is a resection of the tumor and effected duct or ducts achievable. If so, reconstruction with end-to-end ductal anastomosis or duct-to-jejunum anastomosis will provide for physiological drainage of the bile. In most cases, curative or palliative resection will be impossible, and one of the various methods of providing bile drainage must be attempted. The preferred procedure involves forcible dilatation of the malignant stricture, followed by placement of a firm stent connecting the dilated proximal ducts and the distal duct or the duodenum.

4. Radiotherapy

Surgery is the mainstay of treatment of these rare tumors; indications for radiation therapy are limited to certain selected cases:

- Adjuvant treatment following surgical resection in locally advanced tumors, especially in cases where microscopic residual disease is suspected.
- Malignant obstructive jaundice due to the presence of enlarged metastatic lymph nodes at the porta hepatis. Relief of the obstruction could be attained in a certain percentage of cases, especially if the cell type is that of a relatively radiosensitive tumor (e.g., lymphoma).
- For palliation of pain resulting from advanced nonresectable neoplasms.

Patients receiving adjunctive treatment with chemotherapy or radiation therapy are reported to live longer than those treated exclusively by surgery, and clinical trials are needed to substantiate such an approach.

5. Chemotherapy

Because of the small number of cases, systematic investigations of chemotherapeutic prospects in biliary tree cancer are not readily available. Furthermore, the locally infiltrative nature of this disease makes clinical evaluation with respect to objective measurement difficult in most cases. Consequently, available information is derived mainly from small series of cases.

Among active single agents are 5-FU, mitomycin, Adriamycin, and the nitrosoureas. Response rates of more than 20% have been claimed for individual agents in several small series. These claims are somewhat open to question, and it is still necessary to consider these cancers as relatively resistant to chemotherapy.

Several regimens of combination chemotherapy have been reported including 5-FU plus Streptozotocin and 5-FU plus mitomycin plus CCNU. Objective responses are frequent, but benefits to the patient are minimal and survivals are usually quite short. A 30% response rate has been claimed for the FAM combination, though it is not established as yet whether that response will necessarily lead to prolongation of survival. The median duration of response in the FAM series from Georgetown University was 8.5 months, and it was claimed that 6 of 13 patients achieved stable disease without having an objective response. The FAM regimen may thus be recommended for use if there is no other active ongoing clinical trial available that appears to be more relevant. It should be kept in mind that for patients with obstructive jaundice, the dose of

Adriamycin must be severely curtailed, if not entirely eliminated, since Adriamycin is excreted via the biliary system.

SUGGESTED READINGS

Pancreas

1. Brooks, J. R., and Culebros, J. M. Cancer of the pancreas. Palliative operation, whipple procedure or total pancreatectomy? *Am. J. Surg.* **131,** 516 (1976).
2. Cubilla, A. L., Fortner, J., and Fitzgerald, P. J. Lymph node involvement in carcinoma of the head of the pancreas. *Cancer* **41,** 880 (1978).
3. Fonkalsrud, E. W., Dilley, R. B., and Longmire, W. P., Jr. Insulin secreting tumors of the pancreas. *Ann. Surg.* **159,** 730 (1964).
4. Howard, J. M., and Jordan, G. L. Cancer of the pancreas. *Curr. Probl. Cancer* **2,** 1 (1977).
5. MacDonald, J. S., Widerlite, L., and Schein, P. S. Biopsy, diagnosis, and chemotherapeutic management of pancreatic malignancy. *Adv. Pharmacol. Chemother.* **14,** 107 (1977).
6. Rosch, J., Kelhr, F. S., and Bilbao, M. K. Radiologic diagnosis of pancreatic cancer. *Semin. Oncol.* **6,** 318 (1979).
7. Smith, F. P., and Schein, P. S. Chemotherapy of pancreatic cancer. *Semin. Oncol.* **6,** 368 (1979).
8. Stadelmann, P., Sofrany, A., Loffler, A. *et al.* Endoscopic retrograde cholangio pancreatography in the diagnosis of pancreatic cancer: Experience with 54 cases. *Endoscopy* **6,** 84 (1974).

Hepatobiliary

1. Adson, M. A., and Beart, R. W. Elective hepatic resections. *S. Clin. North Am.* **57,** 339 (1977).
2. Arnaud, J. P., Graf, P. *et al.* Primary carcinoma of the gallbladder: Review of 25 cases. *Am. J. Surg.* **138,** 403 (1979).
3. Bismuth, H., and Molt, R. Carcinoma of the biliary tract. *N. Engl. J. Med.* **301,** 704 (1979).
4. Fisher, R. L., Schever, P. J., and Sherlock, S. Primary liver cell carcinoma in the presence or absence of Hepatitis B antigen. *Cancer* **38,** 901 (1976).
5. Sherman, D. M., Weichselbaum, R. *et al.* Palliation of hepatic metastases. *Cancer* **41,** 2013 (1978).
6. Smoron, G. L. Radiation therapy of carcinoma of gallbladder and biliary tract. *Cancer* **40,** 1422 (1977).
7. Terblanche, J., Saunders, S. J., and Louw, J. H. Prolonged palliation in carcinoma of the main hepatic duct junction. *Surgery (St. Louis)* **71,** 728 (1972).

Section 11. Carcinomas of the Alimentary Tract

Part D: Malignant Tumors of the Liver

I. Early Detection and Screening   529
 A. Detection and Screening
 B. Predisposing Factors
 C. Early Signs of Liver Tumors
II. Pretreatment Evaluation and Work-Up   529
 A. Physical Evaluation
  1. Performance Status
  2. Bleeding
  3. Ascites
  4. Jaundice and Other Signs of Liver Failure
 B. Laboratory Findings
  1. Complete Blood Count
  2. SMA-12
  3. Serum Markers
 C. Radiological Studies and Imaging Techniques
  1. Chest X-Ray or CAT Scan
  2. Barium Swallow
  3. Imaging of the Liver
   a. Liver Scan
   b. Sonography
   c. CAT Scan of the Abdomen
  4. Celiac Axis Arteriography
   a. Hepatoma
   b. Cholangiocarcinoma
   c. Metastatic Tumors

  5. Cholangiography
  6. Venacavography and Portal Venography
  7. Laparoscopy
 D. General Medical Evaluation
III. Pretreatment Preparation   532
IV. Therapeutic Management   532
 A. Pathological Considerations
  1. Metastatic Tumors
  2. Primary Tumors
   a. Benign Tumors and Tumorlike Conditions
   b. Malignant Primary Tumors
 B. Surgery
  1. Criteria for Operability
  2. Surgical Approach
  3. Results
  4. Hepatic Artery Ligation or Cannulation
   for Infusion
  5. Special Hepatic Malignancies
   a. Hepatoblastomas
   b. Hemangioendotheliomas
 C. Radiotherapy
 D. Chemotherapy
  1. Systemic Chemotherapy
  2. Hepatic Artery Infusion
  3. Treatment of Metastatic Liver Disease

I. EARLY DETECTION AND SCREENING

A. Detection and Screening

As a result of the rarity of primary malignant tumors of the liver, there is no logical program for early diagnosis or screening. Fortunately, in nearly all hospitalized patients and in patients going through cancer-screening clinics, a battery of automated blood tests is carried out. This battery includes a number of different liver function tests; follow-up on abnormal liver function tests may lead to the diagnosis of a liver tumor. Because hepatic cell carcinoma is usually found in cirrhotic patients, careful observation of these patients and systematic screening for cancer will yield a number of patients with liver tumors.

B. Predisposing Factors

Hepatocellular carcinoma is very frequent in some parts of Africa, Hawaii, and among the Chinese in Singapore. It is less frequent in Japan and Denmark and rather rare elsewhere. In the United States the tumor develops in about 5–10% of cirrhotic livers. In Mosambique it is found in 40% of patients with liver cirrhosis.

The main risk factors recognized as predisposing to liver cancer are diet and liver cirrhosis. Other environmental factors have also been incriminated:

- Viruses, particularly hepatitis type B virus.
- Chemical carcinogens: mycotoxins (alfatoxin), nitrosamines, androgenic compounds.
- Parasitic infestation by *Clonorchis sinensis* also called *Opisthorcis sinensis*.

There seems to be solid evidence that persistent infection of the liver with hepatitis B virus (HBV) is an important etiologic factor of primary hepatocellular carcinoma in humans. It has been suggested that immunization of high-risk populations with the hepatitis B vaccine and prevention of mother-to-child transmission of HBV with immunoglobulins should decrease the chances of developing hepatocellular carcinoma.

C. Early Signs of Liver Tumors

Unfortunately, there are no early identifiable symptoms of liver cancer except where pain is a presenting symptom; most primary hepatic cancers are discovered late, when the patient presents with cachexia, ascites, jaundice, or GI bleeding resulting from esophageal varices.

II. PRETREATMENT EVALUATION AND WORK-UP

The management of patients with liver cancer and the results of treatment depend to a great extent on accurate stratification of patients in various groups where selected treatment options may be contemplated depending on the patients condition, the extent of the disease, and the complications that have already occurred. An extensive preoperative evaluation is thus mandatory.

A. Physical Evaluation

1. Performance Status

Patients who are beridden as a result of cancer cachexia or hepatic coma are not candidates for any treatment other than supportive and symptomatic relief.

2. Bleeding

Bleeding esophageal varices or intraperitoneal bleeding from the tumor itself is also a contraindication to surgery.

3. Ascites

Ascites is seen in 40% of patients, and it should only be tapped for symptomatic relief lest severe protein depletion occur. Besides its indication of the extent of liver damage, ascites raises formidable difficulties for the surgeon in terms of maintaining proper body fluid homeostasis and achieving primary wound healing.

4. Jaundice and Other Signs of Liver Failure

These are generally ominous signs that are indicative of poor prognosis.

B. Laboratory Findings

1. Complete Blood Count

Erythrocytosis is often noted, and anemia is frequent. White blood cells and platelets may be deficient.

2. SMA-12

Hypercalcemia and hypoglycemia may be noted. Liver function tests may be altered, and the alkaline phosphatase is a useful indicator of the progress of the disease.

3. Serum Markers

Hepatitis B surface antigen is commonly present. Levels of AFP are elevated in 78–98% of the cases, depending on the method of identification used. Serum AFPs, which are normally found in the serum of human fetuses, should not be present in children or adults. An elevation of the AFP level in the serum can be used to help make the diagnosis of carcinoma of the liver preoperatively and to follow the patient after total resection of the tumor. Also elevated in patients with hepatic cancer are CEAs.

C. Radiological Studies and Imaging Techniques

1. Chest X-Ray or CAT Scan

Superiorly situated tumors will frequently result in an elevation of the diaphragm, basal effusion, or linear right lobe atelectasis. In addition, 20% of patients will already have pulmonary metastases that must be identified prior to instituting any therapy.

2. Barium Swallow

The barium swallow is useful in documenting esophageal varices.

3. Imaging of the Liver

Imaging of the liver has undergone significant changes during recent years because of the rapid advances in the nonin-

vasive imaging modalities. The radiographic techniques available for the evaluation of hepatic masses include

- Radionuclide scintigraphy.
- Ultrasound.
- CAT scan.
- Angiography.
- PTC.
- ERCP.

a. Liver Scan

Radionuclide scintigraphy is quick to obtain, easy to perform, and relatively inexpensive. It has an accuracy of approximately 85%, but lesions must be at least 2 cm in diameter to be detected. However, all lesions that lack Kupffer's cells are photon deficient, and therefore cold areas on scanning are nonspecific in their appearance; radionuclide imaging is thus associated with a significant number of false positive, as well as false negative, examinations. These false negative and false positive studies require further verification.

b. Sonography

The accuracy of ultrasound in detecting liver tumors is approximately 85%; it is also quick and inexpensive. Approximately 10–25% of hepatic sonograms are technically suboptimal due to interfering intestinal gas and difficult anatomic liver locations.

c. CAT Scan of the Abdomen

The most accurate method of evaluating the liver noninvasively is the CAT scan. Masses must be approximately 1 cm in size to be detected with reliability; however, comparison of the three screening techniques (radionuclide scintigraphy, ultrasound, and CAT) demonstrates that CAT is the best single examination for determining the presence and extent of a hepatic mass. It is superior in sensitivity, specificity, and accuracy of diagnosis, and it is also the procedure of choice to define and differentiate intra- and extrahepatic masses. Suboptimal CAT examinations may result from paucity of fat in the cachetic patient and the presence of artifacts due to surgical clips, motion, etc. The most accurate combination of screening tests is that of CAT scan and scintigraphy; even in combination, however, they may at times be insufficient to differentiate benign lesions (hepatic adenoma, focal nodular hyperplasia) from malignancy, and this may have to be resolved by angiography.

4. Celiac Axis Arteriography

The accuracy of angiography in the diagnosis of hepatic tumors depends on their vascularity and size. It has a high rate of accuracy in the diagnosis of hypervascular tumors, and it may identify a tumor 5–10 mm in diameter. Hypovascular lesions, however, must be at least 2 cm in diameter to be detected. At times, CAT and angiography make a more accurate combination for specific purposes.

A thorough mapping of the vascular anatomy and the relationship of the neoplasm to the anatomic compartments is essential prior to surgery in those cases where resection is contemplated. Selective arteriography is also of great value when dearterialization or occlusion is desired or when selective infusion of cytostatic agents is contemplated.

The following features are useful in interpreting angiography for hepatic tumors:

a. Hepatoma

Hepatoma may present as a massive solitary tumor, multiple nodules, or a diffuse infiltrative tumor. Enlargement of the feeding hepatic arteries, deformity of the hepatic branches, rich tumor neovascularity, tumor stain, and infiltration of portal radicles are characteristic angiographic features of hepatoma. Enlargement of the feeding arteries and displacement of arterial branches adjacent to the tumor occur mainly with large, solitary hepatomas; vascular lakes and arteriovenous shunts with early filling of the veins are also frequently present in a solitary hepatoma. Distortion, straightening, irregular narrowing, direct invasion, or even obstruction of intrahepatic arteries are more often prominent features of the multinodular or diffuse form of hepatoma.

b. Cholangiocarcinoma

This presents in a solitary or infiltrative form. The solitary form has a predominantly expansive growth and displaces surrounding hepatic vessels. It is slightly hypervascular, and its vascularity consists of fine, tortuous vessels. The infiltrative form of cholangiocarcinoma is poorly vascularized and presents as infiltration, distortion, irregular narrowing, or even complete obstruction of hepatic arteries.

c. Metastatic Tumors

These may have variable angiographic appearances depending on their vascularity. Metastases of hemangiosarcoma, hypernephroma, choriocarcinoma, and islet cell and carcinoid tumors are highly vascular. Metastases from colonic, breast, or adrenal carcinoma show moderate vascularity with few small tumor vessels. Metastases from lung, gastric, esophageal, or pancreatic carcinoma are hypovascular, and they are diagnosed by deformity of the intrahepatic branches and defects in liver opacity. With multiple metastases, the capillary phase shows multiple radiolucent defects and may have a "Swiss cheese" appearance.

5. Cholangiography

The adequacy of the diagnostic information provided by CAT and angiography usually obviates any additional preoperative invasive diagnostic techniques such as PTC or ERCP. The only exception to this involves patients who require interventional procedures to decompress the biliary tree, either as definitive treatment or in preparation for a subsequent operation. Another exception in which PTC may follow a diagnostic CAT study is in the patient with a high obstruction near or involving the junction of the right and left hepatic ducts. If surgical decompression is planned, knowledge of the exact location and extent of the ductal obstruction can be extremely valuable and is best provided by PTC.

6. Venacavography and Portal Venography

These procedures may be indicated in rare circumstances where surgical resection is considered, to identify the presence and extent of involvement of these structures prior to surgery.

7. Laparoscopy

Laparoscopy is a highly effective and safe method to diagnose liver disease because 80% of the liver surface can be visualized with ease, and small lesions of a few millimeters in diameter can be identified. Direct biopsy can be obtained with precision, and evaluation of the rest of the peritoneal cavity can be performed to assist in the staging and to determine operability.

In experienced hands, this procedure is an extremely useful method of identifying liver tumors. It is well tolerated with a 0.1% morbidity and a 0.03% mortality and can be performed under local anesthesia. Patients are fully recovered within 2–3 hours.

D. General Medical Evaluation

Surgical treatment of patients with hepatic carcinoma is fraught with danger and carries a high morbidity and mortality for a very low yield in terms of survival. It is thus imperative to select patients for surgery with great discrimination. A complete systemic physical examination with all the supportive laboratory investigations (CBC, SMA-12, EKG, renal function tests and cardiopulmonary function tests, etc.) must be performed to assess the surgical risk as well as the anticipated longevity of the patient. A metastatic survey should also be carried out to rule out any spread of the disease, and the performance status of the patient must be established.

III. PRETREATMENT PREPARATION

The majority of patients with liver tumors are malnourished, anemic, and in poor homeostatic balance; their proteins and vitamins may be depleted, and their blood coagulation factors may be deficient. They often have associated liver cirrhosis and portal hepatofibrosis, which results in further hepatocellular insufficiency. Correction of these various deficiencies must always be undertaken preoperatively or, even when surgery is contraindicated, supportively.

- Hyperalimentation, either enteral with a high-calorie high-protein diet rich in vitamins or parenteral.
- Blood transfusions, as necessary.
- Correction of fluid and electrolytes.
- Correction of any coagulopathy; injections of vitamin K; infusion of any deficient factors or fresh frozen plasma.
- Diuretics for ascites, with careful fluid replacement.
- Antibiotics.

Resections of the liver are demanding procedures; the surgeon must have the patient and the team physically and mentally ready for this major undertaking.

IV. THERAPEUTIC MANAGEMENT

A. Pathological Considerations

1. Metastatic Tumors

The most commonly seen tumors in an otherwise normal liver are metastases from a primary malignant tumor elsewhere; these are usually multiple. The most common primary tumors to spread to the liver are malignant tumors of the alimentary tract, which spread through direct venous drainage via the portal vein. Other common sources of metastatic foci are bronchial and mammary carcinomas and melanomas of the skin. A tumor seen in a cirrhotic liver, however, is more likely to be a primary hepatic cancer.

Patients with metastatic cancer of the liver have a very poor prognosis. Most of them will only be treated symptomatically or with chemotherapy. In rare instances a patient will be found with only one or few localized metastases originating in an otherwise potentially curable tumor. These can be treated by limited hepatic resection but only after a very careful diagnostic investigation has been carried out to rule out all possible metastases elsewhere in the body.

2. Primary Tumors

a. Benign Tumors and Tumorlike Conditions

i. Cavernous Hemangiomas. These may be single or multiple lesions measuring 2.0 cm in diameter or smaller and rarely attaining larger sizes. The tumor is a well-circumscribed, dark-red, soft lesion, usually subcapsular; part of it may be thrombosed and calcified. Hemangiomas of the liver are more common in older people and may be associated with hereditary telangiectasia; they never become malignant.

ii. Hepatocellular Adenomas. This is a very rare, slowly growing, clinically silent lesion that never becomes malignant. It appears as a pale, ill-defined area in an otherwise normal liver. Microscopically it consists of thick plates or hepatic cells that are usually abnormally large. Portal triads are missing. The lesion is usually solitary and does have a capsule. It may show focuses of hematopoiesis.

iii. Bile Duct Adenomas. This tumor presents as a sharply circumscribed, white or grayish nodule. Microscopically it consists of small ductlike structures and may be mistaken for an adenocarcinoma. It is also rare.

iv. Intrahepatic Bile Duct Cystadenomas. This is a benign cystic mucus-containing tumor, usually multiloculated with a fibrous capsule. The tumor is rare and has to be differentiated from its malignant counterpart.

v. Hamartomas. Mesenchymal hamartomas are composed of loose connective tissue, tortuous bile ducts, and numerous blood vessels; these are usually solitary, well-defined lesions that present mostly in children under the age of 1 year.
Biliary hamartomas (Meyenburg's complex) are multiple, small cystic lesions formed by the collection of several cystically dilated bile ducts.

vi. Congenital Biliary Cysts. These cysts are solitary or multiple lesions, part of polycystic disease.

vii. Focal Nodular Hyperplasia. These tumors are composed of nodules of hyperplastic liver parenchyma and fibrous septa in the form of stellate scars. Microscopically they may resemble macronodular cirrhosis. The septa contain bile ducts.

viii. Compensatory Lobar Hyperplasia. This condition is seen in livers that have undergone atrophy.

ix. Peliosis Hepatis. Multiple blood-filled spaces appearing as red dots on the surface of the liver.

x. Other Tumors

- Heterotopic adrenal or pancreatic tissue.
- Pseudolipomas.
- Tertiary syphilis (gumma).
- Amebic abscess.
- Echinococcus cysts.

b. Malignant Primary Tumors

i. Hepatocellular Carcinoma (Hepatomas). Hepatomas occur in three morphological types:

- Multifocal nodular carcinoma, the most common (about two-thirds of cases). The nodules are firm or soft, yellow, brown, red, or hemorrhagic. They vary in size from 1 mm to several centimeters.
- A massive, solitary tumor that may be confined to one lobe only (about one-third of cases).
- Diffuse carcinoma, which can be differentiated from liver cirrhosis only microscopically (a very rare form).

Microscopically, the cells may be well differentiated hepatocytes producing bile (about two-thirds of cases). In 10% of cases they are composed of pleomorphic cells forming solid, irregular masses or glandlike structures. Necrosis is frequent, and some cells (the clear-cell variety) may contain large amounts of glycogen. The trabeculae of the tumor cells may bulge into the sinusoidlike spaces. The tumor grows rapidly and spreads intravascularly. It may first manifest itself as a metastasis in lymph nodes or bones.

ii. Cholangiocarcinomas. This type of tumor is about 14 times less frequent than hepatocellular carcinoma. It is rarely seen below the age of 50. Alfa-fetoprotein is not found in the serum. The tumors are usually composed of well-differentiated columnar epithelium of bile duct type and have a dense, fibrotic stroma. They grow slowly and metastases are rare.

iii. Hepatoblastomas. This type of tumor is a rare type of embryonal tumor, highly malignant, usually seen in the first few years of life. If diagnosed later in life, it seems to be of lesser malignancy and has a rather good prognosis after resection.

iv. Angiosarcomas. These are malignant tumors arising from the blood vessels. They occur in infants and adults. In infants the disease presents with enlargement of the abdomen along with heart failure; lung metastases often follow. In adults some cases have been attributed to oncogenic substances (thorium dioxide and vinyl chloride). They may be solitary or multicentric. Histological confirmation of the diagnosis prior to

therapy is most desirable, particularly if treatment is to be nonsurgical. This may be accomplished by percutaneous liver biopsy under sonographic guidance or by laparoscopy and direct biopsy. Needle biopsy may be dangerous in cases of jaundice or whenever a coagulopathy exists and could result in serious bleeding if the tumor is vascular. One must be prepared to operate should any serious complication occur.

B. Surgery

1. Criteria for Operability

The overall results of hepatic resections are rather disappointing, and the morbidity and mortality of the surgery is formidable. Only the exceptional patient should be considered for surgery, and the following criteria must all be met.

- No evidence of distant metastases.
- Reasonably good general health.
- No signs of severe hepatic insufficiency.
- No ascites, jaundice, or portal hypertension.
- Disease localized to a single area of the liver.

Less than 20% of primary liver cancers are considered operable, and cure rates are dismally low.

A large variety of hepatic resections have been described:

- Partial hepatectomy.
- Hepatic lobectomy.
- Hemihepatectomy.
- Subtotal hepatectomy.

Resections of the left lobe of the liver are relatively easily performed and well tolerated by the patient. Resections of the right lobe, or the right and medial portion of the left lobe, are major, complicated operations and should be performed only if strict operative criteria are met. Resectability seems to be slightly higher in children than in adults, and results are better in this group.

2. Surgical Approach

- A generous thoracoabdominal incision must be performed.
- Access and control of all major vessels is essential. The recent claims that one can achieve a total vascular isolation of the liver for periods of up to .0–1.5 hours, even in normothermic patients, would allow for a relatively easy and bloodless resection of the liver along anatomic planes, with acceptable morbidity and mortality. However, these claims are not yet widely substantiated.
- Up to 80% of the liver can be removed with minimal alteration in hepatic function. Significant regeneration occurs in the remaining segment, provided it is not cirrhotic.

- The use of an ultrasound device to cut through the liver (the Cavitron knife) has been reported to cut through parenchyma but leave all tubular structures (biliary radicles and vessels) intact. These can then be ligated individually.
- Care must be exercised not to compromise the portal or systemic circulation to and from the segment of liver that is preserved and to preserve its biliary drainage.
- Hemostasis must be secured at completion of the operation. The use of fibrinogen glue prepared by cryotherapy from the patient's own serum has recently been described as stopping troublesome bleeding.
- Generous drainage is imperative.
- Secure closure must be ascertained.

Resections of the type described above can be used for all types of primary malignant tumors and for resection of one or more metastatic deposits in carefully selected patients. Several dozen patients have been reported cured following resection of hepatic metastases; these have been usually from primary colon carcinoma.

3. Results

The prognosis for malignant tumors of the liver is not good. The overall 5-year survival is approximately 3%. However, in the hands of a number of surgeons worldwide, the 5-year survival following major hepatic resections for cancer has approached 20%; surgery is the only possible hope for cure and should probably be utilized in a far greater number of patients than is presently done.

4. Hepatic Artery Ligation or Cannulation for Infusion

Ligation of the main hepatic artery or its branches has been investigated as a modality of treatment for primary malignant tumors of the liver during the last 10 years. This can be combined with infusion of cytostatic agents in the distal end of the vessel as regional chemotherapy. The overall results are discouraging. Hepatic necrosis is more frequent than was originally suspected (over 50% of patients in a series from Hong Kong died of hepatic failure), and the salutary results reported are questionable.

Two techniques of hepatic artery cannulation for infusion have been described in order to permit the delivery of high-dose chemotherapy to the liver: direct surgical insertion of a catheter, which is preferred for long-term infusion, and percutaneous catherization of the hepatic artery via the femoral artery for short-term administration of chemotherapy. Both methods have been improved by the use of a self-contained unit and pump that can be totally implanted in the subcutaneous tissues of the patient for long-term ambulatory therapy.

5. Special Hepatic Malignancies

a. Hepatoblastomas

These malignant tumors of children are a rare disease that must be treated surgically whenever possible. Radiotherapy pre- and postoperatively has been claimed to be of some value, and some inoperable patients have been rendered operable by combination chemotherapy with Adriamycin. When resection is possible, results are quite rewarding, and in recent years total hepatectomy with liver transplantation has been attempted with what seems to be early favorable results.

b. Hemangioendotheliomas

These are also tumors of children that respond well to radiotherapy.

C. Radiotherapy

Radiation therapy has a limited role to play in the management of hepatic carcinoma, whether it be primary or metastatic disease. Because of the relatively low tolerance of the liver to radiation, adequate radiation doses cannot be delivered to liver tumors with a curative intent.

Low-dose radiation therapy alone or in combination with chemotherapeutic agents (5-FU, procarbazine, or hydroxyurea) can be employed for palliation in patients with extensive liver carcinoma, whether primary or metastatic. In a certain percentage of such patients, there will be some reduction in the size of the tumor and some pain relief. Moderate daily doses of radiation have to be employed with radiation fields limited only to the area of involvement. None of these approaches has actually been demonstrated to result in significant increases of the median survival time.

More recently, low-dose radiotherapy to the entire liver as an adjuvant in the treatment of carcinoma of the colon has been utilized in an attempt to control subclinical metastases. The results of these clinical trials are eagerly awaited.

D. Chemotherapy

Chemotherapy for carcinoma of the liver can be divided into systemic chemotherapy and intra-arterial chemotherapy.

1. Systemic Chemotherapy

Evaluation of chemotherapy agents in hepatocellular carcinoma is hampered by its relative rarity. Nevertheless, multiple agents have been studied, and some have been found to be marginally active. Of these, 5-FU and Adriamycin have been the agents most commonly employed. Response rates to systemic chemotherapy for hepatoma are highly variable and are based on small series. The best single agent is Adriamycin, even though reported response rates have ranged from 0 to 23%. Single-agent 5-FU is probably ineffective when given systemically, though it has been reported as having a response rate of about 40% when administered intra-arterially by continuous infusion. Various reports in the literature seem to claim response rates varying anywhere from 0 to 100%; a realistic expectation would be in the range of 15–30%. It should be kept in mind that the highest response rates were reported from Africa; most American reports claim much lower response rates.

Combination chemotherapy, including 5-FU and nitrosoureas, 5-FU and Adriamcyin, or 5-FU and mitomycin, etc. have not significantly improved the reported response rate. A reasonable choice for patients with advanced disease who cannot be entered on clinical trials might be the use of FAM.

The association of systemic chemotherapy with low-dose local radiation to the liver is undergoing investigation at the present time, and no conclusions can be drawn.

2. Hepatic Artery Infusion

Most of the available information relative to hepatic artery infusion concerns the use of 5-FU or FUDR. Once again, the reported series tend to have small numbers of patients, and statistical evaluation may, therefore, be unreliable. The rationale in favor of hepatic artery infusion as compared with systemic therapy is discussed below. It must be stated, however, that the logistics required to insert and maintain hepatic artery catheters is now available in many community hospitals in the United States, and the technique is thus no longer as formidable a challenge as it was in the past.

3. Treatment of Metastatic Liver Disease

Systemic chemotherapy for metastatic liver tumors should, of course, be based on the sensitivity of the primary tumor to chemotherapy.

Most patients who present themselves for cancer chemotherapy have either demonstrable disseminated disease or a great likelihood of developing such systemic spread. It is, therefore, reasonable that they be considered for treatment by systemic means, which is most often accomplished by the oral or intravenous administration of anticancer drugs. Depending on the particular protocol employed, intravenous medication may be given by a bolus type of injection over a short period of time or as a continuous infusion over a longer span. There are, however, a number of clinical situations in which the patient's disease is apparently localized to one organ (e.g., the liver) such that all or most of the neoplastic tissue derives its blood supply

from definable arterial sources. Such situations are not at all uncommon. As many as one-third of patients with metastatic colorectal cancer for example, present initially with liver metastases. Most of these patients are destined to die of liver failure, and in many of them, generalized metastatic disease never becomes an important problem. Other examples of clinical situations where intra-arterial chemotherapy has been found to be useful include

- Recurrent melanoma presenting with in-transit metastases on the involved extremity; this can be effectively treated with intra-arterial chemotherapy.
- Advanced or recurrent head and neck cancer that has become inoperable.
- Sarcomas, particularly osteogenic sarcomas of the extremities.

Intra-arterial chemotherapy (IACT) has been attempted and reported on for more than 20 years. Until recently, it has always been a formidable undertaking requiring admission to the hospital (sometimes in an intensive care unit), not only for catheterization of the vessel, but for long periods of time during which the chemotherapeutic agents had to be infused. Complications resulting from the catheter were frequent, including sepsis, dislodgement or thrombosis, and the need to remove the catheter and reinsert it for repeat infusions. More recently, some of the problems that once required inpatient treatment have been resolved as a result of the availability of portable, ambulatory infusion pumps. Drawbacks of this technique include the need to have an external arterial catheter exit from the groin, axilla, or abdominal wall, with the constant risk of infection and dislodgement, and the fact that the infusion device, although relatively small, still has to be carried and requires frequent battery changes, making the patient's quality of life and catheter acceptance less than ideal.

Simplified delivery systems have been achieved in recent years by the development of totally implantable infusion systems that eliminate the need for prolonged hospitalization and are superior to any external portable infusion pump. No external catheter is required, resulting in a significant decrease in infectious complications. Pump refills with the chemotherapeutic agents are required as infrequently as every other week and are expeditiously accomplished on an outpatient basis. The device consists of 2.8 × 8.5-cm pump made of titanium and powered by vaporization of fluorocarbon, which compresses a bellows within it. As the chamber is filled with fluid containing the anticancer drug, the charging fluorocarbon is compressed beneath a membrane; once the loading needle is removed, the charging fluid expands against the membrane, thereby forcing the chemotherapeutic fluid through a catheter that has been previously connected to an angiographic catheter placed in the artery to be infused. Thus, the system is self-charging, requires no battery changes, has no complicated electronics, and has proven reliable. Continuous flow of 2–3 ml per day for more than 2 weeks can be regularly achieved and remains constant during the infusion period.

As a result of these advances, interest in IACT, which waned during the 1970s, has been rekindled. Although most reports claimed higher response rates compared with IV chemotherapy for metastatic liver disease, the effects on overall survival were difficult to evaluate. Some remarkable remissions, however, have resulted from IACT. (For example, although only 20–40% of patients with osteogenic sarcoma respond to IV chemotherapy, 80% respond to intra-arterial infusion to the primary tumor site).

Several clinical situations now appear to be well suited for IACT. Foremost among those being presently investigated is that of liver metastases, particularly in the case of colorectal cancer. When the liver is apparently the only organ to have tumor involvement, several considerations seem to point to the desirability of IACT:

- Hepatic metastases seems to derive most of their blood supply from the arterial circulation, whereas normal hepatocytes receive portal vein circulation in addition.
- Some drugs are metabolized in the liver, resulting in lower systemic levels and less general toxicity after the drug has passed through the liver.
- Response rates in excess of 50% are often cited for hepatic artery infusion chemotherapy as compared with 20% or less for systemic chemotherapy. Furthermore, at least, one report suggests interesting efficacy for *cis*-platinum when given by the intra-arterial route; this drug is inactive for colorectal cancer when given by the standard IV route.

For most patients, insertion of the device and hepatic artery catheterization requires laparotomy. A recently developed transaxillary angiographic catheter placement technique, with simultaneous pump insertion under local anesthesia, has been used and may obviate the need for laparotomy in some patients.

Other clinical settings that might also benefit from IACT using the totally implantable pump include

- Extremity malignancies (sarcomas and recurrent melanomas).
- Pelvic malignancies. Some reports of IACT in pelvic malignancies are available; it has been attempted in situations where all other modalities have already been employed. Pain relief appears to be regularly achievable even if objective tumor responses are difficult to assess.
- Research efforts are underway to study IACT in head and neck cancer (external carotid) and CNS malignancies (internal carotid).
- One interesting report describes the use of subarachnoid continuous infusion of 1 mg of morphine to alleviate otherwise recalcitrant pain, using the totally implantable infusion pump.
- The technique is also available for various research projects. For example, the combination of continuous IACT with radiation, hyperthermias, etc. These, however, remain unexplored as of this writing.

In summary, many of the technical problems connected with IACT have been overcome. It still remains to be established what its final role will prove to be and which subsets of patients will derive benefit from the procedure. As with all other new technologies, estimates of the cost/benefit relationship will increasingly come into play. Thus, despite its initially high cost ($2000–$3000 for the pump in addition to the cost of hospitalization for insertion), the subgroup of patients who benefit from its use may prove to be less of a burden on the system if they can be restored to better functioning as outpatients for longer periods of time.

Section 12

Gynecologic Malignancies

RICHARD CALAME

With Contributions By

Kapila Parikh	Radiotherapy
Hosny Selim	Radiotherapy
Samuel Kopel	Oncology
Bernard Gussof	Hematology-Oncology
Randi Moskowitz	Nursing Oncology

Section 12. Gynecological Malignancies

I. Early Detection and Screening   541
  A. Patient Education
  B. Risk Factors and Predisposition
    1. Age
    2. Parity
    3. Sexual Activity
    4. Socioeconomic Status
    5. Predisposing Factors
    6. Exogenous Estrogens
  C. Early Signs and Symptoms
  D. Gynecologic Screening
    1. Cancer of the Cervix
    2. Cancer of the Vagina and Vulva
    3. Cancer of the Uterus
    4. Cancer of the Ovaries
II. Pretreatment Evaluation and Work-Up   543
  A. Physical Evaluation
    1. History
    2. Clinical Examination
  B. Diagnostic Radiology
    1. Intravenous Urogram
    2. Lymphangiogram
    3. Sonogram
    4. Upper GI Series and Barium Enema
    5. Pelvic and Abdominal CAT Scans
  C. Special Investigative Procedures
    1. Colposcopy
    2. Conization of the Cervix
    3. Dilatation and Curettage
    4. Endoscopy
    5. Laparoscopy
    6. Abdominal Paracentesis
  D. Metastatic Evaluation
  E. Multidisciplinary Evaluation
  F. Site-Specific Data Forms
    1. Vulva and Vaginal Cancer
    2. Cervical Cancer
    3. Uterine Cancer
    4. Ovarian Cancer
III. Pretreatment Preparation   545
IV. Therapeutic Management: Carcinoma of the Vulva   546
  A. In-situ Carcinoma
  B. Infiltrating Carcinoma
    1. Stages I and II
    2. Stages III and IV
  C. Verrucous Carcinoma
  D. Recurrent Carcinoma
V. Therapeutic Management: Carcinoma of the Vagina   555
  A. Radiotherapy
  B. Surgery
    1. Stages I and II

    2. Stage IVA
  C. Adjuvant Chemotherapy
  D. Treatment of the Advanced Vaginal Cancer
  E. Clear-Cell Carcinoma
VI. Therapeutic Management: Carcinoma of the Cervix   556
  A. Notes Pertaining to Staging
    1. Stage I (T1)
    2. Stage II (T2)
    3. Stage III (T3)
    4. Stage IV (T4)
  B. Therapeutic Guidelines
    1. Severe Dysplasia and Carcinoma In-situ
    2. Infiltrating Carcinoma of the Cervix
    3. Special Considerations
    4. Management of Failures of Primary Therapy
    5. Role of Chemotherapy
    6. Treatment of Advanced Cervical Cancer
VII. Therapeutic Management: Carcinoma of the Uterus   560
  A. Staging Considerations
  B. General Outline and Therapeutic Guidelines
  C. Management of Endometrial Carcinoma
    1. Stage I
    2. Stage II
    3. Stage III
    4. Recurrent Carcinoma
  D. Surgery for Carcinoma of the Corpus Uteri
  E. Chemotherapy for Endometrial Cancer
    1. Hormonal Therapy
    2. Cytotoxic Agents
VIII. Therapeutic Management: Carcinoma of the Ovary   562
  A. Natural History
  B. Treatment of Epithelial Tumors
    1. Surgery
    2. Adjunctive Therapy
    3. Second-Look Operation
  C. Specific Situations
    1. Ovarian Carcinoma in the Premenopausal Patient
    2. Nonepithelial Ovarian Carcinoma
  D. Treatment of Advanced Ovarian Cancer
IX. Postoperative Care, Evaluation, and Rehabilitation   566
  A. Postoperative Care
  B. Rehabilitation
  C. Evaluation
X. Management Algorithms   566
  A. Cancer of the Cervix
  B. Cancer of the Uterus
  C. Cancer of the Ovary

Suggested Readings   567

I. EARLY DETECTION AND SCREENING

The contribution of early detection through screening and patient education is nowhere as evident as in the case of cancer of the cervix and has resulted in marked improvement in survival by virtue of early presentation at the time of treatment.

A. Patient Education

Education of the patient is primarily the responsibility of the physician; it may be carried out on an individual basis through office contact or on a community basis. The latter could be a function of a medical center through its department of community services, of the local or county gynecologic society through its pelvic malignancy committee, or of the American Cancer Society. The nurse oncologist may also make significant contributions to patient education through the establishment of educational programs within the individual hospitals or clinics. The understanding and enthusiastic support of the media is also often helpful.

Education of the public may be pursued in three directions:

- Identification of the risk factors.
- Encouragement of the high-risk patients to submit to screening on a regular basis, utilizing regular, periodic gynecologic examinations, including cytological examination.
- Instruction to patients regarding the early signs of gynecologic cancers.

B. Risk Factors and Predisposition

Multiple factors are recognized as being of importance in gynecologic cancer.

1. Age

Women at any age can be affected by carcinoma of the cervix, although those in the fourth and fifth decades seem to be at a greater risk. Carcinoma of the vagina and vulva is a disease of older women, the latter being extremely rare in women under 50 years of age, except in the nonwhite population. Carcinoma of the uterus occurs mainly in the postmenopausal female, particularly in those who reach menopause after age 50.

2. Parity

The risk of carcinoma of the cervix is higher in women of high parity, whereas carcinoma of the endometrium is more prevalent in nulliparous or low-parity women.

3. Sexual Activity

The incidence of carcinoma of the cervix is higher in patients whose sexual activities started before the age of 15 and in females who have had multiple sex partners.

4. Socioeconomic Status

Patients of lower socioeconomic status, particularly among minorities (black and Hispanic), are at greater risk of cervical carcinoma. Carcinoma of the ovary and of the uterus are seen more often in the more affluent patients.

5. Predisposing Factors

- Genital herpes or the papilloma virus may increase the risk of cervix cancer.
- Chronic vulvar pruritis is often noted in patients with vulvar carcinoma.
- Diethylstilbestrol (DES). *In-utero* exposure of the fetus to DES administered to the mother during pregnancy carries a risk of the development of vaginal or cervical carcinoma in the young female offspring many years later.
- Obesity, hypertension, and diabetes mellitus seem to be associated with a higher incidence of endometrial carcinoma.
- Patients with endometrial polyps or hyperplasia are also at greater risk for uterine cancer.
- Estrogen-secreting ovarian tumors.
- Anovulatory females are at greater risk.

6. Exogenous Estrogens

Prolonged uninterrupted administration of exogenous estrogens may be associated with a greater risk of carcinoma of the endometrium.

C. Early Signs and Symptoms

- Bleeding. Bleeding is probably the most important early sign of gynecologic cancers. It can be variably described as
  - Contact bleeding (i.e., bleeding following coitus or douches) is most often seen in *cervical or vaginal cancers.*
  - Postmenopausal bleeding. This is a frequent presentation of *vaginal carcinoma,* where the bleeding is often in the form of a brownish, foul smelling discharge. Postmenopausal bleeding of pure blood, however, is the most common early sign of *endometrial carcinoma.* It should be recognized as extremely significant and should lead to prompt attention by the physician. The index of suspicion should be particularly high in women with other risk factors previously described.
- Pruritis of the vulva.
- A "sore" or "lump" or "white patch" in the vulva.
- Urinary symptoms.
  - Dysuria.
  - Urethral obstruction.
  - Ureteral obstruction, flank pain.
  - Sepsis.
- Bowel symptoms. Bowel symptoms, though evidence of advanced disease, are occasionally presenting symptoms of ovarian cancers.
  - Bloating and feeling of fullness (ovarian carcinoma).
  - Constipation.
  - Tenesmus.
- Inguinal lymphadenopathy or umbilical nodules. Ovarian carcinoma may occasionally present with one of these.

D. Gynecologic Screening

Screening for gynecologic cancer in the form of routine periodic examinations is strongly recommended. Many gynecologic cancers can be identified early during routine gynecologic examination and after cervical and vaginal cytological examinations (the so-called Pap smear). Although mass screening may be carried out and has, at times, been conducted as part of various mass cancer detection programs, screening for gynecologic cancers is usually conducted on a one-to-one basis by the gynecologist with the patient. A complete

gynecologic examination should be carried out on a yearly basis on all women over 20 years of age. This must include

- Thorough visualization of the vulva, vagina, and cervix.
- Adequate speculum examination.
- Vaginal palpation.
- Evaluation of the uterus and adnexa by bimanual and rectovaginal examination.
- Periodic Pap smears (cervical cytology).
- Colposcopy, when indicated.

Cervical cytology, the most important gynecologic screening procedure, should be done on an annual basis. In high-risk patients, it may even be performed at more frequent intervals. It has been suggested, however, that patients at low risk for cervical carcinoma, in whom two negative smears have been obtained at annual intervals, could have cervical cytology omitted from their annual gynecologic examination and carried out at intervals of 3 years. The Pap smear is the mainstay of cervical cancer screening. It is a highly accurate, reproducible, specific, and inexpensive screening procedure that results in an accuracy of detection in the range of 95% when properly performed. Colposcopic examination may be added to the above procedure whenever it is felt to be indicated.

1. Cancer of the Cervix

Cervical cancer may be identified extremely early on routine gynecologic examination. Cervical cancer could even be considered a preventable disease since characteristic cellular changes that herald its onset are easily identified by cytological examination. Such cervical carcinoma precursors identified on Papanicolaou smears include the dysplasias and cervical intraepithelial neoplasia. The early detection and treatment of those precursors will prevent the development of invasive carcinoma. Abnormal cytology in itself is, however, insufficient for diagnosis and demands histological confirmation. This may be obtained by the use of colposcopically directed biopsies or by cervical conization. No therapy should be instituted until a complete and accurate diagnosis has been established.

2. Cancer of the Vagina and Vulva

Vaginal carcinoma is also easy to detect in the patient who submits to regular, periodic gynecologic examination. Lesions involving the mucosa are easily visualized with a careful speculum examination of the vagina. Even those lesions that may be primarily submucosal will be noted by careful palpation. The important point to remember is that rotation of the speculum blades is essential to visualize the otherwise obscured anterior and posterior vaginal walls. The routine cytological examination of the vagina during Pap smears also permits early detection of carcinoma of the vagina and its precursors, which are also detectable by cytological or colposcopic examination of the vagina. Abnormal cytological or colposcopic findings require biopsy prior to the institution of therapy.

3. Cancer of the Uterus

Screening methods have not been very satisfactory for the detection of endometrial cancer in the asymptomatic patient; routine cervical and vaginal cytology has a low detection rate. In symptomatic patients, multiple enhancing techniques using cytological and histological studies have been designed for office diagnosis. These include jet washer techniques with cytology and endometrial biopsy. The formal fractional curettage of the endometrium remains, however, the definitive diagnostic procedure for endometrial carcinoma.

4. Cancer of the Ovaries

Ovarian carcinoma is probably the one gynecologic tumor in which there are no identifiable risk factors, no early signs, nor any available method for screening. Early symptoms are absent or vague in most cases; the patient is usually aware only of a feeling of fullness and bloating and may complain of "quick filling" such that even small amounts of food may cause discomfort. Only after a pelvic mass is noted or ascites develops is the true nature of the problem suspected. The unfortunate result of the above combination of facts is that ovarian carcinoma is rarely diagnosed in its early stages. Surgery is the primary modality of therapy, yet at the time of diagnosis, 65% of the patients already have nonresectable disease. The inability to make an early diagnosis of ovarian cancer is reflected in the overall survival rate, which is rarely more than 30%.

II. PRETREATMENT EVALUATION AND WORK-UP

A. Physical Evaluation

1. History

The following symptoms are indicative of one or another gynecologic tumor and should be elicited. The duration of symptoms should also be noted.

- Bleeding, staining, brown discharge, foul-smelling discharge, hypermenorrhea, or intermenstrual bleeding.
- Vulvar pruritis, lump, or sore.
- Herpetic lesions.

- Pain, dyspareunia.
- Urinary frequency, urinary retention, dysuria.
- Diarrhea or constipation.
- Other GI symptoms: dyspepsia, bloating, increased abdominal girth, etc.
- Weight loss, weakness.

In addition, the gynecologic history of the patient is extremely important and must include the following:

- Menstrual history.
- Age at first coitus.
- Sexual habits.
- Contraceptive practices.
- Obstetric history, number and ages of children.
- Family history, particularly as pertains to cancer, is essential. Past medical history must also be obtained; prior malignancies and their treatment, exposure to irradiation, particularly when directed to the pelvis, and a history of diabetes or other systemic medical illness are all of great importance. The patient's occupation may also have significance.

2. Clinical Examination

a. Gynecologic Examination

A complete visualization and palpation of the cervix, vagina, and vulva is mandatory. One must identify the following features:

- The size of the primary tumor and its exact location.
- Its type: ulcerating or exophytic.
- Its extension: vaginal wall, urethra, anus, perineum, clitoris.

On palpation, one must evaluate the following features:

- Parametrial regions.
- Size of the uterus and its mobility.
- Fixation to the lateral wall of the pelvis.
- Rectovaginal septum and vesicovaginal septum evaluation.

b. Lymph Node Involvement

Inguinal and femoral node examination with assessment of the number, size, confluence, or fixation of nodes should be an integral part of any comprehensive gynecologic examination.

Supraclavicular node evaluation is also important to identify distant spread of the disease, which occasionally involves these nodes.

c. Abdominal Examination

- Abdominal or umbilical masses.
- Abdominal girth.

- Presence of ascites.
- Examination of the liver.

d. Breast Examination

Careful assessment of the breasts should be done in all patients.

e. Extremities

Edema, erythema, or tenderness of the lower extremities should be identified.

B. Diagnostic Radiology

1. Intravenous Urogram

This is an essential examination of all patients suspected of having a pelvic malignancy. Identification of the ureters and their displacement or obstruction is of the greatest importance. Involvement of the bladder may also be identified, and renal function must be ascertained.

2. Lymphangiogram

This test might be indicated in selected cases to evaluate the aortoiliac lymphatics. It may be of particular interest in poorly differentiated cervical or endometrial tumors beyond Stage II, though more recently it has been largely replaced by computerized axial tomography (CAT) scans of the pelvis and abdomen.

3. Sonogram

A sonogram may be utilized for the evaluation of pelvic masses of uncertain nature, although laparotomy is usually essential for the definitive diagnosis and surgical staging of ovarian carcinoma. It would thus seem reasonable to proceed directly to laparotomy to identify the lesion and document the extent of the disease in the majority of pelvic masses of a gynecologic nature.

4. Upper GI Series and Barium Enema

Ovarian carcinomas are often metastatic in nature. It is, therefore, often desirable to try to identify a GI primary before laparotomy, especially in bilateral tumors of the ovaries. Likewise, a barium enema is often indicated to distinguish a colorectal carcinoma from an ovarian primary tumor or to identify involvement of the large bowel by an ovarian tumor.

5. Pelvic and Abdominal CAT Scans

These studies have been able to define with considerable accuracy the nature and extent of the disease within the pelvis,

the presence of enlarged para-aortic nodes, and the presence or absence of renal and ureteral involvement. Although not always essential, they can offer the gynecologic surgeon valuable information.

C. Special Investigative Procedures

Several investigative procedures are extremely useful in identifying the actual extent of the local disease and its spread by contiguous growth. They also frequently permit tissue diagnosis in rather inaccessible areas.

These examinations are particularly important if urethral or anal involvement by the tumor is suspected. When radiotherapy is being contemplated, such tests will also help localize organs at risk.

1. Colposcopy

Colposcopy is an important diagnostic aid in carcinomas of the cervix or vagina. Cytology, endocervical curettage, cervical biopsy, or biopsy of a vaginal lesion may be performed during colposcopic examination.

2. Conization of the Cervix

Where colposcopic examination is unsatisfactory or inconclusive, cervical conization is indicated to further evaluate abnormal cytology.

3. Dilatation and Curettage

Fractional curettage is the definitive diagnostic procedure in all cases of suspected endometrial carcinoma. Cervical biopsy should be included, should the cervix appear suspicious.

4. Endoscopy

- Proctosigmoidoscopy.
- Cystoscopy.

5. Laparoscopy

This procedure is extremely useful to visualize the pelvic structures, identify the existing pathology, and allow for a direct biopsy of the tumor when appropriate.

6. Abdominal Paracentesis

Where ascites is present, this procedure is indicated.

D. Metastatic Evaluation

No metastatic work-up is warranted when treating noninvasive cancer. In most cases of invasive cancers, a basic metastatic evaluation is usually sufficient unless the disease is far advanced. This evaluation should include a biochemical profile (SMA-12 or SMA-18) with liver function tests and a chest x-ray. In those cases of advanced gynecologic cancers, or whenever further evaluation is specifically indicated by symptoms or aberrant serum chemistries, the following tests should be selectively obtained:

- Liver scan.
- Bone scan.
- Selective CAT scans.

Furthermore, the patient who is about to undergo any major surgical procedure should have a thorough medical evaluation including

- Complete physical examination.
- Hemogram and coagulation profile.
- Cardiovascular evaluation.
- Pulmonary assessment.
- Renal evaluation.

E. Multidisciplinary Evaluation

A multidisciplinary approach to the patient with a gynecologic malignancy is desirable. Input from the pathologist, radiologist, gynecologic oncologist, internist, and radiation oncologist is important in the therapeutic planning. The nurse oncologist, psychiatric liaison, and rehabilitation medicine group are particularly helpful when radical surgical procedures are contemplated, and the ostomy team should participate whenever applicable. In ovarian carcinomas, the multidisciplinary approach is most helpful after the laparotomy, surgical staging, and resection, to plan subsequent therapy.

F. Site-Specific Data Forms

It is desirable to have available on the patient's record a site-specific data form containing all the pertinent information, including a classification and staging of the tumor. The following are suggested samples of such forms for the various gynecologic cancers, with diagrams for mapping of the tumor and instructions for accurate staging.

1. **Vulva and Vaginal Cancer Data Form (see pp. 547–548)**

2. **Cervical Cancer Data Form (see pp. 549–550)**

3. **Uterine Cancer Data Form (see pp. 551–552)**

4. **Ovarian Cancer Data Form (see pp. 553–554)**

III. PRETREATMENT PREPARATION

The patient with noninvasive or early carcinoma of the cervix (Stage I) who is being managed by a primary surgical approach is generally a young individual in reasonably good physical condition or she would not have been considered for surgery. Antiembolic measures, including stockings and possibly minidose heparin, are recommended as for most major pelvic operations. No other preparation is necessary preoperatively.

Most other patients with gynecologic malignancies will be in an older age group and may be facing extended surgical procedures. They will therefore require careful preoperative preparation and correction of any physiological aberration prior to surgery. The patient with carcinoma of the ovary, for example, is often in a depleted nutritional state prior to surgery, as she may have experienced weeks, or even months, of intolerance to an adequate food intake, and the associated bloated and quick-filling feeling may even have produced nausea or vomiting, which further complicates the nutritional status. Attention to fluid and electrolytes and blood volume, with preoperative correction of any deficit, is thus extremely important in these patients.

Preoperative preparation must take several parameters into account, and these should be approached and corrected as indicated:

- Electrolyte and fluid replacement.
- Blood volume replacement.
- Nutritional assistance.
- Antibiotics.
- Antiembolic measures: elastic supports, anticoagulants (miniheparin, etc.).
- Psychological counseling. The removal of the external genitalia, as in the case of vulvectomy, might require psychotherapy pre- and postoperatively; preoperative counseling and visits by the ostomy team is also of great value in the patient who is scheduled for pelvic exenteration or colostomy.
- Bowel preparation should always be done preoperatively in patients where bowel resection or colostomy might be required; a mechanical bowel prep is most important. Intestinal antibiotics are today believed to be of questionable value.

Patients receiving radiation therapy as primary therapy will require support during the prolonged course of treatment. The patient should be instructed in proper skin care during therapy. Since the success of radiation therapy is partially dependent upon adequate oxygenation of the irradiated tissue, attention to maintenance of adequate hemoglobin and hematocrit is essential. Those individuals who are troubled with excessive diarrhea during therapy must be monitored in regard to their electrolytes, especially prior to any contemplated surgical procedure, including radium or cesium insertions. It is important to recognize that radiation reaction is dose dependent in most cases; therefore a patient developing early or unexpectedly severe symptoms must be investigated for possible other etiologies. Colitis, diverticulitis, and bladder sepsis are among the most common etiologies.

IV. THERAPEUTIC MANAGEMENT: CARCINOMA OF THE VULVA

A. *In-Situ* Carcinoma

Although previously managed by vulvectomy, increasing attention has recently been paid to more conservative surgical measures in smaller lesions. If local excision is contemplated, however, the multifocal character of the lesion must be recognized, and identification of all the sites of disease should be clearly established. This may be accomplished by the stain-wash technique with toluidine blue and acetic acid (see § 1.I.C, Vol. 1) or by colposcopic examination. Biopsy of all suspicious areas may be accomplished by Keyes punch biopsy.

Truly focal lesions have been successfully treated by the local application of 5-fluorouracil (5-FU), and more recently, CO_2 laser therapy has been utilized. Surgery, however, remains the mainstay of therapy.

If the lesion is extensive or bilateral, a ''skinning'' vulvectomy (i.e., the removal of the skin of the vulva) may be the wiser approach. In Paget's disease, where local recurrence is so common, a wide resection is essential.

B. Infiltrating Carcinoma

While previously treated exclusively by extensive surgical procedures, radiation therapy and chemotherapy have recently assumed a more important role in the management of vulvar cancer.

1. Stages I and II

The usual surgical procedure for carcinomas of the vulva is a radical vulvectomy with bilateral superficial and deep inguinal and femoral node dissection. The management of the deep pelvic nodes is dependent on the identification of metastases within the superficial lymph nodes. If this is found to be the case, there are then two points to consider:

a. *Choice of Therapy*

One may elect to treat the deep pelvic nodes by external beam therapy, or one might chose to carry out surgical resection.

b. *Timing of the Surgery*

If the superficial nodes are positive and surgery is the therapeutic modality selected, some would elect to proceed directly with a retroperitoneal node dissection. Others would allow the patient to recover from the first procedure and then do a transperitoneal deep pelvic node dissection some weeks later.

2. Stages III and IV

The management of the more advanced lesions requires individualization. The morbidity associated with the exenterative procedures usually necessary for the more advanced lesions has somewhat restricted their use in the age group generally associated with vulvar carcinoma. However, when the lesion extensively involves the anus or urethra, the only curative attempt would be by exenteration, though results are far from satisfactory.

More recently, a combination of radiotherapy and surgery is assuming a larger role in the treatment of extensive local lesions. Radical vulvectomy in combination with radiotherapy to the regional nodes has been advanced as one approach.

Where the lesion is so extensive that surgery and/or radiotherapy appears not to be immediately applicable, combination chemotherapy has occasionally resulted in enough local regression as to allow subsequent interventions by radiation or surgery. The agents used include methotrexate, *Cis* Platinum (DDP), and bleomycin. High-dose chemotherapy is generally needed, and morbidity may be substantial; careful planning of treatment by a multidisciplinary team is, therefore, essential.

C. Verrucous Carcinoma

This lesion, much like the verrucous carcinoma in the mouth, is a low-grade, well-differentiated squamous cell cancer that is minimally infiltrative, rarely spreads to lymph nodes, and is of low radiation sensitivity. In fact, radiotherapy has been reported to be detrimental in these patients, resulting in a more aggressive lesion. Radical vulvectomy is the treatment of choice; the need for regional lymphadenectomy in these cases has not been established.

D. Recurrent Carcinoma

The patient with recurrent carcinoma of the vulva may present with local disease or distant metastases. Such patients are particularly difficult to treat, and the lesion has a tendency to recur, seemingly despite any therapeutic measure. Exenteration, wide excision, radiation therapy, cryotherapy, and local and systemic chemotherapy have all been tried, and in a few instances, each has been reported to be of benefit. The overall

SITE-SPECIFIC DATA FORM—VULVA AND/OR VAGINAL CANCER

HISTORY

Age: _____

Symptoms
- _____ Vaginal bleeding
- _____ Foul discharge
- _____ Dysuria
- _____ Pain or dyspareunia
- _____ Diarrhea
- _____ Weight loss _____ lbs.
- _____ Pruritis
- _____ Vulvar sore
- _____ Vulvar nodule

Duration: _____

Social history
Occupation: _____
Race: ____ White ____ Black ____ Oriental ____ Other
Previous history of carcinoma
- _____ No ____ Yes   Site: _____
Treatment (describe): _____
DES exposure: ____ No ____ Yes
Abnormal cytology: ____ No ____ Yes
Family history of carcinoma
Relation: _____ Site: _____
Obstetric history
- _____ Parity
- _____ Catamenia
- _____ Last menstrual period

PHYSICAL EXAMINATION

Tumor (see below
Size: _____
Mobility : _____

Pelvic examination

	Normal	Abnormal
Vulva	_____	_____
Cervix	_____	_____
Corpus	_____	_____
Abdomen	_____	_____

LOCATIONS

	Primary site	Extends to
Carcinoma *in situ*	_____	_____
Anterior wall of vagina	_____	_____
Posterior wall of vagina	_____	_____
Upper third of vagina	_____	_____
Middle third of vagina	_____	_____
Lower third of vagina	_____	_____
Paravaginal extension	_____	_____
Rectovaginal septum	_____	_____
Vesicovaginal septum	_____	_____
Rectal mucosa	_____	_____
Anterior vulva	_____	_____
Posterior vulva	_____	_____
Anus	_____	_____
Perineum	_____	_____
Urethra	_____	_____
Clitoris	_____	_____

Regional lymph nodes (check)

	Neg.	Enlarged
Femoral	_____	_____
Inguinal	_____	_____

	No	Yes
Suspicious	_____	_____
Confluent	_____	_____
Hard	_____	_____
Fixed	_____	_____
Ulcerated	_____	_____

PRETREATMENT WORK-UP (Check, if done)

	Neg.	Pos.	Suspicious		Neg.	Pos.	Suspicious
CBC	_____	_____	_____	Optional	_____	_____	_____
Liver chemistry	_____	_____	_____	CAT scan	_____	_____	_____
Chest x-ray	_____	_____	_____	Liver scan	_____	_____	_____
IVP	_____	_____	_____	Bone scan	_____	_____	_____
Barium enema	_____	_____	_____	Lymphangiogram	_____	_____	_____
(patients over 45)				Sonogram	_____	_____	_____
Proctosigmoidoscopy	_____	_____	_____	Biopsy	_____	_____	_____
Cystoscopy	_____	_____	_____	Other: _____			
Colposcopy	_____	_____	_____				

Classification

Distant metastases: _____ No ____ Yes   Specify: _____
Histologic diagnosis: _____ Adenocarcinoma ____ Adenosquamous ____ Squamous cell
_____ Clear cell ____ Verrucous ____ Paget's disease
Grade: _____ Well-differentiated _____ Moderately differentiated
_____ Poorly differentiated _____ Undifferentiated

Staging: ____ T ____ N ____ M

Stage: _____

Signature: _____
Countersignature: _____
Date: _____

Classification of Vaginal Cancer

FIGO Nomenclature

Stage 0 (TIS)   Carcinoma *in situ*

Stage I (T1)   Carcinoma limited to vaginal wall

Stage II (T2)   Carcinoma involves subvaginal tissues but does not extend to pelvic wall

Stage III (T3)   Carcinoma extends to pelvic wall

Stage IV (T4)   Extension beyond true pelvis or invading bladder or rectum
  IVA (T4a)   Spread to adjacent organs
  IVB (M1)   Spread to distant organs

Uniform TNM Classification

Primary tumor
(As above for FIGO classification)

Nodes (N)

  NX   Not possible to assess regional nodes
  N0   No evidence of regional node involvement
  N1   Evidence of regional node involvement
  N2   Fixed or ulcerated regional nodes
  N3   Juxtaregional node involvement

Distant metastases (M)

  MX   Not assessed
  M0   No (known) distant metastasis
  M1   Distant metastases present (specify site)

Residual tumor (R)

  R0   No residual tumor
  R1   Microscopic residual tumor
  R2   Macroscopic residual tumor

Karnofsky Performance Status

100   Normal, no complaints, no evidence of disease
 90   Able to carry on normal activity, minor signs or symptoms of disease
 80   Normal activity with effort, some signs or symptoms of disease
 70   Cares for self, unable to carry on normal activity or to do active work
 60   Requires occasional assistance, but is able to care for most personal needs
 50   Requires considerable assistance and frequent medical care
 40   Disabled, requires special care and assistance
 30   Severely disabled, hospitalization is indicated, although death not imminent
 20   Very sick, hospitalization necessary, active support treatment is necessary
 10   Morbidity, fatal process progressing rapidly
  0   Dead

SITE-SPECIFIC DATA FORM--CERVICAL CANCER

HISTORY

Age: _____

Symptoms

_____ Vaginal bleeding
_____ Postcoital bleeding
_____ Foul discharge
_____ Pruritis
_____ Abdominal pain
_____ Weight loss _____ lbs.
_____ Pregnancy-related history
_____ GI symptoms
_____ GU symptoms

Duration: _____

Obstetrical history:
_____ Parity
_____ Catamenia
_____ Last menstrual period

Social history
   Occupation: _____
   Race: ____ White ____ Black ____ Oriental ____ Other
   Age at first coitus: _____
Previous history of carcinoma
   ____ No ____ Yes   Site: _____
   Treatment (describe) _____
   _____
Abnormal cytology: ____ No ____ Yes
Family history of carcinoma
   Relation: _____ Site: _____
Contraceptive practices
   ____ Oral ____ Duration ____ IUD ____ Barrier

PHYSICAL EXAMINATION

Size of tumor: _____
Site of involvement and extension
Carcinoma *in situ*: _____
Cervix lesion: _____

	Left	Right
Extends to		
Corpus	_____	_____
Parametrial		
tissues (nonfixed)	_____	_____
Pelvic wall (fixed)	_____	_____
Vagina, upper two-thirds	_____	_____
Vagina, lower one-third	_____	_____
Rectal mucosa	_____	_____
Bladder mucosa	_____	_____
Adjacent organs	_____	_____

	Neg.	Pos.	Suspicious
Pelvic exam			
Vulva	_____	_____	_____
Vagina	_____	_____	_____
Abdomen	_____	_____	_____
Uterus	_____	_____	_____
Size: _____			
Mobility: _____			
Regional nodes			
Parametrial	_____	_____	_____
Hypogastric	_____	_____	_____
Obturator	_____	_____	_____
Presacral	_____	_____	_____
Ext. iliac	_____	_____	_____
Common iliac	_____	_____	_____

PRETREATMENT WORK-UP (Check, if done)

	Neg.	Pos.	Suspicious
CBC	_____	_____	_____
Liver chemistry	_____	_____	_____
Chest x-ray	_____	_____	_____
IVP	_____	_____	_____
Barium enema	_____	_____	_____
(patients over 45)			
Proctosigmoidoscopy	_____	_____	_____
Cystoscopy	_____	_____	_____
Colposcopy	_____	_____	_____

	Neg.	Pos.	Suspicious
Optional			
CAT scan	_____	_____	_____
Liver scan	_____	_____	_____
Bone scan	_____	_____	_____
Lymphangiogram	_____	_____	_____
Sonogram	_____	_____	_____
Biopsy	_____	_____	_____
Other: _____			

Classification

Distant metastases: ____ No ____ Yes   Specify: _____
Histologic diagnosis: ____ Adenocarcinoma ____ Adenosquamous ____ Squamous cell
   Subtype: _____
Other _____
Grade: ____ Well-differentiated ____ Moderately differentiated ____ Poorly differentiated
   ____ Undifferentiated

Staging: ____ T ____ N ____ M
Stage: _____

Signature: _____
Countersignature: _____
Date: _____

Classification of Cervical Cancer

FIGO Nomenclature

Stage 0 (TIS)	Carcinoma *in situ*
Stage I (T1)	Carcinoma confined to cervix
IA (T1a)	Microinvasive carcinoma
IB (T1b)	All other cases of Stage I with invasive cancer identified clinically or occult (IB occ)
Stage II (T2)	Carcinoma extends beyond cervix, but not to pelvic wall or lower one-third of vagina
IIA (T2a)	No obvious parametrial involvement
IIB (T2b)	Obvious parametrial involvement
Stage III (T3)	Carcinoma to pelvic wall or lower vagina, ureteral obstruction
IIIA (T3a)	No extension to pelvic wall
IIIB (T3b)	Extension to one or both pelvic walls, or ureteral obstruction
Stage IV (T4)	Carcinoma beyond true pelvis or invading bladder or rectum
IVA (T4a)	Spread to adjacent organs (invading bladder or rectum).
IVB (T4b)	Spread to distant organs

Uniform TNM Classification

Nodes (N)

NX	Not possible to assess regional nodes
N0	No evidence of regional node involvement
N1	Evidence of regional node involvement
N3	Fixed or ulcerated regional nodes
N4	Juxtaregional node involvement

Distant metastasis (M)

MX	Not assessed
M0	No (known) distant metastasis
M1	Distant metastasis present

Residual tumor (R)

R0	No residual tumor
R1	Microscopic residual tumor
R2	Macroscopic residual tumor

SITE-SPECIFIC DATA FORM—UTERINE CANCER

HISTORY

Age: _____

Symptoms
- _____ Hypermenorrhea
- _____ Polymenorrhea
- _____ Postmenopausal bleeding
- _____ Pain
- _____ Dysuria
- _____ Rectal symptoms

Other _____
Duration: _____

Social history
Occupation: _____
Race: ____White ____Black ____Oriental
____ Other

Menstrual history
First menses: _____
Menopause: _____
Parity: _____
Estrogen exposure: ____Yes____No   Duration: _____

Endometrial polyps: _____ Yes _____ No
Ovarian tumors: _____Yes _____ No
Other: _____
Previous history of carcinoma: ____Yes____No
Site: _____
Treatment (describe): _____
Family history of carcinoma:
Relation: _____
Site: _____
Contraceptive practice
- _____ Oral   Duration: _____
- _____ IUD   Barrier: _____

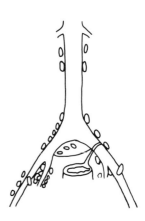

PHYSICAL EXAMINATION

Abdominal mass: ____Yes ____ No
Pelvic or inguinal nodes: ____ Yes ____No

	Neg.	Pos.
Pelvic examination		
Vulva	_____	_____
Vagina	_____	_____
Cervix	_____	_____

Uterine examination
Size (in centimeters): _____
Uterine sound: ____ ≤8 cm ____ >8 cm

	Yes	No
Extension to		
Parametria	_____	_____
Pelvic wall	_____	_____
Rectum	_____	_____
Bladder	_____	_____
Beyond pelvis	_____	_____

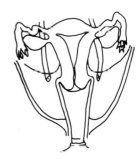

PRETREATMENT WORK-UP (Check, if done)

	Neg.	Pos.	Suspicious
CBC	_____	_____	_____
Liver chemistry	_____	_____	_____
Chest x-ray	_____	_____	_____
IVP	_____	_____	_____
Barium enema (patients over 45)	_____	_____	_____
Proctosigmoidoscopy	_____	_____	_____
Cystoscopy	_____	_____	_____
Colposcopy	_____	_____	_____

	Neg.	Pos.	Suspicious
Optional			
CAT scan	_____	_____	_____
Liver scan	_____	_____	_____
Bone scan	_____	_____	_____
Lymphangiogram	_____	_____	_____
Sonogram	_____	_____	_____
Biopsy	_____	_____	_____
Other:			

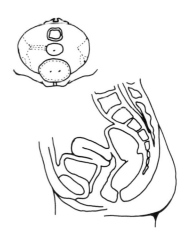

Classification
Staging: _____ T ____ N ____ M
Histologic diagnosis: _____

Grade: ____Well-differentiated (G1)____ Moderately differentiated (G2)
____ Undifferentiated (G3)____ Other

FIGO Stage: _____
Signature: _____
Countersignature: _____
Date: _____

Classification of Uterine Cancers

FIGO Staging Classification

Stage 0 (TIS)   Carcinoma *in situ*
Stage I (T1)   Carcinoma confined to the uterus
  IA (T1a)   Uterine cavity 8 cm or less
  IB (T1b)   Uterine cavity over 8 cm

It is desirable that stage I cases be subgrouped with regard to the histologic grade of the tumor.

Grading

G1   Well differentiated adenocarcinoma
G2   Moderately differentiated adenocarcinoma with solid parts
G3   Undifferentiated carcinoma or predominately solid tumor

Stage II (T2)   Carcinoma involving the cervix, but no outside extension
Stage III (T3) Carcinoma has extended outside the uterus, but is confined to the pelvis
Stage IV (T4)   Carcinoma has extended outside the pelvis or has involved the mucosa of the bladder or rectum
  IVA (T4a)   Carcinoma spread to adjacent organs
  IVB (T4b)   Carcinoma spread to distant organs

Uniform TNM Classification

Primary tumor
(TIS to T4b as identified above)

Nodal involvement (N)

N0   No involvement of regional nodes
N1   Evidence of regional node involvement

Distant Metastases (M)

M0   No known distant metastases
M1   Distant metastases present (specify organ)

Staging

The FIGO staging is identical to the T classification. The American Joint Committee on Cancer Staging groups the TNM as follows:

Stage I   T1 NX M0
Stage II   T2 NX M0
Stage III   T3 NX M0
            T1–T3 N1 M1
Stage IV   Any T or N with M1
            T4

SITE-SPECIFIC DATA FORM—OVARIAN CANCER

HISTORY

Age: _____

Symptoms
_____ Bleeding
_____ Weight gain _____ lbs.
_____ Increased abdominal girth
_____ Dyspepsia and bloating
_____ Constipation
_____ Defeminization or masculization
Duration _____

Social history
    Occupation: _____
    Race: ____ White ____ Black ____ Oriental ____ Other
Previous history of carcinoma: ____ No ____ Yes
    Site: _____
    Treatment (describe): _____
Family history of carcinoma
    Relation: _____ Site: _____
Abnormal cytology: ____ No ____ Yes

PHYSICAL EXAMINATION

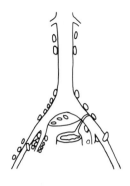

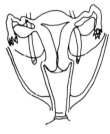

Abdomen
Girth at umbilicus (cm): _____

	Yes	No
Fluid wave	_____	_____
Masses	_____	_____
Umbilical nodule	_____	_____

Regional nodes	Yes	No
Inguinal	_____	_____
Distant	_____	_____
Supraclavicular	_____	_____

Pelvic exam	Normal	Abnormal
Vulva	_____	_____
Vagina	_____	_____
Cervix	_____	_____
Uterus	_____	_____
Rectovaginal septum	_____	_____

Ovaries	Right	Left
Palpable	_____	_____
Enlarged	_____	_____
Fixed	_____	_____
Cystic	_____	_____
Solid	_____	_____
Size____cm		

PRETREATMENT WORK-UP (Check, if done)

	Neg.	Pos.	Suspicious
CBC	_____	_____	_____
Liver chemistry	_____	_____	_____
Chest x-ray	_____	_____	_____
IVP	_____	_____	_____
Barium enema (patients over 45)	_____	_____	_____
Bone scan	_____	_____	_____
Proctosigmoidoscopy	_____	_____	_____
Cystoscopy	_____	_____	_____
Colposcopy	_____	_____	_____

	Neg.	Pos.	Suspicious
Paracentesis	_____	_____	_____
Thoracentesis	_____	_____	_____
Optional			
CAT scan	_____	_____	_____
Bone scan	_____	_____	_____
Liver scan	_____	_____	_____
Lymphangiogram	_____	_____	_____
Sonogram	_____	_____	_____
Biopsy	_____	_____	_____
Other	_____		

LAPAROTOMY ASSESSMENT

Ascites: ____ Yes ____ No
    Amount ____ cc
    Cytology: ____ Positive ____ Negative

Cell washings
    Cytology: ____ Positive ____ Negative

Extent of tumor
Para-aortic nodes
    Palpated: ____ Yes ____ No
    Suspicious: ____ Yes ____ No
    Sampled: ____ Yes ____ No
    ____ Positive ____ Negative

Undersurface of diaphragm
    Palpated: ____ Yes ____ No
    Suspicious: ____ Yes ____ No
    Sampled: ____ Yes ____ No
    ____ Positive ____ Negative

Omentum
    ____ Positive ____ Negative
    Omentectomy: ____ Yes ____ No

Extent of tumor (cont.)
Appendix
    ____ Positive ____ Negative
    Appendectomy: ____ Yes ____ No

Viseral peritoneum
    Site: _____

Parietal peritoneum
    Site: _____

Ovary
    ____ Right ____ Left

Uterus: _____

Tube
    ____ Right ____ Left

Liver
    Palpated: ____ Yes ____ No
    Suspicious: ____ Yes ____ No
    Sampled: ____ Yes ____ No
    ____ Positive ____ Negative

Classification
Histologic diagnosis: ____ Serous ____ Mucinous ____ Endometrioid ____ Clear cell
    ____ Other
Distant metastases: ____ No ____ Yes. Site: _____
Stage: ____ T ____ N ____ M   Signature: _____
FIGO stage: _____   Countersignature: _____
    Date: _____

Classification of Ovarian Cancers

FIGO Nomenclature

Stage 0 (T0)   Carcinoma *in situ*

Stage I (T1)   Carcinoma confined to the ovaries
  IA (T1a)   Carcinoma involves one ovary only, without ascites, with
                  (IAii) or without (IAi) tumor present on the external
                  surface or capsule rupture
  IB (T1B)   Carcinoma involves both ovaries, without ascites, with
                  (IBii) or without (IBi) tumor present on the external
                  surface or capsule rupture
  IC (T1C)   Tumor stage IA or IB, with ascites

Stage II (T2)   Growth involving one or both ovaries, with pelvic extension
  IIA (T2a)   Extension and/or metastases to the uterus and/or tubes
                  without ascites
  IIB (T2b)   Extension to other pelvic tissues, without ascites
  IIC (T2c)   Tumor either stage IIA or stage IIB, but with ascites present
                  or with positive peritoneal washing

Stage III (T3)   Growth involving one or both ovaries, with intraperitoneal
                  metastases outside the pelvis, or with positive retroperitoneal
                  nodes or both
                  Tumor limited to the true pelvis, with histologically proven
                  malignant extension to small bowel or omentum

Stage IV (T4)   Growth involving one or both ovaries with distant metastases.
                  If pleural effusion is present, there must be positive cytology
                  to allot a case to stage IV. Parenchymal liver metastasis
                  equals stage IV

---

picture, however, is that of persistently recurring local disease that reappears despite all methods. The discomfort for the patient is usually enormous and consists primarily of a burning sensation. Supportive care is extremely important in these cases and includes intensive nursing care, attempts at relieving pain, and pastoral and psychiatric assistance. Home health services can be of help if the family feels the patient can be managed at home.

The treatment of the patient whose problem is distant metastases would require individualization. For example, if the distant metastasis were osseous, radiotherapy would be the treatment of choice for palliation; in other cases, chemotherapy might be indicated if palliation is needed.

V. THERAPEUTIC MANAGEMENT: CARCINOMA OF THE VAGINA

Surgery and radiotherapy remain the principal methods of therapy for invasive carcinoma of the vagina. The literature provides no series, or collection of series, large enough to demonstrate a clear advantage of one modality over the other. The younger individual with a favorable small lesion is more likely to be considered for surgery; where advanced age or serious medical problems exist, the choice might be clearly for radiotherapy.

A. Radiotherapy

Radiotherapy usually involves internal and external irradiation in order to accomplish effective control of the local disease as well as the potentially involved regional nodes. The radiotherapist is involved in the pretreatment staging of the tumor as well as in the planning and distribution of the therapy. Individualization of therapy is essential to the successful management of the disease. The radiation fields are determined, in part, by the levels of vaginal involvement, and dosages have to be carefully calculated to achieve the highest success rate with the lowest morbidity. Attention must be given to the dangers of exposure of the bladder and rectum to the radiation and the potential side effects that might ensue (cystitis, proctitis, diarrhea, etc.).

For early-stage disease the treatment is usually external irradiation using ^{60}CO beam or an accelerator beam. The latter is of particular advantage in the obese patient, where energies up to 10 (or more) MeV are used. Treatment is usually supplemented by intracavity insertions of radioactive material (radium or cesium-137). Occasionally an (interstitial) implant of radioactive gold (^{198}Au), iodine (^{125}I), or iridium is used.

B. Surgery

1. Stages I and II

Surgical management of disease in Stages I and II (no extension to pelvic walls) involves total excision of the vagina and uterus. Regional node dissection would depend on the level of vaginal involvement; a lower-third vaginal lesion requires bilateral inguinal and femoral node dissection, while an upper-third lesion would necessitate a deep pelvic node dissection. Middle-third lesions might spread to either inguinal or deep pelvic nodes, and if the selected management is surgical, it would probably entail a deep pelvic and inguinofemoral node dissection. This type of surgery is primarily indicated in the young patient with Stage I disease (carcinoma limited to the vagina) and occasionally in Stage II (involvement of subvaginal tissues).

Stage III disease is preferably treated by radiotherapy, and radiotherapy is often selected for the treatment of Stage II disease as well, because of the extent of morbidity of the necessary surgery in these cases.

2. Stage IVA

Where the lesion involves the mucosa of the bladder or rectum without any evidence of systemic metastases (i.e., Stage IVa), an exenterative procedure is necessary if one intends to achieve a surgical cure. Whether a vaginectomy or an exenteration operation is carried out in a sexually active female, construction of a new vagina must be considered, either at the time of the initial surgery or as soon as is possible thereafter.

An alternative approach would be radiotherapy. Carefully planned and executed radiotherapy delivering high doses to sites of maximum disease has the potential of controlling the disease while avoiding exenterative surgery. Many of these patients are in an advanced age group, and the surgical risk may be unacceptable; radiotherapy, even if not curative, will often palliate symptoms and control growth.

C. Adjuvant Chemotherapy

Chemotherapy has had little role in the primary management of vaginal carcinoma. The lesions in this area are almost exclusively squamous cell carcinomas, and squamous carcinomas in the genital tract have historically been resistant to chemotherapeutic agents. There is some more favorable experience with newer chemotherapy programs, particularly those incorporating *cis*-platinum. Results, however, are sketchy, and the number of cases, limited.

D. Treatment of the Advanced Vaginal Cancer

Advanced vaginal carcinoma (Stage IVB) with distant metastases is not unusual. It has been reported that over 25% of all primary vaginal carcinomas have metastases present at the time of diagnosis. Patients whose advanced disease is manifested by distant metastases require decision by a multidisciplinary group on an individual basis. Palliation is available in the forms of radiation therapy for the primary and for identifiable osseous metastases; chemotherapy at the present time has little to offer.

E. Clear-Cell Carcinoma

Clear-cell carcinoma of the vagina is a specific tumor of the vagina with several unusual characteristic features. The two main features of this entity are the unusually young age incidence and a clearly identifiable risk factor. Both of these factors pose unique problems in detection and management.

The realization of the role that the mother's exposure to DES plays in this disease has helped identify a very specific population at risk. Education of women to alert them to this risk and to ascertain whether they or their mothers might have taken the drug during pregnancy is essential. Here, the cooperation of the media is important, and the message must be clear, though not alarming. The number of patients who received the drug is unknown, and in many instances records are not available. Patients who had pregnancy wastage problems and who received medication in subsequent pregnancies should be encouraged to try to recover their records and identify which medications they received. If they did receive DES, or if they cannot rule it out, all female offspring of those pregnancies should be considered at risk for vaginal or cervical cancer and should have regular, periodic screening examinations. Vaginal and cervical inspection, coupled with cytological examination and maybe even colposcopic examination should be performed at 6-month intervals. Benign changes in the cervix or vagina are often identifiable and would confirm the risk potential.

Treatment of this type of vaginal cancer is also somewhat different. Most patients with early stages are managed surgically as defined above, and in view of the patient's young age, a new vagina should be constructed at the time of the original procedure. In the more advanced lesions, radiotherapy may be the treatment of choice or combination therapy may be advised.

VI. THERAPEUTIC MANAGEMENT: CARCINOMA OF THE CERVIX

A. Notes Pertaining to Staging

1. Stage I (T1)

Stage I is carcinoma confined to the cervix. Stage IA (microinvasive carcinoma) represents those cases of carcinoma *in situ*

in which histological evidence of early stromal invasion is unambiguous. The diagnosis is based on microscopic examination of the tissue removed by biopsy, conization, partial amputation of the cervix, or examination of a removed uterus.

The remainder of Stage I cases should be allotted to Stage IB. As a rule, these cases can be diagnosed by routine clinical examination. The "occult" cancer is one that cannot be diagnosed by routine clinical examination but that is histologically invasive; it is, as a rule, diagnosed on a cone or on the amputated portion and should be included in Stage IB, designated as "Stage IB, occ."

2. Stage II (T2)

Carcinoma beyond the cervix but not involving the lower one-third of the vagina or the pelvic wall is classed as Stage II cancer. As a rule, it is impossible clinically to estimate whether a cancer of the cervix has extended to the corpus or not; extension to the corpus should therefore be disregarded. A patient with a growth that seems to be fixed to the pelvic wall by a short and indurated, but not nodular, parametrium should be allotted to Stage IIB. It is impossible at clinical examination to decide whether a smooth and indurated parametrium is truly cancerous or only inflammatory; therefore, the case should be placed in Stage III only if the parametrium is nodular or if the growth itself extends out onto the pelvic wall.

3. Stage III (T3)

Carcinoma involving the pelvic wall, the lower one-third of the vagina, or causing ureteral obstruction is classed as Stage III cancer. The presence of hydronephrosis or a nonfunctioning kidney due to stenosis of the ureter by cancer permits a case to be allotted to Stage III even if, according to the other findings, the case might have been allotted to Stage I or Stage II.

4. Stage IV (T4)

Carcinomas invading the bladder or rectum and those extending beyond the pelvis constitute Stage IV cancers. The presence of a bullous edema as such does not permit a case to be allotted to Stage IV. Ridges and furrows into the bladder wall, however, should be interpreted as signs of submucosal involvement of the bladder if they remain fixed at palposcopy (i.e., examination from the vagina or the rectum during cystoscopy). A cytological finding of malignant cells in washings from the urinary bladder requires further examination and a biopsy from the wall of the bladder before classifying the tumor as a Stage IV.

B. Therapeutic Guidelines

1. Severe Dysplasia and Carcinoma *In Situ*

Those patients under age 35 with carcinoma *in situ* of the cervix who express a desire for further childbearing may be followed by repeated examinations, cervical cytology, and colpomicroscopic examination. Patients are accepted for the follow-up program only after the nature of their disease and its implications have been explained to them and only if they are considered to be reliable individuals. In all other cases where therapy is indicated or desired, the definitive procedure is hysterectomy.

The following guidelines may be used in the management of intraepithelial neoplasia of the cervix, but keen judgment must be exercised in the selection of cases:

• Where the biopsy procedure has completely excised the lesion, the patient may be followed with no further therapy.
• If residual intraepithelial disease is present, therapy may be either destructive (cryotherapy or CO_2 laser) or ablative (hysterectomy).
• In postmenopausal women, the removal of the ovaries would be routine in combination with the hysterectomy. The removal of the ovaries in the premenopausal woman is optional and left to the discretion of the attending surgeon and the patient. If the ovaries are removed in the premenopausal woman, estrogen replacement may be instituted postoperatively.

2. Infiltrating Carcinoma of the Cervix

Radiation therapy in the form of internal (intracavitary) and external radiotherapy is the most widely accepted modality of treatment for infiltrating carcinoma of the cervix. Radical surgical procedures can, however, be equally effective in the early stages of the disease (Stages IA, IB, and selected instances of IIA), and patients in this category with no medical contraindications may be managed by surgery.

a. Radiotherapy

Treatment of cervical carcinoma by radiotherapy should be, to a large extent, individualized and adapted to the clinical and anatomic situation of each case. It should be planned jointly by the radiotherapist and gynecologist since the initial staging of the clinical disease is fundamental in determining the extent of treatment. Staging should be done by both specialists following the criteria established by the Cancer Committee of the International Federation of Gynecology and Obstetrics in collaboration with the International Union against Cancer, and the American Joint Committee for Cancer Staging and End Results Reporting. It should be remembered that many variations of the tumor exist within the same stage of the disease; the clinician should recognize this fact and manage the patient according to all the pertinent findings; individualized therapy will yield the best results. The following is a broad outline:

i. Stages I and IIA. For carcinoma of cervix only or with involvement of a portion of the adjacent two-thirds of the

vagina wall, the principles of treatment are those that apply to the management of the local disease. The main emphasis is given to radium or cesium insertions that irradiate a relatively small volume of tissue to a high dose without exceeding the tolerance of the normal mucosa. The preferred method of radium or cesium insertion is the afterloading apparatus of the Fletcher-Suit type. With the Fletcher system the dosage is calculated to a plane passing through the internal os of the cervix and the center of the vaginal colpostats that bisects the lower uterine segment and the paracervical area. Radium or cesium insertion are usually employed following external irradiation by a rest period of 7–10 days. Two insertions are recommended 2 weeks apart. When two insertions are impractical or not feasible for medical reasons, treatment can be given by one insertion; the risk of complications with a single insertion is higher, and the effectiveness of the irradiation is decreased. Additional external irradiation (the parametrial boost) can be administered between radium or cesium insertions or, preferably, after completion of the intracavitary insertions.

ii. Stages IIB–IV. For the patient with more advanced disease (carcinomas involving the parametrium and beyond), the treatment is basically that of widespread local and regional disease. Larger doses of external radiation are given prior to the cesium insertion; the purpose is to control regional extensions of the tumor in the pelvic lymph node–bearing areas. When the lesions are very bulky, whole pelvic external irradiation is effective in controlling the disease at the surface of the tumor mass (away from the center or core) and, by reducing the volume of tumor, may facilitate a good radium or cesium application.

In those lesions where secondary symptoms such as pain, leg swelling, or hydronephrosis are more prominent than the local manifestations of bleeding or discharge, external irradiation is of primary importance.

Patients who are to receive radiation therapy as a definitive modality may be subjected to exploratory laparotomy prior to the institution of therapy in order to determine the status of the para-aortic lymph nodes. If these nodes are found to contain metastatic disease, they can then be included in the radiation field.

b. Surgery

Although the majority of patients with carcinoma of the cervix will be treated by radiotherapy, surgery may be equally effective in well-selected early cases.

i. Stage IA. The extrafascial modified radical hysterectomy may be utilized in cases of microinvasive cancer. The ovaries need not be removed in the premenopausal patient unless they are abnormal.

ii. Stage IB. Radical hysterectomy and bilateral pelvic lymph node dissection can be used in this stage of the disease. Ovarian conservation is permitted in the premenopausal patient at the discretion of the attending surgeon and the patient.

iii. Stage IIA. If the vaginal extension and the overall bulk of the tumor is limited, radical hysterectomy with bilateral pelvic lymph node dissection and excision of the upper vagina may be considered.

iv. Stage IV. Patients with Stage IV disease may be considered for a primary surgical approach if the lesion is restricted to the pelvis and the spread is essentially anterior and/or posterior. Pelvic exenteration (removal of the internal genitalia with bladder and/or rectum) may be considered for these patients if it appears that the lesions can be completely resected. Exenteration is, however, associated with considerable morbidity and even mortality and should be undertaken by experienced surgeons with adequate supportive services and only when the likelihood of success is high.

3. Special Considerations

Certain clinical situations present therapeutic problems of a very specific nature that will require some modification of the guidelines discussed above. The specific modification of the therapeutic approach as a result of the peculiar characteristic of the primary lesion itself or of the clinical settings should be determined jointly by the gynecologic oncologist and the radiotherapist when the selection of treatment is discussed. The following are a few such situations:

a. Carcinoma of the Cervical Stump

Carcinomas occurring in the cervical stump of a previously resected uterus are frequently discovered late when they have already extended widely, since the prior disturbance of the fascial planes seems to encourage such an incident. Treatment in these cases is similar to that of cervical carcinoma in an intact uterus, though the effectiveness of radiation may be reduced as a result of the absence of the uterus and the consequent inability to utilize intracavitary irradiation. Surgery is also more difficult and sometimes less effective because of the prior operative intervention. Treatment of these cases can only succeed if it is well tailored with close cooperation between the radiation oncologist and the gynocologic oncologist.

b. Management of the Incidental Invasive Cervical Carcinoma

Occasionally, invasive carcinoma is discovered incidentally in hysterectomy specimens where the indication for hysterectomy was presumed to be benign disease. Such incidents are rather rare, and management will depend on the cell type and the extent of invasion. The presence of lymphatic or vascular invasion is an important factor to be considered. The patient must undergo a full evaluation and metastatic work-up before further treatment. Therapeutic options include pelvic lymph node dissection or external and internal radiotherapy to the pelvis and para-aortic nodes if these are judged to be at risk.

c. Pelvic Inflammatory Disease

Traditionally the presence of pelvic inflammatory disease in a patient with cervical carcinoma is a deterrent to the use of radiotherapy and would sway management decisions toward surgery. Radiotherapy is associated with several complications that are essentially related to the presence of adherent intestinal loops in the pelvis. Surgery, too, in these cases, is not without increased complications, and treatment decisions should be coordinated closely between the gynecologist and the radiation therapist since the extent of the infection and its subsequent effect varies widely from patient to patient.

d. Perforation of the Uterus during Intracavitary Insertions

This is not an uncommon occurrence since the uterus invaded with malignancy is rather soft; even careful instrumentation may result in such an incident. Usually, no serious untoward complications follow, but it is strongly recommended that the procedure be abandoned and that an alternate method of treatment be instituted.

e. Patients with a High-Risk for Local Recurrence

Patients considered at high risk for local recurrence include

- Patients whose primary tumor is in excess of 5 cm in diameter, whether endocervical (barrel-shaped) or exocervical.
- Patients with endometrial extension of their cervical carcinoma.
- Patients with tumors that have a tendency to early lymph node metastases.

In these patients, combined therapy should be used. The external radiation therapy will be directed at control of the regional disease (lymph nodes), while the local disease in the cervix can be managed by a combination of radium or cesium and surgery. The surgical procedure in these cases must be the extrafascial hysterectomy.

f. Carcinoma of the Cervix in Pregnancy

The treatment of carcinoma *in situ* of the cervix identified during pregnancy is much the same as that of the carcinoma *in situ* described above and can be carried out 6 weeks after delivery. There is no need for repeat investigation of the cervix by biopsy, colpomicroscopic examination, or conization, unless a visible lesion appears or cervical cytology is once again abnormal. The patient may be permitted to deliver vaginally.

The treatment of invasive carcinoma of the cervix during pregnancy depends on several factors including the time of pregnancy and the stage of the disease.

i. First Trimester. Stage I and IIA lesions should be individualized; therapy will be instituted without delay; and the pregnancy will have to be sacrificed. Treatment will be surgical or radiotherapeutic. Surgery is usually the preferred modality, and the microscopic picture is a major factor in determining the extent of the operative procedure. For example, a Stage IA lesion with early stromal invasion that is well differentiated may be treated by modified radical hysterectomy, whereas one with a highly anaplastic appearance, even though still showing only early stromal invasion, must be treated by more radical surgery (i.e., radical hysterectomy and bilateral pelvic lymph node dissection). Radical surgery is carried out routinely for Stage IB and selected IIA lesions with radical hysterectomy and bilateral pelvic lymph node dissection. If radiotherapy is the modality selected, external irradiation is given to the whole pelvis. If the patient aborts, this is followed by intracavitary radiotherapy; if no abortion occurs, one should proceed with an extrafascial hysterectomy.

For Stage IIB and III lesions, radiation therapy is the treatment of choice. External therapy is administered first and usually produces abortion. Cesium therapy is to follow immediately. If abortion has not occurred by the completion of the external radiotherapy, the evacuation of the uterus can be accomplished at the time of the intrauterine cesium insertion, or a radical hysterectomy (without lymph node dissection) may be performed instead of the cesium insertion.

ii. Second Trimester. Stages IA and IB are again managed surgically, if feasible. The extent of the surgery is to be determined by the tissue diagnosis, and therapy must proceed without delay.

In Stage II and III lesions, radiation therapy is the treatment of choice. The uterus should be evacuated abdominally prior to the radiotherapy to prevent delivery through the carcinomatous cervix. External radiation is used first, followed by cesium implants.

iii. Third Trimester. In selected cases of Stage IA lesions and depending on the histology (particularly in well-differentiated tumors), delay in instituting therapy in the interest of fetal salvage may be permitted. It is only in this trimester that saving the pregnancy is permitted in selected early cases. The usual approach would then be to deliver the baby by classical cesarean section first and then carry out definitive tumor surgery as indicated by the histological picture.

With Stage IB and IIA lesions, classical cesarean section, radical hysterectomy, and bilateral pelvic lymph node dissection must be carried out not later than 3 weeks after the diagnosis is established, regardless of the viability of the fetus. Radiation therapy may be used instead of radical surgery after delivery of the baby by cesarean section. This must include external radiotherapy and intracavitary cesium implants.

Stage IIB and III lesions require classical cesarean section followed by radiation therapy. There should be no delay in instituting therapy with the hope of delivering a viable fetus in these patients.

iv. Postpartum. When invasive carcinoma is diagnosed in the first 6 weeks following delivery, therapy will be individualized and outlined by the radiotherapist and gynecologic oncologists just as in the nonpregnant patient. History of a recent pregnancy does not change the management per se, but supportive therapy is often necessary.

4. Management of Failures of Primary Therapy

a. Recurrent Carcinoma

This is defined as the presence of active malignant disease that appears more than 6 months after the completion of therapy. The treatment of patients with recurrent disease must be individualized.

In cases of recurrence following radiation therapy where there is no evidence of distant metastases, early surgical exploration is carried out to determine the resectability of the lesion. Resection might involve a radical hysterectomy or pelvic exenteration, depending upon the site and extent of the recurrence.

In cases of recurrence following surgery, each case will be evaluated in light of the findings on tumor survey and physical examination. The treatment recommended may be radiotherapy, repeat surgery of a more radical nature, or a combination of both.

b. Persistent Carcinoma

This is defined as evidence of active disease within 6 months of completion of therapy. Therapy for these patients is generally along the lines stated above for recurrent carcinoma.

5. Role of Chemotherapy

a. Adjunctive Chemotherapy

The role of adjunctive chemotherapy in the management of cervical carcinoma has been limited by two factors: the lack of a clearly demonstrable effective agent or combination of agents and the effect of the advancing tumor on the urinary tract with the eventual compromise of renal function, which limits the use of drugs that require good renal excretion to avoid toxicity.

Many chemotherapeutic regimens have been utilized, and recent reports of combinations of bleomycin and mitomycin C and of single-agent therapy with intermittent doses of *cis*-platinum provide some hope for an eventual breakthrough in this disease.

b. Palliative Chemotherapy

Patients with recurrences who are no longer candidates for further surgery or radiation therapy may be placed on chemotherapy. The management of carcinoma of the cervix by chemotherapy must, at the present time, be considered investigational. Decisions on agents and regimens must be individualized, and whenever possible, patients should be included in clinical trial protocols.

6. Treatment of Advanced Cervical Cancer

Advanced cervical cancer may present in two forms: advanced local disease or distant metastases.

A multidisciplinary approach with the radiotherapist and gynecologic oncologist acting as a team is important. It must be recognized that, for the most part, the treatment objective is palliative; the following guidelines are suggested:

- Patients with para-aortic or supraclavicular node involvement may be managed by including those areas in the irradiated fields.
- Patients with locally extensive disease, such as spread to bladder or bowel, might be considered candidates for a primary exenterative procedure if the age and general medical condition of the patient would permit.
- Individuals whose disease has clearly extended beyond a surgical or radiotherapeutic approach might be candidates for one of the chemotherapy protocols.
- In the extremely advanced disease, palliative therapy is limited primarily to the relief of symptoms by radiation therapy for osseous metastases. No attempt to alleviate uremia, either by surgery or dialysis, is considered sensible in a patient with incurable cervical carcinoma. Attention should, however, be paid to the relief of any distressing symptom (e.g., pain) and to other supportive measures.

VII. THERAPEUTIC MANAGEMENT: CARCINOMA OF THE UTERUS

A. Staging Considerations

The classification of malignant tumors of the uterus that is generally accepted and commonly utilized is that of the Federation of International Gynecologic Oncologists (FIGO):

Stage 0   Carcinoma *in situ*.
Stage I   Carcinoma confined to the corpus uteri.
Stage IA   Length of the uterine cavity is 8 cm or less.
Stage IB   Length of the uterine cavity is over 8 cm.

Stage I patients can be further subdivided according to the degree of differentiation of the tumor into three grades:

G1   Highly differentiated adenocarcinoma.
G2   Moderately differentiated adenocarcinoma with partially solid areas.
G3   Predominately solid or undifferentiated carcinoma.

Stage II   Carcinoma involves the corpus and the cervix but has not extended outside the uterus.
Stage III   Carcinoma has extended beyond the uterus but is confined to the pelvis.
Stage IV   Carcinoma has extended beyond the pelvis or has involved the bladder or rectal mucosa.
Stage IVA   Spread to adjacent organs.
Stage IVB   Spread to distant organs.

Grading is very important in staging the patients. The main prognosticators in endometrial carcinoma are the clinical stage and the histological grade of the tumor. The depth of invasion of the tumor in the myometrium is intimately related to the grade of the carcinoma. The higher the grade, the more likely the tumor is to be deeply invasive, and this is associated with an increase in the incidence of nodal spread. The histological grade of the tumor coupled with clinical stage becomes the main determinate of adequate therapy prior to hysterectomy.

B. General Outline and Therapeutic Guidelines

As in other gynecologic tumors, patients with endometrial carcinoma will benefit from a team approach. A close cooperation between the primary care physician, the gynecologist, the gynecologic oncologist, and the radiotherapist is mandatory. The therapeutic approach will be determined by

- Stage of the tumor.
- Size of the uterus.
- Site of the tumor and its local extension.
- Histological type and degree of differentiation.
- Medical condition and potential operability of patients.

The majority of patients with endometrial carcinoma (75%) present with Stage I disease. The standard therapy for women with Stage I endometrial cancer has been hysterectomy with bilateral salpingo-oophorectomy, with or without radiotherapy. Unfortunately, due to their age, obesity, and other medical problems such as cardiovascular disease, not all the patients are able to undergo such surgery; in such cases, radical radiotherapy has been used. The number of such patients is not large, however, and all reasonable efforts should be made to include a hysterectomy as the major component of therapy in Stage I carcinoma of the uterus.

Regional lymph node metastases have been found to occur in 20% of all operable patients with uterine cancer and more frequently in those patients with high-grade tumors and advanced lesions in the vicinity of the cervix. Surgery alone in these cases will tend to fail, and preoperative radiotherapy plays an important role in the treatment of carcinoma of the endometrium. The rate of vaginal recurrence is significantly lower when postoperative or preoperative radium or cesium is used. When surgery is used as the first modality of treatment, one must identify the poorly differentiated tumors, those tumors involving the cervix, and those with deep myometrial involvement. All three situations would be associated with a higher incidence of pelvic node disease and a poorer prognosis. In such situations, postoperative radiotherapy should always be recommended. At present, surgery combined with radiation therapy preoperatively or postoperatively has become the most common form of therapy for endometrial carcinoma in the United States.

C. Management of Endometrial Carcinoma

1. Stage I

a. Group I: Medically and Technically Operable Patients

i. Stage IA, Grade 1. In these patients, surgery is the primary mode of therapy; the chances of pelvic failure are few; and survival is excellent with surgery alone. Postoperative radiotherapy is reserved for those cases where unexpected cervical involvement or deep myometrial invasion is demonstrated in the hysterectomy specimen. Vaginal cuff irradiation with radium alone, or combined with external beam radiation, depends upon the degree of myometrial invasion.

ii. Stage IA, Grade 2 and 3, and Stage IB. These patients are generally treated with preoperative radiotherapy followed by total hysterectomy and bilateral salpingo-oophorectomy. In general, one insertion with radium or cesium is sufficient. Both intracavitary sources and contracervical vaginal applicators are utilized, and about 4000 mg hours are delivered. If there is myometrial invasion through more than half of the thickness of the wall of the uterus and in cases of Grade 3 tumors, the incidence of pelvic lymph node metastases as well as parametrial failure will increase. In these patients, additional radiotherapy with an external megavoltage beam should be administered in doses capable of erradicating the tumor. The whole pelvis should be irradiated with split fields to protect areas previously treated.

b. Group II: Medically or Technically Inoperable Patients

These patients can be treated with radiotherapy alone. The dose delivered must be high enough to eradicate the tumor.

i. Stage IA and IB, Well Differentiated. Intracavitary radiation by means of tandem and ovoids delivering 9000–10,000 mg hours is the treatment of choice. This is divided into two insertions with a 2-week interval between them. Considerations for external radiotherapy will depend on the presence of risk factors.

ii. Stage IB, Grades 2 and 3. These patients are treated with both external radiotherapy and intracavitary radium. A dose of 4000 rads is delivered with external radiation and supplemented by intracavitary insertions of radium to allow the delivery of adequate doses to all points of interest. Heyman capsules are used if the uterine cavity is large or irregular.

2. Stage II

When the endocervix is involved by endometrial carcinoma, the incidence of pelvic and nodal involvement is rather high. If a patient is medically operable, the therapeutic approach should be combined with surgery following a course of preoperative radiotherapy. A dose of 4000 rads to the whole pelvis would be delivered, followed by radium or cesium insertions with a dose of 3000–4000 mg hours. Following this, a total hysterectomy with bilateral salpingo-oophorectomy is performed. If the patient is medically inoperable, she is treated with radiation alone. In this case, a second intracavitary radium insertion is carried out after a 3-week interval.

An alternative approach to the combined management of Stage II cancer of the uterus is

a. Pre-operative cesium/radium insertion.
b. Total abdominal hysterectomy with salpingo-oophorectomy, peritoneal washings, and node sampling.
c. External radiotherapy if Stage II is confirmed or other risk factors exist.

3. Stage III

These patients with extensive disease are considered technically inoperable and should be treated primarily with radiotherapy. The usual treatment consists of external radiation in doses of 4000–6000 rads followed by one or two intracavitary insertions.

4. Recurrent Carcinoma

Vaginal recurrence can be treated with radiotherapy. Usually vaginal recurrence is an indication of extensive pelvic disease; thus the whole pelvis and the entire length of the vagina should be treated. The whole pelvis is treated to a total dose of 5000 rads, followed by local vaginal radiation, either in the form of intravaginal or interstitial brachytherapy, which should then be used to boost the minimum tumor dose to a sufficiently high level.

D. Surgery for Cancer of the Corpus Uteri

The surgical treatment of endometrial carcinoma consists of total abdominal hysterectomy and bilateral salpingo-oophorectomy. More radical procedures do not appear to improve the survival rate in these patients. Prior to performing the hysterectomy, peritoneal washings of the pelvis and abdomen should be obtained for cytological studies. The liver and bowel should be carefully examined. Pelvic and para-aortic lymph nodes are selectively sampled.

The place of surgery in the various stages of the disease and its combination with radiotherapy is as previously presented.

E. Chemotherapy for Endometrial Cancer

1. Hormonal Therapy

For many years, progestational agents have been the treatment of choice in patients with metastatic endometrial carcinoma. In general, it may be expected that one patient out of three will have objective evidence of tumor regression. The response appears to be related to the histological grade of the tumor: well-differentiated tumors respond more readily than anaplastic tumors. Relatively high doses of progestational agents are necessary to achieve remission; the most commonly used agents have been 17-hydroxyprogesterone caproate (Delalutin) and medroxyprogesterone acetate (Provera). More recently, the oral agent megestrol acetate has been used with similar effectiveness. Although the response rate is relatively low, a significant proportion of patients will derive substantial benefits from the use of hormonal therapy; in fact, the median survival of patients who respond to progesterone therapy is in the neighborhood of 2 years, as compared with 6 months for those patients who do not respond. Furthermore, the virtual absence of serious side effects makes these agents the first-line treatment of choice of metastatic endometrial carcinoma.

The recent discovery of estrogen and progesterone receptor proteins in endometrial cancer specimens suggests that, very much as is the case in breast cancer, this information may be useful in the choice of therapy to be applied. In general, well-differentiated tumors have a higher chance of having measurable amounts of estrogen receptor protein than poorly differentiated tumors, and it is hoped that these studies will, in the future, permit more rational judgments to be made in the selection of hormonal versus cytotoxic agents. The estrogen–progesterone receptor studies, however, can only be performed on the unirradiated uterus.

Although efficacious in the treatment of advanced disease, progestational agents have, to date, not been shown to be effective as adjuvant therapy following radiation and surgery. Although some have advocated their use in high-risk patients, controlled clinical trials have not shown definitive benefits.

2. Cytotoxic Agents

In the evaluation of chemotherapeutic agents in endometrial carcinoma, several classes of drugs have proven to be active. These include alkylating agents (cyclophosphamide and nitrogen mustard) with response rates in the neighborhood of 20–25%, antimetabolites (such as 5-FU) with similar response rates, and antitumor antibiotics (mainly consisting of Adriamycin) with a reported response rate of about 35%. Of these, Adriamycin, either alone or in combination with other agents and/or progestational hormones is the chemotherapeutic drug of choice. Because of the very limited number of well-conducted, controlled clinical studies available, it is not possible, at the present time, to offer firm chemotherapy guidelines. Generally, the recommendation would be to use progestational agents as the first-line treatment, especially in patients with well-differentiated primary tumors. For patients with poorly differentiated or anaplastic carcinomas, or for those who fail to respond to hormonal therapy, chemotherapy alone or in combination with progestational agents seems reasonable.

Finally, there have been some recent early reports suggesting that *cis*-platinum may well have significant activity in this disease.

VIII. THERAPEUTIC MANAGEMENT: CARCINOMA OF THE OVARY

A. Natural History

The treatment considerations in carcinoma of the ovary differ from those of other gynecologic malignancies because of the fairly unique natural history of the former. For instance, the spread of ovarian carcinoma occurs via direct extension to the peritoneal cavity and via the lymphatics but not usually to other local gynecologic organs. At laparotomy, when the disease is diagnosed, it is often far advanced. The few patients who present with early disease are either those in whom a routine examination discloses an asymptomatic ovarian mass (or cyst) or those where the disease manifests itself as a large, smooth-walled cyst and only microscopic examination reveals the neoplastic involvement.

The prognosis of ovarian carcinoma depends on the stage of the disease; within each stage, it apparently depends on the degree of differentiation of the tumor, particularly in the advanced Stages (III and IV). The 5-year surgical survivals reported in the literature are

Stage I   50–60%   (IA 65%, IB 55%, IC 50%)
Stage II   40–50%   (IIA 60%, IIB and IIC 40%)
Stages III and IV <5%

It is thus obvious that a significant fraction of patients with carcinoma of the ovary will require adjuvant treatment. Such treatment is indicated both in the subclinical residual disease (all fully resected Stage III patients and some selected patients with Stage I and II disease) and in patients with bulky residual disease.

B. Treatment of Epithelial Tumors

1. Surgery

The primary management of carcinoma of the ovary is by surgery, and the recommended surgical procedure is total hysterectomy with bilateral salpingo-oophorectomy. For Stage III disease, an attempt is also made to remove all extrapelvic disease.

Prior to exploration, any ascites should be evacuated for cytological analysis. Should no ascites be present, irrigating fluid may be introduced and cell washings taken, separately, from the colic gutters, the pelvis, and the upper abdomen.

Since the staging of ovarian carcinoma is surgical, it is important that thorough inspection and palpation of all areas of anticipated spread be carried out during the operative procedure. Inspection of the undersurface of the diaphragm, visceral and parietal peritoneum, and para-aortic nodes is essential. Biopsy specimens are to be obtained from all suspicious areas.

Where the tumor appears resectable, all reasonable efforts should be made to complete the total hysterectomy and bilateral salpingo-oophorectomy. This is to be accomplished in combination with an omentectomy and appendectomy.

The abdomen should be rendered as free of bulky disease as possible at the completion of surgery; small tumor seedings affecting the visceral or parietal peritoneum need not be excised. The most important variable is the amount of disease left behind and not the amount removed. Patients with minimal residual disease have potentially curable situations, and all reasonable attempts to achieve this state are recommended.

2. Adjunctive Therapy

Additional therapy in the form of chemotherapy or radiation therapy is almost always advisable in the total management of ovarian carcinoma, especially for Stage II, III, and IV patients; adjuvant therapy may be withheld in a Stage I case with favorable histology. Decisions on which modality should be used and when it should be instituted are made upon consideration of all factors available: the surgical findings, the histological type of the tumor, its grading, and its staging.

a. Chemotherapy

At the present time, where epithelial tumors of the ovary are concerned, the principal approach following surgery is usually chemotherapy, especially in Stage III and IV lesions; there have been reports of effective local control in patients with Stage II disease with adjuvant radiotherapy. Combination chemotherapy, including Adriamycin and *cis*-platinum, with or without the addition of cyclophosphamide, is presently the regimen of choice in most patients. This has largely replaced the single-agent alkylating drugs originally used as first-line therapy in epithelial tumors of the ovaries.

i. Stage III and IV Disease. In the single-agent alkylating drugs era (1950s to late 1970s), less than 5% of patients with Stage III disease survived 5 years. A significant fraction of patients (approximately 40%) had objective remissions, and these were occasionally quite durable. Enough women had been treated for extended periods with alkylating agents (chlorambucil, cyclophosphamide, or melphalan—all interchangeable as regards their activity) to establish that such patients have a significant risk of aquiring secondary acute leukemias. Nevertheless, it was recognized early on that ovarian carcinoma is a chemotherapy-responsive neoplasm.

Combination chemotherapy programs have been investigated for about a decade and are now considered superior to single-agent treatment. In a randomized trial, the National Cancer Institute compared melphalan to a multidrug program (Hexa-CAF) consisting of hexamethylmelamine, cyclophosphamide (Cytoxan), Adriamycin, and 5-FU. Results were published in 1979 and established the four-drug program to be superior in all patients except those with well-differentiated tumors. Most importantly, survival curves showed a higher plateau phase for the patients treated with the combination, suggesting that long-term remissions, possibly even cures, were achievable in 15–25% of patients with advanced disease.

More recently, the most significant observation has been that *cis*-platinum is a very active agent in ovarian cancer. As this drug has very little myelotoxicity in conventional doses, it is ideally suited to be included in combination programs with alkylating agents and/or Adriamycin. The combination of Cytoxan (CTX), Adriamycin (ADR), and *cis*-platinum yields significant objective responses in 60–85% of treated patients, with complete clinical remissions in as many as 30–40%. At second-look laparotomies, approximately one-half the patients judged to be in complete clinical remission are found to be in pathological complete remission and potentially cured. Among the remainder, who are found to have residual disease at second-look laporatomy, several further avenues are available, including whole abdominal radiation, peritoneal chemotherapy, investigative approaches, etc.

Chemotherapy with the aforementioned agents is quite toxic and should only be administered by a gynecologic or medical oncologist. Toxicities include myelosuppression (CTX, ADR), alopecia (CTX, ADR), cardiac failure (ADR), renal failure, neuropathy and hearing loss (cis-platinum), cystitis (CTX), severe soft-tissue damage in the advent of paravenous infiltration (ADR), and nausea and vomiting (all three agents). Courses of therapy are generally given every 3–4 weeks as tolerated. Attention must be paid to adequate hydration in order to reduce the likelihood of renal damage secondary to cis-platinum and to avoid CTX-related cystitis. One aims for 9–12 courses, though some patients are unable to tolerate a full year of therapy.

Patients with bulky disease do not achieve complete remission as frequently as those patients who have only minimal residual disease. There is some correlation between bulkiness of disease and histological grade: those patients with anaplastic histology tend to have massive disease and tend to do less well with any treatment, including combination chemotherapy. If a complete remission is achieved, however, a second-look procedure may be advocated.

In some patients, bulky masses shrink with the initial course of chemotherapy but fail to shrink further as the chemotherapy proceeds. Such patients may benefit from a second attempt at surgical debulking after an initial chemotherapy-induced response. Removal of residual disease in these instances may result in significant palliation; subsequent chemotherapy and radiation may then be employed with better results.

ii. Stage I and II Disease. The value of adjuvant chemotherapy in Stage I and II ovarian carcinoma is less clear. Some patients with Stage II disease have incomplete resection and are obvious candidates for adjuvant measures. Since most of the disease in such cases will be in the pelvis, both local and extended irradiation to the entire abdomen have been used in the past. In view of the good results obtained with cis-platinum–based combinations in Stage III and IV disease, it is reasonable to employ these programs in patients with Stage II incompletely resected disease as well. Another category of patients who may benefit from adjuvant chemotherapy are those with Stage IC and IIC completely resected disease (with an approximately 50% cure rate with surgery alone); both radiation and chemotherapy have been advocated. Randomized clinical trials have these options under active investigation, and no clear recommendations can be made at present. The place and ultimate value of second-look procedures in these cases is also not clearly established.

Immunotherapy using intraperitoneal tumor-associated antigens in combination with chemotherapy is, at present, investigative in nature, as is the use of high-dose intraperitoneal chemotherapy.

b. Radiotherapy

The role of adjuvant radiotherapy in the treatment of ovarian cancer is presently receiving more attention, especially in the management of small-volume residual disease. Moreover, the high incidence of relapse after apparent early success of cytotoxic agents has prompted the use of radiation therapy immediately after (or sandwiched in between) several courses of chemotherapy, to "consolidate" the gains obtained. The moving-strip technique of pelvic and abdominal radiotherapy, with extension of the field to include the undersurface of the diaphragm, has been introduced in some centers as an alternative to chemotherapy.

c. Intraperitoneal Radioisotopes

Radioisotopes, principally phosphorous and gold, have been used over the years by several investigators. Their use intraperitoneally has suffered from problems in distribution within the peritoneal cavity.

3. Second-Look Operation

Upon completion of a planned course of chemotherapy, a second-look operation should be contemplated. The following criteria have been suggested as indications for a second-look operation:

- The patient has completed a course of chemotherapy and appears to be clinically free of disease.
- Sonogram, abdominal and pelvic CAT scans are negative.
- The patient has had 10 or more courses of chemotherapy.
- The tumor has had almost complete clinical remission and may have now become resectable.

The various steps taken at the second-look operation should be systematic and include the following:

- Midline incision.
- Cytological washings from several areas of the pelvis and abdomen.
- Inspection of pelvic organs and peritoneum.
- Omental inspection and removal, if present.
- Inspection of all peritoneal surfaces.
- Retroperitoneal inspection of pelvic and para-aortic lymph nodes and biopsies whenever indicated.
- Biopsy of all adhesions.
- Multiple biopsies including biopsies or brushings of both diaphragmatic cupolas.

The second-look procedure permits the discontinuation of chemotherapy when gross microscopic and cytological evidence of tumor is absent and dictates a change in therapy if progression of the disease is identified.

C. Specific Situations

1. Ovarian Carcinoma in the Premenopausal Patient

In the young female desirous of retaining childbearing function who comes to laparotomy with a clinical suspicion of carcinoma of the ovary, the recommended procedure is a unilateral oophorectomy. Only after paraffin sections have confirmed the presence of an epithelial carcinoma should total hysterectomy and bilateral salpingo-oophorectomy be considered.

2. Nonepithelial Ovarian Carcinoma

Germ cell tumors, stromal tumors, and other ovarian tumors are rather infrequent in comparison with the epithelial tumors of the ovary. Because of their relative infrequency and the fact that several of these tumors affect young girls or young women in their childbearing years, they pose some difficult problems in management.

- Conservation of the uterus, or even of the uninvolved ovary, in many of these tumors may be considered.
- The unique responsiveness of some dysgerminomas to radiotherapy and the equally unique responsiveness of other tumors (e.g., endodermal sinus tumors) to combination chemotherapy make the prognosis of these tumors much less guarded than was previously believed.
- The presence of tumor markers—alpha-fetoprotein (AFP) for the endodermal sinus tumor and human chorionic gonadoptropin (HCG) for the choriocarcinomas—makes for much more accurate monitoring of therapy in those categories of tumors.

a. Ovarian Stromal Tumors

These rare tumors (<3% of ovarian carcinomas) tend to grow very slowly. Some cases produce estrogens with resultant feminization, and an increase in endometrial carcinoma has been observed. The treatment is primarily surgical, though unresectable lesions, or those stages at high risk, may be referred for radiation therapy to the pelvis and whole abdomen. There is very little experience with chemotherapy in this disease. It appears that alkylating agents are not very active. Adriamycin has been reported to be somewhat active, and there is not enough information available regarding cis-platinum.

b. Ovarian Germ Cell Tumors

These neoplasms often have a mixed histological pattern incorporating elements of endodermal sinus tumor, embryonal carcinoma, and teratoma much as is seen in germ cell tumors in young men. Before the advent of intensive combination chemotherapy programs, most patients failed to be cured by surgery and/or radiotherapy.

In treating endodermal sinus tumors, several reports have emphasized high response rates with the VAC (vincristine, actinomycin D, and cyclophosphamide) regimen. More than 60% of patients so treated have negative second-look laparotomies and are probably cured.

Malignant teratoma is a rare tumor that has also demonstrated responsiveness to the VAC regimen.

Dysgerminoma, the histological counterpart of seminoma in young males, is seen in young girls; is frequently bilateral; and like seminoma, is exquisitely sensitive to radiation therapy. As is true for seminoma, the tumor tends to spread to regional lymph nodes, and these should be included in the radiation ports. Surgery alone may be adequate therapy for disease confined to one ovary with intact capsule. If bilateral involvement is found, bilateral salpingo-oophorectomy is indicated and should be followed by radiotherapy. Radiotherapy should include irradiation of the whole pelvis, para-aortic nodes as well as one nodal region beyond any identifiable area of disease (e.g., addition of the mediastinum if the para-aortic nodes are involved). Other germ cell tumors such as embyonal carcinomas, while exquisitely sensitive to chemotherapy, are also responsive to radiotherapy, but at high doses (4500 rads); radiation therapy is thus reserved in these cases for either palliation of bone metastases or as an adjuvant in early (Stage I) cases.

If careful pathological examination of a dysgerminoma discloses elements other than pure dysgerminoma, more aggressive therapy is indicated (i.e., combination chemotherapy). Recent reports emphasize that recurrent germ cell tumors respond favorably to intensive chemotherapy similar to that used for germ cell tumors in males (vinblastine, cis-platinum, and bleomycin).

Decisions on the management of nonepithelial tumors of the ovary, subsequent to the removal of the involved ovary are best elicited following a multidisciplinary discussion of their various prognostic features and available therapeutic modalities.

D. Treatment of Advanced Ovarian Cancer

Patients with advanced ovarian carcinoma that has ultimately become unresponsive to the usual radiotherapy or chemotherapy are among the most difficult to manage. As the disease progresses, it is characterized by intermittent bouts of intestinal obstruction and progressive inanition. The picture is often further complicated by repeated episodes of massive fluid accumulation in the peritoneal and/or pleural cavities. The following guidelines are suggested:

- Ascites and hydrothorax often require repeated surgical drainage for reliaf of the patient's distress. The introduction of various agents such as Atabrine or nitrogen mustard has helped to reduce the rate of fluid accumulation in some patients.
- Intestinal obstruction is best handled conservatively by long-tube decompression, intravenous fluid and electrolyte replacement, and occasionally by hyperalimentation. The points of obstruction are often multiple, and surgical intervention rarely helps for more than a short time.
- Pain relief is mandatory, and any available treatment for relief of pain should be carried out.
- Supportive measures should be used at all times, and pastoral care is of primary importance in the final phases of this disease.

IX. POSTOPERATIVE CARE, EVALUATION, AND REHABILITATION

A. Postoperative Care

Postoperative care for those individuals who have undergone radical pelvic procedures must include

- Strict monitoring of the patient's vital signs, hematologic and electrolyte picture, and urinary output.
- Pulmonary toilet and assistance with various respirators to avoid atelectasis.
- Close observation for hemorrhage or other acute wound complications.
- Early mobilization and observation for deep-vein thrombosis or pulmonary embolus.
- Anastomotic leaks, fistulas, or stomal problems must be quickly identified and corrected appropriately.
- Those patients who have been operated on for ovarian carcinomas with ascites must have their fluid shifts adjusted. The loss of large amounts of ascitic fluid could result in shock and loss of proteins that may require correction.
- Wound care, especially when radical vulvectomy and/or inguinal or femoral node dissection has been performed, is imperative. Drains and catheters must be kept patent and removed when indicated by the decreasing amounts of drainage. Wound necrosis, infection, and dehiscences should be watched for. Separate vulvar and groin incisions and meticulous attention to asceptic techniques and wound dressings have decreased these wound complications.

- Elastic support and leg elevation to minimize lymphedema following lymphadenectomy are important.

B. Rehabilitation

All patients completing therapy for vaginal or vulvar carcinomas, whether by radiation or surgery, require significant adjustment. Pastoral care, nursing support, and psychiatric counseling are essential. The operative procedure is considered mutilating by many patients in the same sense as a mastectomy procedure, and rehabilitation from a physical and psychiatric standpoint is extremely important. Where a new vagina has been created, attention to prevention of cicatrix and stenosis is important, and the use of dilators may be necessary. The use of skin grafts or myocutaneous flaps is often necessary to close surgical defects and should be completed without delay.

Sexual counseling is also important from this standpoint; patients who have been sexually active prior to therapy are encouraged to continue sexual activity upon completion of healing. This is not only to prevent coital difficulties but also to allow for a more adequate posttherapy visualization of the vagina and/or cervix for follow-up purposes.

When exenteration has been performed, the assistance of the ostomy nurse will be necessary to rehabilitate the patient.

C. Evaluation

Whether a patient has been treated by surgery or radiotherapy, a systematic follow-up of the patient in an attempt to identify local recurrences or distant spread of the disease must be carried out at appropriate intervals. Such follow-up is also important to identify any late complications (e.g., superficial lymphangitis in the operative field, lymphedema, strictures, etc.) and correct them as early as possible.

Table I is a suggested schedule for such an evaluation.

X. MANAGEMENT ALGORITHMS

A. Algorithm for Cancer of the Cervix
(see p. 568)

B. Algorithm for Cancer of the Uterus
(see p. 569)

C. Algorithm for Cancer of the Ovary
(see p. 570)

Table I

Long-Term Follow-Up Schedule for Gynecologic Malignancies

Management	First two years			Two-to-five years		Thereafter, annually
	Every 2 months x3	Every 6 months	Annually	Every 6 months	Annually	
History						
Pain or local discomfort, pruritis, etc.	X			X		X
Bleeding	X			X		X
Palpable masses	X			X		X
Dysuria	X			X		X
Rectal bleeding	X			X		X
GI distress, bloating, etc.	X			X		X
Weight loss	X			X		X
Eating ability	X			X		X
Leg edema	X			X		X
Other						
Physical						
Complete[a]		X			X	X
Vagina	X			X		X
Cervix	X			X		X
Rectal	X			X		X
Abdomen/liver	X			X		X
Lower extremities	X			X		X
Investigation						
Pap smear	X			X		X
CBC		X		X		X
SMA-12		X	X		X	X
Chest x-ray			X		X	X
Cystoscopic exam			As indicated			
Proctoscopic exam			As indicated			
Colposcopic exam			As indicated			
Peritoneoscopy			As indicated			
Bone scan			As indicated			
CAT scan			As indicated			

SUGGESTED READINGS

1. Ballon, ed. Controversies in cancer treatment. *Gynecol. Oncol.*

2. Nelson. "Atlas of Radical Pelvic Surgery," 2nd ed. Appleton, New York, 1976.

3. Di Saia, P. J., and Creasman, W. T. "Clinical Gynecologic Oncology." Mosby, St. Louis, Missouri, 1981.

ALGORITHM FOR CANCER OF THE CERVIX

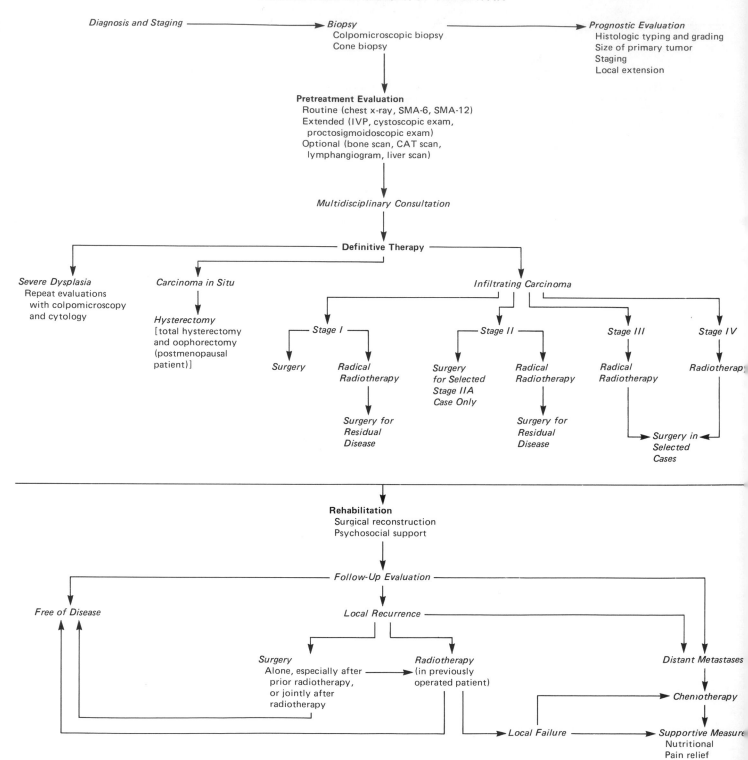

Diagnosis and Staging ──────────────► *Biopsy*
Colpomicroscopic biopsy
Cone biopsy ──────────────► *Prognostic Evaluation*
Histologic typing and grading
Size of primary tumor
Staging
Local extension

Pretreatment Evaluation
Routine (chest x-ray, SMA-6, SMA-12)
Extended (IVP, cystoscopic exam,
proctosigmoidoscopic exam)
Optional (bone scan, CAT scan,
lymphangiogram, liver scan)

Multidisciplinary Consultation

Definitive Therapy

Severe Dysplasia
Repeat evaluations
with colpomicroscopy
and cytology

Carcinoma in Situ

Hysterectomy
[total hysterectomy
and oophorectomy
(postmenopausal
patient)]

Infiltrating Carcinoma

Stage I

Surgery   *Radical Radiotherapy*

Surgery for Residual Disease

Stage II

Surgery for Selected Stage IIA Case Only   *Radical Radiotherapy*

Surgery for Residual Disease

Stage III

Radical Radiotherapy

Stage IV

Radiotherapy

Surgery in Selected Cases

Rehabilitation
Surgical reconstruction
Psychosocial support

Follow-Up Evaluation

Free of Disease

Local Recurrence

Surgery
Alone, especially after
prior radiotherapy,
or jointly after
radiotherapy

Radiotherapy
(in previously
operated patient)

Distant Metastases

Chemotherapy

Local Failure

Supportive Measures
Nutritional
Pain relief
Radiotherapy for
bone metastases

ALGORITHM FOR CANCER OF THE UTERUS

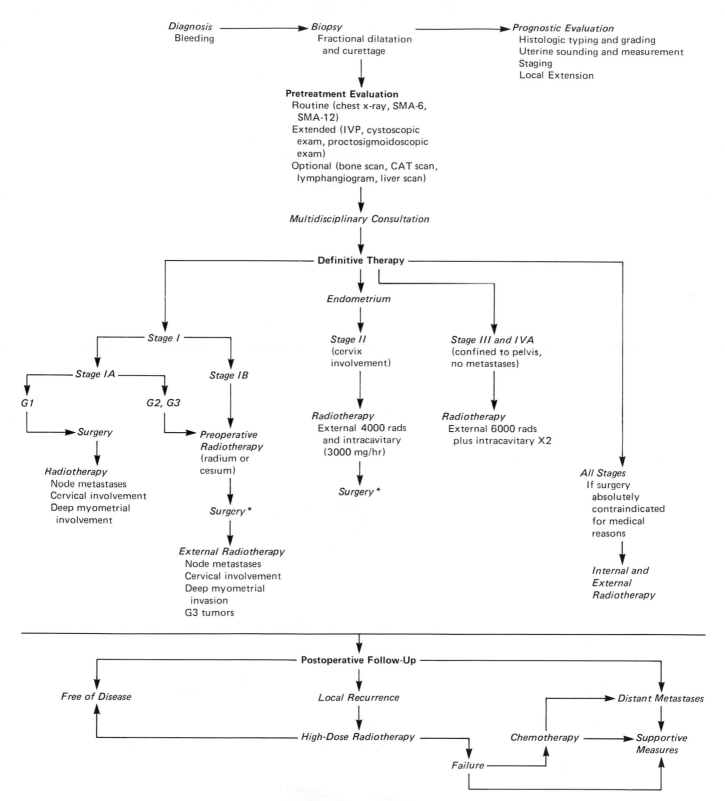

Diagnosis ⟶ *Biopsy* ⟶ *Prognostic Evaluation*
Bleeding   Fractional dilatation   Histologic typing and grading
             and curettage   Uterine sounding and measurement
                                   Staging
                                   Local Extension

Pretreatment Evaluation
Routine (chest x-ray, SMA-6, SMA-12)
Extended (IVP, cystoscopic exam, proctosigmoidoscopic exam)
Optional (bone scan, CAT scan, lymphangiogram, liver scan)

Multidisciplinary Consultation

Definitive Therapy

Endometrium

Stage I

Stage IA — *Stage IB*

G1   *G2, G3*

Surgery ⟶ *Preoperative Radiotherapy* (radium or cesium)

Radiotherapy
Node metastases
Cervical involvement
Deep myometrial involvement

*Surgery **

External Radiotherapy
Node metastases
Cervical involvement
Deep myometrial invasion
G3 tumors

Stage II (cervix involvement)

Radiotherapy
External 4000 rads and intracavitary (3000 mg/hr)

*Surgery **

Stage III and IVA (confined to pelvis, no metastases)

Radiotherapy
External 6000 rads plus intracavitary X2

All Stages
If surgery absolutely contraindicated for medical reasons

Internal and External Radiotherapy

Postoperative Follow-Up

Free of Disease

Local Recurrence

High-Dose Radiotherapy

Failure

Chemotherapy

Distant Metastases

Supportive Measures

*Total hysterectomy with bilateral salpingo-oophorectomy (extrafascial). Peritoneal washings and selected para-aortic and pelvic node sampling.

ALGORITHM FOR CANCER OF THE OVARY

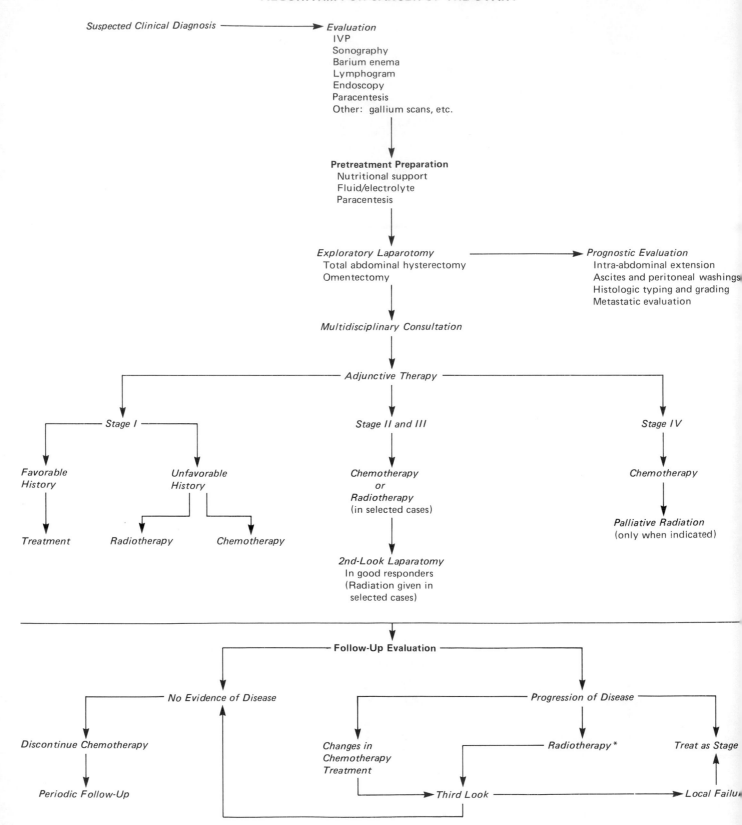

*Treatment depends on prior therapy.

Section 13

Tumors of the Genitourinary System

GILBERT WISE
KRISHNARAJ G. LINDSAY

With Contributions By

Samuel Kopel	Medical Oncology
Aurelia Cacatian	Medical Oncology
Ezzat Youssef	Radiation Oncology
Carolyn Dickson	Nursing Oncology

CURRENT GUIDELINES
FOR THE MANAGEMENT OF CANCER

Section 13 Tumors of the Genitourinary System

Part A: Tumors of the Kidney

I. Early Detection and Screening   575
  A. Detection
    1. Physical Evaluation
    2. Urinalysis
    3. Other
  B. Early Signs
  C. Screening
II. Pretreatment Evaluation and Work-Up   576
  A. Comprehensive History and Physical Examination
    1. History
      a. History of Present Illness
      b. Social History
      c. Past Medical History
    2. Physical Examination
  B. Laboratory Studies
    1. Urinalysis
    2. Routine Blood Work
    3. Routine Chest X-Ray
    4. Electrocardiogram
  C. Definitive Diagnostic Procedures
    1. Intravenous Urogram
    2. Sonography
    3. CAT Scan of the Abdomen
    4. Angiography
    5. Cystoscopy and Retrograde Pyelography
    6. Radionuclide Scan of the Kidney
  D. Metastatic Evaluation
  E. Multidisciplinary Evaluation and Consultation
  F. Site-Specific Data Form for Renal Tumors

III. Preoperative Preparation   578
  A. Nutritional Support
  B. Hematologic Considerations
  C. Cardipulmonary Considerations
  D. Antibiotics
  E. Psychiatric Considerations
  F. Preparation of the Abdomen
IV. Therapeutic Management   581
  A. Surgery
    1. Choice of Procedure
      a. Renal Cell Carcinoma
      b. Transitional Cell Carcinoma (TCC)
         of the Renal Pelvis
    2. Factors Affecting the Choice
      a. Age
      b. Social Factors
      c. Presence of Metastatic Disease
      d. Status of the Contralateral Kidney
    3. Complications of Surgical Treatment
    4. Prognosis
  B. Radiotheraphy
  C. Chemotherapy
V. Postoperative Care and Evaluation   583
  A. Postoperative Care
  B. Evaluation and Follow-Up
VI. Management Algorithm for Renal Tumors   585

This section is designed to provide guidelines for the student in medicine, the family practitioner, the oncologist, the internist, and the urologist in a practical approach to the early identification, the treatment, and the management of patients with carcinoma of the kidney.

These guidelines will address themselves primarily to two tumors that affect the kidneys in adults: renal cell carcinoma (RCC) and transitional cell carcinoma (TCC) of the renal collecting system. We will not attempt to cover those rare tumors that are at times found in adults (leiomyosarcomas or lymphomas) or those renal tumors that affect children (nephroblastomas or Wilms's tumors); this latter entity is discussed separately in §8A.VI.A, Vol. 20.

Neoplasms of the kidney vary in histological type. The RCC is also known as adenocarcinoma, papillary adenocarcinoma, hypernephroma, or Grawitz's tumor; this tumor primarily affects patients in their fifth and sixth decades of life and affects both sexes with some predilection to males. Other neoplasms that affect the kidney are those arising from the pelvis or the collecting system; they originate in the transitional epithelial lining cells and hence their name transitional cell carcinomas.

I. EARLY DETECTION AND SCREENING

A. Detection

Renal cell carcinoma is by far the most prevalent carcinoma of the kidney. The classical manifestations include the triad of flank pain, renal mass, and hematuria. These findings, however, indicate a tumor that has already progressed to a large size and usually invaded the renal pelvis; the physician should not depend on these findings for the early detection of carcinoma of the kidney. Early symptoms are often vague flank pain and a host of apparently unrelated symptoms such as general malaise, anemia, and fever of undetermined origin.

Transitional cell carcinoma of the renal pelvis, on the other hand, manifests itself very early by hematuria and flank pain. Rarely, does it present as a renal mass.

1. Physical Evaluation

It is rare that a routine physical examination can detect kidney tumors at an early stage; it can be helpful, however, especially if a careful history related to flank pain is elicited. Such history should also include inquiries as to weight loss, abdominal pain, or back discomfort; a history of fever of unknown origin unrelated to infection may also suggest the presence of carcinoma of the kidney. A thorough physical evaluation should include palpation of the cervical and supraclavicular lymph nodes, abdominal examination, and genital and rectal examination. The blood pressure should be accurately assessed, since abnormality of blood pressure, particularly in the young patient, may be related to the neoplasm that often results in numerous arteriovenous fistulas seen within the tumors; this could eventually lead to high-output cardiac failure.

2. Urinalysis

Urinalysis is one of the most cost-effective clinical methods and is widely used because of its ease and availability. It may be instrumental in the early detection of renal tumors. Microscopic and chemical tests will determine the presence or absence of blood, and urine cytology may be helpful in identifying the presence of malignant cells that are usually indicative of a TCC. It is not a very sensitive test, however, and should not be depended upon; urine cytology, for example, is of little value in detecting RCC, as these tumors usually develop in the periphery or parenchyma of the kidney without involvement of the renal pelvis.

3. Other

Intravenous urography (IVU), renal sonography, or computerized axial tomography (CAT) scans are much more effective in determining the presence or absence of renal masses. These procedures are not ''cost effective'' as mass screening techniques but are the only known methods by which an early carcinoma of the kidney can be detected. Although it has been suggested that it is not cost effective to do routine IVUs in patients with ''simple'' urinary tract infections or even in those with an initial episode of hematuria, this procedure has been the only method in which early neoplasms of the kidney have been identified.

B. Early Signs

Renal cell carcinoma or TCC is often a silent tumor. The following clinical findings and laboratory data, however, should arouse the clinician's suspicion:

- Flank or abdominal pain of unknown cause.
- Blood in the urine.
- Flank mass.
- Fever of unknown origin.
- Weight loss, weakness, or fatigue.
- Anemia of unknown cause.
- Polycythemia or erythrocytosis.
- Other laboratory data such as hypercalcemia or elevated alkaline phosphatase might also indicate a kidney tumor and should prompt an evaluation by means of x-ray studies.

C. Screening

As indicated above, there is no cost-effective screening method to rule out the presence of renal tumors. The routine annual physical examination recommended in general with the usual urinalysis comes as close to a screening approach as is available for renal tumors. Patient and physician education should be encouraged to promote early consultation and identification of the warning signs enumerated above. Rapid institution of a work-up at the slightest suspicion is the greatest hope for early detection of renal tumors.

II. PRETREATMENT EVALUATION AND WORK-UP

Pretreatment evaluation of the patient with a renal mass, or one suspected of having a renal tumor, should include the following.

A. Comprehensive History and Physical Examination

1. History

a. History of Present Illness

- Pain.
- Hematuria.

- Fatigue.
- Weakness or weight loss.
- Fever.
- Anemia.

b. Social History

- Sex and Race.
- Occupation, exposure to chemicals, industrial toxins, etc.

c. Past Medical History

- History of other carcinomas (particularly bladder tumors or previous kidney tumors).
- Previous surgical procedures (particularly if related to the urinary tract, e.g., transurethral resection [TUR]).
- Metabolic dysfunctions (i.e., thyroid disease or diabetes) or other medical problems, that may represent the paraneoplastic effects of the tumor (e.g., anemia, cardiac decompensation, polycythemias).
- Family history of carcinoma.

2. Physical Examination

Physical examination should stress the following:

- Vital signs with attention to blood pressure.
- Head and neck examination with special attention to lymph nodes.
- Neurological examination, particularly of the lower extremities.
- Abdominal examination, masses, pain and tenderness, liver size.
- Genital and rectal examination.

B. Laboratory Studies

1. Urinalysis

A complete urinalysis should be the first test done. Hematuria can be identified, and urine cytology examination should be carried out.

2. Routine Blood Work

A blood urea nitrogen (BUN) and serum creatinine as well as a check of the serum cholesterol (recent reports suggest the presence of a decreased serum cholesterol in most patients with RCC) and serum acid phosphatase are most important. Liver function tests should be performed, and a serum calcium, albumin, and alkaline phosphatase should also be obtained. A multichannel profile—SMA-12 or SMA-20—is actually indicated, taking in all of the above tests.

3. Routine Chest X-Ray

Chest x-ray or a CAT scan is mandatory on all patients with definitive renal masses to determine the presence or absence of metastatic disease as well as to assess the general fitness of the patient.

4. Electrocardiogram

An electrocardiogram is routinely performed to ensure adequate physical status.

C. Definitive Diagnostic Procedures

1. Intravenous Urogram

The IVU is the mainstay of the evaluation of the urologic patient and particularly of the patient suspected of having a renal tumor. It will identify a mass within the kidney, displacement or distortion of the kidney, filling defect in the pelvis or calyces, or other unrelated renal pathology. If a renal abnormality is noted on the IVU, the following procedures should then be performed in sequence.

2. Sonography

A renal sonogram is indicated in the presence of a mass to determine whether it is sonolucent (cystic) or echogenic (solid). If the sonogram identifies a cyst, cyst puncture under sonography and fluid study should be considered. This includes examination of the fluid by cytology and the determination of its protein and lipid content. The presence of blood in the fluid or a high protein or lipid content is highly suspicious of a renal tumor, and further diagnostic studies are then indicated. If the cytology is suggestive or if the sonogram is echogenic, further evaluation is indicated.

3. CAT Scan of the Abdomen

Abdominal CAT scan will confirm the presence or absence of a renal mass and define, with great accuracy, its extent and its relation to the adjacent structures (liver, abdominal wall, paravertebral muscles, etc.). Lymph nodes can also be identified, and on occcasion, vena cava involvement, extrinsic or intraluminal, may be demonstrated. If the abdominal CAT scan is negative and if the sonogram is suspicious, the patient may then be admitted for renal arteriography. Even if both the sonogram and the cyst fluid are positive, a CAT scan is still necessary to identify the extent of the disease before exploration.

4. Angiography

Arteriographic studies by selective catheterization are sometimes indicated to further assist in establishing the diagnosis; occasionally, selective arterial angiography is the only test that succeeds in identifying small tumors. Angiography may be desirable even when the diagnosis has already been established by the presence of a positive sonogram and CAT scan; it can be extremely useful in identifying the blood supply and neoplastic vascular pattern of the kidney. Inferior venacavography is also important, particularly in right-sided tumors, to determine the presence or absence of tumor extension in the vena cava.

5. Cystoscopy and Retrograde Pyelography

Patients in whom the IVU suggests a filling defect in the pelvis or collecting system compatible with a renal pelvis tumor are candidates for cystoscopy and retrograde intravenous pyelography (IVP). Cystoscopy is indicated to rule out the presence of other urothelial tumors in the bladder, since multicentricity in these tumors is not unusual. Retrograde pyelography is necessary to evaluate the presence or absence of other urothelial tumors in the course of the ureter. At the time of the retrograde IVP, a more definitive evaluation may be made of the renal mass or the filling defect within the renal pelvis or collecting system, and cells may be obtained from the affected kidney by irrigation with saline solution, and these may be submitted for cytological study. In addition, a brush biopsy using brush techniques should yield some cellular material from the collecting system to be submitted for pathological study.

If the diagnosis of TCC of the renal pelvis is clearly established by retograde IVP, no other diagnostic tests are indicated. Arteriography is not mandatory unless there is a large renal mass and the surgeon wishes to define the extent of the renal tumor and its vascular supply.

6. Radionuclide Scan of the Kidney

Scans of the kidney with blood flow studies are particularly useful in assessing the status and functional capacity of the contralateral kidney.

D. Metastatic Evaluation

After the diagnosis is established and prior to the planning of the definitive therapy, a metastatic survey is indicated. In addition to the chest x-rays and SMA-12, a chest CAT scan and at times a liver and bone scan may be selectively indicated. An abdominal CAT scan and even lymphangiography may be desirable to assess the extent of the local disease and its lymphatic spread accurately. A brain scan should be carried out in the presence of any neurological symptom.

E. Multidisciplinary Evaluation and Consultation

A multidisciplinary approach to the diagnosis and management of renal tumors is strongly recommended. Patients with a suspected renal tumor require consultation with the radiologist, who will advise and assist the urologist in selecting the indicated radiological procedures and in interpreting them. In addition, the experienced interventional radiologist skilled in sonography with percutaneous renal cyst puncture and percutaneous needle biopsy is extremely helpful. He or she will also assist in carrying out a thorough metastatic evaluation: bone scan, bone survey, liver scans, and CAT scans. If metastatic disease is suspected and there are bone lesions, the assistance of a medical oncolgist and/or orthopedist may be required to obtain a biopsy from the bone to ascertain the diagnosis. Fine-needle biopsy may also be used to obtain tissue, if the diagnosis is in doubt.

Prior to definitive therapy, a multidisciplinary evaluation with the urologist, radiotherapist, and medical oncologist is desirable to plan the best course of treatment for each specific case. This is necessary in the advanced cases or when metastases are identified in order to address the questions of adjuvant therapy (especially radiotherapy), the sequence of therapeutic modalities, the advisability of surgical resection in the face of solitary metastases, etc. Orthopedic, neurosurgical, or thoracic surgery consultations are required to evaluate the possibility of surgical removal of these peripheral tumors.

F. Site-Specific Data Form for Renal Tumors (see pp. 579–580).

III. PREOPERATIVE PREPARATION

Preoperative preparation of the patient with renal tumors (RCC or TCC) can best be managed by the urologist in conjunction with his or her consulting internist and, if metastatic disease is suspected, with the oncologist.

A. Nutritional Support

Most patients in the early stages (Stage I or II), are in a reasonable nutritional state. However, if the patient has evidence of weight loss, persistent hematuria, fever, or a rapidly growing mass or if the patient's hemoglobin, blood volume, serum albumin, or serum cholestrol are reduced, it is suggested that nutritional support be instituted prior to surgery. This can

best be offered by means of oral or enteral tube supplementation. At the time of surgery, a jejunal line may be inserted to provide the patient with enteral feedings immediately postoperatively. If the patient is severely depleted or when there is a question of bowel dysfunction, a peripheral or central line may be inserted for intravenous hyperalimentation.

B. Hematologic Considerations

Patients with renal tumors may be anemic, although at times RCC may present with polycythemia. The anemia is due to chronic blood loss, to the adverse effect of the tumor on bone marrow production, or to other undetermined factors. Prior to major surgery, the patient's hematocrit should be checked; any patient with a hematocrit lower than 30 should be transfused in preparation for surgery. A coagulation screening is also advised, and adequate blood component replacement should be ordered prior to radical surgery for RCC or nephroureterectomy for TCC.

C. Cardiopulmonary Considerations

Since most patients with renal or urothelial cancers are in the older age group, there may be serious associated cardiac problems related to arteriosclerotic heart disease. An EKG and a thorough evaluation by an internist should be done prior to surgery. Pulmonary function studies, as well as arterial blood gases, should be performed on all patients. Corrective measures for any identifiable problem should be initiated preoperatively.

High-output cardiac failure may be present as a result of arteriovenous shunts that frequently occur within an RCC. These patients may have hypertension, and the blood pressure should be carefully evaluated and corrected prior to surgery.

D. Antibiotics

Patients undergoing radical nephrectomy for carcinoma of the kidney do not generally require antibiotic treatment unless the patient has had a thoracoabdominal approach. Here again, good pulmonary hygiene and pulmonary toilet during the postoperative period may be as important as any antibiotic to prevent pulmonary infection. Patients undergoing nephroureterectomy for renal pelvis tumors will require a bladder tube, either a Foley catheter or a cystostomy tube; in these cases, urinary antimicrobial therapy is indicated. If the patient has documented urinary tract infection or some other infectious site (i.e., pulmonary), appropriate antibiotic therapy should be utilized as indicated by the *in-vitro* sensitivity of the offending bacteria.

SITE-SPECIFIC DATA FORM—KIDNEY CANCER

HISTORY

Age:_____

Symptoms

_____ Flank pain

_____ Hematuria

_____ Fever of unknown origin

_____ Weight loss, fatigue

_____ Abdominal discomfort

_____ Back pain

_____ Others_____

Duration:_____

Social history

Occupation:_____

Race:____White____Black____Oriental____Other

Smoker:____Yes____No. How much?_____

Drinker:____Yes____No. How often?_____

Environmental factors: chemical exposure ?_____

Detail:_____

Family history of carcinoma

Relation:_____ Site:_____

Previous history of carcinoma

_____ No____Yes Site:_____

Rx:_____

Previous treatment (describe):

_____

_____

PHYSICAL EXAMINATION

	Neg.	Pos.	Suspicious
General examination			
Evaluation of lymph nodes (neck)	_____	_____	_____
Heart	_____	_____	_____
Masses in flank	_____	_____	_____
Bruit over kidney	_____	_____	_____
External genitalia	_____	_____	_____
Rectal exam	_____	_____	_____
Extremities	_____	_____	_____
Neurological	_____	_____	_____

	Right	Left
x-Ray findings		
Mass in kidney	_____	_____
Filling defect	_____	_____

Size:_____

Describe:_____

_____

PRETREATMENT WORK-UP (Check, if done)

	Neg.	Pos.	Suspicious		Neg.	Pos.	Suspicious
SMA-20	_____	_____	_____	Chest tomograms or CAT scan	_____	_____	_____
Urinalysis	_____	_____	_____	Bone scans	_____	_____	_____
IVP	_____	_____	_____	Liver scan	_____	_____	_____
Sonogram	_____	_____	_____	Bone marrow biopsy	_____	_____	_____
CAT scan	_____	_____	_____	Cystoscopy— retrograde pyelography	_____	_____	_____
Nuclear imaging	_____	_____	_____	Retrograde brushing	_____	_____	_____
Chest x-ray	_____	_____	_____				

Classification

Histologic diagnosis:_____

Staging:____T____N____M

Stage:_____

Signature:_____

Countersignature:_____

Date:_____

Renal Cell Carcinoma (TNM classification)

Primary tumor (T)

TX   Minimum requirements cannot be met

T0   No evidence of primary tumor

T1   Small tumor, minimal renal and caliceal distortion or deformity. Circumscribed neovasculature surrounded by normal parenchyma. Tumor confined within the renal capsule

T2   Large tumor with deformity and/or enlargement of kidney and/or collecting system. Tumor extending through the capsule but within Gerota's fascia

T3a   Tumor involving the perinephric tissues

T3b   Tumor involving the renal vein

T3c   Tumor involving renal vein and infradiaphragmatic vena cava

> Note: Under T3, tumor may extend into perinephric tissues into renal vein and into vena cava as shown on cavography. In these instances, the T classification may be shown as T3a, b, c, or some appropriate combination, depending on extension, for example, T3a,b if tumor in perinephric fat and extending into renal vein.

T4a   Tumor invasion of neighboring structures (e.g., muscle, bowel)

T4b   Tumor involving supradiaphragmatic vena cava

Nodal involvement (N)

NX   Minimum requirements cannot be met

N0   No evidence of involvement of regional nodes

N1   Single, homolateral regional nodal involvement

N2   Involvement of multiple regional or contralateral or bilateral nodes

N3   Fixed, regional nodes (assessable only at surgical exploration)

N4   Involvement of juxtaregional nodes

Staging of RCC

I	T1–T2, N0
II	T3a
III	T3b and T3c
	N1–N3
IV	T4
	N4 with any T
	M1 with any T and any N

Distant metastasis (M)

MX   Not assessed

M0   No known distant metastasis

M1   Distant metastasis present (specify)

Residual tumor (R)

R0   No residual tumor

R1   Microscopic residual tumor

R2   Macroscopic residual tumor

Tumor grade

G1   Well differentiated

G2   Moderately well differentiated

G3   Poorly differentiated

G4   Very poorly differentiated

Use whichever indicator is most appropriate (term or G number)

Collecting System Tumors Involving the Kidney
(Urothelial Tumors of the Renal, Pelvic, or Calyceal System)

Stage 0   Benign papillomas, no involvement of stalk

Stage A   Tumor with submucosal infiltration

Stage B   Tumor presenting with invasion of the muscularis of calyx, pelvis, or ureter

Stage C   Tumor extension beyond the muscularis into the parenchyma or the peripelvic tissue

Stage D1   Extension of the tumor outside the kidney into adjacent tissue

Stage D2   Metastatic disease

E. Psychiatric Considerations

Patients who require extensive surgery, particularly renal surgery, may be emotionally depressed. If this depression is significant (i.e., causing the patient anxiety, difficulty in sleeping, poor appetite, etc.), psychiatric consultation may be advised. It should be pointed out that this type of surgery will not compromise the patient's potency or lifestyle. Patients with metastatic disease in whom the prognosis is guarded may benefit from psychiatric evaluation and treatment to assist the family and the patient in dealing with the life-threatening disease. In some instances, mild tranquilizers or mood elevators may be indicated for patients who are severely depressed. If, on the other hand, the tumor is confined to the kidney and the prognosis following surgery is favorable, the patient and the family must be reassured about the need for surgery and the hopeful short- and long-term outcome.

F. Preparation of the Abdomen

Routine presurgical procedures (i.e., shaving, washing with antiseptic soap, and use of antiseptic solutions such as iodophor) will be used at the time of surgery. A bowel preparation is not necessary unless it is anticipated that the bowel may be involved and will require resection in the course of the radical nephrectomy. If involvement of the bowel is suspected, a barium enema should be done preoperatively; in the case of potential small-bowel involvement, a small-bowel series and GI series should be performed. If a bowel resection is anticipated, then bowel preparation in the form of oral neomycin or erythromycin is recommended (1 g daily for 3 days). A mechanical preparation is also desirable by means of a liquid diet and enemas until clear.

IV. THERAPEUTIC MANAGEMENT

The most effective treatment for RCC or TCC is radical surgery. No other modality available today appears to offer any chance of cure.

A. Surgery

1. Choice of Procedure

a. Renal Cell Carcinoma

The treatment of choice for RCC is a radical nephrectomy. This can be performed either through a transperitoneal or a thoracoabdominal approach. The kidney and all surrounding tissues within Gerota's fascia, including the adrenal gland, are removed; a ureterectomy need not to be performed. There is some question as to whether radical lymph node dissection is advisable. It is suggested that the perirenal and great vessel lymph nodes be removed for staging purposes; some authors even believe that a radical lymphadenectomy does in fact improve the end result of treatment.

In the case of a massive RCC, it is advisable to consider preoperative renal artery embolization. This may be done in conjunction with the radiologist during arteriography; Gelfoam or an intravascular coil may be inserted, or an injection of 25% alcohol may be used to infarct the kidney; following these, the nephrectomy may be done within a day or two. It should be noted that renal embolization is a painful procedure that can make the patient febrile and toxic; it will however, decrease the vascularity of the kidney considerably and presumably reduce the incidence of hematogenous spread.

In those patients with RCC in whom there is extension of the tumor into the renal vein and vena cava, a joint effort with a vascular surgeon may be advisable so that venacavotomy, or resection of the vena cava, may be performed at the time of the radical nephrectomy. In some instances, the tumor may extend all the way to the right atrium, and in these cases, a surgical team with a cardiac pump will be necessary to remove the tumor from the inferior vena cava and right atrium.

b. Transitional Cell Carcinoma (TCC) of the Renal Pelvis.

In the case of TCC, total nephrectomy, ureterectomy, and resection of a cuff of bladder is mandatory. Some urologists believe that the nephrectomy should be as radical as that done for RCC; others believe that just the kidney and the collecting system need be removed. Surgery may be carried out through one incision via a transperitoneal or a modified extraperitoneal paramedian incision, or by a combined flank and inguinal approach so that the entire ureter and a cuff of bladder can be removed.

It is imperative to ensure the effectiveness of the surgical margins at the time of resection in order to achieve the best results. In the case of RCC, the transected renal vein and Gerota's fascia must be free of tumor. In the case of carcinoma of the renal pelvis, the best results are achieved when the tumor has not penetrated through the renal pelvis or outside of the kidney itself; where a nephroureterectomy is performed, the bladder cuff should be free of tumor, and one must be sure that all satellite tumors within the ureter are completely extirpated. Generous use of perioperative frozen-section examinations by the pathologist is mandatory.

2. Factors Affecting the Choice

a. Age

Age is no contraindication to appropriate surgical treatment for the management of carcinoma of the kidney. However, if the patient has severe cardiovascular problems, pulmonary disease, or other problems that might contraindicate radical surgery, or if the patient's prognosis is such that his or her anticipated survival is no more than 6 months, nephrectomy should not be performed unless it is necessary for palliation (i.e, done to alleviate the patient's pain or continued bleeding). In the elderly, debilitated patient who is not a candidate for radical surgery and where the kidney is a source of pain and discomfort, a simple nephrectomy may be done.

b. Social Factors

There are no social factors that should influence the choice of surgical procedure in the treatment of carcinoma of the kidney. However, patients with religious scruples against blood transfusions may not be suitable for radical surgery since this type of surgery almost always requires blood transfusions. Today, however, with the help of some of the blood substitutes available, it might even be possible to proceed with surgery in this category of patients.

c. Presence of Metastatic Disease

In those patients in whom metastatic disease is suspected, a primary nephrectomy may be indicated in the hope of decreasing the total volume of tumor tissue, though there is no substantial evidence that removal of the primary tumor will cause the metastatic disease to regress. Nephrectomy in the presence of metastatic disease, however, is necessary when symptoms of pain or hematuria exist.

d. Status of the Contralateral Kidney

Adequate assessment of the contralateral kidney is essential prior to nephrectomy.

Approximately 3–5% of patients with RCC may have synchronous bilateral tumors. In such cases, radical nephrectomy should be done on the side that has the major carcinoma, and a partial nephrectomy should be done on the side with the smaller synchronous tumor. In these patients, renal consultation should be obtained prior to radical surgery to assure adequacy of subsequent renal function. In addition, every effort should be made preoperatively to identify the exact extent of the disease and to rule out the possibility of metastases. An alternative modality of treatment would be bilateral radical nephrectomy and placement of the patient on renal dialysis; this, however, should be done only after careful discussion with the patient's family and a renal consultation. Whenever possible, kidney function must be preserved; this is particularly so in the elderly, debilitated patient. In these cases, it might be feasible to remove the primary large tumor and leave the patient with the synchronous contralateral tumor, as the patient's anticipated long-term survival may be less than the time it would take this tumor to cause serious problems.

In those patients with solitary kidneys or those in whom the contralateral "uninvolved kidney" is seriously diseased (e.g., by pyelonephritis, vascular disease, dysplasia, etc.), the tumor surgery should be moderated to preserve "normal" renal parenchyma whenever possible. In the case of RCC, a partial or segmental nephrectomy should be performed if technically feasible. In patients with renal pelvis tumors, fulguration of the tumor or partial nephrectomy should be performed to maintain the integrity of normal kidney function. Intensive medical treatment following the removal of the tumor is of the greatest importance; diet, medications, and at times, hemodialysis will be necessary to keep the patient well after the surgery. If the tumor is extensive, a decision has to be made whether to "cure" the patient by creating an anephric state. The only alternative would be to leave the tumor-involved kidney "in situ" and hope that radiation (or chemotherapy) treatment will slow the growth rate of the neoplasm. The prognosis in such cases is generally poor, even when surgery is feasible.

3. Complications of Surgical Treatment

Of the common early postoperative complications, hemorrhage is the most frequent. This is apt to occur more with RCC in so far as these are extremely vascular tumors with multiple venous collaterals, and the tumor often impinges upon the great vessels (i.e., the vena cava or aorta). Meticulous surgery is necessary to control operative bleeding. Postoperatively, however, in so far as numerous venous channels have been sutured, ligated, or clipped, the patient has to be observed very carefully lest some small vessel begin to bleed and result in extensive retroperitoneal hemorrhage.

Other complications such as infection, prolonged intestinal ileus, pulmonary infection, deep-vein thrombosis, etc., may also occur.

4. Prognosis

The prognosis of renal carcinoma is dependent on the extent of the tumor. Factors affecting survival are extensive local invasion, intraluminal tumor embolization of the inferior vena cava, lymph node metastases, and hematogenous spread. Moreover, there is a certain unpredictability in the behavior of tumors with metastases that appear at a late date. Tumor growth displays wide variability with some patients surviving for long periods of time without intervention.

In patients with renal pelvis TCC, the prognosis is generally much worse, with 5-year survivals in the range of 15%, as compared with 40% for RCC. The prognosis is more favorable if the tumor is confined to the kidney without extension to the collecting system or when there has not been any penetration through the muscularis of the collecting system. In addition, the prognosis appears to be much worse when the tumor is a squamous cell cancer.

B. Radiotherapy

The two main functions of radiotherapy in the management of RCC are palliative or adjuvant. While the indications and application of the former are widely accepted, the adjuvant role of radiation is still controversial.

Palliative radiation is successful in alleviating hemorrhage (necessitating only modest doses of 3000–4000 rads in 2–3 weeks) and pain. The latter responds to treatment more readily when there is no nerve involvement; bone pain and pain due to capsular tension usually respond well to radiotherapy.

Adjuvant radiotherapy can be delivered either preoperatively or postoperatively. Preoperative radiation is given in the hope of reducing tumor size and incidence of metastases, the latter being achieved through the impairment of viability of malignant cells that are displaced during the definitive surgery; however, clinical experience is still too limited to allow confirmation of these theoretical advantages. Postoperative adjuvant radiotherapy was demonstrated to be instrumental in reducing local recurrences and in improving survival in cases where there is invasion of the renal capsule by the tumor or where the renal pelvis is involved. It may also be helpful when there is evidence of lymph node involvement or invasion of lymphatics.

The role of adjuvant radiotherapy in the treatment of tumors of the renal pelvis is much less clear in view of the rarity of these lesions. Tumor radiosensitivity is very similar to that of bladder lesions, and as such, postoperative radiotherapy is expected to be of benefit when there is limited invasion of the renal pelvis wall or the lymphatics. However, for this effect to be instrumental in reducing recurrence, adequate doses (5,000 rads in 5 weeks) have to be delivered to the region of the renal pelvis, ureter, and ipsilateral bladder region. Technically, this is not easy and needs meticulous planning.

C. Chemotherapy

There is no known chemotherapeutic agent that is efficacious in the management of metastatic cancer from the kidney. There have been many reports that RCC responds to progesterone (Provera); this response has been noted at best in less than 15% of the patients. Chemotherapeutic agents evaluated in RCC include essentially all the standard drugs. Claims of response rates as high as 20–30% have been made for vinblastine, but most reports suggest that the true response rate is less than 20%. All other single agents have essentially no activity (i.e., < 10%).

This dismal state of affairs has led many oncologists to the conclusion that patients with metastatic renal cancer should be treated initially with new agents, in the hope of identifying drugs with definite activity.

At the present time, treatment should not be dependent on the basis of successful chemotherapy. Whenever possible, the patient's metastatic disease should be managed with surgery or local radiotherapy, and most of all, the patient should be kept comfortable with analgesics or narcotics. If necessary, the patient may require supplemental nutritional support and other supportive care, and the assistance of a well-organized support care team is invaluable (see §1.VII.D.4, Vol. 1).

V. POSTOPERATIVE CARE AND EVALUATION

A. Postoperative Care

Following radical surgery for either carcinoma of the kidney, the patient will require intravenous fluids and gastric drainage for approximately 4–5 days, as these patients invariably have an intestinal ileus, which will delay their ability to eat by mouth. A premature attempt to feed the patient may result in that patient's developing significant nausea, gastric dilatation, and vomiting. Most recently the availability of peripheral or central vein hyperalimentation has helped maintain the patient's nutritional status, and the use of a jejunal catheter at the time of surgery will enable the patient to be fed with an enteral mixture 1 day following surgery.

In the immediate postoperative period, the patient's vital signs and physical findings should be carefully monitored. In so far as these tumors are extremely vascular, the patient must be followed very carefully for the possible development of postoperative bleeding. It is advisable to do daily hematocrits and follow the patient's venous pressure and urine output closely. If there is any suggestion of hypovolemia (e.g., drop in hematocrit, poor urinary output, or development of a retroperitoneal mass, etc.), the patient should get blood replacement as necessary.

In so far as these patients have required general anesthesia with intubation and because in many of them a trans- or extrapleural approach has been used, the patient's pulmonary status should be observed very carefully. Chest films should be obtained in the recovery room right after surgery and daily thereafter for several days. If there is any question of pneumothorax or atelectasis, it is also advisable that the patient be placed on a respirometer to ensure adequate breathing exercises and prevent the development of atelectasis.

The patient's urine output should be carefully monitored, and daily BUN and serum creatinine should be obtained, as the patient's remaining kidney may not be able to sustain normal renal function. As previously indicated, it is imperative to have had the "normal" kidney assessed prior to the surgery to evaluate its ability to maintain adequate renal function life support.

In patients with renal pelvis tumors, a urethral catheter and cystostomy tube is placed. This should remain *in situ* for at least 1 week, until adequate healing of the bladder has been ascertained and there is no evidence of wound leakage. If the patient has had evidence of poor nutrition prior to surgery, the cystostomy tube should be kept in longer to ensure adequate drainage. In addition, the surgical field should have been adequately drained so that any urinary leakage that might occur will not accumlate into a urinoma.

The use of a drain in the nephrectomy site is a matter of the surgeon's choice. If it is a radical nephrectomy for RCC or TCC and the area has been secured with good hemostasis and no danger of a urine leak, a drain need not be placed. However, if there is a question about the effectiveness of vascular control or a question of possible urinary leakage, it is prudent to leave a drain in this surgical area; this drain can be removed 7–10 days later if there is no evidence of urinary or bloody drainage.

In those cases where a thoracoabdominal approach has been used, a chest tube should be inserted and kept in until such time as the lung is maintained in a fully expanded position. Chest x-ray should be done following all major kidney surgery; if a rib has been resected, there is a possibility that the pleura may have been inadvertently damaged during the course of surgery.

Once the patient is taking diet by mouth, all intravenous lines are removed; the sutures can be removed within 7–10 days following surgery. At that time, if the patient is eating well and clinical and laboratory parameters are within normal limits, the patient may be discharged home and followed by the primary physician and the urologist.

Table I

Long-Term Follow-Up Schedule for Renal Cell Carcinoma

Management	First year				Second year		Third year and thereafter, annually
	3 months	6 months	9 months	12 months	6 months	12 months	
History							
Change in urinary habits	X	X	X	X	X	X	X
Blood in urine	X	X	X	X	X	X	X
Abdominal, suprapubic, perineal, genital, or back pain	X	X	X	X	X	X	X
Bone or muscular pain	X	X	X	X	X	X	X
Physical							
Examination for neck nodes	X	X	X	X	X	X	X
Abdominal examination	X	X	X	X	X	X	X
Blood pressure	X	X	X	X	X	X	X
Genital examination	X	X	X	X	X	X	X
Rectal examination	X	X	X	X	X	X	X
Extremities	X	X	X	X	X	X	X
Cystoscopy (in TCC)	X	X	X	X	X	X	X
Investigation							
CBC	X	X	X	X	X	X	X
SMA-12	X	X	X	X	X	X	X
Urine and cytology (TCC)	X	X	X	X	X	X	X
Chest x-ray, chest tomography		X		X	X	X	X
IVP				X		X	X
CAT scan				Optional			
Sonogram				Optional			
Bone scan (indicated earlier if bone pain develops, alkaline phosphatase rises or anemia develops)				X		X	X

B. Evaluation and Follow-Up

In all cases of renal carcinoma, the patient should have regular follow-up and a chest x-ray at least twice a year for several years. In addition, patients who had a TCC of the renal pelvis should have a cystoscopy at least two or three times a year for the first 2 years as well as cytological studies from the urine to ascertain the presence or absence of recurrent urothelial tumor, which could develop in the bladder or in the contralateral kidney. For this reason, annual IVPs are also advised in patients with either TCC or RCC. If there is any question of a recurrent lesion, either in the area of surgery or in a contralateral kidney, CAT scans and sonography should be done.

A bone scan should be done on a yearly basis or whenever symptoms exist. In case of doubt, evidence of development of metastases can further be documented by arteriography and flush study of the vascular supply to the area of suspected metastasis, since RCC will have a classical hypervascular pattern. If metastatic disease is documented, then management is as indicated in §13A.IV.

Table I suggests a schedule of follow-up evaluation for patients with cancer of the kidney.

VI. MANAGEMENT ALGORITHM FOR RENAL TUMORS (see p. 586)

ALGORITHM FOR RENAL TUMORS

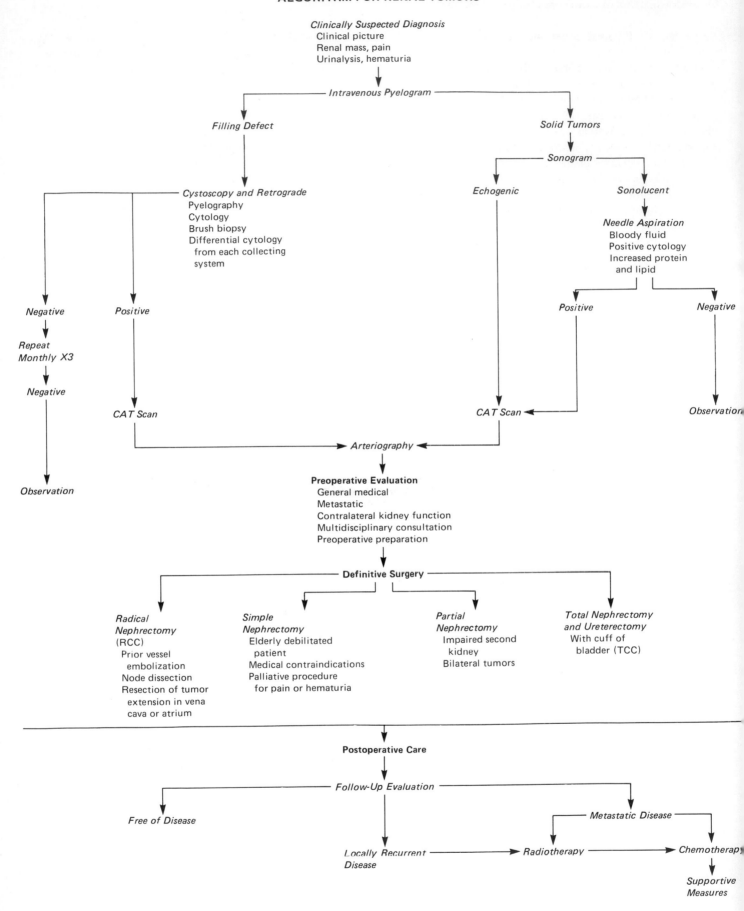

Section 13. Tumors of the Genitourinary System

Part B: Tumors of the Bladder

I. Early Detection and Screening   589
  A. Predisposing Factors
    1. Carcinogenicity of Tobacco
    2. Occupational Bladder Carcinogens
    3. Dietary Factors
      a. Sweeteners
      b. Nitrites and Nitrates
    4. Chronic Bladder Irritation
  B. Early Detection
    1. Clinical Presentation
      a. Hematuria
      b. Bladder Irritability
      c. Recurrent Urinary Tract Infections
      d. Complaints Attributable to Distant Metastases
    2. Urine Cytology
  C. Screening
II. Pretreatment Evaluation and Work-Up   590
  A. Complete History and Physical Examination
  B. Urologic Work-Up
    1. Intravenous Urogram

    2. Cytoscopy and Bladder Biopsy
  C. Medical Evaluation
  D. Staging Evaluation
  E. Site-Specific Data Form for Bladder Tumors
III. Pretreatment Preparation   591
IV. Therapeutic Management   592
  A. Therapy for Superficial Bladder Neoplasms
    1. Surgical Therapy
      a. Transuretheral Resection and Fulguration
      b. Partial Cystectomy
      c. Total Cystectomy
    2. Radiotherapy
      a. Interstitial Implants
      b. External Megavoltage Radiotherapy
    3. Intravesical Chemotherapy
  B. Treatment of the More Aggressive Bladder Cancer
  C. Role of Systemic Chemotherapy
V. Postoperative Care, Evaluation, and Rehabilitation   597
VI. Management for Bladder Tumors   597

I. EARLY DETECTION AND SCREENING

Bladder cancer is the most frequently encountered malignant tumor of the urinary tract. The most common age group affected by bladder cancer is that between 50 and 70 years. Approximately 27,000 new cases are diagnosed annually, and 8000 deaths are attributed to bladder cancer annually. The disease is mainly seen among males (M : F = 4 : 1), and the rate of occurrence is greater in whites. The risk of bladder cancer has been positively associated with the socioeconomic standing of the individual; special white-collar occupational groups are at a higher risk for bladder cancer.

A. Predisposing Factors

1. Carcinogenicity of Tobacco

Numerous authors have shown statistical evidence incriminating tobacco as a definite factor in bladder cancer, and several reports have shown an increased death rate from bladder cancer in cigarette smokers as opposed to nonsmokers. The exact mechanism by which tobacco smoking causes bladder cancer is unclear, but beta-naphthylamine and tryptophan metabolites—known to be carcinogens—have been identified in smokers. Recent evidence suggests that the combination of smoking and hazardous occupations substantially increases the risk of developing bladder cancer.

2. Occupational Bladder Carcinogens

The following substances to which workers are exposed in certain specific industries have been suspected to be important causative agents in bladder cancer:

- Aniline dyes (in the rubber and cable industries) have been found to result in an increased incidence of bladder cancer after long latent periods of 6–20 years. The real carcinogenic agent in these dyes has been actually identified to be an aromatic amine: 2-naphthylamine.
- Beta-naphthylamine and 4-aminodiphenyl are tryptophan

metabolites often present in dye and pigment industries. These chemicals conjugate into 2-amino-1-naphthol, which is concentrated in the urine and is responsible for bladder cancer. Animals fed with diets high in beta-naphthylamine and 4-nitrodiphenyl develop bladder cancers. If the urine is diverted from the bladder, the animals will develop ureteral or renal pelvis cancer.

3. Dietary Factors

a. Sweeteners

No firm conclusions can be arrived at as to the toxicity of nonnutritive sweetners (saccharin and cyclamate) and their relationship to bladder cancer. Cyclamates were found to convert, in laboratory mice, into cyclohexylamine, which is a definite carcinogen. Even though extremely high doses are necessary to demonstrate the carcinogenic effects of cyclamate, this sweetener was banned as a food additive in the United States.

b. Nitrites and Nitrates

These agents, used as preservatives in smoked meats, have been implicated as causative agents for bladder cancer. There is, however, no conclusive evidence to support this claim.

4. Chronic Bladder Irritation

Calculus disease, chronic cystitis, schistosomiasis, and extrophy of the bladder all have a close causal relationship to the development of bladder cancer.

B. Early Detection

1. Clinical Presentation

Early detection actually depends on a high degree of suspicion in any patient who presents with either microscopic or gross, painless hematuria. These patients, as well as those with dysuria or chronic urinary tract infections, should not be ignored. Complete work-up should be done, particularly in the high-risk group as previously indicated.

a. Hematuria

Gross, painless hematuria, often occurring throughout the entire voiding phase, is the most common presenting symptom of bladder cancer. It is noted in 70% of patients and usually brings the patient to the physician.

Microscopic hematuria, on the other hand, is a common, often insignificant phenomenon. It should, however, be thoroughly investigated, especially in the high-risk older age group, in order to rule out bladder cancer or detect it at an early stage. The bleeding may be intermittent, and the patient and physician must not be lulled into a feeling of false security that may delay the work-up.

b. Bladder Irritability

Approximately 25% of patients with bladder tumors will have signs and symptoms of bladder irritability with dysuria or polyuria.

c. Recurrent Urinary Tract Infections

Recurrent urinary tract infections in males in whom prostatitis and urethritis has been ruled out must be suspected of having a bladder tumor and should have a complete work-up.

d. Complaints Attributable to Distant Metastases

Approximately 70% of bladder cancers are localized at the time of first diagnosis; but a minority (7%) are highly aggressive and invasive at the onset, and the patient may present with symptoms other than urinary.

2. Urine Cytology

Routine urinalysis is an essential component of any routine physical examination, whether it be done periodically or as part of admission testing for patients entering the hospital for other causes. Urine cytology of the exfoliated urinary cells is an important diagnostic and screening tool for bladder cancer; the accuracy of the procedure is directly related to the method of collection and the promptness with which the urine specimen is fixed, as well as to the expertise of the cytologist. Detection may range from 60 to 95%. Exfoliated transitional cancer cells are more frequently seen with sessile high-grade tumors and in widely spread carcinoma *in situ*.

C. Screening

Screening for bladder tumors is done on the basis of the urinalysis that is routinely ordered in a large number of circumstances. In populations that are at high risk for bladder cancer (e.g., those with occupational hazards), routine physical examination with urinalysis must be performed at frequent, regular intervals.

II. PRETREATMENT EVALUATION AND WORK-UP

A. Complete History and Physical Examination

This is an essential part of the evaluation of the urologic patient. The physician should attempt to identify the signs and symptoms of the tumor within the urinary tract; its extension within the urinary tract; resultant local complications such as obstruction, infection, renal damage, etc.; and signs and symptoms related to local invasion (e.g., rectal symptoms) or distant metastases. Symptoms that must be elicited include

- Hematuria.
- Dysuria.
- Urinary tract obstruction.
- Infection, fever, or flank pain.
- Tenesmus and rectal symptoms.
- Abdominal mass, etc.

Rectal examination, pelvic examination, and bimanual palpation in the female are most important to assess the degree of fixation of an empty bladder. Bimanual examination under general anesthesia should be repeated after transurethral resection of the tumor to permit accurate clinical staging. The size, location, and mobility of any palpable mass should be noted, and the degree of induration of the bladder wall, the extension to adjacent organs, and the fixation to the pelvic walls must be assessed.

B. Urologic Work-Up

1. Intravenous Urogram

The IVU is a vital tool in evaluating the entire urinary tract. The entire urothelium is considered as one single unit, and the incidence of multicentric tumors elsewhere in the urinary tract associated with a bladder carcinoma is approximately 10%. Filling defects on IVU may be misleading, however, since they may result from any space-occupying lesion (e.g., blood clots or calculi) and must be interpreted carefully. Computerized axial tomography scan of the pelvis and abdomen with the use of dye is a more accurate way of identifying additional tumors. The main value of the IVU is in the evaluation of the upper urinary tract and the assessment of renal function and the patency, size, and position of the ureter. Locally invasive bladder cancer of the ureterovesical junction will often reveal a hydroureteronephrosis.

2. Cystoscopy and Bladder Biopsy

Cystoscopy and urethroscopy is the most effective method of identifying the presence of bladder tumors. This procedure can be done under local, regional, or general anesthesia; it must be done in a meticulous fashion; and all areas of the lower urinary tract should be evaluated.

The location and number of lesions must be noted, as must their gross pathological appearance and the appearance of the adjacent bladder mucosa; and the urethral and trigone areas should be carefully assessed.

If the tumor is extensive, several representative biopsies should be taken from various areas of the tumor and normal adjacent mucosa. Biopsies should be deep enough to enable an accurate assessment of the depth of invasion and the presence of lymphatic or vascular involvement. If the tumor is small enough, total excision biopsy should be done.

Bladder irrigation and cytology is a useful modality in cases of subclinical disease.

C. Medical Evaluation

Because of the patient's usual advanced age, a complete system evaluation of the patient is essential prior to therapy. This must include

- Complete blood count (CBC) and urinalysis with culture and sensitivity.
- SMA-12.
- Chest x-ray.
- EKG.

Pulmonary function, cardiac reserve, and renal function must be carefully assessed whenever pertinent, and the operative risk should be established, particularly if a major ablative procedure is contemplated (for example, total cystectomy with ileal bladder operation).

A metastatic evaluation is also important preoperatively and should include a bone scan and skeletal survey and, whenever liver function tests are abnormal, a liver scan.

D. Staging Evaluation

The most important determinants of the management of bladder cancer are

- The stage of the disease.
- The grade of the tumor.

- The depth of invasion.
- The presence of carcinoma *in situ* along with the size and extent of the lesions.

The physical examination, cystoscopy, and biopsy of the tumor are aided in this respect by lymphangiography and CAT scan of the abdomen and pelvis.

Lymph nodes are rarely involved in the superficial low-grade tumors but reach an incidence of 40% involvement in the more infiltrative and extensive disease. Lymphangiograms and CAT scans will detect over 75% of these cases, and when positive, they are over 90% accurate. Often times, however, accurate staging can only be completed at the time of exploratory laparotomy.

The revised World Health Organization classification of bladder tumors (see Table I) takes into account several parameters such as

- Pattern of growth.
- Histology.
- Grade.
- Depth of infiltration.
- Lymphatic invasion.
- Mode of spread.

E. Site-Specific Data Form for Bladder Tumors (see pp. 593–594)

III. PRETREATMENT PREPARATION

For patients with early bladder cancer (small, noninvasive, papillary, well-differentiated), little or no preparation is necessary since endoscopic surgery of a minor nature is the only required treatment.

Careful preparation is essential for the patient requiring major surgery. Most of them are elderly and debilitated, often suffering from a variety of intercurrent illnesses. Preparation must take into account the following parameters:

- Any previous illness that requires compensation: diabetes, cardiac disease, pulmonary insufficiency, or chronic obstructive disease, renal disease, etc. All must be brought under the best possible control prior to surgery.
- Hyperalimentation may be desirable for 1–2 weeks prior to surgery.
- Fluid and electrolyte balance, blood volume, and hemoglobin and hematocrit should be attended to.
- Bleeding tendencies must be corrected.
- Psychosocial preparation is essential, particularly for patients who will have ostomies and urinary diversion and for

Table I

Revised Histological Classification of Bladder Tumors

I. Pattern of growth
     Not determinable
     Papillary
     Infiltrating
     Papillary and infiltrating
     Nonpapillary noninfiltrating
II. Histology
     Not determinable
     Transitional
     Squamous
     Adenocarcinoma
     Undifferentiated
     Any mixture of the above
III. Grade
     Not determinable
     Grade 1 (well-differentiated)
     Grade 2 (moderately differentiated
     Grade 3 (poorly differentiated)
     Any admixture—specify
IV. Depth of infiltration
     1. Not determinable
     2. Carcinoma *in situ* (nonpapillary, noninfiltrating)
     3. Papillary tumor without invasion of subepithelial connective tissue
     4. Tumor not extending beyond subepithelial connective tissue
     5. Tumor with infiltration of superficial muscle (not more than halfway through the muscle)
     6. Tumor with infiltration of deep muscle (more than halfway through the muscle)
     7. Tumor with infiltration of perivesical tissue
     8. Tumor with invasion of prostate or other extravesical structures
V. Lymphatic invasion
     Not determinable
     Not present
     Superficial lymphatics
     Deep lymphatics
     Lymphatic invasion present but depth not determinable
VI. Mode and location of spread
     Not determinable
     Subjacent
     Lateral
     Tentacular
     Broad front

the younger patient who might suffer from loss of libido and potency.

IV. THERAPEUTIC MANAGEMENT

Local and regional control of bladder cancer is of the greatest importance since the disease rarely results in early failure due to distant spread. Treatment decisions require great care and judgment and are best approached in a multidisciplinary fash-

ion by the urologist, radiotherapist, and medical oncologist simultaneously. Several factors will affect the choice of treatment.

- Tumor stage (see Table II) and size.
- Histological grade.
- Multicentricity and anatomic characteristics of the tumor.
- Tumor location.
- Age and general medical condition.
- Considerations of functional preservation.

Table II

Staging of Bladder Cancer

TNM classification	Marshall staging	Jewett staging	Jewett and Strong staging
Primary tumor 0: no evidence of tumor in the biopsy specimen T1S: sessile carcinoma *in situ* TA: papillary noninvasive cancer	0	A	A
T1: Papillary cancer without invasion (beyond the lamina propria; mass freely mobile by bimanual palpation, which is gone after TUR)	A		
T2: microscopic invasion of superficial muscle layers (induration of bladder wall, which is mobile)	B1	B1	B
T3: Induration and mass in bladder wall, persistent after TUR T3a: invasion deep into muscle	B2	B2	
T3b: through-and-through invasion of bladder wall	C	C	C
T4: tumor fixed or invading neighboring structures T4a: prostate, vagina, uterus T4b: fixation to pelvic wall Nodal involvement N1: involvement of single homolateral regional lymph node N2: bilateral or multiple regional pelvic nodes involved N3: fixed pelvic nodes	D1	D	D
N4: juxtaregional node involvement	D2		

SITE-SPECIFIC DATA SHEET—BLADDER CANCER

HISTORY

Age:_____

Symptoms

_____ Hematuria

_____ Frequency

_____ Dysuria

_____ Fever

_____ Weight loss____ lbs.

_____ Pain

_____ Mass

_____ Other_____

Duration:_____

Social history

Occupation:_____

Race:____White____Black____Oriental____Other

Smoker:____Yes____No   How much?_____

Drinker:____Yes____No   How often?_____

Environmental factors: Chemical exposure?_____

Detail:_____

Family history of carcinoma

Relation:_____ Site:_____

Previous history of carcinoma

_____ No____Yes   Site:_____

Rx:_____

Previous treatment (describe):

(surgery, radiation, chemotherapy, etc.)

_____

_____

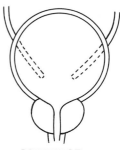

POSTERIOR WALL

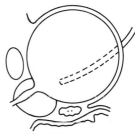

PATIENT'S RIGHT WALL (MALE)

PHYSICAL EXAMINATION (and cystoscopy)

Site:_____

Number of tumors:____ 1 ____ 2 ____ 3 ____ 4 ____ >4

Size in centimeters:____ 1 ____ 2 ____ 3 ____ 4 ____ >4

	Yes	No
Papillary	_____	_____
Sessile	_____	_____
Infiltrating	_____	_____
Bullous edema	_____	_____

	Yes	No
Bimanual exam		
Anesthesia	_____	_____
Induration	_____	_____
Mass	_____	_____
Mobile	_____	_____
Fixed to pelvic wall	_____	_____
Invading neighboring structure	_____	_____
Name of structure:_____		

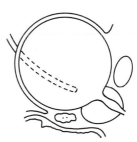

PATIENT'S LEFT WALL (MALE)

PRETREATMENT EVALUATION

	Neg.	Pos.	Suspicious
CBC	_____	_____	_____
Urinalysis	_____	_____	_____
IVP	_____	_____	_____
Cystoscopy	_____	_____	_____
Cystogram	_____	_____	_____
Other	_____	_____	_____

	Neg.	Pos.	Suspicious
Chest x-ray	_____	_____	_____
Lymphangiogram	_____	_____	_____
CAT scan	_____	_____	_____
Liver scan	_____	_____	_____
Bone scan	_____	_____	_____
Skeletal survey	_____	_____	_____

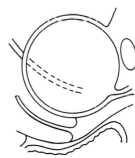

PATIENT'S LEFT WALL (FEMALE)

Staging classification

Histologic diagnosis:_____

Grade:____G1 ____ G2 ____ G3 ____G4

_____ T ____ N ____ M

Marshall classification:_____

Signature:_____

Countersignature:_____

Date:_____

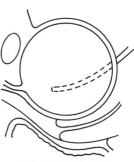

PATIENT'S RIGHT WALL (FEMALE)

TNM Classification

Primary tumor (T)

TX   Minimum requirements cannot be met
T0   No evidence of primary tumor
TIS   Sessile carcinoma *in situ*
T1   Papillary noninvasive carcinoma
      On bimanual examination, a freely mobile mass may be felt; this should not
        be felt after complete transurethral resection of the lesion and/or if there is
        papillary carcinoma without microscopic invasion beyond the lamina propria
T2   On bimanual examination, there is induration of the bladder wall, which is
        mobile. There is no residual induration after complete transurethral resection
        of the lesion and/or there is microscopic invasion of superficial muscle of bladder
T3   On bimanual examination, there is induration or a nodular mobile mass is
        palpable in the bladder wall, which persists after transurethral resection
T3a   Microscopic invasion of deep muscle
T3b   Invasion through the full thickness of bladder wall
T4   Tumor fixed, or invading neighboring structures, and/or there is microscopic
        evidence of invasion of the prostate, and in the other circumstances listed below,
        at least muscle invasion
T4a   Tumor invading substance of prostate, uterus, or vagina
T4b   Tumor fixed to the pelvic wall and/or infiltrating the abdominal wall

Nodal involvement (N)

The regional lymph nodes are the pelvic nodes just below the bifurcation of the common
iliac arteries. The juxtaregional lymph nodes are the inguinal nodes, the common iliac, and
para-aortic nodes.

NX   Minimum requirements cannot be met
N0   No involvement of regional lymph nodes
N1   Involvement of a single homolateral regional lymph node
N2   Involvement of a contralateral, bilateral, or multiple regional lymph nodes
N3   There is a fixed mass on the pelvic wall, with a free space between this and the tumor
N4   Involvement of juxtaregional lymph nodes

Distant metastases (M)

MX   Not assessed
M0   No (known) distant metastasis
M1   Distant metastasis present (specify)

Histopathology

Predominant cancer is a transitional cell cancer.

Stage grouping

No stage grouping is recommended at this time.

Grade

Well-differentiated, moderately well differentiated, poorly differentiated, or very poorly
differentiated (grade numbers 1, 2, 3, or 4, respectively).

Residual tumor (R)

R0   No residual tumor
R1   Microscopic residual tumor
R2   Macroscopic residual tumor (specify)

Performance status of host (H)

H0   Normal activity
H1   Symptomatic but ambulatory, cares for self
H2   Ambulatory more than 50% of time, occasionally needs assistance
H3   Ambulatory 50% or less of time, nursing care needed
H4   Bedridden, may need hospitalization

A. Therapy for Superficial Bladder Neoplasms

Tumors that are *in situ* (T1S or T0 or Stage 0) or those that are papillary with invasion of the lamina propria only (T1 or Stage A) can be treated by any one of several modalities that allow preservation of bladder function while achieving high rates of success with minimum morbidity and mortality.

1. Surgical Therapy

a. Transurethral Resection and Fulguration

Transurethral resection of the bladder (TURB) with fulguration is the method of treatment ideally suited for the small, superficial low-grade tumor that is easily accessible and has well-delineated margins. The entire tumor should be removed, together with the underlying muscularis and a 5-ml mucosal margin. Results of TURB are excellent, yet local recurrences or appearance of new lesions elsewhere in the bladder will occur in over 80% of cases; repeat examinations by cystoscopy and cytology of bladder washings must therefore be pursued at regular and close intervals. A substantial percentage of all bladder tumors are suited for TURB, but multistage electroresections are often required.

b. Partial Cystectomy

This procedure becomes necessary for the larger solitary lesion that is distant from the bladder base and neck. It is particularly indicated in the limited T2 (Stage B1) tumor with invasion of the superficial muscularis layer, where a 2- to 3-cm margin can be resected without compromising function. Segmental cystectomy should not be contemplated in cases of large or multifocal lesions, recurrent tumors, or extensively impaired bladders. Whereas TURB is ideal for appropriate lesions of the posterior and lateral walls of the bladder, partial cystectomy is more suited for tumors of the anterior wall and dome of the bladder.

c. Total Cystectomy

Total cystectomy with urinary diversion should be reserved for more extensive and multifocal or high-grade tumors or for persistent and recurrent lesions. The morbidity and mortality of the operaion are significant, with complications such as prolonged ileus, urinary or fecal fistulas, anastomotic leaks, bleeding, etc. occurring in over one-third of the patients. The results are only satisfactory in the relatively limited tumor (Stage B1 or T2 lesions), and external radiotherapy is therefore usually preferred as the primary modality of treatment for the extensive T2 lesion, with surgery reserved for the radiation failures.

Rehabilitation following cystectomy necessitates a urinary diversion operation. An ileal loop is the safest and most commonly employed method of diversion. Other methods include colonic implantation or ureterocutaneous anastomosis.

2. Radiotherapy

Radiation therapy has been used as an alternative to surgery in the treatment of selected cases of bladder cancers, particularly as it permits functional preservation. Various methods are used to deliver effective doses.

a. Interstitial Implants

Radium needles and radon, gold (^{198} Au), or iodine (^{125} I) seeds are all effective in the treatment of the small T1 tumor (less than 5 cm in size). This modality is preferred over the TURB for the higher grade lesions and is as effective in controlling the local disease. It is also an excellent alternative to segmental resection when the lesion is situated near the bladder base or trigone. Results are improved when supplemented by short courses of external radiotherapy.

b. External Megavoltage Radiotherapy

This modality is recommended under several circumstances:

- Preoperatively, to reduce seeding or dissemination by tumor spillage.
- For multifocal or recurrent superficial (T1 or T2) tumors, particularly when not suitable for segmental resection.
- In association with radium implantation in the more aggressive T2 lesions, or to prevent wound implantation.
- For extensive high-grade tumors, as a substitute for total cystectomy. In this application, radiotherapy has the distinct advantage of maintaining bladder function and preserving sexual function.

Radiotherapy in the treatment of T2 bladder tumors is expected to achieve 5-year survival rates in the range of 50–60%. Furthermore, 20–30% of the radiation failures can still be salvaged by surgery (total cystectomy with ileal conduit), though with a somewhat increased incidence of postoperative complications.

The usual radical dose of 6500–7000 rads in 6.5 to 7 weeks is very well tolerated when carefully planned. Occasionally patients will suffer from dysuria with urgency and burning during urination and mild diarrhea. Late complications of radiation cystitis with contracture and hemorrhage, radiation proctitis, and enteritis are more serious but fortunately uncommon.

3. Intravesical Chemotheraphy

Several agents have been employed for intravesical instillation in the treatment of the superficial bladder cancer (particularly the T1S and T1 cases, especially when they are multiple). Thiotepa, mitomycin C, doxorubicin, and BCG have all been employed at one time or another. The most commonly employed agent today is thiotepa in instillations of 60 mg in 60 cc of distilled water weekly for 4 weeks. The response rate is poor, and toxicity is almost as high as that of systemic chemotheraphy.

Intravesical chemoprophylaxis in the high-risk patient with multicentric or recurrent lesions has been recommended by some, but its salutory effects have not been clearly established. Chemotherapy should not be considered as a substitute for surgery or radiotherapy in the potentially curable bladder cancer.

B. Treatment of the More Aggressive Bladder Cancer

Few patients with T3 (Stage B2 and C) tumors that are deeply infiltrative are suitable for partial cystectomy or interstitial implants. Half of these patients will have lymph node metastases and/or extensive intramural spread. Available methods of treatment in these cases are

- Surgery. Radical total cystectomy and complete urethrectomy, including resection of all prevesical fat as well as all the regional lymph nodes (obturator, hypogastric, and external iliac). In the female, resection of the anterior vaginal wall, uterus, fallopian tubes, and ovaries should also be performed to obtain a more effective tumor margin.
- Radiotherapy. External radiotherapy to a dose of 6500–7000 rads in 6.5–7 weeks. The volume treated should include the bladder and the lymphatic drainage; it will usually encompass the entire pelvis.

The 5-year survival rates are poor with either modality (15–25% for Stage B2 or C lesions). Combined preoperative radiotherapy followed by total radical cystectomy has yielded slightly higher survival rates (35–40% 5-year survivals) but a significantly greater incidence of morbidity and mortality. The pattern or irradiation suggested in these cases is either as a short intensive course (2000 rads in 5 days) immediately before surgery or as a 4-week course (1000 rads per week) followed in 4–6 weeks by cystectomy.

Patients with T4 (Stage D1) disease have a dismal prognosis, with a 5-year survival rate of less than 10%. Significant palliation can, however, be achieved with external radiotherapy.

The use of other adjuvant modalities in the treatment of T3 and T4 bladder cancer is still experimental; systemic chemotherapy, immunotherapy, radiation sensitizers, and hyperthermia are all presently under investigation. Surgery and radiotherapy still remain the mainstay of therapy for the patient with advanced bladder cancer, whether it be for cure or merely for palliation.

The following guidelines are recommended in order to achieve the optimum results with minimum morbidity:

- Careful assessment and evaluation of the patient.
- Thorough preoperative preparation; fluid and electrolytes, blood coagulation functions, and cardiac and pulmonary capacity must all be assessed and optimized. Hyperalimentation, digitalization, preoperative antibiotics, adequate hydration, and bowel preparation should be instituted as needed.
- Psychological assessment and preparation is essential. The quality of life must be considered in patients who will have urinary diversion operations. A skilled ostomy therapist should see the patient prior to surgery and familiarize him or her with all the external devices used and their application. Supportive psychiatric care to the patient and the family is often useful.
- Meticulous attention to details during the operative procedure is mandatory. Careful construction of ureteroileal anastomoses and the ileostomy stoma is extremely important.
- Feeding enterostomy and postoperative anticoagulation are useful in avoiding troublesome postoperative complications.
- Careful planning and delivery of radiotherapy with attention to the requirements for proper patient management during the course of radiation.

C. Role of Systemic Chemotherapy

Antitumor drug therapy in bladder carcinoma has been disappointing at best. Most patients are older and chronically sick and have a poor tolerance for chemotherapy; renal insufficiency is not uncommon, further complicating the administration of the drugs. Furthermore, most failures seem to be locoregional, therefore apparently lending themselves better to local methods such as surgery or radiation rather than chemotherapy. Several agents have been employed both singly or in combinations: cis-platinum, Adriamycin, 5-fluorouracil (5-FU), methotrexate, and vinblastine have all been reported to yield variable response rates in bladder cancer. The responses are small in numbers and usually short in duration. The most active agent to date appears to be cis-platinum, with a 50% response rate, though responses are usually shorter than 6 months in duration. Combinations of drugs are currently being actively investigated in an attempt to identify an effective therapeutic regimen; no clear-cut conclusion can yet be drawn. Several combinations are actively being tried:

- Cyclophosphamide and Adriamycin.
- Cyclophosphamide and cis-platinum.
- Adriamycin and 5-FU.
- Cis-platinum, Adriamycin, and 5-FU.

In practice, they do not appear to yield any higher response rates than their most active individual agent. Further data are necessary in the form of randomized, controlled prospective studies before any firm conclusions can be drawn regarding the value of combined systemic chemotherapy in bladder cancer.

V. POSTOPERATIVE CARE, EVALUATION, AND REHABILITATION

The postoperative care of the patient following radical bladder surgery is identical to that of any other patient with radical intra-abdominal surgery:

- Monitoring of vital signs, fluid and electrolytes, blood gases intake and output, cardiopulmonary parameters, blood volume, etc. Immediate correction of any deviation must be carried out.
- Inhalation therapy.
- Gastrointestinal drainage until resumption of intestinal mobility.
- Meticulous ostomy care.
- Antibiotics.
- Anticoagulation; early ambulation.
- Alimentation, intravenous or via enterostomy tube when appropriate.

Rehabilitation of the patient is of utmost importance and must include

- Psychological support.
- Stoma care. The patients should be instructed as to the vari-

ous types of external appliances available and how to use them. Participation in a stoma clinic and an ostomy club should be encouraged.
- Prevention of urinary tract infection and early treatment if not prevented.

The follow-up evaluation of patients with a bladder tumor is essential for a variety of reasons:

- Multicentricity of the disease throughout the urogenital epithelium.
- High incidence of local recurrences, with increase in grade of the tumor and progressive invasion even in superficial early tumors.
- Detection of regional or systemic spread.
- Early identification of stoma complications or renal damage.

The evaluations should be frequent (every 3 months for the first 2 years and then spaced semiannually) and must include a thorough history, physical examination, and various selectively chosen laboratory tests including IVU, cystoscopy, bladder washings and cytology, proctosigmoidoscopy, sonography, and CAT scan of the abdomen and pelvis, in addition to the more routine tests: CBC, SMA-18, chest x-ray, etc.

IV. MANAGEMENT ALGORITHM FOR BLADDER TUMORS (see p. 598)

ALGORITHM FOR BLADDER TUMORS

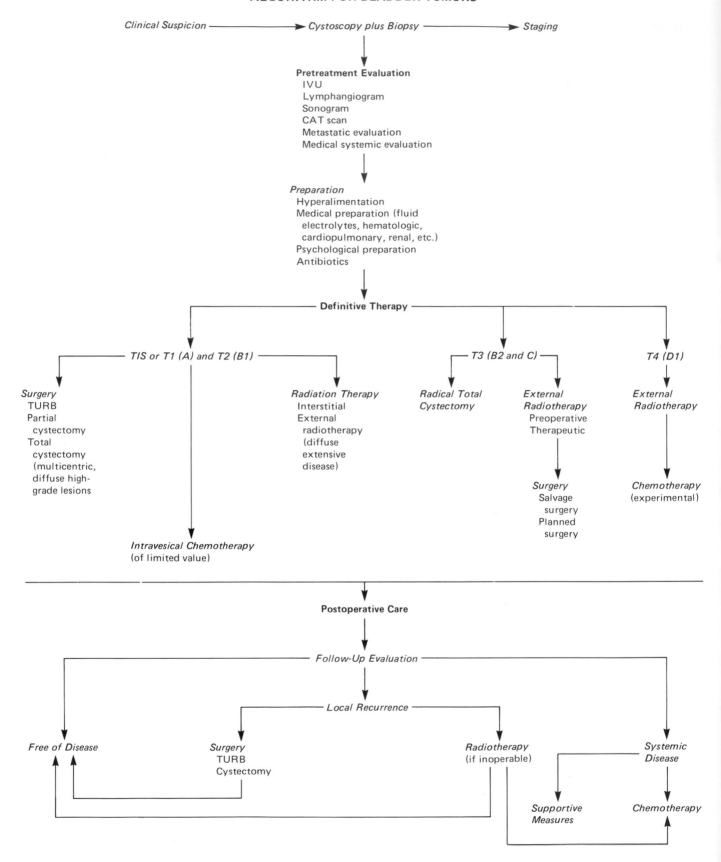

Section 13. Tumors of the Genitourinary Tract

Part C: Tumors of the Prostate

I. Early Detection and Screening   601
   A. Regular Physical Examinations
      and Laboratory Studies
   B. Early Signs
   C. Screening
II. Pretreatment Evaluation and Work-Up   601
   A. History
   B. Clinical Examination
   C. Office Cystoscopy
   D. Diagnostic Radiology
   E. Cytology
   F. General Medical Evaluation
   G. Operative Endoscopy and Biopsy
   H. Staging
      1. Stage A
         a. Stage A1
         b. Stage A2
      2. Stage B
         a. Stage B1
         b. Stage B2
      3. Stage C
      4. Stage D
         a. Stage D1
         b. Stage D2
      5. Prognosis
   I. Multidisciplinary Evaluation and Consultation
   J. Site-Specific Data Form for Prostate Cancer
III. Preoperative Preparation   604
   A. Nutritional Support
   B. Metabolic Considerations
   C. Cardiopulmonary Considerations
   D. Antibiotic Usage
   E. Psychiatric Considerations
   F. Preparations of the Lower Abdomen and Genitalia

IV. Therapeutic Management   607
   A. Early Diagnosis and Biopsy
   B. Modalities of Treatment
   C. Criteria for Adequate Surgery
   D. Radiotherapy
   E. Complications of Treatment
   F. Factors Determining Therapy
      1. Staging
      2. Social Factors
      3. Age
      4. Psychological Factors
      5. Preexisting Tumors
      6. Location of Tumor
V. Treatment of Advanced Prostate Cancer   610
   A. Obstructive Uropathy
   B. Metastatic Disease
      1. Hormonal Therapy
      2. Cytotoxic Chemotherapy
      3. Radiotherapy
   C. Systemic Support and Relief of Pain
VI. Postoperative Care, Evaluation, and Rehabilitation   611
   A. Evaluation and Care of the Postoperative Patient
   B. Care of the Patient following Radical
      Radiation Therapy
   C. Rehabilitation
      1. Urinary Incontinence Due to the Removal
         of the Internal Sphincter
      2. Sexual Impotence
      3. Loss of Wholeness and Attractiveness
         Caused by Treatment or Disease
   D. Follow-Up for Cancer of the Prostate
VII. Management Algorithm for Prostate Cancer   613

I. EARLY DETECTION AND SCREENING

All male patients, particularly those over the age of 40, should be advised to undergo an annual physical examination that must include a rectal examination and evaluation of the prostate; this is the only effective screening method to identify tumors in the prostate. Patients should be instructed that a change in urinary habits, discoloration of the urine, or systemic manifestations such as weight loss or backache may be signs of prostate neoplasm. Patients with any of these signs should be encouraged to consult their physician, or a urologist especially if findings point to a prostatic abnormality.

The cause of carcinoma of the prostate is not known, and no prevention is available. Early detection by routine examinations is thus the only valid recommendation that can be made.

A. Regular Physical Examinations and Laboratory Studies

Annual physical examinations should be carried out on every patient, particularly males, above the age of 40. This should include a thorough abdominal examination, evaluation of the genitalia, and a rectal examination to identify the size, consistency, and any abnormalities or nodules in the prostate. The finger should be extended as far as possible so as to evaluate the ampulla of the rectum and detect any perirectal masses. The rectal sphincter tone should also be evaluated.

B. Early Signs

Carcinoma of the prostate is often a silent tumor; therefore, routine rectal examination is mandatory to try and achieve early detection. The following symptoms should arouse suspicion:

- Changes in urinary habits.
- Frequency.
- Nocturia or Dysuria.

- Any persistent pain in the back, legs, or perineum.
- Anemia of unknown cause.
- Unusual fatigue or weakness.
- Weight loss.

These warning signs are usually indicative of prostatic disease and should prompt the patient to consult his physician and/or urologist.

C. Screening

As females have been alerted to the importance of annual cervical Pap smears, so males should be alerted to the importance of annual rectal examinations and prostatic acid phosphatase studies. Screening thus includes

- Routine rectal examination, which should be done by the physician on all patients.
- Mass screening programs may be sponsored by medical centers, health fairs, clinics, etc. and publicized in men's magazines, social centers, places of employment, or other media.
- Serum acid phosphatase can also be used for screening at the time of physical examination, but its value as a screening tool remains in doubt.

II. PRETREATMENT EVALUATION AND WORK-UP

The pretreatment evaluation of the patient with prostate cancer should include the following comprehensive work-up prior to making any definitive decision.

A. History

- History of present illness
  - Change of urinary habits: dysuria, polyuria, nocturia, hematuria.
  - Back, leg, pelvic, or perineal pain.

- Weakness or fatigue.
- Weight loss.
- Social history
  - Race.
  - Occupation.
  - Exposure to chemicals.
- Sexual history
  - Single.
  - Married.
  - Celibate.
  - Other.
- Family history of carcinoma
- Past medical history
  - History of Carcinoma.
  - Previous therapy.
  - Other.

B. Clinical Examination

A complete examination of the genitalia, groin, and abdomen as well as a thorough rectal examination are mandatory to identify the extent of the tumor, the presence or absence of obstructive signs, and any evidence of spread of the disease. The physical examination must pay particular attention to the following steps:

- A thorough evaluation of the lymph node areas, particularly the femoral, inguinal, and supraclavicular regions.
- A complete abdominal examination to identify tenderness or rigidity, vesical distension, or renal masses.
- Detailed examination of the external genitalia to detect abnormalities of the penis or testicles (induration or nodules). Observation of the urinary stream, preferably with objective measurements on a uroflometer, could be very useful.
- The rectal examination is the most important part of the physical. It should include evaluation of the sphincter tone and hemorrhoids. The physician should search for any masses, examine the seminal vesicles (for consistency, distension, etc.), and make a thorough assessment of the prostate, its consistency (hard, soft, firm), the presence of localized nodules, their location (one lobe, both, midline), number and multicentricity, etc.

C. Office Cystoscopy

If any abnormality of the prostate is suspected, a cystourethroscopy may be indicated to note any changes in the bladder, enlargement of the prostate, anomalies of the trigonal area, or other changes. Such office endoscopy may be useful as part of the preliminary office evaluation of the patient; it is optional, however, since it may have to be repeated at the time

of biopsy and, when done without anesthesia, offers limited data.

D. Diagnostic Radiology

- Intravenous pyelography, including cystomgram and postvoid films.
- Abdominal and pelvic CAT scans.
- Sonography.

E. Cytology

Cytological studies of seminal fluid are unrevealing and constitute a poor screening test for prostatic carcinoma.

F. General Medical Evaluation

- Complete physical examination.
- CBC.
- SMA-12 including alkaline phosphatase and serum calcium.
- Other pertinent studies such as serum acid phosphatase done by the radioimmunoassay (RIA) method.
- EKG (in patients over the age of 40).
- Chest x-ray.
- Search for metastases
  - Bone scan and x-ray skeletal survey of any suspicious area.
    - If there are abnormal liver chemistries, then a liver scan is indicated.

G. Operative Endoscopy and Biopsy

Cystourethroscopy under general anesthesia should be performed in conjunction with prostatic biopsy on all patients suspected of having prostatic pathology; tissue diagnosis must be obtained in all cases prior to definitive treatment. Repeat biopsies may be indicated if clinical suspicion persists in spite of a negative initial biopsy. Different methods are available to obtain tissues for pathological examination:

- Needle biopsy. This is usually performed under anesthesia by means of a transrectal or perineal route. In some institutions, the Franzen small-needle biopsy may be used as an office procedure; most urologists, however, are more successful using the transrectal or percutaneous perineal biopsy using a biopsy needle such as the Travenol Tru-cut or a similar needle (e.g., Vim Silverman needle). The Veemema perineal punch can also be utilized.
- Open biopsy. This procedure, carried out via a perineal

route, may be necessary if previous biopsies are unrewarding in proving carcinoma in patients where the diagnosis is strongly suspected as a result of local findings or the presence of metastases thought to be related to a primary prostate cancer.

- Biopsy of other areas. Biopsy of a suspected metastatic site, such as palpable suspicious lymph nodes or an accessible bone site, may be done in selected cases.
- Bone marrow aspiration and biopsy. This may also be performed if metastatic carcinoma is suspected.

It is not unusual to make the diagnosis of carcinoma of the prostate as an incidental finding on tissues obtained following prostatectomy for "obstructive disease" presumed to be caused by benign prostatic hypertrophy. Approximately 30% of prostate cancer is diagnosed from specimens obtained following transurethral resection of the prostate (TURP) or open prostatectomy for relief of obstructive uropathy. If, however, there is evidence of induration or abnormality of the prostate gland on rectal examination, every effort should be made to determine the presence of cancer prior to the surgery intended to relieve the obstructive uropathy; in many instances, such a patient may require a different surgical approach for definitive therapy (i.e., radical prostatectomy, with or without lymph node dissection) or might benefit from radiation therapy that would obviate the need for palliative conservative prostatic surgery. In some cases, however, immediate relief of the obstructive uropathy in the form of TUR or open prostatectomy is indicated (e.g., to reverse renal failure resulting from bladder neck obstruction). Even in the presence of carcinoma, it must be left to the judgment of the urologist to determine the best method of treatment of the obstructive uropathy. This should be individualized, and no firm guidelines can be set down.

H. Staging

The currently accepted staging system for prostate cancer is cumbersome and confusing for most nonspecialists. This is due, in part, to the fact that early-stage cancer (A) is not associated with any abnormality detectable on physical examination and that certain later stages can only be identified after a pelvic lymphadenectomy is performed, a procedure frequently not considered necessary. In consequence, we will depart from our usual format and describe each stage separately.

1. Stage A

At this stage of the disease, the diagnosis is established only by microscopic examination of tissue removed for apparently benign prostatic hypertrophy.

a. Stage A1

In these cases, there are no symptoms or physical findings to suggest prostatic cancer. The specimen is found to have carcinoma in three (or fewer) high-power microscopic fields and is usually well differentiated. Less than 2% of these patients will ultimately develop metastases, and therefore no further treatment is indicated. The patient should be followed up at regular intervals, however.

b. Stage A2

These are the cases where adenocarcinoma is found in more than three sections or the cancer is *not* well differentiated; the acid phosphatase here is normal. In these patients, further treatment is indicated.

2. Stage B

These patients usually have no urinary symptoms, but a nodule is palpable in the prostate.

a. Stage B1

The nodule is 1.5 cm or less, appears confined to one lobe, and there is no extracapsular or distant spread. Histological confirmation by needle or open biopsy should be done; a TURP may result in a false negative biopsy result if the nodule is peripheral.

b. Stage B2

The abnormality involves both lobes or more than 35% of the gland. The alkaline phosphatase is almost always normal. When lymph nodes are sampled, 20% of B2 cases will have positive nodes, thus making them Stage D1 lesions.

3. Stage C

These patients usually have symptoms of prostatism. Digital examination reveals spread to the seminal vesicles, the bladder neck, or the pelvic walls. In contrast to patients with benign prostatic hypertrophy (BPH), who usually have a slowly progressive history, these patients tend to have a relatively brief period of urinary obstructive problems. Transurethral resection of the prostate is generally diagnostic and relieves the urinary obstruction at the same time. If it does not yield a positive diagnosis, a needle biopsy may be indicated. The serum acid phosphatase is elevated in 20–30% of cases with Stage C prostate cancer. The bone scan is negative, however, and there is no evidence of distant spread. In clinical Stage C disease, a staging lymphadenectomy will demonstrate positive involvement in 40–50% of cases, changing the stage to D1. If lymph nodes are not examined, Stage D1 cannot be confirmed.

4. Stage D

In this advanced stage of the disease, rectal exam reveals a hard, nodular gland; bladder neck obstruction is usually prominent, and the serum acid phosphatase is elevated in most patients. Needle biopsy is almost always positive, and a TURP is generally both diagnostic for the carcinoma and therapeutically necessary for the urinary obstruction.

a. Stage D1

Stage D1 includes those patients in whom pelvic lymphadenectomy reveals positive nodes, only *below* the aortic bifurcation.

b. Stage D2

Stage D2 includes patients with distant spread (usually to bones) or those where lymphatic involvement is above the aortic bifurcation.

5. Prognosis

Of patients with involved nodes, 80% will go on to develop distant metastases within 5 years. Of patients with negative nodes, only 20% will develop distant spread. For each stage of disease, the histological grade of the tumor has a prognostic significance; poorly differentiated tumors have a higher incidence of lymph node involvement and a poorer overall prognosis.

I. Multidisciplinary Evaluation and Consultation

For the most part, the urologist will be primarily responsible for the diagnosis, work-up, and treatment of patients with early-stage (i.e., A1, A2, B1, B2, and C) carcinoma of the prostate. A radiotherapist should be consulted even in the early clinical stages, in so far as adjuvant radiotherapy (in the form of external megavoltage radiation) or definitive therapy with radioactive seed implants may be indicated in selected situations; total management planning in a cooperative fashion is essential at the onset. Consultation with the pathologist as to the tumor type and the differentiation grade is necessary in order adequately to project the prognosis and select the best course of therapy.

As a general rule, medical oncology consultations will not be necessary unless the patient has Stage D1 or D2 carcinoma. The urologist will often utilize hormonal therapy in the form of estrogens or orchiectomy in the management of these advanced cases, but oncologic consultation should be sought when hormonal therapy fails to control the patient's disease.

J. Site-Specific Data Form for Prostate Cancer (see pp. 605–606)

III. PREOPERATIVE PREPARATION

A. Nutritional Support

The preoperative preparation of the prostate cancer patient can best be managed by the urologist in conjunction with a consulting internist. As a rule, most patients with Stages A, B, or even C and D1 carcinoma are in a good nutritional state; some patients with advanced D2 carcinoma may be anemic and in a poor nutritional status, but their surgery, usually orchiectomy, can be performed under local anesthesia. Nutritional support is thus generally not required in patients with carcinoma of the prostate.

B. Metabolic Considerations

Patients with extensive carcinoma of the prostate (i.e., D1 or D2) will often develop obstructive uropathy, resulting in hydronephrosis and, at times, nitrogen retention. Techniques such as ureteral stenting or percutaneous renal pelvis drainage, which can be done under spinal or local anesthesia, may minimize the need for any preoperative preparation in these cases. More major procedures such as nephrostomy or ureteral implantation may occasionally be needed. In these cases, as well as in those slated to undergo radical surgery, a thorough evaluation of the patient and correction of any metabolic aberrations, fluid and electrolyte disturbances, blood volume deficits, and any coagulopathy should be rigorously undertaken.

C. Cardiopulmonary Considerations

Most patients with prostatic cancer are older individuals, many with cardiopulmonary diseases; if the patient is to be a candidate for radical surgery, medical consultation and additional studies (i.e., EKG, chest films, etc.) will be indicated to evaluate the patient's suitability for major prostatic surgery. Regional anesthesia may be utilized for most operations on the prostate whenever the medical condition of the patient precludes a general anesthesia.

D. Antibiotic Usage

As a rule, all patients requiring surgery of the urinary tract require antibiotic therapy to reduce the incidence of urinary

SITE-SPECIFIC DATA SHEET—PROSTATE CANCER

HISTORY

Age:_____

Symptoms
_____ Change in urinary habits
_____ Frequency
_____ Slow stream, dripping
_____ Nocturia
_____ Dysuria
_____ Hematuria
_____ Abdominal pain
_____ Perineal pain
_____ Back pain
_____ Bone pain

Systemic symptoms
_____ Weakness
_____ Fatigue
_____ Fever
_____ Weight loss____ lbs.
_____ Others

Duration _____

Social history
Occupation:_____
Race:____White____Black____Oriental____Other
Smoker: ____Yes____No.   How much?_____
Drinker: ____Yes____No.   How often?_____
Environmental factors: chemical exposure?_____
Detail: _____
Family history of carcinoma
Relation: _____ Site:_____
Previous history of carcinoma
_____ No____Yes   Site:_____
Rx:_____
Previous treatment (describe):
(surgery, radiation, chemotherapy, etc.)
_____
_____

PHYSICAL EXAMINATION

Rectal (prostate)
Size of prostate (estimate in grams) _____
Consistency:____ Hard____ Firm____ Mixed____ Nodular
_____ Diffuse induration
Site:____ Right lobe____ Left____ Both
Extracapsular spread _____
Other rectal findings:____ Ampulla____ Sphincter tone
Abdomen:____ Kidney____ Palpable____ Nonpalpable
_____ Bladder_____ Distended_____ Involved

Genitalia: Yes   No
Penis
Circumcised   _____   _____
Indurated   _____   _____
Edema   _____   _____
Scrotum
Normal   _____   _____
Describe:_____

PRETREATMENT EVALUATION

	Neg.	Pos.	Suspicious		Neg.	Pos.	Suspicious
Serum creatinine	_____	_____	_____	Chest x-ray	_____	_____	_____
Acid phosphatase (prostatic)	_____	_____	_____	Liver enzymes	_____	_____	_____
				Liver scans	_____	_____	_____
Alkaline phosphatase	_____	_____	_____	Bone scans	_____	_____	_____
IVP	_____	_____	_____	Bone marrow biopsy	_____	_____	_____
Cystoscopy	_____	_____	_____	Renal scan	_____	_____	_____
				CAT scan	_____	_____	_____
				Lymphangiogram	_____	_____	_____

Biopsy:____ No____ Yes.   Type:_____
Diagnosis:_____
Grade:_____

Stage:_____
Signature:_____
Countersignature:_____
Date:_____

Prostate Tumor Classification

Stage A   Tumor diagnosed by microscopic exam of tissue
          removed for apparently BPH

   A1   Tumor shows fewer than 3 foci of malignant tumor
          identified by the pathologist

   A2   Tumor greater than 3 foci (multiple), or diffuse
          areas of tumor noted (prostate gland was not
          necessarily thought to have malignancy on
          rectal exam)

Stage B   Patient has a nodule on physical examination
   B1   Isolated nodule 1.5 cm (discrete) noted on
          rectal examination, or tumor appears to be
          confined to one lobe of prostate

   B2   Both lobes of prostate involved with carcinoma,
          or more than 35% of gland is involved

Stage C   Carcinoma extends beyond prostate and involves
          seminal vesicles, bladder neck, or pelvic walls

Stage D   Carcinoma has extended to nodes or distant organs
   D1   Carcinoma has extended to pelvic lymph nodes
   D2   Carcinoma has manifested distant metastases

tract infection. Preoperative antibiotics are advised for those patients who have previously had urinary tract infections; perioperative antibiotics are indicated in those patients who have excessive instrumentation such as TUR, cystoscopy, or biopsy; postoperative antibiotics are indicated in all patients who undergo radical prostate and lymph node surgery. Other surgical procedures such as urinary diversion in the form of nephrostomy, conduits, ureteral implantations, or endoscopic ureteral stenting should also be covered by antibiotic therapy. Orchiectomy does not require antibiotic coverage.

E. Psychiatric Considerations

Patients with cancer of the prostate, particularly those in the younger age groups (i.e., below the age of 70), usually have a fully active sexual life. The prospect of impotence that follows radical prostatic surgery (in almost all cases) or radiation (in about one-third of patients) is of great importance. This matter should be fully discussed with the patient prior to any surgical or radiotherapeutic procedures. The use of hormones (i.e., estrogens) or hormonal surgery (i.e., orchiectomy) will also compromise sexual function and requires a candid discussion with the patient and his spouse. Psychiatric counseling is sometimes necessary to help the patients reach an accommodation with his disease and the potential affects of treatment.

F. Preparation of the Lower Abdomen and Genitalia

Routine surgical preparation (i.e., shaving, washing with antiseptic soap, and solutions such as Betadine) is suitable for all urologic procedures.

A bowel preparation prior to rectal biopsy and certainly prior to any procedure that may utilize the bowel for urinary diversion (i.e., ileal conduit) or that may include a resection of a segment of large intestine, should be carried out preoperatively.

IV. THERAPEUTIC MANAGEMENT

There is no single correct way by which all patients with cancer of the prostate can be treated. Management of the disease may vary from no treatment and observation of the "quiescent" nodule in the elderly patient to extensive pelvic lymphadenectomy and radical prostatectomy followed by orchiectomy. In between these extremes, the therapeutic approach that is best suited to the patient's individual needs will be determined primarily by the clinical stage of the disease and by several prognostic factors (age, general condition, histological grade and differentiation of the tumor, etc.). In addition, availability of treatment modalities and the attitude of the patient and family will affect the final decision.

The biologic behavior of prostatic carcinoma is unpredictable in most patients. Some patients may live many years without therapy and with very slow progression of the disease. No one, however, can predict with confidence which tumor is likely to become biologically aggressive; early diagnosis and appropriate therapy is, therefore, advised in all patients with suspected cancer of the prostate.

The goals of therapy must relate to the potential behavir of a particular tumor and the anticipated longevity of the patient. For example, radical prostatectomy is not advised in an 80-year-old patient with a low-grade tumor; on the other hand, radical surgery is recommended in the 65-year-old male whose life expectancy may exceed 10–15 years and who has a resectable carcinoma.

The urologist must weigh the risks of surgery and the potential complications (i.e., urinary incontinence and impotence) against the potential longevity of the patient and then recommend the therapeutic approach he believes will best control the disease with the least morbidity (i.e., radical surgery, radiotherapy, hormonal therapy, and/or combinations of these three) consistent with the best quality of life in each specific instance.

A. Early Diagnosis and Biopsy

Although there are no rigid criteria for the management of prostatic cancer in most patients, aggressive diagnosis and treatment should be implemented in most cases of suspected cancer of the prostate. In the extremely elderly patient with a short life expectancy due to other medical problems (e.g., severe cardiac disease, other neoplasms, vascular disease, etc.), it may be prudent not to pursue aggressive diagnostic steps. In the younger patient in good general condition, however, an aggressive diagnostic approach with early adequate treatment must be carried out.

Prostatic biopsies should be performed in all patients in whom symptoms suggest prostatic carcinoma or in whom there are other abnormalities (such as elevation of the serum acid phosphatase) that cannot be accounted for by benign prostatic conditions (i.e., infarct, inflammation, or recent massage). Biopsies should also be performed in those patients in whom metastatic disease is found and where the primary may be in the prostate. Insofar as carcinoma of the prostate can be controlled for long periods of time by various modalities, diagnosis should be made as expeditiously as possible.

B. Modalities of Treatment

Carcinoma of the prostate can be managed by multiple methods of treatment:

- Radical prostatectomy with or without combined pelvic lymphadenectomy.
- Conservative surgery in the form of TURP or enucleation.
- Orchiectomy.
- External beam radiation.
- Radioactive seed implantation.
- Estrogen therapy.
- Chemotherapy.

Other modalities have been used in patients with extensive metastatic carcinoma, namely, adrenalectomy and hypophysectomy. Those treatments, however, have poor results and have largely been abandoned.

C. Criteria for Adequate Surgery

If radical surgery is to be performed, the operation must include a total removal of the prostate gland and seminal vesicles. It should be recognized that there is a high risk of postoperative urinary incontinence associated with radical prostatectomy (approximately 10%), and the patient should also be alerted to the likelihood of postoperative impotence. Every effort must be made to protect the sphincter mechanisms during the procedure, though total surgical excision of the tumor must be the first priority. A pelvic lymphadenectomy may be indicated in order to stage the pathological extent of the disease accurately; the lymph node dissection may be modified to include the internal iliac nodes, the obturator nodes, the common iliac nodes, or all of them. The degree and extent of the node dissection is best judged by the urologist.

If surgery is indicated only for the relief of obstructive uropathy, (i.e., TUR or open conservative enucleation), the urologic surgeon must determine how much tissue should be removed to improve the patient's urinary symptoms. It is understood that such surgery in itself will not cure the tumor and is only palliative in nature.

D. Radiotherapy

Radiotherapy in the form of external beam radiation or radioactive seed implants is an accepted modality in the treatment of carcinoma of the prostate.

External beam radiation, using different energy sources, must reach the area of the prostate; insofar as the prostate is situated deep within the pelvis and adjacent to the rectal area, the dosage and depth of penetration must be such that the prostate will receive adequate irradiation without excessive exposure of the surrounding tissues (i.e., rectum, abdominal skin, and perineum). Surgery in the form of TURP or orchiectomy will often be done in conjunction with external beam radiation. Radiation must be carried to a high dose, and treatment volume should include the draining pelvic nodes. The dose directed at the prostate itself should be in the range of 6500–7000 rads.

If radioactive seed implants are used, this is done in conjunction with the urologist. The latter will do a staging pelvic lymphadenectomy, at which time, the radiotherapist will insert the radioactive seeds. Iodine-125 seeds are the preferred radioactive material for surgical implants, inasmuch as they provide a long half-life (60 days) and high-intensity radiation (approximately 15,000–20,000 rads) to the area of the prostatic malignancy.

E. Complications of Treatment

Complications of surgery include

- Postoperative Infection.
- Urinary incontinence (in about 10% of cases).
- Impotence in those patients undergoing lymphadenectomy or radical prostatectomy (in about 90% of cases).
- Lymphocele and lymphedema.

Although many of these complications can be corrected, incontinence and impotence contribute to a compromised lifestyle, and their high incidence must be seriously taken into account when selecting the appropriate therapeutic modality for a specific patient.

Complications associated with radiotherapy include

- Edema, particularly if staging lymphadenectomy has been performed.
- Radiation proctitis (in 10–15% of cases).
- Radiation cystitis (in 10–15% of cases).
- Impotence (in approximately 40% of cases).

F. Factors Determining Therapy

1. Staging

If the carcinoma is confined to the prostate (i.e., Stages A and B1), radical surgery may be the treatment of choice, though radiation therapy will yield equally good results. In A2, B2, or C lesions with tumors of high histological grade, there is a greater than 30–40% incidence of lymph node involvement, and this goes up to as much as 90% in the poorly differentiated Stage C lesions. Staging lymphadenectomy, therefore, should be considered to rule out the presence of metastatic lymph nodes before proceeding with a radical prostatectomy. If the lymph nodes are found to be positive, placing the disease in a Stage D, radical prostatectomy is not indicated, and pelvic external beam irradiation should be considered instead. Radical prostatectomy with radical lymphadenectomy has not resulted in significant cure rates in these cases.

An alternate approach would recommend the use of external beam radiotherapy for all patients with poorly differentiated high-grade tumors, irradiating the pelvic nodes to 5000 rads and the prostate to 6500–7000 rads. This approach is also preferred for patients with Stage C disease. The degree of differentiation of a tumor is thus as important a determination of prognosis and therapy, as is the stage of the disease. Recent methods of classifying prostatic cancers according to their degree of differentiation have been developed by Gleason, with a resultant score varying from 1 to 10. Generally speaking, surgery is the preferred treatment modality for the better differentiated tumors, whereas radiotherapy is preferred in the higher grades of histology.

In patients with D1 tumors, radiotherapy in the form of ^{125}I seed implants may be used to control the primary tumor. External radiotherapy is also frequently used as an adjuvant to palliative surgery (TURP or enucleation). Hormonal therapy, orchiectomy, and chemotherapy are also indicated in these advanced stages of the disease.

The following is a summary of the suggested guidelines for the management of prostate cancer according to stage.

Stage A1 • Close follow-up.
Stage A2 • Radical prostatectomy or radiation therapy.
Stage B • Radical prostatectomy (10-year survival is in excess of 50%).
• Radiation therapy—external or interstitial—followed by external radiotherapy (long-term results similar to surgery).
Stage C • Symptoms of obstruction are treated with TURP, followed by radical prostatectomy (20–30% 10-year survival).
• TURP, followed by radiation therapy (5-year survival of 40%).
Stage D1 • Treatment must be individualized; approaches include
• Radiation to pelvis and para-aortic areas.
• Surgery to remove the nodes, followed by radiation.
• Adding hormonal therapy after local measures are completed.
Stage D2 • The obstructive component is managed by TURP.
• Painful bony metastases are treated with local radiation and/or diethylstilbestrol (DES), 1–3 mg per day. Higher doses of DES do not in-

crease antitumor effects but significantly increase the likelihood of cardiovascular and thrombotic complications; low-dose radiation to the breast prevents painful gynecomastia caused by the chronic use of DES.
• If DES is contraindicated, orchiectomy, which can be performed under local anesthesia in debilitated patients, is an effective endocrine treatment.
• Cytotoxic chemotherapy is only indicated for patients whose disease becomes resistant to endocrine treatments.

The optimal management of patients with Stage D disease is still not clearly defined. It will be discussed in greater detail in a subsequent section on the management of the patient with advanced cancer of the prostate.

2. Social Factors

One must evaluate the patient as to marital status. The patient may have a second wife or a social liaison that provides him with a comfortable sexual relationship, irrespective of age; this matter should not be neglected in discussing various modalities of treatment with the prostate cancer patient. It is also most important to assess the potential effect of postoperative urinary incontinence on the patient's lifestyle.

3. Age

As indicated earlier, if the patient is over the age of 75, radical surgery is not advisable, irrespective of the focal nature of the tumor, since the risk of surgery may be greater than the advantages of a cancer cure by radical operations. Each patient, however, must be judged on his own merits irrespective of age; general medical problems such as cardiovascular disease, pulmonary disease, vascular disease, and metabolic abnormalities may be more important than the patient's age per se in deciding on an overall approach.

4. Psychological Factors

The psychological impact of total impotency associated with pelvic surgery and radical prostatectomy may be devastating to the patient. Although radiotherapy can also result in impotency, the incidence with this modality is significantly less, and it may be the choice of the patient if he is presented with the facts.

5. Preexisting Tumors

Patients may manifest preexisting tumors either in the genitourinary system or elsewhere. Coexistence of bladder carcinoma associated with prostate carcinoma may dictate the choice of therapeutic modality. Radical surgery in these cases entails urethrocystectomy and prostatectomy with urinary diversion, a rather formidable procedure that should only be undertaken if the prospects for cure are high and the patient's general status is suitable. Here again, radiotherapy may be a reasonable alternative in the management of both tumors, which could be treated concomittantly through the same portals. Upper GU tract neoplasms (i.e., kidney, ureter, etc.) should be managed on their own merits but may affect the prognosis of the patient and would thus limit survival even if a radical prostatectomy were to be performed.

Other malignancies (e.g., stomach, lung, or head and neck) should be appropriately treated. Their presence may limit the patient's prognosis and thus effect the urologist's decision as to the best mode of therapy for the treatment of the patient's carcinoma of the prostate.

6. Location of Tumor

At the present time, there is no evidence that the location of the tumor (whether lateral, posterior, or near the apex) affects the prognosis of the disease. As long as the tumor is confined to the prostate, satisfactory cure rates can be achieved with radical surgery, provided the lymph nodes are free of tumor. The location of the tumor will not influence the effectiveness of radiotherapy either; since the prostate is a small gland, variations in the location of the tumor within the gland should not make it less vulnerable to external beam or radioactive seed implants.

V. TREATMENT OF ADVANCED PROSTATE CANCER

Patients with advanced prostate cancer may present with obstructive uropathy caused by enlargement of the prostate or by obstruction of the upper GU tract from subtrigonal or pelvic extension of the carcinoma, or with metastatic disease causing systemic manifestations.

A. Obstructive Uropathy

Obstructive uropathy caused by extensive carcinoma of the prostate may be managed by TUR plus radiotherapy and hormonal manipulation. Ureteral or upper GU tract obstruction can be managed by a variety of means in addition to hormonal manipulation. Some cases will require ureteral stenting by means of the J stent or an indwelling ureteral stent; if this fails, the patient may require ureteral reimplantation in the bladder

or, if necessary, nephrostomy. Temporary dialysis may be needed to stabilize the patient's renal function in order to prepare him for surgical intervention to correct the obstructive uropathy. Cancer of the prostate is often a slow-growing neoplasm that might respond to hormonal manipulation or chemotherapy; it is advisable not to let the patient expire because of acute renal failure, and every effort should be made to improve the kidney function by the methods described above.

B. Metastatic Disease

1. Hormonal Therapy

Patients with metastatic carcinoma of the prostate (Stage D2) have a guarded prognosis. Patients with bone metastases may live for several years without complaints and be quite stable; hormonal therapy, in the form of estrogens or orchiectomy, becomes indicated only as the metastatic lesions become symptomatic. There is no evidence that such hormonal therapy or chemotherapy will prolong life, and each patient should be evaluated according to the severity of his symptoms and his general condition, rather than according to radiological or laboratory findings alone. As a rule, metastatic carcinoma of the prostate is best managed with hormonal treatment (i.e., orchiectomy, estrogens, or both), and these modalities are effective in approximately 60% of the patients with symptomatic bone disease. In many instances, hormonal therapy will cause a shrinkage of the primary tumor as well. If a patient develops regrowth of the carcinoma in the prostatic area following a TURP and radiotherapy, orchiectomy and/or estrogens may induce shrinkage of the tumor; thus hormonal manipulation is used even in the absence of bone metastases.

2. Cytotoxic Chemotherapy

At the present time, hormonal therapy offers the best mode of treatment for metastatic disease. Combinations of chemotherapy and hormonal therapy (estrogenous compounds) have been introduced , though helpful in controlling the disease in some cases, the overall success rate with these agents has not been encouraging. Other chemotherapeutic agents, namely, cyclophosphamide, Adriamycin, and 5-FU, have been found by some to be useful in the management of metastatic disease resistant to hormonal measures. Objective response rates of 30–40% have been reported with combinations including cyclophosphamide and Adriamycin. Most patients with metastatic disease, however, have blastic bone lesions as the only available parameter—a situation in which *objective* response is not readily measurable. One is then required to judge the efficacy of therapy by subjective criteria such as relief of bone pain (quantifiable indirectly by measuring changes in narcotic

VI. POSTOPERATIVE CARE, EVALUATION, AND REHABILITATION

611

analgesic use, for instance) and reversal of constitutional symptoms (such as weight loss, anorexia, etc.). Thus, clinically gratifying but objectively inevaluable remissions are sometimes achieved.

Many prospective patients referred for chemotherapy are elderly, with serious cardiac disease. Such patients should be carefully evaluated before commencing a course of Adriamycin. *Cis*-platinum, thought to be synergistic with both Adriamycin and cyclophosphamide, has also been reported to have activity in this disease, but its nephrotoxicity and the hydration measures required to minimize that toxicity limit its usefulness in this population of patients.

Chemotherapy research is hampered by a number of factors. The frequent inaccuracy of clinical staging, the fact that most patients are elderly and cannot safely receive effective chemotherapy, that most of them do not have objectively measurable disease (blastic bone metastases), and that most have been previously treated with extensive courses of radiation therapy to the primary site, as well as to sites of symptomatic metastatic spread, all make prospective randomized studies extremely difficult to design and carry out to completion.

3. Radiotherapy

The role of radiotherapy in palliating symptoms from the local effects of the tumor is well established. The response of pain (especially when due to bone metastases) to radiation is most gratifying, and soft-tissue masses causing pressure symptoms will also respond well to palliative radiotherapy.

C. Systemic Support and Relief of Pain

For patients who are systemically ill with metastatic carcinoma (i.e., weight loss, anemia, etc.), nutritional support is helpful. The use of blood transfusions, although immediately helpful, offers no long-term improvement; if the patient has a severe cardiac condition, blood replacement may be indicated to alleviate the cardiac symptoms.

If the patient has severe bone pain refractory to orchiectomy, radiotherapy, estrogens, or chemotherapy, consideration should be given to the possibility of steroid therapy or the use of newer, perhaps experimental, drugs that inhibit the adrenal gland (such as aminoglutamide). It should be noted that these drugs are at best experimental and have an uncertain role in the management of carcinoma of the prostate. Adequate doses of narcotic analgesics become the mainstay of treatment of the patient with advanced metastatic prostate cancer.

Involvement of the spine is very common, and spread to the epidural space with consequent spinal cord compression is a constant threat. It is a grave mistake to ignore complaints of leg weakness or to ascribe sphincteric problems to any other

cause, unless spinal cord compression has been ruled out by careful physical examination and urgent neurological consultation in cases of doubtful findings. Cord compression, if diagnosed in a timely fashion, is treatable and reversible by laminectomy and/or radiation therapy.

VI. POSTOPERATIVE CARE, EVALUATION, AND REHABILITATION

A. Evaluation and Care of the Postoperative Patient

For the patients who have undergone radical urologic surgery as described above, the following steps are advised:

- The urethral catheter should be sutured to the penis or securely taped to the leg.
- Urine output must be carefully monitored. Extensive pelvic surgery may cause obstruction of the ureter, and decreased urinary output should not be ascribed solely to hypovolemia but could be due to obstruction.
- Catheter care is extremely important; metal cleansing and use of urinary antimicrobials during the initial post surgical period are essential.
- The surgical site may be drained by either surgical drains or closed-system suction (e.g., Hemovac). The dressing should be changed daily around the area of the drain site.
- All patients undergoing major urologic surgery require prophylactic antibiotics. Often these patients will be given the antibiotics prior to and even during the urologic procedure. The choices of antibiotics should be dictated by results of urine culture and sensitivity studies.
- The other genital areas should be kept clean, and betadine or other antiseptic solutions or cream must be applied around the urethral catheter on a daily basis.
- Frequently, following extensive ureteral manipulation, the ureter is stented with ureteral catheters; these are often removed at the time of surgery, but in some instances they may be kept indwelling. If this is so, their urinary output should be closely watched, and antiseptic care must be used at the connecting point of the ureteral stent and the draining tube.
- Following radical urologic surgery, most patients will be placed on an oral diet within a few days. Ileus may occur and, if it persists, the patient requires careful evaluation to detect any extravasation of intraperitoneal fluid or infection; intravaneous fluid and nutritional support must then be maintained until the patient is able to eat.

B. Care of the Patient following Radical Radiation Treatment

For the most part, these patients require minimal care, though they may develop bladder irritation and rectal discomfort. If this be the case, urinary antiseptics and analgesics should be used. If rectal discomfort persists, the patient may require suppositories and sitz baths. Rarely do these patients develop evidence of radiation sickness (nausea and vomiting).

C. Rehabilitation

The following problems need to be addressed when caring for the patient treated for prostate cancer. Most of the problems have been discussed briefly throughout this section.

1. Urinary Incontinence Due to the Removal of the Internal Sphincter

Goal: Control of incontinence.
Intervention: Instruct the patient to expect some leakage of urine when changing position after removal of the Foley catheter. Apply and instruct the patient about the use of an external appliance and determine the efficacy of the appliance during follow-up visits. Help the patient deal with frustrations if the incontinence becomes permanent.

2. Sexual Impotence

Goal: Adjustment to impaired sexual functioning.
Intervention: Assess the patient's readiness to discuss his concerns regarding sexuality. Encourage interaction between the patient and his partner. Reinforce the information given and include the partner in all teaching sessions and discussions. Provide opportunities for the patient to discuss his feelings.

3. Loss of Wholesomeness and Attractiveness Caused by Treatment or Disease

Goal: Establishment of self-image: ability to control bodily functions.
Intervention: Convey an attitude of acceptance when caring for the patient. Encourage the patient to express his feelings. Be alert to verbal and nonverbal cues. Instruct the patient

Table I

Long-Term Follow-Up Schedule for Prostate Cancer

Management	First year				Second year	
	3 months	6 months	9 months	12 months	6 months	12 months
History						
Change in urinary habits	X	X	X	X	X	X
Blood in urine	X	X	X	X	X	X
Abdominal, suprapubic, perineal, genital, or back pain	X	X	X	X	X	X
Any bone or muscular pain	X	X	X	X	X	X
Physical						
Abdominal exam	X	X	X	X	X	X
Blood pressure	X	X	X	X	X	X
Genital exam	X	X	X	X	X	X
Rectal exam	X	X	X	X	X	X
Extremities: edema	X	X	X	X	X	X
Investigation						
CBC	X	X	X	X	X	X
SMA-12	X	X	X	X	X	X
Acid phosphatase (may be performed more often in stage D disease)	X	X	X	X		X
IVP			As indicated			
CAT scan			As indicated			
Sonogram			As indicated			
Nuclear Study			As indicated			
Bone scan (indicated if bone pain develops and acid phosphatase rises or anemia develops)			As indicated			

regarding methods of maintaining bodily functions and rein-force the information given. Include the family, community agencies, and spiritual counselors in the support process, and encourage the patient to discuss his fears and concerns with his physician.

D. Follow-Up for Cancer of the Prostate

See Table I for a schedule for the first 2 years.

VII. MANAGEMENT ALGORITHM FOR PROSTATE CANCER (see p. 614)

ALGORITHM FOR CANCER OF THE PROSTATE

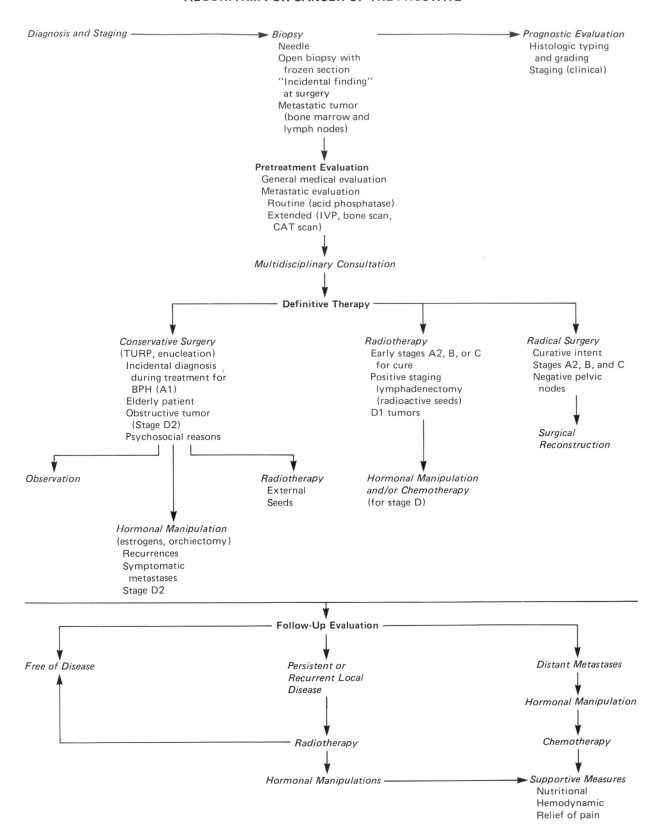

Section 13. Tumors of the Genitourinary Urinary System

Part D: Testicular Tumors

I. Introduction 617
  A. Incidence
  B. Classification
    1. Seminomas
    2. Nonseminomatous Tumors
  C. Prognosis
II. Early Detection and Screening 618
  A. Predisposing Factors
    1. Dysgenetic Testes
    2. Other Predisposing Factors
  B. Early Detection
  C. Screening
III. Pretreatment Evaluation and Work-Up 619
  A. History and Physical Examination
  B. Laboratory Evaluation
    1. Routine Preoperative Evaluation
    2. Serologic Markers
  C. Evaluation of the Scrotum and Testicle

  D. Radiological Evaluation
    1. Intravenous Urogram
    2. Lymphangiography
    3. Computerized Axial Tomography
    4. Venacavography
  E. Metastatic Survey
  F. Multidisciplinary Evaluation
  G. Site-Specific Data Form for Testicular Tumors
IV. Preoperative Preparation 620
V. Therapeutic Management 620
  A. Seminomas
    1. Stage I
    2. Stage II
    3. Stage III
  B. Nonseminomatous Tumors
VI. Chemotherapy for Advanced Testicular Tumors 624
VII. Postoperative Care, Evaluation, and Rehabilitation 625
VIII. Management Algorithm for Testicular Tumors 625

I. INTRODUCTION

A. Incidence

Testicular cancer affects young adults primarily between the ages of 15 and 40 and constitutes the third leading cause of death in this age group. The incidence of testicular tumors is approximately 2–3 per 100,000 males per years. A higher incidence of testicular tumors has been noted in the Scandanavian countries (6.3 per 100,000 per year), whereas they are rarely seen in the black population, especially in the younger age group. Accounting for 1% of all neoplasms in males, testicular tumors have a trimodal distribution with yolk sac tumors or infantile embryonal carcinoma most commonly seen in infancy; embryonal cell carcinomas and teratocarcinomas occurring primarily between 15 and 30 years of age; and seminomas tending to appear more commonly in a slightly older age group (25–40 years).

B. Classification

1. Seminomas

The most common type of testicular tumor, seminoma, constitutes 40–50% of all cases. These are less aggressive lesions than the nonseminomatous group (often called "malignant teratomas"), and only about 25% of them will have lymphatic metastases at the time of diagnosis. Grossly, the tumor usually affects the entire testis, is pale in color, uniform in appearance, and often lobulated by the presence of fibrous intersections. In the classical form, the cells are uniform and round with little anaplasia; a small percentage of cases though fall in one of several variants:

- Anaplastic seminomas (marked nuclear pleomorphism and more than three mitoses per high-power field) constitute 3–5% of cases.
- Spermatocytic seminoma (5% of cases) occurs in the older age group and has an excellent prognosis.

- Mixed seminomas (10–15% of cases) show various cellular elements representing one or more of the other testicular tumors (e.g., embryonal carcinomas). In these cases, the course of the disease is defined by the tumor element that has the most aggressive course.

2. Nonseminomatous Tumors

Embryonal cell carcinoma, teratoma, teratocarcinoma (teratomas with carcinoma), and choriocarcinoma are all considered to be nonseminomatous tumors. The most common variety is the embryonal cell type (20–30% of cases), followed by teratocarcinoma; the least prevalent type is the choriocarcinoma (less than 3% of cases). Of patients with these tumors, 60–70% are found to have retroperitoneal lymph node metastases when initially seen.

Nongerminal tumors of the testis (Leydig's cell tumors, gonadal tumors, and Sertoli cell tumors) constitute less than 5% of testicular tumors and are benign in 90% of the cases.

C. Prognosis

As the major pathway of tumor dissemination is the lymphatic system, the retroperitoneal lymphatics constitute the primary focus of the staging system. Advances in the evaluation of the retroperitoneal nodal system by the use of CAT scan and lymphangiogram and in the assessment of the presence or absence of distant disease by the use of tumor markers has led to more accurate postoperative staging prior to deciding on a definitive treatment modality.

Early-stage tumors (Stages 1 and 2), particularly seminomas, have a 90–95% 3-year survival, whereas patients with Stage 3 lesions have a less favorable picture. The prognosis in cases of embryonal carcinomas is not as good even in Stages 1 and 2, where cure rates are, 75 and 55%, respectively. Recent advances in chemotherapy, however, have significantly increased the survival in patients with advanced testicular tumors especially embryonal carcinoma.

II. EARLY DETECTION
AND SCREENING

A. Predisposing Factors

1. Dysgenetic Testes

Cryptorchidism and dysgenetic testes are the best recognized predisposing factors in the genesis of testicular tumors. The probability of developing a malignant tumor in a cryptorchid or dysgenetic testis is 35 times greater than in a normally descended testis. It is strongly recommended that children with undescended testes be explored prior to age 10 and that the testis be brought down to the scrotum. There is no evidence, however, that orchiopexy materially influences the chances of developing testicular cancer. In fact, carcinoma of the testis often affects the contralateral rather than the undescended testis, and it is believed that it is not the maldescent that predisposes to cancer, but rather a common underlying factor that results both in the failure of the testis to migrate and in a predisposition to testicular malignancy.

2. Other Predisposing Factors

There have been several reports suggesting the possibility of various environmental factors or degenerative changes playing a role in the genesis of testicular tumors:

• Prior history of orchitis (mumps).
• History of trauma (a doubtful influence).
• Bilaterality of testicular cancer. The individual who has had one testicular lesion seems to be at a higher risk for a contralateral tumor than the male population at large.

B. Early Detection

The presence of a testicular mass is, by and large, the all-important sign indicating the possible presence of a testicular tumor. There is almost always a delay in the diagnosis of testicular tumors, and 4–6 months often elapse before the patient alerts the physician to the development of a mass in his testicle. At the time of their first visit, 10% of patients present with symptoms of metastatic disease. A high degree of suspicion in testicular masses will reduce this delay and should bring the patient to treatment at an earlier stage of his disease.

The differential diagnosis facing the clinician includes

• Epididymitis or epididymo-orchitis.
• Trauma with Hemorrhage.
• Hydroceles or other scrotal lesions.

Initially, 20% of testicular tumors are misdiagnosed as epididymo-orchitis or other inflammatory diseases of the testicle.

Likewise, hydrocele associated with a testicular tumor is not uncommon and may present as the primary finding; scrotal transillumination is mandatory in these cases to rule out the presence of a tumor, and the use of ultrasound is likewise helpful in its identification. Thermograms, scrotal scans with technetium-99, and soft-tissue radiology are at times used to identify testicular from other scrotal masses.

Gynecomastia in young males is a rather common and insignificant occurrence, often noted around puberty or in the later teen years. It can, however, be an early sign of a chorionic gonadotrophin–producing tumor, and the astute clinician must keep this possibility in mind. A thorough examination of the testes is required, and beta human chorionic gonadotrophin (HCG) levels should always be obtained when evaluating a young patient with gynecomastia. A chest x-ray may also uncover an extragonadal choriocarcinoma that may present as a mediastinal mass (see §10B).

Changes in libido or secondary sex characteristics should also alert the physician to a hormonally active tumor and initiate an appropriate work-up.

If a clinical examination does not absolutely exclude a testicular tumor, it is strongly recommended that an inguinal exploration of the testis be performed. In such instances, the spermatic cord is first secured at the level of the internal inguinal ring with a noncrushing vascular clamp, and the testicle and fascial contents are then mobilized and brought into the open groin wound. After proper wound draping, the testicle is identified, the tunica vaginalis is opened, and the diagnosis is confirmed. Biopsy of the testis during such exploration is rarely needed, and exploring the patients with epididymitis or epididymo-orchitis does not complicate or lengthen the clinical course of that disease entity. On the other hand, identification of a tumor at an early stage is of utmost importance to the outlook of the patient.

C. Screening

The best screening method for evaluation of testicular neoplasms is routine clinical examination of children and young adults, especially in the age group between 15 and 35 years. Any suspicious testicular masses as described above must be investigated in detail.

Education of the public at large as to the importance of a testicular mass must be encouraged and promoted. Likewise, physician education, especially that of pediatricians and primary care physicians who are most likely to be examining these otherwise healthy young individuals, must be directed toward arousing a high degree of suspicion and "cancer consciousness."

III. PRETREATMENT EVALUATION AND WORK-UP

A. History and Physical Examination

A complete history and physical examination should be done. Particular attention should be paid to the following:

- The age of the patient, weight, and vital signs.
- Familial history.
- Prior illnesses (mumps, undescended testis, etc.).
- Prior surgical procedures.
- History of prior surgery, radiation, or chemotherapy.
- Inflammatory diseases or trauma to the testicle.
- Changes in libido.

A thorough examination of the genitalia is most important:

- Symmetry, size, consistency, and location of the testes must be noted.
- Transillumination must be used to identify fluid and any masses within the hydrocele.
- Tenderness should be elicited.
- Masses must be thoroughly evaluated as to the size, consistency, borders, exact location (epididymis, testis, or skin), and involvement of adjacent structures.

An examination of the groins and abdomen should be done to identify the presence of nodes, abdominal masses, or liver enlargement. In addition, a complete physical examination of all systems must be carried out prior to any therapy.

B. Laboratory Evaluation

1. Routine Preoperative Evaluation

- Urinalysis and CBC.
- Blood chemistries (SMA-12, serum electrolytes).
- Chest x-ray with tomograms or chest CAT scan, if indicated.

2. Serologic Markers

- Serum beta-HCG; elevated in choriocarcinomas.
- Alpha fetoproteins (AFP); elevated in teratomas and in embryonal carcinoma.

C. Evaluation of the Scrotum and Testicle

In addition to a good physical examination and transillumination, several modalities may be valuable in establishing a differential diagnosis of a scrotal mass:

- Soft-tissue radiology and CAT scan.
- Thermography.
- Scrotal scan with technetium-99.

The final diagnosis, however, will require scrotal exploration with identification and examination of the testes as described in §13D.2.B. It is important to stress several technical points in the scrotal exploration in order to minimize the chances of local failure of the definitive treatment:

- Exploration must always be carried out through an inguinal rather than a scrotal approach.
- Early control of the spermatic cord by clamping or high ligation (whenever an orchiectomy is being performed) is most important.
- Needle biopsy of scrotal masses must be avoided since they are associated with a high incidence of tumor implantation and local recurrences.
- If an open biopsy is carried out (in lesions that are strongly suggestive of nonneoplastic disorders at exploration), frozen section should be obtained in order to avoid replacing the testis in the scrotum if it is neoplastic.
- An orchiectomy as a total excisional biopsy is the procedure of choice if one strongly suspects a malignant tumor.

D. Radiological Evaluation

Following removal of the tumor and establishment of the histological diagnosis, a complete radiological evaluation is necessary to identify the status of the lymphatics and properly stage the disease.

1. Intravenous Urogram (IVU)

The IVU is rarely useful in identifying nodes located at the level of the renal pedicle. Nodes can only be identifiable if they are large enough to distort the kidney or ureter.

2. Pedal Lymphangiography

This is helpful in assessing the status of the ilioinguinal and para-aortic nodes. Enlarged nodes can usually be identified, and a foamy appearance or filling defects within the node are indications that these nodes are involved.

3. Computerized Axial Tomography

This is undoubtedly the simplest and least invsasive method to identify bulky disease or retroperitoneal nodes larger than 2 cm.

4. Venacavography and Angiography

These are occasionally indicated in some cases of Stage 2 and 3 disease, though they have largely been supplanted by CAT scan examination.

E. Metastatic Survey

The incidence of metastases in testicular tumors is rather high, and a complete metastatic survey is thus indicated in any patient prior to definitive therapy.

The most common site of metastases is undoubtedly the lymphatics, and these are evaluated as described above in order to stage the disease and plan a rational therapeutic approach. The commonest extranodal metastatic site is the lung, followed by the liver and the bones. Metastatic disease may be suspected on clinical grounds in patients who present with

- Diffuse lumbar pain (nodal disease).
- Breathlessness, chest pain, or hemoptysis (lung metastases).
- Anorexia, weight loss.
- Central nervous system symptoms.

The incidence of blood-borne metastases is much less frequent in seminomas as opposed to nonseminomatous tumors where it may affect other organs (e.g., mesentery).

Investigation for distant metastases should include a minimum of a good chest x-ray and SMA-12. In addition, further work-up should be instituted at the slightest suspicion of distant metastases and may include

- Chest tomograms or CAT scan.
- CAT scan of the brain.
- Bone scan and skeletal survey, if indicated.
- Liver scan.

F. Multidisciplinary Evaluation

The multidisciplinary approach to patients with testicular cancers has resulted in markedly improved survival. A multidisciplinary evaluation prior to definitive therapy is therefore essential in all cases of testicular tumors. The urologic surgeon, radiotherapist, and medical oncologist must map out a joint plan of treatment. Postoperatively, psychosocial rehabilitation is of great importance, and the social worker, nurse oncologist, and psychiatric liaison nurse should be involved in the postoperative care, and at times, even the psychiatrist will be necessary to the rehabilitation of the patient.

G. Site-Specific Data Form for Testicular Tumors (see pp. 621–622)

IV. PREOPERATIVE PREPARATION

Most patients with testicular tumors are young and otherwise healthy, requiring little or no preparation before surgery. Since orchiectomy is indicated in all these patients and since the addition of chemotherapy will almost always result in sterilization, psychosocial preparation may be useful. The patients must be informed of the consequences of the treatment and must be helped in accepting them. From patients who are likely to be sterilized by the treatment, semen samples may be taken, frozen, and stored in sperm banks for possible use at a later date. This approach does not, however, guarantee reproductive success.

V. THERAPEUTIC MANAGEMENT

Treatment of testicular tumors is totally different for seminomas and for nonseminomatous tumors, the latter being considerably more aggressive and requiring radical multimodality therapy. Mixed seminomatous tumors behave as their most aggressive component, and it is important to identify these tumors and modify therapy accordingly. Measurement of the AFP and HCG can be helpful in identifying mixed tumors, since pure seminomas do not produce either marker. A raised level of AFP is definite evidence of a nonseminomatous component, whereas moderate elevations of HCG can be seen rarely in pure seminomas, particularly in bulky disease, though in such instances, it is usually believed that the tumor contains some choriocarcinoma elements not readily appreciated by pathological examination.

A. Seminomas

Pure seminomas are extremely radiosensitive and are treated primarily by radiotherapy following removal of the primary tumor.

1. Stage I

Most patients will already have had an orchiectomy, and additional treatment is exclusively by radiotherapy. Therapy should include the ipsilateral inguinal, pelvic, and paraortic lymph nodes. Radiotherapy should be delivered with a supervoltage beam, preferably a 6- to 8-MeV linear accelerator. A dose of 3000 rads in 3 weeks is adequate. The scrotal sac is only irradiated if there has been a transscrotal needle biopsy or a scrotal orchiectomy.

Cure rates should be in excess of 95%, and a survival beyond 2 years is associated with normal life expectancy.

SITE-SPECIFIC DATA FORM—TESTICULAR TUMORS

HISTORY

Age: _____

Symptoms

_____ Testicular mass

_____ Pain

_____ Change in libido

_____ Gynecomastia

_____ Urinary symptoms

_____ Other: _____

Duration: _____

Social history

Occupation: _____

Race: ____ White ____ Black ____ Oriental ____ Other

Smoker: ____ Yes ____ No. How much? _____

Drinker: ____ Yes ____ No. How often? _____

Environmental factors: chemical exposure? _____

Detail: _____

Family history of carcinoma

Relation: _____ Site: _____

Previous history of carcinoma

Cryptorchidism ____ No ____ Yes

Treatment: _____

Age of treatment: _____

Previous history of orchitis

____ No ____ Yes

Torsion: ____ No ____ Yes

Trauma: ____ No ____ Yes

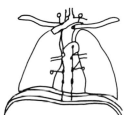

PHYSICAL EXAMINATION

Testicle

Size (in centimeters) _____

Consistency: ____ Firm ____ Hard ____ Nodular

Involvement of	Yes	No
Epididymus	_____	_____
Tunica	_____	_____
Skin	_____	_____
Cord	_____	_____
Edema	_____	_____
Extremities	_____	_____
Neurological	_____	_____

Nodes: _____ Yes _____ No. Size: _____

	Right	Left
Inguinal	_____	_____
Iliac	_____	_____
Aortic	_____	_____
Renal pedicle	_____	_____
Supraclavicular	_____	_____

	Yes	No
Soft	_____	_____
Hard	_____	_____
Mobile	_____	_____
Fixed	_____	_____
Single	_____	_____
Multiple	_____	_____

Abdomen: ____ Negative ____ Positive

Describe: _____

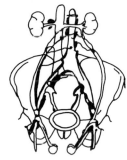

PRETREATMENT WORK-UP

	Neg.	Pos.	Suspicious
Urinalysis	_____	_____	_____
CBC	_____	_____	_____
SMA-12	_____	_____	_____
Beta HCG	_____	_____	_____
AFP	_____	_____	_____
Urinary AFP	_____	_____	_____
Chest x-ray and/or CAT scan	_____	_____	_____

	Neg.	Pos.	Suspicious
IVP	_____	_____	_____
Lymphangiogram	_____	_____	_____
CAT scan of abdomen	_____	_____	_____
Vena cavogram	_____	_____	_____
Bone scan	_____	_____	_____
Liver scan	_____	_____	_____

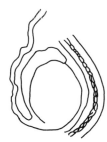

Exploration of testis: ____ Yes ____ No

Histologic diagnosis: _____

Abdominal exploration: ____ Yes ____ No

Finding: _____

Staging and classification

____ T ____ N ____ M (Site: _____)

Stage: _____

Grade: _____

Signature: _____

Countersignature: _____

Date: _____

Testicular Tumor Classification

TNM Classification (AJC System)

Primary tumor (T)

TX   Minimum requirements cannot be met (in the absence of orchiectomy)
T0   No evidence of primary tumor
T1   Limited to body of the testicle
T2   Extends beyond the tunica
T3   Involvement of the rete testis or epididymis
T4   Invasion of spermatic cord (4a) or invasion of scrotal wall (4b)

Nodal involvement (N)

N0   No evidence of involvement of regional lymph nodes
N1   Involvement of a single homolateral regional lymph node which,
         if inguinal, is mobile
N2   Involvement of contralateral or bilateral or multiple regional lymph
         nodes which, if inguinal, are mobile
N3   Palpable abdominal mass present, or fixed inguinal lymph nodes
N4   Involvement of juxtaregional nodes (supraclavicular)

Distant metastases (M)

MX   Not assessed
M0   No (known) distant metastasis
M1   Distant metastasis present (specify site)

Staging (Walter Reed General Hospital System)

Stage IA   Confined to testis, no clinical or x-ray evidence for spread
       IB   Same as IA, but at lymph node dissection, metastases to iliac
               or para-aortic lymph nodes are found
Stage II   Disease below diaphragm, no spread to visceral organs; clinical
               or x-ray evidence of metastases to para-aortic, femoral, inguinal
               or iliac lymph nodes
Stage III   Disease above diaphragm, or spread to other body organs
               (clinical or x-ray), stage III should be subdivided as follows:
                     A   Disease confined to supraclavicular lymph nodes
                     B   Gynecomastia ± elevation in biological markers
                     B—2   Minimal pulmonary disease (<5 lesions in each lung
                               field, with none >2 cm in diameter)
                     B—3   Advanced abdominal disease (palpable abdominal mass,
                               ureteral displacement, or obstructive uropathy)
                     B—5   Visceral disease (excluding lung), liver, GI tract, CNS, IVC

2. Stage II

Clinical or radiological evidence of subdiaphragmatic node metastases requires a modification of the plan of treatment by enlarging the radiation portals to include the mediastinal and left supraclavicular nodes. If the disease is bulky, induction chemotherapy is sometimes used before irradiation. High-dose cyclophosphamide or regimens such as those used for nonseminomatous tumors (CPVB: *cis*-platinum, vinblastine, and bleomycin) have been used prior to irradiation. However, the use of a radiation dose of 3500 rads, with additional boosts to areas of large tumors, is usually sufficient. Cure rates of 80–90% can be expected in patients with Stage II disease, depending on the volume of disease. Some have questioned the need to treat the mediastinum and supraclavicular areas prophylactically, noting that patients who relapsed in such sites are frequently salvaged by subsequent radiation and/or chemotherapy.

3. Stage III

Local and regional disease is treated as in Stage II. Patients with systemic metastases (IIIB) must be aggressively treated with chemotherapy (CPVB), although localized, isolated, distant metastases are still amenable to control by radiotherapy.

B. Nonseminomatous Tumors

In the treatment of nonseminomatous testicular tumors, it is important to assess the stage of the tumor and identify the extent of retroperitoneal metastatic disease with accuracy; thus, retroperitoneal lymph node dissection carried out through either an anterior transabdominal approach or an extraperitoneal thoracoabdominal route has been routinely used in the United States as part of the preliminary treatment of all patients with nonseminomatous testicular tumors in whom no visceral or metastatic lesions are identified above the diaphragm. Following the surgery, radiation therapy, chemotherapy, or both may be selectively employed as adjuvant modalities. Orchiectomy with retroperitoneal node dissection alone, wothout any adjunctive therapy, has been shown to result in a 5-year survival rate of 75–80% in Stage I and early Stage II nonseminomatous tumors of the testis.

In some centers, radiotherapy to the lymphatic drainage areas (para-aortic nodes) is used just as in seminomas, and protection of the contralateral testis with a 1-cm-thick lead cup has been effective in preserving an effective sperm count postirradiation. The dosage of radiotherapy should be in the range of 4000–5000 rads according to the size of the nodes. The results of orchiectomy and adjuvant radiotherapy for Stage I cases are similar to those of radical surgery.

Adjuvant chemotherapy with actinomycin D—1.0 mg intraoperatively and 3 mg in the first 4 days postoperatively—has also been recommended by some for patients with Stage II nonseminomatous tumors. The disadvantage of such an approach is the inability to identify those patients whose retroperitoneal nodes are histologically involved, though clinically negative. When lymphadenectomy is done in patients with Stage I disease, 25–33% will be found to have nodal metastases (thus making them really Stage IB or II). It is therefore recommended that all patients be referred for retroperitoneal lymphadenectomy.

If involved nodes are identified and found to contain very little tumor, and if postoperative tumor markers return to normal values, no further therapy is necessary. Patients are observed closely and followed up every 2 months with chest x-ray, tumor markers, and physical examination and every 6 months with abdominal-pelvic CAT scan for 2 years. At the first sign of relapse, identified clinically, radiologically, or by elevation of the tumor marker, the patient is referred for chemotherapy. Such an approach should lead to (high) cure rates in (almost 90%) patients with early Stage II cancer.

Patients who have more than minimal lymph node involvement (more than five positive nodes or macroscopically involved nodes) who undergo complete resections and whose tumor markers return to normal after surgery constitute a difficult problem. Some adovcate "adjuvant" chemotherapy in this subgroup; others feel that close observation, with chemotherapy instituted at the first hint of recurrence, is indicated instead.

Patients who have bulky but resectable disease or those whose tumor markers remain elevated even though all gross disease has been removed are candidates for adjuvant chemotherapy used postoperatively. Likewise, patients who have unresectable disease should receive postoperative chemotherapy. Retroperitoneal lymph node radiation should be withheld if chemotherapy is planned, as the radiation may compromise bone marrow tolerance for intensive chemotherapy.

If there is no evidence of recurrence (radiological or clinical) and if the tumor markers remain within normal limits for 2 years, the chances for cure are excellent. It should be kept in mind that the half-life of HCG is less than 24 hours and that of AFP is about 5 days. The presence of (abnormal) quantities of either or both markers after a suitable number of half-lives (following treatment) indicates the presence of active disease. Occasionally, a falsely elevated HCG value is reported; it should be kept in mind that some assays for HCG cross-react with LH and that the latter may be elevated as a result of the lack of feedback inhibition produced by chemotherapy-induced testicular failure in the remaining gonad.

In patients with Stage III disease or those with extensive abdominal node metastases, chemotherapy is imperative. Initiation of chemotherapy using *cis*-platinum, vinblastine, and bleomycin as induction regimen is often used. Following four cycles of chemotherapy, if there is residual tumor, surgery may be contemplated to remove all gross disease; otherwise (or postoperatively), the patient should receive 4000–5000 rads to the original site of disease below or above the diaphragm. If tumor markers remain elevated, two additional courses of chemotherapy are administered.

Patients with extensive visceral metastases are treated by chemotherapy alone.

VI. CHEMOTHERAPY FOR ADVANCED TESTICULAR CANCER

In perhaps no other disseminated adult cancer has as much recent progress been achieved as in germ cell tumors of the testis. As far back as the early 1960s, it was appreciated that these tumors respond to a variety of agents of different classes:

Vinblastine	50%
Dactinomycin	50%
Melphalan	55%
Bleomycin	40%
Mithramycin	35%
Adriamycin	20%

It was further noted that the combination of vinblastine and bleomycin induced a rate of complete remission around 30%. The most important event for curative treatment, however, was the development of cis-platinum in the middle 1970s; this drug had a dramatic impact and yielded a response rate in excess of 65% when used as a single agent; when combined with vinblastine and bleomycin, it resulted in a regimen with unprecedented efficacy.

In the most common regimen, the cis-platinum is given in a dose of 20 mg per square meter per day for 5 days with around-the-clock saline hydration to prevent renal damage. Vinblastine, in a dose of 0.15 mg per hour, is given on days 1 and 2 of the cis-platinum infusions. Bleomycin, in a dose of 30 mg, is given once a week for 12 weeks. Courses of cis-platinum and vinblastine are repeated every 3 weeks for four courses. The anticipated toxicity with this regimen can be rather formidable and includes myelosuppression, muscle aches, and neuropathy (from the vinblastine); fevers, chills, skin rashes, and possible lung fibrosis (from bleomycin); and renal failure, neuropathy, tinnitus, hearing loss, paresthesias, hypomagnesemia, nausea, vomiting, anorexia, and alopecia, etc. (from cis-platinum). Some patients will experience severe leukopenia and associated fever; such patients must be presumed to have sepsis and must be treated with intravenous broad-spectrum antibiotics until the granulocytes recover. Most patients will lose 20–30 pounds in weight during the course of treatment.

Results, now confirmed by several centers, are that about 65–75% of patients are induced into a complete remission with disappearance of all measurable disease and normalization of previously elevated tumor markers. An additional 10–15% of patients will have residual mass(es) at the end of the chemotherapy course. Every attempt should be made to resect all such masses; some of these will be found to consist merely of fibrous tissue, presumably reflecting destroyed tumor; others will consist of mature benign teratoma, an interesting phenomenon perhaps indicating "maturation" of malignant elements to a benign state consequent to the chemotherapy. The outcome for both these groups is favorable, and their survival is comparable to that of the patients in complete remission without residual masses. The remainder of the patients will have active tumor in the residual resected mass, occasionally with elevated markers. Such patients require further treatment, as only a fraction of them enters a durable complete remission. Thus, these patients, along with any patient who does not achieve a complete remission with the initial treatment course, are candidates for alternate chemotherapy programs. Sometimes patients may also benefit from a course of radiation directed at the residual tumor site.

It has recently been recognized that VP-16, an epipodophyllotoxin, is a very active agent in germ cell tumors and that it may be synergistic in combination with cis-platinum. A "rescue" regimen consisting of these two drugs has produced some complete remissions in patients resistant to the "standard PVB regimen." A number of other regimens, incorporating a variety of drugs in combination, have been explored. The Memorial Sloan-Kettering Institute has published similar results with their VAB5 and VAB6 regimens, which include dactinomycin, Adriamycin, and other agents in a complex scheme. Others have suggested using bleomycin by continuous infusion.

Most nonseminomatous germ cell tumors contain embryonal carcinoma elements with variable amounts of teratoma and/or choriocarcinoma. The latter has a marked propensity for early hematogenous dissemination, and tumors rich in choriocarcinoma elements tend to present with widespread, massive metastatic disease. Such circumstances, as much as any other inherent biologic resistance, may account for the observation that the prognosis appears to be worse in pure choriocarcinoma, or in mixed tumors with a major chorio component. Additionally, this histological type tends to produce CNS metastases with distressing frequency, generally a catastrophic development resistant to all treatment. Some investigators have thus suggested incorporating VP-16 from the outset into the standard chemotherapy program for these high-risk patients (those with a major choriocarcinoma component or massive liver and lung metastases).

Patients who enter complete remission gain back the weight they lost during treatment. Long-term sequelae of treatment are relatively rare, but an occasional patient will develop irreversible lung fibrosis secondary to bleomycin. Almost all patients develop azoospermia, though in time a fraction of these patients will recover spermatogenesis and may be able to father children.

Less information is available regarding chemotherapy of advanced or recurrent seminoma, reflecting the high cure rates achieved by surgery and radiation in this disease. About half the patients who relapse will have nonseminomatous elements in the metastatic tumor, and many of these will have elevated serum markers. Available data suggest that these cases respond similarly as their nonseminomatous counterparts to chemotherapy programs mentioned above. Because of extensive prior radiation, however, some of these patients do not tolerate intensive chemotherapy.

VII. POSTOPERATIVE CARE, EVALUATION, AND REHABILITATION

The postoperative care is the same as for patients undergoing major abdominal or retroperitoneal operations. Drains, suction tubing, thromboembolism prevention, pulmonary care, ambulation, fluid and electrolyte and hemodynamic balance, etc. must all be attended to. Attention must be paid to prevent, identify, and treat any complications, whether they be from surgery, radiotherapy, or chemotherapy.

Psychosocial rehabilitation is most important because of the psychological and physical impact of the loss of a sex organ. Clear explanations and counseling must be undertaken both pre- and posttherapy. Patients should be encouraged to resume sexual activity as soon as possible, and younger patients must be advised as to their ability to father a child.

Since additional treatment may still cure a certain percentage of failures of the primary therapy, follow-up evaluation of the patient with a testicular tumor is extremely important. It should include

- Physical examination.
- CAT scanning of the abdomen and chest.
- Serial measurements of the tumor markers (AFP and HCG) in nonseminomatous tumors.

All these should be performed at frequent, regular intervals during follow-up examinations.

VIII. MANAGEMENT ALGORITHM FOR TESTICULAR TUMORS (see p. 626)

MANAGEMENT ALGORITHM FOR TESTICULAR TUMORS

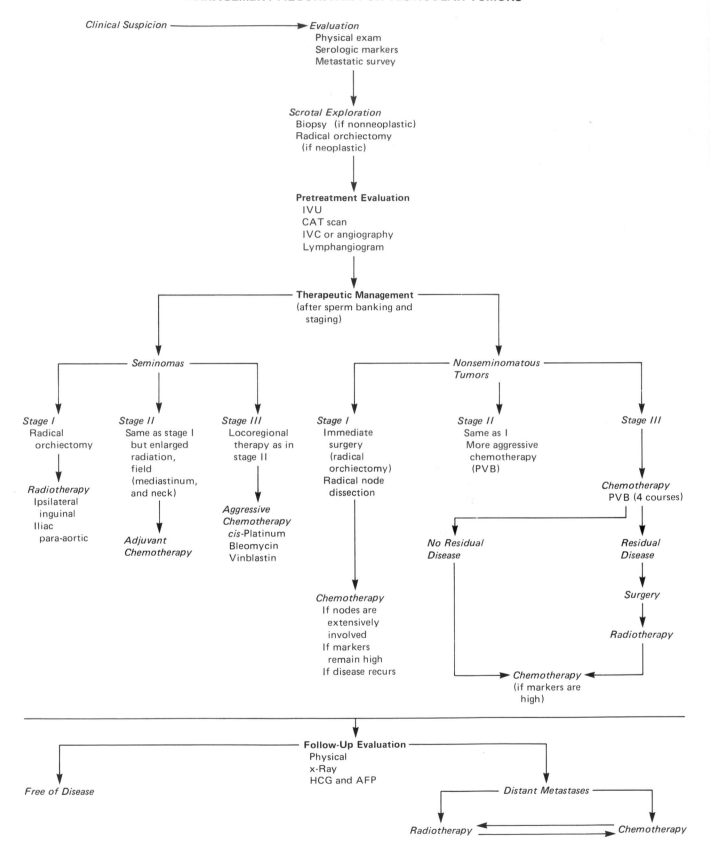

Section 13. Tumors of the Genitourinary System

Part E: Penile Tumors

I. Early Detection and Screening 629
  A. Predisposing Factors
    1. Erythroplasia of Queyrat
    2. Bowen's Disease
    3. Buschke-Löwenstein Tumor
    4. Balanitis Xerotica Obliterans
    5. Leukoplakia of the Glans Penis
  B. Early Detection and Screening
II. Pretreatment Evaluation and Preparation 629
  A. Pretreatment Evaluation and Work-Up
  B. Preoperative Preparation
  C. Staging
    Sentinel Node Biopsy
III. Therapeutic Management 630
  A. Local Treatment
    1. Surgery
      a. Partial Amputation
      b. Total Amputation

    2. Radiotherapy
    3. Other Modalities
  B. Lymph Node Dissection
  C. Treatment of Advanced Penile Cancer
IV. Postoperative Care 631
  A. Penile Surgery
  B. Node Dissection
  C. Nutritional Support
  D. Psychological Support
  E. Reconstructive Surgery
V. Management for Penile Tumors 632

Suggested Readings 632

I. EARLY DETECTION
AND SCREENING

Carcinoma of the penis is a rare malignancy in the United States, resulting in less than 1% of deaths. However, it constitutes 10–20% of tumors seen in males in some Third World countries. The onset of the disease is generally in the sixth or seventh decades, and 35–50% of patients seen initially will have clinically palpable inguinal nodes. Carcinoma of the penis metastasizes primarily to regional lymph nodes. The prepuce and the skin of the penis are drained primarily by the lymphatics that empty into the superficial inguinal nodes; the corpora and the glans penis drain into the deep inguinal and external iliac nodes. There is often crossover of the lymphatics, and nodes on either side may be involved. Invasion of the corpora can lead to blood-borne metastases.

A. Predisposing Factors

Development of penile carcinoma is associated with the uncircumcised male and is believed to be related to poor hygiene and exposure to some undefined irritants or carcinogens in the smegma of the uncircumcised patients. It is important to understand some of the premalignant lesions of the penis, as the awareness of the physician will enhance earlier diagnosis and maybe even prevention.

1. Erythroplasia of Queyrat

The dorsum of the glans penis is the usual site of involvement of this painful lesion, which presents as a flat, red skin condition with poorly defined margins and velvety erythema. There may be periods of regression, but recurrences are very common. These are highly premalignant lesions, and in their evolution to frank malignancy, they often pass through a phase of carcinoma *in situ*.

2. Bowen's Disease

These are painless lesions on the glans penis and are similar to this intraepithelial carcinoma (Bowen's disease) presenting elsewhere.

3. Buschke-Löwenstein Tumor

This destructive giant penile condyloma acuminata has a distinct potential to develop into a frank malignancy. They are unpredictive in their history and difficult to differentiate from penile carcinoma.

4. Balanitis Xerotica Obliterans

This disease affects the foreskin, glans, and urethral meatus. It is found in both the circumcised and the uncircumcised male and may be associated with prior trauma. Pruritis is a frequent symptom.

5. Leukoplakia of the Glans Penis

This is a premalignant change that mandates local excision and repeat biopsy as indicated.

B. Early Detection and Screening

The best screening technique is based on routine physical examination of the penis; in the uncircumscised male, a complete withdrawl of the foreskin and careful examination of the glans, urethral meatus, and shaft of the penis should be done. Patients with any kind of genital sores, areas of irritation or induration, or any recent color changes of the glans penis must be encouraged to seek early medical attention, and the physician should be alert to the risk of malignant changes in such situations.

II. PRETREATMENT EVALUATION
AND PREPARATION

A. Pretreatment Evaluation and Work-Up

All persistent abnormal lesions of the penis should be biopsied. Biopsy should include the adjacent normal tissue as well as a generous sampling of the lesion.

The evaluation of the patient with carcinoma of the penis should include

- Complete physical examination, including an abdominal examination to note the presence of enlarged intra-abdominal nodes. Special attention should be paid to the inguinal nodes on both sides. A detailed note of the lesion, penis, urethra, and perineal region should be made. A rectal examination should be done to identify any rectal masses, and the lower extremities should be examined for lymphedema.
- Laboratory work-up should include CBC, SMA-12, serology for syphilis annd lymphogranuloma venereum, urinalysis, and urine culutre and sensitivity.
- Chest x-ray is usually sufficient as a metastatic screen since penile carcinoma rarely spreads by hematogenous dissemination. Liver scan is necessary if the SMA-12 shows evidence of hepatic damage, and bone scans are ordered selectively.
- Computerized axial tomography, lymphangiography, and ultrasound may be helpful in identifying lymph node metstases.
- Intravenous urogram.

B. Preoperative Preparation

The preoperative preparation of the patient includes the above investigations. An informed consent about the nature of the biopsy and the extent of the surgical procedure contemplated is obtained by the physician. This consent should also include "sentinel" node biopsy if there is a palpable inguinal lymph node. A frozen section should be done at the time of the biopsy to confirm the diagnosis; in most instances, however, it is prudent to biopsy just the lesion, as the pathology may not be clearly diagnosed by frozen section.

The patient must be properly advised as to the nature of the treatment and its consequences. Psychosocial counseling might be advisable, and information relevant to penile reconstruction should be given to the patient.

C. Staging

The vast majority (97%) of penile cancers are squamous cell in origin. After the lesion is confirmed, accurate staging of the disease is essential.

Stage I   Tumor limited to the prepuce or glans penis.
Stage II   The tumor involves the shaft of the penis or corpora without nodal or distant metastases.
Stage III   The tumor is confined to the shaft of the penis, with proven regional node metastases.
Stage IV   The tumor involves locally the shaft of the penis

with inoperable regional nodes or distant metastases.

Sentinel Node Biopsy

Cabanas (1a) has reported on the performance of bilateral sentinel node biopsy. This node is located in the vicinity of the junction of the superifcial and deep femoral vein and is believed to be the first echelon of spread of penile cancer. If tumor is noted in these biopsies, then an extensive lymph node dissection should be considered. There have been other reports, however, that indicate that the sentinel node biopsy may not be a true reflection of metastatic disease in carcinoma of the penis.

III. THERAPEUTIC MANAGEMENT

A. Local Treatment

In selecting the treatment for penile carcinoma, the goals of treatment have to be defined. These are

- Totally eradicating the primary lesion.
- Preventing local recurrences.
- Preserving maximum usable penile length.

Other factors such as the general condition of the patient, the psychological impact of organ loss, and overall morbidity of the procedures must be contemplated. The primary modalities for definitive treatment are either surgery or radiotherapy. The latter also plays an adjuvant role in certain cases.

1. Surgery

a. Partial Amputation

Partial amputation is the procedure most frequently employed. A 2-cm margin of normal tissue is removed, and a neourethral meatus is constructed. This produces a useful, functional penis, and the patient is able to stand and urinate. Attempts to locally excise lesions of the glans penis are not advisable as 30–40% of patients will develop subsequent recurrences.

b. Total Amputation

If the tumor occupies the proximal shaft of the penis, or in any instances where the tumor is extensive, a total penectomy with perineal urethrostomy becomes necessary.

2. Radiotherapy

The definitive role of radiation in the treatment of penile tumors stems from the fact that these cancers are essentially epidermoid skin lesions and in their early stages (Stage I) highly curable by radiotherapy alone. This success is reduced when the lesion travels proximally, involving the corpora. The main advantage of radiotherapy is organ preservation, and morbidity can be kept to minimal levels with careful planning and judicious application. The technique usually involves keeping the penis in a snug-fitting wax box to enable homogeneous irradiation of the volume needed. The dose aimed at is usually radical (6500 rads in 6.5 weeks) and must be delivered carefully. Complications such as urethral strictures are kept in abeyance by attention to hygiene and early, gentle dilatation when necessary. Circumcision prior to radiation is mandatory.

Adjuvant postoperative radiotherapy is also selectively indicated, particularly to inguinal nodal regions, especially in Stage II and III cases, where the incidence of lymph node metastases is rather high. The dose aimed at is usually in the vicinity of 5000 rads when the disease is microscopic.

3. Other Modalities

Circumcision as sole therapy is restricted to lesions that are very small, noninvasive, and limited to the foreskin.

Topical chemotherapy, using 5-FU cream, is used only in young patients with *in-situ* cancer. Long-term close follow up is necessary with this treatment plan.

B. Lymph Node Dissection

There is no uniform method of treatment of inguinal lymphadenopathy. In most instances a prophylactic course of antibiotics is first recommended; there are studies to substantiate that 50% of the palpable nodes are inflammatory in nature. Lymph node dissection is reserved for those patients who have been identified to have metastatic lymph nodes after an interim waiting period.

The node dissection for carcinoma of the penis is done through an inguinofemoral approach. Bilateral groin dissections are sometimes necessary due to the fact that there are intercommunications of the lymphatic system. Pelvic node dissection is reserved for the young patient and those where definite inguinofemoral metastases are demonstrated.

The role of radiotherapy in the treatment of regional node metastases has been discussed earlier; inguinal lymphadenectomy is an operation with significant morbidity (limb edema, pain, lymphangitis), and keen clinical judgment must be exercised in the selection of modality of treatment for inguinal lymphadenopathy in penile cancer.

C. Treatment of Advanced Penile Cancer

Metastatic disease requires the use of chemotherapy. The four chemotherapeutic agents that are somewhat effective are

- Bleomycin.
- Methotrexate.
- *Cis*-platinum.
- 5-FU.

The response to either a single drug or multiple drug therapy is temporary and not encouraging. Elderly patients and those with multiple medical intercurrent conditions or infections are not good candidates for chemotherapy.

IV. POSTOPERATIVE CARE

A. Penile Surgery

The penile stump should heal without difficulty unless there is extensive inflammatory reaction or residual neoplasm. Systemic antibiotics, local wound care, and skin flaps (if there was extensive penile surgery) may be indicated.

B. Node Dissection

Various techniques are utilized for inguinal node dissection. Parallel but separate inguinal and femoral incisions, the midline incision, and the S-shaped inguinofemoral incision that transects the inguinal ligament can all be used. Meticulous dissection and postoperative wound care are necessary. Skin necrosis may develop, and skin grafts are used if needed.

C. Nutritional Support

Supplementary nutrition is generally not necessary in patients with early carcinoma of the penis. In patients with advanced carcinoma or in those on chemotherapy, nutritional support is essential.

D. Psychological Support

Loss of the penis is psychologically devastating to the young patient. Furthermore, in most patients, irrespective of age, penile amputation may produce severe depression. Close liaison with a psychiatrist is advisable to provide supportive care.

E. Reconstructive Surgery

If penile carcinoma is controlled, reconstructive plastic surgery with penile prosthesis may be offered to the patient in order to regain some of the functions of the penis.

V. MANAGEMENT ALGORITHM FOR
PENILE TUMORS (see p. 633)

(see p. 633)

SUGGESTED READINGS

1. Glenn, J. "Urologic Surgery." Lippincott, Philadelphia, Pennsylvania, 1983.

1a. Cabanas. *Cancer* **39**, 456 (1977).

2. Harrison, Gittes, Perlmutter, Stamey, and Walsh. "Compbell's Urology." Saunders, Philadelphia, Pennsylvania, 1979.

3. Kaufman, J. J. "Current Urologic Therapy." Saunders, Philadelphia, Pennsylvania, 1980.

ALGORITHM FOR PENILE LESION

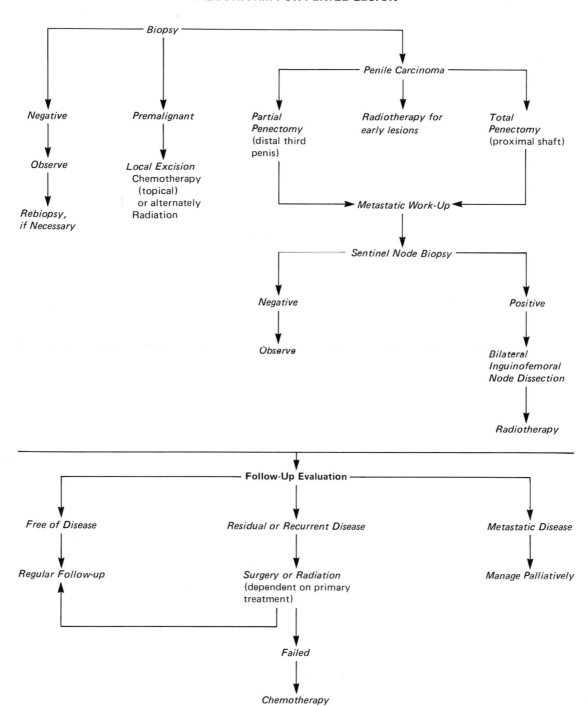

Index

A

Abbe´ flaps, 49
Abdominal lymphoma, non-Hodgkin's, 346, 347
Abdominal mass
    bladder cancer, 590
    colorectal cancer, 490
    gastric cancer, 476
    pediatric, physical findings, 316
Abdominal paracentesis, 544
Abdominoperineal resection, 503
Abscess
    brain, 289
    gastric surgery and, 482
ABVD, in Hodgkin's lymphoma, 346, 367, 368
Accelerator beams, in soft tissue sarcoma, 264
Achalasia, with esophageal cancer, 461
Achlorhydria, 192, 476
Acid-base disorders, 134
    with adrenal tumors
        Cushing's syndrome, 138
        neuroblastoma, preoperative management, 150
        primary aldosteronism, 133, 135
    with leukemias, acute, 386
Acid phosphatase
    with bone tumors, 228
    with kidney tumors, 576
    with leukemias
        acute, 387
        chronic myelocytic, 393
    with prostatic cancer, 602, 604, 612
Acinar adenocarcinoma, lung, 427
Acinar cell carcinoma, pancreas, eccrine, 514
Acinic cell carcinoma, salivary gland, therapy, 39
Acoustic neuromas, 284, 301
Acquired idiopathic hemolytic anemia, 395

Acquired immune deficiency syndrome (AIDS)
    Kaposi's sarcoma, 121-122
    soft tissue sarcoma risk factors, 256
Acral lentiginous melanoma, 102
Acromegaly
    with apudomas, 198
    with brain tumors, 280
        pituitary, 299
        pretreatment management, 283
Acromial flap, 49
Acromiothoracic flap, 49
ACTH
    adrenal tumors
        adrenocortical hyperplasia, 141
        Cushing's syndrome, 139
    apudomas, 199
    carcinoid, 204
    multiple endocrine neoplasia-I, 192
    paraneoplastic syndromes
        diagnostic testing, 185
        oat cell carcinomas of lung, 427
        therapeutic management, 187
    pituitary tumors, 192, 298, 299
ACTH stimulation test, 139
Actinic keratoses, 99, 107
Actinomycin D
    complications of, 320
    head and neck tumors, 46
    Kaposi's sarcoma, 121
    melanoma, 118
    ovarian tumors, germ cell, 565
    rhabdomyosarcoma, 336
    skeletal tumors, Ewing's sarcoma, 243
    soft tissue sarcoma, 265

testicular cancer, 624
toxic reactions, 372
Wilms's tumor, 329
Acute leukemias, *see* Leukemias
Adamantinoma, 219
    age incidence, 219, 225
    anatomic locations, 218
    characteristics of, 222
    histological grades, 231
    versus malignant bone tumors, 226
    site predilection of, 225
    therapeutic approaches, 237
Addison's disease
    brain tumor and, 280
    and hypercalcemia, 175
    as pediatric radiotherapy complication, 320
Adenocarcinomas
    alimentary tract
        colorectal, 492, 495
        esophagus, 461
        gallbladder, 522
        gastric, 478
        pancreatic, 516
    genitourinary tract
        bladder, 592
        kidney, 575
    head and neck
        nasal fossa, 35
        paranasal sinus tumors, 35
        salivary gland, 38, 40
    lung
        brain irradiation in, 433
        chemotherapy, 434-435
        histological evaluation, 427
        metastatic, treatment, 436
        surgery contraindication, 431
    uterus, 560
Adenoid cystic carcinoma
    lung, 427
    salivary gland, 38-39, 40
Adenomas
    adrenal, aldosterone-producing, 136
    colorectal cancer risk, 490, 496
    gallbladder, 522
    lung, 426
    parathyroid, 176
    pituitary, apudomas, 198
    villous, 496
Adenomatous hyperplasia, gallbladder, 522
Adenomatous polyps
    colorectal, 490, 495, 496
    small intestine, 504
Adenomyomatous hyperplasia, gallbladder, 522
Adenosine diphosphate (ADP), 412, 414
Adenosquamous carcinoma
    colorectal, 495
    gastric, 478
    lung, 427
    pancreatic, 516
Adnexal neoplasms, 105

Adrenalectomy, 88
    adrenocortical hyperplasia, 141
    aldosterone-producing adenomas, 136
    bilateral, 141, 142
    breast cancer, 79
    Cushing's disease, 141-142
    in pheochromocytoma , 147
    pheochromocytoma, postoperative care, 147-148
    postoperative care, 142
    postoperative management, 136, 136
    in primary aldosteronism, 135
    with Wilms's tumor, 324
Adrenal heterotopias, liver, 533
Adrenal hyperplasia, *see also* Cushing's syndrome
    bilateral, 135
    therapeutic management, 141-142
Adrenal inhibitors, 88, 187
Adrenal insufficiency
    with brain tumor, pretreatment management, 283
    steroid therapy and, 287
Adrenal steroid inhibitor, 88, 187
Adrenal tumors
    apudomas, 198
    Cushing's syndrome, 136, 143
    liver metastasis, 531
    multiple endocrine neoplasia type I, 192
    multiple endocrine neoplasia type II, 193-194
    neuroblastoma, 148-153
    paraneoplastic syndromes, 184, 187
    pheochromocytoma, 142, 149
    primary aldosteronism, 133-136
Adrenal vein sampling, in Cushing's syndrome, 140
Adrenergic blockers, in pheochromocytoma, 146-147, 194
Adrenergic receptor agonists, in carcinoid surgery, 208
Adrenergic response, with insulinoma, 157
Adrenocortical nodules, 141
Adriamycin (doxorubicin)
    adrenal tumors, 141
        neuroblastoma, 151
        pheochromocytoma, 147
    alimentary tract tumors
        anal, 503
        biliary tree, 524-525
        gastric, 482
        liver, 535
    bladder cancer, 596
    bone tumors
        Ewing's sarcoma, 238
        osteosarcoma, 238, 241, 242, 243
    brain tumors, 290
    breast cancer, dosages and response rates, 87-88
    genitourinary tumors
        bladder, 596
        prostate, 610, 611
        testis, 624
    gynecological tumors
        endometrium, 562
        ovary, 563
    leukemias, acute, myelogenous, 388
    lung cancer, 434, 435

lymphomas
    Hodgkin's, 366, 367
    non-Hodgkin's, 369, 370, 371
  mediastinal germ cell tumors, 450
  melanoma, 118
  mesothelioma, 457
  multiple myeloma, 405, 406
  neuroblastoma, 151, 333
  rhabdomyosarcoma, 336
  in soft tissue sarcoma, 265, 266
  thymoma, 449
  thyroid tumors, 44
  toxic effects of, 373, 564
  in Wilms's tumor, 329
Alfatoxin, liver cancer risk, 529
Alanine aminotransfertase, pancreatic cancer, 510
Alcohol
  and cancer risk
    breast, 67
    head and neck, 5
  intolerance of, in lymphomas, 355
  and nutritional status, 10
  and oral cancer, preoperative considerations, 21-22
  pancreatic tumors, postoperative considerations, 163
  after radiation, 49
Alcohol injection, in pancreatic cancer, 520
Aldosterone levels, 134
Aldosteronism, see Primary hyperaldosteronism
Alimentary tract tumors, see Gastrointestinal tract tumors; specific glands and organs
Alimentation, see Nutritional support
Alkaline phosphatase
  in bone tumors, 228
  in kidney tumors, 576
  in leukemias, acute, 386
  in liver tumors, 530
  in myelofibrosis, 414
  in pancreatic cancer, 510
  in paraneoplastic syndrome, hypercalcemia, 185
  in parathyroid tumors, 174
  in polycythemia vera, 412
  in prostatic cancer, 602
Alkeran, see Melphalan
Alkylating agents, see also specific drugs
  in endometrial cancer, 562
  in lung cancer, 435
  in lymphomas, Hodgkin's, 366
  in mesothelioma, 457
  in multiple myeloma, 406
  in polycythemia vera, 412, 413
Allopurinol
  in leukemias, acute, 388
  in multiple myeloma, 406
Alpha-fetoprotein (AFP)
  brain tumors, 280
  embryonal carcinoma, 337
  liver tumors, 530
  pediatric, 337
  mediastinal tumors, 445, 447, 449
  ovarian tumors, 565
  pancreatic tumors, 510
  pediatric tumors, 316, 337
  testicular tumors, 619, 620, 623, 625
Alpha-naphthyl acetate esterase, 386
Alveolar cell sarcoma, histological grades, 231
Alveolar rhabdomyosarcoma, 267, 335
Alveolar soft-part sarcoma, 267, 269
Amebiasis
  with Kaposi's sarcoma, 121
  liver abscess, 533
Amenorrhea
  with brain tumors, 280, 298
  with Cushing's syndrome, 138
  with pituitary tumors, MEN-I, 192
2-Amino-1-naphthol, and bladder cancer, 589
Amino acid excretion, with brain tumors, 284
Aminocaproic acid, 208
4-Aminodiphenyl, and bladder cancer, 589
Aminoglutethimide
  in breast cancer, 79, 88, 89
  in Cushing's disease, of pituitary origin, 142
  in ectopic ACTH syndrome, 187
  in prostatic cancer, advanced, 611
p-Aminosalicylic acid
  in immunoblastic lymphadenopathy, 377
  in leukemias, acute, 386, 387
  in myeloblasts, 344
Ampulla of Vater, tumors of, 516, 522, 523
Amputation
  with bone tumors, 235-247
  of breast, 76
  of penis, 630
  with skin cancer, trunk and extremities, 112-113
  with soft tissue sarcoma, 262, 270
Amyloid metaplasia, lung carcinoid tumors, 427
Amyloidosis, 405, 407
Anal fissures, colorectal cancer risk, 490
Analgesics, see also Pain relief
  in breast cancer, postoperative, 90
  head and neck cancer patient
    postoperative, 47
    radiation therapy effects and management, 48, 49
  in pancreatic cancer, 520
Anaphylaxis, as chemotherapy side effect, 372, 373, 374
Anaplastic lesions
  breast, 85
  embryonal tumors, 330
  endometrial, 562
  lung, 435-436, see also Oat cell carcinoma
  pancreatic, 516
  seminomas, 617
  thyroid, 41, 44
Anaplastic changes, Wilms's tumor with, 323
Androgens
  in breast cancer, 88, 89
  adrenal tumors excreting, 141
  liver cancer risk, 529
Androstenedione, 141
Andy Gump operation, 30
Anemia
  with alimentary tract tumors
    colorectal, 489, 490

gastric, 476, 478
pancreatic, 515
small intestine, 504
with blood and bone marrow disorders
multiple myeloma, 403, 405, 406
myelofibrosis, 413, 414
polycythemia vera, 413
with carcinoid, 203
with genitourinary tumors
kidney, 576, 578
prostate, 601
with leukemias
acute lymphoblastic, 342, 385
chronic lymphocytic, 394, 395
with lymphoma, 378-379
adult, 355
histiocytic medullary reticulosis, 378
rehabilitation considerations, 378
in pediatric patients, 316, 319
with Waldenstrom's macroglobulinemia, 378
Anesthesia
with brain tumors
neuromas, trigeminal, 301, 302
seizures, 287
for bronchoscopy, 423
in carcinoid surgery, 208
and terminal patient, 47
Aneurysmal bone cysts, 217-228
radiology, 232
Angina, in polycythemia vera, 411
Angiocardiography, in mediastinal tumors, 447
Angiofibroma, nasal fossa, 35
Angiography, see also Arteriography; Venography
in adrenal tumors
Cushing's syndrome, 139
neuroblastoma, 150
pheochromocytoma, 146, 194
primary aldosteronism, 135
in brain tumors, 279
astrocytomas, 292
craniopharyngiomas, 300, 301
hemangioblastomas, 297
meningiomas, 297
oligodendrogliomas, 293
pituitary, 299
in genitourinary tumors
kidney, 577
testicular, 620
in head and neck tumors, 9
in liver tumors, 530-531
in lung cancer, 423
in multiple endocrine neoplasia I, 194
in pancreatic tumors, eccrine, 511, 512
in pancreatic tumors, endocrine
gastrinoma, 162
glucagonoma, 165
insulinoma, 158
vipoma, 166
in soft tissue sarcoma, 257

Angiomatosis, brain hemangioblastomas, 297
Angiosarcoma, 219, 267, 268
characteristics of, 223
histological grades of, 231
in liver, 533
Aniline dyes, bladder cancer risk factors, 589
Animal models, breast tumor, 83-84
Aniridia-Wilms's tumor syndrome, 315
Ann Arbor classification, Hodgkin's lymphoma, 358-359
Antacid therapy, in gastrinoma, 162
Anthracyclines
in leukemias, acute
lymphoblastic, 344
myelogenous, 388
myoblastic, 345
relapsed, 391
in pediatric lymphomas, non-Hodgkin's, 347
Antibiotic prophylaxis
in adrenal tumors, 140
in breast cancer, 90
in head and neck cancer, 22
in leukemia, acute, 388, 389
in lung cancer, 431
with splenectomy, 346
Antibiotics
with alimentary tract tumors
bowel preparation, 319, 491
esophagus, 463, 467
liver, 532
pancreas, 516
stomach, 483
with brain tumors, postoperative management, 304
with genitourinary tumors
bladder, 596, 597
kidney, 578
prostate, 604, 607, 611
with gynecological malignancies, 545
with head and neck cancer, 47
with leukemias
acute, 388
chronic lymphocytic, 398
with lymphomas, Hodgkin's, 366
with pediatric tumors, 321
and pulmonary infiltrates, 422, 423
after radiation, 49
Anticoagulation
bladder cancer, 596, 597
gynecological malignancies, 545
in superior vena cava syndrome, 451
Anticonvulsants, with brain tumors, 283, 287
postoperative management, 304
inadequate management of, 285
Antidiabetics, and immunoblastic lymphadenopathy, 377
Antidiuretic hormone (ADH), paraneoplastic syndromes, 183, 184
oat cell carcinoma of lung, 427
Antidiuretic hormone (ADH)-resistant polyuria, 133
Antiestrogens, 88
Antigenic markers, leukemias, acute lymphoblastic, 342
Antihistamines, carcinoid, 207

Antihypertensive drugs, and breast cancer risk, 67
Antimetabolites, 562, *see also* specific drugs
Anus
  carcinoma, 492, 501, 503
  rhabdomyosarcoma, treatment, 336
Aorta
  kidney tumors and, 582
  lung cancer involvement, surgery contraindication, 431
Aphasia, 278, 293, 296
Apocrine gland carcinoma, 119
Appendectomy, 563
Appendix, carcinoid tumors, 184, 203, 205
APUD cells, 191, 193, *see also* Apudomas; Carcinoid
Apudomas, *see also* Carcinoid
  cell characteristics, 197
  classification, 197-199
    multiple endocrine adenopathy, 199
    orthoendocrine group, 197-199
    paraendocrine group, 199
  oat cell carcinoma of lung and, 427
Arabinoside (ARA-C), *see* Cytosine arabinoside
Arginine vasopressin, 185
Argyrophilia, APUD cells, 197
Arrhythmias
  with adrenal tumors
    in pheochromocytoma surgery, 145, 147
    in primary aldosteronism, 133
  with mesothelioma, 456
Arsenical keratoses, and skin cancer, 99
Arterial blood gases, *see* Blood gases
Arterial blood supply, brain tumor, 288
Arteriography, *see also* Angiography
  in bone tumors, 228, 229
  in brain tumors, glioblastoma multiforme, 291
  in carcinoid, 206
  in paraneoplastic syndrome, 185
  in parathyroid tumors, 175
  in pediatric solid tumors, 318
  in rhabdomyocarcoma, 336
Arteriovenous fistulas, kidney tumors, 575
Arthritis, 226
Arytenoidectomy, 52
Arythenopexy, 52
Asbestos, *see also* Mesotheliomas
  and head and neck cancer, 5
  and lung cancer, 422
Ascites
  in Burkitt's lymphoma, 376
  in colorectal cancer, 490
  in gynecological malignancies, 544, 563, 566
  in liver cancer, 529, 532
  in lymphomas, adult, 355
  in myelofibrosis, 414
  in ovarian cancer, 563, 566
  in pediatric patients, 316
  radiology, 544
L-Asparginase
  in leukemias
    acute lymphoblastic, 343, 389
    chronic myelocytic, 394
  toxicity of, 373

Aspartate aminotransferase, pancreatic cancer, 510
Asthma, with small intestinal tumors, 504
Astrocytic tumors, 291-293
Astrocytomas, 292-293
  glioblastoma multiforme, 291-292
  pediatric, 303
  of spine, 287
  surgical approaches to, 286
  x-ray findings with, 279
Atabrine, in ovarian cancer, 566
Ataxia, with brain tumors, 278
  hemangioblastomas, 297
  meningiomas, 295-296
  metastatic, 293
  neuromas, acoustic, 301
Atelectasis
  gastric surgery and, 482
  lung cancer
    postoperative management, 437
    radiation therapy, palliative, 433
    rehabilitation, 438
    staging criteria, 428
  pediatric patient, postoperative care, 321
Atrophic gastritis, and stomach cancer, 475
Autoimmune disorders, with leukemias, 395, 397
Autologous marrow transplants, 390
Autotransplantation, parathyroid, 194
AV, breast cancer, dosages and response rates, 87
Avitene, brain surgery, 288
Axillary node dissection, in melanoma, 116
Azacytidine
  in mesothelioma, 457
  toxic reactions, 372
Azotemia, in multiple myeloma, 405

B

Back pain
  with bone tumors, sacral chordoma, 239
  with mediastinal tumors, 446
  metastasis and, 219
  with prostatic cancer, 601
  with superior vena cava syndrome, 451
BACOP, in non-Hodgkin's lymphomas, 370, 371
Baker's anastomoses, 496
Balanitis xerotica obliterans, 629, 629
Barbiturates, with brain tumor, 287
Basal cell carcinoma
  anal, 501
  arsenic and, 99
  benign appendage tumors associated with, 119
  biopsy, 101
  chemotherapy, 110
  histological types, 106
  Mohs's surgery for, 109
  skin, 102, 105
  treatment guidelines, 110
  trunk and extremities, 112
Basal metabolic rate, in pheochromocytoma, 145

Basophils, in chronic myelocytic leukemia, 392
Batson, venous plexus of, 284
B-CAVe, in lymphomas, Hodgkin's, 367
B-cell leukemias, 341
    chronic lymphocytic, 394, 395
    hairy cell, 398
B-cell lymphomas
    non-Hodgkin's, 360, 361
    pediatric, 346
B-cells
    immunoblastic lymphadenopathy, 377
    Waldenstrom's macroglobulinemia, 378
BCG
    bladder cancer, 596
    melanoma, 117, 118
BCNU (bichloroethyl nitrosourea; Carmustine)
    in brain tumors, 290, 292
    in lymphomas, Hodgkin's, 366, 367
    in multiple myeloma, 405, 406
    in mycosis fungoides, 120
    in pheochromocytoma, 147
    toxicity, 374
BCVPP, in lymphomas, Hodgkin's, 367
B-DOPA, in lymphomas, Hodgkin's, 367, 368
Behavioral changes, see also Psychiatric and psychological considerations
    with brain tumor, 279
    with breast cancer, advanced, 86
    with hyperparathyroidism, 173
    with pituitary disorders, 298
Bence Jones proteins, 227, 378
Benign bone tumors, 217
Benign breast disease, and breast cancer risk, 67
Benign clear-cell tumors, lung, 427
Benign familial hypocalciuric hypercalcemia, 175
Benign juvenile melanomas, 113, 114
Benign prostatic hypertrophy (BPH), 603
Benign pulmonary tumors, 426
Betatron radiation, in skin cancer, 109
Bichloroethyl nitrosourea, see BCNU
Bilateral adrenal hyperplasia, therapeutic management, 135-136
Biliary decompression, 515, 517
Biliary drainage, liver surgery, 534
Biliary ducts, tumors of, 522
Biliary tree, see Gallbladder and biliary tree
Bilirubin, pancreatic cancer, 510
Billroth II gastrectomy, 481
Biochemical markers, see Markers
Biogenic amines, 197, 203
Bipedicle flap, 49
Birth control pills, 67, 70
Bitemporal hemianopsia, 296
Bladder dysfunction
    with brain tumor, 306
    cancer risk factors, 589
    cervical cancer involvement, 556, 560
    colon surgery and, 499
    colorectal cancer metastasis, 496
    cyclophosphamide and, 333
    with prostatic cancer, 604
    radiotherapy and, 546, 555
    spinal cord compression and, 295

Bladder tube, with nephrectomy, 578
Bladder tumors, 589-597
    rhabdomyosarcoma, 335, 336
Blast cells, in leukemia, 341, 386
Blastic crisis, in chronic myelocytic leukemia, 392
Blastomas, lung, 427
Bleeding, 542, see also Gastrointestinal tract; Hemorrhage
    bladder cancer, preoperative management, 591
    carcinoid, 206
    colorectal cancer, 489
    fiberoptic bronchoscopy and, 424
    gastric cancer, 476
    gynecological malignancies, history taking, 543
    leukemias
        acute, 385, 388
        chronic hairy cell, 398
    liver cancer, 529
    lymphoma patient, rehabilitation considerations, 379
    small intestinal tumors, 504
    after thyroidectomy and parathyroidectomy, 48
Bleomycin
    in alimentary tract tumors
        anal carcinoma, 503
        esophageal cancer, 467
    complications of, 320
    in genitourinary tract tumors
        penile, 631
        testicular, 623-624
    germ cell tumors
        mediastinal, 450
        ovarian, 565
        testis, 623, 624
    in gynecological tumors
        ovarian, germ cell, 565
        vulvar, 546
    in head and neck tumors, 44-45, 46
    in Kaposi's sarcoma, 121
    lung cancer, 434
    in lymphomas, Hodgkin's
        adult, 366, 367
        pediatric, 346
    in lymphomas, non-Hodgkin's, 371
        diffuse, 370
        nodular, 369
    in melanoma, 118
    in multiple myeloma, 406
    in skeletal tumors, metastatic, 243
    toxic reactions, 372
Blindness, with brain tumor, 280, 296
Blom-Singer tube, 50, 52
Blood-brain barrier, 290
Blood cell separation, in multiple myeloma, 407
Blood disorders, see also Leukemias; Lymphomas; Multiple myeloma
    myelofibrosis, acute, and myeloid metaplasia, 413-415
    polycythemia vera, 411-413
    thrombocythemia, essential, 415
Blood group A
    gastric cancer risk, 475
    and thyroid cancer, 42
Blood grouping, leukemias, acute, 386
Blood pressure, see also Hypertension

brain surgery complications, 286
  with kidney tumors, 575, 576, 578
Blood sugar, in insulinoma, 158
Blood urea nitrogen
  kidney tumors, 576, 583
  leukemias, acute, 386
  lymphomas, non-Hodgkin's, pediatric, 347
Blood vessel tumors, 219, 231, 237-269, 534
  localization, 218
  pediatric, 337
  small intestine, 504
  with Waldenstrom's macroglobulinemia, 378
Blue nevus, malignant potential, 113
Blumer's shelf, gastric cancer, 476
Body image, *see also* Psychiatric and psychological considerations
  colorectal surgery and, 500
  prostate surgery and, 612-613
Bone cancer, *see* Bone metastasis; Skeletal system tumors
Bone cysts, 217-219, 222, 225-228, 236-237
Bone flaps, in brain surgery, 286, 288
Bone marrow, *see also* Leukemias; Lymphomas; Multiple myeloma; Myelosuppression
  fibrosis, 413
  in histiocytic medullary reticulosis, 378
  in histiocytosis, 348
  in immunoblastic lymphadenopathy, 377
  in leukemias, acute, 385
    chemotherapy complications, 388
    lymphoblastic, 342
  in leukemias, chronic, lymphocytic, 395, 396
    hairy cell, 398
    myelocytic, 392-393
    myelogenous, 398
  in lung cancer, 424
  in lymphoma
    Hodgkin's, pediatric, 346
    staging work-up, 357
  in lymphoma, non-Hodgkin's
    Burkitt's, 377
    pediatric, 346-347
  in multiple myeloma, 403
  in mycosis fungoides, 377
  in pediatric tumors, metastatic evaluation, 318
  in polycythemia vera, 412
  radiosensitivity of lesions, 233
  suppression of, chemotherapy and, 320, 367
  in thrombocytopenia, essential, 415
  in Waldenstrom's macroglobulinemia, 378
Bone marrow transplant, in leukemias
  acute, 390
    lymphoblastic, 344
    myeloblastic, 345
  chronic
    hairy cell, 398
    myelocytic, 345, 393, 394
Bone metastasis, 217
  age incidence, 225
  age predilection, 219
  anatomic locations, 218
  breast cancer, 72
    management of, 88

  and prognosis, 86
  scintigraphy, 73
  carcinoid, 204
  colorectal cancer, diagnostic studies, 491
  esophageal cancer, 462, 463
  lung cancer
    evaluation of, 424
    radiotherapy, 433
  lymphomas, radiotherapy, 375
  neuroblastoma, 332
  pain relief, radiotherapy for, 46
  pancreatic cancer, evaluation, 515
  paraneoplastic syndrome, hypercalcemia, 185
  pathological fractures with, 227
  pediatric tumors, evaluation techniques, 318
  prostatic cancer
    acid phosphatase in, 228
    advanced, 611
    chemotherapy, 611
    hormonal therapy, 610
  radiology, diagnostic clues, 231
  radiosensitivity of, 233
  site predilection of, 225
  soft-tissue sarcomas, bone scan in, 257
  therapeutic management
    chemotherapy, 243
    radiotherapy, 240
    surgery, 240
  Wilms's tumor, treatment of, 330
Bone necrosis, after radiation, 49
Bone resorption, in parathyroid tumors, 174
Bone tumors, *see also* Bone metastasis; Skeletal system tumors
Bony stenosis, spinal lesions, 288
Botryoid sarcoma, 317, 523
Botryoid tumors, pediatric, 319
Bowel dysfunction
  brain tumor, rehabilitation considerations, 306
  spinal cord compression and, 295
Bowel involvement, *see also* Intestinal obstruction
  in cervical carcinoma, 560
  in kidney tumors, 578, 581
  in prostate cancer, 607
Bowel preparation
  in colorectal cancer, 491
  in gynecological malignances, 545
  with kidney surgery, 578, 581
  with pediatric tumors, retroperitoneal, 319
  with prostate surgery, 607
Bowen's disease, 629
  anal, 501
  arsenic and, 99
  penis, 629
  skin lesions, treatment of, 106, 110
Brachial plexus
  radiation and, 433
  scalene node biopsy and, 426
Brachytherapy, soft-tissue sarcoma, 264
Bradykinin, 203, 204, 208
Brain cancer, *see* Central nervous system tumors
Brain irradiation
  complications of, 391

leukemias, sequelae, 343
lung cancer, 436
with lung tumors, 433
lymphomas, pediatric, 347
Brain metastasis, 293-294
breast cancer, 73, 88
chemotherapy, 290
esophageal cancer, 463
lung cancer
evaluation of, 424
radiotherapy, palliative, 433
small cell, 427
melanoma, adjuvant radiotherapy, 117
Wilms's tumor, treatment of, 330
Brainstem lesions
pediatric gliomas, 304
surgical approaches, 286
Brain tumors, *see* Central nervous system tumors
Breast, lymphomas, 355
Breast cancer, 67-94
ectopic hormone production, ACTH, 184
metastasis
to bone, 72, 73, 86, 88, 240
to brain, 73, 88, 294
to liver, 531
to lung, 72, 73, 83, 86, 88, 436
to small intestine, 504
in pregnancy, 80-82
Breast examination
in brain tumor, 280
with gynecological malignancies, 544
self-examination, 68-69
Breathing exercises
lung cancer, postoperative management, 437
pancreatic cancer, preoperative management, 516
pediatric tumors, postoperative care, 321
Breath sounds, with mesothelioma, 456
Breslow's micromeasurements, 102, 116
Brodie's abscess, 218, 224
Bromocriptine, pituitary tumors, 299
Bronchial adenoma, ectopic hormone production, ACTH, 184
Bronchial carcinoid, 205-210
and Cushing's syndrome, 136
ectopic ACTH syndrome, 187
multiple endocrine neoplasia (MEN-I), 192
pulmonic value fibrosis, 204
Bronchial gland carcinoma, histological evaluation, 427
Bronchial obstruction, palliative resection indications, 432
Bronchial stenosis, open-tube bronchoscopy in, 423
Bronchioalveolar adenocarcinoma, lung, 427
Bronchitis, with esophageal cancer, 463
Bronchodilators
in esophageal cancer, 463
in lung cancer, 431
in superior vena cava syndrome, 451
Bronchogenic cancer
bone marrow biopsy in, 424
ectopic gonadotrophin production, 184
Bronchogenic cysts, 443, 444
Bronchoscopy
in carcinoid, 206

esophageal cancer, 462
in head and neck tumor, 9
lung cancer, 422, 423-424
mesotheliomas, 456
Bronchospasm
carcinoid, 205
fiberoptic bronchoscopy and, 424
in superior vena cava syndrome, 451
Brown-Sequard's syndrome, 296, 297
Brown tumor, 227, 232
Budd-Chiari syndrome, 411
Burkitt's lymphoma, 361, 362, 376-377
chemotherapy, 371
chromosomal abnormalities, 343
pediatric, 346
prognosis, 343
Buschke-Lowenstein tumor, 629
Busulfan (Myleran)
in leukemias, chronic myelocytic, 345, 393
in polycythemia vera, 413
in thrombocythemia, essential, 415
toxic reactions, 372
BVAS, in lymphomas, Hodgkin's, 367, 368
Bypass operations, esophageal cancer, 466

C

Cadaver bone graft, 235
CAF
in breast cancer, 87
in salivary gland tumors, 40
Cafe´-au-lait lesions, 144, 227
Caffeine, pancreatic cancer risk, 509
Calcifications, brain tumor and, 279
Calcinosis circumscripta, 226
Calcitonin
apudomas, 199
in breast cancer, with hypocalcemia, 89
in head and neck tumor, 9
in hypercalcemia
acute, 176
paraneoplastic PTH-secreting syndromes, 186
in mediastinal tumors, 447
in medullary carcinoma of thyroid, 41, 194
in oat cell carcinomas of lung, 427
Calcium density, brain tumors, 293
Calcium infusion test
in carcinoid, 206
in parathyroid tumors, 174
in Zollinger-Ellison syndrome, 162
Calcium levels, 178, *see also* Hypercalcemia; Hyperparathyroidism
with bone tumors, 227
in hyperthyroidism, MEN-II, 194
with leukemias, acute, 385
with mediastinal tumors, 447
with multiple myeloma, 404
with parathyroid tumors, 173, 174, 178
with prostatic cancer, 602
after thyroidectomy and parathyroidectomy, 48, 178

Calculi, urinary
  bladder cancer risk factors, 589
  in hyperparathyroidism, MEN-II, 194
  parathyroid tumors and, 173
CALLA, 342, 343
Callus, 219
CAMP, lung cancer, 434
Campanacci's disease, 236-237
Candida, in nutritional deficiencies, 21
CAP, in salivary gland tumors, 40
Carbenicillin, 388, 389
Carbon dioxide laser, *see* Laser surgery
Carboxyhemoglobin, in polycythemia vera, 412
Carcinoembryonic antigen (CEA)
  brain metastasis, 294
  brain tumor, 280
  colorectal cancer, 490
  liver tumors, 530
  pancreatic cancer, 510
Carcinogens, *see also* Diet; Occupational exposures;
    Smoking and tobacco use
  bladder cancer risk, 589
  liver cancer risk, 529
Carcinoid, 203-212
  alcohol ingestion test, 206
  APUD cells, 191, 193
  apudomas, 198
  ectopic ACTH syndrome, 187
  ectopic hormone production, ACTH, 184
  gastric, 478
  liver metastasis, 531
  lung, histological evaluation, 427
  mediastinal, 446
  multiple endocrine neoplasia-I, 192
  small intestine, 504
  versus vipoma, 166
Carcinoma in *situ*
  breast
      in pregnancy, 81
      treatment of, 77, 79
  cervical, 556-557
  gastric, 475
  penis, 630-631
  skin, *see* Bowen's disease
  uterus, 560
  vocal cord, 32-33
  vulva, 546
Carcinomatosis, meningeal, 279, 290, 294
Carcinosarcoma
  esophagus, 461
  lung, 427
Cardiac lesions
  in carcinoid syndrome, 204, 205
  in small intestinal tumors, 504
Cardiotoxicity, of chemotherapeutic agents, 265, 373, 374
Carmustine, *see* BCNU
Carotid body, APUD cells, 197, 198
Cartilaginous tumors, 217
Catecholamines
  after adrenalectomy, 148
  with carcinoid, 206, 208

  with mediastinal tumors, 447
  with neuroblastoma, 150, 316
  with pheochromocytoma, 145, 146, 194
CAT scan, 630
  adrenal tumors
      Cushing's syndrome, 139-140
      neuroblastoma, 150
      pheochromocytoma, 146
      primary aldosteronism, 135
  alimentary tract tumors
      biliary tree, 523
      colorectum, 491
      esophagus, 462
      liver, 530, 537
      pancreas, eccrine, 511, 515
      stomach, 477
  bone tumors, 228, 229
      chordoma, 239
      follow-up, 244
      osteosarcoma, metastatic, 238-239
  brain tumors, 279, 280
      astrocytoma, 292
      craniopharyngioma, 300-301
      glioblastoma multiforme, 291
      hemangioblastoma, 297
      lymphoma, 301
      meningioma, 297
      metastatic, 293-294
      oligodendroglioma, 293
      osteocytoma, 292
      pediatric, 303, 304
      pituitary, 299
  breast cancer, 73, 86
  endocrine syndromes
      carcinoid, 206
      multiple endocrine neoplasia II, 194
      paraneopastic syndrome, 185
  genitourinary tumors
      bladder, 591, 597
      kidney, 575, 577, 585
      prostate, 602, 612
      testis, 617, 619, 620, 623, 625
  gynecological malignancies, 544, 545, 564
  head and neck tumors, 9
      paranasal sinus tumors, 35
      parathyroid tumors, 175
      lung cancer, 423, 424, 425
      lymphomas
          Hodgkin's, pediatric, 346
          staging work-up, 357
          Burkitt's, 377
          pediatric, 347
      mediastinal tumors, 425, 446
      mesothelioma, 456
      multiple myeloma, 406
      mycosis fungoides, 120
      versus nuclear magnetic resonance, 280
      ovarian cancer, second-look operation indications, 564
      pancreatic tumors, endocrine, 512
          gastrinoma, 162
          glucagonoma, 165

insulinoma, 158
VIPoma, 166
pediatric tumors, 317-318
    brain, 303, 304
    liver, 337
    lymphomas, 346, 347
    metastatic evaluation, 318
    as radiotherapy complications, 320
rhabdomyosarcoma, treatment considerations, 336
soft-tissue sarcoma, 257
    metastatic evaluation, 258
    for radiotherapy, 264
in superior vena cava syndrome, 451
teratoma, 337
CAV, in salivary gland tumors, 40
Cavernous hemangioma, 337, 532
Cavernous sinus
    meningiomas, 296
    nasopharyngeal carcinoma invasion of, 37
    pituitary tumors, 298
Cavitron, 288, 534
CCNU (chloroethyl chlorohexyl nitrosourea; Lomustine)
    adrenal tumors, 141
    biliary tree carcinoma, 524
    brain tumors, 290
    colorectal cancer, 499
    gastric cancer, 483
    lung cancer, 434
    lymphoma, Hodgkin's, 366, 367
    toxicity, 374
Cecal tumors, with chronic lymphocytic leukemias, 398
Cecostomy, 492
Celestin tube, in esophageal cancer, 466
Celiac angiography
    in carcinoid, 206
    in liver tumors
        adult, 530-531
        pediatric, 337
Celiac plexus injection, in pancreatic cancer, 520
Celiotomy, in lung cancer, 426
Cell cultures, 386, 406
Cell kinetics, breast tumor, 83-84
Cell-mediated immunity, in nutritional deficiencies, 21
Central nervous system prophylaxis, see Brain irradiation
Central nervous system symptoms, see Neurological symptoms
Central nervous system tumors, 277-308
    chemotherapy intra-arterial, 536
    colorectal tumors with, syndromes found in, 496
    incidence of, 6
    leukemias, 385, 386, 342, 391
    lymphomas, non-Hodgkin's
        Burkitt's, 377
        pediatric, 346, 347
        radiotherapy, 376
    multiple myeloma, 405
    pediatric, see also Neuroblastoma
        histological types, 303, 304
        lymphomas, 346, 347
        symptoms, 316
    specific types of, 291-304

astrocytic, 291-292
astrocytomas, pediatric, 303
brainstem gliomas, pediatric, 304
chordomas, 303
craniopharyngiomas, 300-301
cysts, colloid, 302-303
cysts, epidermoid, 302
ependymomas, pediatric, 304
hemangiblastomas, 297
lymphomas, 301
medulloblastomas, pediatric, 303-304
meningiomas, 295
metastatic, to brain, 293-294
metastatic, meningeal carcinomatosis, 294
metastatic, to spinal cord, 294-295
neuromas and neurofibromas, 301-302
oligodendrogliomas, 293-294
pediatric, 303-304
pineal region, 300
pituitary, 297-300
Cerebellar astrocytomas, pediatric, 303
Cerebellar fits, 288
Cerebellar signs, with meningiomas, 296
Cerebellar syndrome, with pediatric brainstem gliomas, 304
Cerebral edema, see also Increased intracranial pressure
    with glioblastoma multiforme, 292
    radiotherapy and, 288-289
Cerebral hemorrhage
    in acute leukemias, 385
    in pheochromocytoma, 145
    as surgery complication, 286
Cerebrospinal fluid
    in bone tumors, 233
    in central nervous system tumors, 279
        medulloblastomas, pediatric, 303
        meningeal carcinomatosis, 294
        pituitary, 298
    in histiocytosis, 348
    in leukemias, acute, 342, 386
    in lymphomas, non-Hodgkin's, 347, 377
Cerebrum
    breast cancer metastasis, 88
    cortex tumors, radiotherapy, 289
    glioblastoma, 291
    herniation, brain tumors and, 285
    vasculature, brain surgery goals, 287
Cervical carcinoma, see Cervix, carcinoma of
Cervical esophagus, carcinoma of
    annual incidence of, 6
    five-year relative survival, 23
    follow-up schedule, 51
    spread of, 461
Cervical exploration, in benign parathyroid tumor, 176
Cervical flap, 49
Cervical lymph nodes
    dissection of, see Radical neck dissection
    head and neck cancer
        skin lesions, 112, 116
        in thyroid cancer, 43-44
        treatment of, 27-29

in lymphomas
  adult, 355
  pediatric, 346
Cervical plexus, in radical neck dissection, 29
Cervical stump, carcinoma of, 558
Cervical tracheal cancer, 6, 35
Cervix, carcinoma of, 542-568
  endometrial carcinoma and, 561
  radiology, 544
  risk factors, 541
Cesarean section, with breast cancer in pregnancy, 81
Chediak-Higashi syndromes, 315
Chemodectoma, 198, 444
Chemosurgery
  Mohs's, 109
  skin cancer
    head and neck, 111
    postoperative care, 122
Chemotherapy, *see also* individual chemotherapeutic agents and
    specific tumors
  adrenal tumors, 141
    neuroblastoma, 151
    pheochromocytoma, 147
  alimentary tract tumors
    anus, 503
    colorectum, 499
    esophagus, 467
    gallbladder and biliary tree, 524-525
    liver, 534-536
    pancreas, eccrine, 519-520
    stomach, 482-483
  bone marrow and blood disorders, *see also* Chemotherapy, leukemias;
      Chemotherapy, lymphomas
    histiocytosis, 348
    multiple myeloma, 404-406
    polycythemia vera, 412, 413
    Waldenstrom's macroglobulinemia, 378
  bone tumors, 241-243
    chondrosarcomas, 239
    Ewing's sarcoma, 238
    osteosarcomas, 238
  brain tumors, 290-291
    complications of treatment, 305
    lymphomas, 301
    meningeal carcinomatosis, 294
    pediatric medulloblastomas, 304
    pineal region, 300
    therapeutic goals, 286
  breast cancer
    adjuvant, 83-85
    in advanced disease, 87-88
    menopause and, 86
    in pregnancy, 81
    recurrent, 89
    stage and, 77, 78
  endocrine tumors
    carcinoid, 210
    ectopic ADH syndrome, 187
    hypoglycemia, 187

genitourinary tumors
  bladder, 595-597
  kidney, 582, 583
  penis, 631
  prostate, 608, 609, 610-611
  testis, 619, 623, 623-625
gynecological tumors
  cervix, 559-560
  endometrium, 562
  ovary, 563-564, 565
  vagina, 555
head and neck tumors
  adjuvant, 44-45
  in advanced disease, 45-46
  salivary glands, 40
  thyroid, 44
histiocytosis, 348
leukemias
  acute lymphoblastic, 343
  hairy cell, 398
  chronic lymphocytic, 396-397
  chronic myelocytic, 392, 393, 394
lung cancer, 433-436
lymphomas, 371
  Hodgkin's, 366-368
  toxic reactions, 372-374
lymphomas, non-Hodgkin's, 375-376
  Burkitt's, 377
  diffuse, 370
  nodular, 369
  pediatric, 347
mediastinal tumors, 448-449
mesothelioma, 456, 457
and nutritional status, 10
pancreatic tumors, endocrine
  gastrinoma, 163
  glucagonoma, 166
  insulinoma, 159
  VIPoma, 166
in paraneoplastic syndrome, 187
pediatric leukemias, 343-345
pediatric lymphomas, 347, 348
pediatric solid tumors
  adjuvant, 320
  neuroblastoma, 333
  Wilms's tumor, 324, 329
polycythemia vera, 412, 413
skin cancer
  complications of , 106
  indications, contraindications, and disadvantages, 108, 111
  Kaposi's sarcoma, 121
  melanoma, 117
  mycosis fungoides, 121
soft-tissue sarcoma, 265, 270
spinal metastases, 295
in superior vena cava syndrome, 451
toxic reactions and special considerations, 372-374
Chest tumors, 445, *see also* Lung cancer; Lung metastasis;
    Mediastinal tumors; Mesotheliomas

Chest wall invasion, lung cancer, surgery contraindication, 431
Childbearing, and breast cancer risk, 67, 70
Chloracetate esterase, 386, 387
Chlorambucil
    in leukemias
        hairy cell, 398
        lymphocytic, 396
    in lymphomas
        Hodgkin's, 346, 366
        non-Hodgkin's, 369, 371
        Waldenstrom's macroglobulinemia, 378
    in mycosis fungoides, 121
    in polycythemia vera, 413
    toxic reactions, 372
Chloride levels, in Cushing's syndrome, 138
Chloroethyl chlorohexyl nitrosourea, see CCNU
Chlorophenols, soft tissue sarcoma risk factors, 256
Chloroquine, 397
Chlorozotocin, toxic reactions, 372
Cholangiocarcinoma, 531, 533
Cholangiography, liver tumors, 531
Cholecystectomy
    gallbladder lesions, 524
    pancreatic cancer, 517
Cholecystogram, 523
Cholecystojujunostomy, 517
Cholecystokinin, 510
Choledocojejunostomy, 517, 524
Cholelithiasis, with apudomas, 198
Cholera, pancreatic, see Vipoma
Cholesteatomas, brain, 302
Cholesterol intake, and colorectal cancer risk, 490
Cholesterol levels, with kidney tumors, 576, 578
Cholesterol scans, in Cushing's syndrome, 140
Cholestyramine, in carcinoid, 207
Cholinesterase, APUD cells, 197
Chondroblastoma, 217
    age incidence, 225
    age predilection, 219
    anatomic locations, 218
    characteristics of, 220
    versus malignant bone tumors, 226
    regional predilection of, 224
    therapeutic approaches, 237
Chondrocalcinosis, in parathyroid tumors, 173
Chondroma, 219, 220, 225
Chondromatous hamartomas, lung, 427
Chondromyxoid fibroma, 217, 219, 226
    age incidence, 225
    behavior of, 224
    characteristics of, 220
    regional predilection of, 224
    site predilection of, 225
    therapeutic approaches, 237
Chondrosarcoma, 217, 237, 267
    age incidence, 225
    age predilection, 219
    arteriography in, 229
    behavior of, 224
    biopsy of, 232
    characteristics of, 223

follow-up, 244
histological grades, 231
radiology, diagnostic clues, 231
site predilection of, 225, 225
therapeutic approaches, 237, 239
CHOP, in lymphoma, 369, 370, 371
Chordoma, 217
    age predilection, 219
    anatomic locations, 218
    central nervous system, 302
    characteristics of, 224
    histological grades, 231
    therapeutic approaches, 239
Choriocarcinoma
    gastric, 478
    liver metastasis, 531
    mediastinal, 445, 449
    nonseminomatous germ cell tumors, 624
    testis, 617
Chorionepithelioma, pineal region, 300
Chorionic gonadotrophins, 294
Chromaffinity, APUD cells, 197
Chromophobe adenoma, 280
Chromosomal abnormalities
    increased cancer risk, 315
    in leukemias, 341, 388, 392
        acute lymphoblastic, 343
        chronic myelocytic, 345
    as radiotherapy complication, 320, 366
Chronic irritation and cancer risk
    skin cancer, 99
    bladder cancer, 589
Chronic lymphocytic leukemia, 394-398
Chronic myelocytic leukemia, 341, 345, 391-394
Chvostek's sign, 133, 178
Chylothorax, mediastinal tumors, 446
Chylous fistula, scalene node biopsy and, 426
Cribriform plate involvement, paranasal sinus tumors, 36
Cimetidine
    gastrinoma, 162, 163
    in vipoma, 166
Circumcision, 631
Cirrhosis, liver cancer risk, 529
cis -platinum (Cisplatin)
    esophageal cancer, 467
    genitourinary tumors
        bladder, 596
        penis, 631
        prostate, 611
        testis, 623, 624
    gynecological tumors
        endometrium, 562
        ovary, 563
        vagina, 555
        vulva, 546
    germ cell tumors
        mediastinal, 449-450
        ovary, 565
        testis, 623, 624
    head and neck cancer, 44-45
    intra-arterial route, 536

lung cancer, 434, 435
melanoma, 118
multiple myeloma, 406
skeletal tumors, metastatic, 243
soft tissue sarcoma, 265
thymoma, 449
toxic effects of, 372, 564
Cisternal myelography, in spinal metastases, 295
Citrovorum rescue, 344
Clark's levels, 102
Claudication, in polycythemia vera, 411
Clear-cell carcinoma
liver, 533
lung, 427
vagina, 556
Clear-cell chondrosarcomas, 223
Clear-cell sarcomas, 223, 267
histological grades, 231
pediatric, follow-up, 322
therapeutic guidelines, 269
therapy, 269
Wilms's tumor, 323, 330
Clonorchis sinensis, 529
Clotting, *see* Coagulation
Clubbing
with bone tumors, 227
with lung cancer, 422
with mesothelioma, 455
CMF, breast cancer
adjuvant therapy, 84
dosages and response rates, 87
in recurrent cancer, 90
CMF, in salivary gland tumors, 40
CMF(P), breast cancer, 87
CMFVP, breast cancer, 87
C-MOPP, in lymphomas, 369, 370, 371
Coal tars, skin cancer in, 99
Cobalt therapy
in skin cancer, 109
in soft tissue sarcoma, 264
Cocaine, with Kaposi's sarcoma, 121
Codman's triangle, 226
Codman's tumor, 218, 226
Coexisting tumors, 26, *see also* Second malignancy
Coin lesion, lung cancer, 423
Colectomy, 497
Colitis, versus radiation symptoms, 546
Collagen, in myelofibrosis, 414
Colloidal gold, in mesothelioma, 457
Colloid carcinomas, *see* Mucinous carcinomas
Colloid cysts, central nervous system, 302
Colloid goiter, 192
Colonic transposition, 34
Colonoscopy, 489, *see also* Endoscopy
Colorectal cancer, 489-503
ectopic ACTH production, 184
liver metastasis, 531, 535
lung metastasis, treatment of, 436
pathological considerations, 492, 495
Colostomy, *see* Ostomy
Colposcopy, 542, 544

Coma, *see also* Consciousness
hypercalcemic, 176
with insulinoma, 157
Common duct tumors, 522
Companacci's disease, 219
Compensatory lobar hyperplasia, liver, 532
Compression syndromes, *see also* Spinal cord compression
with leukemia, 398
with pediatric ependymomas, 304
with pituitary tumor, 298
with spinal lesions, 241, 288
Condemned mucosa, head and neck cancer, 24
Condylomata
colorectal, cancer risk, 490
giant malignant, anal, 501
gynecological, cancer risk, 541
with Kaposi's sarcoma, 121
Congenital anomalies
and increased cancer risk, 315
neuroblastoma with, 330
as pediatric radiotherapy complication, 320
Congenital biliary cysts, liver, 532
Congenital nevi
malignant potential, 113, 114
and skin cancer, 99
Congestive heart failure
lung cancer surgery evaluation, 428
with mesothelioma, 456
with Waldenstrom's macroglobulinemia, 378
Conization, cervical, 542, 544
Conpadri 1, 242
Consciousness, with brain tumors, 278
colloid cysts, 303
glioblastoma multiforme, 291
Consolidation radiotherapy, Hodgkin's lymphoma, 366
Constipation, 542
with colorectal cancer, 489, 490
with gynecological malignancies, 543
Consumption coagulopathy, with leukemias, acute, 385, 388
Contact bleeding, 542
Contraceptive practices, and gynecological malignancies, 543
Contractures
with brain tumor, rehabilitation considerations, 306
as skin cancer treatment complication, 106
Contralateral disease, lung cancer, 428
Coombs's test, 396
COPP, lymphomas, non-Hodgkin's, 371
Cordectomy, vocal cord, 33
Corpus callosum glioblastoma, 291
Cortical desmoid, behavior of, 219
Corticosteroid therapy, 166
with adrenal inhibitors, 187
after adrenal surgery, 140, 148
with brain tumors
complications of treatment, 305
glioblastoma multiforme, 291, 292
increased intracranial pressure management, 283
metastatic, 294
pediatric, 304
postoperative management, 304
therapeutic goals, 286

in breast cancer
   with hypercalcemia, 73, 89
   metastatic, 88
in carcinoid, 207
in cerebral edema, postirradiation, 289
in head and neck cancer, adjuvant therapy, 45
in hypercalcemia
   in breast cancer, 73, 89
   in hyperparathyroidism, ectopic, 186
in leukemias, acute
   adult lymphoblastic, 389
   lymphoblastic, 343
in leukemias, chronic lymphocytic, 396, 397
in lymphomas, Hodgkin's, 366
in prostate cancer, 611
with spinal lesions, 287, 295
in superior vena cava syndrome, 451
after thyroidectomy and parathyroidectomy, 48
Corticotrophinoma, carcinoid, 204
Cortisol levels
   in Cushing's syndrome, 138
   in paraneoplastic syndromes, 142, 185
   with pituitary tumors, 299
Cortisol therapy after adrenal surgery, 136, 142, 147, 148
Cortisone infusion test, in parathyroid tumors, 174
Corynebacterium parvum, 118
Cosmegen, *see* Actinomycin D
Cosmetic rehabilitation
   head and neck surgery patient, 52
   skin cancer, 122-123
CPVB, testicular tumors, 623
Craig needle biopsy, bone tumors, 232
Cranial irradiation, *see* Brain irradiation
Cranial nerves
   with brain tumors, 278
      epidermoid and dermoid cysts, 302
      lymphomas, 301
      meningiomas, 296
      pediatric brainstem gliomas, 304
      pituitary, 298
   with head and neck tumors, 8
      nasopharyngeal carcinoma, 37
      salivary gland, 40
   with leukemias, acute lymphoblastic, 342
   with lymphomas, Burkitt's, 377
Craniofacial resections, 37
Craniopharyngiomas, 300-301
   endocrine evaluation with, 280
   radiosensitivity of, 290
   x-ray finding with, 279
Craniotomy, 287
   in astrocytoma, 293
   frontal, 303
   in pituitary tumors, 299
Creatinine
   with kidney tumors, 576, 583
   with lymphomas, non-Hodgkin's, 347
   with multiple myeloma, 404
   with parathyroid tumors, 174
Cribriform plate involvement, paranasal sinus tumors, 36
Cronkhite-Canada syndrome, 478
Cryoglobulinemia, 397, 407

Cryosurgery
   bone tumors, giant-cell, 237
   cervical carcinoma *in situ*, 557
   head and neck cancer, 26-27
   nasopharyngeal tumors, 37
   skin cancer, 106, 108
      head and neck, 111
      histology and, 110
      postoperative care, 122
      postsurgical edema, 105
      trunk and extremities, 112
Cryptorchidism, 618
Curettage
   bone lesions, 222, 234, 236, 237
   dilatation and, 544
   skin cancer, 106, 110
Cushing's syndrome, 136-144
   apudomas and, 198
   brain tumor and, 280
   with ectopic ACTH production, 183
      diagnosis, 185
      therapeutic management, 187
   localization of cause, 139-140
   with multiple endocrine neoplasia syndrome (MEN-I), 192
   pituitary tumors, 192, 299
Cutaneous recurrence, breast cancer, management of, 89
Cutaneous syndrome, glucagonoma, 165
CVB, in lymphomas, Hodgkin's, 367, 368
Cyclamate, bladder cancer risk factors, 589
Cyclic AMP, 174, 204
Cyclohexylamine, bladder cancer risk factors, 589
Cyclophosphamide (Cytoxan)
   adrenal tumors, 141
      neuroblastoma, 151
      pheochromocytoma, 147
   bone tumors, 242
      Ewing's sarcoma, 238, 243
      metastatic, 243
   breast cancer
      adjuvant therapy, 84
      dosages and response rates, 87-88
   carcinoid, 210
   genitourinary tumors
      bladder, 596
      prostate, 610, 611
      testis, 623
   gynecological tumors
      endometrium, 562
      ovary, 563, 565
   and immunoblastic lymphadenopathy, 377
   leukemia, chronic lymphocytic, 397
   lung cancer, 434, 435
   lymphomas, Hodgkin's, 366, 367
   lymphomas, non-Hodgkin's, 371
      Burkitt's, 377
      diffuse, 370
      nodular, 369, 369
      pediatric, 347
      Waldenstrom's macroglobulinemia, 378
   melanoma, 118
   mesothelioma, 457

multiple myeloma, 405, 406
mycosis fungoides, 121
neuroblastoma, 151, 333
soft tissue sarcoma, 265
rhabdomyosarcoma, 336
thymoma, 449
toxic effects of, 372, 564
Wilms tumor, 329
Cylindromas
paranasal sinus, 35
salivary gland, 38-39, 40
Cyproheptadine
in carcinoid, 207, 208
in Cushing's disease of pituitary origin, 142
Cyst, bone, *see* Bone cysts
Cystadenocarcinoma (mucinous), pancreatic, 516
Cystectomy, 591
bladder cancer, 595, 596
in genitourinary cancer, bladder, 591
Cyst formation, in parathyroid tumors, 174
Cystic astrocytomas, in children, 303
Cystic basal cell carcinoma, 106
Cystic duct, tumors of, 522
Cystic mastitis, 70
Cystic tumors, radiotherapy, 289
Cystitis
bladder cancer, risk factors, 589
chemotherapy and, 564
cyclophosphamide and, 333
radiation, 555, 595, 608
Cystosarcoma phyllodes, 79
Cystoscopy
with bladder cancer, 591
follow-up evaluation, 597
after transurethral resection, 595
with gynecological malignancies, 544
with kidney tumors, 577, 585
with prostate tumors, 602-603, 607
Cysts, 141
central nervous system, 302-303
mediastinal, 444-445
incidence and location of, 443
radiological findings, 446
pineal region, 300
Cytochemical properties
acute leukemia cells, 386
APUD cells, 197
Cytogenetic abnormalities, in leukemias, 341
acute, 386
acute lymphoblastic, 343
chronic myelocytic, 345
Cytology
bladder cancer, 590
follow-up evaluation, 597
after transurethral resection, 595
brain metastasis, 294
cervical, 542
esophageal cancer, 462
head and neck cancer, 9

kidney tumors, 575
lung cancer, 422, 423
mesiotheliomas, 456
pancreatic carcinoma, eccrine, 512
prostate cancer, 602
Cytomegalovirus, 356, 395
Cytopenia, in chronic leukemias, 395, 398
Cytosine arabinoside (ARA-C)
in brain tumors, 290
in breast cancer, metastatic, 88
in carcinoid, 210
in leukemias, acute
lymphoblastic, 344
myelogenous, 388
myoblastic, 345
relapsed, 391
in lymphoma, Burkitt's, 377
toxic reactions, 372
Cytotoxic chemotherapy, *see also* specific agents
in carcinoid, 210
in endometrial cancer, 562
in prostatic cancer, advanced, 610-611
in endocrine tumors, carcinoid, 210
Cytoxan, *see* Cyclophosphamide
CYVADIC, in soft tissue sarcoma, 265

D

Dacarbazine, *see also* DTIC
in lymphomas, Hodgkin's, 366, 367
toxic reactions, 372
Dactinomycin, *see* Actinomycin D
Daunorubicin (daunomycin, rubidomycin)
leukemias, acute
adult lymphoblastic, 389
myelogenous, 388
toxicity, 373
DAV, breast cancer, dosages and response rates, 87
DCNU, toxic reactions, 372
o'p' DDD
with adrenal tumors, 141
and Cushing's syndrome, 142
in ectopic ACTH syndrome, 187
in pheochromocytoma, 147
DDP, lung cancer, 434
Debulking
brain tumors
pediatric medulloblastomas, 303
therapeutic goals, 286
mediastinal tumors, 447
ovarian tumors, 564
pancreatic tumors, insulinoma, 160
thymomas, 449
Decerebration, 287-288
Decompression, spinal lesions, 288
Decubiti, with brain tumor, 306
Dedifferentiated tumors

age incidence, 225
    chondrosarcoma, 219, 223
Deep-vein thrombosis, 566, 582
Deglutition, postsurgical rehabilitation, 51
Delautin, endometrial cancer, 562
Deltopectoral flap, 49
Demeclocycline, in ectopic ADH syndrome, 187
Dementia, 278
    with craniopharyngioma, 300
    with glioblastoma multiforme, 291
    with meningiomas, 295, 296
    with neuromas, acoustic, 301
Dental prophylaxis, with head and neck tumors, 51, 52
Deoxycorticosterone test (DOC), 134
Deoxynucleotidyl transferase, 342, 386
Depo-Medrol, bone cysts, 236
Depression
    with craniopharyngioma, 300
    kidney patient, 581
Dermatitis, and skin cancer, 99
Dermatofibroma, therapy, 269
Dermatofibrosarcoma protuberans, 266, 267, 268
Dermatophytin, in nutritional deficiencies, 21
Dermoid cysts
    central nervous system, 302
    mediastinal, incidence and location of, 443
Desmoid tumors, 267-268
    behavior of, 224
    therapy, 269
Desmoplastic fibromas, 237
Dessication and curettage, 106, 108
    histology and, 110
    indications, contraindications, and disadvantages, 108, 109
Dexamethasone
    with brain tumors, 290
        increased intracranial pressure management, 283, 288
        metastatic, 294
    in hyperparathyroidism, ectopic, 186
    with spinal lesions, 287, 295
Dexamethasone suppression test, 138-139, 185
Diabetes insipidus
    brain tumors
        pineal region, 300
        postoperative management, 304
        pretreatment management, 283
    in histiocytosis, 348
Diabetes mellitus
    apudomas, 198
    gynecological malignancies, 541, 543
    and pancreatic cancer risk, 509
    with pancreatic tumors, eccrine, 509
        postoperative, 520
        preoperative management, 515
    with pancreatic tumors, endocrine, 158
        insulinoma, 160
        glucagonoma, 163, 166, 192
Dialysis, 73, 176, 610
    in leukemia, 388
    in multiple myeloma, 406

Diamox, in multiple myeloma, 406
Diaphragm, resection and reconstruction, 263
Diaphynography, 71
Diarrhea
    with apudomas, 198
    in carcinoid syndrome, 204
    chemotherapy and, 372-374
    with colorectal cancer, 489, 490
    with gynecological malignancies, 543
    with mediastinal tumors, 446
    with pancreatic cancer, 510
    radiation therapy and, 545-546, 555
    with small intestinal tumors, 504
Diazepam, for bronchoscopy, 423
Diazoxide, 158, 159, 160, 187
Dibenzyline, in adrenal angiography, 146
Dibromodulcitol, 87
Diet
    with adrenal tumors
        neuroblastoma, preoperative management, 150
        primary aldosteronism, 133, 135
    for colon endoscopy, 489
    after esophageal surgery, 468
    after gastric surgery, 483
    after pancreatic surgery, 163, 520
    after prostate surgery, 611
    and renin levels, 134
    as risk factor
        in bladder cancer, 589
        in breast cancer, 67
        in colorectal cancer, 490
        in esophageal cancer, 461
        in liver cancer, 5293
        in pancreatic cancer, 509
        in stomach cancer, 475
Diethylstilbestrol (DES)
    in breast cancer, recurrent, 89
    and gynecological malignancy, 541, 556
    in prostatic cancer, 609
Diffuse anaplastic changes, Wilms's tumor with, 323
Diffuse histiocytic lymphoma, 360, 361, 362, 371
Diffuse lymphomas, 360, 361, 362, 370, 371
Diffuse mixed lymphoma, 371
Diffuse poorly differentiated lymphoma, 360, 361, 362, 371
Digitalization, in bladder cancer, 596
Di Guglielmo's syndrome, 344
1, 25-Dihyroxyvitamin D, 174
Dilantin, 283, 286, 2827
Dilatation and curettage, 544
Dimethyl triazeno imidazole carboxamide, see DTIC
Dinitrochlorobenzene, 118
Diphenylhydantoin, 286
Diplopia
    with brain tumors, 280, 296
    with insulinoma, 157
    in pediatric patients, 316
Disease-free interval, in breast cancer, 86, 90
Disseminated intravascular coagulation, 414
Distal blind pouch, 497

Distention, small intestinal tumors, 504
Diuretics
    for ascites, 532
    and hematocrit elevation, 412
    in hypercalcemia
        acute, 176
            with breast cancer, 73, 89
            with multiple myeloma, 406
    in increased intracranial pressure management, 283
    in primary aldosteronism, 133
    renin stimulation with, 134
    in superior vena cava syndrome, 451
Diversion without resection, esophageal cancer, 466
Diverticulitis, versus radiation symptoms, 546
DNCB, melanoma, 118, 118
DOC test, 134
Dopamine, 197, see also Apudomas
Dopamine agonists, pituitary tumors, 299
Dorfman classification, 360
Doubling time, breast tumor, 83
Doxorubicin, see Adriamycin
Drainage, 584
    after brain surgery, 304
    after breast surgery, 90
    gallbladder lesions, 524
    after gastric surgery, 483
    after gynecological surgery, 566
    after head and neck surgery, 48
    after liver surgery, 534
Drug abuse, as risk factor, 121, 256
Drugs
    and breast cancer risk, 70
    and immunoblastic lymphadenopathy, 377
    liver metablism of, 536
DTIC (dimethyl triazeno imidazole carboxamide)
    adrenal neuroblastoma, 151
    glucagonoma, 166
    Kaposi's sarcoma, 121
    in lymphomas, Hodgkin's
        adult, 366
        pediatric, 346
    melanoma, 117, 118
    neuroblastoma, 333
    rhabdomyosarcoma, 336
    in skeletal tumors, metastatic, 243
    in soft tissue sarcoma, 265
Duct cell carcinomas, pancreatic, 516
Dukes's classification, colorectal cancer, 495
Dumping syndrome, gastric surgery and, 482
Duodenal drainage studies, with pancreatic tumor, 512
Duodenum, apudomas, 198
Dysgenetic testes, 618
Dysgerminomas
    mediastinal, radiological findings, 446
    ovarian, 565
Dysphagia
    with brain tumors
        meningiomas, 296
        neuromas, acoustic, 301
    with esophageal cancer, 461
    with parathyroid tumors, 174

Dysplasia
    cervical, 556-557
    lung, 426, 426
    mammary, 71
    and stomach cancer, 475
Dysplastic nevus syndrome (DNS), 113-114
Dyspnea
    mediastinal tumors, 446
    mesothelioma, 455
    radiation therapy, palliative, 433
Dysuria, 542
    in bladder cancer, 590
    in gynecological malignancies, 543
    in paraneoplastic endocrine syndromes, 183
    in parathyroid tumors, 173
    in prostatic cancer, 601

E

EAC rosettes, leukemias, chronic lymphocytic, 395
Ear, nose, and throat (ENT) examination, with esophageal cancer, 463
Ears
    examination of, 6
    tumors of
        annual incidence of, 6
        sarcoma botryoides, 334
        skin tumors, treatment of, 111-112
Ecchymosis, in leukemia, 342
Eccrine gland carcinoma
    pancreas, see Pancreatic tumors, eccrine
    skin, 105, 119
ECG, see Electrocardiography
Echinococcus cysts, liver, 533
Ectopic horomone-producing tumors, 183-188, see also Apudomas;
        Carcinoid and Cushing's syndrome, 139, 142
Ectopic meningiomas, 297
Edema
    with brain tumors, surgical goals, 287
    breast, 69
    in carcinoid syndrome, 204, 205
    with gynecological malignancies, 544
    with lymphomas, adult, 355
    in primary aldosteronism, 133
    with prostatic cancer, 608
    skin cancer treatment complications, 105
    spinal, 287
Edema, cerebral, see Increased intracranial pressure
EEG, see Electroencephalography, in brain tumors
EKG, see Electrocardiography
Elastic support stockings, 520, 545
Elbow, bone tumors, 218
Elderly
    bone metastasis, 219
    brain tumors, unwarranted aggressive treatment, 285
    breast cancer
        adjuvant chemotherapy, 84
        chemotherapy, 89
        hormonal therapy, 90
        mastectomy in, 76

colorectal cancer
    evaluation, 490
    signs of, 489
    leukemias, prognosis, 386
    lymphomas, non-Hodgkin's, treatment of, 370
    pancreatic cancer, 509, 517
    skin cancer
        microvascular considerations, 113
        pretreatment evaluation, 102
        treatment modality, 107
        undertreatment of, 105
Electrical nerve stimulation, for pain management, 246
Electrodessication, in skin cancer, 110, 122
Electroencephalography (EEG), in brain tumors, 279
    astrocytomas, 292
    meningiomas, 297
    pediatric, 303
    postoperative, 304
Electrolytes, *see also* Fluids
    with adrenal tumors
        neuroblastoma, 151
        primary aldosteronism, 133, 136
    after brain surgery, 304
    after colon surgery, 499
    after gastric surgery, 483
    with leukemias, acute, 386
    in paraneoplastic syndromes, 188
Electromyography, 279, 297
Electron beam therapy, in mycosis fungoides, 120
Electron microscopy, leukemias, acute, 386
Electrophoresis, 227, 356
Electrosurgery, in skin cancer, 108
    head and neck, 111, 112
    histology and, 110
    indications, contraindications, and disadvantages, 108, 109
    trunk and extremities, 112
Embolism, *see* Thromboembolic complications
Embolization, renal artery, 581
Embryonal carcinoma, 337-338
    mediastinal, 445, 449
    ovarian, 565
    testicular, 617, 619, 624
Embryonal notochord tumors, 217
Embryonal rhabdomyosarcoma, 267, 268, 330
    bile duct, 523
    prognosis, 335
    therapy, 269
Emphysema, with esophageal cancer, 463
Endocervix, in endometrial carcinoma, 561
Endochondroma, 217
    age predilection, 219
    anatomic locations, 218
    behavior of, 224
    characteristics of, 220
    follow-up, 244
Endocrine ablation, in breast cancer, 79, 81-82, 88
Endocrine disturbances, with brain tumors, 278, 279, 283
    craniopharyngiomas, 300
    meningiomas, 296
    pituitary gland, 298
    postoperative management, 304

Endocrine heterotopias, liver, 533
Endocrine therapy, *see* Hormone therapy
Endocrine tumors, *see also* Apudomas; Carcinoid; Paraneoplastic
        syndromes; specific glands
    annual incidence of, 6
    lymphomas, 355
    pediatric, biochemical markers, 316
Endodermal sinus tumor, ovarian, 565
Endometrial carcinoma, 541-562
Endophotocautery, *see* Laser surgery
Endoscopic retrograde cannulation of pancreatic ducts, 158
Endoscopic retrograde cholangiopancreatography, 512, 530
Endoscopic ureteral stenting, 607
Endoscopy
    in alimentary tract tumors
        esophagus, 462
        pancreas, 512
        stomach, 475, 477
    in carcinoid, 206
    in genitourinary cancer
        bladder, 591
        prostate, 602-603, 607
    head and neck cancer, 8, 9
    lung cancer, 423-424, 425
    radiology, 544
Endosteal osteosarcoma, 231
Endosteal sarcoma, 238
Endostosis, characteristics of, 221
Engelmann's progressive diaphyseal dysplasia, 226
Enteric cysts, mediastinal, 443, 444-445, 446
Enteritis, radiation, 595
Enterochromaffin cells, carcinoid, 204
Enteroglucagonoma, 204
Enucleation, prostatic cancer, 608, 609
Environmental factors
    liver cancer risk, 529
    soft tissue sarcoma risk, 256
Enzymes, in chronic myelocytic leukemias, 393
Enzyme supplements, for gastric surgery patient, 483
Eosinophilic granuloma, 217, 347-348
    age predilection and behavior, 219, 225
    characteristics of, 222
    lung, 427
    versus malignant bone tumors, 226
    radiology, 232
    regional predilection of, 224
    therapeutic approaches, 236
Eosinophils
    in immunoblastic lymphadenopathy, 377
    in leukemia, chronic myelocytic, 392
    in lymphoma, Hodgkin's, 359
Ependymoma
    in children, 303, 304
    radiosensitivity of, 290
    spine, 287
    surgical approaches, 286
Epidermoid carcinoma
    colorectal, 495
    head and neck
        metastatic from unknown primary, 27-28
        salivary gland, 39, 40

therapeutic modality selection, 25
lung, 431, 434-435
Epidermoid cysts, central nervous system, 302
Epididymis, with hemangioblastomas, 297
Epididymitis, with testicular tumors, 618
Epidural tumors, spinal, 288
Epinephrine, 157, 412, 414
Epipodophyllotoxin analogue, 344, 366
Epithelial abnormalities, lung, 426
Epithelial cell carcinomas
esophageal, 461
lung, 426-427
lung metastasis, treatment, 436
Epithelial mesothelioma, *see* Mesotheliomas
Epithelial sarcoma, 267
histological grades, 231
therapy, 269
Epithelioid cell nevus, malignant potential, 113
Epithelioid sarcoma, *see* Epithelial sarcoma
Epsilon-aminocaproic acid, 208
Epstein-Barr virus, 376
Erythema
in carcinoid, 204
with gynecological malignancies, 544
in mycosis fungoides, 120
as treatment complication
in head and neck cancer, 48-49
in skin cancer, 106
Erythrocytosis, kidney tumors, 576, *see also* Polycythemia
Erythroid precursors, in acute lymphoblastic leukemias, 342
Erythroleukemia, 341, 344
Erythroplasia, inadequate biopsy, 24
Erythroplasia of Queyrat, 629
Erythropoietin, in polycythemia vera, 411, 412
Esophageal resection, 481
Esophageal varices, 529, 530
Esophagectomy, 466
Esophagogastrectomy, 466, 481
Esophagogastrostomy, 466
Esophagojejunostomy, 482
Esophagoscopy, 9, 462
Esophagostomy, 46
Esophagrams, 9, 468
Esophagus
enteric cysts, 443, 444-445
injury to, in mediastinoscopy, 425, 426
invasion of in lung cancer, 431
Esophagus, cancer of, 461-469
annual incidence of, 6
Bantu, cancer incidence in, 461
China, esophageal cancer incidence in, 461
ectopic hormone production, ACTH, 184
epidemiology, 461
five-year relative survival, 23
liver metastasis, 531
Essential hypertension, after adrenalectomy, 148
Essential thrombocythemia, 415
Esterases
APUD cells, 197
leukemias, acute, 387

Estlander lip-switch flaps, 49
Estrogen receptors
breast cancer, 72
adjuvant therapy, 84, 85
and management, 89-90
in pregnancy, 81
and prognosis, 86
recurrent, 90
endometrial cancer, 562
Estrogen replacement therapy, and breast cancer risk, 67, 70
Estrogens
in adrenal tumors, 141
and breast cancer, in pregnancy, 80
and endometrial cancer, 542
Estrogen therapy, 88
breast cancer, recurrent, 89
in endometrial cancer, 562
in prostatic cancer, 604, 608, 609
advanced, 610
psychiatric complications of, 607
Ethnic factors, and skin cancer, 99
Etoposide, 434, *see also* VP-16
Ewing's sarcoma, 217, 219, 267, 330
age incidence, 225
age predilection, 219
anatomic locations, 218
behavior of, 225
characteristics of, 224
fever in, 227
metastatic evaluation, 228
onionskin appearance, 226
radiology, diagnostic clues, 231
regional predilection of, 224
surgery, 234
therapeutic approaches, 238
therapeutic management
chemotherapy, 243
radiosensitivity of, 233
radiotherapy, 241
Exophthalmos
with brain tumors, 280, 296
in Burkitt's lymphoma, 376
in histiocytosis, 348
Exostoses, 217, 244
External beam radiation
prostatic cancer, 608
in skin cancer, 109
Extended-field radiation, in Hodgkin's disease, 365
External megavoltage radiotherapy, in bladder cancer, 595
Extra-adrenal paragangliomas, 145
Extrahepatic retrograde cholangiopancreaticoduodenography (ERCP), 523, 530
Extramedullary disease, multiple myeloma, 405
Extremity tumors
bone, types with predilection for, 218-219
chemotherapy intra-arterial, 536
Eyes, *see also* Exophthalmos; Optic nerve; Retina; Vision disturbances; Visual fields
brain tumors and, 279, 302
prostheses, 50

sella turcia enlargement and, 141
tumors
    annual incidence of, 6
    meningiomas, ectopic, 297
    skin, treatment of, 110-111

F

Facial nerve, 284
    palsy, rehabilitation, 52
    salivary gland tumor excision, 38, 39
Facial nerve involvement
    with acoustic neuromas, 301
    cranial nerve removal and, 284
    meningiomas and, 296
    in polycythemia vera, 411
Fallopian tubes, in bladder cancer, 596
FAM
    biliary tree carcinoma, 524
    gastric cancer, 482
    lung cancer, 434
    pancreatic cancer, 519
Familial disorders, *see also* Genetic factors
    bone tumors, 227
    breast cancer risk, 67, 70
    gynecological malignancies, 543
    hemophagocytic lymphohistiocytosis, 348
    melanoma, 113
    polyposis, 490, 495
    soft tissue sarcoma risk, 25
    testicular cancer risk, 619
Fan flaps, 49
Fast neutron beam therapy, 519
Fatty acid levels
    in paraneoplastic syndrome, hypoglycemia, 185
    in pheochromocytoma, 145
Feeding enterostomy, bladder cancer, 596
Feeding test, in Zollinger-Ellison syndrome, 162
Feminizing tumors, adrenal, 141
Fiberoptic endoscopy
    alimentary tract
        in colorectal cancer, 489, 491
        in small intestinal tumors, 504
        in stomach cancer, 475, 476, 477
    bronchoscopy, in lung cancer, 422, 423-424
Fibrillary astrocytomas, 292
Fibrinogen, in histiocytosis, 348
Fibrinolytic agents, in superior vena cava syndrome, 451
Fibroblastic tissue, gastric lesions, 481
Fibroma, 219
    bone, 227
        age incidence, 225
        behavior of, 224
        characteristics of, 222
        therapeutic approaches, 236-237
    small intestine, 504
Fibromatosis, therapy, 269

Fibrosarcoma, 217, 219, 237
    age incidence, 225
    age predilection, 219
    behavior of, 225
    characteristics of, 223
    follow-up, 244
    histological grades, 231
    mediastinal, 445
    radiosensitivity of, 263
    therapeutic guidelines, 267-268
Fibrosarcomatous mesothelioma, *see* Mesotheliomas
Fibrosis
    bone marrow, 413-415
    skin cancer, treatment complications, 106
    in thrombocythemia, essential , 415
Fibrous dysplasia, 217, 217, 219
    age incidence, 225
    age predilection, 219
    behavior of, 219
    regional predilection of, 224
    surgery, 235
    therapeutic approaches, 236, 237
Fibrous histiocytoma, malignant, 223, 267, 268
    age incidence, 225
    fever in, 227
    histological grades, 231
    pathological fractures with, 227
    radiosensitivity of, 263
    therapeutic guidelines, 268, 269
Fibroxanthomas, lung, 427
Fistula
    colorectal cancer risk, 490
    with esophageal cancer, 462
    after gynecological surgery, 566
Flaps
    head and neck surgery, reconstruction, 49-50
    skin cancer, postoperative care, 122
Floor of mouth cancer
    annual incidence of, 6
    five-year relative survival, 23
Florinef administration, 134
Floxuridine (FUDR), 499, 535
Fluid replacement, in breast cancer, with hypocalcemia, 89
Fluids, *see also* Electrolytes
    in adrenal surgery, 148
        for neuroblastoma, preoperative management, 150
        for primary aldosteronism, postoperative care, 136
    in alimentary tract surgery
        for colorectal cancer, preoperative, 491
        for esophageal cancer, postoperative, 468
        for gastric cancer, 483
        for liver tumors, preoperative, 532
    brain tumors, postoperative management, 304
    breast cancer, preoperative assessment, 73
    in genitourinary malignancies
        bladder, 591, 596, 597
        prostate, 604
    in gynecological malignancies
        ovarian, 566

preoperative preparation, 545
postoperative management, 566
in head and neck tumors
  oral cavity cancers, 21
  with radiation therapy, 48
intravenous hyperalimentation and, 21
in leukemia, acute, 386, 389
lung cancer, postoperative management, 437
pancreatic surgery
  eccrine tumors, 510, 520
  endocrine tumors, 162, 163
in paraneoplastic syndromes
  hypercalcemia, 186
  postoperative care, 188
pediatric tumors, postoperative care, 321
prostatic cancer, preoperative preparation, 604
Fluorocortisone, 134, 136, 148
Fluoroscopy
  in gastric cancer, 476-477
  mediastinal tumors, 446
5-Fluorouracil
  in adrenal tumors, 141
  in alimentary tract tumors
    anus, 503
    colorectum, 498, 499
    esophagus, 467
    liver, 534, 535
    stomach, 482
  in breast cancer
    adjuvant therapy, 84
    dosages and response rates, 87
  carcinoid, 210
  genitourinary tumors
    bladder, 596
    penis, 631
    prostate, 610
  in gynecological tumors
    endometrium, 562
    vulva, 546
  in head and neck tumors, 45
  lung cancer, 434
  mesothelioma, 457
  pancreatic tumors
    eccrine, 519
    gastromp,a. 162
    glucagonoma, 166
    insulinoma, 159
  skin cancer, 10
  toxicity, 373
Focal anaplastic changes, Wilms's tumor with, 323
Focal nodular hyperplasia, liver, 532
Focal signs, with brain tumors, 278
  craniopharyngiomas, 300
  glioblastoma multiforme, 291
  metastatic, 293
  oligodendrogliomas, 293
  pituitary gland, 298
Follicle-stimulating hormone, 192, 299
Follicular carcinoma, thyroid, 41, 43
Foramen of Monro, 302

Forbes-Albright syndrome, 192, 198
Forehead flap, 49
Forequarter amputation, 262
Foster Kennedy's syndrome, 296
Fracture, pathological
  with bone metastasis, radiotherapy, 241
  with breast cancer, 73, 88
  with Cushing's syndrome, 138
  with multiple myeloma, 403, 406
  with skeletal tumors, 227, 246
Freezing, see Cryosurgery
Frontal craniotomy, 303
Frontal lobes, oligodendrogliomas, 293
Frontal lobe syndrome, 287, 295
5-FU, see 5-Flurouracil
FUDR, 499, 535
Fulguration, 497
  in bladder cancer, 591, 595
  in head and neck cancer, 26
  in nasopharyngeal tumors, 37
  rectal lesions, 496
Furosemide
  in hypercalcemia
    acute, 176
    with multiple myeloma, 406
    paraneoplastic PTH-secreting syndromes, 186
  in increased intracranial pressure, 288
  renin stimulation with, 134

G

Gaisbock's syndrome, 412
Gait disturbances,
  brain tumors and, 278
    hemangioblastomas, 297
    pediatric brainstem gliomas, 304
  in pediatric patients, 316
Galactorrhea, 192, 280, 298
Gallbladder and bilary tree, 522-525
  ectopic hormone secretion by tumors, 173, 184
  evaluation, 523
  pathological considerations, 522-523
  sarcoma botryoides, 334
  therapeutic considerations, 523-525
Gallium scans, see also Scintigraphy
  bone tumors, 226
  gastric cancer, 477
  in lymphoma staging, 358
Gamma globulin, 398, 403
Ganglioma, ectopic hormone production, ACTH, 184
Ganglion cyst, characteristics of, 222
Ganglioneuroma, 41
  mediastinal, 443, 446
  neuroblastoma, metastasis maturation to, 332
Ganglionic blockers, and renin levels, 134
Gardner's syndrome, 221, 490, 496
Gastrectomy, 481
  in carcinoid, 208

in pancreatic tumors, gastrinoma, 163
Gastric acid secretory studies, MEN-I diagnosis, 192
Gastric carcinoids, 205, 208
Gastric carcinoma, *see* Stomach, carcinoma of
Gastric pull-up, 34
Gastric secretion
  with carcinoid, 205
  with gastrinomas, 160, 192
  with vipoma, 166
Gastric transposition, head and neck cancer patient, 50
Gastric ulcer, *see* Peptic ulcer
Gastrin
  apudomas, 199
  pancreatic tumors affecting, 158, 163
  MEN-I diagnosis, 192
Gastrinoma, 158, 160-165
  apudomas, 198, 199
  carcinoid, 204
  in MEN-I, 191
Gastrocamera, gastric cancer, 475
Gastroduodenoscopy, 512
Gastrointestinal
  APUD cells, 197
  bleeding, *see also* Rectal bleeding; Stools
    in carcinoid, 203
    chemotherapy side effects, 374
    with Kaposi's sarcoma, 121
    in liver cancer, 529
    with pancreatic tumors, gastrinoma, 162
  chemotherapy and, 320, 374
  in esophageal cancer, preoperative preparation, 463
Gastrointestinal bypass, in pancreatic cancer, 517
Gastrointestinal carcinoid
  early detection and screening, 205
  postoperative care, 210
  therapeutic management, surgical, 208
Gastrointestinal series, *see also* Barium enema; Barium swallow
  with brain tumors, 280
  with carcinoid, 206
  with gastrinoma, 162
  with gynecological malignancies, 544
  with lymphomas, non-Hodgkin's, pediatric, 347
  in multiple endocrine neoplasia, diagnosis, 192
  with pancreatic carcinoma, eccrine, 511, 512
  with paraneoplastic syndrome, 185
  with parathyroid tumors, 175
  with soft-tissue sarcoma, 257
Gastrointestinal symptoms
  with gynecological malignancies, 543
  with pancreatic tumors, insulinoma, 157
  with parathyroid tumors, 173
Gastrointestinal tract tumors, *see also* specific primary sites
  anal lesions, 501, 503
  apudomas, 198
  back pain with, 219
  carcinoid, 204, 205, 208
  ectopic hormone production, 184, 186, 187

Kaposi's sarcoma, 121
  lymphomas
    adult, 355
    radiotherapy, 375
  small intestinal lesions, 504
Gastrojejunostomy, 482, 518
Gastroscopy, 206, 476
Gastrostomy, 46
Gemistocytic astrocytomas, 292
Genetic abnormalities, *see* Chromosomal abnormalities
Genetic factors, *see also* Familial disorders
  in stomach cancer, 475
  in pediatric cancer, 315
Genitourinary tract
  rhabdomyosarcoma, treatment, 336
  sarcoma botryoides, 334
  tumors of, *see* specific primary sites
  with Wilms's tumor, 315
Germ cell tumors
  mediastinal, 445, 448, 449-450
  ovarian, 565
  testis, 623, 624
Giant-cell carcinoma
  lung, 427
  pancreas, 516
Giant-cell tumors, skeletal system, 217, 219
  age incidence, 225
  age predilection, 219
  anatomic locations, 218
  behavior of, 224
  benign, 217
  characteristics of, 221
  follow-up evaluation, 228
  histological grades, 231
  versus malignant bone tumors, 226
  pathological fractures with, 227
  regional predilection of, 224
  therapeutic approaches, 237
    radiotherapy, 241
    surgery, 235
Giant cells, in histiocytosis, 348
Giant congenital hairy nevi, 114
Giant follicle lymphoma, 361
Gigantism
  apudomas, 198
  brain tumors and, 280, 283
  in multiple endocrine neoplasia-I, 192
Gliobastoma mulitiforme, 291-292
Glioblastomas, 288, 289
Gliomas
  chemotherapy, 290
  incurable lesions, 284-285
  pediatric, 303, 304
  pineal region, 300
  radiotherapy, 289
  surgery, 286
Glomus cell, 198

Glottis tumor, 14
Glucagon
    for gastric double contrast studies, 476
    pancreatic tumors affecting, 158
Glucagonoma, 158, 163, 165-166, 169
    apudomas, 198
    versus vipoma, 166
Glucagon provocation test, in pheochromocytoma, 145
Glucocorticoid receptors, leukemia cells, 343
Glucocorticoid remediable hyperaldosteronism, 133
Glucocorticoid-suppressible hyperaldosternism, therapeutic management, 135
Glucose levels
    brain tumor and, 280
    cerebrospinal fluid, in meningeal carcinomatosis, 294
    MEN-I diagnosis, 192
    pancreatic tumors, 158
        insulinoma, 157, 158, 159
        postoperative care, 160
    paraneoplastic syndromes, postoperative care, 188
    in pheochromocytoma, 145
Glucose-6-phosphate dehydrogenase, 413
Glucose tolerance, 134
    in Cushing's syndrome, 136, 138
    in gastrinomas, 192
Glucosuria, pituitary tumors and, 298
alpha-Glycerophosphate dehydrogenase, APUD cells, 197
Gly-Oxide, 48
Goiters
    colloidal, in MEN-İ, 192
    mediastinal, radiological findings, 446
Gold radiotherapy
    in bladder cancer, 595
    in mesothelioma, 457
Gonadotrophins
    in paraneoplastic endocrine syndromes, 183, 184, 188
    pituitary tumors and, 298, 299
Gonads
    brain tumors affecting, 280
        craniopharyngioma, 300
        pituitary gland, 298, 299
        pretreatment management, 283
    lymphomas involving, 346
    radiotherapy complications, 320, 365, 366
    tumors of, 436, 617, see also Gynecological malignancies;
        specific primary sites
Gonorrhea, with Kaposi's sarcoma, 121
Graft, bone, 235, 236, 237
Graft necrosis, 105
Graft versus host disease, 390
Grand mal seizures, 296
Granular cell tumor, malignant, 267, 269
Granulocytes
    chemotherapy toxicity, 624
    in leukemias
        chronic lymphocytic, 394, 395
        transfusions of, 388, 389
Grawitz's tumor, kidney, 575
Great vessels, kidney tumors and, 582

Growth, patient
    with bone tumors, 229
    with brain tumors, pituitary gland, 298
    in histiocytosis, 348
    radiotherapy and, 320
Growth factor, megakaryocytes, 413
Growth hormone, 192, 298
Growth rate, breast tumor, 83-84
Gumma, liver, 533
Gynecological malignancies, 542-570, see also specific sites
Gynecomastia, 141, 618

H

Hair dyes, and breast cancer risk, 67
Hairy cell leukemia, 395, 398-399
Haitians, Kaposi's sarcoma in, 256
Halothane, in pheochromocytoma surgery, 147
Hamartomas
    gastric lesions, 478
    liver, 532
    lung, 427
    pediatric, 337
    small intestine, 504
Hand-Schüller-Christian disease, 347-348
Haptoglobins, 396
Hartman operation, 497
Hashimoto's disease, 192
Headache, see also Increased intracranial pressure
    with adrenal tumors
        Cushing's syndrome, 138
        pheochromocytoma, 142, 144, 145
    with brain tumors
        colloid cysts, 302
        lymphomas, 301
        meningiomas, 295
        pediatric ependymomas, 304
        pineal region, 300
        pituitary gland, 298, 298
    in leukemias, acute lymphoblastic, 342
    in pediatric patients, 316
    in polycythemia vera, 411
Head and neck tumors, 5-61, see also specific sites
    age, 26
    annual incidence of, 6
    bone, chondrosarcoma, 239
    Burkitt's lymphoma, 376
    lymphomas, 357
    neuroblastomas, 150
    pediatric, 337, see also Neuroblastoma; Rhabdomyosarcoma
    rhabdomyosarcoma, 336
    skin, treatment of, 110-112
    soft-tissue sarcomas, 267
    therapy, adjuvant chemotherapy, 44-45
    therapy, advanced disease, 45-47
    therapy, general considerations, 23-29

chemotherapy, intra-arterial, 535, 536
therapy, site-specific, 29-44
Hearing loss
 with brain tumors, 278
  meningiomas, 296
  neuromas, acoustic, 301
 chemotherapy and, 564, 624
 cranial nerve removal and, 284
Heart, *see also* Cardiac status; Cardiopulmonary status
 in carcinoid syndrome, 204
 in pheochromocytoma, 145
 in primary aldosteronism, 133
Heavy-chain disease, 396, 404
Heineke-Mikulicz pyloroplasty, 466
Hemangioblastomas, 297
Hemangioendothelioma, 534
 age predilection, 219
 anatomic locations, 218
 histological grades, 231
 pediatric, 337
 therapeutic approaches, 239
Hemangiomas, 217, 219, 225
 and bone tumors, 227
 small intestine, 504
 therapeutic approaches, 237
Hemangiopericytoma, 217, 219, 267
 histological grades, 231
 malignant, 268
 therapy, 269
Hemangiosarcoma, 267, 269
Hematemesis, in gastric cancer, 476
Hematopoietic stem cells, in polycythemia vera, 411
Hematuria
 in bladder cancer, 590
 colon surgery and, 499
 with kidney tumors, 575, 576, 578
 in pediatric patients, 316
Hemianopsia, 280, 296, 298
Hemicorporectomy, 245-246
Hemiparesis, 293, 296, 304
Hemipelvectomy, 245, 262
Hemispherectomy, in glioma, 285
Hemodialysis, in hypercalcemia, acute, 176
Hemodynamic status, with pancreatic cancer, 515
Hemogram, in gynecological malignancies, 545
Hemolysis, in leukemia, 396
Hemolytic anemia
 autoimmune, 397
 with immunoblastic lymphadenopathy, 377
 with leukemias, chronic lymphocytic, 394, 395
 in myelofibrosis, splenectomy indications, 414
Hemophagocytic lymphohistiocytosis, familial, 348
Hemophiliacs, soft tissue sarcoma risk factors, 256
Hemophilic pseudotumor, radiology, 232
Hemoptysis
 in carcinoid, 203
 in lung cancer, 432, 433
 open-tube bronschoscopy in, 423
 with testicular tumors, 620
Hemorrhage, *see also* Bleeding; Gastrointestinal tract

 after gynecological surgery, 566
 kidney surgery and, 582
 in leukemias, acute lymphoblastic, 342
 lung biopsy and, 424
 mediastinoscopy and, 425, 426
 in myelofibrosis and myeloid metaplasia, 4150
 as pediatric chemotherapy complication, 320
 in polycythemia vera, 411, 413
 scalene node biopsy and, 426
 in thrombocythemia, essential , 415
Hemorrhagic cystitis, 372
Hemorrhagic sarcoma, multipe idiopathic, *see* Kaposi's sarcoma
Heparin
 in gynecological surgery, 545
 in leukemias, acute, 388
 in pancreatic surgery
  postoperative, 520
  preoperative management, 516
Hepatectomy, 533
Hepatic angiomas, 297
Hepatic artery infusion, chemotherapy, 535, 536
Hepaticojejunostomy, 524
Hepatic tumors, *see* Liver tumors
Hepatitis type B, 121, 529, 530
Hepatoblastoma, 533, 534
 ectopic gonadotrophin production, 184
 pediatric, 337
Hepatocellular adenomas, 532
Hepatocellular carcinoma, 533, 537
Hepatoma, 533
 angiography, 531
 ectopic hormone production, hypoglycemia, 184
 paraneoplastic syndrome, diagnosis, 185
Hepatomegaly, in polycythemia vera, 411
Hepatosplenomegaly
 in leukemias, acute lymphoblastic, 342
 in Waldenström's macroglobulinemia, 378
Hepatotoxicity, of chemotherapeutic agents, 372, 374
Herbicides, soft tissue sarcoma risk factors, 256
Hernia, colorectal cancer, 489, 490
Herniation
 with brain tumors, 285
  surgical goals, 287
  therapeutic goals, 286
 pneumonectomy and, 437
Herpes simplex virus infections, 121, 541, 543
Herpes zoster, 395
Heterotopias, liver, 533
Hexa-CAF, ovarian cancer, 563
Hexamethylmelamine
 lung cancer, 434, 435
 multiple myeloma, 406
 ovarian cancer, 563
 toxicity, 373
Hilar node involvement, in lung cancer, 432
Hip disarticulation, 245, 262
Hippel-Lindau disease, 297
Hirsutism
 with brain tumors, 280, 298
 in Cushing's syndrome, 136, 138

Histamine, 203, 205
Histamine provocation test, in pheochromocytoma, 145
Histamine receptor blocker, in gastrinoma, 162
Histiocytic lymphoma, 217, 360, 361, 362
    brain, 301
    chemotherapy, 371
    leukemias, chronic, lymphocytic, 396
    pediatric, 346
Histiocytic medullary reticulosis, 377-378
Histiocytomas, malignant
    age predilection, 219
    therapy, 269
Histiocytoses, 347-348
    lung, 427
    malignant, 377-378
    pediatric, 347-348
Histiocytosis X, 347-348, 427
    age, 348
Histogenesis, of mesenchymal tumors, 218
Hives, chemotherapy side effects, 374
HLA DR-5, with Kaposi's sarcoma, 121
Hodgkin's lymphoma, see Lymphomas
Homer Wright rosettes, 330
Homonymous hemianopsia, 280, 284, 296
Homosexuals, Kaposi's sarcoma risk, 121, 256
Hormone therapy, 88
    bone metastasis, 240
    breast cancer, 85
        adjuvant therapy, 85
        advanced, 88
        recurrent, 89, 90
    endometrial cancer, 562
    genitourinary tumors, prostate, 610
    prostatic cancer, 604, 609
        advanced, 610
        psychiatric complications, 607
Hormone receptors
    breast cancer, 72
        adjuvant therapy, 84, 85
        in pregnancy, 81
        and prognosis, 86
    endometrial cancer, 562
Hormone-secreting tumors, see Endocrine tumors; specific glands
Hormone therapy, 88
    bone metastasis, 240
    breast cancer, 85
        adjuvant therapy, 85
        advanced, 88
        recurrent, 89, 90
    endometrial cancer, 562
    genitourinary tumors, prostate, 610
    prostatic cancer, 604, 609
        advanced, 610
        psychiatric complications, 607
Horner's syndrome, mediastinal tumors, 446
5-HTP, 203
Human chorionic gonadotrophins (HCG)
    brain tumors and, 280, 300
    in germ cell tumors, mediastinal, 445, 449

    in ovarian tumors, 565
    in pediatric tumors, 316
    in testicular tumors, 618, 619, 620, 623, 625
Human T cell virus (HTLV-I), 122
Hutchinson's freckle, 102, 113
Hyaluronic acid, 456
Hydantoin, 377
Hydrea, see Hydroxyurea
Hydrocarbons, and skin cancer, 99
Hydrocele, 618, 619
Hydrocephalus, with brain tumors
    craniopharyngioma, 300
    hemangioblastomas, 297
    meningiomas, 296
    metastatic, 293
    neuromas, acoustic, 301
    pineal region, 300
    therapeutic goals, 286, 287
    colloid cysts and, 302
    decompression surgery, 285
Hydrocortisone, see Corticosteroid
Hydronephrosis, 556, 604
Hydrothorax, 21, 566
Hydroureteronephrosis, bladder cancer, 591
5-Hydroxyindoleacetic acid, 139, 504
17-Hydroxyprogesterone caproate, 562
5-Hydroxytryptamine, 197, 204, see also Apudomas
Hydroxyurea
    in head and neck tumors, 46
    in leukemias, chronic myelocytic, 345, 393
    in liver tumors, 534
    in melanoma, 118
    in polycythemia vera, 413
    toxicity, 373
Hyperaldosteronism, see Primary hyperaldosteronism
Hyperalimentation
    in bladder cancer, 591, 596
    in colorectal cancer, preoperative, 491
    with gastric surgery, 483
    in head and neck cancer, 10, 21, 45
    in kidney tumors, preoperative, 578
    in liver tumors, preoperative, 532
    in ovarian cancer, advanced, 566
    in pancreatic cancer
        postoperative, 520
        preoperative, 515
Hypercalcemia, 41, see also Hyperparathyroidism
    breast cancer, 73, 89
    gastrinomas, 192
    kidney tumors, 576
    liver tumors, 530
    lung cancer, palliative resection indications, 432
    lymphomas, adult, 355
    multiple myeloma, 403, 405
    neoplasms associated with, 184
    paraneoplastic syndromes
        pseudohyperparathyroidism, 184-187
    parathyroid tumors
        differential diagnosis, 175

laboratory tests, 175
    preoperative preparation, 176
Hypercalcitonemia, apudomas, 198
Hyperglycemia
    brain tumor and, 280
    rebound, 159
Hyperglycemic syndrome, 158, 163, 165-167, 169
Hyperkalemia, with paraneoplastic syndromes, 188
Hypernatremia, with paraneoplastic syndromes, 185
Hypernephroma, 297, 531, 575
Hyperostosis, meningiomas and, 296, 297
Hyperparathyroidism, 41, *see also* Parathyroid tumors
    and bone tumors, 227
    multiple endocrine neoplasia type I, 191
    multiple endocrine neoplasia type II, 194
    paraneoplastic endocrine syndromes, 183
Hyperplasia
    gallbladder, 522
    parathyroid, 176
Hyperplastic polyps
    colorectal, cancer risk, 490
    gastric lesions, 478
Hypersplenism, in chronic lymphocytic leukemias, 397
Hypertension
    in adrenal angiography, 146
    after adrenalectomy, 148
    with apudomas, 198
    with brain tumors, 280, 298
    in Cushing's syndrome, 138
    and gynecological malignancy, 541
    with kidney tumors, 578
    with mediastinal tumors, 446
    in pheochromocytoma, 142, 144-145
        surgical management, 146-147
        types of, 144
    in primary aldosteronism, 133
        postoperative care, 136
        preoperative preparations, 135
Hyperthermia
    bladder cancer, 596
    chemotherapy intra-arterial, 536
    melanoma, 118
    skin cancer, treatment complications, 106
Hyperthyroidism
    and hypercalcemia, 175
    versus vipoma, 166
Hypertonic saline, in ectopic ADH syndrome, 187
Hypertrophic osteoarthropathy
    with lung cancer, 422, 427
    with mediastinal tumors, 446
Hyperuricemia
    with leukemia, acute, 385
    with lymphomas, 346, 376
    with multiple myeloma, 406
Hyperviscosity, 405, 407
Hypervitaminoses A and C, and hypercalcemia, 175
Hypocalcemia
    in leukemia, acute, 385
    after parathyroid surgery, 178
Hypocalcemic alkalosis, in primary aldosteronism, 135

Hypochlorhydria, in gastrinomas, 192
Hypogammaglobulinemia
    with leukemias, chronic lymphocytic, 394, 396
    with mediastinal tumor, 446
Hypoglossal nerve, in salivary gland tumors, 40
Hypoglycemia
    with apudomas, 198
    with liver tumors, 530
    with mesothelioma, 456
    with pancreatic tumors, 157, 158, 159, 184
    with paraneoplastic endocrine syndromes, 183, 185-188
Hypogonadism
    with apudomas, 198
    with pituitary tumors, 192, 298
Hypokalemia
    with gastrinomas, 192
    with paraneoplastic endocrine syndromes, 183, 186
    in primary aldosteronism, 133
Hypokalemic alkalosis, 133, 134
Hypomagnesemia, chemotherapy toxicity, 624
Hyponatremia, with paraneoplastic syndrome, 185, 187
Hypopharynx, cancer of
    annual incidence of, 6
    cervical node metastases, occult, 28
    early signs, 7
    examination of, 6
    five-year relative survival, 23
    follow-up schedule, 51
    management algorithm, 57
    site-specific data form, 13-14
    therapeutic guidelines, 34
    tumor classification, 14
Hypophysectomy, 88
    in breast cancer, 79
    transsphenoidal, 141
Hypophysis
    APUD cells, 197
    brain tumor origination in, 284
Hypopituitarism, 300
Hypotension
    in carcinoid surgery, 208
    chemotherapeutic agents and, 372
Hypothalamus
    brain tumors and, 278, 279, 296
    pituitary tumors and, 298
Hypothyroidism, 320, 365
Hypotonic duodenography, 511
Hysterectomy
    in cervical carcinoma, 557
    in ovarian cancer, 565
    on uterine cancer, 560, 561
Hysterovaginectomy, in rhabdomyosarcoma, 336

I

Idiopathic hemorrhagic sarcoma, multiple, *see* Kaposi's sarcoma
Idiopathic thrombocytopenic purpura, 395
Ileal carcinoids, bone metastases with, 204

Ileal conduit
    with bladder cancer, 595
    with prostate surgery, 607
Ileostomy
    bladder cancer, 596
    colorectal cancer, 497
Ilioinguinal node dissection, in melanoma, 116-117
Immune system, *see also* Leukemias; Lymphomas; Multiple myeloma
    in leukemias, chronic, 398, 399
    in lymphoma, Hodgkin's, 359
    nutritional deficiency and, 10
Immunization, with splenectomy, 346
Immunoblastic lymphadenopathy, 377
Immunodeficiency, *see* Immunosuppression
Immunoelectrophoresis
    leukemias, acute, 386
    leukemias, chronic, lymphocytic, 396
    multiple myeloma, 403, 404
Immunoglobulins
    leukemias, chronic lymphocytic, 394, 395, 396
    IgM, in Waldenstrom's macroglobulinemia, 378
    in multiple myeloma, 403
Immunological markers, *see* Markers
Immunologic status, in nutritional deficiencies, 21
Immunoreactive insulin/glucose ratio, in insulinoma,
    in lymphoblastic lymphadenopathy, 377
    in lymphomas
        adult, 355
        brain, 301
        rehabilitation considerations, 379
    with splenectomy, 346
Immunotherapy
    bladder cancer, 596
    head and neck cancer, 27
    Kaposi's sarcoma, 121
    skin cancer, melanoma, 117
Implants, breast, 92
Impotence
    with brain tumor, 280
    colorectal surgery and, 492
    with Cushing's syndrome, 138
    with prostatic cancer, 607, 608, 609, 612
Incontinence, *see also* Sphincteric dysfunction
    brain tumors and, 295
    prostate tumors and, 607, 608, 612
    spinal cord compression and, 295
Increased intracranial pressure, 278
    craniopharyngioma, 300
    glioblastoma multiforme, 291
    hemangioblastomas, 297
    inadequate management of, 285
    meningiomas, 296
    metastatic, 293
    oligodendrogliomas, 293
    osteocytomas, 292
    preoperative control of, 283
    therapeutic goals, 286-287
Inderal, in pheochromocytoma surgery, 147

Indomethacin
    in hypercalcemia, 185, 186
    with vipoma, 166
Industrial hazards, *see* Occupational exposure
Infection
    versus bone tumors, 226
    in brain tumors
        epidermoid and dermoid cysts, 302
        pituitary gland, 298
    with chest surgery, 438
    in genitourinary cancer
        bladder, 590
        kidney, 578
    after gynecological surgery, 566
    in leukemias, acute, 385, 388
        acute lymphoblastic, 342
        chemotherapy complications, 388
    in leukemia, chronic
        hairy cell, 398
        lymphocytic, 394, 397
    in lymphoma
        adult, 355
        Hodgkin's, treatment, 378
        rehabilitation considerations, 379
    in lung cancer, 438-439
    mediastinoscopy and, 426
    in meningeal carcinomatosis, 294
    in multiple myeloma, 403
    in myelofibrosis and myeloid metaplasia, 415
    in prostatic cancer, 608
    and skin cancer, 99-100
    skin cancer treatment complications, 105
    and thrombocytosis, reactive, 415
Infectious mononucleosis, 356
Infiltrating carcinoma
    bladder, 592
    lobular, of breast, 77
Inflammation and inflammatory processes
    brain, 289
    fibroid polyps, gastric lesions, 478
    in Hodgkin's lymphoma, 359
    pseudotumors, lung, 427
    in testicular cancer, 619
Infusion pumps
    in head and neck tumors, 46
    in liver cancer, 534-536
Inguinal lymphadenopathy, 542
Inoperability criteria, with lung tumors, 431
Insulin
    in multiple endocrine neoplasia syndrome (MEN-I), 192
    after pancreatic surgery, 520
    pancreatic tumors affecting, 158
    in paraneoplastic syndrome, 187
Insulinoma, 157-161
    apudomas, 198, 199
    in multiple endocrine neoplasia (MEN-I), 191
Insulin suppression test, 157
Intermediate-cell carcinoma, lung, 427

Intermittent claudication, in polycythemia vera, 411
Internal carotid artery, with pituitary tumors, 298
Interstitial radioactive implants
    bladder cancer, 595
    lung cancer, 432
    mesiotheliomas, 457
    prostate cancer, 609
    skin cancer, 109
    rhabdomyosarcoma, 336
    soft tissue sarcoma, 264
Intestinal carcinoid, 203-205
    multiple endocrine neoplasia (MEN-I), 192
    therapeutic management, surgical, 208
Intestinal obstruction
    in carcinoid, 203
    colon surgery and, 499
    in colorectal cancer, 491, 492
    gastric surgery and, 482
    in leukemia, 397
    in ovarian cancer, advanced, 566
    in pediatric patients, 316
    with small intestine tumors, 504
Intestinal resection, with prostate surgery, 607
Intestine, APUD cells, 197, *see also* Bowel involvement; Colorectal
        cancer; Small intestine tumors
Intracavitary radiotherapy
    colorectal cancer, 498
    endometrial carcinoma, 561
    mesiotheliomas, 457
    ovarian cancer, 564
    perforation of uterus, 558
Intraductal carcinoma, breast, 77, 79
Intradural extramedullary lesions, spine, 287
Intraepithelial carcinoma, penis, 629
Intrahepatic bile duct cystadenomas, 532
Intramedullary lesions, spine, 287
Intraosseous fibrosarcoma, therapeutic approaches, 237
Intraperitoneal bleeding, in liver cancer, 529
Intraperitoneal radioisotopes, *see* Intracavitary radiotherapy
Intravenous hyperalimentation, *see* Hyperalimentation
Intravenous pyelogram/urogram (IUP)
    with adrenal tumors
        Cushing's syndrome, 139-140
        neuroblastoma, 150
        pheochromocytoma, 144
        primary aldosteronism, 135
    with brain tumors, 280, 294
    with colorectal cancer, 491
    with genitourinary tumors
        bladder, 590-591
        kidney, 575, 576, 577, 585
        penis, 630
        prostate, 602
        testis, 619
    with gynecological malignances, 544
    with liver tumors, pediatric, 337
    in lymphomas
        Burkitt's, 377
        pediatric, 347
        staging work-up, 357

    with paraneoplastic syndrome, 185
    with parathyroid tumors, 175
    with pediatric solid tumors, 316, 317
    in polycythemia vera, 412
    with soft-tissue sarcomas, 257
Intussusception, in pediatric patients, 316
In-utero exposure, and gynecological malignancy, 541
Invasive carcinomas, breast, 79
In vitro cultures
    leukemia cells, 386
    myeloma cells, 406
Iodine 131 cholesterol adrenal scan, in Cushing's syndrome, 140
Iodine therapy, radioactive
    in bladder cancer, 595
    in lung cancer, 432
    in mesothelioma, 457
    in thyroid tumors, 44
Iodophendylate, 295
Iridium brachytherapy, soft tissue sarcoma, 264
Iron stores, in polycythemia vera, 413
Irradiation, *see* Radiation; Radiotherapy
Ischemia, brain tumors, surgical goals, 287
Islet cells, APUD cells, 197
Islet cell tumors, *see also* Pancreatic tumors, endocrine
    insulinomas, *see* Insulinomas
    multiple endocrine neoplasia type I, 191-192
Isoniazid, in leukemias, acute, 388
Isotope scans, *see* Scintigraphy
Isthmusectomy, thyroid, 43

J

Jaundice, 523
    with leukemias, chronic, lymphocytic, 395
    with liver tumors, 529, 530
    with lymphomas, adult, 355
    with pancreatic cancer, 509, 510
    radiological diagnostic approach, 523-524
    with small intestinal tumors, 504
Jejunal line, 578
Jejunal loop, 482
Jejunojejunostomy, 482, 517
Jejunostomy feedings, 483
Joint replacement, 235, 240
Junctional nevus, malignant potential, 113
Juvenile polyps, gastrointestinal tract, 478, 490
Juxtacortical osteoma, 221
Juxtacortical osteosarcoma, 217, 219, 232

K

Kallikrein, 208
Kaposi's sarcoma, 267
    in Africans, 256
    histological grades, 231
    skin lesions, 121-122

symptoms, 255
therapeutic guidelines, 268-269
Karyotyping, in leukemias
acute, 386, 388
chronic myelocytic, 392, 393
Keloid, skin cancer treatment complications, 106
Keratoacanthoma, 102, 110
Ketosteroids, in Cushing's syndrome, 139
Kidney function, *see* Renal failure; Renal function
Kidney invasion, adrenal carcinoma, 141
Kidney stones, *see* Calculi
Kidney tumors, 575-586, *see also* Renal cell carcinoma; Wilms's tumor
ectopic hormone production by, 183
ACTH, 184
parathyroid hormone, 173, 175
with hemangioblastomas, 297
and hypercalcemia, 175
pediatric, 316
Kiel classification, lymphoma, 360, 361
Knudsen theory of carcinogenesis, 315
Krukenberg tumor, 481
Kulchitsky cells, 504
Kupffer's cells, and scintigraphy, 530

L

Labeling index, in acute leukemias, 386
Laminectomy, 287
brain tumors, meningiomas, 297
breast cancer, 88
neuroblastoma, 333
Laparoscopy
for liver tumors, 531
in lung cancer, 426
in pancreatic tumor, 512
radiology, 544
Laparotomy
biliary tree carcinomas, 523
gastric cancer, 477
lymphoma, staging work-up, 347, 357-358
neuroblastoma, 333
Large-cell carcinoma
ADH-producing, 184
lung, 427, 434-435
pancreatic, 516
Large intestine, *see* Bowel involvement; Colorectal cancer
Laryngeal edema, 48, 178
Laryngeal nerve paralysis, 428
Laryngectomy
indications for, 32, 33-34
postoperative care, 48
preoperative preparations, 22
rehabilitation after, 51-52
supraglottic, 32
total, 32
Laryngogram, 9

Laryngoscopy, 6, 8, 9, 174
Laryngospasm, 424
Larynx, cancer of
annual incidence of, 6
cervical node metastases, occult, 28
early signs, 7
five-year survival with, 23
follow-up schedule, 51
management algorithm, 57
prostheses, 50
site-specific data sheet, 13-14
therapeutic guidelines, 32-33
tobacco use and, 5
Laser surgery
with brain tumors, 288
in head and neck cancer, 26
in skin cancer, 109-111
in vulvar carcinoma, 546
with vocal cord lesions, 33
Leiomyomas, small intestine, 504
Leiomyomatous hamartomas, lung, 427
Leiomyosarcoma, 267, 268
esophagus, 461
kidney, 575
stomach, 477, 478
symptoms, 255
therapeutic guidelines, 268
Lennert classification, lymphoma, 360
Lentigo maligna, 102, 113, 114
Leptomeninges
brain tumor origination in, 284
metastases, chemotherapy with, 290
Letterer-Siwe disease, 347-348
Leucovorin, in skeletal tumors, 242
Leukemias
age incidence, 225
bone metastasis, 219
brain, chemotherapy, 290
ectopic hormone production, hypoglycemia, 184
with Kaposi's sarcoma, 122
in myelofibrosis and myeloid metaplasia, 415
polycythemia vera treatment and, 413
as treatment complication
with Hodgkin's disease, 367, 368
with radiotherapy, 365, 366
Leukemias, acute, 385-393
bone marrow transplantation, 390
central nervous system involvement, 390
lymphoblastic (ALL), 385
adult, 389-390
cytochemical typing, 386, 387
pediatric, 341-344
myeloblastic, pediatric, 344-345
myelocytic, cytochemical typing, 386, 387
myelogenous (AML), 385, 388-389
myeloid, chronic myleogenous leukemia and, 392, 393
myelomonoleukemia, cytochemical typing, 386, 387
nonmyeloblastic (ANL), 385

promyelocytic, consumption coagulopathy with, 388
relapsed, 390-391
smoldering, 390
undifferentiated (AUL)
  adult, 385
  pediatric, 345
Leukemias, chronic lymphocytic, 394-398
Leukemias, chronic myelocytic, 391-394
Leukemias, hairy cell, 398-399
Leukemias, pediatric, 316
  acute lymphoblastic, 341-344
  acute myeloblastic, 344-345
  acute undifferentiated, 345
  chronic myelocytic, 345
  classification, 341
Leukocyte alkaline phosphatase, 386, 412, 414
Leukocytosis, *see* White cell count
Leukopenia, *see also* Myelosuppression
  chemotherapy and, 372-374, 624
    Adriamycin, 242
    in pediatric patients, 320
  lung cancer patient, 431
  lymphoma patient, 379
Leukophoresis, 393
Leukoplakia
  oral, 24, 29-30
  penis, 629
  vulva, 542
Leydig's cell tumors, 617
Lhermitte's sign, 288, 289
Light-chain excretion, multiple myeloma, 403, 404
Limb-salvage surgery, skeletal tumors, 242
Lineal accelerator sharp beams, spinal cord tumors, 303
Linear tomography, bone tumors, 228
Linitis plastica variant, colon, 495
Lip cancer
  annual incidence of, 6
  five-year relative survival, 23
  treatment, 30, 111
Lipid-soluble drugs, and chemotherapy, 290
Lipoblastic liposarcoma, 267
Lipomas, 256
  mediastinal, 445
  multiple endocrine neoplasia (MEN-I), 192
  small intestine, 504
Liposarcoma
  histological grades, 231
  mediastinal, 445
  radiosensitivity of, 263
  symptoms, 255
  therapy, 267, 268, 269
Lithium, in ectopic ADH syndrome, 187
Liver
  chemotherapy drug toxicity, 372
  in gastric cancer, 476
  hemangioblastomas, lesions with, 297
  in histiocytosis, 348
  in immunoblastic lymphadenopathy, 377

kidney tumors and, 576
in leukemias
  acute, 385
  chronic lymphocytic, 394
with lung cancer, 431
lymphoma staging, 357
in mycosis fungoides, 377
in myelofibrosis, 413
in polycythemia vera, 411
in Waldenström's macroglobulinemia, 378
Liver metastasis
  with adrenal carcinoma, 141
  with alimentary tract tumors
    colorectum, 490, 491, 496
    esophagus, 462, 463
    stomach, 481, 483
  angiography, 531
  with bone metastasis, 240
  with breast cancer, 72
    palliative therapy, 83
    and prognosis, 86
    scintigraphy, 73
  with carcinoid, 204, 210
  CAT scan detection of, 318
  with lung cancer, radiotherapy, 433
  in pediatric tumors
    evaluation techniques, 318
    Wilms's tumor, treatment of, 330
  in soft tissue sarcomas, bone scan in, 257
  treatment, chemotherapy, 535-536
Liver tumors, 529-536
  pediatric, 316, 336
Lobectomy, thyroid, 43
Lobular carcinoma, breast, 79
Local excision, skin cancer, histology and, 110
Lomustine, *see* CCNU
Low-grade central osteosarcoma, 219
Low-grade chondrosarcomas, biopsy of, 232
L-PAM, breast cancer, *see* Phenylalanine mustard
Lukes and Collins classification, lymphomas, 360, 361
Lumbar puncture, *see* Cerebrospinal fluid
Lumpectomy, 76
Lundt test, 510
Lung cancer, *see also* Mediastinal tumors; Mesotheliomas, 421-440
  apudomas, 198
  bone metastasis, 219
  brain metastasis, 293, 294
  bronchial carcinoid, 203
    early detection and screening, 205
    postoperative care, 210
    surgical management, 210
  ectopic hormone production by, 183
    ACTH, 184
    ADH, 184
    and Cushing's syndrome, 136, 142
    PTH-secreting, 173, 175
  and hypercalcemia, 175
  liver metastasis, 531

mediastinal symptoms, 446
melanomas, 427
in superior vena cava syndrome, 451
Lung metastasis
in adrenal carcinoma, 141
with bone metastasis, 240
in bone tumors, 230
diagnostic clues, 231, 232
follow-up studies, 244
radiation therapy of, 240-241
radiological studies, 229
thoracotomy in, 243
in brain tumor, evaluation, 280
in breast cancer, 72
chest x-rays, 73
palliative therapy, 83
pleural effusion management, 88
and prognosis, 86
in carcinoid, 204
in esophageal cancer, 462
in gastric cancer, 481, 483
in leukemias, chronic lymphocytic, 397
in lymphomas, adult, 355
in melanomas, 427
in pediatric tumors, 316, 318
treatment of, 436-437
in Wilms's tumor, treatment of, 330
Lungs
in mycosis fungoides, 377
therapy complications
bleomycin toxicity, 625
chemotherapeutic agents, toxicity of, 373, 374, 625
radiotherapy, 365
Lung scans, see Scintigraphy
Luteinizing hormone, 299
Lye strictures, 461
Lymphadenectomy
in adrenal neuroblastoma, 150
in prostatic cancer, 608
regional, 159
in skin cancer, melanoma, 115-117
with vulvectomy, 546
Lymphadenopathy
immunoblastic, 377
with lung cancer, 422
with lymphomas, adult, 356
in pediatric patients, 316
in Waldenstrom's macroglobulinemia, 378
Lymphangiogram
in bone tumors, 228, 229
in colorectal cancer, 491
in genitourinary tumors
bladder, 591
penis, 630
testis, 619
in gynecological malignancies, 544
with lymphomas, 358
pediatric, 346
staging work-up, 357

in rhabdomyosarcoma, 336
in soft-tissue sarcoma, 257
Lymphangiomas, small intestine, 504
Lymphangiosarcoma, 267, 268, 269
Lymphatic system, see Leukemias; Lymphomas; Multiple myeloma
Lymphedema
after gynecological surgery, 566
after mastectomy, 91-92
with prostatic cancer, 608
Lymph fistula, scalene node biopsy and, 426
Lymph nodes, see specific tumor types and primary sites
Lymphoblastic leukemia, acute
adult, 389-390
pediatric, 341-344
Lymphoblastic lymphoma
chemotherapy, 371
pediatric, 346
Lymphocele, prostatic cancer, 608
Lymphocytes
in leukemias
chronic lymphocytic, 395, 396
acute, surface markers in, 342, 386
in lymphomas, 359
Hodgkin's, pediatric, 346
immunoblastic lymphadenopathy, 377
Lymphocytic leukemia, chronic, 394-398
Lymphoepithelial carcinomas, nasopharyngeal, 37
Lymphohistiocytosis, familial hemophagocytic, 348
Lymphoid hyperplasia, gastric lesions, 478
Lymphomas, 355-381
age incidence, 225
alimentary tract involvement
anus, 501
liver, 357
small intestine, 504
stomach, 477, 478
annual incidence of, 6
behavior of, 225
bone lesions, 217, 219
Burkitt's, 376-377
CNS involvement, brain, 279, 301
chemotherapy, 290
origin of, 284
radiosensitivity of, 290
CNS involvement, spine, 287, 288
ectopic hormone production, hypoglycemia, 184
head and neck
nasopharynx, 37
paranasal sinus, 35
therapeutic modality selection, 25
histiocytic medullary reticulosis, 377-378
immunoblastic lymphadenopathy, 377
with Kaposi's sarcoma, 122
kidney, 575
lung, 427
mediastinal, 444
incidence and location of, 443
radiological findings, 446
symptoms, 446

therapeutic management, 448
mycosis fungoides, 377
pediatric, 345-348
  diagnosis, 316
  histiocytoses, 347-348
  Hodgkin's, 346, 366
  non-Hodgkin's, 346-347
Sézary syndrome, 377
therapeutic management, Hodgkin's disease, 362, 365-369
  basic principles, 362, 365
  chemotherapy, 366-368
  radiotherapy, 233, 365-366
  stage-specific guidelines, 368-369
therapeutic management, non-Hodgkin's lymphoma, 369-376
  central nervous system involvement, 376
  criteria for therapy, 369
  curability, potential, 371
  diffuse lymphomas, 370
  extranodal sites, 375-376
  hyperuricemia, 376
  nodular lymphomas, 369-370
  radiotherapy, 233, 375-376
  stage-specific, 370-371
Waldenström's macroglobulinemia, 378
Lymphoplasmocytic infiltrates, stomach, 481
Lymphoproliferative disease, lung, 427
Lymphosarcoma, 361
Lymphosarcoma cell leukemia, 395

M

MACC, lung cancer, 434
Macroglobulinemia, in multiple myeloma, 407
Mafucci's syndrome, 220
Malabsorption syndromes, 158, 198
Malignant fibrous histiocytoma, 267, 268
  behavior of, 225
  therapeutic guidelines, 268
Malignant fibrous tumors, 268
Malignant giant-cell tumor, 267
Malignant granular cell tumor, 267
Malignant hemangioendothelioma, 239
Malignant hemangiopericytoma, 268
Malignant histiocytosis, 377-378
Malignant hypertension, in pheochromocytoma, 145
Malignant melanoma, *see* Melanoma
Malignant mesenchymoma, 267
Malignant mixed tumor, salivary gland, 39
Malignant pleomorphic fibrous histiocytoma, 267
Malignant schwannoma, 267, 268
Malignant synovioma, 231
Malnutrition, *see* Nutritional status
Mammary dysplasia, 71
Mammography, 69-71, 72, 91

Mandible
  Burkitt's lymphoma, 376
  in parathyroid tumors, 174
  after radiation, 49
Mandibulectomy, prostheses, 50
Mannitol, 283, 288
Marcus Gunn pupil, 298
Marijuana, with Kaposi's sarcoma, 121
Marjolin's ulcer, 99, 106
Markers
  brain metastases, 294
  brain tumors, 280
  colorectal cancer, 490-491
  germ cell tumors, *see* Alpha-fetoprotein; Human
     chorionic gonadotrophins
  leukemias, acute lymphoblastic, 341-342, 343, 348
  leukemias, chronic
    lymphocytic, 395
    myelocytic, 393
  liver tumors, 337, 530
  mediastinal tumors, 445, 449
  ovarian tumors, 565
  pancreatic carcinoma, eccrine, 510
  pediatric tumors, 316, 337
  testicular tumors, 617, 619, 620, 623, 625
Marrow, *see* Bone marrow
Mast cells, 392
Mastectomy
  in carcinoma *in situ*, 77
  clean-up, 73, 78, 85
  lymphedema management, 91-92
  postoperative management, 90-91
  in pregnancy, 81
  prophylactic, 93
  rehabilitation, 91-93
  stage and, 77, 78
  types of
    defined, 76-77
    stages of disease and, 77-78
Maxilla
  in occult cervical node metastases, 28
  in parathyroid tumors, 174
Maxillary sinus tumors
  management algorithm, 58
  TNM classification of cancer, 16
Maxillary tumors
  Burkitt's lymphoma, 376
  follow-up schedule, 51
Maxillectomy
  antibiotic prophylaxes, 22
  postoperative care, 48
  prosthetic rehabilitation, 50
  salivary gland tumors, 40
  types of, 36-37
M-component, multiple myeloma, 404, 405
MEA, *see* Multiple endocrine neoplasia (MEN)
Mechlorethamine, *see* Nitrogen mustard

Mediastinal mass
  in chronic lymphocytic leukemia, 397
  in lymphoma, non-Hodgkin's
    pediatric, 346
    radiotherapy, 366
  neuroblastomas, 150
Mediastinal node involvement, in lung cancer
  radiotherapy, 432
  staging criteria, 428
  surgery contraindication, 431
Mediastinal shift, pneumonectomy and, 437
Mediastinal tumors, 443-451
  lung cancer, 423
  neuroblastoma, 333
  pediatric, teratomas, 337
    superior vena cava syndrome, 450-451
Mediastinoscopy
  in lung cancer, 425-426
  with mediastinal tumors, 447
  in superior vena cava syndrome, 451
Medroxyprogesterone acetate, in endometrial cancer, 562
Medullary carcinoma, of breast, 79
Medullary carcinoma, of thyroid, 41
  apudomas, 198, 199
  ectopic hormone production, ACTH, 184
  multiple endocrine neoplasia type II, 193
  surgery, 43
  versus vipoma, 166
Medullary osteoma, characteristics of, 221
Medullary reticulosis, histiocytic, 377-378
Medulloblastomas
  chemotherapy, 290
  in children, 303
  pediatric, 303-304
  radiosensitivity of, 289, 290
  surgical approaches, 286
Megakaryocytes
  growth factors, 413
  in leukemia, chronic myelocytic, 392
  in thrombocythemia, essential, 415
Megathrombocytes, 392
Megavoltage radiotherapy, bladder cancer, 595
Melanoblasts, as APUD cells, 197
Melanocyte-stimulating hormone, 142, 192, 427
Melanoma, 113-119
  anal, 501
  annual incidence of, 6
  apudomas, 198
  biopsy, 102
  chemotherapy intra-arterial, 535-536
  esophagus, 461
  gastric, 478
  metastasis
    bone, 219
    brain, 294
    liver, 535
    small intestine, 504
  patient evaluation, 114-115

Melanoma *in situ*, 113
Melanotic freckle, 102, 113
Melena, gastric cancer, 476
Melorheostosis, 226
Melphalan
  multiple myeloma, 104, 105, 106
  testicular cancer, 624
  toxicity, 373
  Waldenström's macroglobulinemia, 378
Menetrier's disease, 478
MEN, *see* Multiple endocrine neoplasia
Meningeal carcinomatosis, 279, 290, 294
Meningeal involvement
  breast cancer, 88
  pediatric lymphoma, 346
Meningiomas, 256, 295-297
  chemotherapy, 290
  radiotherapy, 289
  spine, 287
  x-ray finding with, 279
Meningiomatosis, 297
Meningitis, 302, 342, 348
Meningoceles, mediastinal, 444
Meningoencephalitis, 348
Menopausal status, and breast cancer treatment, 89, 90
  chemotherapy, 84, 85, 88
  prognosis, 86
Menstrual history
  and breast cancer risk, 67, 70
  in gynecological malignancies, 543
Mental status, *see also* Psychiatric and psychological considerations
  brain tumors, 277
    colloid cysts, 303
    craniopharyngiomas, 300
    glioblastoma multiforme, 291
    lymphomas, 301
    meningeal carcinomatosis, 294
    nursing care, 304-305
  with endocrine tumors
    Cushing's syndrome, 138
    insulinoma, 157
    paraneoplastic endocrine syndromes, 183
    parathyroid, 173
MER, melanoma, 118
6-Mercaptopurine
  in histiocytosis, 348
  in leukemias
    acute, adult lymphoblastic, 389
    chronic myelocytic, 394
  toxicity, 373
Mercury-based fixatives, for lymphomas, 356
Mesenchymal tumors, 217, 218
  chondrosarcoma, 219, 223
  ectopic hormone production, hypoglycemia, 184, 187
  histogenesis of, 218
  mediastinal, 427, 445
Mesenchymomas, lung, 427
Mesenteric mass, Burkitt's lymphoma, 376

Mesenteric thrombosis, in polycythemia vera, 411
Mesotheliomas, 455-458
    mediastinal, 445
    paraneoplastic syndrome, hypoglycemia, 187
    symptoms, 255
Metabolic abnormalities
    in Cushing's syndrome, 138
    in prostatic cancer, 604, 609
Metabolic rate, in pheochromocytoma, 145
Metachromasia, APUD cells, 197
Metanephrine, in pheochromocytoma, 145, 194
Metaplasia
    lung carcinoid tumors, 427
    and stomach cancer, 475
Metapyrone test, 139
Metastasis, *see* specific primary and metastatic sites
Methadone, 46, 520
Methotrexate
    bladder cancer, 596
    bone tumors, osteosarcoma, 238, 241, 242, 243
    brain tumors, 290
        meningeal carcinomatosis, 294
        pineal region, 300
    breast cancer
        adjuvant therapy, 84
        dosages and response rates, 87
        metastatic, 88
    carcinoid, 210
    esophageal cancer, 467
    in head and neck tumors, 44-45
    leukemia, 391
        acute lymphoblastic, 342, 344, 389
        chronic myelocytic, 394
    lung cancer, 434, 435
    lymphoma, non-Hodgkin's, Burkitt's, 377
    mycosis fungoides, 121
    penile cancer, 631
    skeletal tumors, 242, 243
    soft tissue sarcoma, 265
    toxicity, 373
    vulvar tumor, 546
Methoxamine, carcinoid surgery, 208
Methyl-chloroethyl cyclohexyl nitrosourea (CCNU)
    adrenal tumors, 141
    colorectal cancer, 499
    gastric cancer, 483
Methyldopa, 134, 207
Methylmethacrylate, 235, 238
Methylprednisone, 294
alpha-Methyl-*p*-tyrosine (MPT), in pheochromocytoma, 147
Methysergide, 207, 208
Metrizamide, 288, 297
Metronidazole, 498
Metyrapone, 142, 187
Microadenocarcinoma, pancreatic, 516
Microgliomas, brain, 301
Micrometastases, breast tumor, 83
Microvasculature, in skin cancer treatment, 113

Midbrain tumor, radiotherapy, 289
Milk-alkali syndrome, and hypercalcemia, 175
Mineralocorticoids, after adrenalectomy, 148
Minithoracotomy, mediastinal tumors, 447
Minor salivary gland tumors, 38-40
    nasal fossa, 35
Mithramycin
    in hypercalcemia, 176
        in breast cancer, 73, 89
        paraneoplastic PTH-secreting syndromes, 186
    with testicular cancer, 624
Mitomycin C
    alimentary tract tumors
        biliary tree, 524
        colorectum, 498
        esophagus, 467
        liver, 535
        pancreas, 519
        stomach, 482
    bladder cancer, 596
    breast cancer, 87
    lung cancer, 434, 435
    toxicity, 373
Mitotane, *see* o'p'-DDD
Mixed cellularity lymphoma, 346, 359
Mixed papillary and follicular carcinoma, thyroid, 41
Mixed seminomas, 617
Mixed tumor, salivary gland, 39
Mohs's surgery, in skin cancer, 109
    head and neck, 27, 112
    histology and, 110
    indications, contraindications, and disadvantages, 108, 110
Monoclonal antibodies, 342
Monoclonal hypergammaglobulinemia, 403
Monocytes, 360
Monocytic leukemia, 344
Monocytopenia, 399
Mononuclear cell infiltrate, in melanoma, 102
Monro, foramen of, 302
Mood elevators, 520, 581
Moon facies, in Cushing's syndrome, 136
MOPP, in lymphomas
    Hodgkin's, 366, 367
    non-Hodgkin's, 369
    pediatric, 346
Morphea type basal cell carcinoma, 106, 109
Morphine, pancreatic cancer, 520
Motilin, 203, 204
Mouth, *see also* Oral cavity tumors; Oropharynx
    examination of, 6
    radiotherapy complications, 356, 366
Mucinous carcinomas
    breast, 79
    gastric, 478
    colorectal, 495
    pancreatic, 516
Mucinous cystadenocarcinoma, pancreatic, 516
Mucinous metaplasia, gallbladder, 522

Mucoepidermoid carcinoma
   lung, 427
   paranasal sinus, 35
   salivary gland, therapy, 38, 40
Mucoid stool, colorectal cancer, 489, 490
Mucosal pattern, gastric lesions, 477
Mucous cell carcinoma, nasal fossa, 35
Multicentric osteosarcoma, 219
Multifocal nodular carcinoma, liver, 533
Multinucleated giant cells, in histiocytosis, 348
Multiple endocrine neoplasia
   apudomas, 199
   parathyroid tumors, 174
   thyroid tumors with, 41
   type I (MEN-I, Werner's syndrome), 191-193
      carcinoid, 204
      pancreatic tumors, gastrinomas, 162
      pancreatic tumors, glucagonomas, 165
      pancreatic tumors, insulinomas, 157, 158
   type II (MEN-II, Sipple's syndrome), 193-194
Multiple exostoses, follow-up, 244
Multiple familial polyposis, 490, 497
Multiple idiopathic hemorrhagic sarcoma, see Kaposi's sarcoma
Multiple myeloma, 217, 403-407
   age incidence, 225
   anatomic locations, 218
   behavior of, 225
   and hypercalcemia, 175
   radiology, diagnostic clues, 231
   site predilection of, 225
Multiple polyposis, 490, 497
Multiple spinal lesions, 287
Multiple primaries, head and neck cancer, 24
Mumps, 21, 618, 619
Muramidase, 386
Muscle flaps, 49-50
Muscle relaxants, in carcinoid surgery, 208
Mustargen, see Nitrogen mustard
MVPP, in lymphoma, Hodgkin's, 346, 367
Myasthenia gravis, 444, 446, 447, 449
Mycosis fungoides, 120-121, 377
Mycotoxins, liver cancer risk, 529
Myeloblastic leukemia, acute, 344-345
Myeloblasts, in chronic myelocytic leukemia, 345
Myelocytic leukemia, chronic, 341, 345, 391-394
Myelofibrosis, 413-415
   in hairy cell leukemia, 398
   polycythemia vera and, 413
Myelogenous leukemia, acute, 388-389
Myelographic block, spinal lesions, 288
Myelography, 279
   bone tumors, 229
   central nervous system tumors
      pediatric medulloblastomas, 303
      spinal lesions, 288, 295
   breast cancer, 88
   enteric cysts, 445
   superior vena cava syndrome, 451

Myeloid elements
   in chronic myelocytic leukemia, 345
   precursors, in acute lymphoblastic leukemia, 342
Myeloid metaplasia, 413-415
   polycythemia vera and, 413
Myelolipomas, 141
Myeloma, 219
   bone metastasis, 219
   versus bone metastasis, 240
   radiology, diagnostic clues, 231
   radiosensitivity of, 233
   spine, 287
Myelomonocytic leukemia, 344
Myelophthisic anemia, 394
Myelosuppression, see also Bone marrow; Leukopenia
   chemotherapy and, 372-374, 388, 396, 564, 624
   leukemias, acute myoblastic, 345
   radiotherapy complications, 289, 365
   therapeutic, in polycythemia vera, 413
Myelotomies, spine, 287
Myleran, see Busulfan
Myocardial infarction, in polycythemia vera, 411
Myositis ossificans, 222, 226, 227
Myxoid liposarcoma, 231, 267

N

a-Naphthylacetate esterase, 386
b-Naphthylamine, 589
a-Naphtylbutyrate esterase, 387
Narcotics
   after head and neck surgery, 47
   in pancreatic cancer, 520
   in prostate cancer, advanced, 611
Nasal tumors, see also Nasopharynx, cancer of
   early signs, 7
   five-year relative survival, 23
   nasopharyngeal carcinoma, 37, 284
   site-specific data sheet, 15-16
   therapeutic guidelines, 35
   TNM classification of cancer, 16
Nasal polyps, 35
Nasoesophageal intubation, 48
Nasolabial flaps, 49
Nasopharyngeal tumors, brain involvement, 284
Nasopharyngoscopy, 8, 9
Nasopharynx, cancer of
   annual incidence of, 6
   cervical node metastasis, occult, 28
   early signs, 7
   examination of, 6
   five-year relative survival, 23
   follow-up schedule, 51
   management algorithm, 59
   rhabdomyosarcoma, prognosis, 335
   sarcoma botryoides in, 334

site-specific data sheet, 15-16
TNM classification, 16
Waldeyer's ring, 357, 375
Neck, *see also* Head and neck tumors
early signs of cancer, 7
examination of, 6
lymph nodes, *see* Cervical lymph nodes
skin tumors, treatment of, 112
Neck dissection, *see also* Radical neck dissection
Necrolytic migratory erythema, 165
Necrosis
brain, 289
chemotherapy side effect, 372, 373, 374
colon surgery and, 499
in histiocytosis, 348
liver, 534
after radiation, 49
skin cancer treatment complications, 105, 106
Nelson's syndrome, 141, 142
Neoglottic methods, 52
Nephrectomy, 581, 582, 584
Nephroblastoma, *see* Wilms's tumor
Nephrolithiasis, *see* Calculi, urinary
Nephrostomy, 604, 607, 610
Nephrotoxicity, *see* Renal function
Nephroureterectomy, 578, 581
Nerve cells, brain tumor origination in, 284
Nerve compression, *see* Compression syndromes
Nerve-root syndromes, with pediatric ependymomas, 304
Nerve stimulation, for pain management, 246
Nesidioblast, in MEN-I, 191
Neural crest cells, in MEN-I, 191
Neural crest neoplasms, ectopic ACTH production, 184
Neurilemmoma, 217, 302
age predilection, 219
mediastinal, 443
small intestine, 504
Neuroblastoma, 148-153, 217, 316-333
age predilection, 219
mediastinal, 443-444, 448
metastatic evaluation, 318
Neuroepithelium, brain tumor origination in, 284
Neurofibroma, 302
central nervous system, 287, 302
mediastinal, 443
and pheochromocytoma, 144
small intestine, 504
Neurofibromatosis, 301, 302, 330
Neurofibrosarcoma, 231, 267, 268, 269
Neurogenic bladder, colon surgery and, 499
Neurogenic tumors, *see also* specific tumors
mediastinal, 443-444, 446
pediatric, biopsy of, 319
Neurological symptoms, *see also* Sensory deficits
in bone metastases, 241
in brain tumors
astrocytomas, 292
evauation of, 278-279
surgery and, 286, 287

in breast cancer, 86, 88
chemotherapy and, 342, 374, 564, 624
with endocrine tumors
carcinoid, 205
insulinoma, 157
in kidney tumors, 576
in leukemias, acute, 385
in lymphomas, adult, 355
in mediastinal tumors, 446
in pediatric patients, 316
with testicular tumors, 620
Neuromas, 41, 301-302
Neuropathic joints, 228
Neurosarcoma, 302
Neurosecretory cells, *see also* Oat-cell carcinoma
APUD cells, 191, 193
carcinoid, *see* Carcinoid
small-cell lung carcinomas, 427
Neutrophils, *see also* Myelosuppresion; White cell count
chemotherapy complications, 388
in immunoblastic lymphadenopathy, 377
in leukemias
acute, 385
chronic, hairy cell, 399
Nevi, benign, 113-114
malignant potential, 99. 113
patient education, 100
Nevus sebaceus, 119
Nickel, as carcinogen, 5, 422
Nicotinamide deficiencies, in carcinoid, 204
Night sweats
in leukemias, chronic
lymphocytic, 394, 395
myelocytic, 392
in lymphomas, adult, 355, 359
with mediastinal tumors, 446
in myelofibrosis and myeloid metaplasia, 414
Nipple changes, 69, 71
Nitrates and nitrites, bladder cancer risk, 589
Nitrogen balance, in pancreatic cancer, 510
Nitrogen mustard
in endometrial cancer, 562
in Kaposi's sarcoma, 121
in leukemia, chronic lymphocytic, pleural effusion, 397
in lymphomas, Hodgkin's
adult, 366, 367
pediatric, 346
in lymphomas, non-Hodgkin's, 369
in melanoma, 118
in mycosis fungoides, 120
in ovarian cancer, advanced, 566
toxicity, 373
Nitroprusside (Nipride), in pheochromocytoma surgery, 147
Nitrosamines, as cancer risk, 475, 589
Nitrosoureas, 290
brain tumors, glioblastoma multiforme, 292
liver tumors, 535
lung cancer, 434, 435
lymphomas, Hodgkin's, 366

melanoma, adjuvant, 117
Nocturia
    in primary aldosteronism, 133
    in prostatic cancer, 601
Nodular basal cell carcinoma, 106
Nodular lymphomas, 369-370
    histiocytic, 360, 361, 362, 371
    mixed, 361
    pediatric, 346
    treatment, 371
Nodular melanoma, 102
Nodular sclerosis lymphoma, 346, 359
Nodular ulcerative basal cell carcinoma, 106
Non-B, non-T-cell acute lymphoblastic leukemia, 342
Nonmalignant osseous tumors, 217
Nonossifying fibroma, 217, 219, 236
Nonsuppressible insulinlike activity (NSILA), 185
Normetanephrine, 145
Nose, see Nasopharynx, cancer of
    examination of, 6
    skin tumors, treatment of, 111
Nuchal rigidity, 342
Nuclear magnetic resonance, 279
Nuclear studies, see Scintigraphy
Nutrition, 584
Nutritional support
    with alimentary tract tumors
        colorectal cacner, 491
        gastric cancer, 483
        liver cancer, 532
    in carcinoid, 211
    with central nervous system tumors, 283
    with genitourinary surgery
        kidney, 578, 583
        penis, 631
        prostate, 604
    with head and neck cancer, 10, 21, 45, 46
    in lymphoma, Hodgkin's, 378

O

Oat cell carcinoma, see also Small-cell carcinomas
    apudomas, 198, 199
    brain metastasis, 293, 294
    chemotherapy, 435-436
    and Cushing's syndrome, 136, 142
    ectopic hormone production, ADH, 184
    surgery, contraindication, 431
    treatment, 433
Obesity
    with brain tumors, 280
        craniopharyngioma, 300
        pituitary gland, 298
    and breast cancer risk, 67, 70
    colorectal cancer risk, 490
    in Cushing's syndrome, 136
    and gynecological malignancy, 541

lung cancer surgery evaluation, 428
    in paraneoplastic endocrine syndromes, 183
Obstetric history, in gynecological malignancies, 543
Obstruction, bowel, see Intestinal obstruction
Obstructive jaundice, 523-524
Obstructive uropathy
    with bladder cancer, 590
    with gynecological cancer, 542
    with prostatic cancer
        advanced, 610
        preoperative preparation, 604
Occipital lobectomy, 284
Occupational exposure, see also Mesotheliomas
    and bladder cancer, 589
    and head and neck cancer, 5
    and liver cancer, 529
    and lung cancer, 421, 422
    and skin cancer, 99
Ocular plethysmography, in head and neck tumors, 9
Oculomotor nerve palsy, with brain tumors, 278, 280
    meningiomas, 296
    pituitary gland, 298
    urgent situations, 287
Olfactory nerve, transection of, 284
Oligodendroglioma, 279, 290
Ollier's disease, 220
Omentectomy, in ovarian cancer, 563
Ommaya reservoir, 290, 294
Oncovin, see Vincristine
Onionskin appearance, bone lesions, 226
Oophorectomy, see Ovariectomy
Oophoropexy, 358, 368
Open-wedge resection, in lung cancer, 432
Ophthalmologic evaluation, central nervous system tumors, 279
Ophthalmoparesis, trigeminal neuromas and, 302
Ophthalmoplegia
    with Burkitt's lymphoma, 376
    sella turcica enlargement and, 141
Opisthorcis sinensis, 529
Optic chiasm
    pineal tumors and, 300
    pituitary tumors and, 298
Optic discs, with brain tumor, 280
Optic nerve, brain tumors and
    craniopharyngioma, 300
    meningiomas, 296
    pituitary gland, 298
Optic nerve glioma
    nerve transection in, 284
    x-ray findings with, 279
Oral antidiabetics, 377
Oral cavity preparation, in head and neck cancer, 22
Oral cavity tumors, see also Oropharynx
    annual incidence of, 6
    cervical node metastases, occult, 28
    early signs of, 6-7
    five-year relative survival, 23
    follow-up schedule, 51
    management algorithm, 56
    pediatric, 319

postsurgical rehabilitation, 51
site-specific data sheet, 11-12
therapeutic guidelines, 29-31
tobacco use and, 5
Oral contraceptives, 67, 70
Oral hygiene, in head and neck cancer patient, 47, 48, 49
Orbit
    in histiocytosis, 348
    lymphomas, 376
    meningiomas, 296, 297
    in nasopharyngeal carcinoma, 37
    neuroblastomas, 150
    paranasal sinus tumors, 35, 36
    rhabdomyosarcoma, 335
Orbital exenteration, 37
Orchiectomy
    prostatic cancer, 604, 608, 609
        advanced, 610
        psychiatric complications, 607
    testicular cancer, 336, 619, 620, 623
Orchitis, 618
Oropharynx, cancer of, *see also* Oral cavity tumors
    with esophageal cancer, 463
    examination of, 6
    sarcoma botryoides in, 334
    therapeutic guidelines, 31
Orthoendocrine group, apudomas, 197-199
Orthopedic complications, multiple myeloma, 406
Ossifying fibroma
    behavior of, 219, 224
    site predilection of, 225
    therapeutic approaches, 236-237
Ossifying soft tissue tumor, fever in, 227
Osteitis fibrosa cystica, in parathyroid tumors, 173, 174
Osteoarthropathy
    with lung cancer, 432
    mesothelioma, 455
    multiple myeloma, 406
Osteoblastoma, 217, 219
    age incidence, 225
    age predilection, 219
    behavior of, 224
    characteristics of, 221
    regional predilection of, 224
    site predilection of, 225
    therapeutic approaches, 237
Osteochondroma, 217, 219
    age incidence, 225
    age predilection, 219
    biopsy of, 232
    characteristics of, 220
    site predilection of, 225
Osteoclast activator factor, 186
Osteogenic sarcoma, *see* Osteosarcoma
Osteoid metaplasia, lung carcinoid, 427
Osteoid osteoma, 217, 219
    age incidence, 225
    age predilection, 219

anatomic locations, 218
behavior of, 219
characteristics of, 221
regional predilection of, 224
surgery, 235
therapeutic approaches, 237
Osteoma, 219, 221
Osteomyelitis, 99
    onionskin appearance, 226
    radiology, 232
    regional predilection of, 224
Osteoporosis
    in Cushing's syndrome, 136, 138
    in parathyroid tumors, 173
    with pituitary tumors, 298
Osteosarcoma, 217, 219, 267
    Adriamycin, 242
    age incidence, 225
    age predilection, 219
    anatomic locations, 218
    arteriography in, 229
    behavior of, 224
    biopsy of, 232
    bone scans in, 230
    characteristics of, 223
    chemotherapy, intra-arterial, 535
    extraskeletal, 267
    follow-up, 244
    histological grades, 231
    lung metastasis, treatment, 436
    metastatic evaluation, 228
    radiology, diagnostic clues, 231, 232
    regional predilection of, 224
    site predilection of, 225
    therapeutic approaches, 238-243
Ostomy
    in bladder cancer, 591, 596, 597
    in colorectal cancer, 492, 496, 500
    with gynecological malignancies, 545, 566
Otitis, in histiocytosis, 348
Ototoxicity, of chemotherapeutic agents, 372
Ovarian tumors, 541-566
    carcinoid, 203
    ectopic hormone production by, 183, 184
    management algorithm, 570
    metastatis
        from bladder cancer, 596
        from gastric cancer, 481
        from colorectal cancer, 496
    paraneoplastic syndrome, diagnosis, 185
    pediatric, teratomas, 337
Ovariectomy
    breast cancer, 79, 81-82, 88, 89, 90
    cervical carcinoma *in situ*, 557
    ovarian cancer, 563, 565
    uterine cancer, 560, 561
Ovulation, and gynecological malignancy, 541
Oxygen saturation, in polycythemia vera, 412

P

Paget's disease, 219, 228
  age incidence, 225
  anal, 501
  anatomic locations, 218
  versus bone metastasis, 240
  bone tumor risk factor, 227
  breast, 79
  characteristics of, 224
  histological grades, 231
  and osteosarcoma, 238
  regional predilection of, 224
Pain relief, *see* specific primary tumors
Palatal fenestration, in nasopharyngeal tumors, 37
Palate lesions, therapeutic guidelines, 31
Palpitations
  with pancreatic tumors, insulinoma, 157
  with paraneoplastic endocrine syndromes, 183
Palsies, *see* Neurological symptoms
PAM, *see* Phenylalanine mustard
Pancreas
  APUD cells, 197
  apudomas, 198
  brain tumors, hemangioblastomas, 297
  colorectal cancer metastasis, 496
  gastric lesions, 477
Pancreatectomies, 166, 518, 519
Pancreatic cholera, *see* Vipoma
Pancreatic heterotopias, liver, 533
Pancreaticoduodenectomy, 524
Pancreatic oncofetal antigen, pancreatic cancer, 510
Pancreatic polypeptide, 158
Pancreatic scanning, *see* Scintigraphy
Pancreatic tumors, eccrine, 509-521
Pancreatic tumors, endocrine
  ACTH-producing, 184
  back pain with, 219
  gastrinoma (Zollinger-Ellison syndrome), 160-163
  glucagonoma (hyperglycemic syndrome), 163-166
  insulinoma, 157-160
    early detection and screening, 157-158
    management algorithm, 160, 161
    postoperative care, 160
    pretreatment work-up, 157-158
    therapeutic management, 158-160
  liver metastases, 531
  multiple endocrine neoplasia type I, 191-192
  vipoma, 167, 169
Pancreatitis, 41, 173, 373
Pancreatoduodenectomy, 166, 518, 519
Pancreatojejunostomy, 518
Pancuronium bromide, in carcinoid surgery, 208
Pancytopenia, leukemias
  acute, chemotherapy complications, 388
  chronic, hairy cell, 398
Pancytopenia, lymphomas, adult, 355
Panje button, 50, 52

Papillary adenoma, gallbladder, 522
Papillary (adeno)carcinoma
  bladder, 592
  breast, 79
  gallbladder, 522
  kidney, 575
  lung, 427
  stomach, 478
  thyroid, 41
    occult cervical metastases, 28
    surgery, 43
Papilledema
  brain tumors, 280, 287
    colloid cysts, 303
    craniopharyngioma, 300
    glioblastoma multiforme, 291
    meningiomas, 296
    neuromas, acoustic, 301
    pineal region, 300
  decompression surgery, 285
Papillomas
  and gynecological malignancy, 541
  lung, 426
  nasal fossa, 35
  villous, 496
Para-aortic node involvement, in cervical carcinoma, 560
Parachlorophenylalanine, carcinoid, 207
Paraendocrine tumors, *see* Ectopic hormone-producing tumors
Paraganglia, brain tumor origination in, 284
Paraganglioma
  ectopic ACTH syndrome, 187
  ectopic hormone production, ACTH, 184
  extra-adrenal, 145
  lung, 427
  mediastinal, 444
Paralysis, *see also* Neurological symptoms; Paraplegia
  with pancreatic tumors, insulinoma, 157
  in primary aldosteronism, 133
Paranasal sinus cancer
  annual incidence of, 6
  early signs, 7
  five-year relative survival, 23
  management algorithm, 58
  meningioma, ectopic, 297
  site-specific data sheet, 15-16
  therapeutic guidelines, 35-37
  TNM classification of cancer, 16
Paraneoplastic endocrine syndromes, 183-188, see *also* Ectopic hormone-
      producing tumors
  apudomas, 199
  and Cushing's syndrome, 142
Paraparesis, brain tumors and, 278
Paraplegia
  in bone metastasis, radiotherapy, 241
  with brain tumors, meningiomas, 297
  with Burkitt's lymphoma, 377
Paraprotein, 396
Parapsoriasis en plaque, 120
Parasite infections, liver, 529, 533

Parasitic granuloma, gastric, 478
Paratesticular rhabdomyosarcoma, 336
Parathyroid hormone (PTH)
    ectopic production of
        diagnosis, 184-185
            preoperative management, 185-186
    in head and neck tumors, 9
    mediastinal tumors producing, 445, 447
    in multiple endocrine neoplasia-II, 193
Parathyroid tumors, 173-180
    mediastinal, 445, 447
    multiple endocrine neoplasia type I, 191, 192
    multiple endocrine neoplasia type II, 193, 194
    pancreatic tumors, gastrinoma, 162
Parenteral hyperalimentation, see Hyperalimentation
Paresis
    brain tumors, meningiomas, 297
    pancreatic tumors, insulinoma, 157
Paresthesias
    with brain tumors, 278, 301
    chemotherapy toxicity, 624
    after parathyroid surgery, 178
Parietal sarcomas, 263
Parinaud's syndrome, 300
Parity, 81, 541
Parosteal osteosarcoma, 219
    age incidence, 225
    arteriography in, 229
    histological grades, 231
    site predilection of, 225
    therapeutic approaches, 238
Parotid tumors
    classification, 18
    follow-up schedule, 52
    head and neck, therapeutic modality selection, 25
    occult cervical node metastasis, 28
    therapy, 25, 39-40
Patch-plaque lesions, in mycosis fungoides, 120
Paterson-Kelly syndrome, 461
Pautrier's microabscesses, 120
Peau d'orange skin, 69, 71
Pediatric tumors, 315-320
    central nervous system, 300, 303-304
    leukemias and lymphomas, see Leukemias, pediatric; Lymphomas,
        pediatric
    liver, 336
    mediastinal, 443-444
    neuroblastomas, 330, 332-333
    rhabdomyosarcomas, 333-336
    teratomas, 337-338
    Wilms's tumor, 322-331
Pel-Ebstein fever, 446
Peliosis hepatis, 532
Pellagra, carcinoid, 204
Pelvic exenteration
    cervical cancer, 558
    preoperative preparation, 545
    vaginal cancer, 555

Pelvic inflammatory disease, radiotherapy with, 558
Pelvic lymphadenectomy, prostatic cancer, 608
Pelvic malignancies, intra-arterial chemotherapy, 536
Pelvic node dissection, cervical cancer, 558
Pelvic wall, cervical cancer involvement, 556
Pelvis
    bone metastasis, 228
    rhabdomyosarcoma
        prognosis, 335
        treatment, 336
Penile tumors, 629-633
Peptic ulcer
    carcinoid, 205
    enteric cysts, 445
    gastric cancer risk, 475
    in parathyroid tumors, 173
    in polycythemia vera, 411
    and stomach cancer, 475
    Zollinger-Ellison syndrome, 160
Percutaneous biliary decompression, 523-524
Percutaneous renal pelvis drainage, 604
Percutaneous transhepatic cholangiography (PTC)
    biliary tree carcinomas, 523
    liver tumors, 530, 531
    pancreatic carcinoma, eccrine, 511-512
Percutaneous transhepatic portal splenography (PTPS), 162
Pericardial cysts, 443, 444
Pericardial effusion, with mesothelioma, 456
Perimyocarditis, radiotherapy complications, 365
Periosteal chondroma, 225
Periosteal osteosarcoma, 219, 232
Periosteal sarcoma, 231
Peripheral nerve neuromas, 302
Peripheral nerves, brain tumor origination in, 284
Peripheral neuropathy
    chemotherapy side effect, 372, 373
    Waldernstrom's macroglobulinemia, 378
Peripheral vascular disease, in skin cancer treatment, 113
Peristalsis, gastric lesions and, 477
Peritoneal cavity radiation therapy, ovarian cancer, 564
Pernicious anemia, 475, 476
Peroxidase stains, in leukemias, 344, 387
Personality changes, brain tumors and, 278
Petroleum products, skin cancer in, 99
Peutz-Jeghers syndrome
    colorectal cancer risk, 490
    small intestine lesions, 504
    stomach lesions, 478
Pharyngograms, 9
Pharyngotomy, 37
Pharynx, see Nasopharynx; Oropharynx
Phenobarbital, with brain tumors, 283
Phenol injection, pain relief, 520
Phenothiazine, 520
Phenoxybenzamine, 147, 207
Phentolamine, 146-147
Phentolamine suppression test, 146
Phenylalanine mustard (PAM)

in breast cancer, 84, 87
in skeletal tumors, 242
Phenylephrine, in carcinoid surgery, 208
Pheochromocytoma, 41, 142-149
apudomas, 198, 199
with brain tumors, hemangioblastomas, 297
ectopic ACTH syndrome, 184, 187
mediastinal, 444
laboratory findings, 447
symptoms, 446
multiple endocrine neoplasia type II, 193-194
paraneoplastic syndrome, 184, 185, 187
Philadelphia chromosome, 341, 343, 345, 391, 392
Phlebotomy, in polycythemia vera, 413
Phosphatases, see Acid phosphatase; Leucocyte alkaline phosphatase
Phosphates
in breast cancer, with hypocalcemia, 89
in hypercalcemia, 176, 186
in hyperparathyroidism, 174
tubular reabsorption of (TRP), 184
Phosphorus, radioactive, in polycythemia vera, 412, 413
Phosphorus levels
in acute leukemia, 385
with bone tumors, 227
mediastinal tumors, 447
in parathyroid tumors, 174
Photocautery, see Laser surgery
Photosensitivity, skin cancer treatment complications, 106
Phrenic nerve injury
lung cancer
staging criteria, 428
as surgery contraindication, 431
scalene node biopsy and, 426
Physiotherapy, see also Pulmonary physiotherapy
after esophageal surgery, 468
terminal patient, 47
Pigmentation
apudomas, 198
with para-endocrine tumors, 142
skin cancer treatment complications, 106
small intestinal lesions and, 504
Pigmented basal cell carcinoma, 106
Pigmented lesions, malignant potential, 114
Pig skin, 69
Pineal gland, tumor origination in, 284
Pineal region tumors, 300
Pituitary gland
APUD cells, 197
endocrine dysfunction
brain tumors and, 280, 283, 296
and Cushing's syndrome, 136
in histiocytosis, 348
Pituitary tumors, 297-300
adrenocortical hyperplasia, 141, 142
apudomas, 348
multiple endocrine neoplasia type I, 192
radiosensitivity of, 290
surgical approaches, 286
x-ray finding with, 279

Plasma cell granulomas, lung, 427
Plasma cells, see also Multiple myeloma
in Hodgkin's lymphoma, 359
in immunoblastic lymphadenopathy, 377
in multiple myeloma, 403, 404, 405
in Waldernstrom's macroglobulinemia, 378
Plasmacytoma, 217
radiation therapy, 406
radiology, diagnostic clues, 231
Plasmapheresis, in multiple myeloma, 407
Platelets, see also Thrombocytopenia
leukemias, chronic
lymphocytic, 395
myelocytic, 345, 392
in multiple myeloma, 403
in myelofibrosis, 413, 414
in polycythemia vera, 411, 412
thrombocythemia, essential, 415
Platelet transfusions, 388
Pleomorphic carcinoma, salivary gland, 39, see also Malignant mixed tumor
Pleomorphic fibrosarcoma, 267
Pleomorphic fibrous histiocytoma, 267
Pleomorphic infiltrate, in Hodgkin's lymphoma, 359
Pleomorphic liposarcoma, 231, 267
Pleomorphic rhabdomyosarcoma, 267, 268
Pleural effusion
breast cancer metastasis, 88
leukemias, chronic lymphocytic, 397
lung cancer
staging criteria, 428
surgery contraindication, 431
lymphomas, adult, 355
mediastinal tumors, 446
mesothelioma, 456
in superior vena cava syndrome, 451
Pleural shock, lung biopsy and, 424
Pleural tumors, see Mesotheliomas
Pleurectomy, mesothelioma, 456, 457
Pneumococcal vaccine, 346, 358
Pneumoencephalography, 279, 299
Pneumomediastinum, 447
Pneumonectomy, 437, 456
Pneumonia
kidney surgery and, 578, 582
leukemias, chronic lymphocytic, 394
lung cancer
postoperative management, 437
staging criteria, 428
Pneumothorax
fiberoptic bronchoscopy and, 424
intravenous hyperalimentation and, 21
lung biopsy and, 424
mediastinoscopy and, 425, 426
metastasis from osteosarcoma and, 232
scalene node biopsy and, 426
Poikilocytes, 392
Poikiloderma, 120
Polyclonal hypergammaglobulinemia, 377
Polycystic kidneys, 316

Polycythemia
    with brain tumors, 284, 297
    with kidney tumors, 576, 578
Polycythemia vera, 411-413
Polypoid carcinomas, esophagus, 461
Polyps
    and bone tumors, 227
    colon and rectum, 495-496
        cancer risk, 490
        colectomy with tumors arising from, 497
        Gardner's syndrome, 496
        prognosis of malignant lesions, 495
        Turcot syndrome, 496
    gallbladder, 522
    gastric lesions, 478
    and gynecological malignancy, 541
    and stomach cancer, 475
Polytomography, 35, 299
Polyuria, 183
Poorly differentiated lymphocytic lymphoma, 360, 361, 362
Portal circulation, with liver surgery, 534
Portal hypertension, 414
Portal splenography, 162
Portal venography, 531
Posterior fossa lesions, 285
Posterior occipital flap, 49
Postmenopausal bleeding, 542
Potassium levels
    in Cushing's syndrome, 138
    in leukemias, acute, 385
    in paraneoplastic syndromes, 188
    in primary aldosteronism, 135-136
PPD, 21, 356
Ppoma, 158, 198, 199
Precocious puberty, 300
Prednisone, 46, see also Corticosteroids
    in breast cancer, dosages and response rates, 87
    in histiocytosis, 348
    in hypercalcemia
        hyperparathyroidism, ectopic, 1869
        with multiple myeloma, 406
    in leukemias, acute
        lymphoblastic, 343, 344, 389
        myelogenous, 388
        myoblastic, 345
    in leukemias, chronic
        lymphocytic, 397
        myelocytic, 393, 394
    in lymphoblastic lymphadenopathy, 377
    in lymphoma, Hodgkin's
        adult, 366, 367, 367
        pediatric, 346
    in lymphoma, non-Hodgkin's, 371
        diffuse, 370
        nodular, 369
        pediatric, 347
    in multiple myeloma, 404, 405, 406
Pregnancy
    breast cancer in, 80-82

    and breast cancer risk, 70
    cervical carcinoma in, 558-559
Primaries, multiple, see Multiple primaries; Second malignancy
Primary aldosteronism, 133-137
Procarbazine
    and chemotherapy, 290
    in liver tumors, 534
    in lung cancer, 434
    in lymphomas, Hodgkin's
        adult, 366, 367
        pediatric, 346
    in lymphomas, non-Hodgkin's, 369, 371
    in melanoma, 118
    in multiple myeloma, 406
    toxicity, 374
Prochlorperazine, 207
Proctitis, radiation, 555, 595, 608
Proctosigmoidoscopy
    anal cancer, 503
    bladder cancer, follow-up evaluation, 597
    in carcinoid, 206
    in colorectal cancer, 489, 491
    in gynecological malignancies, 544
Progestational agents, and endometrial cancer, 562
Progesterone, 562
    with breast cancer, 88
    with kidney tumors, 583
Progesterone receptors, in breast cancer, 72
    adjuvant therapy, 84
    in pregnancy, 81
    and prognosis, 86
Proinsulin, 158
Prolactin
    apudomas, 199
    pituitary tumors, 192, 298, 299
Prolymphocytic leukemia, 395
Promyelocytic leukemia, 344
Prophylactic mastectomy, 76
Propranolol, 134, 147
Proptosis, see Exophthalmos
Prostaglandins, 203
    carcinoid, 204
    in paraneoplastic syndrome, hypercalcemia, 185
    in vipoma, 166
Prostatectomy, 603, 608, 609
Prostate tumors, 601-615
    bone metastasis
        acid phosphatase in, 228
        hormone therapy in, 240
        radiotherapy, 241
    ectopic ACTH production, 184
Prostatic hypertrophy (BPH), 603
Protein electrophoresis
    leukemias, acute, 386
    leukemias, chronic, lymphocytic, 396
    lymphomas, adult, 356
    multiple myeloma, 403
Protein levels
    with bone tumors, 227

cerebrospinal fluid, in meningeal carcinomatosis, 294
    after gynecological surgery, 566
Prothrombin, in myelofibrosis, 414
Protoplasmic astrocytomas, 292
Protuberans, therapy, 269
Provera, 562, 583
Provocative tests
    in adrenal disorders
        Cushing's syndrome, 139
        pheochromocytoma, 145-146
    in carcinoid, 206
Proximal subtotal gastrectomy, 481
Pruritus, 542
    gynecological malignancies, 541, 543
    lymphomas, adult, 355
    pancreatic cancer, 509
    in polycythemia vera, 411
    skin cancer treatment complications, 106
Pseudogout, 173
Pseudohyperparathyroidism, 175
    paraneoplastic endocrine syndromes, 183
    therapeutic management, 186-187
Pseudolipomas, liver, 533
Pseudolymphoma, gastric lesions, 478
Pseudomalignant ossifying soft tissue tumor, 227
Pseudosarcoma, esophagus, 461
Psychiatric and psychological considerations
    with adrenal surgery, 140
    with bone cancer, 246-247
    with breast cacner, 90-91
    with carcinoid tumors, 211
    with colorectal cancer, 491
    with genitourinary tumors
        bladder, 591, 596, 597
        kidney, 578, 581
        penis, 631
        prostate, 607, 609
    with gynecological malignancies, 545
    with head and neck cancer, 22, 26, 50
    with lung cancer, 438
    with lymphoma, 378
    with parathyroid tumors, 173
    with skin cancer, 107, 123
    with soft-tissue sarcoma, 261, 269
    terminal patient, 47
Puberty, paraneoplastic endocrine syndromes, 183
Pull-up operation, gastric, 50
Pulmonary embolus
    after gynecological surgery, 566
    in lung cancer, 423
Pulmonary fibrosis, chemotherapeutic agents causing, 320, 372, 625
Pulmonary infection, see Pneumonia
Pulmonary infiltrates, in lung cancer, 422-423
Pulmonary physiotherapy, see also Respiratory therapy
    preoperative
        in esophageal cancer, 463
        in lung cancer, 431
        in pancreatic cancer, 515

postoperative
    after esophageal surgery, 468
    after gynecological surgery, 566
Pulmonary ventilation, gastric surgery patient, 483
Pulmonic valve fibrosis, with carcinoid, 204
Pupil reactivity, with brain tumors, 298, 300
Pure mucinous carcinoma, breast, 79
Purpura, with myelofibrosis, 413
PUVA, in mycosis fungoides, 120
Pyeloureterectasis, rhabdomyosarcoma and, 317
Pyloric obstruction, in gastric cancer, 476
Pyloromyotomy, 466
Pylorus-preserving operations, 518
Pyriform sinus, 34

                    Q

Quarterectomy, 76
Queyrat, erythroplasia of, 629

                    R

Radiation
    as risk factor
        in bone cancer, 217, 219, 227, 231
        in breast cancer, 67, 70
        in skin cancer, 99
        in testicular cancer, 619
        in thyroid cancer, 42
    and nutritional status, 10
Radiation sarcoma, 219, 231
Radiation sensitizers
    in bladder cancer, 596
    in colorectal cancer, 498
Radical hysterectomy, cervical cancer, 558
Radical mastectomy, stage and, 77, 78
Radical neck dissection, 29
    with cervical node metastasis, occult, 28
    with salivary gland tumors, 39, 40
    in medullary carcinoma of thyroid, 194
    with parathyroid tumors, 176
    in skin cancer, 112, 116
    in thyroid cancer, 43-44
Radical prostatectomy, prostatic cancer, 609
Radicular pain, with meningiomas, 297
Radioactive isotope scans, see Scintigraphy; specific organ scans
Radioactive phosphorus, in polycythemia vera, 412
Radioimmunoassay
    paraneoplastic syndrome, hypercalcemia, 185
    prostatic cancer, 602
Radiotherapy, 85, 239-240
    adrenal tumors, 141
        neuroblastoma, 151
        pheochromocytoma, 147

alimentary tract tumors
  anal lesions, 503
  colorectal cancer, 497–499
  esophagus, 466–467
  gallbladder and biliary tree, 524
  liver, 534
  pancreas, eccrine, 518–519
  stomach, 482
bone tumors, 240–241
  metastasis, 240
brain tumors, 288–290
  astrocytomas, 293, 303
  complications of treatment, 305
  lymphomas, 301
  metastatic, 294
  pediatric, 303, 304
  pineal region, 300
  pituitary gland, 141, 142
  therapeutic goals, 286
breast cancer, 82–83
  in pregnancy, 81
  recurrent, 89
  stage and, 77, 78
endocrine tumors, *see also* specific glands
  carcinoid, 210
  ectopic ACTH syndrome, 187
genitourinary tumors
  bladder, 595, 596
  kidney, 582, 583
  penis, 630–631
  prostate, 608, 609, 610, 611, 612
  testis, 620, 623
gynecological tumors
  cervix, 557
  endometrium, 561–562
  ovary, 563, 564, 565
  vagina, 555
head and neck tumors, 44
  advanced, 46
  cervical node metastasis, occult, 28
  inadequate, 24
  larynx and adjacent sites, 32, 33, 34, 35
  nasopharyngeal, 37
  nose, nasopharynx, and paranasal sinus sites, 35, 36, 37
  oral cavity and oropharyngeal sites, 29, 30, 31, 32
  posttreatment care, 48–49
  salivary glands, 39, 40
  thyroid, 43, 44
histiocytosis, 348
Kaposi's sarcoma, 121–122
leukemias
  acute, 391
  acute lymphoblastic, 342
  chronic lymphocytic, 397, 398
lung cancer, 432–433

lymphomas
  Hodgkin's, 365–366
  non-Hodgkin's, 369, 375–376
  pediatric, 346, 347
  staging laparotomy and, 358
mediastinal tumors, 448
mesiotheliomas, 456, 457
multiple myeloma, 406
pain relief with bone metastasis, 46
pancreatic tumors, insulinoma, 160
pediatric solid tumors
  adjuvant, 320
  neuroblastoma, 333
  Wilms's tumor, 324
skin cancer, 106, 108–109
  appendage tumors, 119
  complications of, 106
  head and neck, 111, 112
  histology and, 110
  indications, contraindications, and disadvantages, 108, 109–110
  melanoma, 117
soft-tissue sarcoma, 263–265
  postoperative, 270
  radical resection, 261
spinal lesions, 287, 288, 295, 303
  in superior vena cava syndrome, 451
Radium needles, bladder cancer, 595
Radon 222 implants
  bladder cancer, 595
  lung cancer, 432
Rappaport's classification, lymphoma, 360–361, 362
Rash
  in histiocytosis, 348
  with lymphomas, adult, 355
Reactive bone, biopsy of, 232
Reactive thrombocytosis, 415
Rebound hyperglycemia, 159
Receptors, *see* Hormone receptors; Markers
Reconstructive surgery
  breast, 92
  in nasopharyngeal tumors, 37
  in penile cancer, 631
Rectal biopsy, with prostate surgery, 607
Rectal bleeding, *see also* Stools
  in carcinoid, 203
  in colorectal cancer, 489, 490
  in pediatric patients, 316
  with small intestinal tumors, 504
Rectal carcinoid, 208
Rectum
  carcinomas of, 496, *see also* Colorectal cancer
  cervical cancer involvement, 556
  radiotherapy and, 555
Recurrence interval, in breast cancer, 86
Recurrent laryngeal nerve palsy, 431

Red blood cell transfusions
    in esophageal cancer, 462
    in myeloma, 406
Reed-Sternberg cells, 359
Reflexes, *see also* Neurological symptoms
    with brain tumors, 298, 300, 304
    in primary aldosteronism, 133
Regional lymphadenectomy, 159
Regional node dissection, vaginal cancer, 555
Regitine, 146
Remission, leukemias
    acute myelogenous
        defined, 389
        karyotypic abnormalities, 388
    chronic
        lymphocytic, 396
        myelocytic, 392
Renal artery embolization, 581
Renal cell carcinoma, 575
    follow-up schedule, 584, 585
    metastasis,
        bone, 219, 240
        lung, treatment of, 436
    paraneoplastic syndrome, 184, 185
    prognosis, 582
    surgery, 581
Renal dialysis, *see* Dialysis
Renal failure
    and bone tumors, 227
    chemotherapy and, 564
    with leukemias, acute, 385, 388
    in multiple myeloma, 403
    in primary aldosteronism, 133
    with prostatic cancer, 603
Renal function
    chemotherapy complications, 320, 372, 373, 374
    in hyperparathyroidism, 176
    with leukemias, acute, 385, 386
    with lymphomas, adult, 355
    with multiple myeloma, 404, 406
    with pediatric tumors
        postoperative care, 321
        radiation therapy complications, 320
    radiotherapy complications, 320, 365
Renal scans, with kidney tumors, 577
Renal stones, *see* Calculi
Renal transplant, and lymphoma, 301
Renal tumors, *see* Kidney tumors
Renin levels, 134, 185
Reserpine, 134
Respiratory distress
    with lymphomas, 355
    with meningiomas, 296
    after parathyroid surgery, 178
    in superior vena cava syndrome, 451
    after thyroidectomy and parathyroidectomy, 48
Respiratory therapy, *see also* Pulmonary physiotherapy
    brain tumor, pretreatment management, 283
    colorectal cancer, preoperative, 491

gastric cancer, preoperative management, 478
    lung cancer patient, 431
Reticular cells, 360
Reticuloendothelial tumors, brain, origin of, 284
Reticulosis, medullary histiocytic, 377-378
Reticulum cell sarcomas, 217, 301, 361
Retina
    in brain tumors, 280, 297
    breast cancer metastasis, 86, 88
    hemangioblastomas, 297
    in pheochromocytoma, 144, 145
    in polycythemia vera, 411
    Waldenstro"m's macroglobulinemia, 378
Retinoblastoma, 315, 319
Retrograde cystogram, 317
Retrograde pyelography, 577
Retro-orbital tumors, pediatric, 319
Retroperitoneal nodes, testicular tumors, 617, 623
Retroperitoneal tumors
    Burkitt's lymphoma, 376
    neuroblastoma, 150, 333
    pediatric, 316
        preoperative preparation, 319
        teratomas, 337
    sarcomas, 263
Rhabdoid sarcoma, Wilms's tumor with, 323
Rhabdomyosarcomas, 267, 268
    histological grades, 231
    metastatic evaluation, 318
    pediatric, 333-336
        intravenous pyelogram in, 317
        pathological considerations, 334
        physical findings, 316
        prognostic features, 335
        staging and classification, 334-335
        therapeutic management, 335-336
    therapeutic guidelines, 266-267, 269
Rheumatoid arthritis, 397
Richter's syndrome, 396
Roux-en-Y procedures
    in gastric cancer, 482
    in pancreatic cancer, 163, 517
Rubidazone, toxicity, 374
Rubidomycin, *see* Daunorubicin

S

Saccharin, bladder cancer risk factors, 589
Sacrococcygeal teratoma, pediatric, 337
Saline, in ectopic ADH syndrome, 187
Salivary gland tumors
    annual incidence of, 6
    cervical node metastasis, occult, 28
    ectopic hormone production, ACTH, 184
    five-year relative survival, 23

lymphomas, adult, 355
management algorithm, 60
site-specific data sheet, 17-18
therapeutic guidelines, 37-40
therapeutic modality selection, 25
Salpingo-oophorectomy, *see* Ovariectomy
Salt-loading test, 134
Sarcoidosis, and hypercalcemia, 175
Sarcoma, 302
chemotherapy intra-arterial, 536
chordomas, 303
head and neck, therapeutic modality selection, 25
pancreatic, eccrine, 516
pediatric, physical findings, 316
radiosensitivity of, 233
Sarcoma botryoides, 267, 334
intravenous pyelography in, 317
pediatric, symptoms, 316
prognosis, 335
Sarcomatous degeneration, meningioma, 290
Sarcomatous variants, neurogenic tumors, 443
Satellitosis, in melanoma, 102
Scalene nodes, in lung cancer, 426, 431
Scalloping, bone lesions, 226
Scalp
meningioma, ectopic, 297
skin tumors, treatment of, 112
Schistosomiasis, 589
Schneiderian papilloma, 35
Schwann cells, neurofibromas, 302
Schwannoma, 267, 268
histological grades, 231
MEN-I, 192
Schwartz-Bartter syndrome, 198
Sciatic nerve palsy, 286
Scintigraphy, *see also* specific sites
adrenal
Cushing's syndrome, 140
pheochromocytoma, 146, 194
primary aldosteronism, 135
alimentary tract tumors
colorectum, 491
liver, 337, 530
pancreas, 165
stomach, 477
bone tumors, 226, 228, 229, 233
follow-up, 245
brain metastasis, 294
breast cancer, 73
advanced, evaluation of, 86
follow-up schedule, 91
endocrine
multiple endocrine neoplasia-II, 194
pancreatic tumors, 165

parathyroid tumors, 175
genitourinary tumors
bladder, 591
kidney, 577, 585
testis, 619
head and neck tumors, thyroid, 42
lung cancer, 423, 428
lymphoma, staging work-up, 358
mediastinal tumors, 446-447
pediatric tumors
liver, 337
metastatic evaluation, 318
soft-tissue sarcoma, metastatic evaluation, 257
Sclerosing hemangioma, lung, 427
Scopolamine, in pheochromocytoma surgery, 147
Scrotal scan, in testicular cancer, 619
Seabright bantam syndrome, 227
Sebaceous gland carcinoma, 105, 119
Secondary chondrosarcoma, histological grades, 231
Secondary operations, brain tumors, 286
Secondary sex characteristics, testicular tumors and, 618
Second-look operation
embryonal carcinoma, 338
ovarian cancer, 564-565
Second malignancy
head and neck cancer, 26
leukemias
acute, 386
chronic lymphocytic, 398
in myelofibrosis and myeloid metaplasia, 415
polycythemia vera treatment and, 413
radiotherapy and, 366
Secretin tests, 510, 512
with carcinoid, 206
in Zollinger-Ellison syndrome, 162
Sedimentation rate, in bone tumors, 227
Segmental resection, lung, 437
Segmentectomy, lung, 432
Seizures
with brain tumors, 278
astrocytomas, 292
epidermoid and dermoid cysts, 302
glioblastoma multiforme, 291
lymphomas, 301
meningiomas, 296
metastatic, 293
pituitary gland, 298
postoperative, 285, 304
therapeutic goals, 286
with insulinoma, 157
Selenium, colorectal cancer risk, 490
Self-examination, breast, 68-69
Self-healing lesions, bone, 219, 225, 236
Sella turcica, 141, 279, 298

Seminomas
   classification, 617
   mediastinal, therapeutic management, 450
   therapeutic management, 620, 623
Sensory deficits, *see also* Neurological symptoms
   with central nervous sytem lesions, 278
      neuromas, trigeminal, 301, 302
      nursing care, 305
      spinal cord compression, 295
   with insulinoma, 157
Sentinel node biopsy, 630
Sepsis, 542
   intravenous hyperalimentation and, 21
   in leukemia, acute myoblastic, 345
   with lung cancer, palliative resection indications, 432
   as pediatric chemotherapy complication, 320
Serology, 630, *see also* Markers
   lymphomas, 356
   pancreatic tumors, 510
Serotonin, 197, *see also* Apudomas
   APUD cells, 197
   carcinoid, 204, 208
   oat cell carcinomas of lung and, 427
Serotonin antagonists
   in carcinoid, 207, 208
   in Cushing's disease, 142
   with small intestinal tumors, 504
Sertoli cell tumors, 617
Serum markers, *see* Markers
Sex prevalence, bone tumors, 220-224
Sexual history, in gynecological malignancies, 541, 543
Sexuality, with prostatic cancer, 609, *see also* Impotence
Sexually transmitted diseases, with Kaposi's sarcoma, 121
Se´zary syndrome, 120-121, 377
SGOT and SGPT, in pancreatic cancer, 510
Shoulder
   bone tumors, 218, 228
   disarticulation of, in soft-tissue sarcoma, 262
   in lung cancer rehabilitation, 438
Shoulder flap, 49
Shunts, ventricular, 286, 287
Sialography, 9
Sickle cell trait, and Burkitt's lymphoma, 376
Sigmoidoscopy, *see* Proctosigmoidoscopy
Signet-ring cell adenocarcinoma, gastric, 478
Silver staining, hemangioendothelioma, 239
Simple cyst, 219, 224
Simple mastectomy, 76-77
Sinuses, *see* Paranasal sinuses
Sipple's syndrome (MEN-II), 193-194
Sjögren's disease, 397
Skeletal survey
   bladder cancer, 591
   multiple myeloma, 404
   parathyroid tumors, 175

   pediatric tumors, metastatic evaluation, 318
   prostatic cancer, 602
Skeletal system tumors, 219-249, *see also* Bone metastasis
   leukemias, acute lymphoblastic, 343
   lymphomas, radiotherapy, 375
   in histiocytosis, 348
   metastatic evaluation, 318
   metastases to, *see* Bone metastasis
   multiple myeloma, 403-407
Skin cancer, 99-122
   anal region, 501
   of appendages, 118-119
   apudomas, 198
   breast cancer recurrence, 78, 89
   head and neck
      cervical node metastasis, occult, 28
      early signs, 7
      therapeutic modality selection, 25
   Kaposi's sarcoma, 121-122
   with leukemias, chronic lymphocytic, 398
   melanoma, 113-120, 123, *see also* Melanoma
   mycosis fungoides, 120-121
   Se´zary syndrome, 120-121
   therapeutic modalities, nonmelanoma lesions, 107-110
      chemotherapy, 110
      cryosurgery, 108
      dessication and curettage (electrosurgery), 108
      excision surgery, 108
      laser surgery, 109-110
      Moh's surgery, 109
      radiotherapy, 108-109
Skin flaps, 48
Skin grafts
   after mastectomy, 91
   in skin cancer, postoperative care, 122
Skin metastasis
   gastric cancer, 481, 483
   treatment of, 112, 483
Skin ulcers, breast, 69
Skinning vulvectomy, 546
Sleep disturbances, 279, 298
Sleeve resection, lung cancer, 432
Small-cell carcinomas, *see also* Oat cell carcinoma
   lung
      chemotherapy, 435-436
      ectopic ADH production, 184
      histological evaluation, 427
      radiotherapy, 433
   nasal fossa, 35
   pancreatic, 516
   radiosensitivity, 233, 433
   thyroid, radiotherapy, 44
Small intestine tumors, 504
   apudomas, 198
   carcinoid, 204
      early detection and screening, 205
      surgical management, 208
   with kidney tumors, 581

SMF, pancreatic cancer, 519
Smoking and tobacco use, 163
   and bladder cancer, 589
   and head and neck cancer, 5
   and lung cancer, 421, 422, 438-439
   and nutritional status, 10
   and pancreatic cancer, 509
   after radiation, 49
Smoldering leukemias, acute, 386, 390
Social factors
   in head and neck cancer treatment, 26
   kidney cancer treatment, 581, 582
   prostatic cancer, 609
   in breast cancer, 67, 81
   in gynecological cancer, 541
Sodium bicarbonate, in multiple myeloma, 406
Sodium intake, in primary aldosteronism, 133, 134
Sodium levels
   in ectopic ADH syndrome, 187, 188
   in primary aldosteronism, postoperative care, 136
Sodium nitrite, gastric cancer risk, 475
Soft-tissue sarcomas, 255-272
   Adriamycin, 242
   age, risk factor, 256
   CAT scan, 318
   annual incidence of, 6
   cure rates, 320
   intravenous pyelography, 317
   lung, histological evaluation, 427
   lung metastasis, 436
   lymphomas, 355
   pancreas, eccrine, 516
   pediatric, see Rhabdomyosarcoma
Somatomedins, 185
Somatostatin, 158, 204
Somatostatinoma, 158, 198, 199
Sonography,
   adrenal
      in Cushing's syndrome, 139
      in pheochromocytoma (MEN-II), 194
      in primary aldosteronism, 135
   in alimentary tract tumors
      biliary tree, 523
      liver, 337, 530
      pancreas, 511, 512
   breast, 71, 78
   genitourinary tumors
      bladder, 597
      kidney, 577, 585
      penis, 630
      prostate, 602
   gynecological malignancies, 544, 564
   pancreatic tumors, eccrine, 511, 512
   pancreatic tumors, insulinomas, 158
   pediatric tumors, 317, 337
   soft tissue tumors, 229, 264
   in superior vena cava syndrome, 451
   teratoma, 337
   thyroid, 42

Speech difficulties, with brain tumors, 278, 296, 301
Speech rehabilitation, 51-52
Spermatocytic seminoma, 617
Sphenoid sinus, pituitary tumors and, 298
Sphincteric dysfunction, see also Incontinence
   brain tumors and, 278, 279
   with Burkitt's lymphoma, 377
Spinal accessory nerve, in radical neck dissection, 29
Spinal cord, see also Central nervous system tumors; Spine
   meningiomas, 296-297
   metastatic tumors, 294-295
   neuromas, 302
   radiation sequelae, 289
   surgery, 286-287
   urgent situations, 288
Spinal cord compression
   in breast cancer, 86, 88
   epidural metastasis, 294-295
   in lymphomas, adult, 355
   in mediastinal tumors, 446
   in meningiomas and, 297
   in prostatic cancer, advanced, 611
   radiation therapy, palliative, 433
   in superior vena cava syndrome, 451
Spinal cord metastasis, 294-295
Spinal neuromas, 302
Spinal tap, see Cerebrospinal fluid
Spindle cell carcinoma, lung, 426-427
Spindle cell components, in squamous cell carcinoma, skin, 101
Spindle cell nevus, malignant potential, 113
Spine, see also Spinal cord
   bone metastasis, 228
   bone tumors
      myelography, 229
      palliation, 235
      types, with predilection for, 218
   chordomas, 303
   lung cancer metastasis
      staging criteria, 428
      radiotherapy, palliative, 433
   myeloma, 406
Spironolactone, 135-136
Spitz's nevus, 113
Spleen
   in histiocytosis, 348
   in immunoblastic lymphadenopathy, 377
   in leukemias
      acute, 385
      chronic, hairy cell, 398
      chronic lymphocytic, 394, 395, 397
      chronic myelocytic, 392
   in lymphoma, 357, 358
   in myelofibrosis, 413
   in polycythemia vera, 411, 412
   in Waldenstrom's macroglobulinemia, 378
Spleen scan
   in lymphoma, staging work-up, 358
   pediatric tumors, metastatic evaluation, 318
Splenectomy

in leukemias, 393, 397, 398
in lymphoma, Hodgkin's, 346
Splenography, 162
Spurious polycythemia, 412
Sputum cytology
  with brain tumors, 280, 294
  with lung cancer, 422, 422
  with mesiotheliomas, 456
Squamous cell carcinomas
  bladder, 592
  colorectal, 495
  ectopic hormone production, ADH, 184
  esophagus, 461
  gastric, 478
  lung, histological evaluation, 426-427
  lung metastasis, treatment, 436
  nasal fossa, 35
  nasopharyngeal, 37
  skin, 105
    biopsy, 102
    treatment, 106, 110
  vulva, 546
Squamous cell papilloma, lung, 426
Staging laparotomy, see Laparotomy
Steatorrhea, in pancreatic cancer, 509
Sterility
  chemotherapy and
    in Hodgkin's lymphoma, 368
    in germ cell tumors, 450
  radiotherapy complications, 365
Sternum, malignancy of 231
Steroid therapy, see Corticosteroid therapy
Stoma, see Ostomy
Stomach, APUD cells, 197
Stomach, carcinoma of, 475-485
  apudomas, 198
  carcinoid, 205
  ectopic hormone production, 184
  liver metastasis, 531
Stomatitis, chemotherapy and, 372-374
Stones, see Calculi
Storage pool defect, in polycythemia vera, 412
Streptozotocin
  biliary tree carcinoma, 524
  carcinoid, 210
  in lymphomas, Hodgkin's, 367
  pancreatic tumors, eccrine, 519
  pancreatic tumors, endocrine
    gastrinoma, 163
    glucagonoma, 166
    insulinoma, 159, 160
    vipoma, 166
  in paraneoplastic syndrome, hypoglycemia, 187
  in pheochromocytoma, 147
  toxicity, 374
Stress polycythemia, 412
Striae
  brain tumor and, 280
  in Cushing's syndrome, 138

Stroke
  brain surgery complications, 286
  in polycythemia vera, 411
Stromal tumors, ovarian, 565
Subcutaneous mastectomy, 76
Subglottis, tumor classification, 14
Submaxillary gland
  in neck dissection, 29
  tumors, 38, 40
Subphrenic abscess, 482
Substance P, 203, 204
Substernal goiters, 445
Subtotal gastrectomy, 481
Subtotal maxillectomy, 36
Sudan black, leukemia cells, 387
Sulfonamides, and immunoblastic lymphadenopathy, 377
Sun exposure, and skin cancer, 99
Superficial basal cell carcinoma, 106
Superior mesenteric arteriography, in carcinoid, 206
Superior vena cava syndrome
  chemodectomas and, 444
  with leukemias, chronic lymphocytic, 398
  lung cancer, 422, 423, 426, 431
  lymphomas, adult, 355
  mediastinal tumors, 446, 450-451
  radiation therapy, palliative, 433
  scintigraphy, 446
Super-voltage beam, spinal cord tumors, 303
Supraclavicular lymph nodes
  in cervical cancer, 560
  in gastric cancer, 476
Supraglottic laryngeal tumors, 14, 28
Surface antigens, see Markers
Surgery, see specific operations and primary sites
Surgicel, brain surgery, 288
Swan-Ganz catheter, 467, 516
Sweat gland carcinoma, 119
Sweeteners, and bladder cancer, 589
Sympathetic nervous system tumors, mediastinal, 444
Synovial chondromatosis, 219, 222, 228
Synovial cyst, 222
Synovial sarcoma, 219, 267-269
Synovioma, histological grades, 231
Syphilis, 121, 533
Syringocystadenoma papilliferum, 119
Systemic disease, breast cancer, 85, 89-90

T

Tamoxifen, in breast cancer, 79, 88
  adjuvant therapy, 84
  in recurrent disease, 89
T-cell leukemias, 341-342, 395
T-cell lymphomas, 346, 360, 361
T-cells
  in Hairy cell leukemia, 399
  in Se´zary syndrome, 377

Technetium scans
    bone tumors, 226
    brain metastasis, 294
    testicular cancer, 619
Tegretol, 283, 286, 287
Telangiectasia
    in carcinoid, 205
    in mycosis fungoides, 120
    skin cancer treatment complications, 106
Telangiectatic osteosarcoma, 219, 223
Temporal lobes tumors, 291, 298
Tendosynovial sarcoma, 267, 268
Tenesmus, 542
    in bladder cancer, 590
    in colorectal cancer, 490
Tentorial lesions, surgical approaches, 286
Teratocarcinoma, testis, 617
Teratodermoids, mediastinal, 444
Teratogenesis, 315, 366
Teratoma
    lung, 427
    markers (AFP), 620, *see also* Alpha-fetoprotein
    mediastinal, 444
        chemotherapy, 449, 450
        radiological findings, 446
    nonseminomatous germ cell tumors, 624
    ovary, 565
    pediatric, 316, 337-338
    pineal region, 300
    testis, 617, 619
Terminal deoxynucleotidyltransferase (TDT), 342, 386, 393
Testicular tumors, 618-626
    carcinoid, 203
    classification, 617
    ectopic hormone production, ACTH, 184
    incidence, 617
    leukemias, acute lymphoblastic, 343
    lung metastasis, treatment of, 436
    lymphomas, radiotherapy, 376
Testosterone level, pituitary tumors and, 299
Tetany, 133, 178
Thallium scans, lung cancer surgery evaluation, 428
Therapy-related leukemia, 386
Thermography, 71, 619
Thiazides, and immunoblastic lymphadenopathy, 377
6-Thioguanine, in leukemias, 345, 374, 388
Thiotepa, bladder cancer, 596
Thoracentesis, mesiotheliomas, 456
Thoracoscopy, 424, 456
Thoracotomy
    lung cancer, 424
    mediastinal tumors, 447
    mesiotheliomas, 456
    neuroblastoma, 333
    in skeletal tumors, metastatic, 243
Thrombocythemia, essential, 415
Thrombocytopenia, *see also* Platelets
    autoimmune, 397
    histiocytic medullary reticulosis, 378

    in leukemias
        acute, 385, 388
        chronic lymphocytic, 394, 395
        chronic myelocytic, 345
    in lymphoma patient, 379
    in myelofibrosis, 414
    as pediatric chemotherapy complication, 320
Thrombocytosis, in myelofibrosis, 414
Thromboembolic complications
    with brain tumor, 306
    after colon surgery, 499
    after gynecological surgery, 566
    after kidney surgery, 582
    after lung surgery, 437
    in myelofibrosis and myeloid metaplasia, 415
    of pancreatic cancer, 516, 520
    in polycythemia vera, 411, 413
Thrombophlebitis
    with lung adenocarcinomas, 427
    with pancreatic cancer, 509
Thymic carcinoma, 184
Thymoma, 444
    ectopic ACTH syndrome, 184, 187
    incidence and location of, 443
    laboratory findings, 447
    multiple endocrine neoplasia (MEN-I), 192
    radiological findings, 446
    symptoms, 446
    therapeutic management, 448, 449
Thymus, carcinoid tumors, 203
Thyroidectomy, 48
Thyroid gland
    APUD cells, 197
    central nervous system lesions and, 280, 283, 298
    parathyroid tumors and, 174
Thyroid hormones, 192, 299, 447
Thyroid scans, 42
Thyroid-stimulating hormone (TSH), 298
    in multiple endocrine neoplasia type I, 192
    and thyroid cancer, 42
Thyroid-stimulating hormone (TSH)-suppression therapy, 44
Thyroid tumors
    apudomas, 198
    annual incidence of, 6
    bone metastasis, 219, 240
    cervical node metastasis, occult, 28
    classification and staging, 20
    ectopic hormone production, 184
    five-year relative survival, 23
    follow-up schedule, 52
    management algorithm, 61
    mediastinal, 445
        laboratory findings, 447
        radioisotope scans, 446
    multiple endocrine neoplasia type I, 192
    multiple endocrine neoplasia type II, 193
    and pheochromocytoma, 144
    site-specific data sheet, 14-15
    therapeutic guidelines, 40-44

treatment, 25, 43-44
versus vipoma, 166
Thyrotoxicosis, 192
Thyrotrophin-releasing hormone, 299
Thyroxine, 299
Tissue culture, 386, 406
Tobacco, see Smoking and tobacco use
Todd's phenomenon, 285
Tolbutamide test, in insulinoma, 158
Toludine blue staining, 6, 546
Tomography
    bone tumors, 228, 229
    brain metastasis, 294
    brain tumor, 280
    breast cancer, 73, 86
    central nervous system tumors, 279
    esophageal cancer, 462
    head and neck cancer, 8
    lung cancer, 423
    mediastinal tumors, 446
    paranasal sinus tumors, 35
    testicular tumors, 619, 620
Tongue cancer, 6, 23, 31, 357, 375
Tongue flaps, 49
Tonsil lesions, 28, 31, 357, 375
Toxoplasmosis, 356
Tracheal cancer
    annual incidence of, 6
    cervical, therapeutic guidelines, 35
    lung cancer spread to, 431
Tracheal obstruction
    compression after parathyroid surgery, 178
    open-tube bronschoscopy in, 423
Tracheostomy, 33, 47
Transcobalamine III, 412
Transcutaneous electrical nerve stimulation (TENS), 246, 306
Transfusions, see Blood component transfusions; Blood transfusions
Transillumination
    testicular cancer, 619
    thyroid cancer, 42
Transitional cell carcinoma
    bladder, 590, 592
    follow-up schedule, 584, 585
    kidney, 575
    prognosis, 582
    surgery, 581
    symptoms, 575, 576
Transitional cell papilloma, lung, 426
Transurethral resection, in bladder cancer, 591, 595
Transurethral resection of prostate (TURP), 603, 607, 608, 609, 610
Transverse colostomy, 496
Transverse myelitis, 365
Trasylol, 208
Trauma
    and bone tumors, 227
    and skin cancer, 99, 114
    and soft tissue sarcoma, 256
    and testicular cancer, 618, 619
Tracheobronchograms, 9
Trigeminal neuralgia, 296

Trigeminal neuromas, 301-302
Trousseau sign, 133
Tryptophan metabolites, and bladder cancer, 589
Tube feeding, see Hyperalimentation
Tuberculosis, 388, 398
Tubular adenocarcinoma, gastric, 478
Tubular adenomas, see Adenomatous polyps
Tubular carcinomas, breast, 79
Tumor antigens, see Immunotherapy; Markers
Tumor burden, in multiple myeloma, 404, see also Debulking
Tumor cell kinetics, breast tumor, 83-84
Tumor lysis syndrome, 362
Turcot's syndrome, 490, 496
Tylosis, with esophageal cancer, 461
Tyramine provocation test, 145

U

Ulcer, gastric, see Peptic ulcer
Ulceration, skin
    breast, 69
    in melanoma, 102
    and skin cancer, 99-100
Ulcerative colitis
    and biliary tree cancer, 522
    colectomy with tumors arising from, 497
    colorectal cancer risk, 489-490
Ulnar nerve palsy, 286
Ultrasound, see Sonography
Ultrasound surgery, brain tumors, 288
Ultraviolet radiation, and skin cancer, 99
Uncal herniation, 285, 287
Unclassified carcinoma, gastric, 478
Undifferentiated carcinoma
    bladder, 592
    gastric, 478
    head and neck, therapeutic modality selection, 25
    thyroid, 20, 44
Undifferentiated leukemia, acute, 345
Undifferentiated lymphoma, 361, 362, 371
Unicameral bone cyst, 219
    age incidence, 225
    characteristics of, 222
    therapeutic approaches, 236
Unifocal fibrous dysplasia, behavior of, 219
Uranium, and lung cancer, 422
Ureteroileal anastomoses, bladder cancer, 596
Ureterovesical junction, lesions of, 591
Ureters
    in bladder cancer, 596
    colon surgery and, 499
    in gynecological cancer, 542
    in lymphoma, 355
    in prostate surgery
        implantation of, 607, 610
        stenting, 604, 607
    in Wilms's tumor, 324

Urethral obstruction, *see* Obstructive uropathy
Urethrectomy, bladder cancer, 596
Urethroscopy, bladder cancer, 591
Urinary diversion
    bladder cancer, 591, 595
    in prostate surgery, antibiotic coverage, 607
Urinary frequency, gynecological malignancies, 543
Urinary hydroxyindole acetic acid, 139
Urinary incontinence, *see* Incontinence
Urinary ketosteroids, in Cushing's syndrome, 139
Urinary normetanephrine and metanephrine, in pheochromocytoma, 145
Urinary tract obstruction, *see* Calculi; Obstructive uropathy
Urine cytology, 590
Urine light-chain component, multiple myeloma, 404
Urine output
    brain tumors, postoperative management, 304
    after gynecological surgery, 566
    kidney tumors, postoperative, 583
    prostatic cancer, postoperative, 611
Urogenital tract, *see* specific primary sites
Uterine carcinoma, 542-569
Uterus
    in bladder cancer, 596
    conservation of, in ovarian cancer, 565

V

VAB, chemotherapy toxicity, 624
VAC
    in Ewing's sarcoma, 243
    in ovarian tumors, germ cell, 565
Vagina, in bladder cancer, 596
Vaginal bleeding, in pediatric patients, 316
Vaginal tumors, 541-556
    endometrial cancer recurrence, 561-562
    rhabdomyosarcoma, 336
Vaginectomy, 555
Vanillylmandelic acid (VMA)
    in neuroblastomas, 316
    mediastinal tumors, 443, 447
    in neuroblastomas, 316
    in pheochromocytoma, 145, 194
Vanous catheterization, in pheochromocytoma, 146
Varidase, 21
Vascular complications, *see also* Thromboembolic complications
    pheochromocytoma, 144-145
    prostatic cancer, 609
    skin cancer treatment complications, 105
Vasoactive intestinal polypeptide, *see also* Vipoma
    carcinoid, 203, 204
    pancreatic tumors affecting, 158
Vasoactive drugs, *see* specific agents
Vasoactive substances, *see* Apudomas; Carcinoid; Vipoma
VBAP, multiple myeloma, 406
VCR, leukemias, acute lymphoblastic, 343
Velban, *see* Vinblastine
Vena cava, *see* Superior vena cava syndrome

Venacavography
    liver tumors, 531
    pediatric solid tumors, 318
    soft-tissue sarcoma, 257
    testicular tumors, 620
Venacavotomy, with nephrectomy, 581
Venography, *see also* Angiography
    bone tumors, 228, 229
    lung cancer, 423, 426
    in primary aldosteronism, 135
Venous catheterization
    with head and neck tumor, 9
    with pancreatic tumors, insulinomas, 158
    with paraneoplastic syndrome, ACTH-producing, 185
    with parathyroid tumors, 175
    with pheochromocytoma, 146, 194
Venous sampling, adrenal, 135, 146, 194
Venous sinuses, meningiomas, 297
Ventricle drainage, brain tumors, therapeutic goals, 286
Ventricular crisis, colloid cysts and, 302
Ventricular shunts, with brain tumors, 286, 287
Vermillion flaps, 49
Verner-Morrison syndrome, *see* Vipoma
Verrucous carcinomas, 33, 546
Vertebral disease, *see* Spine
Vertical hemilaryngectomy, 33
Villous adenomas, 495, 496
Vinblastine
    adrenal tumors, 141
    bladder cancer, 596
    germ cell tumors, mediastinal, 450
    in head and neck tumors, 45
    in histiocytosis, 348
    kidney tumors, 583
    lymphoma, Hodgkin's, 346, 366, 367
    melanoma, 118
    ovarian tumors, germ cell, 565
    testicular tumor, 623, 624
    toxicity, 374
Vinca alkaloids
    esophageal cancer, 467
    lung cancer, 434, 435
    in lymphomas, Hodgkin's, 366
    melanoma, 118
    in soft tissue sarcoma, 265
Vincristine
    adrenal tumors
        neuroblastoma, 151
        pheochromocytoma, 147
    bone tumors
        Ewing's sarcoma, 238
        osteosarcoma, 238
    breast cancer, dosages and response rates, 87
    head and neck tumors, 45
    leukemias, acute
        lymphoblastic, 342, 344, 389
        myelogenous, 388
        myoblastic, 345
    leukemias, chronic

lymphocytic, 397
  myelocytic, 393, 394
lymphoma, Hodgkin's
  adult, 366, 367
  pediatric, 346
lymphoma, non-Hodgkin's, 371
  Burkitt's, 377
  diffuse, 370
  nodular, 369, 369
  pediatric, 347
multiple myeloma, 405, 406
neuroblastoma, 333
ovarian tumors, germ cell, 565
rhabdomyosarcoma, 336
skeletal tumors, 242, 243
soft tissue sarcoma, 265
toxicity, 374
Wilms's tumor, 329
Vipoma, 158, 167, 169
apudomas, 198
in MEN-I, 191
Viral infections
and gynecological malignancy, 541
in leukemias, chronic lymphocytic, 395
liver cancer risk, 529
in lymphoblastic lymphadenopathy, 377
Vision disturbances
with brain tumors
  craniopharyngioma, 300
  meningiomas, 296
  pituitary gland, 138, 298
with endocrine disturbances
  Cushing's syndrome, 138
  pancreatic tumors, insulinoma, 157
Visual acuity, with brain tumor, 280
Visual fields
with brain tumors, 278, 280
  metastatic, 293
  pituitary, 298
  sella turcica enlargement and, 141
  trigeminal neuromas, 302
in multiple endocrine neuropathy (MEN-I) diagnosis, 192
Vitamin B12
after gastrinoma surgery, 163
in leukemias, chronic myelocytic, 393
in polycythemia vera, 412
Vitamin K
deficiencies of, in leukemia, 388, 389
liver tumors, preoperative, 532
pancreatic cancer, preoperative management, 515
VM-26
in leukemias, acute lymphoblastic, 344
in lymphomas, Hodgkin's, 366
toxicity, 374
Vocal cord paralysis
arytenoid cartilage surgery in, 52
after parathyroid surgery, 48, 178
in parathyroid tumors, 174
after thyroidectomy, 48

Vocal cord tumors
cervical node metastasis, occult, 28
rehabilitation, voice, 50
therapeutic management, 32-33
Volume disorders, see Blood volume; Fluids and electrolytes
Von Recklinghausen's disease, 302, 443
mediastinal tumor, 446
meningeal meningiomatosis, 297
Von Willebrand's knee, 298
VP-16 (Etoposide)
chemotherapy toxicity, 624
lung cancer, 434, 435
toxicity, 374
Vulvar carcinoma, 541-555

W

Waldenstrom's macroglobulinemia, 378, 396
Waldeyer's ring, 357, 375
Water restriction, in ectopic ADH syndrome, 187
WDHA syndrome, see Vipoma
Wedge resection, lung, 437
Welders, skin cancer in, 99
Well-differentiated lymphocytic lymphoma, 360, 361, 362
Werner's syndrome (MEN-I), 191-193
Wheezing, in carcinoid syndrome, 204
Whipple's disease, mediastinal tumor, 446
Whipple's operation, 518, 518
White cell count, see also Leukopenia; Myelosuppression
in leukemias, acute, 386, 388
  lymphoblastic, 342, 343
  myelogenous, remission, 389
in leukemias, chronic
  hairy cell, 398
  lymphocytic, 395
  myelocytic, 345, 392
in lymphoma, 379
in myelofibrosis, 414
in polycythemia vera, 411, 413
White patch, 542, see also Leukoplakia
Whole-brain irradiation, 436, see also Brain irradiation
Wide-field laryngectomy, 33
Wilms's tumor, 575
congenital anomalies with, 315
cure rates, 320
follow-up schedule, 322
intravenous pyelogram in, 317
intravenous pyelography, 317
metastatic evaluation, 318
pathology, 322-323
physical findings, 316
site-specific data form, 323, 325, 326, 327, 328
surgical management, 319
Wiskott-Aldrich syndrome, 315
Witzelsucht syndrome, 296
Wolfe's classification, breast cancer, 71

Wood dust, as carcinogen, 5
Wood preservatives, as carcinogens, 256

X

Xanthomas, mediastinal, 445
133-Xenon ventilation perfusion scan, 428
Xeroderma pigmentosa, 113, 114, 315
Xerography, 229
X-ray exposure, and cancer risk, 70, 99

Y

Yttrium implants, 141

Z

Zollinger-Ellison syndrome, 41, 160, 162-163, 164
    apudomas, 198
    pancreatic tumors producing, 158
    versus vipoma, 166